Disorders of the Cervical Spine

Disorders of the Cervical Spine

Edited by

Martin B. Camins, M.D., F.A.C.S.
Associate Clinical Professor of Neurosurgery
Mount Sinai Hospital School of Medicine
New York, New York

Patrick F. O'Leary, M.D., F.A.C.S.
Associate Clinical Professor of Surgery
Cornell University Medical College
Chief, Spine Section
Hospital for Special Surgery
Associate Director, Chief of Spine
Lenox Hill Hospital
New York, New York

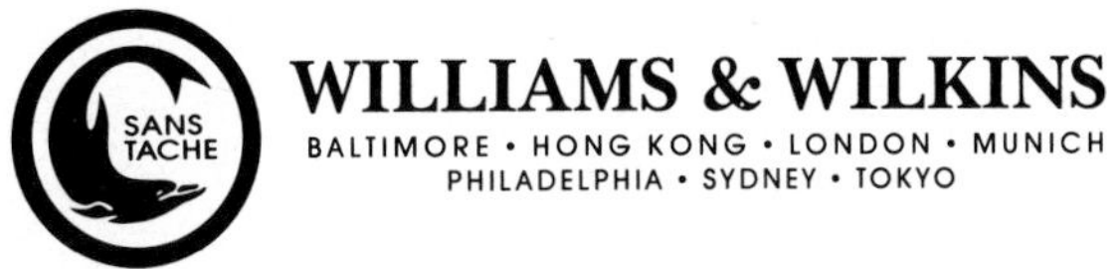

WILLIAMS & WILKINS
BALTIMORE • HONG KONG • LONDON • MUNICH
PHILADELPHIA • SYDNEY • TOKYO

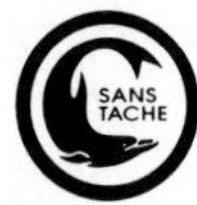

Editor: Charles W. Mitchell
Managing Editor: Victoria M. Vaughn
Copy Editor: Mary Kidd
Designer: Karen Klinedinst
Illustration Planner: Lorraine Wrzosek
Production Coordinator: Kathleen C. Millet
Cover Designer: Dan Pfisterer

Williams & Wilkins
428 East Preston Street
Baltimore, Maryland 21202, USA

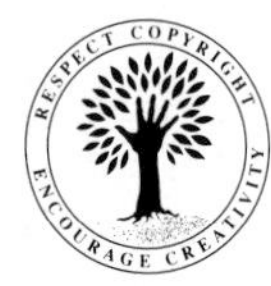

Accurate indications, adverse reactions, and dosage schedules for drugs are provided in this book, but it is possible that they may change. The reader is urged to review the package information data of the manufacturers of the medications mentioned.

Printed in the United States of America

Library of Congress Cataloging in Publication Data

Disorders of the cervical spine / edited by Martin B. Camins, Patrick F. O'Leary
p. cm.
Includes bibliographical references and index.
ISBN 0-683-01401-3
1. Vertebrae, Cervical—Diseases. 2. Vertebrae, Cervical—Wounds and injuries. 3. Vertebrae, Cervical—Surgery. I. Camins, Martin B. II. O'Leary, Patrick F.
[DNLM: 1. Cervical Vertebrae. 2. Cervical Vertebrae—injuries. 3. Spinal Diseases—diagnosis. 4. Spinal Diseases—therapy. 5. Spinal Injuries—diagnosis. 6. Spinal Injuries—therapy. WE 725 D613]
RD533.D57 1992
617.3'75--dc20
DNLM/DLC
for Library of Congress 91-27785
CIP

DEDICATION

To my parents, Ruth and Hyman Camins, who have continually served as a source of encouragement and inspiration in fulfilling my dreams as a neurosurgeon.

M.B.C

My sincere appreciation to Dr. Michael Alexiades for his many hours of work devoted to reviewing the chapters with me for this publication.

P.F.O'L.

FOREWORD

Joseph A. Epstein, M.D.

Dr. Camins and Dr. O'Leary are to be congratulated for successfully assembling a group of esteemed authors to present a most comprehensive review of current concepts and practices of the management of disorders of the cervical spine. Each chapter has been carefully selected to provide in considerable detail current techniques of both diagnosis and management, oriented both surgically and nonsurgically. The methods of diagnosis, including the proper taking of a detailed history, the neurological examination, and when and how to select ancillary radiological studies, are all presented with clarity and brevity. The various authors emphasize those studies with the greatest yield, avoiding time-consuming diversions that are scarcely justified on a clinical, financial, and legal basis. Included are chapters on surgical technique that have survived the test of time, with the appropriate indications concerning the purpose and the anatomical bases justifying either the anterior or the posterior approaches. This includes problems related to herniated cervical discs, spondyloarthrosis with and without the associated stenosis, congenital stenosis, and problems related to patients with ossification of the posterior longitudinal ligament. Chapters on the management of traumatic lesions provide proper directions in the use of conservative care and management using both internal and external fixation. The text is actually a vade mecum concerned with the treatment of major as well as minor disorders related to cervical spine pathology. Included are chapters covering the various medical-legal issues that plague the managing physician. Advice is provided as to the means of avoiding the concern and harassment that beset all of us who willingly or, often, unwillingly are drawn into judgmental situations wherein one is "damned if he does and damned if he doesn't." Both the patient and the concerned physician are entitled to equal protection under the law which unfortunately does not often treat each in an egalitarian manner.

PREFACE

This textbook focuses on a wide variety of aspects concerning the treatment of cervical spine disorders with an emphasis on presenting discussions of the latest advances made toward their treatment. Each individual chapter provides an expert's opinion on the treatment of a specific problem. In aggregate, the text represents a compendium of knowledge on which to build better comprehension of the disorders of the cervical spine.

The contributing authors are recognized experts in the topics on which their chapters are based. Each author is uniquely well-qualified to recommend appropriate treatment, whether surgical or nonsurgical, for specific cervical spine disorders and to summarize the treatment alternatives and modalities relevant to his specific topic. In combination, the contributing authors' opinions represent the best experience and expertise on disorders of the cervical spine available internationally.

Choices of alternative surgical procedures and nonsurgical treatment, pre- and postoperative care regimens, and comprehensive postoperative rehabilitation programs are detailed. Illustrations, radiographs, and clinical photographs are included to assist the reader in following the diagnostic and therapeutic processes discussed. The medical student, house staff officer, neurologist, neurosurgeon, orthopaedic spinal surgeon, and physiatrist will each find this text an invaluable tool.

Acknowledgment

Ms. Vicki Vaughn and Ms. Carol-Lynn Brown, our editors, have been the catalyst for the completion of this text. Without their insights, encouragement, and reinforcement this text's publication date would have been significantly delayed. Ms. Maria Ojeda-Acevedo and Ms. Ruth Kortright have provided excellent secretarial assistance to the editors, as well as soothing ruffled feathers when delays occurred in preparation of the text. To each of them we give our deepest thanks.

Contributors

Paul A. Anderson, M.D.
Assistant Professor, Department of Orthopaedics
Harborview Medical Center
University of Washington School of Medicine
Seattle, Washington

J. Lobo Antunes, M.D.
Professor and Chairman, Department of Neurosurgery
University of Lisbon
Libson, Portugal

Ronald I. Apfelbaum, M.D., F.A.C.S.
Professor of Surgery (Neurosurgery)
University of Utah Health Sciences Center
Salt Lake City, Utah

Robert E. Barrett, M.D.
Clinical Professor of Neurology
Columbia University College of Physicians and Surgeons
Attending Neurologist
Neurological Institute of New York
New York, New York

Scott D. Boden, M.D.
Assistant in Orthopaedic Surgery
Department of Orthopaedic Surgery
George Washington University Medical Center
Washington, DC

Henry H. Bohlman, M.D.
Professor, Department of Orthopaedics
Case Western Reserve University School of Medicine
Cleveland, Ohio

Mark R. Brinker, M.D.
Research Fellow, Department of Orthopaedic Surgery
Tulane University School of Medicine
New Orleans, Louisiana

Alexander E. Brodsky, M.D.*
Medical Director, Texas Institute for Spinal Disorders
Associate Clinical Professor of Orthopaedic Surgery
Baylor College of Medicine and University of Texas School of Medicine
Houston, Texas

Roy Buchsbaum, M.D.
Assistant Professor, Department of Radiation Oncology
University of Pittsburgh School of Medicine
Joint Radiation Oncology Center
Pittsburgh Cancer Institute
Pittsburgh, Pennsylvania

Martin J. Buckingham, M.D.
Clinical Instructor, Department of Neurosurgery
Rockford School of Medicine
University of Illinois
Rockford, Illinois

Stephen W. Burke, M.D.
Associate Attending Surgeon
The Hospital for Special Surgery
Associate Clinical Professor of Surgery (Orthopaedics) and Pediatrics
Cornell University Medical College
New York, New York

Martin B. Camins, M.D., F.A.C.S.
Associate Clinical Professor of Neurosurgery
Mount Sinai Hospital School of Medicine
New York, New York

Frank P. Cammisa, Jr., M.D.
Assistant Attending Surgeon
The Hospital for Special Surgery
Assistant Professor of Surgery (Orthopaedics)
Cornell University Medical College
New York, New York

*deceased

DAVID R. CHANDLER, M.D.
Clinical Assistant Professor, Department of Orthopaedics
University of Southern California
Los Angeles, California
Consultant, Spinal Cord Injury Service
Rancho Los Amigos Medical Center
Downey, California

WILLIAM F. CHANDLER, M.D.
Professor of Surgery
Section of Neurosurgery
University of Michigan Medical Center
Ann Arbor, Michigan

JONATHAN Z. CHARNEY, M.D.
Assistant Clinical Professor Neurology
Mount Sinai Hospital and Medical School
New York, New York

IN SUP CHOI, M.D.
Assistant Professor of Radiology
New York University School of Medicine
New York, New York

CHARLES L. CHRISTIAN, M.D.
Physician-in-Chief
The Hospital for Special Surgery
Professor of Medicine
Cornell University Medical College
New York, New York

DAVID H. CLEMENTS, M.D.
Instructor of Orthopaedics
Department of Orthopaedic Surgery
Temple University Hospital
Philadelphia, Pennsylvania

PAUL R. COOPER, M.D.
Associate Professor of Neurosurgery
New York University Medical Center
New York, New York

H. ALAN CROCKARD, M.D., F.R.C.S.
Consultant Neurosurgeon
Department of Surgical Neurology
The National Hospitals for Nervous Diseases
Honorary Senior Lecturer
Institute of Neurology and University College
London, England

WILLIAM H. DILLIN, M.D.
Orthopaedic Surgeon Kerlan-Jobe Orthopaedic Clinic
Inglewood, California

SOHEI EBARA, M.D., PH.D.
Assistant Professor, Department of Orthopaedic Surgery
Osaka University Medical School
Osaka, Japan

FRANK J. EISMONT, M.D.
Professor of Orthopaedic Surgery and Neurosurgery
The University of Miami School of Medicine
Co-Director, The Acute Spinal Injury Service
Jackson Memorial Medical Center
Miami, Florida

SANFORD E. EMERY, M.D.
Assistant Professor, Department of Orthopaedics
Case Western Reserve University School of Medicine
Cleveland, Ohio

MAHMOOD FAZAL, M.D., F.R.C.S.C.
Co-Director, Acute Spinal Cord Injury Unit
Division of Neurosurgery
Sunnybrook Medical Centre
Toronto, Ontario, Canada

J. WILLIAM FIELDING, M.D.
Emeritus Attending Surgeon
Saint Luke's-Roosevelt Hospital
Professor of Orthopaedic Surgery, Emeritus
Columbia University College of Physicians and Surgeons
New York, New York

WILLIAM R. FRANCIS, M.D.
Reconstructive Spine Surgeon
Private Practice
Houston, Texas

NANCY ANN FRANTZ, R.N., B.S.N.
Clinical Specialist
Infectious Disease Service
Metrohealth Medical Center
Case Western Reserve University
Cleveland, Ohio

WILLIAM A. FRIEDMAN, M.D.
Associate Chairman and Professor
Department of Neurological Surgery
University of Florida School of Medicine
Gainesville, Florida

STANLEY D. GERTZBEIN, M.D.
Director of Education and Research
Texas Back Institute
Associate Professor
University of Texas
Houston, Texas

STEVEN G. GLASGOW, M.D.
Assistant Professor of Orthopaedic Surgery
University of Pennsylvania School of Medicine
Philadelphia, Pennsylvania

BARTH A. GREEN, M.D.
Professor, Department of Neurological Surgery
University of Miami School of Medicine
Miami, Florida

BRUCE G. HABIAN, ESQ.
Senior Partner
Martin, Clearwater and Bell
New York, New York

MARK N. HADLEY, M.D.
Assistant Professor of Surgery
Division of Neurosurgery
University of Alabama at Birmingham
Birmingham, Alabama

VAN V. HALBACH, M.D.
Assistant Professor of Radiology and Neurological Surgery
Diagnostic and Interventional Neuroradiology Section
University of California School of Medicine
San Francisco, California

GRANT B. HIESHIMA, M.D.
Professor of Radiology and Neurological Surgery
Diagnostic and Interventional Neuroradiology Section
University of California School of Medicine
Los Angeles, California

JULIAN T. HOFF, M.D.
Head, Section of Neurosurgery
University of Michigan Medical Center
Ann Arbor, Michigan

BARRY JORDAN, M.D.
Assistant Attending Neurologist
The Hospital for Special Surgery
Assistant Professor of Neurology and Public Health
Cornell University Medical College
New York, New York

SHALOM KALNICKI, M.D.
Associate Professor, Department of Radiation Oncology
University of Pittsburgh School of Medicine
Joint Radiation Oncology Center and Pittsburgh Cancer Institute
Pittsburgh, Pennsylvania

MOMTAZ A. KHALIL, M.D.
Director, Orthopaedic Research Center
Saint Luke's Episcopal Hospital
Houston, Texas

K. JOHN KLOSE, M.D.
Research Assistant Professor
Department of Neurological Surgery
University of Miami School of Medicine
Miami, Florida

ROBIN KOELEVELD, M.D.
Resident, Department of Neurosurgery
Tufts-New England Medical Center
Boston, Massachusetts

MICHAEL A. KROPF, M.D.
Resident, Rancho Los Amigos Medical Center
Downey, California

CHARLES F. LANZIERI, M.D.
Associate Professor, Director of Neuroradiology
Case Western Reserve University
University Hospital of Cleveland
Cleveland, Ohio

RICHARD LECHTENBERG, M.D.
Chief, Department of Neuroscience
Division of Neurology
Long Island College Hospital
Brooklyn, New York

GRAHAM LEE, M.D.
Assistant Professor of Radiology
Yale University School of Medicine
New Haven, Connecticut

ALAN M. LEVINE, M.D.
Associate Professor of Orthopaedic Surgery and Oncology
Division of Orthopaedic Surgery
University of Maryland School of Medicine
Baltimore, Maryland

STEPHEN J. LIPSON, M.D.
Associate Clinical Professor of Orthopaedic Surgery
Harvard Medical School
Brigham and Women's Hospital
Boston, Massachusetts

JOSEPH C. MAROON, M.D.
Chairman, Department of Neurosurgery
Allegheny General Hospital
Pittsburgh, Pennsylvania

CHRISTIAN MAZEL, M.D.
Assistant
Service de Chirurgie Orthopédique et Traumatologique
Centre Hospitalier Pitié-Salpétrière
Paris, France

R.J. MCBROOM, M.D., F.R.C.S
Division of Orthopaedics
The Wellesley Hospital
University of Toronto
Toronto, Ontario, Canada

J. MICHAEL MCWHORTER, M.D.
Associate Professor of Neurosurgery
Bowman Gray School of Medicine of Wake Forest University
Winston-Salem, North Carolina

ARNOLD H. MENEZES, M.D.
Professor and Vice Chairman
Division of Neurosurgery
University of Iowa Hospitals
Iowa City, Iowa

HANNO MILLESI, M.D.
Head, Department of Plastic and Reconstructive Surgery
First Surgical University Clinic
Director of Ludwig-Baltzmann Institute for Experimental Plastic Surgery
Vienna, Austria

STUART E. MIRVIS, M.D.
Associate Professor of Radiology
University of Maryland Medical Center
Director of Radiology
Shock Trauma Center
Maryland Institute for Emergency Medical Services Systems
Baltimore, Maryland

PASQUALE X. MONTESANO, M.D.
Assistant Professor, Department of Orthopaedic Surgery
University of California at Davis
Sacramento, California

CHARLES R. NEBLETT, M.D.
Clinical Associate Professor of Surgery
University of Texas Health and Science Center
Houston, Texas

JEFFREY Y.F. NGEOW, M.D.
Director, Pain Management
Hospital for Special Surgery
New York, New York

PATRICK F. O'LEARY, M.D., F.A.C.S.
Associate Clinical Professor of Surgery
Cornell University Medical College
Chief, Spine Section
Hospital for Special Surgery
Associate Director, Chief of Spine
Lenox Hill Hospital
New York, New York

KEIRO ONO, M.D., PH.D.
Professor and Chairman
Department of Orthopaedic Surgery
Osaka University Medical School
Osaka, Japan

HELENE PAVLOV, M.D.
Professor of Radiology
Cornell University Medical College
Attending Radiologist
Hospital for Special Surgery and New York Hospital
New York, New York

R.G. PERRIN, M.D., M.SC., F.R.C.S.(C), F.A.C.S.
Division of Neurosurgery
The Wellesley Hospital
University of Toronto
Toronto, Ontario, Canada

KRISTJAN T. RAGNARSSON, M.D.
Chairman, Department of Rehabilitative Medicine
Mount Sinai Hospital Medical School
New York, New York

BRUCE R. ROSENBLUM, M.D.
Department of Neurosurgery
Bayshore Community Hospital
Holmdel, New Jersey

MICHAEL ROTHMAN, M.D.
Assistant Professor of Radiology
Department of Radiology
Division of Neuroradiology
University of Maryland Medical Center
Baltimore, Maryland

RAYMOND ROY-CAMILLE, M.D.
Professeur de Chirurgie Orthopédique et Tramatologique à la Faculté Pitié-Salpétrière
Université Pierre et Marie Curie à Paris
Chef, Service de Chirurgie Orthopédique et Tramatologique
Centre Hospitalier Pitié-Salpétrière
Paris, France

JONATHAN M. RUBIN, M.D.
Professor of Radiology
Department of Radiology
University of Michigan
Ann Arbor, Michigan

THOMAS G. SAUL, M.D.
Associate Professor of Clinical Neurosurgery
University of Cincinnati Medical Center
Chairman, Section of Neurosurgery
Good Samaritan Hospital
Cincinnati, Ohio

MICHAEL L. SCHWARTZ, M.D., M.SC., F.R.C.S.C.
Director, Neurotrauma Program
Division of Neurosurgery
Sunnybrook Medical Centre
Toronto, Ontario, Canada

SHASHI K. SHAH, M.D.
Pacific Physician Services
Redlands, California

WILLIAM A. SCHUCART, M.D.
Professor and Chairman, Department of Neurosurgery
Tufts-New England Medical Center
Boston, Massachusetts

VOLKER K.H. SONNTAG, M.D., F.A.C.S.
Vice Chairman, Division of Neurological Surgery
Barrow Neurological Institute
Phoenix, Arizona
Clinical Professor of Surgery (Neurosurgery)
University of Arizona

THOMAS A. SWEASEY, M.D.
Private Practice
Anderson, South Carolina

GEORGE W. SYPERT, M.D., F.A.C.S.
Overstreet Professor and Eminent Scholar
University of Florida College of Medicine
Southwest Florida Neurosurgical Institute
Fort Myers, Florida

YOSHIHIRO TAKEBE, M.D.
Department of Neurosurgery
Fukui Red Cross Hospital
Fukui, Japan

JUJI TAKEUCHI, M.D.
Department of Neurosurgery
Utano National Hospital
Kyoto, Japan

JOHN M. TEW, JR., M.D.
Chairman and Professor, Department of Neurological Surgery
University of Cincinnati College of Medicine
Mayfield Neurological Institute, Inc.
Cincinnati, Ohio

THOMAS TOLLI, M.D.
Resident in Orthopaedic Surgery
Saint Luke's-Roosevelt Hospital Center
New York, New York

JOSEPH S. TORG, M.D.
Professor of Orthopaedic Surgery
University of Pennsylvania School of Medicine
Director, University of Pennsylvania Sports Medicine Center
Philadelphia, Pennsylvania

ENSOR E. TRANSFELDT, M.D.
Assistant Professor, Department of Orthopaedic Surgery
University of Minnesota School of Medicine
Minneapolis, Minnesota

PETER TSAIRIS, M.D.
Director of Neurology, Emeritus
The Hospital for Special Surgery
Associate Professor of Neurology
Cornell University Medical Center
New York, New York

JOHN J. WASENKO, M.D.
Assistant Professor, Department of Radiology
State University of New York Health Science Center
Syracuse, New York

ROBERT L. WATERS, M.D.
Clinical Professor of Orthopaedics
University of Southern California
Los Angeles, California
Medical Director
Rancho Los Amigos Medical Center
Downey, California

ROBERT G. WATKINS, M.D.
Orthopaedic Surgeon
Kerban-Jobe Orthopaedic Clinic
Inglewood, California

T.S. WHITECLOUD, III, M.D.
Professor of Orthopaedic Surgery
Department of Orthopaedic Surgery
Tulane University School of Medicine
New Orleans, Louisiana

SAM W. WIESEL, M.D.
Professor of Orthopaedic Surgery
Department of Orthopaedic Surgery
Georgetown University Medical Center
Washington, DC

R. GEOFFREY WILBER, M.D.
Assistant Professor of Orthopaedics
Director, Orthopaedic Spine Service
Metrohealth Medical Center
Case Western Reserve University
Cleveland, Ohio

JACK WILBERGER, M.D.
Vice Chairman, Department of Neurosurgery
Allegheny General Hospital
Pittsburgh, Pennsylvania

DAVID G. WILDER, PH.D., P.E.
Research Assistant Professor
Department of Orthopaedics and Rehabilitation Medicine
University of Vermont College of Medicine
Burlington, Vermont

CHARLES B. WILSON, M.D.
Tong-Po Kan Professor and Chairman
Department of Neurological Surgery
University of California School of Medicine
San Francisco, California

THOMAS A.S. WILSON, JR., M.D.
Resident, Department of Neurosurgery
Bowman Gray School of Medicine of Wake Forest University
Winston-Salem, North Carolina

J. GEOFFREY WIOT, M.D.
Assistant Professor of Radiology
Department of Neuroradiology
University of Cincinnati College of Medicine
Cincinnati, Ohio

FREMONT P. WIRTH, M.D.
Clinical Associate Professor of Surgery (Neurosurgery)
Medical College of Georgia
Augusta, Georgia

Contents

INTRODUCTION: CERVICAL SPINE SURGERY—PAST, PRESENT, AND FUTURE POTENTIAL

J. William Fielding

Cervical spine surgery had its foundations in antiquity. It developed extremely slowly through the Middle Ages when advances in medicine and science in general were meager. It was not until the 19th century that medicine in general and cervical spine surgery in particular developed rapidly. One of the first physicians contributing to cervical spine surgery was Imhotep of the third Egyptian Dynasty. Not only was he a physician but also an architect, building the step pyramid at Sakkara during the reign of Pharoah Djoser (2686–2613 BC). This was the largest building ever until the pyramids at Giza (24). The Edwin Smith Papyrus, the first treatise on surgery, is attributed to this individual, rendering his name synonymous with the dawn of medicine (24). This papyrus described 48 mainly osseous lesions, some involving the cervical spine (12). Considering that this document was written about 4635 years ago, its observations were surprisingly accurate, identifying vertebral subluxations and dislocations and also differentiating between lower and upper cervical spine injuries. Surprisingly, Tutankhamen (King Tut), the famous 18th Dynasty pharoah, had the first recorded cervical laminectomy, which was actually part of the mummification process to remove the brain (26).

Greece also produced some outstanding physicians. Hippocrates, born in 460 BC, realized that vertebral injuries cause paralysis, but was unable to explain the reason. The traction principle developed by him for the spine was used in some form until the 19th century. In the 2nd century AD, Galen, the physician to the Roman Emperor Marcus Aurelius, became a sports medicine specialist when the emperor officially appointed him as the official doctor of the gladiatorial ampitheater, providing a bonanza for anatomic research (31). Among his experiments was to divide the spinal cord at varying levels noting the effect on the muscular structures (31, 54). Surprisingly, the first laminectomy was attributed to Paul of Aeginia, who lived between 625 and 690 AD (1). The first laminectomy in America was performed in 1828 (47).

Ambrose Pare probably did the first operation on the spinal cord, removing bony pressure and reducing dislocations with traction (37). In 1646, fracture reduction by a forceps clamped in soft tissue of the neck was attempted by Fabricus Hildanus (29). It was not until the 19th century that significant advances in medicine were made. Anesthesia was introduced in 1848 by William Morton (7, 8). Louis Pasteur discoverd that microorganisms caused infection (17, 38). Lister was the first to develop antiseptic surgery (17, 33), but perhaps the greatest medical development of all time had to wait until 1896 when Conrad Roentgen develop x-rays (43). Surprisingly, Hippocrates (40) spoke strongly on the significance of head injuries, especially those of an intracranial nature. He did not realize, however, that the majority of injuries to the neck occurred as a result of head trauma with the force transferred to the cervical area. Henry Bohlman (10) studied 300 patients with neck injuries, 11 of whom died or were paralyzed as the result of an injury to the cervical spine that was not identified. In 1974 George Alker (2) was able to x-ray the necks of 200 individuals killed in automobile accidents. Surprisingly, 25% had occult cervical spine damage quite capable of causing the death of the individual. Indeed the incidence of cervical spine injuries may never be fully appreciated, since autopsies do not always include the cervical region. An important study was carried out at the Naval Biodynamics Laboratory in New Orleans by Professor Unterharnscheidt (51). This experiment consisted of rapidly accelerating, then rapidly decelerating monkeys in a specially designed sled. The inertia of the unrestrained head caused the neck to markedly elongate and into sudden violent flexion with resultant fatality from occiput–C1 dislocation and cord and vertebral artery disruption. Surprisingly, roentgenograms were essentially normal, because the displacements, spontaneously reduced. Damage was only demonstrated at autopsy.

This head-neck relationship is well exemplified by the whiplash injury, a term coined by Crowe (16) in 1928, believed to be due to ligamentous injury caused by neck hyperextension beyond physiological range produced by the inertially moving head. The symptoms include neck pain of short or long duration. Surgical intervention rarely occurs in these individuals, and there are no supporting autopsy studies to correlate with the cause of the complaints, therefore the etiology is often conjectural.

Hippocrates probably introduced traction over 2000 years ago. In 1887, Bontecou (11) provided traction using adhesive tape attached to the patient's face to reduce a cervical fracture. The introduction of head halter traction can be attributed to Taylor in 1929 (49). Professor Edward Gallie of Toronto University in 1937 described his method or treatment of fractures and dislocations of the neck by skeletal traction (22). The use of tongs for traction was introduced by Crutchfield in 1933 (18). Wires were placed through holes drilled in the skull by Hoen in 1936 (30). In 1938 Barton (5) and in 1948 Vinke (53) introduced tongs that prevented intracranial protrusion of the traction device. In 1973 Gardner and Wells introduced a very efficient form of skull tong, but the most effective immobilizing device remains the halo. This was reported by Nickel, Perry, and Heppenstall in 1968 (36).

The subspecialty of biomechanics is valuable in assessing stability of the cervical spine as it relates to stabilizing surgical intervention. In an attempt to elucidate this, studies were carried out at St. Luke's Hospital in New York City in 1974 (21). In this experiment the stability of the C1 and C2 ligament complex was correlated with the strength of this motion segment using fresh adult anatomic specimens of C1 and C2. In this experiment to test the strength of the supporting ligaments, the second cervical vertebra was firmly mounted in epoxy, and C1 was pulled forward against ligament resistance. Forward displacements of up to 3 mm were essentially normal, but when the transverse ligament, the first line of defense, ruptured, the atlanto-dens interval was from 3 to 5 mm. The alar ligaments were the second line of defense, surprisingly these did not rupture, but gradually stretched out in elastic fashion under the load. They were considered completely deficient with a forward displacement of 5 to 10 mm and no longer able to stabilize the atlanto-axial segment and enclosed spinal cord. The experiment also indicated that the transverse ligament and alar ligaments were of equal strength, thus an individual may not be able to withstand a second episode of trauma equal to the first.

White, Punjabi, and Southwick biomechanically analyzed the clinical stability of the subaxial cervical spine. The conclusion from their experiments was that when one segment shifted 3.5 mm more or tilted in excess of 11° more than other interspaces, the motion segment is unstable and should be fused (55).

In another study by Stauffer and Kelly (48) 16 patients with posterior ligament disruption were fused by the interbody technique. This resulted in soft tissue disruption, not only anteriorly, but also posteriorly. As a result of this, every one of the 16 patients underwent an angular deformity following surgery, some with progressive neurologic deficit. Further surgical attempts to stabilize these spines were needed in 11 individuals who needed two or more operative procedures, and in spite of immobilization and skeletal traction the angulation continued. The message is not to fuse on the intact side, but proceed with a posterior fusion for posterior disruption and vice versa. Surgery on the intact side will remove the remaining ligamentous stability and may result in spinal collapse.

The posterior elements of the cervical spine are very applicable for fusion through the posterior approach. In 1891, 5 years before the introduction of x-rays, Hadra wired the spinous processes of C6 and 7 in order to treat a fracture of the 7th cervical vertebra. In 1900 he was unsuccessful in reducing an atlantoaxial displacement. He did not attempt fusion; however, a mass of callus developed as a result of the surgical trauma, serendipitously resulting in a fusion between the occiput and the 2nd cervical vertebra. The first successful atlantoaxial fusion took place in Brooklyn, New York, by Louis Pilcher (39) in 1910.

Mixter and Osgood (35) from Boston understood the need to reduce and fix atlantoaxial displacements. In one of their early procedures the posterior elements were exposed surgically, a silk thread was looped beneath the posterior C1 arch while the other surgeon went beneath the table and pushed backward on the pharynx. The atlantoaxial fusion was probably popularized by Professor W. Edward Gallie, Professor of Surgery at the University of Toronto, the technique bearing his name, Gallie fusion (22, 23). Professor Gallie realized the danger of catastrophic cord and vertebral artery damage, noting that this may develop later due to glacier-like displacement of C1 on C2, stating that although no neurologic signs may be present at the time of injury they may indeed develop later.

Numerous methods of grafting and wire fixation have followed, but they all adhere to the Gallie principle that uses the wire for simultaneous reduction and fixation on the graft in place (13, 42). In performing this procedure a fixation wire is usually passed beneath the arch of C1 and C2, or alternatively, under the arch of C1 and through the spine of C2. A graft is then cut to fit astride the spine and lamina of C2 and curved to fit over the convexity of the posterior arch of C1. The wire is then tied over the graft. Other methods of atlantoaxial fusion have been described but generally adhere to the principles put forward by W. Edward Gallie. Atlantoaxial fusion can also be carried out by alternative means. In Australia, Barbour (4) used transarticular C1–C2 screws. These were inserted laterally, first through the inferior facet of C1, and across the joint and into the superior facet of C2. Concern with the loss of rotation with a C1–2 fusion led George Jorg Bohler to develop a method of fixing the odontoid process with a screw (9). Through an anterior approach the screw was inserted into the body of the second cervical vertebra and upward into the odontoid process (see chapter by Apfelbaum).

William A. Rogers (44), pioneer among cervical spine surgeons, is probably responsible for our modern principles and techniques utilizing surgery with corrective traction during open reduction and utilizing the spinous processes to maintain fixation wires. Dr. Roger addressed not only cord protection but also complete reduction and adequate fixation restoring stability of the cervical spine allowing the patient to ambulate earlier.

Innumerable methods of cervical spine fusion have been spawned by the increasing interest in this area, these include facet fusion for the laminectomised spine in which longitudinal grafts are held in place by drill holes through facets binding them to the underlined individual facet masses extending onward and upward through the adjacent intact spinous processes (14).

Among the many problems assocated with cervical spine surgery are those related to congenital anomalies. The majority are probably at the upper portion of the cervical spine and may involve other structures as the vascular supply, the cerebellum, the brain stem, or the cord. A galaxy of sometimes confusing symptoms may result. Some of these somatic abnormalities include low cerebellar tonsils, progressive dural bands, and vascular and neurologic anomalies which may not be fully appreciated. Mechanical problems can be managed generally by fusion, neurogenic problems such as a high riding odontoid may require a transpharyngeal approach. This approach was first used in 1896 by Auffert, and it was proven feasible in dogs, then in humans. Samuel Crowe, Professor of Otolaryngology, at Johns Hopkin's Hospital drained tuberculous abscesses through this approach. The use of the operating microscope has widened the surgical field considerably, especially in surgical procedures such as odontoid and clivus resection.

Congenital anomalies, especially those that are nonsymptomatic, may remain undetected throughout the life of an individual. The Klippel-Feil syndrome, however, was known in antiquity and takes its name from the two individuals who first adequately described the problem in 1912 (32). Hensinger, Lang, and MacEwen, 62 years after its initial description, studied a series of 50 patients reporting a multitude of congenital anomalies, some of which were occult. Among these are scoliosis, renal anomalies, Sprengel's deformity, impaired hearing, synkinesia, and congenital heart disease (27). They concluded that those individuals with fewer open interspaces were under higher mechanical demand and should avoid stressful situations. A delicate balance can be drawn between the loss of mobility from a fusion and potential damage to neurologic structures from a catastrophic displacement.

Prior to 1954, anterior approaches to the cervical spine were infrequently used and only occasionally reported. In 1964 Boudot used an approach posterior to the sternomastoid muscle to approach the cervical apophyses. In 1930 it was used by Dickson Wright of Toronto who approached cervical tuberculosis. Subsequent to this, anterior cervical approaches were rarely used or reported. A resurgence of interest was stimulated in February of 1954, however, when for the first time an anterior cervical disc removal and fusion was carried out by Robinson and Smith (41). Use of this approach rapidly spread, which allowed exposure from the clivus to the chest. It was used to fuse the skull to the upper portion of the cervical spine, done by DeAndrade and MacNab (19). Interest in this approach led to a multitude of graft constructs, as well as instrumentation. In 1958, Cloward reported a circular bony graft implant (15). In 1960, Bailey and Badgley reported a longitudinal anterior graft for multilevel fusions (3). John Tew and Frank Mayfield of Cincinnati and others have questioned the necessity of performing a fusion at the time of removal of a herniated intervertebral disc. Their conclusions were based upon the undesirability of bone graft related complications (50). Their thoughts were based upon a comparison study of 20 herniated intervertebral discs with and without fusion. They observed that fusion took place within 6 months with a graft and 2–3 years without; however, some of those without grafting had slight anterior kyphotic deformity. They concluded equally good or excellent results in 90% of each group.

The anterior approach to the cervical spine is particularly useful to salvage kyphotic collapse following laminectomy. This problem is of particular concern in children, where biologic plasticity may alter the contour of the vertebral bodies, making it extremely difficult to correct the deformity. Stabilization is best carried out by a strong strut graft, preferably fibula, inserted in a longitudinal slot, cut in the vertebral bodies and countersunk into a normal vertebra above and below holding the vertebra apart like a prop.

Cervical osteotomy for ankylosing spondylitis is infrequently performed and may be hazardous. Mason et al. (34) and Herbert (28) reported only 3 cases. Marshal Urist (52) reported a single case in 1958 setting forth the surgical principles, anatomy, and safeguards in this procedure. Urist recommended that the patient be seated, that the condition be performed under local anesthesia at the C7–T1 interspace where the canal is widest and an osteotomy is less likely to damage the cord. At surgery the lamina of C7 is completely removed together with the facets, with the laminectomy extending upward into the C6 lamina, caudad to the T1 lamina. Temporary general anesthesia is then administered, as the pressure is applied beneath the chin, C7 separates from T1, and the head is placed in the selected position and maintained by a halo. Marshall Urist introduced the operative technique, but its continued clinical application goes to Edward Simmons (46) who has performed more than anyone in history.

The future anticipations of this rapidly developing subspecialty are many. Such indispensable tools as computed tomography (CT scanning) and magnetic resonance imaging (MRI) may evolve rapidly in three ways (45). MRI may be used for prolonged visualization, and in the case of CT, a lower dosage scan also may be possible for prolonged visualization without damage to the patient. Surgery may in the future be done under continuous MRI or CT scanning. Myelography in many instances has already been replaced by MRI. Myelography and even MRI may become obsolete with enhancement of neurologic structures by giving a systemic agent that localizes the nervous tissue. Three dimensional computerized modeling is already available demonstrating soft tissue, bone, spinal cord, and nerve roots.

Spinal fusion may decrease in its technical uncertainty also in three ways. First, the electrotherapeutic methods of Bassett (6) and Brighton in the appendicular skeleton may be used to enhance fusion, especially in conditions such as tumors and rheumatoid arthritis. Second, bone morphologic factor may be available, and this protein may be utilized in preference to iliac grafts to stimulate bone growth. Fusion may be obtained without surgery by injecting synthetic enzymes into the disc, intraspinous, or annular ligaments, producing an ankylosing spondylitic-like change in selected areas. Plate fixation, now commonly used in the thoracic and lumbar area, is now increasingly being used in the cervical spine. Screws have already been used successfully across the cervical pedicles in hangman's fracture, eliminating the necessity for a fusion with it's potential for decreasing cervical motion. Anterior cervical plates transfixed with screws are becoming increasingly popular as a method of stabilizing the cervical spine especially in instances of wide laminectomy. A more general understanding of pain syndromes may develop, and the management of chronic pain is already moving away from destructive techniques, such as rhizotomy and cordotomy (20). Methylmethacrylate, in preference to bone graft and total excision of vertebral bodies, is becoming more common for use with such destructive lesions as tumors.

Fantastic, perhaps, but who in the 19th century would have predicted that x-rays were possible, and who could have even imagined the dramatic change in medicine that occurred as a result of their use.

REFERENCES

1. Adams F. Paulus aeginata, Vol 2. London: Sydenham Society, 1816:155–156, 193, 197.
2. Alker GJ, Oh YS, Leslie EB. High cervical spine and craniocervical function injuries in fatal traffic accidents: a radiologic study. Orthop Clin North Am 1978;9:1003.
3. Bailey RW, Badgley CE. Stabilization of the cervical spine by anterior fusion. J Bone Joint Surg 1960;42A:565.
4. Barbour JR. Screw fixation in fractures of the odontoid process. S Austral Clin 1971;5:20.
5. Barton LG. The reduction of fracture dislocations of the cervical vertebrae by skeletal traction. Surg Gynecol Obstet 1938;67:94.
6. Basset AC. Personal communication, 1985.
7. Bigelow HJ. Insensibility during surgical operations produced by inhalation. Boston Med Surg J 1846;35:309.
8. Bigelow HJ. History of the discovery of modern anesthesia. Am J Med Sci 1876;141:164.

9. Böhler J. Anterior stabilization for acute fractures and non-unions of the dens. J Bone Joint Surg 1982;64A:18.
10. Bohlman H. Acute fractures and dislocations of the cervical spine. J Bone Joint Surg 1979;61A:1119.
11. Bontecou RB. Trans. New York M.A., Concord N.H. 1887;III:317.
12. Breasted JH. The Edwin-Smith surgical papyrus (The University of Chicago Oriental Institute Publications, Vol 3). Chicago: The University of Chicago Press, 1933.
13. Brooks AL, Jenkins EB. Atlantoaxial arthrodesis by the wedge compression method. J Bone Joint Surg 1978;60A:279.
14. Callahan RA, Johnson RM, Margolis RN, Keggi KJ, Albright JA, Southwick WO. Cervical facet fusion for control of instability following laminectomy. J Bone Joint Surg 1977;59A:991.
15. Cloward RB. The anterior approach for ruptured cervical disks. J Neurosurg 1958;15:602.
16. Crowe HL. Injuries to the cervical spine. Paper presented at the meeting of the Western Orthopaedic Association, San Francisco, 1928.
17. Crowther JG. Six great doctors: Harvey, Pasteur, Lister, Pardee, Riss, Fleming. London: H. Hamilton, 1957:207.
18. Crutchfield WG. Skeletal traction for dislocation of cervical spine. South Surg J 1933;2:156.
19. De Andrade JR, Macnab I. Anterior occipitocervical fusion using an extra-pharyngeal exposure. J Bone Surg 1969;51A:1621.
20. Epstein J. Changing trends in the neurosurgical management of chronic pain. Spine 1982;10:100.
21. Fielding JW, Cochran GVB, Lawsing JR III, Hohl M. Tears of the transverse ligament of the atlas. A clinical and biomechanical study. J Bone Joint Surg 1969;56A:1621.
22. Gallie WE. Skeletal traction in the treatment of fractures and dislocations of the cervical spine. Ann Surg 1937;106:770.
23. Gallie WE. Fractures and dislocations of the cervical spine. Am J Surg 1939;46:495.
24. Hamada G, Rida A. Orthopaedics and orthopaedic diseases in ancient and modern Egypt. Letter editor. Clin Orthop 1972;89:253.
25. Harris JE. Personal communication, 1982.
26. Harris RI. New investigations: instrument for tightening knots in steel wire. Lancet 1944;1:504.
27. Hensinger RN, Lang JE, MacEwan GD. Klippel-Feil syndrome. J Bone Joint Surg 1974;56A:1246.
28. Herbert JJ. Reflexions sur la technique et les résultats de 42 osteotomies vertebrales. Rev Chir Orthop 1954;73:357.
29. Hildanus, F. Opera (1672). *In*: Walker, AE. A history of neurological surgery. New York, Hatner Publishing Company, 1967:366.
30. Hoen, TL. A method of skeletal traction for treatment of fracture dislocation of cervical vertebrae. Arch Neurol 1936;36:158.
31. Howorth, B, Petrie G. Injuries to the spine. Baltimore: Williams & Wilkins, 1964.
32. Klippel M, Feil A. Un cas d'absence des vertebres cervicales. Avec cage thoracique remontant jusqu' à la base du crane (cage thoracique cervicale). Nouv Icon Sal 1912;25:223.
33. Lister J. On the antiseptic principle in the practice of surgery. Lancet 1867;12:353.
34. Mason C, Cozen, L, Adelstein L. Surgical correction of flexion deformity of the cervical spine. Cal Med 1953;79:244.
35. Mixter SJ, Osgood RB. Traumatic lesions of the atlas and axis. Ann Surg 1910;56B:193.
36. Nickel VL, Perry, J, Garret, A, Heppenstall, M. The halo: a spinal skeletal traction fixation device. J Bone Joint Surg 1968;50A:1400.
37. Paré A. Oeuvres Paris. 1958:528, 551, 559.
38. Pasteur L. Etudes sur le vin; ses maladees, causes qui provoquent, procedes nouveaux pour le conserver et pour le vieiller. L'Imprimerie Imperiale, 1866;8:32.
30. Pilcher LS. Atlo-axoid fracture dislocation. Ann Surg 1910;51:208.
40. Pott P. Observations on the nature and consequences of those injuries to which the head is liable from external violence. *In*: Hawes L, Clarke W, Collins R. eds. London, 1768.
41. Robinson RA, Smith GW. Anterior disc removal with fusion. Anterolateral cervical disk removal and interbody fusion for cervical disk syndrome. Bull Johns Hopkins Hosp 1955;96:223.
42. Robinson RA, Southwick WO. Indications and techniques for early stabilization of the neck in some fracture-dislocations of the cervical spine. South Med J 1960;53:565.
43. Röentgen WC. Über eine Neve Art Von Strahlen: Sitzungsberichte der Physik Wurzburg: Med. Gesellschaft, 1895:132.
44. Rogers WA. Treatment of fracture-dislocation of the cervical spine. J Bone Joint Surg 1942;24:245.
45. Rothman R. Personal communication, 1982.
46. Simmons EH. The surgical correction of flexion deformity on the cervical spine in ankylosing spondylitis. Clin Orthop 1972;86:132.
47. Smith AG. Account of a case in which portions of three dorsal vertebrae were removed for the relief of paralysis from fracture, with partial success. 1829;8:94.
48. Stauffer ES, Kelly EG. Fracture-dislocations of the cervical spine. J Bone Joint Surg 1977;59A:45.
49. Taylor AS. Fracture dislocation of the cervical spine. Ann Surg 1929;90:321.
50. Tew JM, Jr, Mayfield FH. The anterior interbody approach in the treatment of herniated cervical disc, spondylosis, and fracture dislocation. Presented at the 22nd Annual Meeting of the Congress of Neurological Surgeons, Denver, Colorado, October 19, 1972.
51. Unterharnscheidt HF. Morphologic findings in Rhesus monkeys undergoing $-G_3$ impact acceleration. Presented at the Cervical Spine Research Society meeting. Palm Beach, Florida, December 7, 1983.
52. Urist MR. Osteotomy of the cervical spine. J Bone Joint Surg 1958;40A:833.
53. Vinke TH. A skull traction apparatus. J Bone Joint Surg 1948;30A:522.
54. Walker EA. A History of neurological surgery. New York: Hafner Publishing, 1967.
55. White AA, Johnson RM, Panjabi MM, Southwick WO. Biomechanical analysis of clinical stability in the cervical spine. Clin Orthop 1975;109:85.

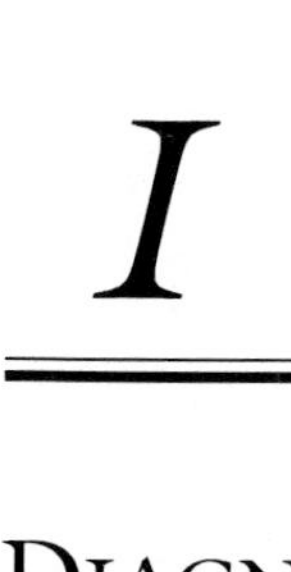

I

Neurologic and Diagnostic Evaluation

1

Cervical Spine Biomechanics

David G. Wilder

Introduction

The cervical spine protects the spinal cord while providing a stable and mobile platform for the head. It can be considered a mechanism consisting of links (vertebrae) that are stiffer than the flexible connections (discs or articulating surfaces) between them. As with any mechanism, it operates best when the demands placed upon it are within its "design" limits. When excessive loads and torques are applied, its active and passive components begin to fail. There are limits to the cervical spine's motion and load-bearing capacity, based not only upon geometric, elastic, and strength characteristics, but also on material and muscular fatigue properties. While the most apparent concerns for the neck relate to impact and trauma, long-term maintenance of large, continuous static muscle efforts is also important.

Much has been written about the biomechanics of the cervical spine (7, 26, 66). This writer hopes to provide a helpful introduction to the subject.

The cervical spine consists of mechanical elements that play passive and active roles. "Passive" refers to those elements whose primary function is to provide load transmission, distribution, and interconnections (such as ligaments, discs, and vertebrae). "Active" refers to those elements that can generate force on demand. The active stabilizers of the cervical spine are its surrounding muscles. Such a long, slender, and mobile column depends on its peripheral muscular supports. Without them, it would collapse.

Most mechanical environments that humans experience do not overload the body. When considering how the cervical spine is affected mechanically, one needs to describe carefully the direction and magnitude of the loads and torques (twisting or bending moments) applied to it. Loads and torques can be applied to the cervical vertebrae in many ways; they have properties of both orientation and magnitude (and as such are called vector quantities). Sources and types of loads and torques vary.

Static loads can originate from ligamentous and capsular tensions, load of the head and gear on top of the head, the effect of gravity or local acceleration field (tight turns in a vehicle or plane), and normal muscle tone or forces due to a constant muscle contraction exerted to maintain a posture. Dynamic forces are those that change with time and can occur either once or repetitively. "One-shot" loads would compromise the following examples: a "whiplash" event, a diving accident where the head hits a solid object, and a "spearing" type tackle in football. Repetitive loads are applied to the body quite often these days due to vehicular vibration. Kelsey and Hardy (29) and Heliovaara (24) have shown that exposure to driving affects not only the lumbar spine but also the cervical spine (30). Those loads can be either steady state sinusoidal vibrations or non-steady state random vibrations. Depending on the road and vehicular conditions, vertical impacts can also occur.

Anthropometric Aspects

One of the challenging aspects of studying the body as a machine is the "reverse engineering" involved. In building a machine, the designer specifies what it should do and then builds it toward that end. The body is a "found" machine that generally runs quite well. To help it get over some of its occasional difficulties, such as recovering from mechanical trauma, we study its rules of mechanical behavior. The first step in evaluating a mechanism's function is to look at the size and shape of its pieces, how they are arranged, and how they interact. Avoiding spinal cord and blood vessel impingement while providing protection for the cord and allowing the necessary range of motion is the basic requirement of the cervical spine.

Francis (15) performed a systematic study of the cervical vertebrae to establish dimensional range, and mean and standard deviation in a sample with known age, gender, and race. He measured the overall and foraminal anterior-posterior and lateral diameters of the seven cervical vertebrae from 100 young adult white males, 100 young adult black males, 27 young adult white females, and 57 young adult black females. In addition, centra were measured for their anterior-posterior, lateral, and vertical diameters. No significant differences were found due to race. Although the dimensions of the female vertebrae were smaller than the male, significance was not clear.

In another study to determine basic dimensional relationships, Mazzara and Fielding (38) looked at the effect of odontoid tilt and rotation on the narrowing of the spinal canal between the atlas and the axis. Using a mean cord diameter of 100 mm as the limit, they found that the atlanto-axial complex could rotate up to 64° before the narrowing was too great. In 57% of the specimens tested, facet dislocation occurred before that limit was reached. The limit was exceeded in 39% of the cases, after which facet dislocation occurred. As long as the limit of 10 mm was not exceded, cord damage would not have been likely.

Geometric measurements taken by Pal and Routal (47) show that vertical loads are transmitted down the cervical spine (C2–C7) not only by means of the discs and centra, but also via postero-lateral columns comprised of the engaged articular processes. This kind of arrangement is inherently more stable than one requiring a single, slender column to accommodate the load. A comparison could be made to a milking stool. A three-legged stool is more difficult to tip over than a stool with one leg.

It is difficult to test certain experimental hypotheses using in-vivo and in-vitro humans. In order to use animals as experimental models, it is necessary, for both physical and ethical reasons, to know how well the animal matches the human. Huang and Suarez (25) reported a comparison between a 10-week-old female pig and a 3-year-old female child. Computed tomography (CT) scans were obtained of the pig before and after sacrifice and of the child, who had died of leukemia. The measured area and calculated mass of the neck was larger in the pig than in the child, whereas the opposite was true using the same measures of the head. If 10-week-old pigs are then used to design safety limits for children, the limits may be underestimates. The human child supports a relatively larger head on a relatively smaller neck. The pig, with a smaller head on a larger neck, should be able to withstand larger accelerations and decelerations than the child.

KINEMATIC ASPECTS

Kinematic analysis is another way to evaluate the cervical spine. Kinematics is the study of the motion of an object without consideration of the forces involved. As an object moves, it can change its position and orientation with the passage of time. The basis of this method can be made apparent using a camera flash to "freeze" a moving object in space and time or by using a (blinking) stroboscopic light to "freeze" the object's position at regular time intervals. A variety of methods are available for recording motion: film, videotape, or computer-linked cameras sensitive to emitted or reflected light or to infra-red radiating markers. Mechanical pointers and linkages containing displacement and/or rotation indicators can also be used to sense motion (3) and to provide an objective correlate to radiography.

Unconstrained, a rigid body has the potential to move in six different directions, one at a time or in combination. The rigid body is then said to be able to move with six degrees of freedom. In the spine, the rigid body is the vertebra, and the six degrees of freedom consist of three translations (anterior-posterior shear, right and left lateral shear, and caudo-cephalad compression and distraction) and three rotations (flexion-extension, right and left lateral bend, and right and left axial rotation). In-vitro and in-vivo studies have determined ranges of motion for different regions of the cervical spine.

Dimnet et al. (11) discuss a method for obtaining both kinematic and geometric parameters from a minimum number of radiographs. Dunsker, Colley, and Mayfield (12) provide a review with x-rays of the motion of the cervical spine from 25 normal patients. Lind et al. (33) obtained range of motion data from a large number of normal subjects, both male and female of widely varying ages (12–79). Lateral bend and flexion-extension extremes were monitored radiographically. Axial rotation was sensed nonradiographically, using a compass placed on the head. Tests were performed twice for reliability. Only in flexion-extension were intervertebral movements measured and ranged from 10°–16°. Gross, main motion from the occiput to C7 was measured during flexion-extension, lateral bend, and axial rotation. Both men and women had the largest range of motion in axial rotation (ranging from 80°–200°) and the least in lateral bend (ranging from 22°–81°), with flexion-extension in between (ranging from 24°–114°). Range of motion data were compared to age via linear regression and showed that with age, all motion decreased.

COUPLED MOTION

Due to the cervical region's complex mechanical characteristics and interactions, it is difficult for the region to exhibit a single motion type alone. Most of the time, when the region moves in one way it also exhibits another motion coupled with the primary motion. For example, coupled axial rotation can occur as a result of a primary lateral bend motion.

In 1969, Lysell published his findings on the range and type of motion exhibited in the cervical spine and the effect of degenerative changes (35). He looked at motion in the region from several views in order to determine three-dimensional behavior. His observations included the ranges of flexion-extension, lateral bend, and axial rotation; he noted the existence of simple and coupled motion.

Penning (53) superimposed radiographs of 20 healthy young adults and graphically analyzed the motion possible in the cervical spine. His observations of the coupled motion behavior in the region led him to speculate on cervical muscle function. The article also provided some convenient paper templates (to be cut out) to assist in visualizing the motion there.

From biplanar radiographs of axial rotation extremes in 20 normal subjects, Mimura et al. (40) found that most of the motion in the cervical spine occurred between the occiput and C2 (averaging 70°). From C2 to C7, the average intervertebral axial rotations ranged from 4.2–7.2°. There was also evidence of coupled motion (in the flexion-extension and lateral bend modes) resulting from the imposed axial rotation. Coupled responses were sensitive to the level rotated. For instance, coupled lateral bending occurred in the same direction as the imposed axial rotation from the occiput to C3, but the bending response was reversed from C3 to C7. Similar responses were observed for coupled flexion-extension, with the transition between flexion and extension occurring at C5.

Biomechanics

The study of the mechanics of the cervical spine includes theory regarding the applied and reactive forces and torques involved in cervical spine behavior. Active and passive elements have stiffness (resistance to motion) and damping characteristics (the ability to reduce actively occurring movement) that affect their behavior. Muscles exhibit additional characteristics due to their force-generating capacity.

Many studies have performed load-deflection or torque-rotation evaluations of all or portions of the cervical spine. Basically, a load-deflection evaluation involves pushing or pulling on an object with increasing amounts of force and measuring the resulting motion. The rotational analog is called a torque-rotation test and measures the rotation occurring in response to increasing levels of twist or torque. These are basic techniques for mechanically characterizing the properties of materials, structures, and mechanisms. A load-deflection or stress-strain test to failure can indicate an item's stiffness, elastic limit, point at which irreversible plastic deformation begins, point of failure, and whether it is brittle or ductile (17, 46, 54).

In an early review of spinal mechanics, Schultz (61) provided an overview of regional motion ranges and tissue properties. Another productive spinal research group, Panjabi et al. (50), have performed extensive multidirectional intact segment testing measuring main, coupled, load-deflection, and rotation responses. Raynor et al. (57) found that there was a significant decrease in main and coupled motion following facetectomy, except when applying distraction loads. Moroney et al. (41) studied 35 fresh adult cadaveric cervical motion segments (from C2 to T1) by testing them in compression, shear, flexion, lateral bend, and axial rotation, both with and without posterior elements and under different states of degeneration. They found effects of both posterior element removal and degeneration. When rotating the C0–C1–C2 to failure, Goel et al. (21) observed that maximum torsional resistance occurred at the point of complete bilateral dislocation of C1–C2 facets (at 55°–70°). If the segment was released before that point, the imposed rotation was reversible, beyond that point it was irreversible.

As shown above, much in-vitro work has evaluated the load-deflection and strength properties of the motion segments in the neck under various conditions. Results of these types of tests have practical value beyond knowledge of basic biomechanics. Use of these data can, for example, aid in helmet design such that helmet impingement on the back of the neck will result in minimal applied forces and bending moments. Vehicle windshields could be designed to "pop out" at certain loads, below the buckling loads in the neck. Vehicle and occupant seat suspensions could be designed to minimize the vibration loading transmitted to the neck, deleterious to the cervical spine (30).

Biomechanics—Components

It is important to know the overall behavior of the cervical spine. Knowledge of the mechanics of the components that make up the neck is also valuable. Preventive and corrective measures can be adopted in treatment and in situations where the cervical spine is at risk.

Fielding et al. (14), evaluated the in-vitro load needed to produce a tearing failure of 20 transverse ligaments using a deflection rate of 12 mm over 0.1 seconds (equivalent to 120 mm per second). These results were correlated to 11 clinical cases surviving traumatic disruption and anterior subluxation of the atlas on the axis due to trauma to the head. They found that the in-vitro failure load ranged from 40–180 kilopounds and resulted in no odontoid process failures. As a result, they advocate fusion of the atlanto-axial joint as conservative treatment. Using a much lower deflection rate (1.5 mm per second), Dvorak et al. (13) performed an in-vitro, mechanical, and histological study of the alar and transverse ligaments (using a sample size of seven). Load was applied until failure of the tissue occurred. The failure was always at bone-cartilage interface, probably because of the lower deflection rates than in the study by Fielding et al. (14). They found that the odontoid failed before the transverse ligament did (at 350 Newtons) which appeared able to accommodate physiologic loads. In contrast, they found that the alar ligament was weaker, failing at 200 Newtons and suggesting that this failure may need more stabilization than previously thought.

Yoganandan et al. (69) tested 68 ligaments (anterior longitudinal ligaments and ligamentum flavum) from 28 cadavers, and corroborated the effects of viscoelasticity. Their tensile tests used dynamic loads produced by deflection rates ranging from 2.5–2500 mm per second. The ligaments became stiffer, and failure loads increased with higher loading rates. Because "elongation to failure" did not correlate with increasing deflection rate, the tissue failures appeared to be sensitive to a length threshold. Tissues can withstand high deflection and load rates as long as they are of a short duration. In an evaluation of the tensile strengths of the ligaments of the upper cervical spine, Myklebust et al. (44) found that the alar and anterior atlanto-occipital membrane were the strongest (with means of 500–600 Newtons) and the tectorial the weakest (at 100 Newtons).

Component transection studies are helpful because they reveal just how much of the region must be disrupted before catastrophic failure occurs. Panjabi et al. (49) studied 17 motion segments to determine basic information on the threshold of stability as function of transection of components. The response was similar regardless of the direction tested. When either a flexion moment was applied and components were cut, proceeding from anterior to posterior, or an extension moment was applied and components were cut from posterior to anterior, there were small incremental increases in motion until there was a sudden complete disruption without warning. Elastic deformation was small overall even after many ligaments were cut. It appears that cervical stability depends most upon ligaments opposite the motion or moment. In addition, removing the facet decreased rotation and increased horizontal displacement. Wetzel et al. (64), trying to develop an in-vivo injury model for the human spine, looked at the effect of serial component transections of ligaments in the rabbit. The response was similar to that found in the human, except there was more motion in the rabbit with incremental transections.

The next level of "component" are the motion segments. Of special interest is the upper cervical region. Panjabi et al. (51) evaluated the three-dimensional movements of upper cervical spine. They found that more flexion, axial rotation, and lateral bend motion occurs in the C1–C2 segment than in C0–C1. However, in extension, the motion is comparable at both levels. In general they found the existence of large neutral zones, regions in the middle of the range of motion, where small loads or torques produce large deflections or rotations. Goel et al. (20), in their in-vitro moment-rotation studies (sample size of 8) of the occipito-atlanto-axial complex, found a nonlinear response, corroborated the existence of a large neutral zone, where small moments produce large rotations, and also observed that lateral bend and axial rotation were highly coupled. With so much complex motion possible in the region, it is important that the muscles behave properly and are not compromised by fatigue, injury, or disease.

Nolan and Sherk (45) dissected and physically modelled the semispinalis cervicis and capitis muscles, demonstrating their roles as the primary extensors of the cervical spine. Based on those findings, the authors altered their surgical approach and now minimize the disruption of those muscles.

INSTABILITY/STABILITY

The passive mechanical components of the cervical spine that give it mobility also endow it with the potential for mechanical buckling (65). The potential for buckling instability is a property of slender columns. There is a curious aspect to it also. Long column buckling allows a structure the possibility of having two different orientations at essentially the same applied load (62). Consider the case of a long, narrow wooden dowel held end to end between one's hands. As an increasing compressive load is applied, the rod remains straight, but becomes longitudinally shorter, based on its axial elastic characteristics. The load can increase with little motion between the hands applying the load until the dowel suddenly changes its configuration from straight to curved. It continues to bend rapidly until it either breaks or reaches a configuration that can resist the load in bending. If it does reach that new orientation at which it can resist the applied load, that is its second configuration (bent) at essentially the same load as that resisted just prior to buckling (pure compression).

Unfortunately, many structures and mechanisms are unable to resist the load in bending, which they could accommodate in compression (e.g., Nimitz Freeway columns). Keep in mind that under pure axial compression, all its elements experience compression. If the axially applied load shifts outside of its "base of support" or a noncoaxial load is applied or a moment is applied, buckling can start. During bending, one side of a rod's neutral axis experiences further compression while the other side is subjected to sudden tension. From a different perspective, buckling can be considered that transition which occurs when the peripheral elements of the rod change their roles from all being in compression to some in compression and some in tension. During that change, the material can experience a large strain as one region relaxes from the compression and is then stretched out by the tension. During the buckling transition, there is very little resistance to the applied load. This can allow the mass applying the load to accelerate, gain momentum, and increase the energy and force which the buckling column will eventually need to resist.

Especially difficult for the cervical spine in the buckling transition from a compressive to a bending mode is the fact that the muscles often cannot respond with enough speed or force to prevent, accommodate, or slow its sudden bending. A small imbalance in muscle tension on opposite sides may initiate and accelerate the buckling event. Muscles on the tensile side of the bending neck lie along a longer path and therefore must develop a stabilizing tension faster than those on the compressive side. There is an additional limitation: the speed with which the system can respond to an applied load or acceleration. Muscles have finite response times; they can only "turn on" so fast. If an imposed mechanical event occurs more rapidly than muscles can respond, then the system depends on its passive mechanical properties, such as its base of support (48) for protection.

BIOMECHANICS—INJURY/REPAIR

The awareness of cervical spine injury mechanics has been growing (59). This knowledge has affected athletic (5, 28, 62), vehicular (22, 31, 32), and recreational safety (1, 16). It has also suggested efficient classification of cervical fractures, with a more organized approach to diagnosis and treatment (2). In order to continue to improve awareness of injury potential and to improve trauma prevention and treatment, further injury biomechanics research is needed (63), such as that already conducted on injury mechanisms (27, 37, 43, 52, 56) and repair biomechanics (8, 18).

OCCUPATIONAL CONSIDERATIONS

When evaluating a patient for neck pain, it is wise to keep the demands of his or her job in mind. Although Ramazzini (55) pointed this out 285 years ago, it is still valid today (6). Bendix and Biering-Sorensen (4) pointed out that the neck is quite flexible and can maintain a posture regardless of that dictated by the seat for the lower back, while sitting for 1 hour. This implies that the head and neck can be kept still and stable for prolonged periods. Extreme postures of the head and neck lead to pain, even though muscle activity is low (23). Because work postures affect neck muscle activity, they should be optimized to reduce it (60). In addition, vibration environments such as car and truck driving, which have deleterious effects on the lumbar spine (24, 29), also affect the cervical spine (30) and should be avoided or minimized.

BIOMECHANICS—MODEL

Mathematical and physical models of the cervical spine have been developed in order to gain insight into its workings under different conditions (9, 10, 34, 39, 67, 69). They also allow researchers to study tissue properties and component behavior mathematically and manipulate them, trying to model reality (19, 41, 58). A working model of the cervical spine would allow prediction and avoidance of conditions that could harm the neck, without the use of human or animal research subjects. However, for a model to be helpful, its abilities and limitations must be known and confirmed with reality, such as the model utilized by Moroney, Schultz, and Miller (41). If historical data are not available in the literature, then experiments do need to be carried out to test the model. Although an imposing and challenging task, the validated model would be invaluable.

SUMMARY

Some of the concepts related to the biomechanics of the cervical spine have been introduced. The region is an engineering wonder of strength, flexibility, and function, able to function in many diverse environments ranging from impact and vibration to static postures held for long durations. There are many biomechanical aspects to understanding, controlling, and preventing injury and pain in the cervical spine. It should continue to be a fertile area for study.

ACKNOWLEDGMENTS

The author appreciated the opportunity to express his views on this subject. However, he is especially indebted to his wife, for her patience with the challenges of controlling "chaos central" and the inquisitive, untiring nature of the very young. Carrie Beauchemin was a great help with the "crunches." Gratefully acknowledged is financial support from several sources: The McClure Musculoskeletal Research Center, the National Institute for Occupational Safety and Health (Grant No. 1-K01-0H00090-01), The Whitaker Foundation, the National Institute for Disability and Rehabilitation Research (Grant No. USOE H133E80018), and the National Institutes of Health (Grant No. 1-R23-AM38317-01) all of which embrace the potential that orthopedic biomechanics holds for solving musculoskeletal mysteries.

REFERENCES

1. Albrand OW, Walter J. Underwater deceleration curves in relation to injuries from diving. Surg Neurol 1975;4:461–464.

2. Allen BL Jr, Ferguson RL, Lehmann TR, O'Brien RP. A mechanistic classification of closed indirect fractures and dislocations of the lower cervical spine. Spine 1982;7:1–27.

3. Alund M, Larsson SE. Three-dimensional analysis of neck motion. A clinical method. Spine 1990;15:87–91.

4. Bendix T, Biering-Sorensen F. Posture of the trunk when sitting on forward inclining seats. Scand J Rehabil Med 1983;15:197–203.

5. Carter DR, Frankel VH. Biomechanics of hyperextension injuries to the cervical spine in football. Am J Sports Med 1980;8:302–309.

6. Centers for Disease Control. Leading work-related diseases and injuries—United States. Musculoskeletal injuries. MMWR 32(14):189–191.

7. Cervical Spine Research Society Editorial Committee, Sherk HH, Chairman. The cervical spine. Philadelphia: Lippincott, 1989.

8. Crisco JJ, Panjabi MM, Wang E, Price MA, Pelker RR. The injured canine cervical spine after six months of healing. An in vitro three-dimensional study. Spine 1990;15:1047.

9. Deng YC, Goldsmith W. Response of a human head/neck/upper-torso replica to dynamic loading—I. Physical model. J Biomech 1987;20:471–486.

10. Deng YC, Goldsmith W. Response of a human head/neck/upper-torso replica to dynamic loading—II. Analytical/numerical model. J Biomech 1987;20:487–497.

11. Dimnet J, Pasquet A, Krag MH, Panjabi MM. Cervical spine motion in the sagittal plane: kinematic and geometric parameters. J Biomech 1982;15:959–969.

12. Dunsker SB, Colley DP, Mayfield FH. Kinematics of the cervical spine. Clin Neurosurg 1978;25:174–183.

13. Dvorak J, Schneider E, Saldinger P, Rahn B. Biomechanics of the craniocervical region: the altar and transverse ligaments. J Orthop Res 1988;6:452–461.

14. Fielding JW, Cochran G van B, Lawsing JF, Hohl M. Tears of the transverse ligament of the atlas. A clinical and biomechanical study. J Bone Joint Surg [Am] 1974;56A:1683–1691.

15. Francis CC. Dimensions of the cervical vertebrae. Anat Rec 1955;122:603–609.

16. Francis WR, Fielding JW. Traumatic spondylolisthesis of the axis. Orthop Clin North Am 9(4):1011–1027.

17. Fung YC. Biomechanics. Mechanical properties of living tissues. New York: Springer-Verlag, 1981.

18. Goel VK, Clark CR, McGowan D, Goyal S. An in-vitro study of the kinematics of the normal, injured and stabilized cervical spine. J Biomech 1984;17:363–376.

19. Goel VK, Liu YK, Clark CR, Alexander EJ, Chandra S. Muscles of the cervical spine—a biomechanical approach. Orthop Trans 1985;9:132.

20. Goel VK, Clark CR, Gallaes K, Liu YK. Moment-rotation relationships of the ligamentous occipito-atlanto-axial complex. J Biomech 1988;21:673–680.

21. Goel VK, Winterbotton JM, Schulte KR, et al. Ligamentous laxity across C0-C1-C2 complex. Axial torque-rotation characteristics until failure. Spine 1990;15:990.

22. Gogler H, Athanasiadis S, Adomeit D. Fatal cervical dislocation related to wearing a seat belt: a care report. Injury 1979;10:196–200.

23. Harms-Ringdahl K. An assessment of shoulder exercise and load-elicited pain in the cervical spine. Biomechanical analysis of load—EMG—methodological studies of pain provoked by extreme position. Scand J Rehabil Med Suppl 1986;14:1–40.

24. Heliovaara M. Occupation and risk of herniated lumbar intervertebral disc or sciatica leading to hospitalization. J Chron Dis 1987;40:259–264.

25. Huang HK, Suarez FR. Evaluation of cross-sectional geometry and mass density distributions of humans and laboratory animals using computerized tomography. J Biomech 1983;16:821–832.

26. Huelke DF, Nusholtz GS. Cervical spine biomechanics: a review of the literature. J Orthop Res 1986;4:232–245.

27. Kabo JM, Goldsmith W, Harris NM. In-vitro head and neck response to impact. J Biomech Eng 1983;105:316–320.

28. Kazarian L. Injuries to the human spinal column: biomechanics and injury classification. Exerc Sport Sci Rev 1981;9:297–352.

29. Kelsey JL, Hardy RJ. Driving of motor vehicles as a risk factor for acute herniated lumbar intervertebral disc. Am J Epidemiol 1975;102:63–73.

30. Kelsey JL, Githens PB, Walter SD, et al. An epidemiological study of acute prolapsed cervical intervertebral disc. J Bone Joint Surg 1984;66-A(6):907–914, July.

31. LaRocca H. Acceleration injuries of the neck. Clin Neurosurg 1978;25:209–217.

32. Lesoin F, Thomas CE, Lozes G, Villette L, Jomin M. Has the safety belt replaced the hangman's noose? Lancet 1985;1341, June 8.

33. Lind B, Sihlbom H, Nordwall A, Malchau H. Normal range of motion of the cervical spine. Arch Phys Med Rehabil 1989;70:692–695.

34. Liu YK, Dai QG. The second stiffest axis of a beam-column: implications for cervical spine trauma. J Biomech Eng 1989;111:122–127.

35. Lysell E. Motion in the cervical spine. An experimental study on autopsy specimens. Acta Orthop Scand Suppl 1969;40:123.

36. Macnab I. The "whiplash syndrome." Orthop Clin North Am 1971;2:389–403.

37. Maiman DJ, Sances A Jr, Myklebust JB, et al. Compression injuries of the cervical spine: a biomechanical analysis. Neurosurgery 1983;13:254–260.

38. Mazzara JT, Fielding JW. A dynamic anthropometric study of the atlas and axis. Orthop Trans 1988;12:51.

39. Merrill T, Goldsmith W, Deng YC. Three-dimensional response of a lumped parameter head-neck model due to impact and impulsive loading. J Biomech 1984;17:81–95.

40. Mimura M, Moriya H, Watanabe T, Takahashi K, Yamagata M, Tamaki T. Three-dimensional motion analysis of the cervical spine with special reference to the axial rotation. Spine 1989;14:1135.

41. Moroney SP, Schultz AB, Miller JA. Analysis and measurement of neck loads. J Orthop Res 1988;6:713–720.

42. Moroney SP, Schultz AB, Miller JA, Andersson GB. Load-displacement properties of lower cervical spine motion segments. J Biomech 1988;21:769–779.

43. Mouradian WH, Fietti VG Jr, Cochran GV, Fielding JW, Young J. Fractures of the odontoid: a laboratory and clinical study of mechanisms. Orthop Clin North Am 1978;9:985–1001.

44. Myklebust JB, Pintar F, Rauschning W, Sances A Jr, Cusick JF. Tensile strength of the upper cervical ligaments. Orthop Trans 1985;9:132.

45. Nolan JP Jr, Sherk HH. Biomechanical evaluation of the extensor musculature of the cervical spine. Spine 1988;13:9–11.

46. Olsen GA. Elements of mechanics of materials. Englewood Cliffs, New Jersey: Prentice Hall, 1966.

47. Pal GP, Routal RV. A study of weight transmission through the cervical and upper thoracic regions of the vertebral column in man. J Anat 1986;148:245–261.

48. Pal GP, Sherk HH. The vertical stability of the cervical spine. Spine 1988;13:447–449.

49. Panjabi MM, White AA, Johnson RM. Cervical spine mechanics as a function of transection of components. J Biomech 1975;8:327–336.

50. Panjabi MM, Summers DJ, Pelker RR, Videman T, Friedlaender GE, Southwick WO. Three-dimensional load-displacement curves due to forces on the cervical spine. J Orthop Res 1986;4:152–161.

51. Panjabi M, Dvorak J, Duranceau J, Gerber M, Yamamoto I, Buff U. Three-dimensional movements of the upper cervical spine. Orthop Trans 1988;12:50–51.

52. Panjabi MM, Duranceau JS, Oxland TR, Bowen CE. Three dimensional instability of traumatic cervical spine injuries in a porcine model. Orthop Trans 1989;13:204.

53. Penning L. Normal movements of the cervical spine. Am J Roentgenol 1978;130:317–326.

54. Radin EL, Simon SR, Rose RM, Paul IL. Practical biomechanics for the orthopaedic surgeon. New York: John Wiley & Sons, 1979.

55. Ramazzini B. A treatise of the diseases of tradesmen. English translation: A Bell, R Smith, D Midwinter, et al. London. Quoted in Talbott JH. A biographical history of medicine. New York: Grune and Stratton, 1970:135.

56. Raynor RB, Koplik B. Cervical cord trauma. The relationship between clinical syndromes and force of injury. Spine 1985;10:193–197.

57. Raynor RB, Moskovich R, Zidel P, Pugh J. Alterations in primary and coupled neck motions after facectomy. Neurosurgery. 1987;21:681–687.

58. Reber JG, Goldsmith W. Analysis of large head-neck motions. J Biomech 1979;12:211–222.

59. Sances A Jr, Myklebust JB, Maiman DJ, Larson SJ, Cusick JF, Jodat RW. The biomechanics of spinal injuries. Crit Rev Biomed Eng 1984;11:1–76.

60. Schuldt K. On neck muscle activity and load reduction in sitting postures. An electromyographic and biomechanical study with applications in ergonomics and rehabilitation. Scand J Rehabil Med Suppl 1988;19:1–49.

61. Schultz AB. Mechanics of the human spine. Appl Mech Rev 1974;27:1487–1497.

62. Torg JS, Quedenfeld TC, Burstein A, Spealman A, Nichols C. National football head and neck injury registry: report on cervical quadriplegia, 1971 to 1975. Am J Sports Med 1979;7:127–132.

63. Viano DC, King AI, Melvin JW, Weber K. Injury biomechanics

research: an essential element in the prevention of trauma. J Biomech 1989;22:403–417.

64. Wetzel FT, Panjabi MM, Pelker RR. Biomechanics of the rabbit cervical spine as a function of component transection. J Orthop Res 1989;7:723–727.

65. White AA, Johnson RM, Panjabi MM, Southwick WO. Biomechanical analysis of clinical stability in the cervical spine. Clin Orthop 1975;109:85–96.

66. White AA, Panjabi MM. Clinical biomechanics of the spine. Philadelphia: Lippincott, 1990.

67. Williams JL, Belytschko TB. A three-dimensional model of the human cervical spine for impact simulation. J Biomech Eng 1983;105:321–331.

68. Yoganandan N, Butler J, Pintar F, Myklebust J, Reinartz J, Sances A. Dynamic response of human cervical spine ligaments. Orthop Trans 1989;13:203.

69. Yoganandan N, Sances A Jr, Pintar F. Biomechanical evaluation of the axial compressive responses of the human cadaveric and manikin necks. J Biomech Eng 1989;111:250–255.

2

Neurological Evaluation of Cervical Spinal Disorders

Peter Tsairis and Barry Jordan

Introduction

The fundamental elements for correct diagnosis of cervical spinal syndromes are the history and neurological-musculoskeletal examinations; they should not be minimized or underestimated. If careless or abbreviated, they often provide a shallow basis for understanding the patient's disorder for which no supporting laboratory test will substitute. The application of neuroanatomy and neurophysiology to these clinical disorders affecting the neck is one of the satisfying exercises of neurological practice. The radiological, electrophysiological, and other ancillary investigations should help to confirm or disprove the clinical impression and assist in formulating the differential diagnosis.

The nerve root compression syndromes and the types of myelopathy produced by spondylosis, disc herniation, and space occupying lesions were largely elucidated in the early 1950s (1). In those days surgeons diagnosed and operated on patients on the basis of the clinical examination, aided for the most part by plain radiography and air myelography. Electrophysiological techniques have been of questionable value except in those patients who lack solid evidence of nerve root and/or spinal cord compression, or are in need of a positive test for purposes of economic settlement in an American court or within a compensation system. It is our view, however, that electrophysiological studies do play an essential role in the differential diagnosis, particularly in those cases in which intrinsic neural disease such as brachial plexus neuritis or amyotrophic lateral sclerosis must be differentiated from extrinsic lesions of the spine.

As most of us know, many patients with plain x-ray evidence of osteoarthritis are asymptomatic, and in some symptomatic patients these films may be normal or minimally abnormal. In the last 15 years neuroimaging scans (computed tomography and magnetic resonance imaging) have added tremendously to pinpointing the pathologic substrate in these syndromes and, additionally, have provided surgeons with additional information with which to make a decision about surgical intervention. These scans have also aided clinicians in sorting out the treatable patients formerly denied treatment through clinical misdiagnosis of such disorders as multiple sclerosis, syringomyelia, or spinal neoplasms.

The following sections in this chapter will focus on the key diagnostic elements that should aid clinicians in the evaluation of cervical spine disorders.

Clinical Analysis and Presentations

The patient evaluation has three components: 1) a detailed history and physical examination, 2) neurological and musculoskeletal examinations, and 3) radiological and/or electrophysiological studies.

The primary objective of the *clinical history* is to determine whether the patient's spinal symptoms are consistent with a primary disorder of the cervical spine or a secondary manifestation of a systemic disorder, such as polymyalgia rheumatica. If the history is hurried or abbreviated, it lends to a dangerously shallow basis for understanding the clinical problems for which no amount of ancillary laboratory testing will substitute.

The *general physical examination* should identify any medical complications or cervical spine disease that are potentially life threatening, for example, vascular disease in the neck and/or pulmonary dysfunction. Secondly, this examination should also identify medical diseases that may cause cervical spine symptomology. Medical complications are of particular importance because they often provide helpful clues in distinguishing cord from root involvement. The majority of these are more likely to be associated with cervical myelopathy than radiculopathy. For example, autonomic dysfunction (sphincter dysfunction, sexual dysfunction, decubitus ulcers) is usually associated with cervical cord disease. In some cases one needs to determine if there is lumbar root involvement that might account for the autonomic dysfunction as well. Dysphagia may be a feature of anterior midcervical spondylosis. Pulmonary dysfunction may result from either severe high cervical cord compression or C3, 4 root involvement (phrenic nerve paralysis).

In the *neurological assessment of these patients* the physician requires precise knowledge of the location and function of each spinal cord segment, emergent roots and spinal nerves, and how irritations, compressions, and deficits of these neural structures are expressed. In addition to the neurological assessment, a thorough *musculoskeletal examination* is equally important in the overall evaluation. With this knowledge the clinician learns to see the relationships that point to one neural structure and exclude others, and in addition, helps him to determine if the primary condition is secondary to local disease within the soft tissues or bony structures of the neck.

The *radiological evaluation* begins with plain cervical spine films. Subsequent investigations may include computed tomography (CT), magnetic resonance imaging, nucleide bone scans, and myelography/CT studies.

Electrophysiological studies are useful in assessing whether there is root or peripheral nerve involvement, the degree and extent of the neuropathic deficit, and in sorting out whether limb weakness is functional or organic.

CLINICAL PRESENTATIONS

There are essentially three major *clinical presentations* of cervical spine dysfunction. The first is localized neck pain, soreness, and/or stiffness; the second is a cervical root compression syndrome (radiculopathy) without signs or symptoms of a myelopathy; thirdly, is the syndrome of cord compression (myelopathy) which may not be associated with radiculopathy. At times one may see the clinical presentation of cervical spine dysfunction associated with mechanical impingement of the odontoid on the upper cervical cord or brain stem (rheumatoid neck disease) (2,3). Another less common clinical presentation is one of cerebrovascular insufficiency secondary to compression and/or thromboembolism of the carotid or vertebral arteries caused by severe osteoarthritis and/or cervical spine instability. Vertigo may be the only symptom of this condition. Other forms of vertigo, for example cervical vertigo, are on occasion caused by spondylosis (4). The mechanism has been attributed to sympathetic nerve dysfunction and/or compressive-irritative stimulation of afferent nerve fibers in cervical muscles which integrate with labyrinthine structures.

Localized neck pain, soreness, and/or stiffness without associated radicular or myelopathic symptoms and signs represents the most benign clinical presentation. This symptom complex may be related to soft tissue involvement in the neck secondary to trauma, e.g., whiplash injury or bony disease, as in cervical spondylosis. Patients may have several trigger points and nonspecific complaints suggesting a myofascial syndrome fibromyalgia (5). In such cases, a combination of amitriptyline and oral nonsteroidal anti-inflammatory may be effective in controlling symptoms (6). If the neurological examination is normal, then plain cervical spine radiography is usually sufficient to evaluate for soft tissue disease, fractures, or spondylosis.

Cervical radiculopathy typically presents with motor and/or referred sensory symptoms in the upper extremities or in the scapula. These neural symptoms may or may not be associated with neck pain and/or stiffness. Pain, paresthesias, and other sensory phenomena are usually of less value in precise localization of an affected nerve root than muscle weakness, focal atrophy, and/or reflex hypoactivity. Neck pain or proximal arm pain is often valueless in precise localization of the affected nerve segment. Referred pain to the medial or upper scapula may be the only manifestation of segmental root involvement and typically reflects compression of the posterior primary ramus of the spinal nerve anywhere from C6 to T1.

Pain or other sensory phenomena from a high cervical disorder, for example at the C1 and C2 levels, is usually distributed in a collar-like fashion. Paresthesias in specific fingers provide a better chance for localization of segment root compression, but some patients are incapable of stating exactly where paresthesias are felt, insisting at times that the "whole hand feels numb" even when the eventual clinical diagnosis indicates involvement of only a single root.

The conical pattern of painless hand weakness and/or atrophy without appreciable sensory loss may be seen in patients with lower cervical spondylosis and/or disc herniations (7). These patients may sometimes be misdiagnosed as having motor neuron disease (8) or ulnar neuropathies at the elbow.

Conversion hysteria and psychogenic pain disorders may simulate a cervical radiculopathy syndrome. These patients are usually histrionic in describing their symptoms, have variable weakness (giving-way pattern), excessive flinching, no reflex abnormalities, and nonsegmental sensory loss.

Clinical symptomatology compatible with *cervical myelopathy* includes spastic weakness and/or incoordination of one or both lower limbs, proprioceptive dysfunction, paresthesias in the lower limbs and/or sphincter dysfunction. Neck pain or radicular complaints may or may not be associated with a myelopathy. Myelopathic symptoms are dependent upon the pathophysiology of the etiologic process. Mechanical deformation of the cervical cord may not cause frank pain in the neck or limbs, though L'hermitte's sign (electric shocks or burning sensations in the trunk or limbs) induced by neck movement, usually flexion, may be present. This sensation may be extremely disagreeable. In some patients with only radicular symptoms or signs there may be subclinical signs of a myelopathy and thus, accordingly these patients should always have their lower limbs examined for gait dysfunction, proximal leg weakness, sensory changes, particularly proprioceptive sensory loss; they should be questioned about any change in sphincter functions.

In spondylotic myelopathy, sphincter dysfunction is rarely affected unless the cord is severely involved. Neoplastic compression usually produces urinary retention or incontinence at about the same time the patient develops spastic paresis. In 1952, Brain and his colleagues commented that disturbance of sphincter function was usually absent in spondylitic myelopathy (1). The afferent pathways to the bladder are fairly superficial in the anterior quadrant, and the efferent pathways are more deeply situated adjacent to the dorsal part of the anterior gray matter. Both pathways are in the same quadrant of the spinal cord as the spinothalamic tract. When this area is involved as seen in the anterolateral cordotomy patients, sphincter function is invariably affected. In addition, there may be selective and asymmetrical involvement of motor and sensory pathways. The pyramidal tracts appear to be the most vulnerable to compression. Paresis in the proximal lower legs, mild spasticity or incoordination of the legs, or reflex hyperactivity with or without Babinski signs may be the only findings. Compression of the anterolateral columns, less commonly affected, may produce loss of pinprick and temperature sensations on only one side even when weakness and/or spasticity signs are fairly symmetrical. The dorsal columns may be spared early, but as the cord compression worsens or progresses, proprioception or vibratory loss and/or loss of graphesthesia come to be associated with the spasticity components. In this situation of "combined-system disease," vitamin B12 deficiency should be suspected even in the absence of an abnormal Schilling test. Other non-spondylitis myelopathic syndromes such as primary spinal muscular atrophy (selective involvement of the anterior horn cells), amyotrophic lateral sclerosis (both upper and lower motor neuron deficits), multiple sclerosis, and syringomyelia should be part of the differential diagnosis. Neurosyphilis, particularly tabes dorsalis, should not be confused with a compressive myelopathy, because reflexes and sensation may be significantly impaired or absent in the lower extremities.

A confusing clinical picture may be seen in those patients who also have associated lumbar spondylosis (9, 10). Such patients may have an absence of low back pain and/or radicular symptoms. On examination, hypoactive or absent tendon reflexes and/or mild focal weakness or atrophy distally may be found which may contribute to a confusing clinical picture. In this situation electrophysiological studies are very helpful in defining the extent of the lower motor neuron disease process.

Segmental Root Patterns

Segmental root patterns deserve discussion particularly in the overall understanding of the various clinical cervical spine disorders (see Table 2.1).

The C1 root which lies above the neural arch of C1 and just posterior to the occipital condyle, lacks a posterior primary sensory ramus. The muscles served by the vestigeal C1 motor root are so well supplied by other segments that C1 involvement is not known to generate a characteristic cervical syndrome.

The C2 root has a large sensory component and lies posterior to the diarthrodial joint between the atlas (C1) and axis (C2) which it innervates. There is no disc at this level. Therefore the motor function of C2 like C1 is of no clinical interest. The C2 sensory ramus, however, is clinically important. It serves as a pain pathway from an arthritic atlanto-axial articulation or subluxation. Compression or irritation of this root produces unilateral pain or paresthesias in the upper neck, suboccipital area, or retromastoid region. This pain is usually aggravated by neck motion and is associated with localized tenderness in this region. It is unclear whether these sensory symptoms arise from inflammatory disease communicated to the nerves which lie in contact with the affected arthritic joint or whether the articular nerve branch from the painful joint mediates the pain to the C2 pathway centrally. The literature suggests that the latter is probably the mechanism, since in most cases the pain is not felt throughout the C2 nerve root distribution (11). Occasionally, one may find a small patch of occipital hypalgesia in these patients. Spondylotic arthropathy or instability of the atlanto-axial joint secondary to rheumatoid neck disease with accompanying C2 root irritation should be easily diagnosed with appropriate cervical spine x-rays, including an open mouth and lateral flexion-extension views or by an imaging scan.

Unilateral complaints in the posterior cervical region associated with tenderness higher and medially in the occiput should alert you to the condition of occipital neuralgia due to entrapment of the occipital nerve as it pierces the occipital aponeurosis. In these patients x-rays of the C1–C2 joints will be normal. Whiplash injuries or other forms of trauma which cause twisting of the neck may injure the C2 nerve root as it passes between the C1 and C2 lamina. The neurosurgical literature recommends treating this problem with a rhizotomy of the C2 root (12).

The C3 and C4 roots are rarely involved by cervical disc herniations but may be impinged upon by arthrosis of the posterior articulations. In compression of these roots, there is usually no motor deficit. Pain, however, is characteristic in that it spreads from the side of the neck laterally to the region of the acromioclavicular joint, stopping just short of the deltoid muscle. Sometimes pathology in the C3–C4 area is difficult to see on a plain myelogram and therefore cervical myelography/computerized tomography has become a gold standard in giving more definitive information of this region.

Root compressions of C5 through T1 contribute characteristic motor deficits and sensory phenomenon. Paravertebral and intrascapular pain or paresthesias arising from compression of any of these roots are insufficiently different to pinpoint which root is involved. These roots supply

Table 2.1. Segmental Root Patterns

Nerve Root	Motor	Sensory	Reflex	Comments
C1	—	—	—	Vestigeal nerves
C2	Paraspinal	Suboccipital	—	Sensory loss may not be present
C3/4	Neck muscle weakness	Lateral neck A/C joint area	—	Phrenic nerve paralysis if severely involved
C5	Deltoid	Lateral arm	Bicep	
C6	Wrist extension	Lateral forearm	Brachioradialis	Wrist extension is not pure C6. Pronation may be selectively involved
C7	Triceps	Middle finger	Triceps	May also test strength of wrist flexors and finger extensors
C8	Finger flexors interossei	Medial forearm	Finger flexor	Painless weakness and atrophy may be only signs
T1	Interossei	Medial upper arm	Finger flexor	Check for miosis and/or ptosis. Suspect superior sulcus tumor.

the upper limb via the anterior primary ramus of the spinal nerve and the brachial plexus. The posterior primary ramus innervates the paraspinal muscles and skin.

Pectoral pain simulating angina may be seen occasionally with lesions of the C5 through C8 roots. This pectoral sensation occurs because of upper chest muscle dysfunction which produces a sensory phenomenon.

C5 root pain extends into the region of the deltoid or upper arm. There may be associated paresthesias over the cap of the shoulder or medial to the scapula. On examination, paresis of the supraspinatous, intraspinatous, deltoid, flexor muscles of the elbow, along with a reduction of the biceps reflex may be present. It is important when testing muscle function to examine the belly of the muscle for tone and atrophy. Contraction tensions should also be compared with muscles of the opposite asymptomatic side while the patient resists the physician's effort on power testing. Tests of strength in the flexors of the elbow are important in differentiating C5 and C6 root compressions from idiopathic brachial plexus neuropathy involving the upper trunk, since the elbow flexors are generally spared in the latter case.

C6 root compression causes paraspinal pain indistinguishable from the adjacent root segment. Pain usually radiates into the flexor surface of the upper arm to the level of the elbow; there may be paresthesias in the thumb and distal radial forearm. Motor testing usually reveals weakness of elbow flexion because of paresis of all three elbow flexor muscles. In addition, the brachial radialis reflex is hypoactive, and the extensor carpi radialis muscles may also be weakened. The deltoid is usually spared in these cases even though this muscle may receive partial innervation from the C6 root.

C7 root compression may cause a variety of different patterns of sensory dysfunction and weakness. Pure C7 motor loss seems to affect mainly the triceps muscle where there may be an associated reduction of the triceps tendon reflex. There may be weakness of the latissimus and pectoralis major, all of which are innervated to a much lesser extent by the two adjacent roots. The pectoralis major reflex may be hypoactive as well. Abnormal tendon reflexes may occur with or without weakness or atrophy, because the hypoactivity of these reflexes seems to be largely dependent on involvement of the afferent loop of the reflex arc. A perfectly strong muscle may lose its reflex without showing any signs of atrophy or muscle irritability (fasciculations). The C7 root also innervates extensors and flexors of the wrist. In my experience the weakness will most often affect wrist extension because of the predominance of flexor effort deriving from the C8 root. In general, C7 sensory phenomena are indistinguishable from sensations caused by compression of the C6 or C8 roots in their proximal manifestations. However, the extension of pain down the posterior lateral aspect of the upper arm into the radial forearm complying with paresthesias in the index and neighboring fingers including part of the 4th finger is a characteristic pattern in most C7 root syndromes. C7 radiculopathies may mimic distal median nerve entrapment at the carpal tunnel, but with C7 lesions the fingers are more severely affected than the whole radial surface of the hand as in distal median nerve entrapment. Certainly, if the patient has neck dysfunction and arm pain, this should alert you to a root lesion rather than a peripheral nerve entrapment syndrome. Weakness in other C7 muscles coupled with areflexia is not seen in the latter.

One would expect that lesions of the C5–C6 and/or C7 roots may cause paralysis of the serratus anterior muscle leading to a wing scapula. This is not usually seen in cervical radiculopathies with any degree of frequency. It is more commonly seen in patients with either an idiopathic form of brachial plexus neuropathy or isolated involvement of the long thoracic nerve (13).

The C8 nerve root is not commonly affected by spondylosis or disc herniation, but certainly is more so than the C5 root. Compression of the C8 root causes pain to be felt in the intrascapular area or along the medial scapula. The pain may radiate posteromedially in the upper arm and along the medial aspect of the elbow with paresthesias in the ulnar distribution. Patients may show weakness of the flexor carpi ulnaris, long finger flexors, and intrinsic hand muscles. A Froment's sign may be present; this is usually due to weakness of the adductor pollicis muscle. There is no evidence of a Horner's syndrome in these cases. The finger flexor reflex may be reduced or absent. One differentiating clinical feature between a C8 root lesion and an ulnar entrapment neuropathy at the elbow is preservation of the flexor carpi ulnaris in the latter case.

T1 root lesions are rare and are not in the strict sense part of the cervical motion segment disorders, because this root exits at the T1–T2 level. In those patients with T1 involvement there may be pain in the axilla and along the ulnar aspect of the arm with paresis and atrophy of intrinsic hand muscles almost identical to that produced by C8 root compression. In some, there may be a complete Horner's syndrome, or only one of its components may be present, either ptosis or miosis. Apical pulmonary carcinoma and other neoplasms in this region may simulate a T1 radiculopathy and should be considered in the differential diagnosis.

Muscle dysfunction associated with cervical radiculopathy and the neurological signs of myelopathy are outlined in Tables 2.2 and 2.3 respectively.

LABORATORY EVALUATIONS

The radiological evaluation begins with plain radiographs and may end there, depending on the patient's clinical analysis. The utilization of other specific radiological modalities should be determined by the optimal method of confirming the clinical impression. Each radiological modality has specific indications with various advantages and disadvantages.

Plain radiographs should be the minimal radiological evaluation in any patient initially presenting with cervical spine symptomatology. If trauma is involved, cross-table lateral and anterior-posterior x-rays should be obtained, because all seven cervical vertebrae must be visualized on the lateral film, or the examination is incomplete. In addition these films are important to determine if there are congenital anomalies, dislocations, bony tumors, or subtle infections of bone. Certainly degenerative changes in the discs or apophyseal joints can be assessed by these films. The caudad verebra can best be seen by pulling the patient's arms down either directly or with straps. In some cases this is preferable to swimmer's view which is also an acceptable film. In addition, plain radiographs should determine the stability or instability of the cervical spine. The AP films should include the open-mouth view to look at the odontoid and the C1–C2 articulations for athrosis. In addition, lateral flexion-extension views are important to evaluate upper and lower cervical spine instability. A lateral view will determine the degree of the normal lordotic curve. The cervical spine, however, may be straightened in 70° of the population by depressing the chin 1 inch. The extent of structural instability of the cervical spine may also provide clues as to the status of the associated ligamentous structures. For example, forward dislocation of a vertebral body of more than ½ the anterior posterior diameter of the body below is indicative of bilateral facet dislocation associated with destruction of either the longitudinal, intraspinous, and facet ligaments along with the disc annulus. Prevertebral soft tissue thickness should normally be less than 5 mm at the anterior-inferior border of the C3 vertebral body. Soft tissue swelling greater than 5 mm in adults suggests either hematoma from a fracture or some other soft tissue lesion in the neck.

A normal spinal canal has a ratio of 1, whereas a ratio of less than 0.80 indicates cervical spinal stenosis and suggests a spine that is at risk for spinal cord injury (14). This diameter should be measured as a ratio of the canal diameter to the vertebral body diameter. This eliminates magnification variability. If this measurement suggests cervical stenosis, then a computed tomographic (CT) or magnetic resonance imaging (MRI) scan of the cervical spine is recommended.

The AA interval, measured between the posterior aspect of the anterior arch of C1 and the anterior aspect of the odontoid should normally be less than 3 mm in the adult. An increase in the AA interval should suggest rupture or inflammation of the transverse ligaments.

Oblique views of the cervical spine identify the neural foramina that may be encroached upon by osteophytes which may in turn impinge upon the exiting nerve roots. The oblique views visualize the lamina, lateral masses, pedicles, and facet joints as well. If all these structures are normal and the patient is neurologically intact despite radicular symptomatology, then disc herniation should be suspected.

Specialized tomography is sometimes required to visualize C7–C8 and T1 particularly in stocky, short-necked individuals. Tomography is also useful in identified facet and laminar fractures and also to visualize the cervical occipital junction much better. In this case CT scan may be more useful to evaluate the AA articulation.

Neuroimaging scans have become more precise in defining the pathological substrate. CT scanning provides a means to evaluate the skeletal structures and discs in a more precise manner. In addition, there is better visualization of the spinal cord diameter and assessment of the lateral recesses. In situations where the odontoid is eroded as in rheumatoid neck disease, the CT scan may provide a clearer view of the an-

Table 2.2. Muscles Commonly Tested in the Diagnosis of Root Compression in the Upper Extremities

Muscle	Nerve	Root
Levator scapulae	C3, C4, and dorsal scapular	*C3*, *C4*, *C5**
Rhomboids	Dorsal scapular	C4, *C5*
Supraspinatus	Suprascapular	*C5*, C6
Infraspinatus	Suprascapular	*C5*, C6
Deltoid	Axillary	*C5*, C6
Biceps brachii	Musculocutaneous	*C5*, *C6*
Brachioradialis	Radial	*C5*, C6
Supinator	Deep radial	C5, *C6*
Flexor carpi radialis	Median	*C6*, *C7*
Pronator teres	Median	*C6*, *C7*
Serratus anterior	Long thoracic	*C5*, *C6*, *C7*
Latissimus dorsi	Thoracodorsal	C6, *C7*, C8
Pectoralis major; clavicle	Lateral pectoral	C5, *C6*, C7
sternum	Medial pectoral	C6, *C7*, *C8*
Triceps brachii	Radial	C6, *C7*, C8
Extensor carpi radialis longus	Radial	*C6*, *C7*
Extensor carpi radialis brevis	Radial	C6, C7, C8
Extensor digitorum	Deep radial	*C7*, C8
Extensor carpi ulnaris	Deep radial	*C7*, *C8*
Palmaris longus	Median	C7, *C8*, T1
Flexor carpi ulnaris	Ulnar	C7, *C8*, T1
Flexor digitorum superficialis	Median	C7, *C8*
Flexor digitorum profundus	Median and ulnar	C7, *C8*, T1
Abductor pollicis brevis	Median	*C8*, *T1*
First dorsal interosseous	Ulnar	*C8*, *T1*
Hypothenar group	Ulnar	*C8*, *T1*

*Italic indicates principal root supply

Table 2.3. Neurologic Signs in Cervical Myelopathy

Motor

1) Increased tone or spasticity in the lower extremities;
2) Weakness of the lower extremities;
3) Ataxia or difficulty controlling lower extremities while walking.

Sensory

1) Impaired sensation to pin, light touch, or temperature that may correspond to a level;
2) Impaired position and/or vibration in the lower extremities with dorsal column involvement.

Reflexes

1) Hyperactive deep tendon reflexes in the lower extremities;
2) Hypoactive deep tendon reflexes in the upper extremities in nerve roots C5, C6, or C7 are involved (i.e., associated with cervical radiculopathy);
3) Hyperactive reflexes in the upper extremities if the upper cervical spinal cord (i.e., above C4) is involved;
4) Positive Babinski's.

atomical relationship of these structures. In general, CT scanning is more ideally suitable for the visualization of skeletal structures, but it can also identify soft tissue structures such as discs and surrounding neural tissue and ligaments.

MRI has become the most widely used test in evaluation of cervical spine disorders. Obviously it provides a means of noninvasive visualization of the spinal cord and nerve roots from almost any plane. It also affords the ability to identify intrinsic and extrinsic soft tissue lesions of the spinal cord much better than CT scanning. However, in some instances where one suspects a peripheral lesion causing a radicular pattern, a CT may be a better tool to demonstrate small fractures, especially when it is combined with a contrast agent. In this way the nerve root can be visualized better in close proximity to the suspected bony lesion.

Cervical discography is an invasive diagnostic procedure utilized to evaluate the integrity of cervical disc when other imaging modalities such as CT with or without myelography and MRI are negative or equivocal. The rationale for using cervical discograms today is dependent upon the integrity of the disc or lack of it after the contrast media has been injected into the disc. In interpreting the discogram, attention is paid to the reproduction of the patient's pain, extravasation of the dye, and the extent of disc opacification. The efficacy of the cervical discogram is somewhat limited in patients over the age of forty because the cervical disc offers little resistence to the injection of contrast media and therefore extravasation of contrast material can occur easily, often yielding a false positive result. With the advent of MRI, however, cervical discography will probably lose its value.

Nucleide bone scanning is a diagnostic imaging study utilizing radionucleides to detect pathophysiological abnormalities in the bony structures. Although bone scanning is sensitive in identifying disturbances in the vascularity or osteogenesis of bone, it tends to lack specificity. The scintographic appearance of various pathological processes involving bone are shown in Table 2.4.

ELECTROPHYSIOLOGICAL STUDIES

Clinical electrophysiology can provide an objective measure of the level and degree of cervical root involvement. It also differentiates disorders of the cervical spine from those primarily involving the peripheral nervous system (intrinsic neuropathies and myopathies). In the evaluation of patients with cervical spine diseases, nerve conduction velocities including late responses (F waves), needle electromyography (EMG), and somatosensory spinal evoked potentials (SEPs) may be employed.

Nerve conduction tests are important because they differentiate root from peripheral nerve disease. In essence, they provide objective information regarding the integrity of the peripheral axon. These studies primarily measure the velocity at which the particular nerve in question conducts an impulse and the distal latencies of that nerve. A slowing of motor or sensory conduction velocities is suggestive of demyelination of the peripheral nerve. If there is a loss of amplitude in the evoked muscle action potential, this is suggestive of predominently axonal dropout. The late responses, particularly the F wave latency, which is a measure of retrograde motor conduction through the spinal cord, is sometimes helpful in defining whether the patient has a root compression syndrome, especially when the nerve conduction velocities are normal.

Needle electromyography which is the second part of the nerve conduction/EMG study assessment examines the electrical properties of the muscle much like an EKG examines

Table 2.4. Radionuclide Imaging in Spinal Disorders

Spinal Disorders	Scintigraphic Findings	Comments
Degenerative changes	Mild to moderate increased uptake eccentrically placed and bridging two vertebrae.	Need plain radiographs to distinguish from metastatic disease.
Metastatic bone tumors	Increased radionuclide uptake, but can have a false negative bone scan with slow growing tumors.	Usually from breast, prostate, lung, kidney, thyroid carcinomas.
Myeloma	Preponderance of osteoclastic activity coupled with relatively little osteoblastic response with a negative bone scan in about 40%. Positive scans are related to superimposed pathologic fractures.	Most frequent primary tumor of the spine in adults.
Primary malignant tumors	Markedly increased radionuclide uptake.	Cannot distinguish between various primary malignancies.
Osteoid osteoma	One of the most scintigraphically active bone lesions. Round well demarcated area of intense increased activity (nidus) and less intense surrounding activity (reactive sclerosis).	Differential includes osteoblastoma, aneurysmal bone cyst, metastasis, and fracture.
Paget's disease	Multiple or single areas of increased activity which may be localized to the posterior spinous process or transverse process, appearing concurrently with an enlarged vertebral body.	
Metabolic disease	Usually normal unless associated with a pathologic fracture.	Examples: osteoporosis, primary hyperparathyroidism, renal osteodystrophy, and osteomalacia.
Fractures	Localized increased radioactivity.	Scans are usually abnormal 24 hours after the traumatic event.
Discitis	Intense focal accumulation of activity in the disc space and the two adjacent vertebral bodies.	Needs to be differentiated from Scheuermann's disease (juvenile kyphosis).
Osteomyelitis	Localized increased radioactivity on both the immediate and delayed images.	May be similar to that seen with neoplasm or fracture.

the electrical properties of cardiac muscle. A needle electrode, usually a monopolar or bipolar needle, is inserted into the muscle under sterile conditions. This examination identifies muscles that are either acutely or chronically denervated. In the acutely denervated muscle one will find either positive sharp waves or fibrillations. Depending upon the distribution of muscles denervated, a determination can be made as to whether the neuropathic process affecting the muscles is secondary to a peripheral nerve or nerve root.

The classic EMG signs of acute denervation may not show up until 2 weeks after the time of initial insult to the nerve. In chronically denervated muscle, motor unit action potentials will appear to be large and deformed in amplitude (polyphasic). In addition, the motor unit action potentials may recruit incompletely with attempted maximal voluntary contraction. In addition to polyphasia one examines amplitude of the potential to determine if there is a suspected underlying anterior horn cell disease. Very large amplitude potentials measuring above 10 millivolts is more suggestive of anterior horn cell involvement than root involvement. The presence of fasciculations (discharges of single motor units) is also indicative of injury to the anterior horn cell or nerve root. If present in large numbers or seen diffusely, it should alert you to the possibility of lower motor neuron dysfunction associated with the syndrome of amyotrophic lateral sclerosis or poliomyelitis. On rare occasions, fasciculations associated with large amplitude polyphasic potentials are seen in chronic cervical spondylitic radiculopathy.

Lastly, needle EMG studies can distinguish neuropathic from myopathic disease. The characteristic EMG findings of active or chronic myopathy vary according to the type and stage of the disease process. There may be fibrillation potentials in an active myopathy much like there are in a neuropathic disorder, but the motor unit action potentials during muscle contraction tend to be smaller in amplitude, fragmented and polyphasic, and increased in number during minimal voluntary contractions.

Somatosensory evoked potential studies (SEPs) are used to assess brachial plexus and/or spinal cord dysfunction. They may be useful in assessing patients who may have thoracic outlet syndromes or brachial plexopathies from trauma or tumor compression, especially when peripheral nerve conduction studies may be normal in the early stages of these diseases. They are of particular value in determining whether the patient has evidence of a cervical myelopathy when the clinical signs and/or radiographic findings are equivocal. SEPs are felt to measure the physiological integrity of the dorsal columns. Certainly if there is a myelopathy with no or minimal involvement of the dorsal column these studies may be normal.

Table 2.5. Immunological and Serological Evaluation of Cervical Spine Disease

Laboratory test	Disorders that can affect the cervical spine.
Rheumatoid factor	Rheumatoid arthritis, but may also occur in SLE, sarcoid, and syphilis.
Complement levels	Connective tissue diseases such as SLE and RA.
Antinuclear antibodies	SLE, but may also be positive in scleroderma, Sjögren's syndrome, RA, and mixed connective disease.
HLA typing	Ankylosing spondylitis
VDRL	Syphilis
ESR	Polymyalgia rheumatica

OTHER LABORATORY INVESTIGATIONS

In the overall assessment of patients who have cervical spine disease one should consider hematological, biochemical, immunological, and urological studies when the history and physical examination appropriately indicate it.

A routine immunological evaluation should include an erythrocyte sedimentation rate (ESR) especially if the syndrome of polymyalgia rheumatica is considered. The ESR also provides a nonspecific indication of a systemic disorder such as inflammation, infection, or occult malignancy. The routine CBC may determine if a patient with spine symptoms has leukemia, lymphoma, or an infection. Occasionally sickle cell anemia patients may have cervical spine pain. The immunological/serological studies are also of particular importance in the diagnosis of cervical spine dysfunction. Testing for rheumatoid factor, low complement levels, antinuclear antibodies, HLA typing, and VDRL can detect a variety of disorders that involve the cervical spine (see Table 2.5).

The biochemistry profile is also important because of the disorders of calcium and phosphorus metabolism which may present with cervical spine symptomatology. Hypercalcemia may suggest sarcoid disease or an occult malignancy. Elevation of the serum alkaline phosphate level may be seen in any disease of bone involving increased osteoblastic activity such as Paget's disease or primary and secondary malignancies of bone.

A routine urinalysis may detect renal disease secondary to systemic lupus erythematosus which may cause cervical spine dysfunction. If a patient has cervical myelopathy with bladder dysfunction, the urinalysis may also be useful in detecting an associated urinary tract infection.

A cerebral spinal fluid (CSF) study is useful in diagnosing carcinomatous meningitis that may be affecting the cervical nerve roots. Ten cc of spinal fluid are necessary to do an adequate cytological evaluation. Lumbar puncture may need to be done several times before yielding a positive

Table 2.6. Etiologic and Pathogenic Classification of Cervical Spine Disorders

Congenital disorders
Traumatic injuries
Neoplastic disorders
Infectious diseases
Inflammatory disorders
Vascular disorders
Endocrine and metabolic disorders
Miscellaneous and idiopathic

result. If myelopathy is present and is not felt to be associated with spondylosis or disc herniation, then the patient should have CSF protein studies for oligoclonal bands and immunoelectrophoresis to determine gamma globulin concentration. Abnormalities in any of these two protein studies may indicate a demyelinating disease of the central nervous system (multiple sclerosis). In any case of myelopathy, even in association with cervical spondylosis, the radiologist should be alerted to the fact that he/she should obtain extra spinal fluid in cases where the cervical myelogram proves not to indicate spinal cord compression.

Lastly, multiple myeloma and other myeloproliferative disorders may present with cervical spinal cord dysfunction. Tissue biopsy, particularly a bone marrow biopsy, may be necessary to fully evaluate the condition in question. In some instances where there is a space-occupying lesion that is not felt to be due to a degenerative process, tissue biopsy may be necessary to determine if the patient has an infection or cancerous lesion.

Differential Diagnosis

The diagnosis of cervical spine diseases should exclude other disorders which may display similar clinical presentations or may masquerade as cervical spondylosis with radiculopathy or myelopathy. The etiological classification of disorders to be considered in the differential diagnosis is presented in Table 2.6 and Table 2.7. In general, these clinical entities responsible for similar manifestations of cervical spine disease do in fact recapitulate the history of the condition as well as give the physician more knowledge of the extraordinary variety of manifestations of cervical spondylosis and radiculopathy.

Peripheral neuropathy or brachial neuritis due to specific causes, for example compressive mechanisms in the interscalene triangle or compression of the plexus between the clavicle and the first rib need to be considered (thoracic outlet syndromes).

The symptoms of these conditions are often vague and obscure and the anatomical changes quite varied and at times unpredictable. The symptoms, however, reflect the degree to which particular nerves and vascular structures are compressed as they exit from the neck and mediastinum toward the axilla. In the various types of thoracic outlet syndromes, the close proximity of nerves and vessels to one another as they traverse the outlet causes varying degrees of plexus and/or subclavian artery compression. This combined form of "neurovascular compression" accounts for the myriad of symptoms that one encounters in this syndrome. For example, there may be pain in the face, neck, head, arm, chest, shoulder, axilla, and upper limb and/or paresthesias, numbness, weakness, heaviness, fatigability, swelling, or discoloration and in some instances, Raynaud's phenomenon (15).

Table 2.7. Congenital Malformations of the Cervical Spine

Bony Anomalies of Cervical Spine

1) *Cranio-occipital anomalies*
   - Occipital vertebra
   - Basilar coarction/occipital dysplasia
   - Condylar hypoplasia
   - Assimilation of atlas

2) *Anomalies of atlas and axis*
   - Aplasias of arch of the atlas
   - Aplasia of odontoid

3) *Anomalies below C2*
   - Klippel-Feil syndrome
   - Stenosis of the cervical spinal canal
   - Spina bifida
   - Cervical ribs

Neural Anomalies of Cervical Spine

1) Arnold-Chiari malformation
2) Syringomyelia
3) Meningocele
4) Neurofibromatosis

The most common symptom complex occurs as a manifestation of compression of the lower trunk of the brachial plexus. In this, pain and paresthesias occur along the medial aspect of the arm and ulnar aspect of the forearm with extension into the 4th and 5th fingers. The patient may or may not experience weakness of grasp secondary to intrinsic muscle dysfunction.

Compression of the upper trunk of the brachial plexus is a much less frequent occurrence and results in a symptom pattern that is characterized by complaints of more proximal pain, particularly in the anterior and posterior aspect of the shoulder and neck and occasionally in the face. In this instance, the symptom complex may mimic C5–6 spondylosis or disc herniation. In rare occasions there may be a compression of the arterial and/or venous systems as they exit the thoracic outlet. Venous obstruction may cause edema in the arm and/or cyanotic discoloration of the hand. On physical exam there may be venous collateralization across the shoulder and chest wall. Arterial obstruction produces symptoms of coldness and numbness of the hand and exertional fatigue of the arm. If the outlet compression is significant, mixed symptoms patterns may occur with variable degrees of actual insufficiency and neurologic dysfunction either in the upper or lower trunk distribution.

There are a number of ways in which these large neurovascular structures may be compressed by anomalous musculoskeletal structures in the neck and shoulder girdle. These include cervical ribs or anomalous first thoracic ribs, hypertrophied scalene muscles, and a narrowed costoclavicular space (space between the first rib and the clavicle). Distally there is the possibility of compression just proximal to the axilla as the neurovascular structures pass under the pectoralis minor insertion on the coracoid process. Trauma and dynamic changes in shoulder mechanics are recognized as more common etiologies of the thoracic outlet syndrome.

Brachial neuritis due to inflammation or entrapment of either an isolated branch of the brachial plexus or incomplete or complete involvement of the brachial plexus must be considered in the differential diagnosis of cervical spine disease.

Idiopathic brachial plexus neuropathy, known also as neuralgic amyotrophy, paralytic brachial neuritis, or the Parsonage-Turner syndrome, is a specific nosological entity that dates back to the early 40s when it was initially described by Spillane (16). This type of neuritis has an abrupt onset manifested by severe pain which frequently awakens the patient and is maximized in the shoulder region where it may remain constant for several weeks to a month. Occasionally the limb pain may be bilateral. Following the pain the patient will frequently experience weakness and atrophy particularly in the shoulder girdle muscles or the distribution of the upper trunk of the brachial plexus. These patients are primarily males. In 50% of the patients the condition usually follows an infection or vaccination. Paresthesias are not a prominent complaint. There is no aggravation of the symptoms by neck motion or by Valsalva maneuvers. For the most part cervical myelograms and cerebrospinal fluid analyses are normal. This is a benign self-limiting condition which may be severe and disabling in onset, but 80% of patients will generally improve within 2 years. Twenty percent of patients may have residual deficit persisting beyond 2 years (13). The site of the lesion and its cause are unknown. Because most have involvement of the upper trunk of the brachial plexus, these patients may simulate a C5 or C6 root compression from a space-occupying lesion. This type of idiopathic neuropathy may also cause paralysis of the hemidiaphragm as well as involvement of other muscle groups and may manifest as a winged scapula.

Zoster ganglionitis may cause segmental pain 2–3 weeks before lesions appear in the dermatome. The thoracic and trigeminal distributions are more often affected than cervical roots. The elderly are usually the favorite targets of this disease, and in such cases a suspicion of malignancy should be considered; approximately 40–50% of these patients have an underlying lymphoma. The complaints are usually cutaneous hyperpathia, but on occasion there may be paralysis of selective muscles in the distribution of the lesions within the first 2 days antedating the appearance of the lesions. If the zoster infection is attended by a malignant deposit within the spinal canal or foramen, neck motion may aggravate the symptomatology. Aggravation of pain by cervical motion is rarely present, probably because the pathology is in the sensory ganglion which lies outside the intervertebral foramen.

Table 2.8. Neoplastic Disorders of the Cervical Spine

1. *Extradural: spinal origin*
   Primary bone tumors
2. *Extradural: intraspinal origin*
   Epidural metastasis
3. *Intradural: extramedullary*
   Meningioma
   Schwannoma
4. *Intradural: intramedullary*
   Ependymoma
   Astrocytoma
   Glioblastoma

Multiple myeloma may cause root impingement either by extension of the myelomatous process into the root or by vertebral collapse.

Other *neoplastic disorders* can be classified into four categories (Table 2.8). This classification is dependent upon whether the tumors are primarily extradural or intradural and upon the site of origin. Primary tumors originating from vertebral bodies tend to be extradural. Benign primary tumors include giant cell tumors, osteochondromas, bone cysts, and hemangiomas. The malignant bone tumors include the osteogenic sarcomas and chordomas. Metastatic cervical spine tumors occur more frequently than primary bone tumors. Metastatic lesions from the prostate, breast, kidney, and gastrointestinal tract are the more common sites. Metastatic tumors of the cervical spine will often present as osseous lesions of the spine with epidural extension and manifest themselves as severe pain which is constant and more intense at night, particularly when the patient assumes the supine position. There may be associated tenderness over the vertebral bodies posteriorly.

An intradural tumor of the cervical spine can have either an extramedullary or intramedullary origin. The extramedullary intradural tumors include the meningiomas and benign neurofibromas or Schwannomas. Intramedullary neoplasms represent the ependymomas or gliomas of the spinal cord. Lymphosarcoma and Hodgkin's disease may present as lytic lesions of bone or an epidural mass which may rapidly progress to myelopathy. The features which differentiate these tumors from cervical spondylosis include severe pain at rest and/or associated tenderness over the vertebral body with or without aggravation by cervical

Table 2.9. Inflammatory Disorders

Osteoarthritis
Rheumatoid arthritis
Ankylosing spondylitis
Multiple sclerosis
Transverse myelitis
Sarcoid

spine motion. On the diagnostic side, these patients will have elevated spinal fluid proteins with or without pleocytosis. The myelogram/CT shows characteristic changes in the vertebral bodies and defects uncharacteristic for cervical spondylosis with root compression.

Bacterial, viral, parasitic, and fungal infections can involve the cervical spine, both bony and neural elements. The most common agent of nontuberculous osteomyelitis is staphylococcal aureus. Bacterial and fungal infections may cause epidural abscesses and discitis. Trichinella infestation from eating contaminated or uncooked meat products may present as radiculitis manifesting as flaccid weakness with or without associated sensory involvement. These patients will often have fever, rash, gastroenteritis, and edema of the eyelids. Lastly, bacterial organisms can be introduced into the cervical spine via hematogenous or lymphatic routes, and a variety of viral disorders can directly affect the cervical nerve roots and/or spinal cord (transverse myelitis). Poliomyelitis is seldom encountered today.

In the *acquired immune deficiency syndrome* (AIDS), a variety of spinal cord syndromes and peripheral neuropathies have been described. Cytomegalic virus (CMV) and herpes simplex virus (HSV) have been implicated as causes of myelitis in AIDS. Human T-lymphotropic virus Type I (HTLV-1), a human retrovirus, has been etiologically implicated in tropical spastic paraparesis.

Inflammatory disorders of the cervical spine are listed in Table 2.9. Rheumatoid arthritis does not directly involve cervical roots. This disease causes laxity of the transverse ligaments resulting in, and thereby leading to, malalignment of cervical vertebra, instability at the AA junction or subaxial levels and, thus, root impingement. Associated characteristic deformities in the limbs of rheumatoid arthritis eliminates any chance of confusing this disease with cervical spondylosis, although the two conditions may coexist in the same patient.

Ankylosing spondylitis may affect the cervical cord and present as a myelopathy. Other conditions of the cervical spine which may present as a myelopathy include sarcoidosis and multiple sclerosis.

Neuritis due to heavy metal intoxication or industrial poisons may present as a localized brachial neuritis but should rarely be confused with cervical spine disease secondary to spondylosis. Chronic lead exposure causes a mononeuropathy more affecting the arms and legs, but it is distinguished by its symmetrical appearance in the absence of pain or early sensory involvement.

Disorders of the shoulder, particularly periarthritis or capsulitis and/or the frozen shoulder syndrome, are referred to neurologists for a suspected radiculopathy because the possibility of shoulder pathology is often overlooked. These patients may have major limitations of motor function in the arm, but usually all of the weakness is secondary to pain brought about by efforts to move the shoulder. In these cases the shoulder joint will be tender and restricted in motion with relatively normal reflex, motor, and sensory functions.

Inflammatory lesions or idiopathic entrapment of the suprascapular nerve innervating the supra and infraspinatus causes pain in the posterior shoulder and occasionally extend into the neck and upper arm. This pain may be aggravated by use of the shoulder, particularly moving the shoulder across the body (crossed-adduction test). The electromyogram is helpful in defining the abnormality, thereby eliminating pathology in the C5 root distribution (deltoid and biceps muscles are normal).

Summary

With the advances in radiological technology, the diagnosis of cervical spine diseases has become more accurate and has helped the physician-surgeon deal with the problem more effectively. In spondylitic radiculopathies and/or myelopathies, surgical management should be dictated by the disability of the patient, the nature of his neurologic deficit and his response to conservative therapy. If the patients has a progressive myelopathy over a short time then surgical intervention should be rapid.

References

1. Brain WR, et al. The neurological manifestations of cervical spondylosis. Brain 1952;75:187–225.

2. Ranawat CS, et al. Cervical spine fusion in rheumatoid arthritis. J Bone Joint Surg 1979;61A:1003–1010.

3. Pellicci P, Ranawat CS, Tsairis P. The natural history of rheumatoid arthritis of the cervical spine. J Bone Joint Surg 1981;63A:342–350.

4. Johngkees LB, Cervical vertigo. Laryngoscope 1969;79:1473–1484.

5. Travell J, Simons DG. Myofascial pain and dysfunction, the trigger point manual. Baltimore: Williams & Wilkins, 1983.

6. Goldenberg DL, et al. A randomized, controlled trial of amitriptyline and Naproxen in the treatment of patients with fibromyalgia. Arthritis Rheum 1986;29:1371–1377.

7. Dorsen M, Ehni G. Cervical spondylotic radiculopathy producing motor manifestations mimicking primary muscular atrophy. Neurosurg 1979;5:427–431.

8. Liversedge LA, et al. Cervical spondylosis simulating motorneuron disease. Lancet 1953;2:652–655.

9. Teng P, Pavotheodorow G. Combined cervical and lumbar spondylosis. Arch Neurol 1964;10:298–307.

10. Jacobs B, et al. Coexistence of cervical and lumbar disc disease. Spine 1990;15:1261–1264.

11. Ehni G. Extradural spine cord and nerve root compression from benign lesions of the cervical area. In: Neurological surgery. Philadelphia: WB Saunders Co, 1982.

12. Hunter CR, Mayfield FH. Role of the upper cervical roots in the production of pain in the head. Amer J Surg 1949;78:743–751.

13. Tsairis P, et al: Natural history of brachial plexus neuropathy. Report of 99 cases. Arch Neurol 1972;27:109–117.

14. Pavlov H, et al. Cervical spine stenosis: determination with vertebral body method. Radiology 1987;164:771–775.

15. Karas SE. Thoracic outlet syndrome. Clinics in Sport Medicine 1990;9:297–309.

16. Spillane JD. Localized neuritis of the shoulder girdle. Lancet 1943;2:532–535.

3

Cervical Myelopathy and Root Syndromes

Richard Lechtenberg and Shashi K. Shah

The cervical spinal cord and its associated roots are vulnerable to many types of injury, including trauma, infection, and other destructive processes. Congenital disturbances that produce symptomatic neurologic disorders are also common in the cervical region. Chiari type 1 and type 2 malformations, syringomyelia, and Klippel-Feil syndromes are only a few of the congenital disorders producing static or progressive cervical myelopathies and radiculopathies. Several acquired diseases may produce neurologic syndromes affecting the cervical spinal cord and roots, but most of them do not preferentially target the cervical region. The purely skeletal consequences of spinal arthropathies may be no more severe in the cervical region than elsewhere in the spine, but the neurologic problems associated with cervical neuropathies are quite distinct from the neurologic complications of arthropathies occurring in the remainder of the spine. Neoplastic disease and the consequences of treating neoplastic disease involving the cervical spine are also not unique to this region, but they may have more dramatic consequences because of the greater potential for disability with damage to the cervical, rather than thoracic or lumbosacral, cord. The consequences of vascular injuries, infections, degenerative diseases, and demyelinating diseases are also more significant when the cervical cord is involved. It is the complexity of the cervical cord, rather than the uniqueness of the diseases attacking this part of the spinal cord, which confers special significance on diseases attacking this part of the central nervous system.

Congenital Anomalies

The cervical spine is normally composed of seven unfused vertebrae. The size of each vertebra increases from the first to the seventh. The third, fourth, fifth, and sixth vertebrae have identical features and are called typical vertebrae. The first, second, and seventh vertebrae have distinct anatomic features and are called atypical (1). The height of the body of a typical vertebra is greater posteriorly than anteriorly, and the normal curvature of the neck arises from the shape of the intervertebral discs, rather than that of the vertebral bodies (1).

The vertebral pedicles are short and support superior and inferior articular processes. On either side of the body is a transverse process through which runs a transverse foramen for passage of the vertebral artery (1). Each typical vertebra has a short bifid spinous process. The first cervical vertebra or atlas is atypical in that it possesses no body (1). It is joined to the second vertebra at the odontoid process (dens) of that vertebra. The atlas itself consists of slender anterior and posterior arches and thick lateral masses which support the articular surfaces. The superior facets articulate with the occiput, and the inferior facets articulate with the axis (1). The atlas has a thick transverse ligament which arches across the ring of the atlas and retains the odontoid in contact with the anterior arch of the atlas (2). A series of strong ligaments from the occiput to the second cervical vertebra maintain the normal alignment of the first and second vertebrae (1).

In the cervical region the disc material makes up 22% of the length of the column. The discs permit greater motion between the vertebral bodies than would be allowed by simple joints, and they help absorb shock and distribute weight over the surface of the vertebral body during bending. Each disc consists of four parts: a nucleus pulposus, an anulus fibrosus, and two cartilaginous end-plates (1). The anulus is thicker anteriorly than posteriorly; this, together with the fact that the anterior longitudinal ligament is stronger than the posterior ligament, may be why posterior protrusion of nuclear material is more common than anterior protrusion (1).

Anomalies of the cervical spine are relatively common. In many cases of congenital malformations, the cervical spine and roots are also anomalous or eventually become dysfunctional because of impingement by the bony structures surrounding them. Rarely, anomalous elements inside the cord, such as cysts (syringomyelia), are responsible for progressive cord damage.

Chiari Malformations

Chiari malformations usually involve cervical, as well as cerebellar and brainstem, anomalies (3). These congenital anomalies of the hindbrain are characterized by downward

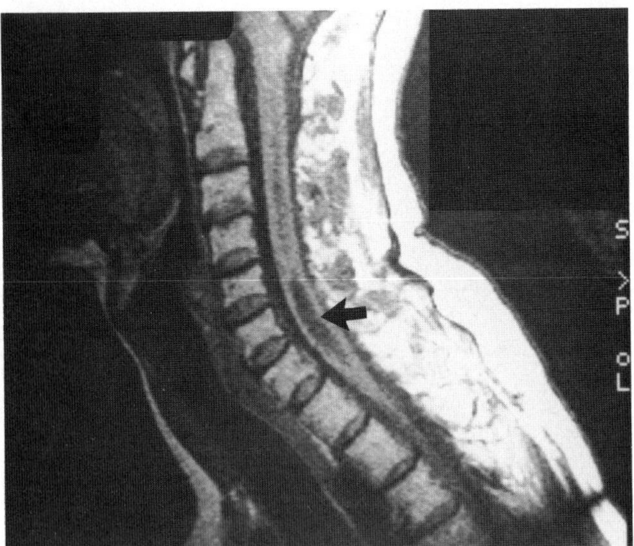

Figure 3.1. MRI of the cervical spine. This 52-year-old woman complained of progressive numbness and paresthesias in both of her arms over the course of 1 year. This MRI reveals a large syrinx in the cervical spinal cord.

elongation of the brainstem and cerebellum into the cervical canal posterior to the spinal cord. The defect is occasionally associated with myelomeningocele or spina bifida occulta, hydrocephalus, and syringomyelia. The cerebellar elements displaced downward into the cervical canal may be the tonsils in the type 1 or the vermis in the type 2 anomalies. The caudad displacement of the brainstem and cervical cord produce anomalous courses for the cervical roots. The first few cervical roots may exhibit cephalad courses on their way to the neural foramina.

Chiari malformations usually become symptomatic when hydrocephalus occurs or when an associated syrinx enlarges (3). The anomaly may not become symptomatic until adult life if hydrocephalus is not part of the syndrome in infancy. The initial symptoms in infancy are ataxia and stupor. In adult life, ataxia, dysmetria, and sensory disturbances in the arms may herald the progression of hindbrain and cervical cord damage.

These types of malformations probably result from disturbed hindbrain development, rather than damage incurred after normal development has occurred. Symptoms may be relieved in part by shunting if hydrocephalus has developed. More complex procedures, such as enlargement of the foramen magnum and cervical laminectomies, may be useful in patients with more focal problems associated with cerebellar, brainstem, or cervical cord compression.

Syringomyelia

Syringomyelia, or cavitation of the cord, may originate in the cervical spinal cord or extend into it from the brainstem or other cord levels (Fig. 3.1). It probably arises from congenital cysts, occult tumors, or perinatal necrosis of the central cord in most individuals affected. In some cases, syringomyelia forms with gradual dilatation of the spinal central canal. This is presumed to occur as cerebrospinal (CSF) pulse waves are directed downward from the fourth ventricle in individuals with a defect in the development of formina in the embryonic rhombic roof (4).

Whatever the cause, syringomyelia of the cervical cord will usually present with sensory deficits over several dermatomes. Impaired pain perception may develop with damage to the anterior decussation of the spinothalamic tracts. The patient may develop burns or abrasions on the fingers because of inadequate pain perception. As the syrinx enlarges, anterior horn cell damage will occur, and focal atrophy will be evident. Enlargement of the syrinx usually occurs, and spontaneous resolution of the cavitation does not occur. Long tract signs evolve along with focal motor and sensory deficits as the cyst enlarges.

There is no one satisfactory treatment for syringomyelia, although a variety of surgical approaches have been attempted. Shunting the cyst may produce transient improvement in some individuals.

Klippel-Feil Anomaly

The Klippel-Feil anomaly occurs when two or more cervical vertebrae fail to segment. Affected patients exhibit a short neck, low posterior hairline, and decreased range of neck motion (5, 6). This anomaly frequently is associated with fascial, osseous, cardiovascular, neurologic, and other nonskeletal abnormalities (7). These defects may arise from an underlying disruption in fetal subclavian artery circulation and may exhibit autosomal dominant or recessive transmission (8, 9). Syringomyelia may develop along with the skeletal anomaly.

The varieties of Klippel-Feil anomalies are sometimes divided into type I and type II. The skeletal anomaly is most prominent in the type I anomaly. Type II anomalies are distinct in having subtle physical findings referrable to the neck associated with prominent neurologic problems such as mental retardation, ataxia, spasticity, synkinesias, extraocular muscle palsies, nystagmus, deafness, breathing and swallowing difficulty, cervical radiculopathy, and myelopathy. The neurologic symptoms associated with Klippel-Feil anomalies are usually ascribed to associated neural anomalies, abnormal cerebrospinal fluid dynamics, or pressure from bony malformations or cervical osteoarthritis adjacent to the fused vertebrae (10). Quadriparesis after trauma and sudden death can occur with either type of Klippel-Feil anomaly (11). Surgical remedies for limited neck mobility do not improve the longevity of the patients.

Congenital Osteopetrosis

In osteopetrosis there is a bilateral symmetrical increase in the density of the bones with loss of the normal trabecular pattern. The thickening of the posterior vertebral elements produces spinal stenosis and secondarily causes spinal cord compression and a myelopathy (12). This is a rare congenital problem which may impose severe limitations on the developing child as the spinal cord is constricted. Relief of the spinal stenosis is an option, but the outcome is poor in most cases.

Trauma

Trauma to the cervical region may produce damage to the cord and roots directly or indirectly. With displacement or fracture of boney elements, the cord or roots are likely to be injured, but even without bone changes the neural tissue may be severely contused. Damage to the central cord, anterior cord, or individual roots may develop with cervical trauma. At worst, the cervical roots may be avulsed or the cervical cord transected.

Root Injuries

The least serious of the root injuries is that in which only a single root is affected. Because of the vulnerability of the cervical region to massive trauma, multiple roots are likely to be affected if any are damaged (13). The various root syndromes which develop with cervical trauma exhibit fairly specific associations of motor and sensory findings along with selective suppression of tendon reflexes (Table 3.1) (13).

Central Cord Syndrome

With whiplash injuries or direct trauma to the cervical spine, the patient may develop a contusion or hematoma in the central area of the cord. This may produce an apparent transection of the cord or focal weakness, depending upon the size of the lesion and associated edema. The deficits will resolve at least partly as the damage to the cord abates. Deficits associated with irreversibly damaged neural structures will persist. The most common permanent sequelae of a central cord injury are focal weakness and atrophy in the distribution of the anterior horn cells that are lost. Surgical remedies are usually counterproductive. Attempts to minimize associated edema with high dose steroids are usually ineffective, if not started within 12 hours of injury. Support of vital functions, such as respiration, is often necessary until the contusion or hematoma resolves.

Anterior Cord Syndrome

With anterior spinal cord injury, there is complete paralysis of the muscles controlled by the anterior horn cells at the level injured, hypesthesia and hypalgesia to the level of the lesion together with preservation of touch, motion, position, and some vibration sense. Strength below the level of the injury is usually profoundly impaired or absent, and spasticity is evident. The posterior columns are spared with this type of injury, thereby preserving position, vibration, and deep pressure perception. More peripheral sensory modalities, such as pain and temperature perception, are compromised to a much lesser degree than is strength (13).

In most cases the anterior cord syndrome results from vascular disease. The anterior spinal artery supplies the areas usually affected. Occlusion of the artery may be a direct consequence of trauma or may develop indirectly with posttraumatic dissection of the aorta or vertebral arteries from which segments of the anterior spinal artery arise. Trauma to the cord may also cause the syndrome without damage to the anterior spinal artery if the resulting contusion is relatively restricted to the anterior cord (13).

Athetoid-Dystonic Cerebral Palsy

Cerebral palsy patients with congenital or early onset neurological deficits, manifested mainly by severe athetoid-dystonic movements of the neck and limbs, may develop progressive cervical radiculomyelopathy during the fourth and fifth decades (14). Radiographic evaluation usually reveals cervical spondylotic changes (14). Compression of the cervical spinal cord and roots occurs, and occasionally substantial cord atrophy develops (14). The constant athetoid-dystonic movements of the neck produce excessive torsion with cumulative injury to the cervical spinal cord and roots (14). In addition, the involuntary movements aggravate degenerative changes of the cervical spinal column which also compress the cord and roots (14). Decompressive cervical laminectomy may minimize the effects of the degenerative spine disease, but this is only useful if

Table 3.1. Innervation of Muscles of the Upper Extremity

Root	Pain	Sensory Loss	Weakness	Hyporeflexia
C5	Neck, shoulder, anterior arm	Deltoid area	Deltoid, biceps	Biceps
C6	Neck, shoulder, medial scapula, lateral arm, dorsum forearm	Thumb and index finger	Biceps	Biceps
C7	Neck, shoulder, medial scapula, lateral arm, dorsum forearm	Index and forefinger	Triceps	Triceps
C8	Neck, medial scapula, medial arm and forearm	Ring and little finger	Intrinsic hand muscles	None

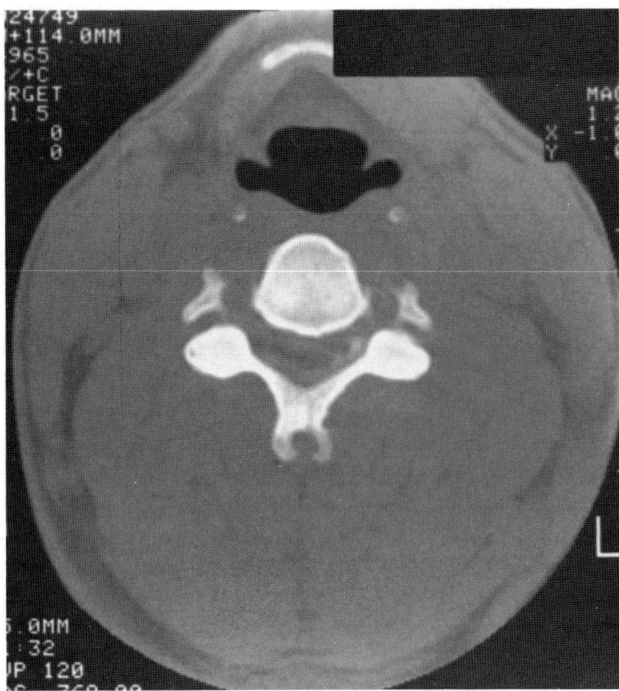

Figure 3.2. CT of the cervical spine at C5–C6 level. There is considerable spinal stenosis.

the movement disorder can be suppressed (15, 16). Athetoid-dystonic movements not suppressed by drugs lead to more instability of the cervical spine following such surgery (14); however, anterior decompression and fusion combined with posterior stabilization and holo may be effective in some cases.

ARTHROPATHIES

Many arthritic disorders produce changes in the cervical spine which eventually affect the cervical cord and roots. Many of these are degenerative or inflammatory, and most cause problems by directly compressing neural tissue. Less frequently, the arthropathy interferes with the vascular supply to the neural structures, and ischemic injuries result. How the cervical cord or root problem should be managed is greatly determined by the underlying cause of the arthropathy which gave rise to the problem.

Degenerative Arthropathies

Osteoarthritis, posttraumatic arthritis, and idiopathic arthritis may produce degenerative changes along the spine which include spur formation and disc disease. Narrowing of the neural foramina will crush cervical spinal roots, just as stenosis of the cervical spinal canal will crush the cord (Fig. 3.2). In addition to these direct manifestations of degenerative disease, more complex problems, such as subluxation of the vertebrae, may develop as the vertebral joints deteriorate. Stabilization of the spine and removal of boney elements impinging on neural structures may minimize the patients neurologic signs and symptoms.

CERVICAL SPONDYLOSIS

Cervical spondylosis denotes progressive degenerative changes in the spine that begin in the cervical intervertebral discs and extend to the surrounding bones and soft tissues (1). This degenerative process occurs to some extent in 98% of people older than 70 years of age (17). Those most severely affected will develop a myelopathy. Contributing to the development of that myelopathy are congenital narrowing of the spinal canal, inexorable progression of the cervical spondylosis, direct spinal cord compression, and encroachment upon the blood supply of the spinal cord (18).

The pattern of cervical spondylosis often starts in the third decade of life. From early life to the 8th decade of life the water content of the intervertebral discs decreases from a level approaching 88% to one of 69% (1). The anulus weakens and nuclear herniation or anulus protrusion may develop. In nuclear herniation the nuclear material is forced through a tear in the anulus and forms a well-circumscribed mass (Fig. 3.3). This often is associated with trauma. If herniation does not occur early in the process, disc degeneration may continue with a progressive decrease in structural mucopolysaccharides and an increase in collagen, causing disc fibrosis and loss of structural integrity.

ATLANTOAXIAL DISLOCATION

A common cause of myelopathy associated with degenerative joint disease is atlantoaxial dislocation. Atlantoaxial subluxation may be divided into two categories: 1. those due to incompetence of the transverse atlas ligament and 2. those due to incompetence of the odontoid process (19). Either of these may be congenital, caused by trauma, or secondary to infection (2). Symptoms of atlantoaxial subluxation include neck pain, torticollis, abnormal gait, quadriparesis, and urinary incontinence. Symptoms appear insidiously and progress slowly. Plain roentgenograms may show C1–C2 subluxation. Myelography with CT or MRI may be necessary prior to surgery. Initial management requires immobilization of the neck to prevent further trauma to the spinal cord (2).

JUVENILE RHEUMATOID ARTHRITIS

Perhaps 25–30% of patients hospitalized with rheumatoid arthritis have radiological involvement of the cervical spine (20). Atlantoaxial subluxation is relatively common in patients with rheumatoid arthritis. The resultant compression of the cervical spinal cord as the axis slips anterior to the atlas produces a progressive cervical myelopathy with characteristic features. Ligamentous laxity and bone destruction produced by synovial proliferation at the facet joints

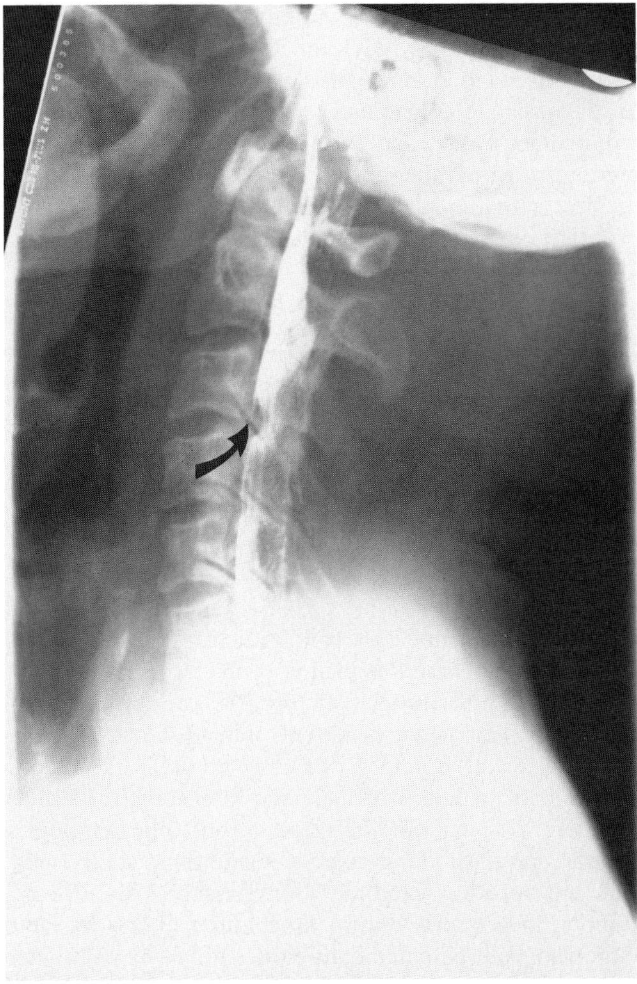

Figure 3.3. Myelogram of the cervical spine. This 59-year-old man complained of neck pain and weakness in his arms and legs progressing over the course of 3 weeks. On examination he had a sensory level at C3 associated with a spastic paraparesis and a plantar extensor response on the left. This myelogram revealed a large defect at the C3–C4 level which proved to be a herniated nucleus pulposus (HNP). At surgery there was considerable cord compression.

and bursal sacs are primarily responsible for the cervical spine instability in these patients.

Posterior, rather than anterior, atlantoaxial subluxation in patients with rheumatoid arthritis is uncommon (21). For posterior atlantoaxial subluxation to occur, certain anatomical abnormalities must be present singly or in combination. These include incompetence of the anterior arch of the atlas, erosion or fracture of the odontoid process, and superior and posterior migration of the atlas (21).

Posterior atlantoaxial subluxation generally has been considered more benign than anterior subluxation (26). The earliest symptoms are usually pain and neck stiffness (22). Pain frequently results from irritation of the second cervical root; classically this involves the occiput and the upper cervical spine and is made worse by sudden or jarring movements. Unilateral atlantoaxial subluxation may cause rotational deformity and stiffness (22). Vertical subluxation of the odontoid is usually painless, but subaxial subluxation is usually accompanied by both pain and neck stiffness.

Myelography with CT or MRI in addition to plain roentgenograms should be performed if compressive cervical myelopathy is suspected in patients with rheumatoid arthritis. The main indications for surgery are progressive neurological impairment and progressive radiographic instability. Occasionally surgery is required as well for intractable pain (23, 24).

TRISOMY 21 (DOWN SYNDROME)

Although asymptomatic subluxation of the atlantoaxial joint occurs in 10–20% of persons with Down syndrome, symptomatic dislocation is rare (25, 26). Atlantoaxial dislocation is diagnosed in children when the distance between the anterior arch of the atlas and the odontoid process is greater than 4.5 mm (27). The age at presentation of symptomatic atlantoaxial dislocation ranges from 5–28 years, with an average age of 12.7 years. The ratio of affected males to females is 5 to 14 (27). The preponderance of females suggests they have greater ligamentous laxity and more tendency to sublux than males (2).

Odontoid abnormalities, especially of the free apical ligament of the odontoid process (orsiculum terminale), and hypoplasia both may occur with Down syndrome. When combined with ligamentous laxity, these two problems increase the risk of dislocation (38).

Ossification of Posterior Longitudinal Ligament

Ossification of the posterior longitudinal ligament in the cervical spine is a rare cause of cervical myelopathy and occurs more commonly among Japanese individuals (39). Ossification may occur anywhere from C1 to C7, but occurs most often between the second and fourth cervical vertebrae (40, 41). The age of affected patients ranges from 42 to 75 years of age, and there is no sex preponderance. The basis for this ossification is unknown. Problems caused by this disorder range from no symptoms to severe compressive cervical myelopathy (39). The calcification of the posterior longitudinal ligament may be demonstrated on plain x-ray films, but CT scanning will routinely define the shape and extent of the ossified ligament (41). Decompressive surgery is appropriate in patients who are symptomatic.

Synovial Cysts

Synovial or ganglion cysts of the spinal facet joints causing nerve root compression occur in both the cervical and lumbar spine (32). The clinical presentation most often imitates that of a herniated intervertebral disc. Hemorrhage within the cystic lesion may initiate acute back and radicular pain or dramatically increase existing chronic pain (32). Symptomatic patients require surgical intervention.

INFECTIONS

The cervical cord and roots are not the favored site for any specific type of infection, but they are as susceptible as the rest of the spinal cord and roots to a variety of infections. Certain types of infections, such as human immunodeficiency virus (HIV) and syphilis, have a predilection for the spinal cord, which makes them suspect when the patient has progressive signs of cord dysfunction. The recent finding that HTLV-1 virus, as well as HIV-1 and HIV-2, cause progressive demyelinating myelopathies increases the probabilities that many unexplained myelopathies will prove to be caused by viruses, with RNA retroviruses accounting for a large share of those unexplained syndromes.

Acquired Immunodeficiency Syndrome (AIDS)

Central nervous system complications occur in approximately 30% of patients with AIDS (33). The brain may be attacked by either opportunistic infections or the the AIDS virus, HIV, directly, but the spinal cord is more likely to exhibit neurologic signs on the basis of HIV invasion rather than as a consequence of opportunistic organisms. A vacuolar myelopathy pathologically resembling subacute combined degeneration may develop in patients with HIV disease, but precisely what causes the vacuolar demyelination that occurs with this myelopathy is still unknown (34). The myelopathy is characterized by spongiform myelin changes predominantly in the dorsal and lateral columns of the spinal cord (35, 36). The lesions develop independently of any opportunistic infection and appear to be a direct consequence of HIV infection of the central nervous system (37, 38). Where vacuolation is most prominent there is little or no evidence of inflammation, and the spongiform changes are confined to the parenchyma of the spinal cord, sparing the anterior horn cells (37). The only treatment for this HIV myelopathy is zidovudine, but patients with extensive signs may show little improvement (34).

Intramedullary Spinal Tuberculoma

Central nervous system involvement by tuberculosis is uncommon compared to the involvement of other systems (39). Intramedullary spinal tuberculoma is especially uncommon in North America, but when it does occur it is usually in association with multiple intracranial tuberculomas; intracranial tuberculomas are found in 10–33% of the patients with intramedullary tuberculomas. This multiplicity of lesions is presumed to occur because of hematogenous spread of the organism (39). Intraspinal tuberculoma is almost always secondary to tuberculous involvement elsewhere in the body, most commonly pulmonary tuberculosis. MRI and CT myelography are especially useful in localizing this type of lesion. Also helpful in diagnosis are an elevated leukocyte count, an elevated sedimentation rate, and an elevated CSF protein with a predominance of mononuclear cells. Triple antituberculous therapy with isoniazid, rifampin, and ethambutol is appropriate as the principal management.

Spinal Epidural Abscess

The most common source for an infection that spreads hematogenously to the epidural space is the skin. Other sources include the urinary tract, lungs, pharynx, and teeth. A contiguous focus, such as a psoas abscess, dermal sinus, or sacral decubitus, also may evolve into an epidural abscess (40). Antecedent trauma may be an important predisposing factor. The organism most commonly isolated is *Staphylococcus aureus*.

Typically the clinical picture of an epidural abscess includes four elements: back pain, radicular pain, weakness, and paralysis. These complaints evolve sequentially; any patient with this characteristic progression must be managed on an emergency basis with spinal CT or MRI, followed by needle aspiration or surgery to drain the abscess. Febrile patients with back pain and local spine tenderness may have a spinal epidural abscess, but other etiologies include spinal subdural abscess, meningitis, acute transverse myelopathy, vertebral or intervertebral disc disease, tumors, and vascular lesions. An epidural abscess warrants treatment with parenteral antibiotics for 3–4 weeks after diagnosis; any concurrent vertebral osteomyelitis should be treated with antibiotics for 6–8 weeks (40).

TUMORS

Several different tumors extend to the spinal cord and spinal roots, but none has an extraordinary proclivity for the cervical region. The most common tumors affecting this region are metastatic lesions or benign tumors, such as neurofibromas and meningiomas. Lesions developing within the cord, such as gliomas, may be benign histologically but lethal because of their location (Fig. 3.4). Resection is appropriate for single masses outside the cord unless the lesion is clearly metastatic. Spinal irradiation is an alternative for lesions sensitive to this modality.

Neurofibromas

Neurofibromas involving the spinal cord presumably derive from sensory or autonomic ganglions, nerve roots, or proximal nerve trunks. These tumors usually grow along the nerves in which they originate and compress the spinal roots at the exit zone or compress the cord if the tumor is large enough (Fig. 3.5) (41). Malignant degeneration of previously benign neurofibromas may

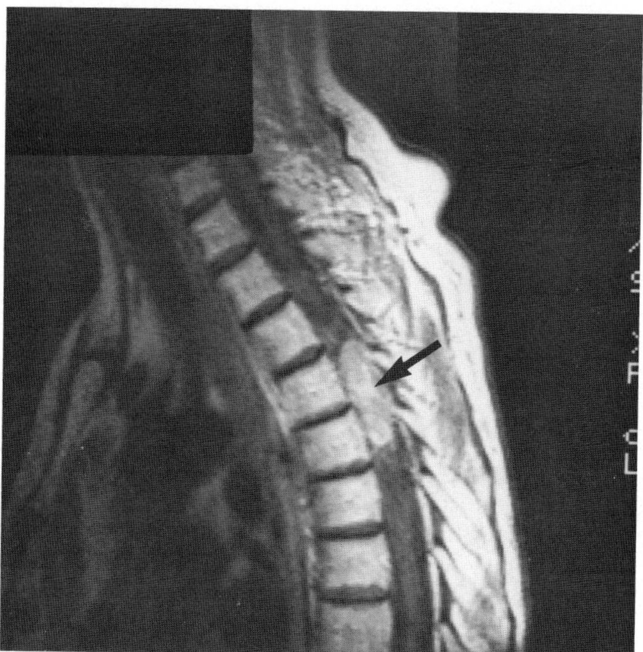

Figure 3.4. MRI of the spinal cord reveals a large intramedullary tumor extending down into the high thoracic cord.

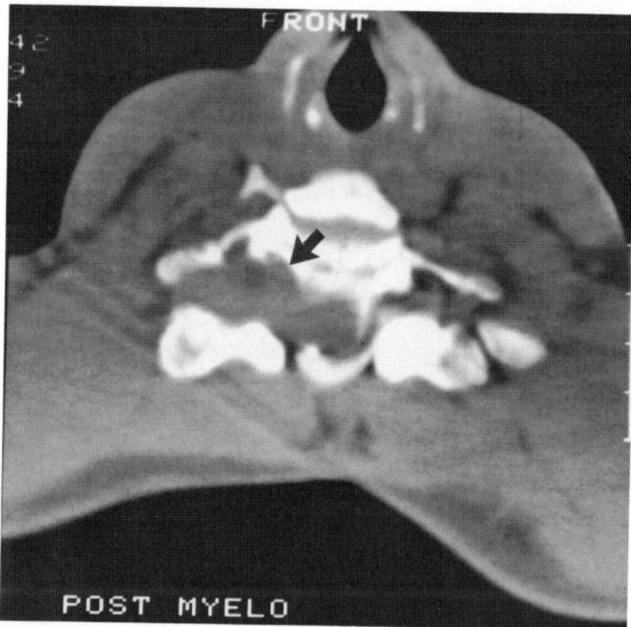

Figure 3.5. Postmyelogram CT scan of C7 vertebra. This 28-year-old man had a progressive history of leg weakness and gait difficulty spanning 6 months. This CT revealed a large epidural and paraspinal mass on the right which has displaced the spinal cord to the left. This proved to be a massive neurofibroma.

occur at any time. The lesions increase in size and number during the second and third decades of life. In many patients the predominant symptom is radicular pain. Whenever a neurofibroma becomes symptomatic, because of either root or cord compression, it should be removed as completely as possible.

Meningiomas

Meningiomas overlying the cervical spine are rare, but must be considered in any patient with complaints suggestive of cervical cord compression. These are benign tumors, but permanent resection of the lesion may be hampered by the tendency of meningiomas to recur (Fig. 3.6). Radiation therapy after resection provides little additional protection against recurrence in most patients and increases the risk of malignant degeneration of the tumor.

Epidural Metastases

Metastatic epidural tumors compressing the spinal cord are common neurological complications of cancer. The primary tumors most often producing spinal cord compression are breast, lung, prostate, and kidney. Spinal cord compression is often manifested by pain, weakness, ataxia, or autonomic dysfunction (42). Pain is either local or radicular. Unlike the pain from a herniated in-

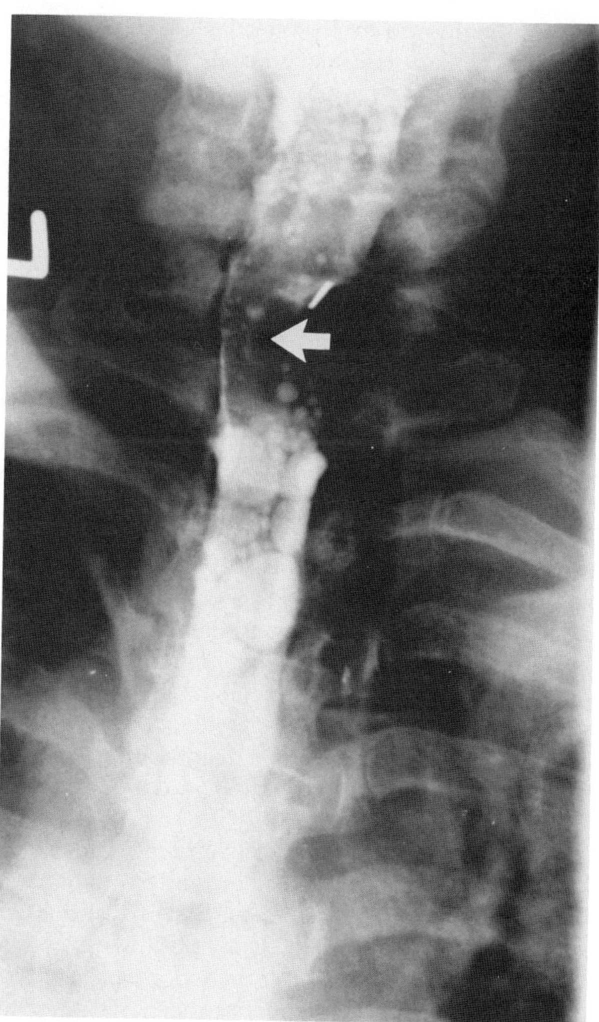

Figure 3.6. Myelogram of the cervical spine. Nearly complete obstruction at the C7–T1 level is consistent with a meningioma or other extramedullary tumor.

tervertebral disc, the pain becomes worse when the patient lies down.

Radiation therapy is often the treatment of choice for most patients with extradural spinal cord compression from systemic cancer. Some decompression may be achieved with high dose steroid treatment. This high dose steroid treatment is only feasible for a few days or weeks before side effects necessitate reducing the dose to 4 mg four times daily. Anterior vertebrectomy, decompressive laminectomy, and stabilization procedures are indicated when the nature of the primary tumor is not known, if the diagnosis is in doubt, if relapse occurs and the patient cannot be given further radiation, if symptoms progress despite radiation therapy, or if spinal instability is present (42). The nature of the primary tumor is as important in determining long-term improvement as the nature of the treatment.

Meningeal Carcinomatosis and Lymphomatosis

Diffuse infiltration of the leptomeninges and subarachnoid space by carcinoma cells metastasizing from a primary tumor outside the central nervous system may be the first evidence of malignant disease. The most common primary tumors that metastasize in this way to the cervical cord and roots are breast, lymphoma, lung, and melanoma. Adenocarcinoma is the most frequent histologic type of carcinoma to metastasize to the meninges.

Tumor cells are presumed to spread into the central nervous system by direct invasion of the cerebrospinal fluid through the choroid plexus, through the leptomeningeal vessels, or from secondary extension of tumors residing in the brain parenchyma or nerve roots. Diffuse infiltration of the leptomeninges with metastatic carcinoma is distinct from the nodular proliferation that characterizes parenchymal and most dural metastatic tumors.

The manifestations of spinal leptomeningeal involvement include meningeal signs in addition to low back pain and pain in the extremities associated with weakness and numbness. Fasciculations, areflexia, and sensory deficits result from carcinomatous infiltration of spinal nerve roots, with those to the lower limbs most often being symptomatic. Presumably this predilection for involvement of the lower limbs results from settling of malignant cells in the CSF into the cul-de-sac about the cauda equina.

Positive identification of malignant cells is crucial, and the yield for an abnormal examination can be increased from 45–80% with repeated spinal taps. Patients with meningeal carcinomatosis or lymphomatosis may prove refractory to therapy, even if their tumor type is sensitive to chemotherapy or radiation elsewhere. Whatever modality works against the primary tumor in other sites should be attempted when the tumor is metastatic to the meninges. Supplementary radiation or intrathecal chemotherapy may be appropriate with specific malignancies.

Intramedullary Subependymoma

Subependymoma is a rare tumor which may develop in the cervical region. Spinal intramedullary subependymomas are routinely symptomatic early in their evolution because of the cord compression that they cause as they enlarge (51, 52). The spinal variety of this tumor primarily affects the cervical cord and usually affects several levels (44).

Subependymomas have a distinctive microscopic pattern characterized by clusters of glial cells separated by wide bands of fibrillary processes. The almost simultaneous onset of subependymomas in identical twins and the association of subependymoma and heterotopic leptomeningeal tissue suggest that this tumor is a type of hamartoma resulting from a developmental defect (45).

There is usually a distinct plane of cleavage between the tumor and the surrounding tissue, allowing the tumor to be totally removed with microsurgery (46). The results of surgery are more variable if the tumor exhibits astrocytic predominance (47).

Chondroma

Chondromas are benign, but rare, tumors in the cervical spine, which appear as firm, well-circumscribed masses. They account for 5% of all bone tumors, but only 4% occur as spinal tumors (48). The spinal chondroma may arise from hyperplasia of immature spinal cartilage with migration outside the vertebral axis or from metaplasia of the connective tissue in contact with the spine or the anulus fibrosus (48). These lesions are only slightly, if at all, responsive to radiotherapy. Surgical resection is often not feasible.

Lipomas

Subdural lipomas of the spinal cord comprise only 7% of all spinal tumors (49). The tumor is more common in the thoracic spine (31%) than at cervical levels (25%). Forty-four percent of high cervical lipomas extend into the posterior fossa (49). This problem generally affects young people. Surgical resection is appropriate when patients are symptomatic.

VASCULAR DISEASE

The cervical spinal cord is less susceptible to vascular injury than is the lumbosacral spinal cord. This is primarily because the vascular supply to the cervical cord is more redundant than that supplying lower levels of the cord. This makes the cervical cord less at risk for infarction than is the lumbosacral cord, but it may still suffer ischemic or hemorrhagic damage.

Stroke

Many types of aortic disease, including dissecting aneurysm, aortic thrombosis, and atheromatous plaque erosion, may produce spinal cord infarction. In many cases the aortic disease is occult and is only suspected after it produces neurological signs and symptoms (50). Hemorrhages occurring in the cervical cord are generally from vascular malformations or vascular tumors, rather than from hemorrhage into an area of infarction. Whether the stroke is ischemic or hemorrhagic, the development of this type of problem in the cervical cord is usually lethal and is not manageable with surgical or medical intervention.

Epidural Varicose Veins

Spinal epidural varices are a rare basis for myelopathy and associated neurological dysfunction, but they must be considered in patients with acutely or subacutely evolving signs of spinal cord damage (51). Signs and symptoms probably develop from thrombosis and progressive venous distension (51). This type of vascular disorder more typically affects the cord at thoracic or lower levels. There is no clearly effective therapy for this disorder.

Epidural Hematoma

Most spinal epidural hematomas occur spontaneously (52–55). Those cases that can be explained usually develop from arteriovenous malformations, coagulation disturbances, and tumors (52–54). With spontaneous spinal epidural hematoma, deficits typically develop with some physical exertion, but they may develop during sleep (56). The primary symptoms of cervical epidural hematoma are radicular pain into the arms and acute cervical or interscapular pain followed within hours by paraparesis, progressive sensory loss, and other signs of myelopathy (56). Treatment consists of prompt laminectomy and decompression along with removal of the hematoma (64). The prognosis is good in younger patients and in those who undergo surgery within a few hours of the appearance of severe neurologic deficits (56). Patients with epidural hematomas overlying the cervical spinal cord not operated upon usually die of respiratory failure (56).

Subdural Hematoma

Spinal subdural hematoma, unlike intracranial subdural hematoma, is rare (57). It usually occurs in patients with coagulation disorders due to anticoagulant therapy or a blood dyscrasia (57). Spinal trauma only rarely produces this type of hematoma. Vascular malformations overlying the cord should be sought whenever this type of hematoma develops in a patient with normal coagulation studies. Some patients develop subdural hematomas after spinal surgery, and some develop hematomas for no apparent reason, but both etiologies are extremely rare (57). Surgical evacuation is essential with this type of lesion.

MOTOR NEURON DISEASE

With motor neuron disease involving the cervical cord the patient exhibits both upper and lower motor neuron signs and symptoms. Lead poisoning was once a fairly common cause of motor neuron disease affecting the cervical cord, but this was largely from industrial exposure which has been greatly reduced. Before the introduction of effective vaccination, poliomyelitis accounted for much of the anterior horn cell disease that occurred in the United States. Many of the other forms of motor neuron disease are adequately similar to poliomyelitis so that they too are presumed to have a viral basis which has yet to be elucidated. Amyotrophic lateral sclerosis is the most common of the motor neuron diseases currently affecting this part of the cord.

Amyotrophic Lateral Sclerosis (ALS)

Amyotrophic lateral sclerosis is a crippling and fatal neurologic disease with a worldwide incidence of 1–2 per 100,000 and a worldwide prevalence ranging from 3–7 per 1,000,000 (58). This disease most often affects men rather than women. Symptoms are always motor in nature and usually present as segmental asymmetric weakness. It presents in adults as progressive muscular atrophy with weakness, wasting, and fasciculations in any of the striated muscles except the extraocular and cardiac muscles. The disease is usually inexorably progressive, but rare patients do have protracted remissions (59).

Almost 95% of patients with classical ALS lack a family history of the disorder, but there are families in which the disease follows an autosomal dominant pattern of inheritance in adult onset disease and both autosomal dominant and recessive patterns in juvenile onset disease (60, 61). This obviously suggests a genetic predisposition in some patients but does not explain the bulk of patients. Increased exposure to lead, mercury, or other heavy metals has been reported in some ALS patients, but the significance of this is uncertain (62).

Motor neurons of the brainstem and spinal cord of patients with ALS show atrophy, shrinkage, and intracytoplasmic lipofuscin associated with neuronal loss and astrocytosis. Intracytoplasmic inclusions and ghost cells are frequent. Central chromatolysis and neuronophagia are rarely seen except in rapidly progressive disease.

Systemic or iontophoretic administration of thyrotropin-release hormone (TRH) to animals increase motor neuron function measured electrophysiologically. Some controlled studies of intravenous TRH administration suggest that this hormone may produce short term clinical benefits (63, 64). There are no consistently effective treatments for this disorder.

METABOLIC DISORDERS

The cervical spine may be involved in metabolic disorders that affect the brain or brainstem, but more typically it is affected by the same problems that affect the remainder of the spinal cord. An excess of cervical cord involvement may be apparent in some demyelinating or degenerative metabolic disorders, but this apparent predominance of cervical involvement simply reflects the increasing number of fibers in the spinal cord tracts at higher levels of the spinal cord.

Combined Systems Disease

Subacute combined degeneration of the spinal cord, also known as combined systems disease, is characterized by parasthesias and weakness of the extremities, spasticity of the legs, loss of position and vibration sense, and gait or limb ataxia. This may develop with insufficient intake of vitamin B12 or from absent intrinsic factor, a problem occurring with pernicious anemia, after gastrectomy, or with small bowel disease. The pathologic changes in the spinal cord are most evident in the white matter and primarily consist of demyelination and axonal loss in the posterior and lateral columns. Vitamin B12 replacement is usually effective in halting the progression of the neurologic deficits, but it may not suffice to correct the damage that occurred before replacement therapy began.

Mucopolysaccharidoses

Several genetically determined disorders characterized by the accumulation of mucopolysaccharides secondary to specific catabolic enzyme deficiencies have been described (65). Cervical myelopathy often occurs in patients with mucopolysaccharidosis, but this is not from neuronal damage secondary to intracellular storage of the mucopolysaccharide. On the contrary, it is usually from ligamentous abnormalities along the cervical spine, which produce instability of the craniocervical or atlantoaxial junctions (66). Hypoplasia of the odontoid process is common in patients with Morquio's syndrome (67). Alternatively, a myelopathy may develop secondary to dural thickening.

No treatment is available to halt the progression of the mucopolysaccharidoses, but the myelopathy developing with these metabolic disorders may be minimized with surgical intervention. This may mean stabilizing the cervical elements which have subluxed in association with skeletal and ligamentous disorders characteristic of the storage diseases. Myelopathy due to dural thickening in mucopolysaccharidoses may respond to surgical decompression (68).

IATROGENIC DISORDERS

Radiation Myelopathy

The major complications of cervical spinal cord irradiation are white matter necrosis and coagulative necrosis secondary to vascular damage (69, 70). This radiation myelopathy is a life-threatening complication of radiotherapy. Cervical cord injuries cause greater and earlier mortality than thoracic cord injuries (71). The survival rate for these patients is poorer than for traumatic myelopathy, possibly because of the poorer health of the patients treated with radiation (71).

The clinical signs of radiation myelopathy are quite variable. The onset of symptoms is usually delayed for several months after the termination of treatment. When they do appear, it is usually in an insidious manner, thus making it difficult to determine on clinical grounds whether the signs and symptoms have developed because of radiation damage or recurrent tumor. Usually the affected individuals complain of numbness or pins and needles sensations affecting the hands and feet. These hypesthesias and parasthesias may be elicited or aggravated by flexion or extension of the neck. In patients with progressive symptoms, the paresthesias are followed by weakness or paralysis of one or more extremities, by a progressive hypalgesia, and subsequently by bowel and bladder dysfunction. Involvement of the sphincters implies a poor prognosis.

The probability of radiation myelopathy increases with cervical cord exposure in excess of 3500 rads over less than 2 weeks. Once the myelopathy has begun, there is no satisfactory treatment to reduce the extent of damage that eventually develops. The cause of radiation myelopathy is unresolved.

OTHER CAUSES OF CERVICAL DISEASE

The cervical spinal cord and spinal roots are vulnerable to many other diseases which affect the spinal cord and roots in general. Multiple sclerosis, Guillain-Barre syndrome, and diphtheritic polyneuropathy are only a few of the many other problems that may produce changes in cervical structure and function. These changes may be disabling or lethal, because much of the spinal cord activity must course through the cervical cord. Because of the diversity of problems that may cause signs and symptoms referrable to the cervical region, any patient with deficits originating in this region should be investigated rapidly and thoroughly.

REFERENCES

1. Lestini WF, Wiesel SW. The pathogenesis of cervical spondylosis. Clin Orthop 1989;239:69–93.

2. Chaudry V, Sturgeon C, Gates J, Myers G. Symptomatic atlantoaxial dislocation in Down's syndrome. Ann Neurol 1987;21:606–609.

3. Gilman S, Bloedel J, Lechtenberg R. Disorders of the Cerebellum. Philadelphia: F.A. Davis, 1981.

4. Gardner WJ. Hydrodynamic mechanism of syringomyelia: its relationship to myelocele. J Neurol Neurosurg Psychiatry 1965;28:247–259.

5. Pizzutillo PD. Klippel-Feil syndrome. In: Baily RW, Sherk HH, Dunn EJ, et al., eds. The cervical spine. Philadelphia: JB Lippincott, 1983:174–188.

6. Winter RB, Moe JM, Lonstein JE. The incidence of Klippel-Feil syndrome in patients with congenital scoliosis and kyphosis. Spine 1984;9:463–466.

7. Brill CB, Peyster RG, Keller MS, Galtman L. Isolation of the right subclavian artery with subclavian steal in a child with Klippel-Feil anomaly. Am J Med Genet 1987;26:933–940.

8. Bavinick JNB, Weaver DD. Subclavian artery supply disruption sequence: hypothesis of a vascular etiology for Poland, Klippel-Feil and Mobius anomalies. Am J Med Genet 1986;23:903–918.

9. Tanaka T, Uhthoff HK. The pathogenesis of congenital vertebral malformations. Acta Orthop Scand 1981;52:423–425.

10. Spillane JD, Pallis G, Jones AM. Developmental abnormalities in the region of the foramen magnum. Brain 1957;80:11–50.

11. Wilkinson M. The Klippel-Feil syndrome. In: Vinken PJ, Bruyns GW, eds. Handbook of clinical neurology. New York: Elsevier-North Hollond, 1978:111–122.

12. McCleary L, Rovit RL, Marali R. Case report: myelopathy secondary to congenital osteopetrosis of the cervical spine. Neurosurgery 1987;20:487–489.

13. Raynor RB, Koplik B. Cervical cord trauma. The relationship between clinical syndromes and force of injury. Spine 1985;10:193–197.

14. Kidron D, Steiner I, Melamed E. Late onset progressive radiculomyelopathy in patients with cervical athetoid-dystonic cerebral palsy. Eur Neurol 1987;27:164–166.

15. Nisihara N, Tanabe G, Nakahara S, Iwai T, Marakawa H. Surgical treatment of cervical spondylotic myelopathy complicating athetoid cerebral palsy. J Bone Joint Surg 1984;66:504–508.

16. Kadoya S, Kwak R, Hirose G, Mamooto T. Cervical spondylitic myelopathy treated by microsurgical anterior approach with or without interbody fusion. In: Brock M, ed. Modern neurosurgery. Berlin: Springer, 1982.

17. Hunt WE. Cervical spondylosis. Natural history and rare indications for surgical decompression. In: Congress of Neurological Surgeons: clinical neurosurgery. Baltimore: Williams & Wilkins, 1980.

18. Ogino H, Tada K, Okada K, Yonenoba K, Yamamoto T, Ono K, Nauiki H. Canal diameter, anteroposterior compression ratio, and spondylotic myelopathy of the cervical spine. Spine 1983;8:1.

19. Greenberg AD. Atlanto axial dislocation. Brain 1968;91:655–684.

20. Matthews TA. Atlantoaxial subluxation in rheumatoid arthritis. Ann Rheum Dis 1969;28:260–266.

21. Lipson SJ. Cervical myelopathy and posterior atlantoaxial subluxation in patients with rheumatoid arthritis. J Bone Joint Surg 1985;67:593–597.

22. Toma A, Sturrock RD, Fisher WD, et al. Surgical stabilization of the rheumatoid cervical spine. A review of indications and results. J Bone Joint Surg 1987;69-B:8–11.

23. Ranawat CS, O'Leary P, Pellici P, Tsairis P, Marchisello P, Dorr L. Cervical spine fusion in rheumatoid arthritis. J Bone Joint Surg 1979;61:3–10.

24. Hamblen DL. Surgical management of rheumatoid arthritis. The cervical spine. In: Harris NH, ed. Postgraduate textbook of clinical orthopedics. Bristol: Wright PSG, 1983;487–497.

25. Diamond LS, Lynne D, Sigman B. Orthopedic disorders in patients with Down's syndrome. Orthop Clin North Am 1981;12:57–71.

26. Pieschel SM, Seola FH, Perry CD. Atlantoaxial instability in children with Down's syndrome. Pediatr Radiol 1981;10:129–132.

27. Tischler J, Martel W. Dislocation of the atlas in mongolism. Radiology 1965;84:904–906.

28. Finerman GAM, Sakai D, Weingarten S. Atlantoaxial dislocation with spinal cord compression in a mongoloid child: a case report. J Bone Joint Surg 1976;58:408–409.

29. Peled R, Harnes BZ, Waisbrod H, Simon J. Cervical myelopathy caused by ossification of the posterior longitudinal ligaments of the spine. Eur Neurol 1982;21:392–395.

30. Chin WS, Oon CC. Ossification of the posterior longitudinal ligaments of the spine. Br J Radiol 1979;52:865–869.

31. Yamamoto I, Kageyama N, Nakamura K, Takahashi T. Computed tomography in ossification of the posterior longitudinal ligaments in the cervical spine. Surg Neurol 1979;12:414–418.

32. Burton M, Onofrio, AD. Synovial cysts of the spine. Neurosurgery 1988;22:642–647.

33. Singh BM, Levine S, Yarrish RL, Myland MJ, Jeanty D, Wormser GP. Spinal cord syndromes in the acquired immune deficiency syndrome. Acta Neurol Scand 1986;73:590–598.

34. Lechtenberg R, Sher J. AIDS in the nervous system. New York: Churchill Livingstone, 1989.

35. Roman GC. Retrovirus-associated myelopathies. Arch Neurol 1987;44:659.

36. Petito CK, Navia BA, Choo ES, et al. Vacuolar myelopathy pathologically resembling subacute combined degeneration in patients with the acquired immunodeficiency syndrome. N Engl J Med 1985;312:874.

37. Johnson RT, McArthur JC. Myelopathies and retroviral infections. Ann Neurol 1987;21:113.

38. de la Monte SM, Ho DD, Schooley RT, et al. Subacute encephalomyelitis of AIDS and its relation to HTLV-III infection. Neurology 1987;37:562.

39. Rhoton EL, Ballinger WE, Omsling R, Sypert G. Intramedullary spinal tuberculoma. Neurosurgery 1988;22:733–736.

40. Baker AS, Ojemann RG, Swartz MN, Richardson EP, Jr. Spinal epidural abscess. N Engl J Med 1975;293:465–468.

41. Riccardi VM. Von Recklinghausen—neurofibromatosis. Med Prog Technol 305:1617–1626.

42. Liebelt SA, Gutin PH, Sneed PK, et al. Interstitial irradiation for the treatment of primary and metastatic brain tumors. Prin Pract Oncol 1989;3:1–11.

43. Gilbert RW, Kim JH, Posner JB. Epidural spinal cord compression from metastatic tumor: diagnosis and treatment. Ann Neurol 1978;3:40–51.

44. Lee KS, Angelo JN, McWhorter JM, Davis CM. Symptomatic subependymoma of the cervical spinal cord. Report of two cases. J Neurosurg 1987;67:128–131.

45. Pluchino F, Loderim S, Lasio G, Allegranza A. Complete removal of a spinal subependymoma. Case Report. Acta Neurochir 1984;73:243–50.

46. Ho KL. Concurrence of subependymoma and heterotopic leptomeningeal neurological tissue. Arch Pathol Lab Med 1983;107:136–140.

47. Salcman M, Mayer R. Intramedullary subependymoma of the cervical spinal cord. Case Report. Neurosurgery 1984;14:608–611.

48. Lozes G, Fawaz A, Perper H, et al. Chondroma of cervical spine—case report. J Neurosurg 1987;66:128–130.

49. Fan CJ, Vurapen RJ, Tn CT. Case report. Subdural spinal lipoma with posterior fossa extension. Clin Radiol 1989;40:91–94.

50. Herrick MK, Mills PE, Jr. Infarction of spinal cord. Two cases of selective gray matter involvement secondary to asymptomatic aortic disease. Arch Neurol 1971;24:228–241.

51. Dickman CA, Zabramski M, Sonntag Volker KM, et al. Myelopathy due to epidural varicose veins of the cervicothoracic junction. Case report. J Neurosurg 1988;69:940–941.

52. Foo D, Chang YC, Rossier AB. Spontaneous cervical epidural hemorrhage, anterior cord syndrome, and familial vascular malformation: case report. Neurology 1980;30:308–311.

53. Muller H, Schramm J, Roggendorf W, Brock M. Vascular malformations as a cause of spontaneous spinal epidural haematoma. Acta Neurochir 1982;62:297–305.

54. Stanley P, McComb JG. Chronic spinal epidural hematoma in hemophilia A in a child. Pediatr Radiol 1983;12:241–243.

55. Beatty RM, Winston KR. Spontaneous cervical epidural hematoma. A consideration of etiology. J Neurosurg 1984;61:143–148.

56. Matsumae M, Shimoda M, Shibuya N, Ieda M, Yamamoto I, Sato O. Spontaneous cervical epidural hematoma. Surg Neurol 1987;28:381–384.

57. Smith RA. Spinal subdural hematoma, neurilemoma and acute transverse myelopathy. Surg Neurol 1985;23:367–70.

58. Milder DW. Clinical limits of amyotrophic lateral sclerosis. In: Rowland LP, ed. Human motor neuron diseases. New York: Raven Press, 1982:15–22.

59. Tucker T, Layzer RB. Subacute reversible motor neuron disease. Neurology 1985;35(suppl 1):108.

60. Alberca R, Castilla JM, Peralta AG. Hereditary amyotrophic lateral sclerosis. J Neurol Sci 1981;50:201–216.

61. Emery AEH, Holloway S. Familial motor neuron diseases. In: Rowland LP, ed. Human motor neuron disease. New York: Raven Press, 1982:139–147.

62. Roelofs-Iverson RA, Mulder DW, Elveback LR, et al. ALS and heavy metals: a pilot case control study. Neurology 1984;34:393–395.

63. Gracco VL, Caligiuri M, Abbs JH, et al. Placebo controlled computerized dynametric measurements of bulbar and somatic muscle strength increase in patients with amyotrophic lateral sclerosis following intravenous infusion of 10 mg/kg thyrotropin releasing hormone. Ann Neurol 1984;16:110.

64. Sufit RL, Beaulieu DA, Sangug M, et al. Placebo controlled quantitative measurements of neuromuscular function following intravenous infusion of 10 mg/kg of thyrotropin releasing hormone in 16 male patients with amyotrophic lateral sclerosis. Ann Neurol 1984;16:110–111.

65. Rosenberg RN. Biochemical genetics of neurologic disease. N Engl J Med 1981;305:1181–1193.

66. Brill CB, Rose JS, Godmilow L, et al. Spastic quadriparesis due to C1–C2 subluxation in Hurler syndrome. J Pediatr 1978;92:441–443.

67. Holzgreve W, Grobe H, von Figura K, et al. Morquio syndrome: clinical findings in 11 patients with MPS IV A and 2 patients with MPS IV B. Hum Genet 1981;57:360–365.

68. Kaufman HH, Rosenberg HS, Scott CI, et al. Cervical myelopathy due to dural compression in mucopolysaccharidosis. Surg Neurol 1982;17:404–410.

69. van der Kogel AJ. Mechanisms of late radiation injury in the spinal cord. In: Meyn RE, Withers HR, eds. Radiation biology in cancer research. New York: Raven Press, 1980:461–469.

70. Reinhold HS, Van Putten WLJ, Hopewell JW, van der Kogel AJ. The latent period in clinical radiation myelopathy. Int J Radiat Oncol Biol Phys 1984;10:2385–2387.

71. Schultheiss TE, Stephens LC, Peters L. Survival in radiation therapy. Int J Radiat Onc Biol Phys 1986;12:1765–1769.

4

Cervical Cord Syndromes

Jonathan Z. Charney, M.D.

Introduction

Syndromes involving the cervical spine are based on a lesion affecting either the spinal cord, nerve roots, or the vertebrae.

The parenchyma of the cervical spinal cord consists of a butterfly-shape-core of gray matter which is surrounded by white matter. The gray matter consists of nerve cells. The white matter consists of fiber pathways both descending from higher centers as well as ascending pathways which carry sensory impulses. In the dorsal funiculus proprioceptive and tactile impulses are carried. In the lateral and ventral areas the spinothalamic tracts carry painful impulses. In the center of the gray matter is the spinal canal. The cells in the gray matter are arranged into the anterior horns, the lateral horns, and the posterior horns. The cells in the anterior horns supply motor function to the arms and legs (lateral cells), trunk, and diaphragm (medial cells). The cells in the lateral horns supply sympathetic and parasympathetic fibers, while the cells in the posterior horns receive terminal synapses from sensory fibers.

Motor deficits are dependent on the level of the lesion in the cervical spinal cord. Thus a lesion at vertebral body C5 produces a C6 spinal lesion. At first there is flaccid paralysis below the lesion followed by spasticity. The head and neck movements (flexion and extension) are dependent on the first three cervical nerves. The fourth cervical nerve innervates the diaphragm, and a lesion at this level causes respiratory paralysis. The remainder of the cervical nerves are responsible for movements of the arms. The fifth cervical nerve innervates the deltoids, rhomboids, supra and infraspinatous muscles, and the teres minor and major. A lesion at this level causes paralysis of these muscles, and the arms are adducted and internally rotated. There is loss of the biceps reflex. The sixth cervical innervates the biceps muscle. A lesion at this level results in paralysis of the biceps muscle and loss of the biceps and brachioradialis reflex. The seventh cervical nerve innervates the triceps and the extensors of the wrist and fingers. With a lesion at this level there is loss of the triceps reflex and there is abduction of the upper arm with flexion of the forearm, wrist, and fingers. Lesions of the eighth cervical nerve cause paralysis of flexion of the fingers and wrist as well as of the small muscles of the hand. There are no changes in the triceps, biceps, or brachioradialis reflexes. This produces a claw hand.

Sensory changes are seen in a determatome distribution at the level of the lesion and tend to be dissociative below this level. Electric-like sensations, with flexion of the neck (Lhermitte's sign), is characteristically seen in diseases of the cervical spine. It may be seen after trauma, in multiple sclerosis, in syringomyelia and cervical cord tumors. The most commonly involved sensory findings below the lesion are loss of pain, temperature, and proprioception.

Autonomic dysfunction may be seen in transverse spinal cord lesions in the cervical spinal cord at any level. This may be manifested by a Horner's syndrome, a loss in sweating, vasodilatation, piloerection, and changes in skin temperature. There can be bowel and bladder dysfunction as well as loss of sexual potency.

Localization of Lesions

Transections of the Spinal Cord

Complete transection of the spinal cord may be associated with trauma or tumors or may have an inflammatory or vascular etiology (14). Functions above the lesion tend to be maintained, while those below are destroyed. When the onset is acute, "spinal shock" ensues. All motor and sensory functions are lost as well as autonomic functions. The paralysis initially is flaccid and is associated with areflexia and loss of all sensory and autonomic functions. After a period of time the lower extremities become spastic with hyperreflexia as well as the appearance of pathological reflexes (Hoffman, Babinski). There is no return of voluntary motor function. The bladder which initially is distended and atonic becomes spastic and small. Spinal reflexes become exaggerated. There are flexor spasms to noxious stimuli and occasional mass response to these stimuli with defecation and urination. The anal sphincter is patulous. The lower extremities are held in flexion. Although sensation is completely lost, the patient may at times experience bizarre and frequently painful sensation below the level of the lesion.

Incomplete lesions may be classified as central, hemisection, anterior, lateral, and posterior syndromes. Incomplete transections of the spinal cord are dependent on the area destroyed. With hemisection of the cord, Brown-Sequard syndrome, there is ipsilateral loss of motor function and proprioception, and contralateral loss of pain and temperature. There is spasticity and hyperreflexia with associated pathological reflexes ipsilaterally. Pain and temperatures are usually impaired one or two levels beneath the lesion. Hyperesthesia may also be seen below the level of the lesion. As an extramedullary lesion increases its size it too may produce a Brown-Sequard syndrome with contralateral loss of pain and temperature and ipsilateral loss of proprioception. At the level of the lesion there is loss of pain and temperature sensation. Pain and temperature sensation loss is prominent in the saddle area with an extramedullary lesion. Ipsilaterally there may also be seen vasomotor paralysis below the level of the lesion.

There are two syndromes associated with acute severe hyperextension injuries of the neck (15). Fractures or subluxations most frequently involve the fifth and sixth cervical vertebral bodies. The first of these is the syndrome of "acute anterior spinal cord injury." It results from compression of the anterior spinal cord or anterior spinal artery. It can be caused by a bony fragment, a herniated disc, or by actual destruction of the vertebral body. The syndrome is characterized by immediate loss of motor function with hypesthesia and hypalgesia from the level of the lesion down, with preservation of position, vibration, and touch sensation. The second syndrome is the syndrome of "acute central cervical spinal cord injury." This may be due to contusion of the cord or compromise of the vasculature of the vertebral arterial blood supply to the cervical spinal cord (6). Here there is disproportionately more motor impairment of the upper than the lower extremities. There is urinary retention and lesser degrees of sensory loss. This syndrome acutely consists of immediate complete paralysis of the extremities with hypesthesia and hypalgesia to the level of the lesion, with preservation of motion, position, and vibratory sensation below. Recovery returns first in the legs, then the arms, and finally the hands.

Extra/Intra Medullary Lesions

Extramedullary and intramedullary lesions of the cervical spinal cord, usually from tumors, may be differentiated by the syndromes they produce (5). Spontaneous pain is characteristic of extramedullary lesions. The pain is an early symptom and radicular in distribution. It is sharp rather than burning. It is made worse with coughing or sneezing and by movement. Extramedullary lesions produce early pyramidal tract changes with increased reflexes and upgoing toes. Spastic paresis occurs early and is more marked distally. Lower motor neuron involvement is segmental with extramedullary lesions but is seen early in intramedullary lesion (tumors and syringomyelia) and is diffuse. Lower motor neuron lesions are characterized by decreased tone, fasciculations, and atrophy.

Cervical intramedullarly lesions, in contrast, rarely have pain early. When pain occurs it is poorly localized and burning in nature. There is spastic paresis of late onset in the lower limbs and early onset of flaccid paresis in the upper limbs. There is prominent atrophy of the muscles of the upper limbs as well as fasciculations. Muscle stretch reflexes are depressed early in the upper limbs, and there is late hyperactivity in the lower limbs. The Babinski sign is a late feature. Root pain is usually absent as is local vertebral pain. Intramedullary lesions cause incomplete and patchy sensory syndromes. There is a dissociated sensory loss, which is maximal at the level of the lesion. There is dissociation of the loss of pain and temperature sensations on the contralateral side and the loss of proprioception on the ipsilateral side. This occurs because the fibers for pain and temperature cross at that level in the spinal cord, while those of proprioception cross higher. By contrast, the loss of pain and temperature sensation is most marked at the level of the lesion with intramedullary lesions. Skin trophic changes are present. There is early incontinence.

CLASSIC LESIONS OF THE CERVICAL REGION

Tabes (tertiary lues) is representative of a posterior column syndrome. This syndrome may also result from trauma. In tabes there is degeneration of the posterior columns. There is loss of position and vibratory sense in the feet. There is loss of reflexes in the legs. Lightning (lancinating) pains are present in the legs. Ataxia, pupillary abnomalities, and bladder and bowel dysfunction are commonly seen in tabes. Tabes is classically treated with penicillin. The degree to which function returns depends upon the level of dysfunction at the time of the initiation of treatment and physical therapy.

Dorsolateral syndromes are seen in Friedreich's ataxia and subacute combined degeneration [B12 deficiency]. Less frequently these findings are associated with an extradural tumor. Lateral cord syndromes seen in cervical spondylosis are usually from anterolateral lesions. Corticospinal findings predominate with lack of sensory findings present. Poliomyelitis presents as an anterior cord syndrome with involvement of the anterior horn cells. There are lower motor neuron findings (flaccidity, atrophy, fasciculations, areflexia in the upper extremities) and upper motor neuron findings (hyperreflexia and spasticity in the lower extremities). Abdominal, cremasteric, and tendon reflexes are diminished or lost. Sensation is practically never involved.

Amyotrophic lateral sclerosis (3, 11, 17) involves both the anterior horns and lateral columns. There is atrophy initially of the hands with hyperreflexia and no sensory findings. Fasciculations are seen. Involvement of the lower extremities occurs late in the disease. There is involvement of the bulbar musculature as well as of the trunk. Corticospinal tract signs are present. The weakness is symmetrical. There is difficulty in swallowing. There is atrophy and weakness of the tongue. Electromyography can distinguish it from cervical spondylosis by the involvement of the tongue. The lack of sensory findings distinguishes it from syringomyelia and spinal cord tumors.

Syringomyelia (4, 10) consists of gliosis and cavitation of the spinal cord. The cavity is usually centrally located dorsally in the gray matter. It tends to extend posteriorly and laterally involving the lateral and posterior columns. It produces a dissociative sensory loss with loss of pain and temperature but preservation of light touch, vibration, and position sense. There are associated hypesthesias. There is involvement of the central sympathetic connections. With anterior spread there is pyramidal tract involvement with spasticity and paralysis below the lesion. A central cord syndrome may result from syringomyelia or intramedullary gliomas. The cavity or tumor lies paracentrally. There are both motor and sensory changes. With anterior horn cell changes there are atrophy and weakness of the hands initially followed by loss of muscle mass and function in the forearm, arm, and shoulder. There are associated fasciculations. The sensory loss is dissociated with interruption of the decussating pain and temperature fibers. There is a capelike loss to pinprick. Involvement of the corticospinal tracts produces upper motor neuron signs including spasticity, hyperreflexia, Babinski signs, and a neurogenic bladder. Involvement of the dorsal columns produces loss of vibratory sensation and proprioception. There is decreased pinprick below the level of the lesion. Trophic changes of the hands are seen. If the lesion involves C8 and T1, a Horner's syndrome will be present.

Cervical spondylosis (2, 7, 8, 16, 18) may present with both spinal cord and cervical nerve root involvement. Compression of the spinal cord occurs posteriorly with loss of posterior column functions (position and vibratory sensation) followed by an increase in reflexes in the lower extremities. Motor deficits include spasticity and weakness in the lower extremities. When there is involvement of spinal roots at the cervical level, radicular and lower motor neurons are present. These consist of weakness, decreased tone, fasciculations and decreased reflexes in the upper extremities. Cervical spondylosis may also give false localizing signs by presenting with a posterior cord syndrome with vibratory and proprioceptive losses in the feet.

Combined systems disease is seen in vitamin B12 deficiency (9, 12), although the onset of neurological symptomatology may occur before the presence of anemia. There is symmetrical involvement of both the dorsal and lateral columns of the spinal cord. Vibratory and position sense may be diminished in the lower extremities. Weakness in the lower extremities is associated with spasticity and pathologic reflexes. The patient's gait is ataxic. There are associated mental changes and visual impairment. Treatment consists of weekly injections of vitamin B12 for 1 to 2 months and then monthly. The anemia responds in a few weeks, but the neurological deficit takes months to recover.

CONCLUSION AND TREATMENT

Lesions of the cervical spinal cord can be secondary to intrinsic or extrinsic involvement of the spinal cord. Correlating the patient's history with his clinical neurologic examination will help us to define the level and location of the lesion. Protein, sugar, cell, and serologic studies of cerebrospinal fluid as well as cytologic evaluation may prove invaluable. Utilizing pre- and post-contrast magnetic resonance imaging, computerized axial tomography, and myelography with post contrast computerized axial tomography will further aid us in visualizing these lesions so that appropriate treatment can be initiated (1, 13).

REFERENCES

1. Adams RD, Victor M, eds. Principles of neurology. 4th ed. New York: McGraw Hill, 1989.

2. Brain WR, Northfield D, Wilkenson M. The neurological manifestations of cervical spondylosis. Brain 1952;75:187–225.

3. Friedman AP, Freedman D. Amyotrophic lateral sclerosis. J Nerv Ment Dis 1950;111:1–18.

4. Gardner WJ, Angel J. The mechanism of syringomyelia and its surgical correction. Clin Neurosurg 1958;6:131–140.

5. Gilbert RW, Kim JH, Posner JB. Epidural spinal cord compression from metastatic tumor. Ann Neurol 1978;3:40–51.

6. Herrick M, Mills PE. Infarction of the spinal cord. Arch Neurol 1971;24:228–241.

7. Hughes JT, Brownell B. Cervical spondylosis complicated by anterior spinal artery thrombosis. Neurology 1964;14:1073–1077.

8. Kahn EA. The role of the dentate ligaments in spinal cord compression and the syndrome of lateral sclerosis. J Neurosurg 1947;4:191–199.

9. Lindenbaum J, Healton EB, Savage DG, et al. Neuropsychiatric disorders caused by cobalamine deficiency in the absence of anemia or macrocytosis. New Engl J Med 1988;318:1720–1728.

10. Logue V, Edwards MR. Syringomyelia and its surgical treatment—analysis of 75 cases. J Neurol Neurosurg Psychiatry 1981;44:273–284.

11. Munsat TL, Andres PL, Finson L, Conlon T, Thiobeau L. The natural history of motorneuron loss in amyotrophic lateral sclerosis. Neurology 1988;38:409–413.

12. Robertson DM, Dinsdale HB, Campbell RJ. Subacute combined degeneration of the spinal cord. Arch Neurol 1971:24:203–209.

13. Rowland L. Merritt's textbook of neurology. Philadelphia: Lea and Febiger, 1989.

14. Satran R. Spinal cord infarction. Stroke 1988;19:529–532.

15. Schneider RC, Cherry G, Pantek H. The syndrome of acute central cervical spinal cord injury with special reference to the mechanisms involved in hyperextension injuries of the cervical spine. J Neurosurg 1954;11:546–577.

16. Spillane JD, Lloyd GHT. The diagnosis of lesions of the spinal cord in association with "osteoarthritic" disease of the cervical spine. Brain 1952;75:177.

17. Tandan R, Bradley WG. Amyotrophic lateral sclerosis: etiopathogenesis. Ann Neurol 1985;18(pt 2):419–431.

18. Yu YL, Woo E, Huang CY. Cervical spondylotic myelopathy and radiculopathy. Acta Neurol Scand 1987;75:367–373.

5

Clinical Neurophysiology: Diagnostic and Monitoring Applications in Cervical Spine Disease

William A. Friedman

Introduction

Surgical diseases of the cervical spine frequently compress the nerve roots or spinal cord. When they do, a variety of neurological syndromes may result. A number of neurophysiological tests have been developed which may, in appropriate cases, be of great aid in reaching the correct diagnosis. Furthermore, they may help exclude neurological diseases which are not surgically correctable.

The purpose of this chapter is to introduce the reader to the following neurophysiological tests: electromyogram (EMG), nerve conduction velocity (NCV), H-reflex, F wave, and somatosensory evoked potential (SEP). The basic physiological and anatomical principles underlying these tests will be reviewed. Specific examples of diagnostic applications and monitoring applications will be presented.

Methods

Cellular Neurophysiology

All neurons have a resting membrane potential (1). That is, if one inserts a measuring electrode through the cell membrane and inside the cell, the electrical potential will be approximately −70 millivolts (mV) compared to the extracellular environment. This resting potential depends on basic principles of physical chemistry. The predominant intracellular ions are potassium and impermeable anions (negatively charged ions). The predominant extracellular ions are sodium and chloride (Fig. 5.1). The resting cell membrane is much more permeable to potassium than sodium. In resting conditions, potassium ions tend to diffuse down the concentration gradient, from intracellular to extracellular. This loss of positive ions (cations) renders the interior of the cell relatively more negative than the exterior. The magnitude of the electrical potential required to prevent further diffusion of ions (the equilibrium potential) is related to the concentration gradient via the Nernst equation. In the resting state, only potassium approaches its equilibrium potential, because the membrane is relatively impermeable to the other important ions. The resting cell potential, therefore, is primarily determined by the potassium concentration gradient.

Neurons transmit information via electrical currents. These currents are generated by changes in the permeability of the cell membrane to the various ions. For example, an excitatory postsynaptic potential (EPSP) is a depolarization of the cell towards less negative interior values, thought to result from increased permeability of the membrane to sodium, potassium, and chloride. An inhibitory postsynaptic potential (IPSP) is a hyperpolarization of the cell towards more negative interior values thought to be primarily related to increases in chloride permeability. These

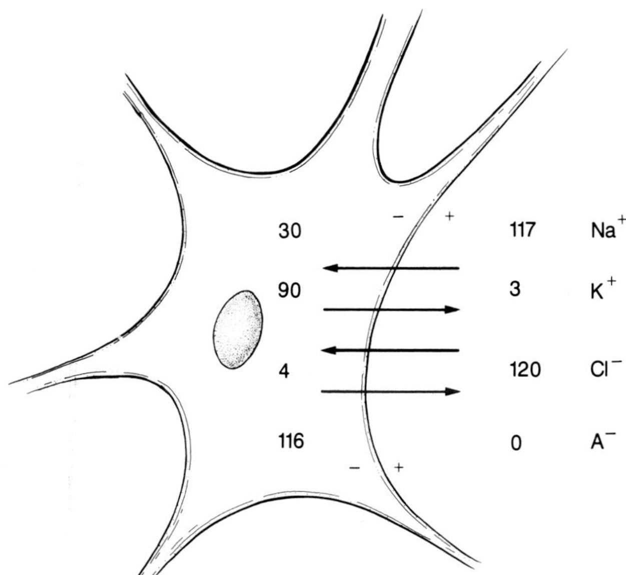

Figure 5.1. The predominant intracellular ions are potassium and negatively charged inorganic anions. The predominant extracellular ions are sodium and chloride. In its resting molecular configuration, the cell membrane is much more permeable to potassium than to the other ions. Potassium tends to diffuse down its concentration gradient until the resulting electrical difference (approximately −70mV) results in electrochemical equilibrium.

permeability changes are generated by the effects of synaptic neurotransmitters on the postsynaptic cell membranes. Because nerves are relatively poor conductors of electricity, EPSPs and IPSPs generally spread very short distances along the nerve.

If the sum of the EPSPs and IPSPs at the nerve cell body reaches a certain critical level of depolarization, a molecular change in the cell membrane leads to a great increase in sodium permeability. This results in the net flow of positive sodium ions into the cell, during which the interior of the cell actually becomes positive (Fig. 5.2). This event, called an action potential, leads to electrotonic currents and self-propagation of the action potential, all the way to the next synapse. Such action potentials give rise to currents which are externally recordable. The classic experiments on volume conduction of these potentials were performed by Lorente de No (22) and are displayed in Figure 5.3. This volume conductor theory nicely predicts the triphasic shape of certain somatosensory evoked potentials, H-reflexes, F waves, and EMG findings (fasciculations and fibrillations). It also predicts the biphasic shape of the so-called "positive sharp waves" seen in an abnormal muscle when the recording EMG electrode damages the muscle fiber, preventing conduction of the action potential past the recording site (see below).

Electromyography (EMG)

Normally, resting muscle is electrically silent. The insertion of an EMG needle electrode mechanically stimulates the muscle fibers, causing a short burst of electrical activity, termed "normal insertional activity." When the muscle under examination is voluntarily contracted, a large number of motor units are eventually recruited, leading to vigorous electrical activity, termed the "interference pattern."

In the abnormal muscle, the following findings may be present: increased or decreased insertional activity, abnormal "spontaneous" activity, abnormalities in the shape of single motor units, and a decrease in the number or amplitude of motor units (4). Special note is usually made on the EMG report if these findings are present. Of particular value is the presence of fibrillations (the sponta-

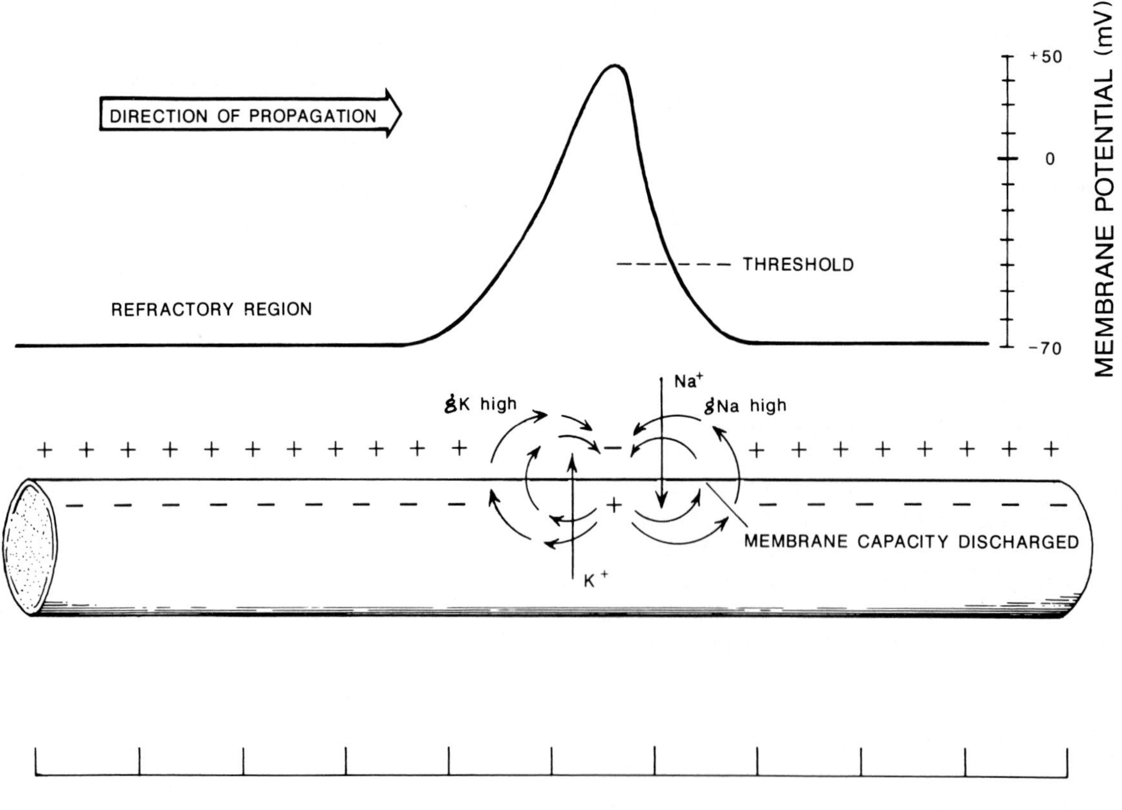

Figure 5.2. When the cell is electrically or chemically depolarized to approximately −60mV (threshold), the membrane changes its molecular configuration. It becomes much more permeable to sodium. As sodium flows down its concentration gradient, it brings positive charge into the cell. This event, called an action potential, generates electronic currents on its leading edge, which are of sufficient magnitude to bring the adjacent patch of cell membrane to threshold. Thus, the action potential is an "all-or-none" event, which self-propagates all the way down the nerve axon.

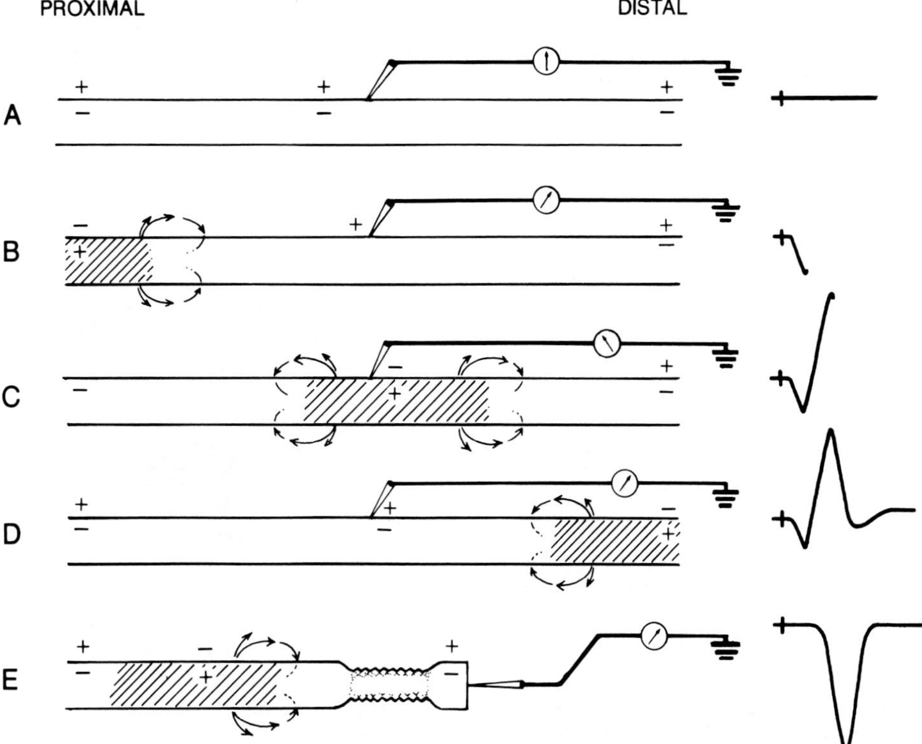

Figure 5.3. These classic diagrams successfully predict the shape of externally recorded neurophysiological events. **A**—At rest, the extracellular electrode records the same potential as the reference. This is 0 voltage, displayed as a straight line on the oscilloscope. **B**—As the action potential approaches the recording electrode, positive extracellular potential is generated, depicted here as a downward deflection on the oscilloscope. **C**—As the action potential reaches the recording electrode, negative extracellular potential is seen, leading to a downward deflection on the oscilloscope. **D**—As the action potential passes the electrode, the electrotonic currents on its trailing edge are recorded as positive extracellular potential (another upward deflection). **E**—If the nerve or muscle is injured, such that the action potential can approach, but cannot reach or pass the recording electrode, only the approach and disappearance of the leading electrotonic potential will be recorded (a biphasic potential). The triphasic recording (**D**) is typically seen in sensory nerve conduction velocity studies, peripheral SEPs, or the abnormal EMG activity called fibrillation and fasciculation. A "positive sharp wave" is a typical biphasic potential.

neous contraction of single muscle fibers) or fasciculations (spontaneous contraction of an entire motor unit, that is, all muscle fibers innervated by one motor neuron). Positive sharp waves are probably fibrillations arising from fibers which have been damaged by the recording electrode (Fig. 5.4). Fasciculations, fibrillations, and positive sharp waves are frequently found in an EMG examination of denervated muscle.

By studying these findings and making note of the pattern of muscles involved, a skilled electromyographer can often localize neurologic disease to the nerve root (8), brachial plexus, peripheral nerve, motor neuron, neuromuscular junction, or muscular level. Of all the neurophysiologic tests, the EMG remains the most valuable diagnostic aid. More recently, the EMG has been increasingly utilized as an intraoperative monitor of nerve root function, especially during selective dorsal rhizotomy for spasticity. In this application, the surgeon dissects and stimulates single dorsal rootlets. Those which produce intense EMG activity

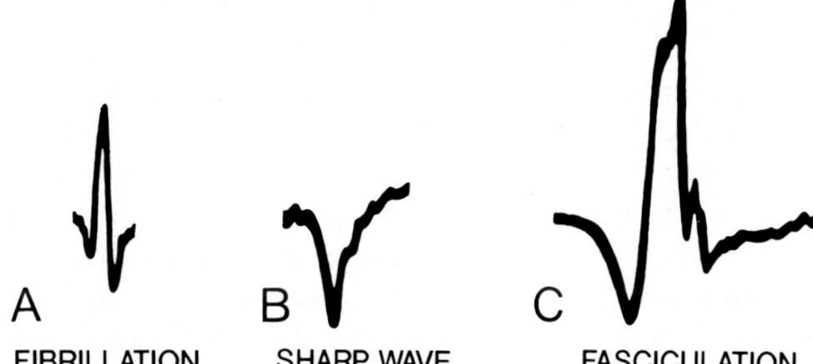

Figure 5.4. Abnormal spontaneous muscular electrical activity often signifies denervation. **A**—Fibrillations are the spontaneous discharge of single muscle fibers. **B**—Positive sharp waves are probably biphasic fibrillations recorded from muscle fibers damaged by the recording electrode. **C**—Fasciculations are the spontaneous discharge of all the muscle fibers innervated by a single motoneuron (a motor unit).

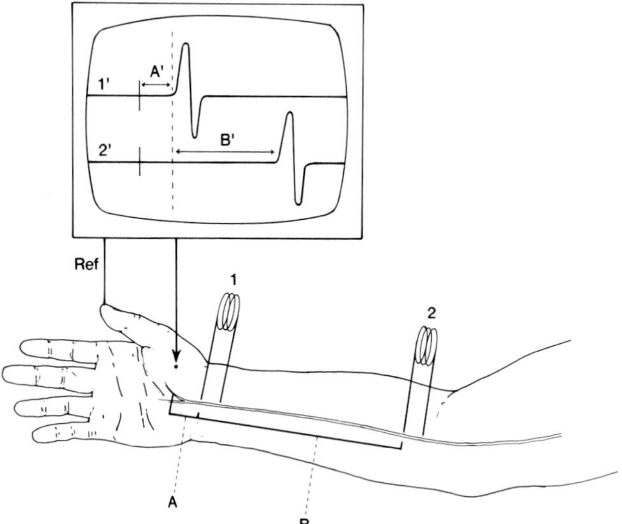

Figure 5.5. A motor nerve conduction velocity is recorded by stimulating the nerve transcutaneously and recording the resultant compound action potential distally. The stimulating electrode is moved from proximal to distal locations. If the distances between the sites of stimulation are known and the "latency" between stimulus and response is recorded, the nerve conduction velocity between the two sites of stimulation can be calculated as follows: Nerve conduction velocity (meters/second) = B − A (cm) / B′ − A′ (msec). The conduction time (not velocity) from the most distal stimulating site to the recording site is called the "distal latency." Each electrophysiology lab determines normal values for NCV and distal latency.

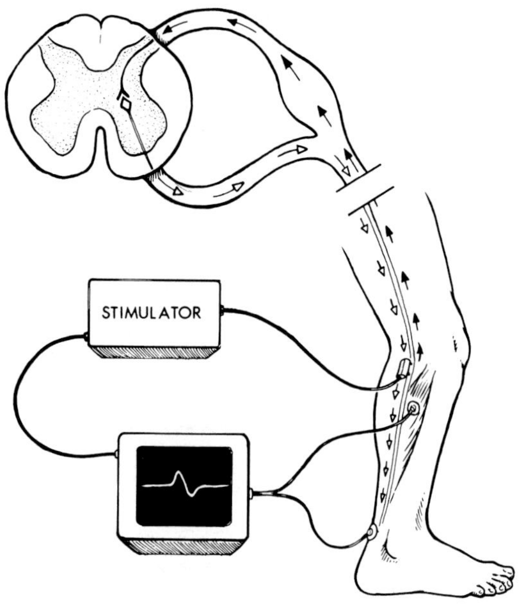

Figure 5.6. The H-reflex is generated by stimulating the posterior tibial nerve. The orthodromic response travels into the dorsal nerve roots and makes a monosynaptic connection with soleus-gastrocnemius motoneurons. The descending motor response is recorded over the soleus muscle.

are sectioned selectively, leading to reduced spasticity with preserved cutaneous sensation.

Nerve Conduction Velocity (NCV)

An accessible nerve is stimulated through the skin by surface electrodes, and the resulting action potential recorded (Fig. 5.5). The conduction time from the most distal stimulating electrode, measured in milliseconds, from the stimulus artifact to the onset of the response, is termed the "distal latency." If a second stimulus is applied to a nerve more proximally, a new and longer conduction time can be measured. When the distance between the two sites of stimulation is divided by the difference in conduction time, a conduction velocity is obtained. These velocities vary from 40–80 m/sec, depending on the nerve examined. Normal values have been established for distal latencies and conduction velocities. For example, the distal latency for conduction through the carpal tunnel to the abductor pollicis brevis is normally less than 4.5 msec. An increased latency is typically found in carpal tunnel syndrome.

In addition to conduction velocity, the amplitude of the muscle or nerve action potentials can be examined. These amplitudes are often more sensitive than conduction velocities in detecting disorders that cause axonal loss. This is true for typical alcoholic, nutritional, carcinomatous,

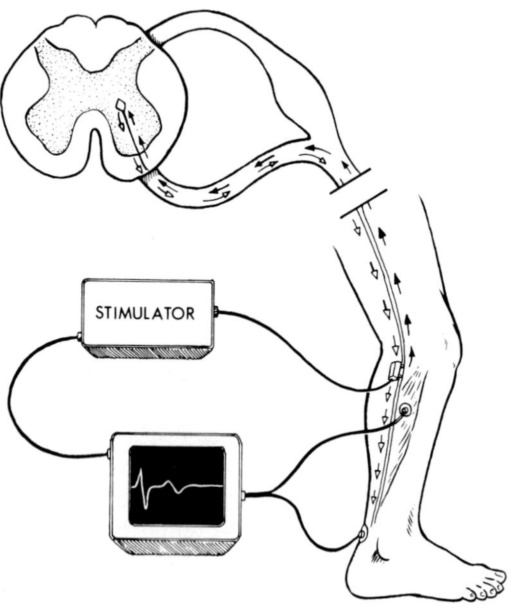

Figure 5.7. The F wave is generated by stimulating a mixed peripheral nerve. An antidromic action potential travels up the motor axons, through the ventral roots, and brings a small percentage of the motorneuronal pool to threshold. The resultant descending motor action potential is recorded.

uremic, and other metabolic neuropathies. In contrast, neuropathies of the Guillain-Barré type and those associated with diphtheria, Charcot-Marie-Tooth disease, Krabbe's disease, or focal nerve injury or compression, affect Schwann cells or myelin primarily and produce slow conduction velocities or complete conduction block.

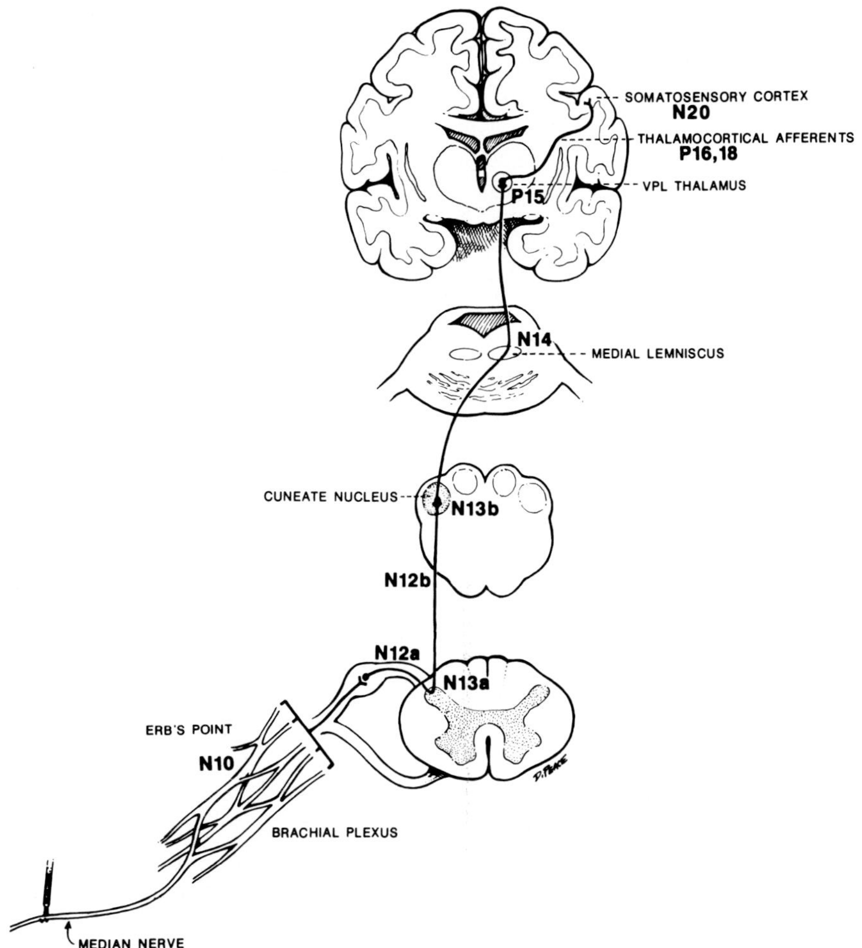

Figure 5.8. Putative sites of generation of the commonly observed components of the median nerve somatosensory evoked potential.

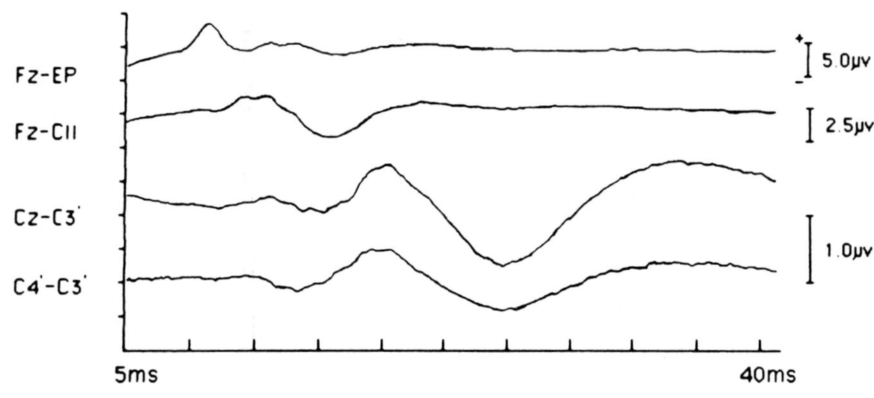

Figure 5.9. Four channels of information are recorded after median nerve stimulation. Fz, CII, Erb's, C3, etc. refer to different recording electrode locations. A combination of two recording electrodes is called a "montage." The top montage (Fz-Erb's) shows the response recorded over the brachial plexus. This verifies that the stimulus has entered the nervous system. The Fz-CII montage shows the response recorded over the cervical spine. This response is typically much more resistant to anesthesia than the cortical potentials. The bottom two traces display two different recording montages for scalp recorded cortical potentials.

Late Responses (H-Reflex and F Wave)

In 1918, Paul Hoffmann demonstrated that a submaximal electrical stimulus delivered to lower extremity nerves produced a late electrical response similar in latency to the compound muscle action potential associated with ankle reflexes (3). Subsequent investigators confirmed his findings and coined the term, H (Hoffman)-reflex. To record H-reflexes, the posterior tibial nerve is stimulated with a surface electrode in the popliteal fossa (Fig. 5.6). This stimulus electrically activates the same sensory nerve fibers which subserve the ankle reflex. They synapse directly with motoneurons innervating the soleus-gastrocnemius muscle complex. A small number of motoneurons are brought to threshold for action potentials by this stimulus. The efferent impulse travels down the motor axons and generates

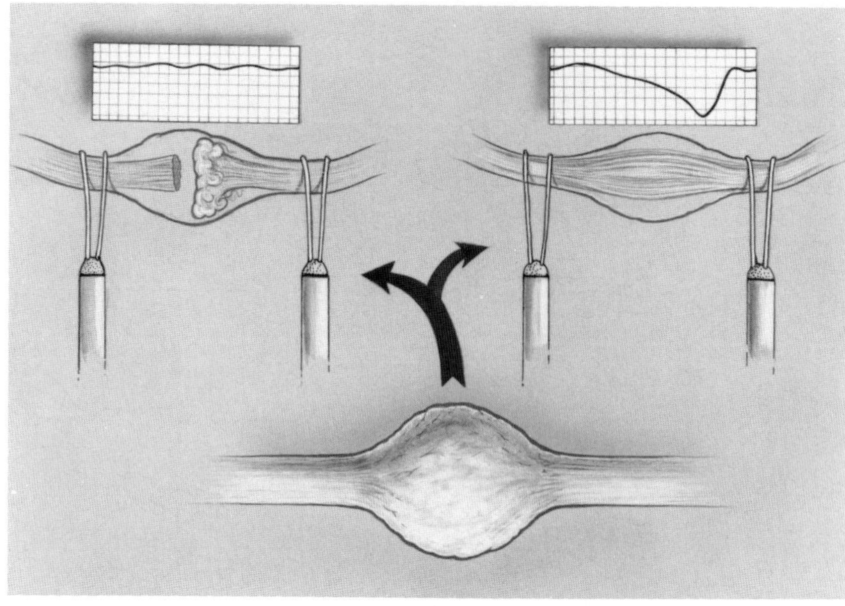

Figure 5.10. Nerve action potential testing can be used intraoperatively to distinguish axonotometic from neurotometic injuries. In the axonotometic situation (left), the connective tissue cylinders remain intact. The axons regrow at approximately 1 inch per month. If explored and tested 3 months postinjury, therefore, a nerve action potential should be recorded. In the neurotometic situation, internal scarring or complete disruption of the nerve prevents axonal regrowth, and no potential is recorded. This nerve will only recover if the neuroma is removed until viable fascicular anatomy is identified and the nerve reanastamosed or grafted.

a muscle action potential which can be recorded from the skin over the soleus muscle. In the adult, the H-reflex can only be recorded reliably from the soleus muscle.

Another type of late response that is not a reflex is the F wave, which can be easily recorded from most distal skeletal muscles. The afferent portion of this response is the antidromic action potential generated in motor axons by surface stimulation of a peripheral nerve (Fig. 5.7). The efferent portion of the pathway is the orthodromic discharge of the small number of the same axons brought to threshold by the stimulus. The resultant muscle action potential is recorded in or near a muscle innervated by that nerve.

Late responses have been used to evaluate peripheral neuropathies, entrapment neuropathies, and radiculopathies. When peripheral nerve conduction velocity (NCV) is normal, a prolonged F wave or H-reflex generally indicates disease of the proximal segment of the nerve or nerve root, an area difficult to evaluate by other electrophysiologic means. Thus, they may be of use in the diagnosis of diseases that involve the proximal nerves, such as disc herniation, thoracic outlet syndrome, and Guillain-Barré syndrome.

Somatosensory Evoked Potentials (SEPs)

The somatosensory evoked potential is typically generated by applying electrical stimuli to an extremity nerve (6). A square wave of .1–.2 msec is most commonly used, at an intensity sufficient to produce motor activity. This stimulus has been shown to preferentially activate the largest peripheral sensory nerve fibers (those mediating vibratory and proprioceptive sensation). The propagated nerve action potentials elicited by this electrical stimulation can be easily recorded more proximally over the peripheral nerve (i.e., Erb's point). Such a recording will show the triphasic shape predicted by volume conductor theory.

Over the lower cervical spine, two potentials are frequently recorded: N12a (meaning negative wave at 12 msec poststimulus), which is thought to correspond to postsynaptic dorsal horn interneuronal activity (Fig. 5.8). Similar potentials can be recorded over the upper cervical spine-lower medullary region, at slightly prolonged latencies corresponding to the spinal cord distance travelled. They are called N12b and N13b. Some labs refer to N12 waves as N11 waves. That these potentials are indeed locally generated within the segmental spinal cord or sensory relay nuclei is supported by the shift of N12 onset latency from lower to upper cervical spinal cord and by a phase reversal of the N13 component when recorded at prevertebral sites (esophageal leads).

Noncephalic referenced scalp recordings consistently reveal three widely distributed far-field positivities: P9, P11, and P14. The P9 potential corresponds to the afferent impulses recorded over the brachial plexus. The P11 potential corresponds to the cervical spinal cord potential. In lesions of the upper cervical spinal cord and medulla, the P9 and P11 potentials persist, but the P14 potential is absent. This supports the generally held view that P14 is a nonspinal component generated above the foramen magnum, perhaps in the medial lemniscus.

The afferent somatosensory fibers eventually terminate in layer IV of the somatosensory cortex (2). Multiple potentials can be recorded from the cortical surface (23). Scalp recorded cortical SEPs represent a combination of these various potentials. After median nerve stimulation, a cortical potential is typically recorded at about 19 msec poststimulus (Fig. 5.9). Of course, these latency values are highly dependent on the subject's age, limb length, and body height.

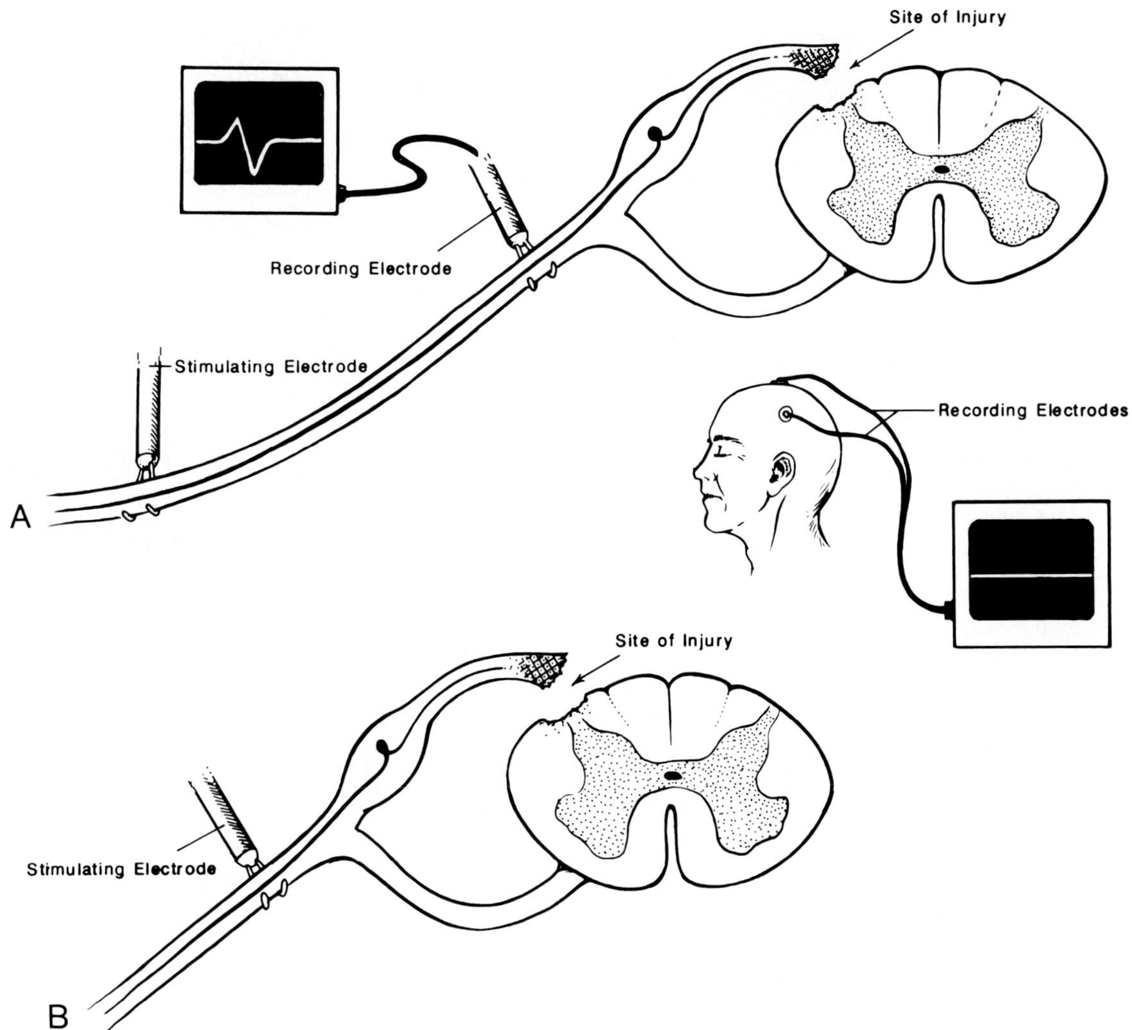

Figure 5.11. Electrophysiological testing can help distinguish preganglionic from postganglionic brachial plexus injuries. **A**—In a preganglionic injury, the nerve roots are generally avulsed from the spinal cord. Since the dorsal root ganglion cell remains in continuity with its distal axon, a peripheral somatosensory evoked potential can be recorded. No cortical response, however, is present. **B**—In a postganglionic injury, the dorsal root ganglion is no longer in continuity with the peripheral nerve. The sensory axon dies, and no peripheral SEP is recorded. Stimulation of the nerve root or trunk will, however, generate a cortical SEP.

Diagnostic Applications—Examples

A comprehensive review of the diagnostic applications of these electrophysiological techniques is beyond the scope of this chapter. Instead, a series of illustrative cases will be presented to reinforce their practical applications in neurosurgical and orthopaedic practice.

Case 1—Cervical Radiculopathy

Patient H.A. is a 45-year-old white male who awakened 3 weeks prior to presentation with right sided cervicobrachial pain. His family physician prescribed antiinflammatory agents and a cervical collar. Plain cervical spine radiographs were unremarkable. Failure of conservative therapy led to neurosurgical consultation. Examination revealed a negative Spurling's maneuver. Neurological findings include −1 right biceps, −2 right triceps, an absent right triceps reflex, and decreased pin sensation over the right middle and ring fingers.

The patient was sent for an electromyogram and a magnetic resonance scan. An EMG survey of the right arm revealed increased insertional activity, positive sharp waves, and fasciculations in the triceps muscle and right sided cervical paraspinous muscles. The EMG report was therefore consistent with C7 radiculopathy. The MRI suggested a disc herniation at C6–7, which was confirmed by myelography. A subsequent anterior cervical discectomy and fusion completely relieved the patient's symptoms.

Comment: In this typical application, the EMG was utilized as an electrophysiological confirmation of the primary clinical diagnosis. The presence of paraspinous denervation indicates involvement of the nerve root proximal to the takeoff of the paraspinous ramus, therefore excluding more distal diseases, such as brachial plexopathy. In cases where the clinical exam is less re-

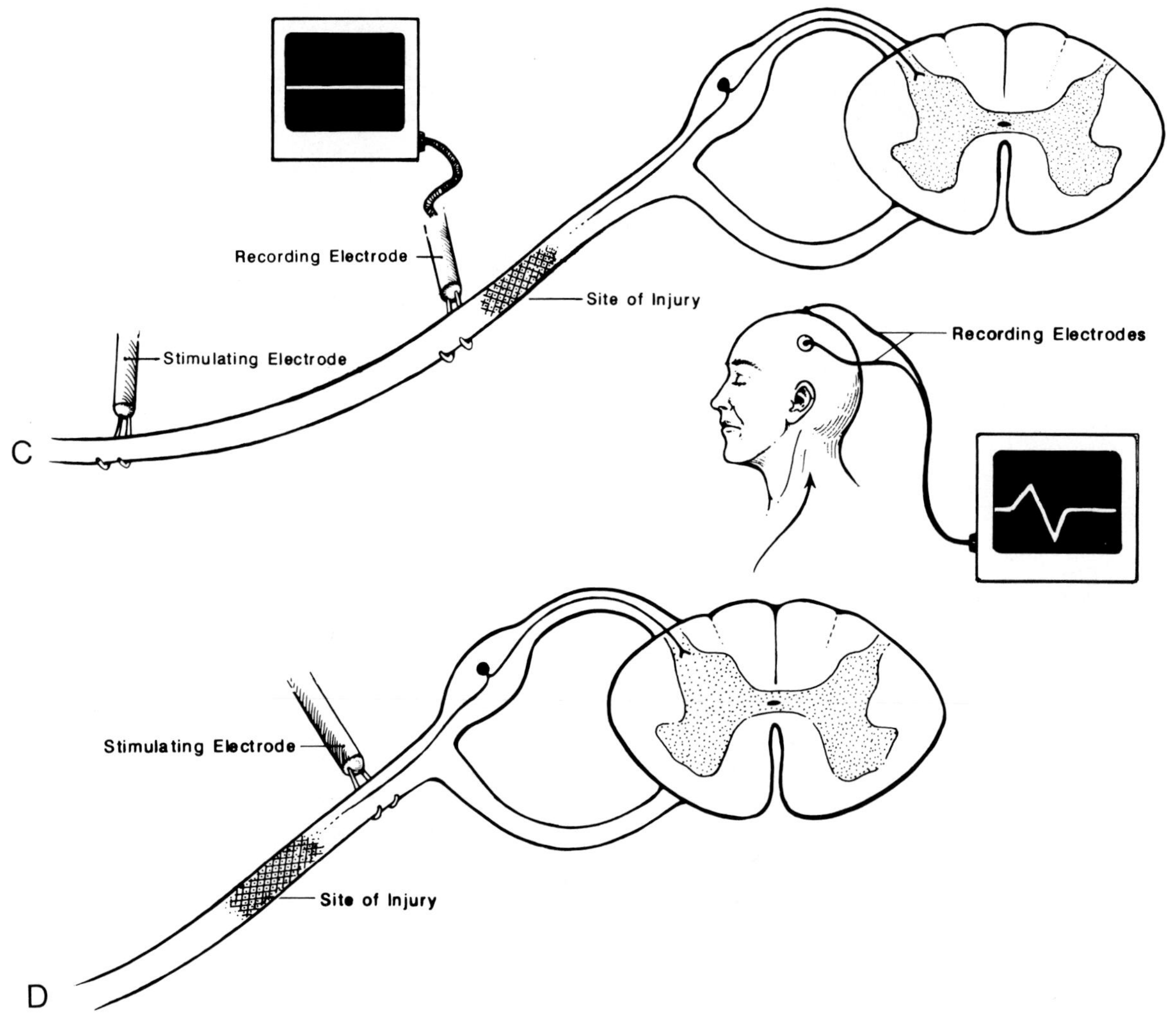

Figure 5.11. C–D.

vealing (as is frequently the case), the EMG data becomes much more important in establishing the diagnosis.

Case 2—Brachial Plexus Injury

Patient A.P. was involved in a motor vehicle accident, sustaining a closed head injury and a stretch injury to the brachial plexus. She made an uneventful and complete recovery from the head injury but, 3 months later, had no evidence of improved arm function. Clinical examination showed a flail, anesthetic right upper extremity. A Horner's syndrome was not present, and phrenic nerve function was normal. An EMG examination disclosed evidence of denervation in the deltoid, biceps, triceps, and hand intrinsic muscles. The rhomboid, serratus anterior, and paraspinous muscles were normal. No sensory nerve conduction velocity could be obtained from median nerve stimulation. A median nerve somatosensory evoked potential study revealed a normal Erb's point potential, but no cervical or cortical response. The patient subsequently underwent a myelogram, which revealed no evidence of nerve root avulsion.

Surgical exploration of the brachial plexus was undertaken. Areas of "neuroma in continuity" were identified in the medial, lateral, and posterior cords. Intraoperative nerve action potential and evoked potential studies disclosed intact trunk function but no conduction through the areas of neuroma formation (Fig. 5.10). The cords were incised until normal fascicular anatomy was identified, then reconstructed with sural nerve grafts. One year postop., partial function had returned to the deltoid, biceps, and triceps muscles.

Comment: Electrophysiological studies are very valuable in the assessment of brachial plexus injuries (18–21). Lack of denervation in the proximal muscles supported the presence of a postganglionic injury, amenable to surgical repair. The lack of a sensory NCV or cortical SEP are also consistent with this diagnosis (Fig. 5.11). Intraoperative SEPs are indispensable in distinguishing axonotometic from neurotmetic lesions, when confronted with a "neuroma-in-continuity."

Case 3—Cervical Spondylotic Myelopathy Versus Amyotrophic Lateral Sclerosis

Patient W.J. presented with a 6-month history of progressive weakness of the hands and arms. He also complained of "stiff" lower extremities, with clumsiness of gait. The neurological exam disclosed mild–moderate weakness of the hands and forearms. Fasciculations and atrophy were noted. Reflexes were increased in the arms and legs, with bilateral Babinski and Hoffmann signs. Sensory exam was normal. A total axis myelogram revealed a

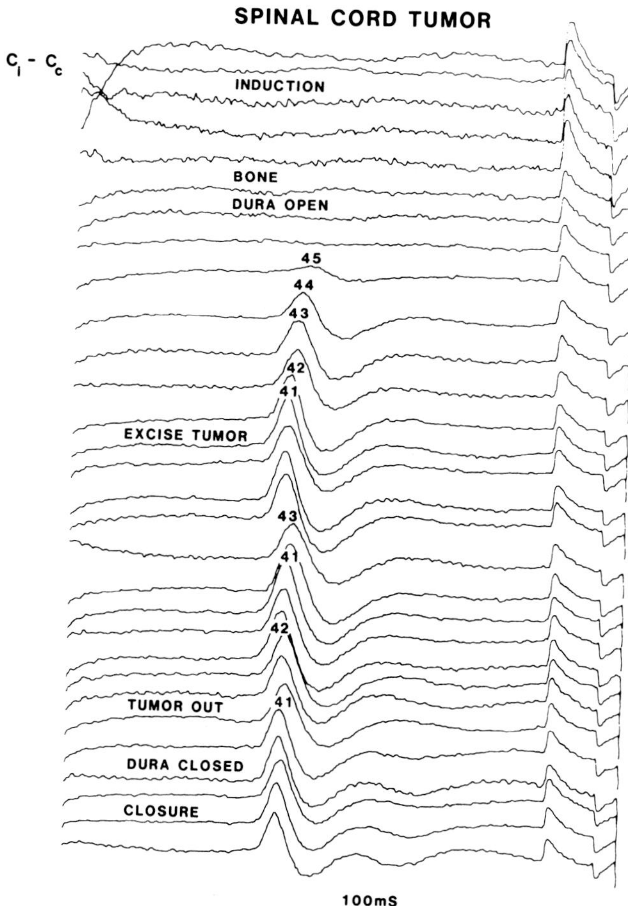

Figure 5.12. This SEP study shows no cortical potential at the beginning of surgery. At the time of pial incision, a good cortical SEP was identified. It remained present until the end of surgery. Postoperatively, the patient had improved sensation but was paraplegic. This study emphasizes this important point: in surgical situations where focal spinal cord injury is likely to occur, the SEP serves as a monitor of dorsal column function only.

normal lumbar spine and moderate spondylotic bars at C5–6 and C6–7.

An EMG was performed. Evidence of denervation was found in the deltoids, biceps, triceps, and hand intrinsics bilaterally. In addition, mild denervation was seen in the few leg muscles sampled. Surgery was not performed.

Comment: In this case, the EMG, by revealing a much more widespread pattern of denervation than was clinically obvious, strongly supported the diagnosis of ALS rather than cervical spondylotic myelopathy.

MONITORING APPLICATIONS

Of the electrophysiologic tests described above, only EMG and SEP have found consistent application as monitoring tools in the intensive care unit or operating room. EMG monitoring is primarily used during selective dorsal rhizotomy and cerebellopontine angle surgery. Selective dorsal rhizotomy is a procedure done for relief of spasticity in cerebral palsy (and other related conditions). The lumbar nerve roots are exposed and the dorsal rootlets individually dissected and stimulated. Multichannel EMG recordings are made from 8–16 lower extremity muscles. Those rootlets which, when stimulated, lead to an EMG response which is qualitatively or quantitatively abnormal, are severed. The remaining roots are preserved. Typically, the patient awakens with preserved cutaneous sensation but reduced spasticity.

Similar monitoring techniques are used to identify the facial nerve during acoustic neuroma surgery. The surgeon touches a stimulating electrode to the tumor capsule until an audible or visible EMG response indicates he has found the facial nerve. Continuous EMG monitoring of the facial muscles during tumor dissection will reveal spontaneous discharge if the nerve is overly manipulated during the procedure. This provides useful feedback to the surgeon and may increase the yield of normal facial function postoperatively. Similar monitoring of cervical or lumbar muscles during segmental surgery may be used to identify roots and reduce root trauma (although this is rarely done).

Four criteria must be satisfied if SEP monitoring is to be of value in the operating room (13, 15, 17). First, the neural pathways at risk must be amenable to monitoring. Second, personnel and equipment must be available for recording and interpreting the EPs correctly. Third, appropriate sites must be available for stimulation and recording. Fourth, the possibility of corrective intervention, if the EPs change, must exist. Failure to satisfy these basic criteria accounts for all of the so-called "false-negative" EPs thus far reported.

In this regard, it is vital to recognize that SEPs are a monitor of sensory pathways (mainly dorsal column) (16, 29). In situations where global spinal cord trauma may occur (such as scoliosis surgery, trauma surgery, etc.), the SEPs will predict both motor and sensory outcome. In situations where focal spinal cord trauma may occur (such as microsurgical dissection of an intramedullary spinal cord tumor), the SEPs will only accurately predict neurologic outcome in the sensory pathways. They may fail to predict motor deficit (10). An example is shown in Figure 5.12. The surgeon subtotally resected an intramedullary cervical cord astrocytoma. The SEP dramatically improved after pial incision and release of the intraspinal pressure. The surgeon, however, damaged the corticospinal tracts while removing tumor but left the dorsal columns intact. The patient awakened with improved sensation, as predicted, but was paraplegic! This is an absolute limitation of SEP monitoring which can only be overcome by developing a practical motor system monitor. Motor evoked potentials, through either magnetic brain stimulation or electrical stimulation of the brain or spinal cord, are in the process of development but, currently, remain experimental.

SEPs have also been monitored during surgery for spinal fractures, scoliosis, congenital or acquired anomalies of the atlanto-axial joints, and cervical spondylosis (24, 25, 27).

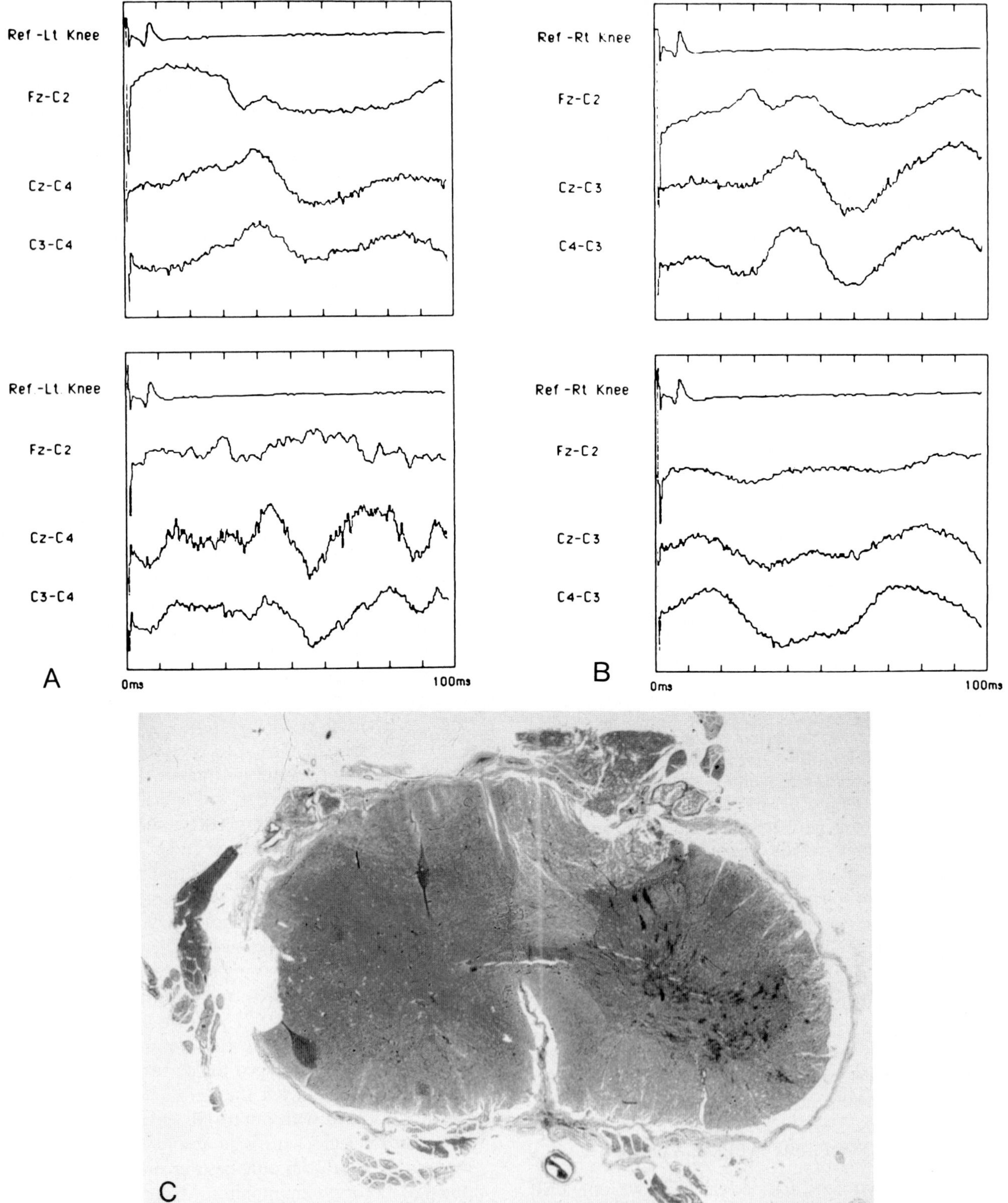

Figure 5.13. **A**—SEPs from left posterior tibial nerve stimulation are normal before and after instrumentation. **B**—SEPs from right posterior tibial nerve stimulation are normal before instrumentation. After instrumentation, only the peripheral potential, recorded at the knee, remains. **C**—Spinal cord pathology shows severe injury to the right hemicord.

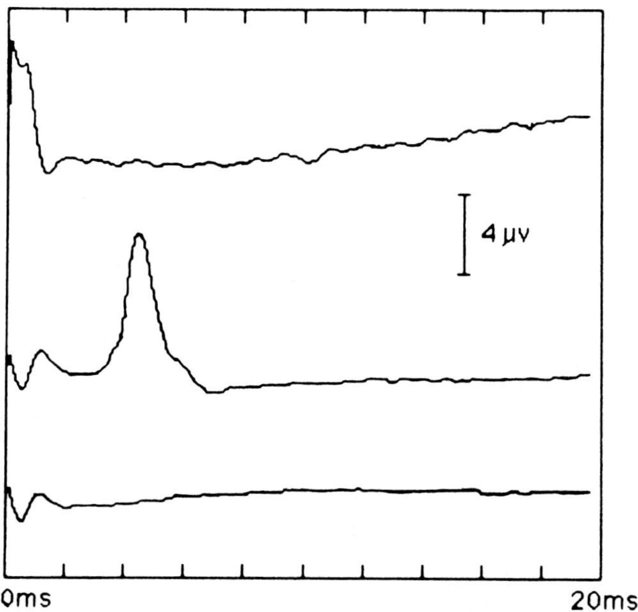

Figure 5.14. During this DREZL procedure for postherpetic neuralgia, a stimulating electrode was placed on the scarified skin area. Recordings were made from three dorsal roots, near the point where they entered the cord. The presence of a large nerve action from the middle root identified it definitively as that root innervating the involved skin area.

We have monitored over 100 cases of spinal trauma (11). Significant changes have been detected in two instances. In the first, the SEP disappeared for 5 minutes after passage of a Luque wire. It subsequently returned to normal, and the patient awakened without deficit. In the second case, the SEP disappeared from the right leg during spinal instrumentation. The SEP remained normal from the left leg (Fig. 5.13). Unfortunately, the patient suffered a myocardial infarction near the end of surgery, arrested, and could not be resuscitated. Though neurological exam was not possible, the spinal cord was obtained at autopsy. Pathology revealed acute hemorrhage and mechanical disruption of the right half of the cord, without significant damage to the left (14). No new neurological deficits were present in those patients without SEP changes.

SEPs have been used during dorsal root entry zone lesions (DREZL) (5, 9). They are helpful in two ways. First, they can be used to electrophysiologically confirm the precise area of the cord to be lesioned. Stimulating electrodes are positioned on the skin in the painful area or over the appropriate intercostal nerves (if the thoracic area is involved). The recording electrode is placed on the nerve root as it enters the cord. When the electrode is positioned on the correct root, a nerve action potential is recorded (Fig. 5.14). Second, the SEP from the ipsilateral lower extremity can be monitored while the dorsal root entry zone lesions are placed. Preservation of the SEP will allow one to confidently continue lesion-making without fear of significant lower extremity sensory proprioceptive loss. This was formerly the most commonly reported complication of DREZL.

We currently do not advocate SEP monitoring during routine anterior or posterior surgery for spondylosis. Individual nerve root function cannot be reliably monitored with SEPs. For example, median nerve SEPs travel via the C5–T1 nerve roots. Complete transection of one root, therefore, would not likely alter the SEP. Attempts to overcome this problem have included stimulation of multiple upper extremity nerves (i.e., ulnar, median, and radial) or dermatomal skin stimulation (7). None have demonstrated, in a statistically valid fashion, any value as a diagnostic or monitoring test for cervical radicular disease (26, 28). Although lower extremity SEPs may be used to monitor spinal cord function during surgery for cervical spondylotic myelopathy, we have found the incidence of neurologic complications too low to justify monitoring every case.

Whatever the clinical diagnosis, accurate intraoperative electrophysiological monitoring requires that the monitoring team be able to distinguish surgical trauma from metabolically induced changes. We have been able to accomplish this with a high degree of reliability by always recording SEPs from a "control" extremity (12). For example, when monitoring thoracic or lumbar spine surgery, posterior tibial nerve SEPs provide information about spinal cord function in the area of surgery. Median nerve SEPs, on the other hand, provide "control" information. They should only change if there is a technical problem, such as equipment malfunction, or a metabolic problem, such as increased levels of anesthetic, hypothermia, or hypotension. If the median nerve SEPs remain normal and the posterior tibial nerve SEPs disappear, one can confidently report a problem to the surgeon, so that he can undertake corrective measures. If the SEPs from the arm and leg change, a metabolic or technical problem is present and the surgeon needn't be bothered.

Conclusions

Neurophysiological tests currently used in the diagnosis and treatment of cervical spine disease include EMG, NCV, late responses, and SEPs. The physiological basis of these tests has been reviewed. Examples of typical diagnostic application have been provided. A brief review of EMG and SEP intraoperative monitoring has been presented. The interested reader is referred to the reference list for more detailed information.

References

1. Aidley DJ. The physiology of excitable cells. London: Cambridge University Press, 1978:7–71.

2. Allison T. Anatomical and physiological foundations of the SEP. In: Starr A, Nudleman K, eds. Sensory evoked potentials. Milan: Centro Richerche e Studi Amplifon, 1984:9–32.

3. Aminoff MJ. Electrodiagnosis in clinical neurology. New York: Churchill-Livingstone, 1980.

4. Basmajian JV. Muscles alive. 4th ed. Baltimore: Williams & Wilkins, 1979.

5. Campbell JA, Miles J. Evoked potentials as an aid to lesion making in the dorsal root entry zone. Neurosurgery 1984;15:951–952.

6. Dawson GD. Cerebral responses to electrical stimulation of peripheral nerve in man. J Neurol Neurosurg Psychiatry 1947;10:137–140.

7. Dvonch V, Scarff T, Bunch WH, et al. Dermatomal somatosensory evoked potentials: their use in lumbar radiculopathy. Spine 1984;9:291–293.

8. Eisen A. Electrodiagnosis of radiculopathies. Neurol Clin 1985;3:495–510.

9. Friedman AH, Nashold BS, Ovelmen-Levitt J. Dorsal root entry zone lesions for the treatment of post-herpetic neuralgia. J Neurosurg 1984;60:1258–1262.

10. Friedman WA. Somatosensory evoked potentials in neurosurgery. Clin Neurosurg 1988;34:187–238.

11. Friedman WA. Evoked potentials in neurosurgery. In: Youmans J, ed. Neurological surgery. Philadelphia: WB Saunders Co, 1990:1005–1032.

12. Friedman WA, Curran MT. Somatosensory evoked potentials after sequential extremity stimulation: a new method for improved monitoring accuracy. Neurosurgery 1987;21:755–758.

13. Friedman WA, Grundy BL. Are the sensory evoked potentials useful in the operating room. J Clin Monit 1987;3:38–45.

14. Friedman WA, Richards R. Somatosensory evoked potential monitoring accurately predicts hemi-spinal cord damage: a case report. Neurosurgery 1988;22:140–142.

15. Friedman WA, Theisen GJ, Grundy BL. Electrophysiologic monitoring of the nervous system. Adv Anes 1989;6:231–290.

16. Grundy BL, Nelson PB, Doyle E, et al. Intraoperative loss of somatosensory-evoked potentials predicts loss of spinal cord function. Anesthesiology 1982;57:321–322.

17. Grundy BL, Friedman W. Electrophysiological evaluation of the patient with acute spinal cord injury. Crit Care Clin 1987;3:519–548.

18. Jones SJ, Wynn-Parry CB, Landi A. Diagnosis of brachial plexus traction lesions by sensory nerve action potentials and somatosensory evoked potentials. Injury 1981;12:376–382.

19. Kaplan BJ, Friedman WA, Gravenstein D. Intraoperative electrophysiology in treatment of peripheral nerve injuries. J Fla Med Assoc 1984;71:400–403.

20. Kline DG, Judice DJ. Operative management of selectre brachial plexus lesions. J Neurosurg 1983;58:631–649.

21. Landi A, Copeland SA, Wynn-Parry CB, et al. The role of somatosensory evoked potentials and nerve conduction studies in the surgical management of brachial plexus injuries. J Bone Joint Surg 1980;4:492–496.

22. Lorente de No, R. Analysis of the distribution of action currents of nerve in volume conductors. Stud Rockefeller Inst Med Res 1947;132:384–477.

23. Luders H, Lesser RP, Hahn J, et al. Cortical somatosensory evoked potentials in response to hand stimulation. J Neurosurg 1983;58:885–894.

24. Mostegl A, Bauer R. The application of somatosensory-evoked potentials in orthopedic spine surgery. Arch Orthop Trauma Surg 1984;103:179–184.

25. Nuwer MR. Evoked potential monitoring in the operating room. New York: Raven Press, 1986.

26. Schmid UD, Hess CW, Ludin HP. Somatosensory evoked potentials following nerve and segmental stimulation do not confirm cervical radiculopathy with sensory deficit. J Neurol Neurosurg Psychiatry 1988;51:182–187.

27. Veilleux M, Daube JR, Cucchiara RF. Monitoring of cortical evoked potentials during surgical procedures on the cervical spine. Mayo Clin Proc 1987;62:256–264.

28. Veilleux M, Stevens JC, Campbell JK. Somatosensory evoked potentials: lack of value for diagnosis of thoracic outlet syndrome. Muscle Nerve 1988;11:571–575.

29. York DH. Somatosensory evoked potentials in man: differentiation of spinal pathways responsible for conduction from the forelimb vs hindlimb. Prog Neurobiol 1985;25:1–25.

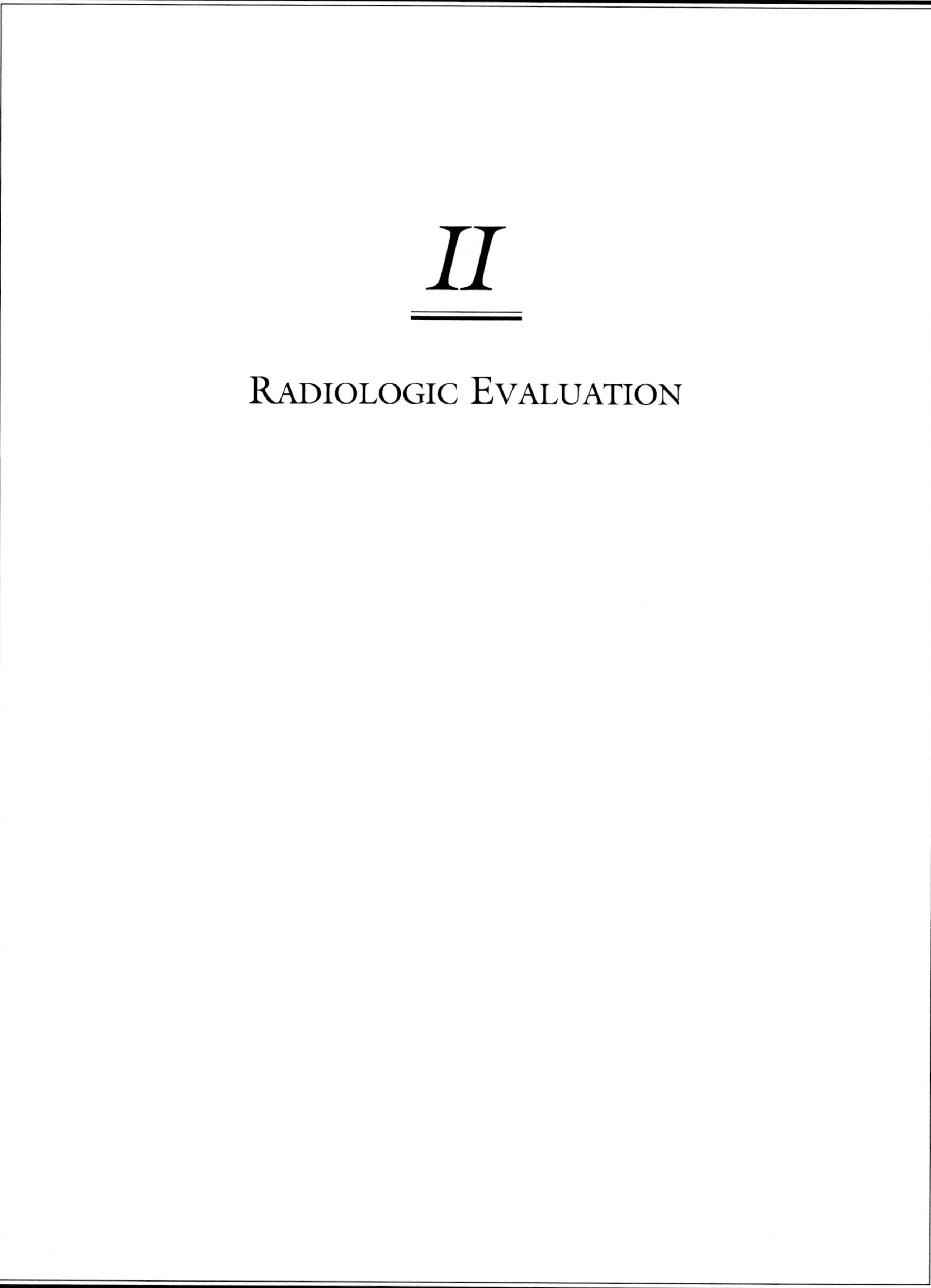

II

Radiologic Evaluation

6

Plain Radiographic Examination in Cervical Spine Trauma

John J. Wasenko and Charles F. Lanzieri

One of the most common complaints following a motor vehicle accident, fall or other trauma is pain referable to the cervical spine. The first physician to see such a patient in the emergency department will request neuroradiologic consultation based on one or more of several questions. Is there a fracture or other disruptive injury of the cervical spine? How is this injury threatening to the patient? Is this a litiginous setting? It falls upon the neuroradiologist to answer these questions in a safe, swift, and economical manner.

In spite of startling advances in neuroradiology within the past decade, the plain radiographic examination remains irreplaceable in these situations. A portable lateral view of the cervical spine can be obtained without moving the patient from the stretcher and without manipulating whatever fixation or intubation devices may be in use. Furthermore, this single film identifies or excludes more posttraumatic pathology than any other sophisticated and expensive test that is subsequently requested. Once this lateral radiograph has been interpreted, evaluation proceeds with the other standard views of the cervical spine and additional special projections at the discretion of the radiologist.

Any questions left unanswered by the plain radiographs are best pursued utilizing linear tomography, computed tomography (CT), and magnetic resonance imaging (MRI). These studies are best used to differentiate artifactual from real findings and to search for small fragments. We believe that linear tomography possesses several advantages over CT in these patients. Entire subunits of vertebrae such as a pedicle can be visualized compared to 2 or 3 mm of a structure on CT. It is far easier to identify a linear fracture through a pedicle when one sees the entire structure than when one sees a small part of it. Relationships of vertebrae to each other are better appreciated. Finally, linear tomography is usually easier to schedule, cheaper to perform, and can be done well in a less than cooperative patient.

The role of magnetic resonance imaging in cervical spine trauma remains unclear. It is certainly the best means of evaluating the neural axis and should probably be obtained in all patients with posttraumatic neurological complaints or deficits.

Normal Cervical Spine

Lateral View

The plain lateral radiograph of the cervical spine remains the single most important imaging study in the postcervical spine trauma patient. The initial examination may be done with the patient still immobilized on a stretcher in the emergency department and interpreted before manipulating or moving the patient for further studies. In this manner, a large percentage of unstable fractures may be identified early. One should insist on a complete lateral study that includes from the skull base to the body of C7. In addition to evaluating the bony structures, one must remember to notice the vertebral soft tissues for evidence of a hematoma, an indication of a fracture that may be occult on the lateral view. There are four imaginary lines which follow an uninterupted lordotic curve from the foramen magnum to the T1 vertebral body. These are the anterior spinal line formed by the anterior margins of the vertebral bodies, the posterior spinal line formed by the posterior margins, the spinolaminar line formed by the anterior cortical margin of the spinous process, and a line connecting the tips of the spinous processes (Fig 6.1).

With this gross examination completed one should proceed to a more detailed study of the film. The vertebral bodies are square in configuration and increase in height from C3 to C7. The intervertebral discs are equal in height throughout the cervical spine. The prevertebral tissues are useful in evaluating the patient with cervical spine injury. The width of the prevertebral soft tissue at the level of C3 is not greater than 7 mm in normal individuals (4). Measurement greater than 7 mm is suggestive of edema or hemorrhage secondary to injury. The apophyseal joints are formed by the articulating facets of the articular masses. The superior articulating facets of the vertebral body below are anterior and inferior to the inferior articulating facets

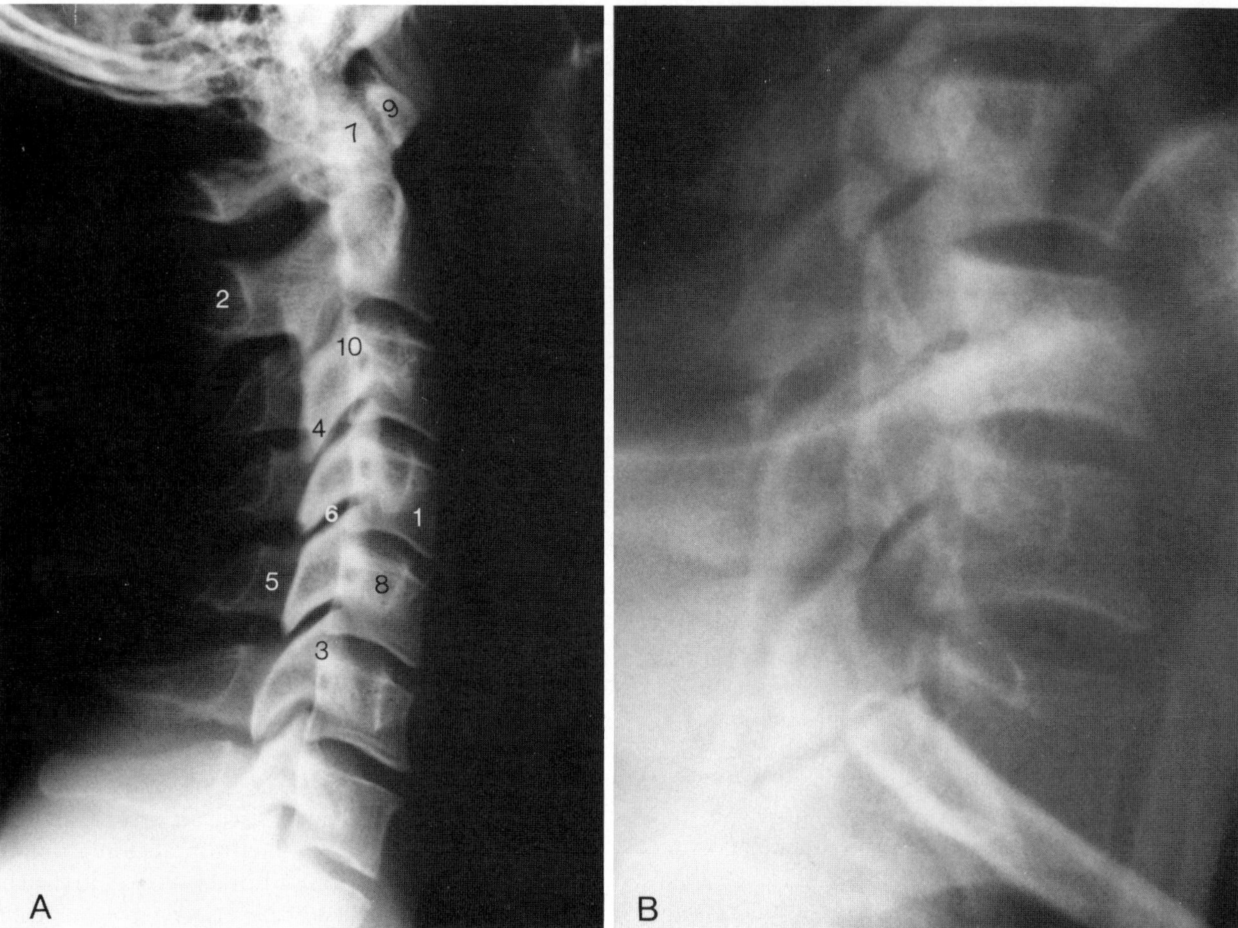

Figure 6.1. Normal lateral projection. **A,** is the initial examination that may be performed without moving the patient. Most of the significant lesions are perceptible in this projection. The cervical/thoracic junction can be seen by forceful inferior movemen of the shoulders or by the swimmer's view (**B**). (1, vertebral body; 2, spinous process; 3, ascending (superior) facet; 4, descending (inferior) facet; 5, lamina; 6, facet joint; 7, dens; 8, transverse foramen; 9, anterior arch of C1; 10, pedicle.)

of the vertebral body immediately above. The joint spaces, site of the capsular ligaments, are equal in height. The laminae are posterior to the lateral masses and unite posteromedially to form the spinous processes. The ligamentum flavum between adjacent laminae are equal in height as well as the interspinous distances, site of the interspinous ligaments. Several relationships are of value in the evaluation of the upper cervical spine. The distance between the anterior arch of C1 and the odontoid process is no greater than 2.5 mm in adults. A line drawn from the clivus should intersect the odontoid process at the junction of its anterior and middle thirds. The posterior margin of the foramen magnum and the spinolaminar line of C1 should be in alignment (2).

Anterior/Posterior Projection

If the portable lateral radiograph fails to demonstrate an unstable injury, then the patient may proceed to a complete radiographic examination including frontal and oblique.

The frontal or anteroposterior projection is performed in two parts because of the difference in attenuation between the infrahyoid and suprahyoid portions of the neck. In addition, if the suprahyoid cervical spine is studied through an opened mouth, an excellent view of the craniocervical junction can be obtained. After the lateral view, the A-P projection is the next important study to obtain.

The Normal A-P Projection

The vertebral bodies have a symmetrical rectangular appearance with a uniform texture. Subtle compression injuries may be identified only by the disruption and superimposition of trabeculae. Such injuries may even be less apparent on CT than plain film. The spinous processes appear as teardrop structures that align themselves in the midline and are regularly spaced. The lateral masses with their articulating apophyseal surfaces line up slightly lateral to the midline. Because the joint spaces are oblique to the central x-ray, the apophyseal joints are poorly seen in the A-P projection (Fig. 6.2).

On the other hand, the transoral or "open-mouth" view is the single most important projection for evaluation of C1 and C2. In this projection, the odontoid process is

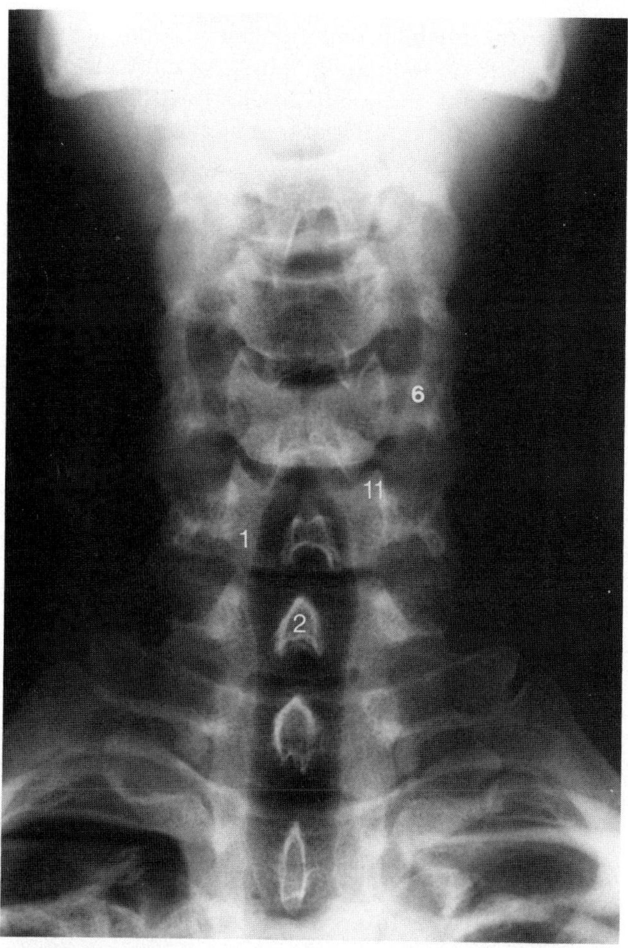

Figure 6.2. Normal frontal projection. This view is most useful as the next step in ruling out unilateral interlocked facets. If the spinous processes are aligned, then a unilateral interlocked facet joint is doubtful. (1, vertebral body; 2, spinous process; 6, facet joint; 11, uncinate process.)

located precisely equidistant from the lateral masses of C1. Strict interpretation of the view requires that no asymmetry is to be allowed between these spaces. Furthermore, the lateral cortical margins of the lateral masses of C1 must line up with the lateral masses of C2. Again, no unexplained asymmetry must be allowed. Any variation must be considered pathological until proven otherwise. There are, of course, normal variations in these relationships. Pseudosubluxation, for example, is seen in adolescent patients. This is characterized by lateral displacement of the lateral masses of C1. It thus mimics a Jefferson fracture and, in uninjured patients, is felt to be due to differences in growth between C1 and C2.

An open mouth view that is rotated is treacherous, because it is both easy to see asymmetry between C1 and C2 and difficult to tell that the film is, in fact, slightly oblique. Tilting or rotation of the head may also result in widening of the distance between the odontoid and the lateral mass of C1. Because of the atlas and the occiput move as a single unit, the margin of the lateral mass of C1 will be lateral to the lateral mass of C2 on the side of rotation (Fig. 6.3).

Oblique Projection

There are few injuries that are exclusively seen or even more apparent on the oblique view than in the lateral and A-P views. This projection best demonstrates the neural foramina, pedicles, laminae, articular masses, and facet joints. The articular mass of the vertebral body above is posterior and superior to the articular mass inferior to it. The laminae are projected over the articular masses as oval densities. This view is helpful for showing compression fractures of the lateral masses or oblique fractures through the neural arches (Fig. 6.4).

Figure 6.3. Open-mouth projection. This is the best way of evaluating the atlantoaxial articulation. It is also one of the more treacherous examinations to interpret because of the many anatomical variations. (1, vertebral body; 3, ascending (superior) facet; 4, descending (inferior) facet; 7, dens; 9, anterior arch of C1; 12, transverse foramen of C1; 13, posterior arch of C2; 14, superior articulating facet of C1.)

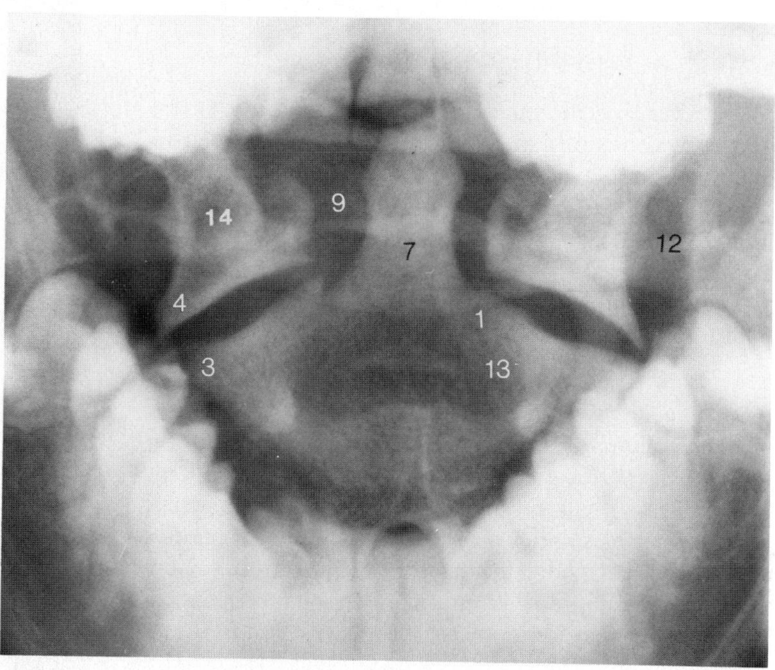

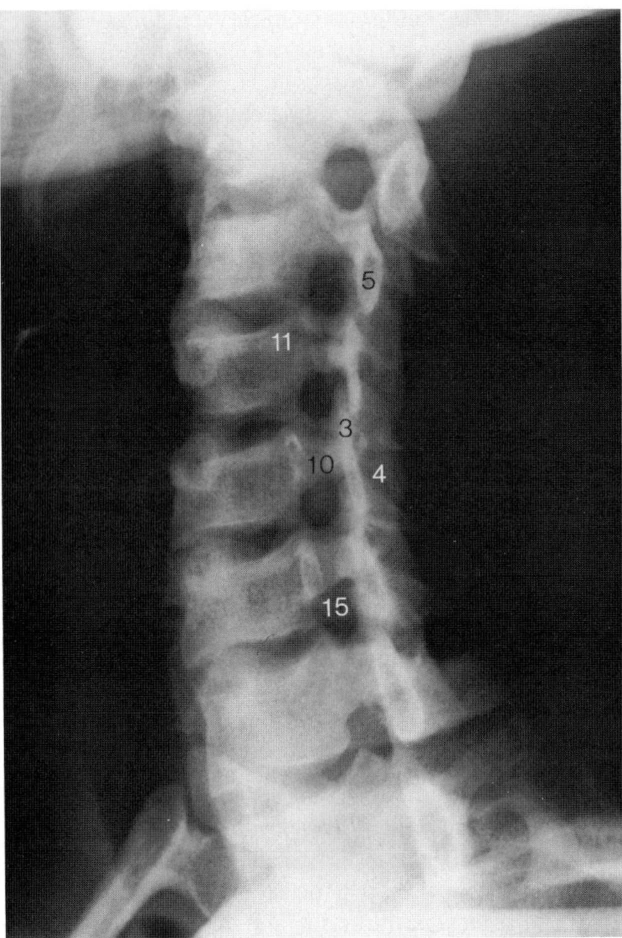

Figure 6.4. Oblique projection. A minority of traumatic lesions are seen exclusively on this view. It is the best projection for evaluating the neural foramina and, therefore, is quite useful in the posttreatment patient who complains of radiculopathy. (3, ascending (superior) facet; 4, descending (inferior) facet; 5, lamina; 10, pedicle; 11, uncinate process; 15, neural foramen.)

Pillar Projection

This is a very specific study designed to evaluate the lateral masses. It consists of an A-P projection angled caudad so that the central ray is parallel to the articulating facets. Its only role is to rule out compression fractures of the lateral masses (pillars) or to rule out extension of a linear fracture into a joint space.

THE ABNORMAL LATERAL PROJECTION

Flexion Injuries

These usually result from rapid forward deceleration or a blow to the vertex or occiput of the skull. The resultant lesions include avulsion injuries to elements of the neural arch such as the spinous process and compression injuries to the vertebral body such as a teardrop fracture. There are also a wide range of accompanying ligamentous injuries which, while beyond the scope of this chapter, contribute mightily to the instability of flexion injuries. Although they do not appear on the radiographs, one must remember that the ligaments and joint capsules hold the spine together and are of far greater importance to the stability of the spine than the osseous structures themselves.

Spinous Process Fracture

An avulsion fracture of the spinous process (clay shoveler's fracture) commonly involves the lower cervical spine. The C6 through T1 levels are usually involved, with C7 the most frequent site of injury. The lateral radiograph best demonstrates this stable fracture (5, 6) (Fig. 6.5).

Compression Fracture

Compression (wedge) fracture results in loss of height of the involved vertebral body anteriorly. The lateral radiograph reveals buckling of the anterior aspect of the cortex. A defect in the superior endplate of the vertebral body may also be seen (1).

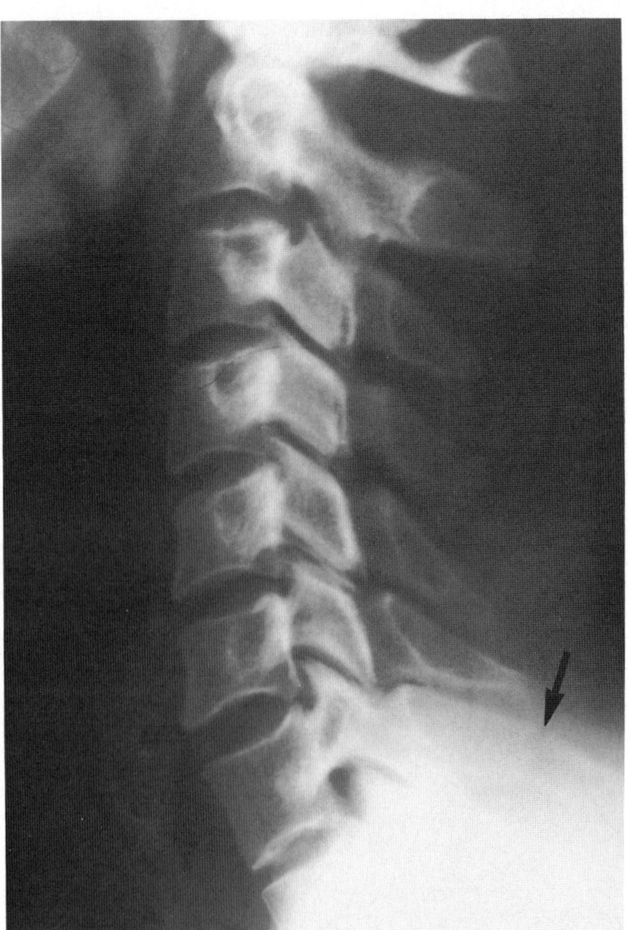

Figure 6.5. Clay shoveler's fracture. This very stable avulsion fracture of the spinous process of C7 (*arrow*) is due to heavy physical exertion rather than direct trauma.

Anterior Subluxation

Disruption of the posterior ligamentous complex results in anterior subluxation. Radiographic findings in this injury include: loss of the normal lordotic curve with kyphotic deformity at the level of injury, widening of the interspinous and interlaminar spaces, widening of the posterior aspect of the disc space, and anterior subluxation of the inferior articulating facet of the vertebral body above with respect to the superior articulating facet of the vertebral body below (7, 8). Flexion and extension views respectively exaggerate and reduce the degree of subluxation (Fig. 6.6).

Bilateral Facet Dislocation

Bilateral facet dislocation (bilateral locked facets) is characterized by disruption of the posterior ligamentous complex as well as the posterior and sometimes anterior spinal ligaments. The inferior articulating facets of the vertebral body above are dislocated anterior to the superior articulating facets of the vertebral body below. The facets lie within the neural foramina. Occasionally, the facets lie immediately above those of the body below resulting in a "perched" facet (3, 6). The vertebral body is displaced anteriorly greater than one-half the A-P diameter of a cervical vertebral body (6) (Fig. 6.7).

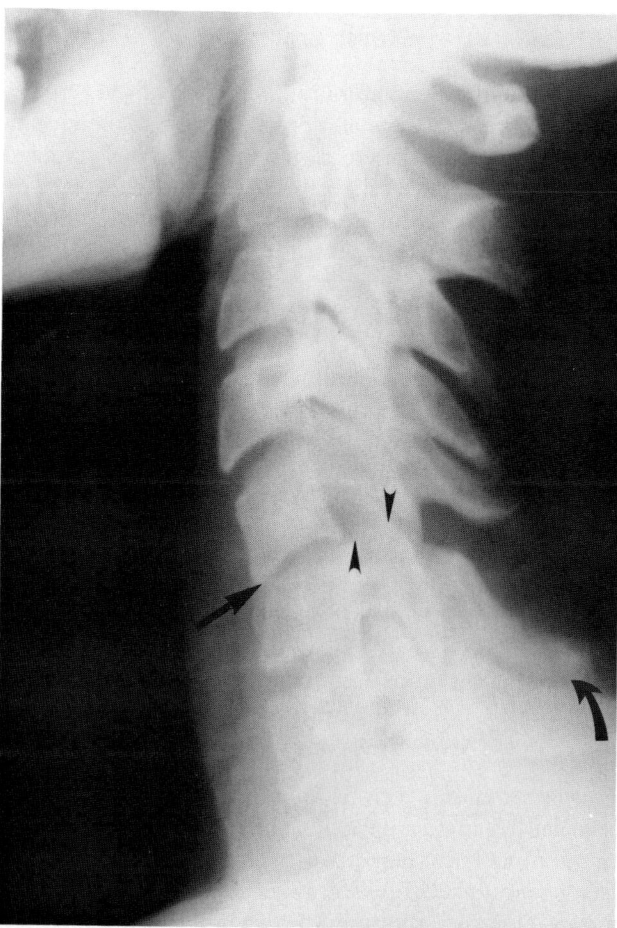

Figure 6.6. Ligamentous flexion injury. The lateral view reveals widening of the interspinous distance (*curved arrow*); partial subluxation of the apophyseal joints (*arrowheads*); and spondylolysthesis at the C5–6 level (*arrow*). These findings suggest rupture of the interspinous ligament, joint capsules, ligamentum flavum, and posterior longitudinal ligament as well as traumatic herniation of the C5–6 disc. Because only the anterior longitudinal ligament remains intact, this is an unstable injury.

Flexion Teardrop Fracture

The name teardrop fracture is derived from the triangular "teardrop" fragment of the anteroinferior aspect of the affected vertebral body (9, 10, 11). The inferior aspect of the posterior fragment is displaced posteriorly while the superior aspect of the posterior fragment is not. There is a kyphotic deformity at the level of the injury with posterior displacement of the cervical spine above the level of injury. The interspinous and interlaminar spaces are wid-

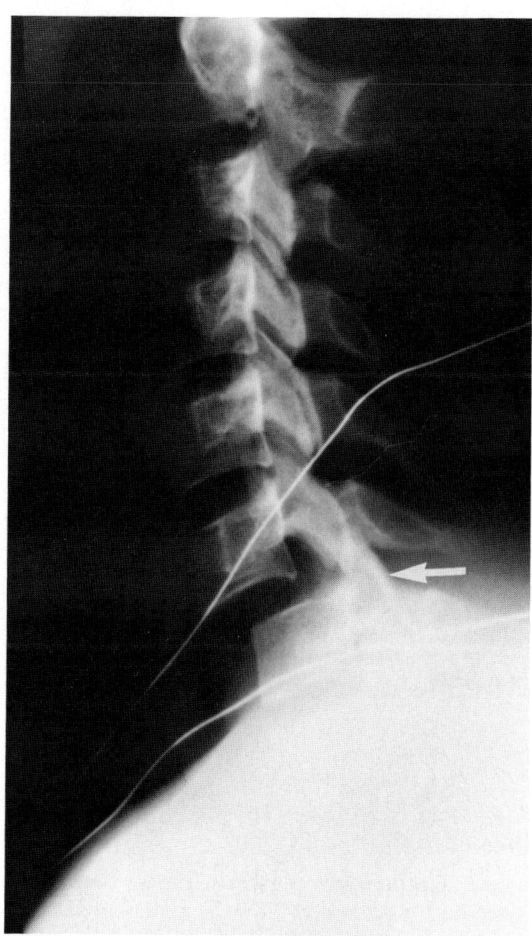

Figure 6.7. Bilateral facet dislocation. The inferior facets of C6 lie anterior to the superior facets of C7. Disruption of the ligamentous complex makes this an unstable injury. (Case courtesy of Dr. Alison Smith, Cleveland Metropolitan General Hospital.)

ened secondary to disruption of the posterior ligamentous complex. Widening of the facet joint is present with posterior displacement of the inferior facet of the vertebral body above with respect to the superior facet of the vertebral body below. Sagittal fracture of the vertebral body and laminar fractures are present in many instances. The most commonly involved level is C5 (11). Flexion teardrop fracture, an unstable injury, may be differentiated from extension teardrop fracture, a more stable injury, when the fragment is wider than it is tall (Fig. 6.8).

FLEXION AND ROTATION INJURES

Unilateral Facet Dislocation

In the lateral projection of the articular masses are superimposed upon each other. With unilateral facet dislocation, the articular mass of the vertebral body above is anteriorly dislocated. The inferior articulating facet of the vertebral body above is dislocated anteroinferior to the superior articulating facet of the vertebral body below. The facet may sometimes be perched on the facet below (3, 12). A "bow tie" configuration of the articular masses is present due to the anterior subluxation of one mass with respect to the other (12). Alteration of the laminar space, a line from the articular masses to the spinolaminar line is present in a large number of cases (13). The vertebral body with the dislocated facet is displaced anteriorly less than one-half the A-P diameter of a cervical vertebral body (1). There may be fractures of the superior and inferior articulating facets. There is disruption of the ligamentous complex on the side of dislocation (Figs. 6.9A and 6.9B).

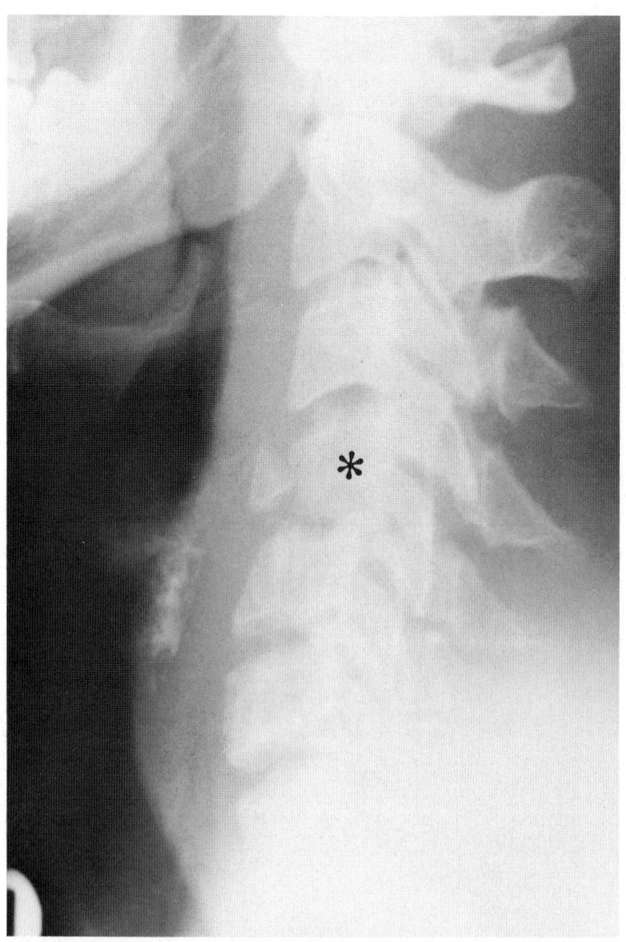

Figure 6.8. Flexion teardrop fracture. The C5 vertebral body is compressed due to the flexion forces. The anterior-inferior aspect was driven inferiorly against the superior-anterior rim of C5, resulting in an avulsion fracture. C4 has also been driven posteriorly into the spinal canal. Note the widening of the prevertebral soft tissues due to hematoma. This feature should prompt a search for an occult fracture when it is the only radiographic finding.

VERTICAL COMPRESSION INJURY

Burst Fracture

A burst fracture is a comminuted fracture of the vertebral body with both anterior and posterior displacement of the fracture fragments. There is variable degree of impingement upon the spinal canal (Fig. 10A). A slight loss of the normal lordotic curve is usually present at the level of injury. The posterior ligamentous complex is intact with no evidence of interlaminar or interspinous widening (7, 14). This feature allows differentiation from the teardrop fracture. Disruption of the posterior margin of the vertebral body, normally a smooth line, is present (15). Fractures of the lamina, though not evident on plain films are present on CT (1) (Figs. 6.10B and 6.10C).

Hyperextension Injuries

In general, the extension injuries are more common than the flexion type injuries to the cervical spine. They are also regarded as slightly more stable than flexion injuries due to the tendency toward lack of disruption of the posterior ligamentous structures and joint capsules.

Anterior Arch Fracture C1

This uncommonly seen fracture of the anterior arch of C1 is visualized as a disruption of the oval-shaped arch on the lateral film. There may be distraction of the fracture fragments and prevertebral soft tissue swelling is present. The distance between the anterior arch and the odontoid process is normal. The transverse ligament and posterior arch of C1 are intact (1, 3).

Posterior Arch C1 Fracture

Fracture of the posterior arch of C1 may be unilateral or bilateral. The fracture occurs posterior to the articular mass. There is no prevertebral soft tissue swelling, and the dis-

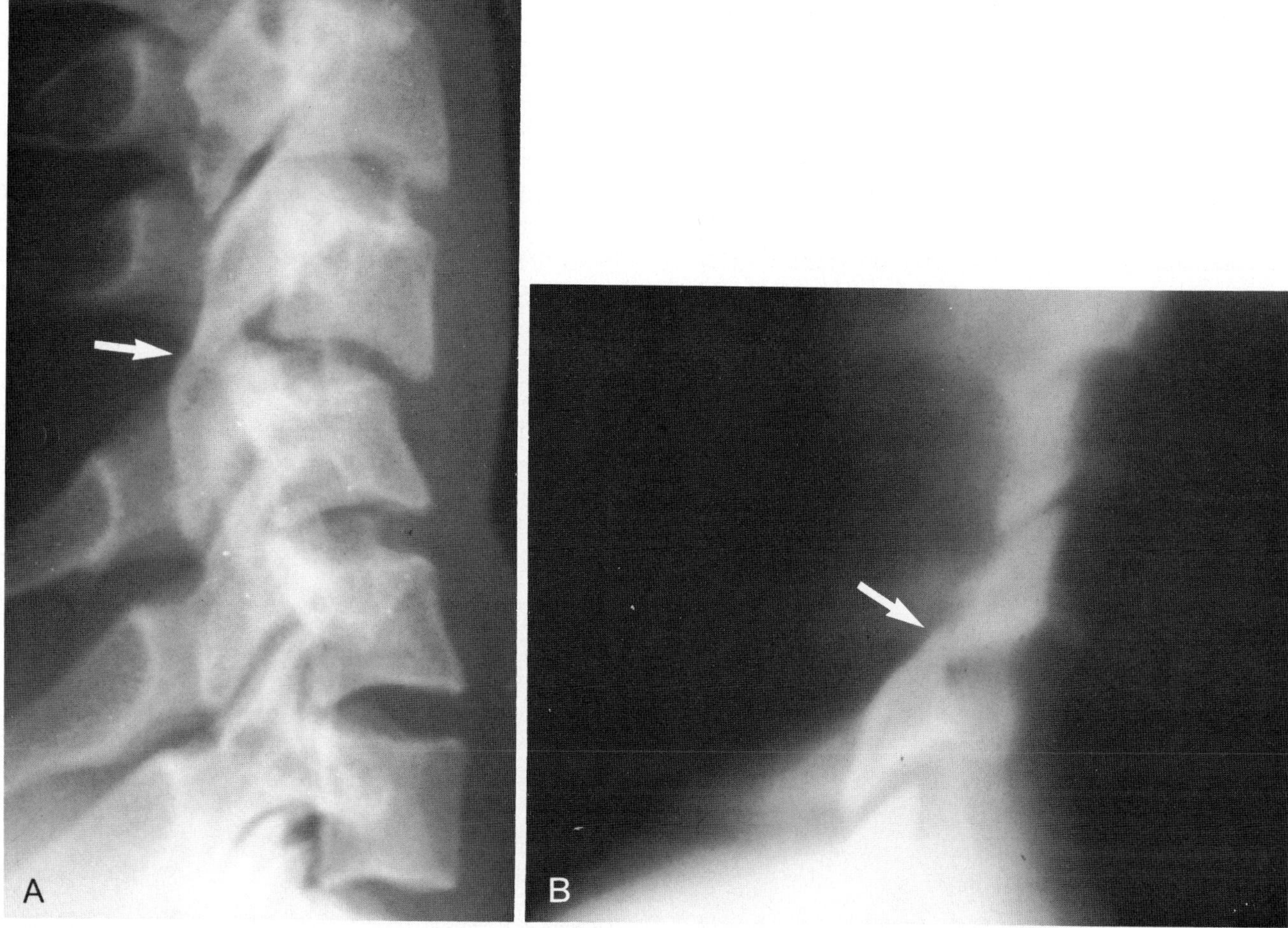

Figure 6.9. Interlocked facet. The lateral radiograph (**A**) demonstrates what appears to be a flexion soft tissue injury with widening of the interspinous distance and anterior angulation. One of the apophyseal joints is not well seen (**B** *arrow*), raising the suspicion of a fracture or interlocked facet. The lateral laminogram confirms the presence of a locked facet joint which is a relatively stable injury.

tance between the anterior arch and odontoid process is normal (1, 3).

Extension Teardrop Fracture

This is a relatively common stable injury resulting from rapid forward acceleration or backward deceleration as seen in patients following "whiplash." An avulsion of the anterior vertebral body margin occurs at the site of insertion of Sharpey's fibers from the anterior longitudinal ligament. The resultant fragment is, therefore, longer in the sagittal plane than in the axial plane. This may help to distinguish this lesion from the flexion type teardrop fracture, a less stable lesion, which is usually wider than it is tall.

Hangman's Fracture

Traumatic spondylolisthesis (hangman's fracture) is a bilateral fracture of the pars interarticularis of C2 (1). This fracture has been classified into 3 types. Type I consists of minimal displacement of the fracture fragments. Type II demonstrates anterior displacement of the vertebral body. Type III is associated with bilateral facet dislocation (16). Radiographic fractures include a high incidence of unilateral or bilateral fracture of the foramen transversarium and Jefferson fractures (17). Soft tissue swelling is present (Fig. 6.11).

Laminar Fracture

Fracture of the lamina is an uncommon isolated injury (3). The fracture is well visualized in the lateral radiograph or with CT (1).

ABNORMAL FRONTAL PROJECTIONS

Flexion Injuries

Because flexion injuries tend to stretch or rupture the posterior ligamentous structures and joint capsules, when the neck recoils, there may be a residual increased distance between the spinous processes. On the frontal projection, one should be sure that the tips of the spinous process are equidistant from one another.

Avulsion fracture of the spinous process may appear as an extra spinous process if it remains in the midline.

Since flexion injuries may result in asymmetrical crushing of the vertebral body, the frontal view is useful because both sides can be compared.

Because the fragments are usually small and overlie many other bony structures, neither flexion nor extension teardrop fractures are reliably evaluated in the frontal projection. Secondary derangement such as widening of the interspinous distance may be seen.

Facet Dislocation

Combined flexion and rotation mechanisms of injury may result in soft tissue disruption of the ligaments and joint capsules without causing a fracture. In these instances, one or both superior articulating surfaces of a given facet joint may travel forward during the rapid deceleration at the onset of the injury. As the cervical spine recoils posteriorly, the posterior corner of the superior facet may be prevented from returning to its normal position by the anterior corner of the inferior facet. The facet joints are then interlocked with narrowing at the spinal canal and neural foramina. In the frontal projection, a unilateral locked facet should be suspected when there is an interruption in the alignment of the spinous processes. Because of the rotation caused by one locked facet, the spinous processes above and below the level of injury will be offset.

Compression/Burst Fracture

A vertical or oblique fracture through the vertebral body may be evident. More often there is subtle widening of the vertebral body.

Fractures of the uncinate process are most often caused by lateral flexion injuries. These are best demonstrated at

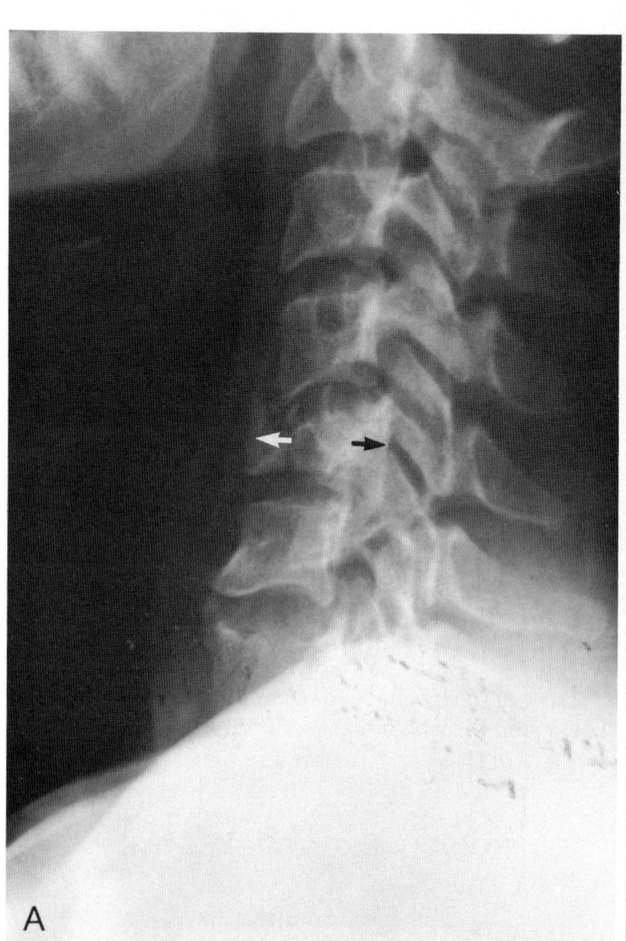

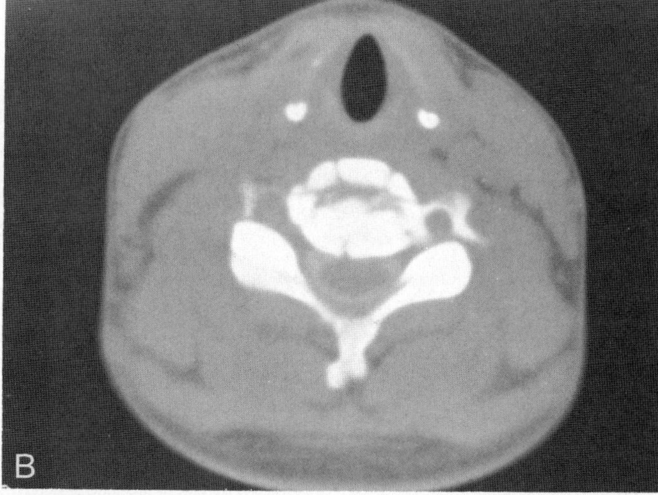

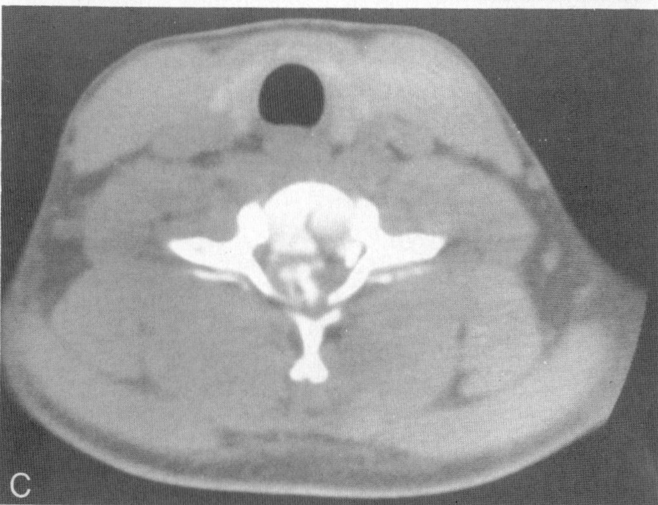

Figure 6.10. Burst fracture. The lateral radiograph (**A**) demonstrates fracture of the C5 vertebral body with displacement of the fracture fragments (*arrow*). CT at the same level (**B**) shows impingement upon the spinal cord. Burst fracture in another patient with transection of the spinal cord (**C**) reveals bony fragments and contrast material within the spinal canal. (Case courtesy of Dr. Alison Smith, Cleveland Metropolitan General Hospital.)

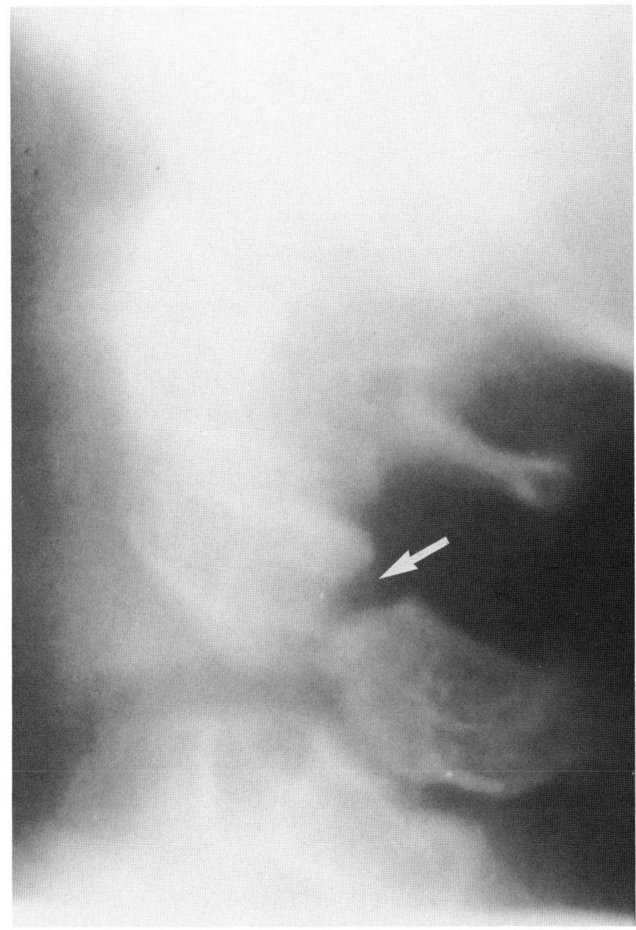

Figure 6.11. Hangman's fracture. As an extension and rotation type of injury, this is a relatively unstable injury. It is well demonstrated by lateral linear tomography (*arrow*).

the A-P projection. These are relatively stable lesions characterized by indistinct visualization of one of the uncinate processes. Linear fractures may be seen through the base of the uncinate process which can extend into the vertical body (3).

Extension Injuries

The majority of these injuries including fractures of the arch of C1, hyperextension dislocation, laminar fractures, and hangman's fractures cannot be seen in the A-P projection.

HYPEREXTENSION AND ROTATION INJURY

Pillar Fracture

Authorities disagree as to the exact mechanisms of injury of the pillar fracture (1, 2, 3). The lateral radiograph demonstrates posterior displacement of the fracture fragment which results in loss of superior position of the articular masses. (Fig. 6.12A) This posterior displacement results in what has been termed the double outline sign (18). The fracture is well visualized with CT (Fig. 6.12B).

Abnormal Open Mouth Projection

Although this view includes the smallest space of any of the views of the cervical spine, it is arguably the image one should spend the most time studying. Differences of a single millimeter must be taken seriously. The number of normal variants, especially of the odontoid, and overlying shadows make this projection one of the most difficult radiological examinations to interpret correctly (Figs. 6.13A, 6.13B, 6.13C, and 6.13D).

Jefferson Fracture

This unstable lesion is most often due to a compression type injury from a direct blow to the vertex of the skull. Typically, these fractures occur following motor vehicle or diving accidents. The compressive force is transmitted downward into the cervical spine. The wedge-shaped lateral masses are narrower medially so that the compressive forces result in a planing effect and the lateral masses are driven laterally with resultant burst fracture of C1. The more elastic ligamentous structures cause some centripetal recoil of the fragments (Fig. 6.14).

Identification of these lesions depends on a careful perusal of the A-P view to be sure that the lateral masses align themselves with the lateral masses of C2. Once head tilt, rotation, and pseudosubluxation have been eliminated as causes, any derangement is considered a fracture until proven otherwise.

Jefferson fractures associated with disruption of the transverse ligament are considered even less stable. If displacement of the anterior arch of C1 from the odontoid is greater than 6.9 mm on the lateral projection, the possibility of disruption of the transverse ligament should be considered (3).

Linear Structure of C1

Fractures through the arch of C1 are relatively stable injuries. The diagnosis depends upon visualization of a curvilinear lucency representing the fracture line. Similar lines can be produced by fractures through the body of C2, overlying interdental spaces, and other artifacts. In addition, these fractures can allow slight lateral displacement of the lateral masses. Additional views or studies are generally required. One should try to differentiate linear fractures from simple nonunion of the posterior arch which is considered a stable cogenital anomaly, Simply put, a congenital lesion should exhibit a white cortical line on either side of the lucency, while an acute fracture has no cortex. Demonstration of this important subtle finding may require additional studies (Figs. 6.15A, 6.15B, and 6.15C).

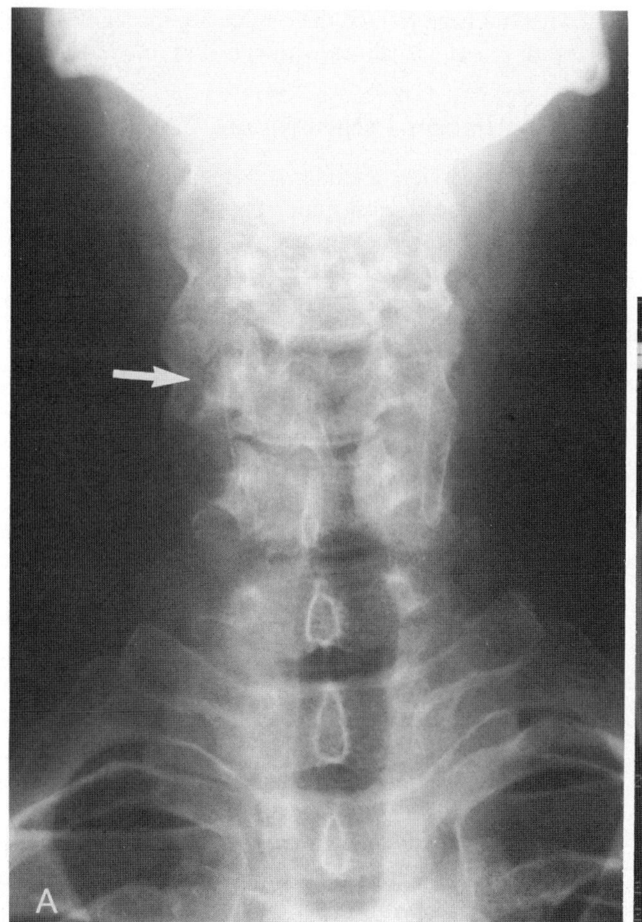

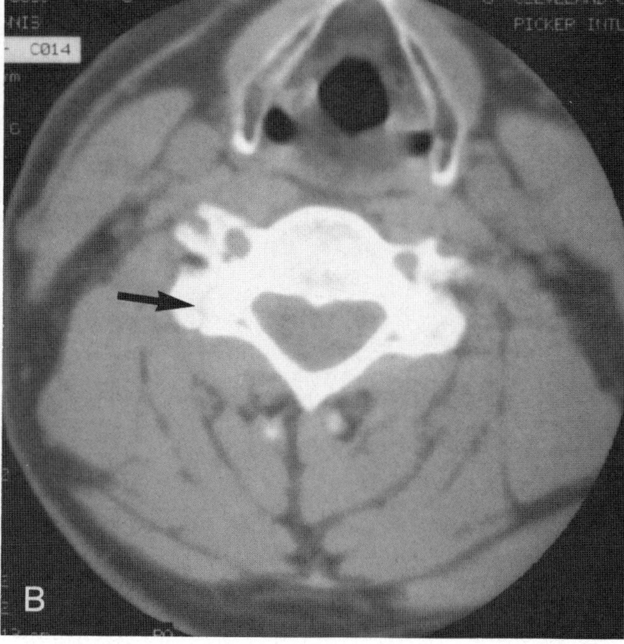

Figure 6.12. Pillar fracture. The A-P projection (**A**) reveals a subtle lucency through the right lateral mass of C5 (*arrow*). A pillar view was not obtained. The axial CT through C5 (**B**) confirms the finding.

Odontoid Fracture

A variety of mechanisms can be postulated for these lesions, including avulsion, rotation, and compression. The open mouth examination is the best projection for evaluating the odontoid. Fracture patterns include the tip of the dens, the base of the dens, and through the dens but extending into the body of C1 (19). In most instances, these are stable fractures with little secondary narrowing of the spinal canal. Flexion and extension lateral views are useful to assess stability and to identify associated disruption of the C-2 relationship.

It may be difficult to distinguish these fractures from congenital nonunion or incomplete ossification of the odontoid. Os odontoideium may, in fact, be posttraumatic or congenital in origin (3, 20). The dystopic type of os odontoideum is located adjacent to the base of the skull where it may mimic an avulsion injury while the orthotopic type is located adjacent to the upper aspect of the dens (3). The differentiation of these depends on the identification of a well-corticated oval or round structure, as opposed to a fracture fragment missing one cortical margin (Figs. 6.16A, 6.16B, 6.16C, and 6.16D).

SUMMARY

The simple and inexpensive plain film examination has survived as one of the most efficient radiographic studies. Nearly every evaluation of cervical trauma begins with plain radiographs and often ends there. One is remiss to ignore or omit them or leave their interpretation to the uninitiated.

ACKNOWLEDGMENTS

The authors are grateful to Ms. Ellen Holly (manuscript preparation), and Mr. Robert Maynard (photography), and to Dr. Paul M. Duchesneau for reviewing the manuscript.

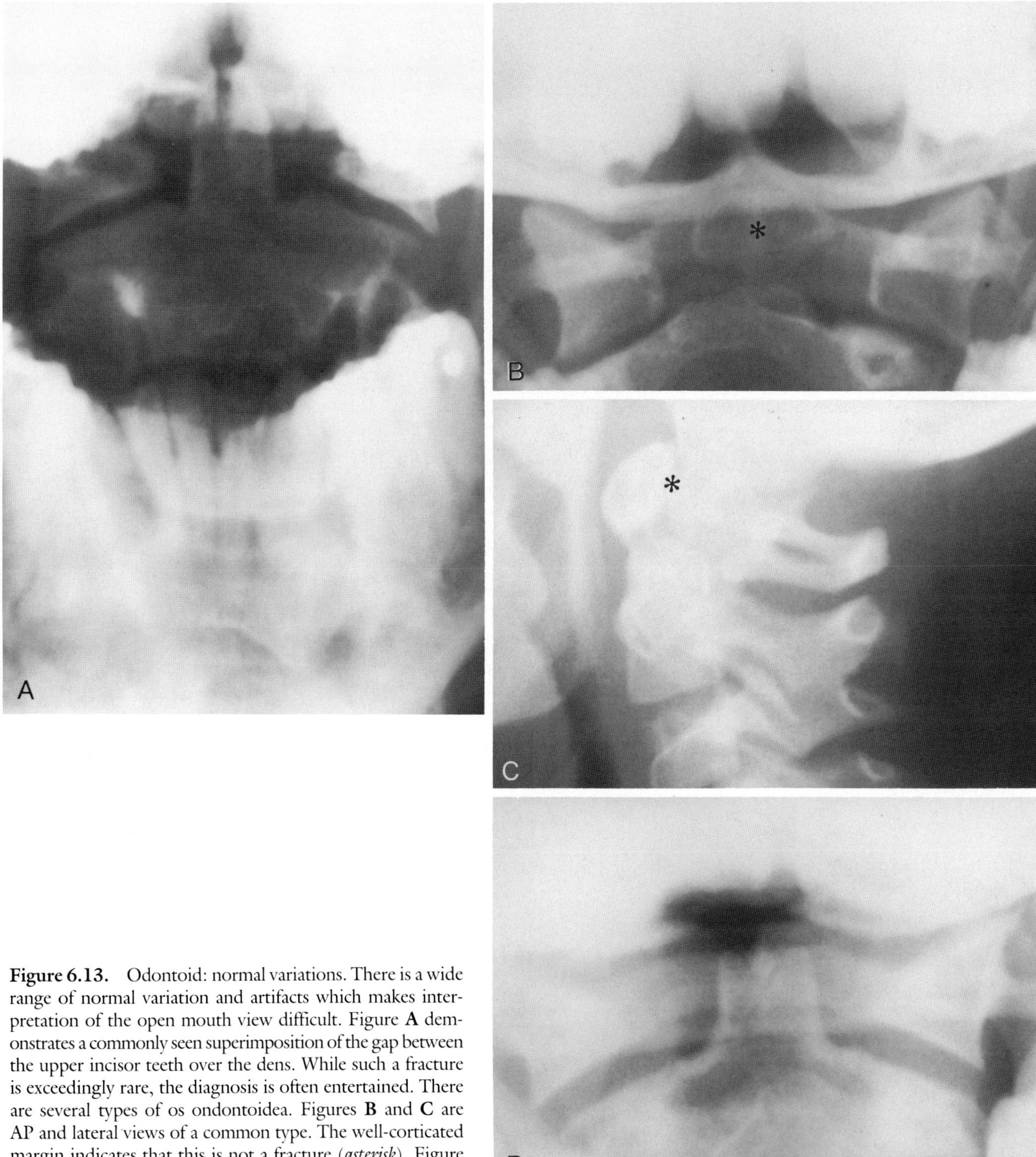

Figure 6.13. Odontoid: normal variations. There is a wide range of normal variation and artifacts which makes interpretation of the open mouth view difficult. Figure **A** demonstrates a commonly seen superimposition of the gap between the upper incisor teeth over the dens. While such a fracture is exceedingly rare, the diagnosis is often entertained. There are several types of os ondontoidea. Figures **B** and **C** are AP and lateral views of a common type. The well-corticated margin indicates that this is not a fracture (*asterisk*). Figure **D** demonstrates a less common type of os.

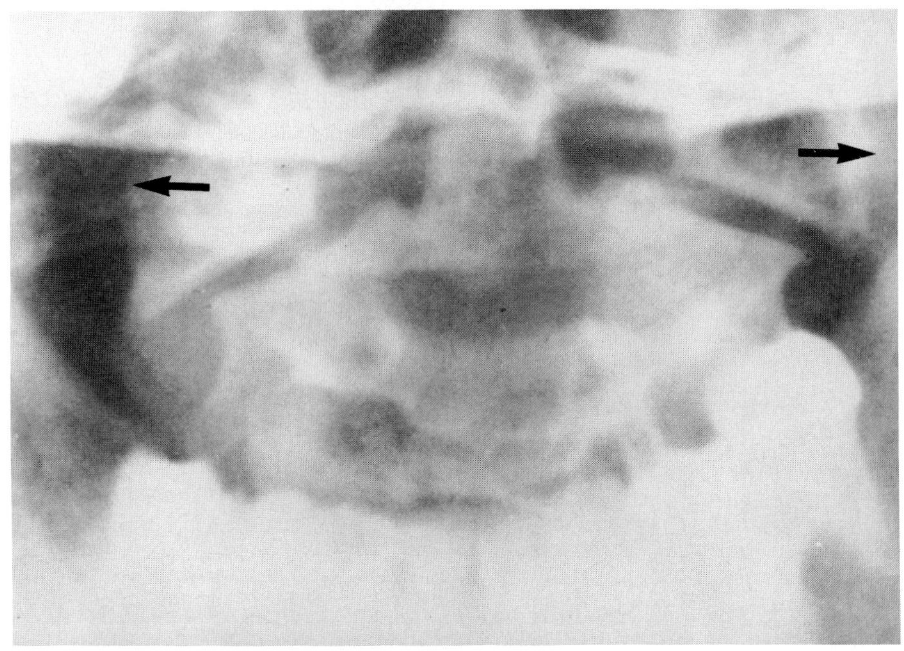

Figure 6.14. Jefferson fracture. Compression force results in disruption of the ring of C1 with lateral displacement (*arrows*) of the articular masses of C1 with respect to C2.

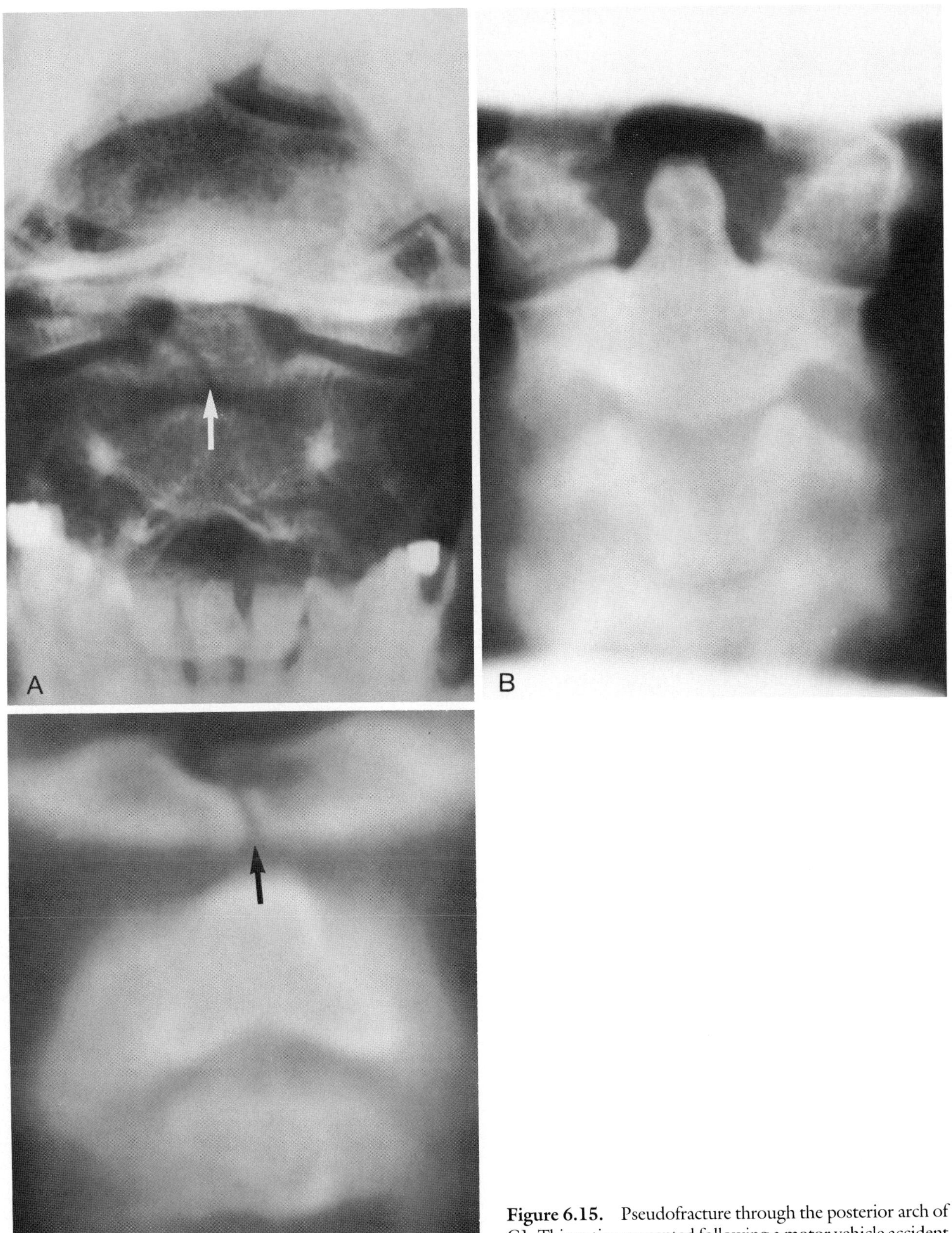

Figure 6.15. Pseudofracture through the posterior arch of C1. This patien presented following a motor vehicle accident complaining of neck pain. The open mouth view demonstrates a lucent line through the body and dens of C2 (**A**, *arrow*). Linear tomography was performed to confirm the finding. There is no fracture through the dens (**B**). More posterior cuts revealed nonunion of the C1 arch. The well-corticated margins (**C** *arrow*) suggest that this is a congenital anomaly.

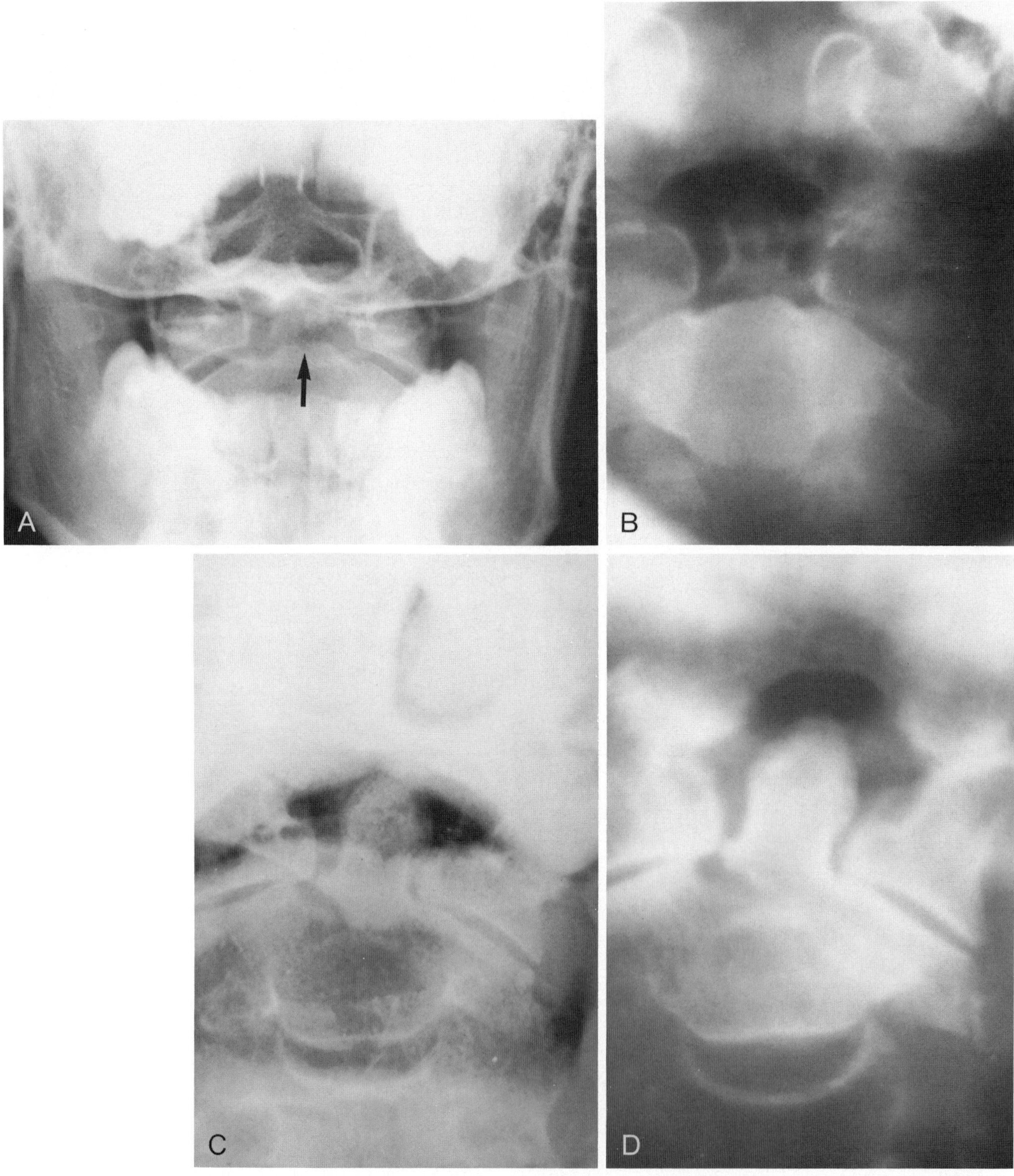

Figure 6.16. Odontoid fractures. These two patients presented following severe cervical spine trauma. The open mouth views are suspicious for fractures through the base of the dens in both patients (**A, C**). The linear tomograms (**B, D**) confirm fractures through the dens in both cases.

REFERENCES

1. Harris JH, Jr, Edeiken-Monroe B. The radiology of cervical spine trauma. 2nd ed. Baltimore: Williams & Wilkins, 1987.

2. Berquist TH. Imaging of orthopedic trauma and surgery. Philadelphia: Saunders, 1986.

3. Gehweiler JA, Jr, Osborn RL, Becker RF. The radiology of vertebral trauma. Philadelphia: Saunders, 1980.

4. Templeton PA, Young JWR, Mirvis SE, et al. The value of retropharyngeal soft tissue measurements in trauma of the adult cervical spine. Skeletal Radiol 1987;16:98–104.

5. Cancelmo JJ, Jr. Clay shoveler's fracture: a helpful diagnostic sign. AJR Am J Roentgenol 1972;115:540–543.

6. Harris JH, Jr. Acute injuries of the cervical spine. Semin Roentgenol 1978;Vol XIII(1):53–68.

7. Holdsworth F. Fractures, dislocations and fracture-dislocations of the spine. J Bone Joint Surg 1970;52A:1534–1551.

8. Green JD, Harle TS, Harris JH, Jr. Anterior subluxation of the cervical spine: hyperflexion sprain. AJNR 1981;2:243–250.

9. Babcock JL. Cervical spine injuries: diagnosis and classification. Arch Surg 1976;111:646–651.

10. Gehweiler JA, Jr, Clar WM, Schaaf RE, et al. Cervical spine trauma: the common combined conditions. Radiology 1979;130:77–86.

11. Kim KS, Chen HH, Russell EJ, et al. Flexion teardrop fracture of the cervical spine: radiographic characteristics. AJNR 1988;9:1221–1228.

12. Berquist TH. Imaging of adult cervical spine trauma. Radiographics 1988;8:667–694.

13. Young JWR, Resnick CS, DeCandido P, et al. The laminar space in the diagnosis of rotation flexion injuries of the cervical spine. AJR Am J Roentgenol 1989;152:103–107.

14. Lee C, Kim KS, Rogers LF. Sagittal fracture of the cervical vertebral body. AJR Am J Roentgenol 1982;139:55–60.

15. Daffner RH, Deeb ZL, Rothfus WE. Fingerprints of vertebral trauma: a unifying concept based on mechanisms. Skeletal Radiol 1986;15:518–525.

16. Effendi B, Roy D, Cornish B, et al. Fracture of the ring of the axis: a classification based on analysis of 131 cases. J Bone Joint Surg 1981;63:319–327.

17. Mirvis SE, Young JWR, Lim C, et al. Hangman's fracture: radiologic assessment in 27 cases. Radiology 1987;163:713–717.

18. Smith RG, Beckley DE, Abel MS. Articular mass fracture: a neglected cause of post traumatic pain? Clin Radiol 1976;27:335–340.

19. Anderson LD, D'Alonzo RT. Fracture of the odontoid process of the axis. J Bone Joint Surg 1974;56A:1633–1674.

20. Fielding JW, Griffin PP. Os odontoideum: an acquired lesion. J Bone Joint Surg 1974;56A:187–190.

7

Magnetic Resonance Imaging of the Cervical Spine

Stuart E. Mirvis and Michael Rothman

Introduction

The role of magnetic resonance imaging (MRI) of the cervical spine has evolved significantly over the past decade. MR imaging offers superior diagnostic sensitivity in evaluation of spinal stenosis, spondylosis, herniated disc, inflammatory and infectious disorders, and neoplasia affecting the cervical spine as compared to CT with and without intrathecal contrast (1–6). Recently, MRI has begun to contribute valuable information towards better management of cervical spine trauma (7–13). This chapter will review some basic physical principles and terminology used in MR imaging. Next, we will consider the normal cervical anatomy as seen on typical imaging sequences and orientations utilized diagnostically, emphasizing the strengths and weaknesses of different image acquisition strategies. We will then evaluate the contribution of MRI to diagnosing nontraumatic pathology of the cervical spine followed by a discussion of the rapidly emerging role of MRI in cervical spine injury.

MRI: Advantages and Disadvantages

MRI offers several advantages over CT of the cervical spine with or without intrathecal myelographic contrast. MRI provides significantly better *contrast resolution* (*lesion conspicuity*) than CT, which improves evaluation of soft tissues, including detailed assessment of the intervertebral discs and ligaments. MRI evaluates the cervical thecal space and shows the effects of adjacent epidural pathology, without the need for invasive instillation of intrathecal contrast material. MRI is highly sensitive in demonstrating and characterizing pathologic processes involving the spinal cord and surrounding epidural soft tissues. MRI can directly acquire images in any orientation to maximize diagnostic potential and can image a larger tissue volume than thin-section axial CT, without requiring a substantial number of axial images. MRI does not utilize ionizing radiation.

MRI has some limitations compared to CT for cervical spine imaging. The technique is more expensive than CT, although the cost difference is minimal when the cost of myelography and CT are considered together. MRI has poorer *spatial resolution* than CT and is therefore less accurate in depicting subtleties of osseous anatomy. MRI can not be performed readily in patients requiring extensive physiologic monitoring and support equipment that may not function properly in close proximity to the magnet or that may generate image artifacts. Currently, many of these limitations are being resolved (14). Metallic foreign bodies or fixation devices that are ferromagnetic, such as stainless steel, interfere with MR image acquisition if near the imaged region, but use of other metals for spinal fixation, which possess a lower magnetic susceptibility, such as titanium, will lessen this difficulty (15). Typically, MRI studies are more time-consuming than CT evaluation, although again, when both CT and myelography are utilized, these studies require more time and physician involvement. Recent technical developments are permitted extremely rapid scan times rivaling and surpassing those of current CT image acquisition (16–18). MRI requires substantial patient cooperation due to great motion sensitivity, but this problem is also receding with development of both motion suppression scanning techniques and faster image acquisition. Finally, about 5% of patients develop severe claustrophobia in the confined space of the magnet bore (19), but this problem is often resolved by administration of anxiolytic medication.

Basic Principles of Magnetic Resonance Imaging

Creating an Image — Method of Spatial Localization

To better comprehend the appearance of the MR image some understanding of the manner in which MR signals are obtained and influenced by different image acquisition techniques is necessary. It is well beyond the scope of this chapter to delve deeply into the physical principles of MRI, but an attempt will be made to relate, in a clinically relevant manner, some of the principles underlying MR imaging.

When the body is placed in a magnetic field certain nuclei will align with or against the orientation of this external field. In the case of most clinical imaging currently performed, the hydrogen atom (proton) is the nucleus of greatest interest, since its abundance in the body makes it a good choice to study. A small excess of protons will align themselves in the direction of the external magnetic field producing a net magnetization within the body. When the protons are placed in the magnetic field they will precess about their magnetic axis, much as the earth precesses around its magnetic axis as it rotates. The velocity of precession is proportional to the strength of the externally applied magnetic field. This relationship is described as: F (precessional frequency) = K (constant) × B_0 (strength of the external field). The constant K is referred to as the Larmor frequency and is unique to different atomic nuclei. In the case of hydrogen K is 42.56 mHz/Tesla (where 1 Tesla = 10,000 gauss).

If a radiofrequency (RF) signal (which can be considered another external magnetic field) is sent into the tissue within the magnet at the Lamor frequency, this energy is absorbed by all protons precessing at that frequency (those spins that are resonant with the radiofrequency). A slice of tissue can be "excited" by the radiofrequency by superimposing a small additional magnetic field gradient on the external magnetic field, so that only a thin band of tissue contains protons precessing at the precise resonance (Larmor) frequency.

Once the excess energy is absorbed by the precessing protons their orientation (net magnetization) is briefly deflected away from the main magnetic field. The rate at which these protons "give up" this excess energy and return to their equilibrium state is greatly influenced by the "molecular environment" (i.e., the type of tissue, motion, external magnetic field homogeneity, adjacent ferromagnetic or magnetically susceptible atoms, etc.). The complex radiofrequency signal arising from excited tissue is detected by an antenna (receiver coil), greatly amplified, and analyzed (Fourier transformation) to sort out the location and intensity of the returning radiofrequency signal. The greater the signal intensity from a given location, the brighter the image appears. The location of the returning signal is further defined by creating an addition "phase-shift" domain that typically divides the tissue into 128 or 256 sections. Finally, the third dimension that defines location of signal strength is created by another superimposed magnetic gradient, referred to as the "read gradient." Thus, the signal address (location) within the volume of the body is determined by the slice selection, phase encoding, and readout gradients. The intensity of the returning signal is also strongly influenced by the number of protons in the tissue sample, predominantly from fat and water molecules.

Tissue Parameters T1 and T2

The vector of magnetization aligned with the main external magnetic field direction (referred to as the longitudinal magnetization) can be altered by applying an external RF signal. The magnetization can be rotated into a another orientation briefly. A 90° RF pulse causes the net magnetization to flip 90° into a transverse plane. Immediately the protons in the transverse plane begin to lose "phase coherence" (dephase) by virtue of imperfections in the external field and local interactions with adjacent nuclei. As time progress, the signal in the transverse plane decays. The rate of signal loss is exponential, with a decay constant referred to as T2. At a time of T2 after the RF pulse the signal strength has decreased by 63.2% of its initial value (Fig. 7.1*B*). T2 varies among tissue types. The longer the tissue T2, the longer the signal takes to decay and the brighter the tissue appears. At the same time that the transverse magnetization is decreasing, the longitudinal magnetization is increasing exponentially with a time constant T1. At time T1 after the RF pulse, the signal has regained 63.2% of its preexcitation value (Fig. 7.1*A*). The shorter the T1, the more rapidly the tissue returns to full longitudinal magnetization. T1 also varies among different tissue types. The inherent differences in the T1 and T2 of different tissues are exploited to create signal intensity differences.

Imaging Parameters TR and TE

In order to optimally differentiate among tissues of different T1 and T2, the selection of imaging parameters is

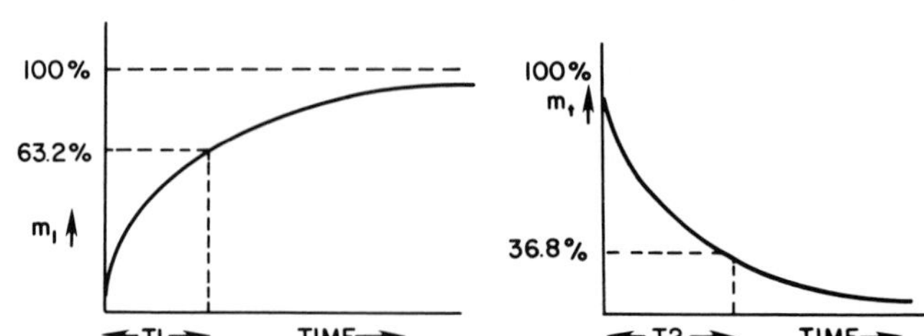

Figure 7.1. **A,** diagram illustrates the exponential regrowth of longitudinal magnetization following radiofrequency pulse. At a time constant (T1) the magnetization aligned with the external magnetic field has reached 63.2% of its pre-excitation value. **B,** diagram illustrates the expnential decay of signal intensity due to loss of transverse magnetization. At a time T2 after the radiofrequency pulse, the signal decays by 63.2% of its initial value. (Adapted from Heiken JP, Glaser HS, Lee JKT, Murphy WA, Gado M, eds. Manual of clinical magnetic resonance imaging. New York: Raven Press, 1986.)

crucial. For instance, two tissues with different T1 time constants will have a different rate of regrowth of longitudinal magnetization (Fig. 7.2) If we wait too long both tissues will be fully remagnetized, and no difference in their signal is discerned. Generally, we should sample the signal arising from the tissue soon after the RF pulse to optimally differentiate tissue based on T1 differences. The time between RF pulses is referred to as TR and is relatively short when we wish is increase *tissue contrast* based on T1 differences. Similarly, as the transverse magnetization decays with a time constant T2, if we sample the signal arising from the transverse magnetization too soon after the RF pulse there will be little difference among tissues with different T2 values (Fig. 7.3). However, if we wait sufficiently long, the signal intensity variation based on tissue T2 differences becomes more marked. However, at very long TR values, these signal differences are lost due to decrease in signal strength and increasing noise. The time we wait to sample the signal strength after the RF pulse is known as the TE (echo time). It should be noted that in order to obtain an echo at time TE after the RF pulse another RF pulse must be applied to the tissue that briefly restores phase coherence to generate a signal of sufficient strength. This pulse referred to as a 180° refocusing pulse, is performed at a time half-way between the RF pulse and the signal acquisition at time TE after the initial 90° RF pulse. The sequence of an initial 90° RF pulse followed by a rephasing 180° pulse is known as a **spin-echo sequence.**

Instead of tipping the longitudinal magnetization through 90°, a RF pulse can be applied that tips the longitudinal magnetization to a lesser extent (tip angle <90°). In addition, the magnetic "read-out" gradients can be reversed soon after this initial RF pulse to refocus the transverse magnetization to achieve an echo signal in a fashion similar to the manner in which the 180° pulse described above reestablishes the phase coherence of the transverse magnetization. This imaging method referred to as **gradient recalled echo** (GRE) acquires signals in less time and emphasizes different tissue characteristics than the spin echo method. However, the gradient echo technique is more sensitive to inhomogeneity in the external magnetic field that leads to increased noise and therefore requires more image samples (acquisitions) to retain image quality.

In general, imaging sequences that maximize T1 tissue differences employ short TR (repetition time) and short TE (echo time). Imaging sequences that employ long TR and long TE are intended to maximize tissue contrast based upon inherent differences in the T2 of tissues. Sequences using long TR and short TE substantially negate both T1 and T2 tissue contrast differences, and signal intensity is determined by the number of protons in the tissue volume (proton density or balanced sequence) (Table 7.1).

Relaxation Enhancement — Pharmacologic Manipulation

Although the inherent T1 and T2 of different tissues is fixed, relaxation can be influenced by substances introduced in close proximity to the tissue of interest. Substances that enhance relaxation (restoration of the equilibrium state) are referred to as paramagnetic. Atoms with numerous unpaired electrons in their outer electron orbitals such as gadolinium with seven unpaired electrons have strong paramagnetic properties, but must be chelated

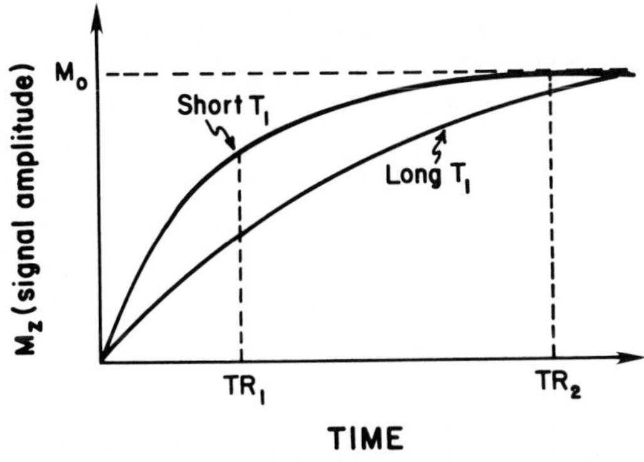

Figure 7.2. Differentiation of tissue based on T1 contrast. Effect of TR. Diagram shows how the signal intensity difference between two different tissues with different T1 values changes with time. Maximal signal difference (contrast) is obtained by sampling the signal at a time before both tissues have regained full magnetization. A short TR is required to maximize T1 contrast differences. (Adapted from Heiken JP, Glaser HS, Lee JKT, Murphy WA, Gado M, eds. Manual of clinical magnetic resonance imaging. New York: Raven Press, 1986.)

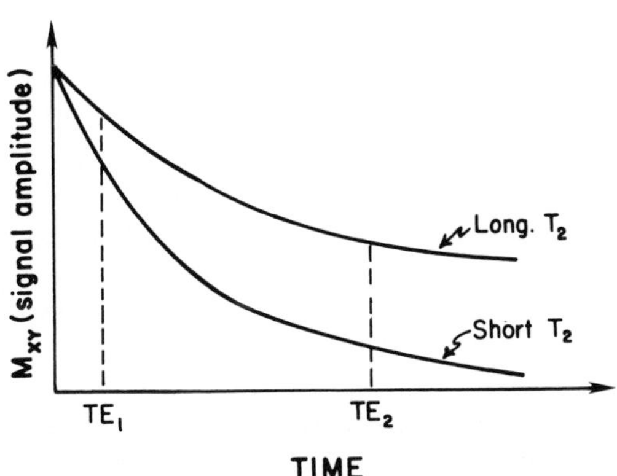

Figure 7.3. Differentiation of tissues based on T2 contrast. Diagram shows how the loss of signal amplitude (decreased intensity) from transverse magentization, which decays with a time constant T2 is maximized with longer TE (echo time). (Adapted from Heiken JP, Glaser HS, Lee JKT, Murphy WA, Gado M, eds. Manual of clinical magnetic resonance imaging. New York: Raven Press, 1986.)

Table 7.1. Relationship of TR, TE, Sequence Weighting, and Signal Intensity for Spin Echo Technique

Weighting	Imaging parameters		Signal intensity
T1 weighting:	Short TR	Short TE	Shorter T1 tissue = brighter
T2 weighting:	Long TR	Long TE	Longer T2 tissue = brighter
Proton density:	Long TR	Short TE	High proton density = brighter

TR = 90° pulse repetition time.
TE = time from 90° pulse to acquisition of rephased transverse magnetization signal.
T1 = time constant for exponential regrowth of longitudinal magnetization.
T2 = time constant for exponential decay of transverse magnetization.

with EDTA to decrease biologic toxicity (20). Although Gd-EDTA decreases both T1 and T2 of adjacent tissues, the T1 shortening effect predominates at the doses currently used clinically. Thus, tissues in close proximity to Gd-EDTA appear brighter or enhanced (shorter T1) on T1-weighted imaging sequences than they otherwise would. Other contrast agents with high magnetic susceptibility (easily induced magnetism) can be utilized to markedly shorten the apparent T2 of adjacent tissues and diminish their signal (darken) on T2-weighted sequences. The safety of gadolinium in pregnancy has not been established. Use of Gadolinium appears safe in patients with severe renal insufficiency (21).

NORMAL MR ANATOMY OF THE CERVICAL SPINE

Sagittal Orientation

The typical MR examination of the cervical spine includes a spin echo (SE) sagittal T1, proton density, and T2-weighted examination. Some centers may perform sagittal GRE images instead of T-2 weighted spin echo studies. On the T1-weighted sequence (Fig. 7.4) the osseous structures appear relatively bright, similar to the subcutaneous fat, due to the presence of fat in the bone marrow, which varies with patient age and hematologic status. Fat has a relatively short T1 constant and thus appears bright on T1-weighted sequences. Pathologic processes that replace the marrow will appear less intense (darker) than the surrounding marrow fat. The cortical bone is low in signal on all sequences due to a lack of free mobile protons to contribute signal; air is dark for the same reason. The intervertebral discs are also relatively high in signal intensity similar to bone marrow, but the surrounding outer annulus fibrosis and ligaments are dark, again due to a lack of mobile protons in their substance. The cerebrospinal fluid (CSF) is of low signal intensity on T1-weighted sequences due to a longer T1 relaxation constant. The spinal cord is of intermediate and homogeneous signal, similar to muscle, and few details of internal architecture can be discerned. The T1-weighted spin echo image provides good anatomic detail, a high signal to noise ratio, and a relatively short examination time (due to a short TR). The sequence provides excellent information regarding invasion of the bone marrow and degenerative changes along the vertebral endplates. The sequence is used with gadolinium enhancement to detect both intra- and extra-medullary pathology and is least susceptible to magnetic field inhomogeneity created by metal implants or foreign bodies [22].

On the proton density sagittal image (Fig. 7.4), the marrow and fat signals are less intense than on T1-weighted images. The very low signal of the cortical bone and ligaments is well displayed, since this sequence depends largely upon mobile proton density that is decreased in these tissues. This sequence provides little contrast between the CSF and spinal cord, but a high degree of contrast between the CSF and extradural space. The intervertebral discs appear somewhat brighter than the marrow fat and are highly contrasted against the adjacent dark ligaments and cortical bone. The longitudinal ligaments cannot be separated from the outer annulus fibrosis and appear as a continuous dark signal.

The T2-weighted sagittal image (Fig. 7.4) provides a "myelographic effect" due to the increased signal of the CSF (long T2) versus the intermediate signal spinal cord and is ideally suited to evaluated impingement of the thecal space as well as intradural lesions. In addition, the T2-

Figure 7.4. Normal sagittal MRI anatomy seen on different signal acquisitions. **A,** mid-sagittal T1-weighted image shows relative bright bone marrow signal, intermediate intervertebral disks, and lower signal from the CSF outlining an intermediate signal intensity cord. The cord has similar intensity to paraspinal muscles, while the bone marrow has similar signal intensity to subcutaneous fat. Note very low signal from interspinous ligaments (*arrows*) and combination of anterior longitudinal ligament and outer fibers of annulus fibrosis (*arrowheads*). **B,** this proton density mid-sagittal image enhances low signal of ligaments and shows increased CSF signal obscuring cord signal. **C,** this T2-weighted mid-sagittal image shows "myelographic effect" of increased CSF signal around lower cord signal. The bone marrow appears lower in signal intensity. Better hydrated intervertebral discs appear brighter than desiccated discs. **D,** this mid-sagittal image produced by a gradient echo, rather than spin-echo, sequence shows marked suppression of bone marrow and fat signal, bright CSF, and bright intervertebral discs. The bright vertical line through the cord (arrows) represent an artifact.

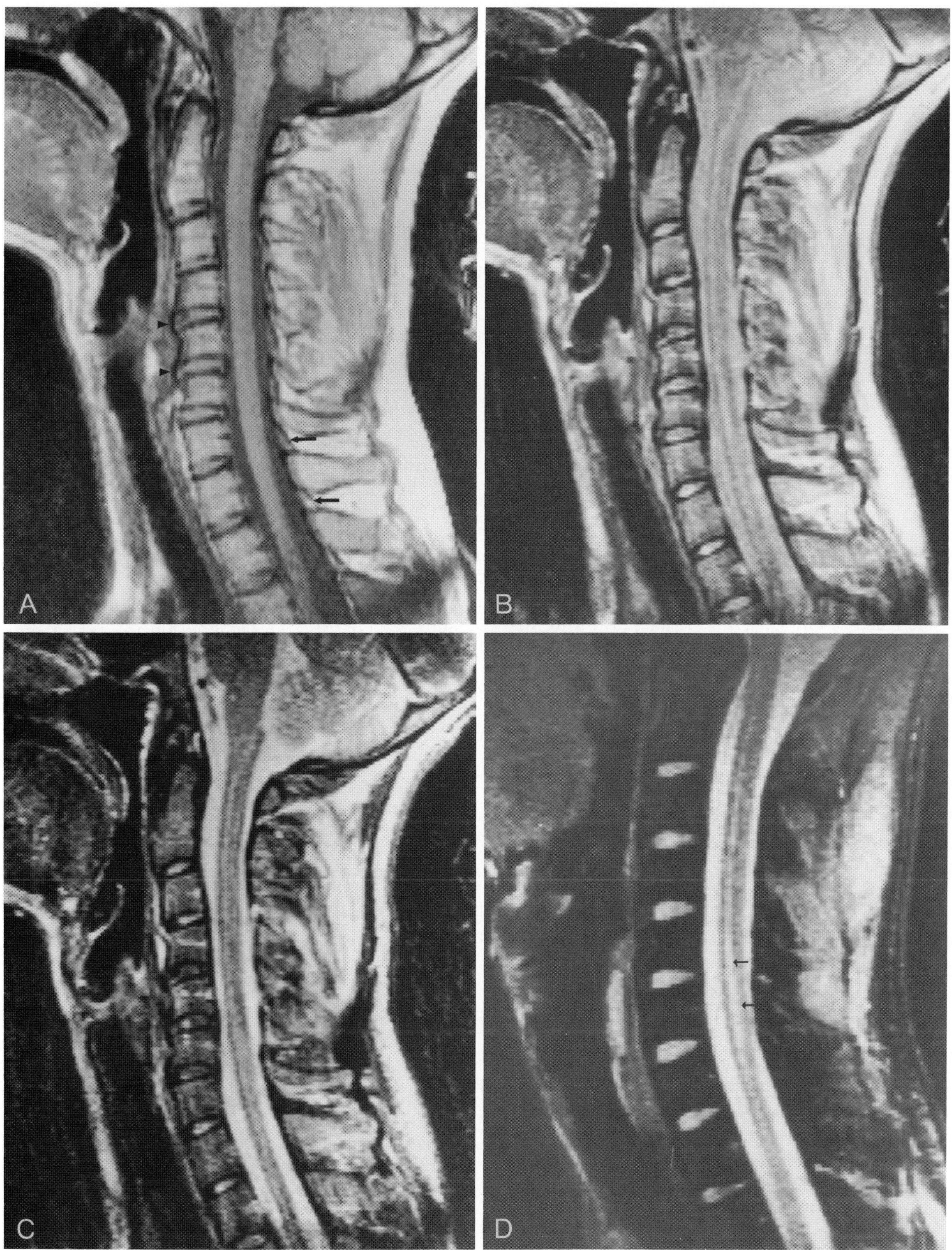
A
B
C
D

weighted sequence has increased sensitivity to intramedullary disease and disc space infection due to the edema (increased water content with longer T2) associated with these pathologic processes. The T2 sequence however is time-consuming (long TR, more signal averages needed due to low signal to noise ratio), and more susceptible to patient motion, CSF pulsation, and field inhomogeneity induced by metal implants or foreign bodies.

The sagittal gradient echo (GE) sequence is also known as FLASH, FISP, GRASS, among others depending on the manufacturer of the MR unit and nuances of the sequence. This sequence also produces a strong myelographic effect particularly when using small flip angles to produce a T2-weighted effect (Fig. 7.4). The marrow signal appears intensely low on GE sequences, while the intervertebral disc signal remains intense. This quality helps differentiate protruding discs from osteophytic spurs better than on other sequences (23). GE images are also ideal for defining the contours of osseous structures. The T1 and T2 weighting of GE images can be altered by changing the tip angle, with smaller angles producing T2-weighting, and larger angles (>30°) leading to T1-weighting effects. While GE images have the advantages of short acquisition time, greater signal to noise and contrast to noise than SE images (22) they are more susceptible to motion and other artifacts (22). The speed of GE sequences permits data to be acquired in a 3-D mode (a volume of tissue, rather than a slice) permitting subsequent reformatting of images in any orientation, including orthogonal to the neural foramen.

Axial Orientation

Axially oriented images mimic the anatomic plane typically acquired in CT imaging. Usually, axial images in MR are obtained through areas of interest identified by sagittal or oblique sagittal imaging. The axial SE T1-weighted image is used to optimize anatomic detail and demonstrates a relatively homogeneous spinal cord surrounded by low signal CSF (Fig. 7.5). Again, the cortical bone is of low signal as are ligaments, and the bone marrow fat appears bright. There is generally a signal void in blood vessels seen on SE sequences due to rapidly flowing blood that moves beyond the imaged slice prior to giving up its signal. The axial plane is well suited for evaluation of the exiting neural foramen.

Gradient echo images are also acquired in the axial plane using both T1- and T2-weighted sequences. The axial T2-weighted GE study again shows decreased signal from bone marrow and fat and enhanced CSF signal intensity producing excellent contrast between bone, CSF, herniated nucleus pulposus, and spinal cord (Fig. 7.5). In addition, the internal anatomy of the spinal cord can be discerned on GE images. The grey matter appears as an H-shaped region of increased signal relative to the surrounding white matter. On gradient echo images, flowing blood generates a signal due, in part, to negation of spin dephasing in flowing blood by the read-out gradient reversal described above, among other reasons (23). The GE axial sequence is also valuable to study the nerve root foramina and may be the only axial image obtained in some institutions.

MRI OF CERVICAL PATHOLOGY

Degenerative Spondylopathy

Degenerative changes involving the cervical spine are common in the later decades of life and principally involve intervertebral disk degeneration and herniation, marginal osteophyte formation, ligament hypertrophy and calcification, and hypertrophic changes involving the facet joints. Degenerative changes may be asymptomatic or may manifest as radiculopathy or myelopathy depending on whether the nerve roots or spinal cord are primarily involved. Plain radiography will demonstrate cervical degenerative pathology and spinal stenosis, but will not display cord or nerve root compression or myelopathic changes directly. CT with intrathecal contrast (CT-M) has been considered the optimal examination for degenerative cervical spondylopathy since the procedure can directly demonstrate spinal cord or thecal sac compression and can better detect neural foraminal encroachment by osteophyte or herniated disk. Recently, MRI has begun to challenge CT-M for several reasons. MRI requires no instillation of intrathecal contrast, has direct multiplanar imaging capability, can create a "myelographic equivalent" appearance, and can detect myelopathy. MRI also appears more sensitive than CT-M in detection of disc abnormalities. Typically, central disc herniation is best detected on sagittal views and confirmed with selected axial images (24) (Fig. 7.6–7.8). Lateral herniations are more subtle and require thin-section axial images, preferably using gradient echo sequences with small flip angles (T2-weighted) (24). Gradient echo sequences enhance contrast between osteophytes and herniated disc material, since bone appears dark relative to the more intense signal of herniated disc material (Fig. 7.7) (24, 25). Chronic spinal cord compression due to cervical spinal stenosis can lead to cervical myelopathy that will manifest as cord atrophy and edema within cord. T2-weighted spin-echo sequences are quite sensitive in detecting cord edema related to compression myelopathy (26) (Fig. 7.9). Gradient echo images best define canal compression due to ossification of the posterior longitudinal ligament (Fig. 7.10).

Infectious/Inflammatory Disease

Infection of the cervical spine may manifest as discitis, osteomyelitis, epidural abscess, or a combination of these

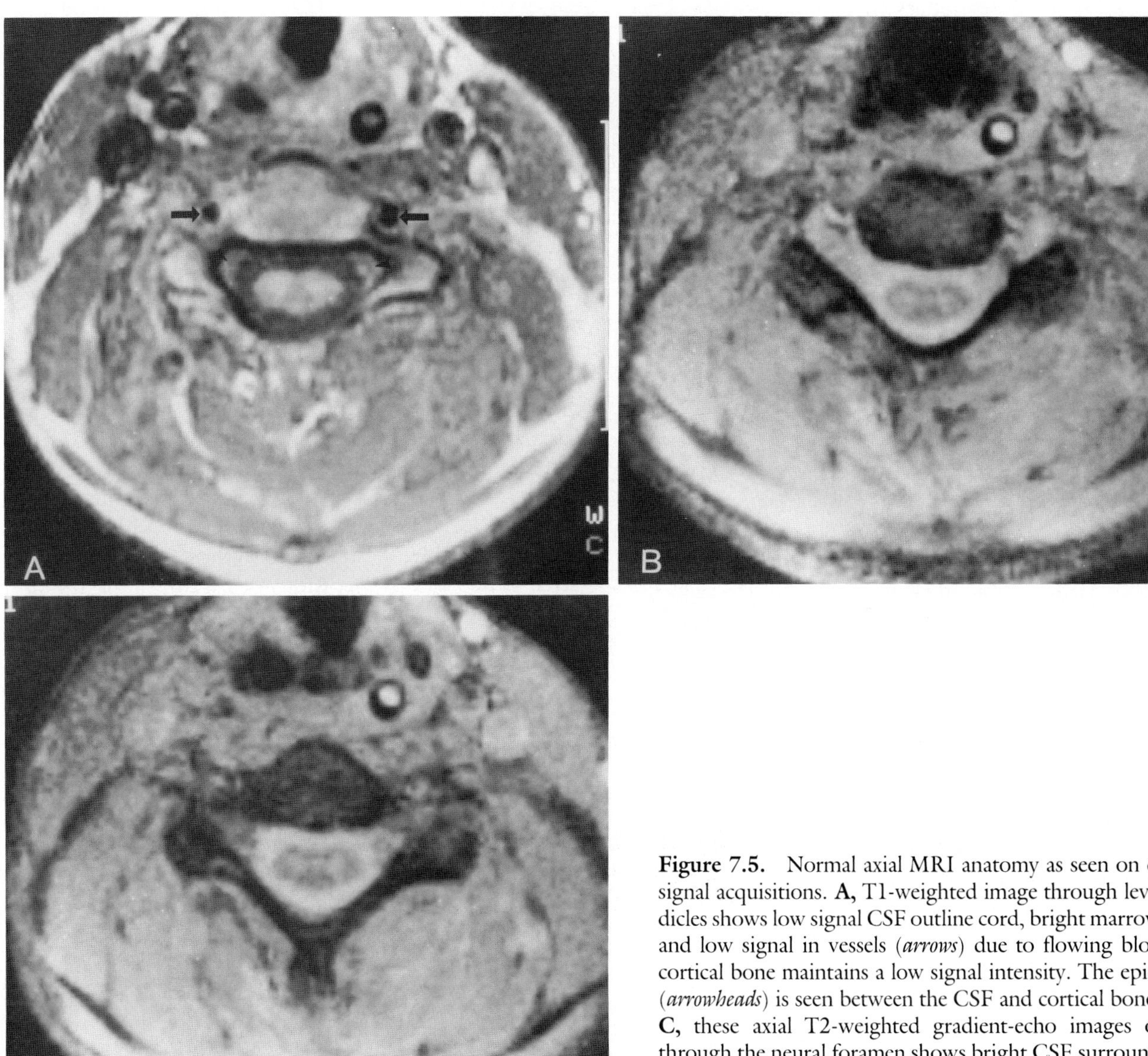

Figure 7.5. Normal axial MRI anatomy as seen on different signal acquisitions. **A,** T1-weighted image through level of pedicles shows low signal CSF outline cord, bright marrow signal, and low signal in vessels (*arrows*) due to flowing blood. The cortical bone maintains a low signal intensity. The epidural fat (*arrowheads*) is seen between the CSF and cortical bone. **B and C,** these axial T2-weighted gradient-echo images obtained through the neural foramen shows bright CSF surrounding the cord. Note higher signal H-shaped grey matter in central cord that is best seen on gradient echo imges. The blood vessels contain bright signals, rather than flow voids with gradient echo acquisitions.

entities. Osteomyelitis results from direct hematogenous spread of organisms or occurs as a result of direct interventions such as penetrating trauma or surgery. Plain radiographs are relatively insensitive to osseous changes accompanying vertebral infection, which include endplate irregularity, fragmentation, soft tissue swelling, loss of disc space height, and vertebral body destruction, but these findings may not become apparent for 2 to 8 weeks after infection ensues. Also, findings of osteomyelitis can be confused radiographically with chronic degenerative changes. CT is more sensitive to the findings described above, and with addition of intrathecal contrast can reveal epidural extension of infection. MRI is more sensitive than CT to detect vertebral body infection, since loss of the replaced bone marrow signal occurs well prior to osseous destruction. MRI findings in osteomyelitis on T1-weighted sequences include a decrease in signal intensity in bone marrow and loss of the distinct vertebral endplate. T2-weighted images show an increase in signal in the vertebral endplates and discs due to an increase in water content in these tissues from edema and ischemia (27) (Figs. 7.11–7.13). MRI has shown a sensitivity of 96%, a specificity of 92% and an accuracy of 94% in the diagnosis of vertebral osteomyelitis. Combined gallium and bone scintigraphy com-

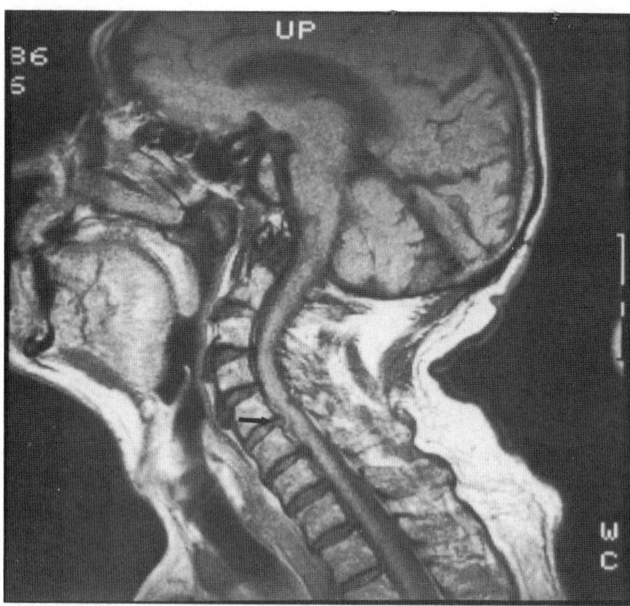

Figure 7.6. MRI of herniated intervertebral disk. This sagittal T1-weighted image obtained in an elderly man with myelopathy shows a herniated disc indenting the spinal cord at the C5/6 level (*arrow*). Several anteriorly herniated discs are observed at more rostral levels.

pares favorably with a sensitivity of 90%, specificity of 100%, and accuracy of 94% (28, 29). In experimental studies in rabbits, MRI was considerably more sensitive than CT for diagnosis of osteomyelitis, 94% versus 66%, and was more accurate, 93% versus 80%. However, CT was more specific than MRI excluding osteomyelitis (30).

On T1-weighted images disc space infection appears as confluent decreased signal from the disc and adjacent endplates relative to the bone marrow. T2-weighted images show increased signal from the same tissues (31) (Fig. 7.12). Typically, degenerative disk disease appears as a decrease in signal on T2-weighted sequences due to desiccation of the disk and neoplastic disease tends to spare the intervertebral disc. MRI appears as sensitive as gallium scan combined with bone scan for detection of discitis and is more sensitive than radiographs (32).

Epidural abscess is rare occurring in 1.96/10,000 hospital admissions (27). Well-established risk factors include diabetes mellitus, intravenous drug use, renal failure, and alcohol abuse (27) and causes mortality in 18–31% of cases. About 25% of epidural abscesses occur in the cervical spine (27). The majority of epidural abscesses are anterior or circumferential and are associated with osteomyelitis or discitis (33). To delineate the extent of epidural involvement myelography may require both a C1–C2 puncture and lumbar puncture. Myelography carries some risk of exacerbating spinal cord compression and in contaminating noninfected spinal compartments. CT can noninvasively visualize a soft tissue epidural mass and reveal the extent of osseous destruction. Intravenous contrast is helpful to enhance the rim of the inflammatory mass and delineate the mass from the thecal sac (34). MRI can show the extent of osseous involvement, paraspinal soft tissue involvement and distinguish the spinal cord from the epidural mass (Figs. 7.11–7.13). MRI is as sensitive as CT with intrathecal contrast in diagnosing epidural abscess but is more specific at distinguishing epidural abscess from other epidural masses and in defining disease extent (33). T1-weighted sequences provide anatomic detail demonstrating the epidural soft tissue mass, cord displacement and compression, bone and paraspinal involvement. T2-weighted images show liquified portions of the infection, while T1-weighted gadolinium-enhanced images show vascularized granulation tissue (Fig. 7.13).

A recent report indicated that gadolinium-enhanced MRI is better than nonenhanced MRI at differentiating epidural abscess from the thecal sac, increased confidence in the diagnosis of discitis and osteomyelitis over noncontrast MRI, better localized portions of paraspinal masses most likely to yield a positive percutaneous biopsy, and better distinguished active infections from those that responded adequately to antibiotic therapy (35).

A number of inflammatory processes of bone can involve the cervical spine including ankylosing spondylitis, psoriatic arthritis, and Reiter's disease. The cervical spine is the second most common location for manifestation of rheumatoid arthritis and can lead to direct spinal cord compression at the craniocervical junction (36) due to inflammatory pannus and atlanto-axial instability. Cervical involvement in rheumatoid arthritis occurs late in the disease and effects the synovial atlanto-occipital, atlanto-axial, and uncovertebral joints. Vascular pannus erodes and fragments bone and cartilage leading to possible ligamentous disruption and instability. CT is probably more sensitive to bony erosive changes than MRI, but MRI can detail the extent of inflammatory pannus and its relationship to the cervicomedullary junction (Fig. 7.14) (37). MRI is also helpful at distinguishing changes related to rheumatoid arthritis from those caused by cervical spondylosis (38). Again, T1-weighted images provide the best anatomic detail, while T2-weighted images show increase signal from pannus and joint effusions. T1-weighted gadolinium-enhanced images show increased signal in vascular pannus. MRI findings such as demonstration of cranial migration of the axis and narrowing of the spinal cord diameter to less than 6mm in cervical flexion indicate the need for surgical intervention (39).

Neoplastic Disease

MRI provides an effective diagnostic modality for the direct noninvasive demonstration and localization of primary and secondary neoplasia involving the cervical spine. MRI

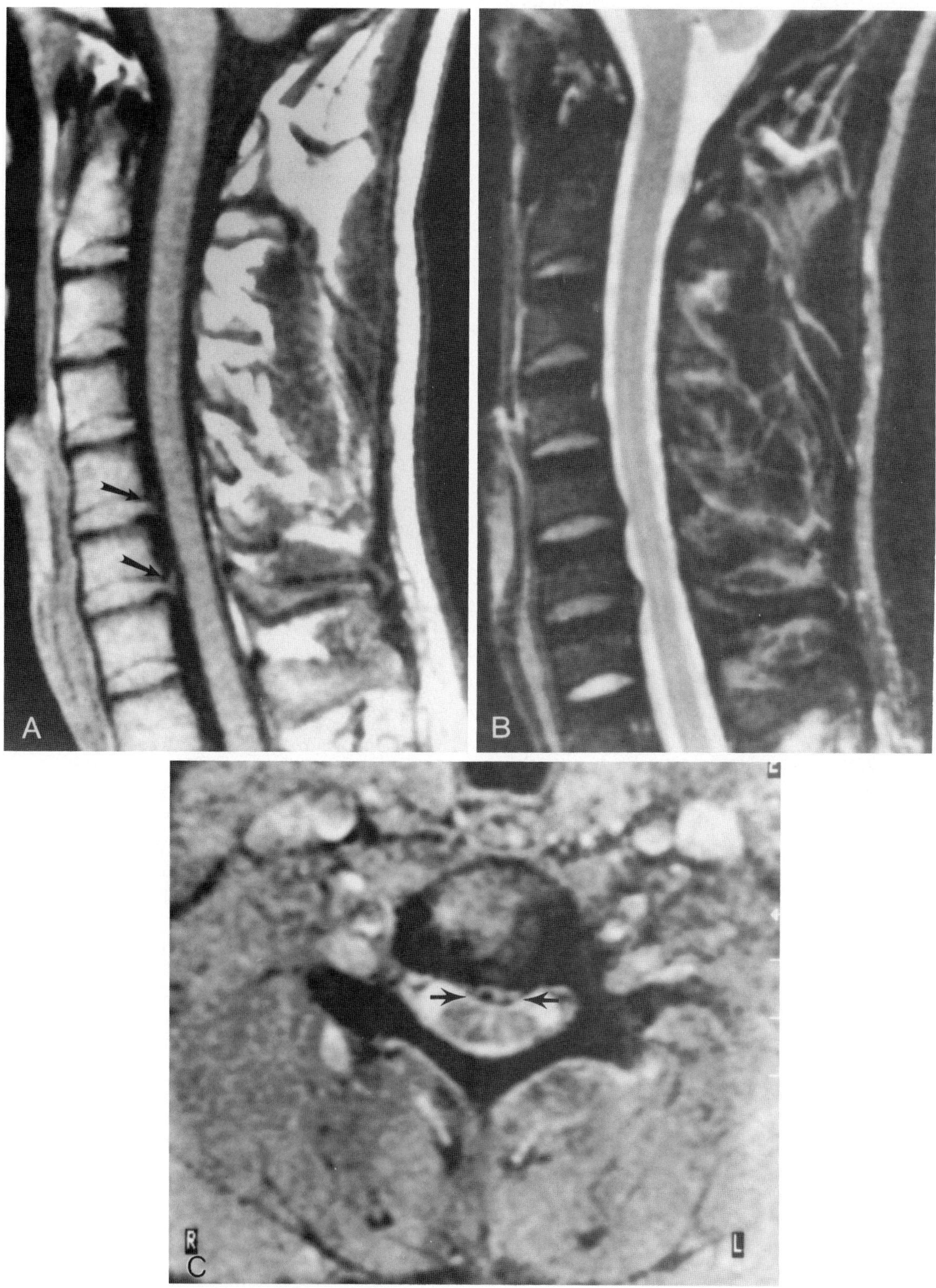

Figure 7.7. MRI multiple disc herniations. **A,** this sagittal T1-weighted spin-echo study shows dorsal disc herniations at C5/6 and C6/7 (*arrows*) in a 40-year-old man who complained of neck pain after an MVA. **B,** this gradient-echo T2-weighted sagittal image shows disc herniations somewhat less well and reveals no direct cord compression or parenchymal signal abnormality. **C,** this axial gradient echo T2-weighted image shows central disc herniation and suggests some flattening of the anterior cord (*arrows*).

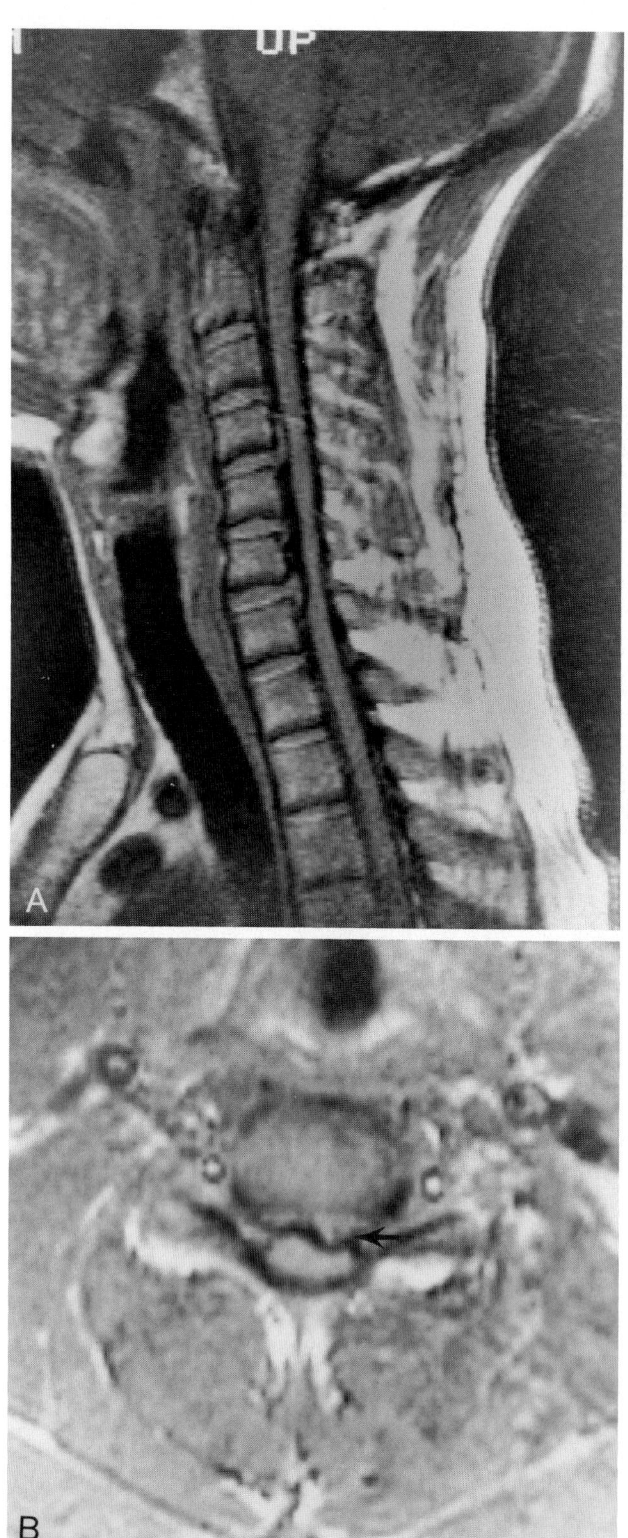

Figure 7.8. MRI of intervertebral disc herniation. **A,** this sagittal T1-weighted spin echo image shows dorsal disc herniations at C3/4 with disk migration, at C5/6 and at C6/7. The cord is most compressed at the C6/7 level. **B,** this axial T1-weighted gradient echo of the same patient through the C6/7 disc level shows lateral disc herniation indenting the cord (*arrow*).

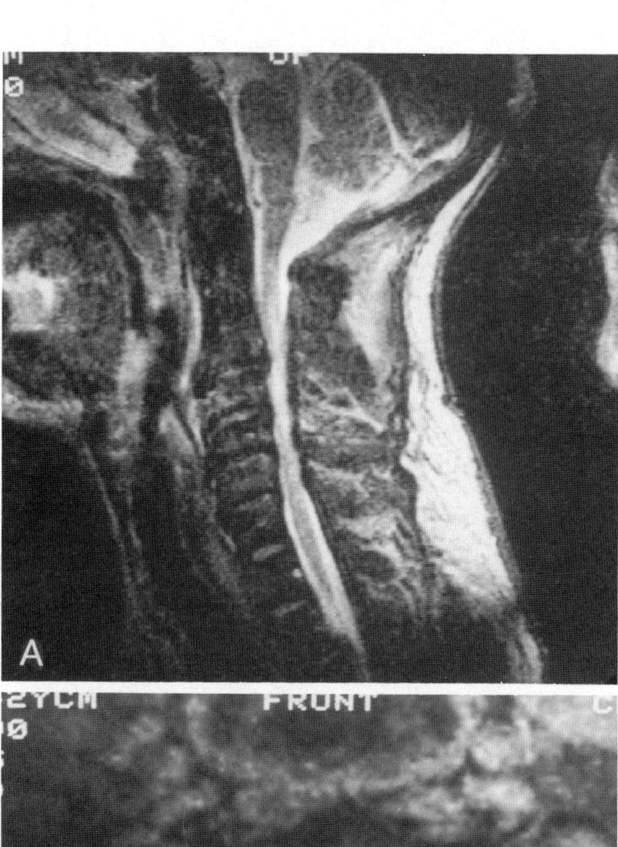

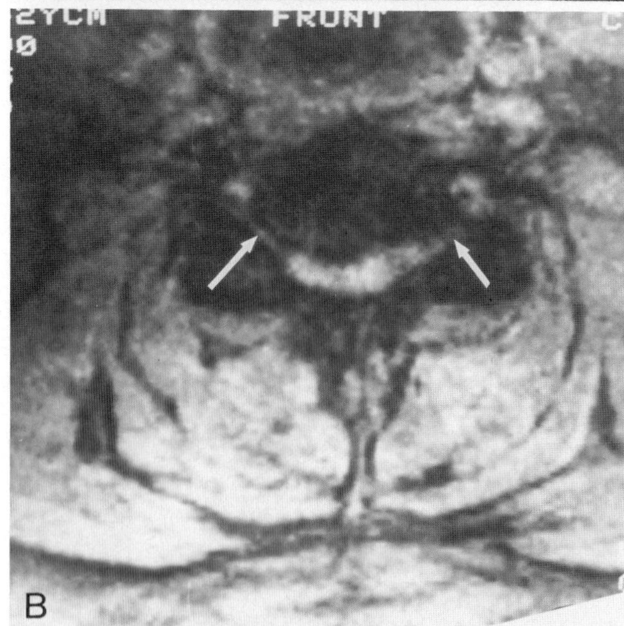

Figure 7.9. MRI of spinal stenosis. **A,** this sagittal T2-weighted spin echo image shows marked compression of the cord at C4 and C5 levels. Faint increased signal in cord represents edema from chronic compression. Note that T2 image tends to be poorer at defining details of anatomy than T1-weighted images. **B,** this axial gradient echo image through the C4/5 level of the same patient reveals marked spinal canal compromise and cord compression. Neural foramen are also severely compromised (*arrows*).

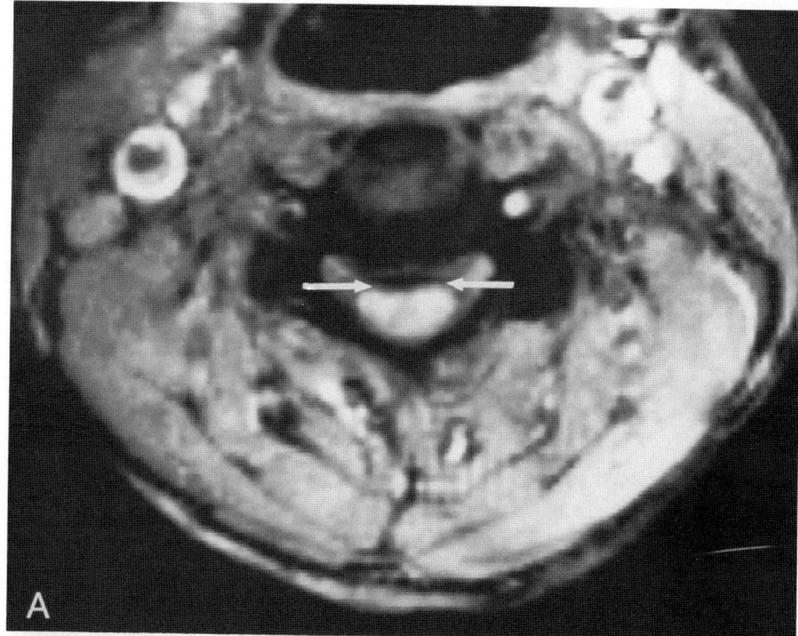

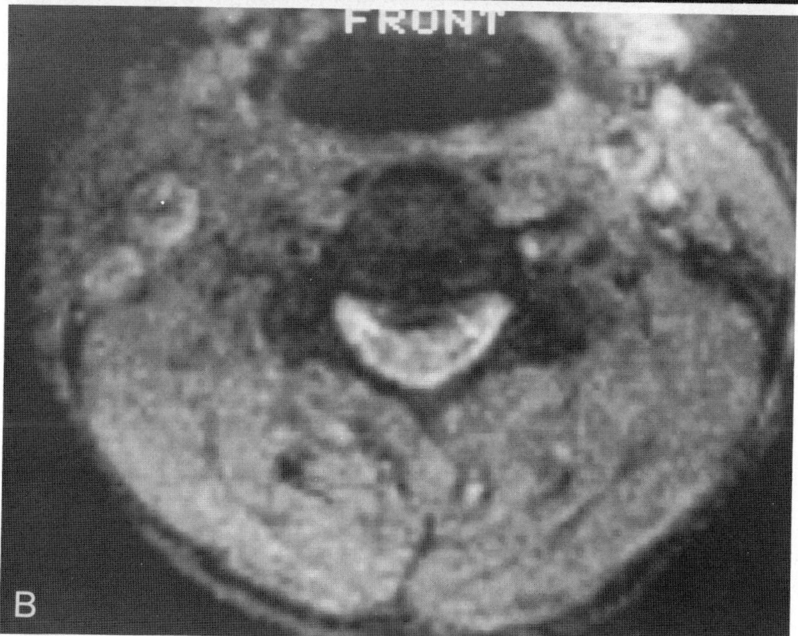

Figure 7.10. MRI of ossified posterior longitudinal ligament. **A,** this axial T1-weighted gradient echo image shows low signal linear structure effacing anterior thecal space (*arrows*). Signal intensity is similar with bone signal. **B,** this axial T2-weighted gradient echo image at the same level better demonstrates compression of cord and obliteration of anterior CSF space. Low signal ossified PLL is again well-visualized.

compares favorably with myelography in demonstrating either intradural or extradural compression of the spinal cord from neoplastic processes but is more accurate at defining the extent of bone and paravertebral soft tissue involvement. MRI can show spinal cord compression without injection of intrathecal contrast material via lumbar puncture, which, in the presence of a complete block, can create CSF pressure shifts that may lead to neurologic deterioration (40). MRI is more sensitive at detecting neoplastic invasion of the spinal cord parenchyma than enhanced-CT with or without intrathecal contrast. Paramagnetic gadolinium agents further enhance MRI's sensitivity in the detection of neoplasia involving the cervical spine. This section will briefly review the MRI appearance of primary and secondary lesions tumors in various locations within the spinal column.

Primary Extradural Tumors

Chordomas, which arise from notochord remnants, are rare spinal tumors, accounting for 3–4% of primary spinal tumors (41). They are quite uncommon in the cervical region per se but often involve the basioccipital region producing myelopathic symptoms. These lesions tend to

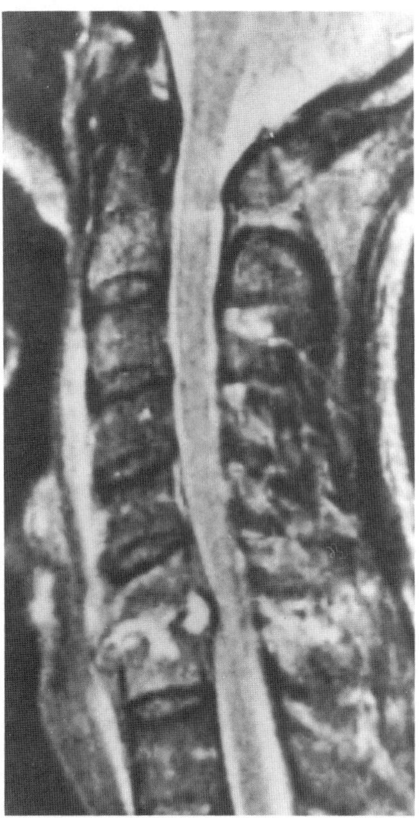

Figure 7.11. MRI of osteomyelitis, discitis, and epidural abscess. This T2-weighted spin echo image shows increased signal in the C6/7 intervertebral disc space with loss of endplate integrity and increased signal in the superior aspect of C7. Note bulging epidural mass at this level corresponding to epidural extension of infection. Increased signal in the prevertebral soft tissue is due to tissue edema.

be expansile and destructive. On MRI, chordomas are usually isointense or hypointense on T1-weighted sequences and hypertintense on T2-weighted studies with internal low signal septa (42). MRI is inferior to CT scan for identifying calcified matrix that typically occurs in these tumors and is less accurate than CT in showing bone destruction.

Hemangiomas are present in 11% of autopsies and histologically are composed of thin-walled vessels or sinusoids lined by endothelium interspersed with thick bone trabeculae and adipose tissue (41). Hemangiomas are most commonly present in the thoracic spine and have a typical plain radiographic appearance of coarsened vertical trabeculae. The MRI appearance is distinctive, demonstrating mottled increased signal due to fat interspersed with bone trabeculae. Extraosseous matrix, when present, displays a lower signal intensity. On T2-weighted sequences both intra- and extraosseous matrix show increased signal intensity, possibly related to the high cellularity of the tumor (43).

Aneurysmal bone cysts (ABC) involve the vertebral column in 20% of cases (40). On MRI they appear as numerous well-defined cystic cavities bounded by a low signal intensity rim and occasionally reveal fluid-fluid levels (44). The MRI appearance of these lesions may be quite complex due to the presence of hemorrhage and blood breakdown products that produce a variety of signal intensities. The MRI appearance is not distinctive and can be mimicked by fibrous dysplasia, malignant fibrous histiocytoma, simple bone cysts, and osteosarcoma, among other lesions.

Secondary Extradural Tumors

Most neoplasms metastasizing to the vertebrae possess a long T1 compared to the T1 of vertebral marrow and for this reason display decreased signal intensity on T1-weighted sequences, appearing dark against the normal marrow intensity (Fig. 7.15). While most neoplasms also have a long T2 time constant, in general, they are less conspicuous relative to normal marrow on T2-weighted sequences. Paramagnetic contrast agents that shorten the T1 of tumors tend to decrease contrast between tumor and normal vertebral marrow, so gadolinium-enhanced T1-weighted images should not be used alone to search for metastatic disease within the spinal column (45). MRI is not specific in characterizing the type of tumor metastasis, which is most commonly from breast, lung, prostate, or lymphoma. MRI can quantify extent of osseous involvement and reveal spinal canal encroachment from extra-osseous spread of disease (Fig. 7.15). Carmody et al. (3) evaluated efficacy of MRI in diagnosing spinal cord compression due to metastatic spinal disease. They found that MRI was 92% sensitive and 90% specific in the diagnosis of epidural metastasis causing spinal cord compression, while myelography was 95% sensitive and 88% specific. For diagnosing extradural metastasis without spinal cord compression MRI was 73% sensitive and 90% specific, versus 49% sensitivity and 88% specificity for myelography. MRI was considerable more sensitive for detection of bone metastasis (90% versus 49%) compared to myelography. Smoker et al. (46) compared MRI with myelography in 22 patients with spinal metastatic disease and found that MRI was more accurate in demonstrating paravertebral tumor extension, additional osseous metastasis, and in evaluating the spinal cord in areas between myelographic blocks. MRI is currently the procedure of choice in evaluating possible metastatic spinal disease.

Intradural-Extramedullary Tumors

Meningioma and nerve sheath tumors together account for about 50% of all adult primary spinal tumors (41). Meningiomas have a four-fold predominance in women, usually present after age 40, and 80% of cases occur in the thoracic spine. Meningiomas also have a predilection for involving the foramen magnum region. Although typically completely intradural, on occasion, meningiomas may be

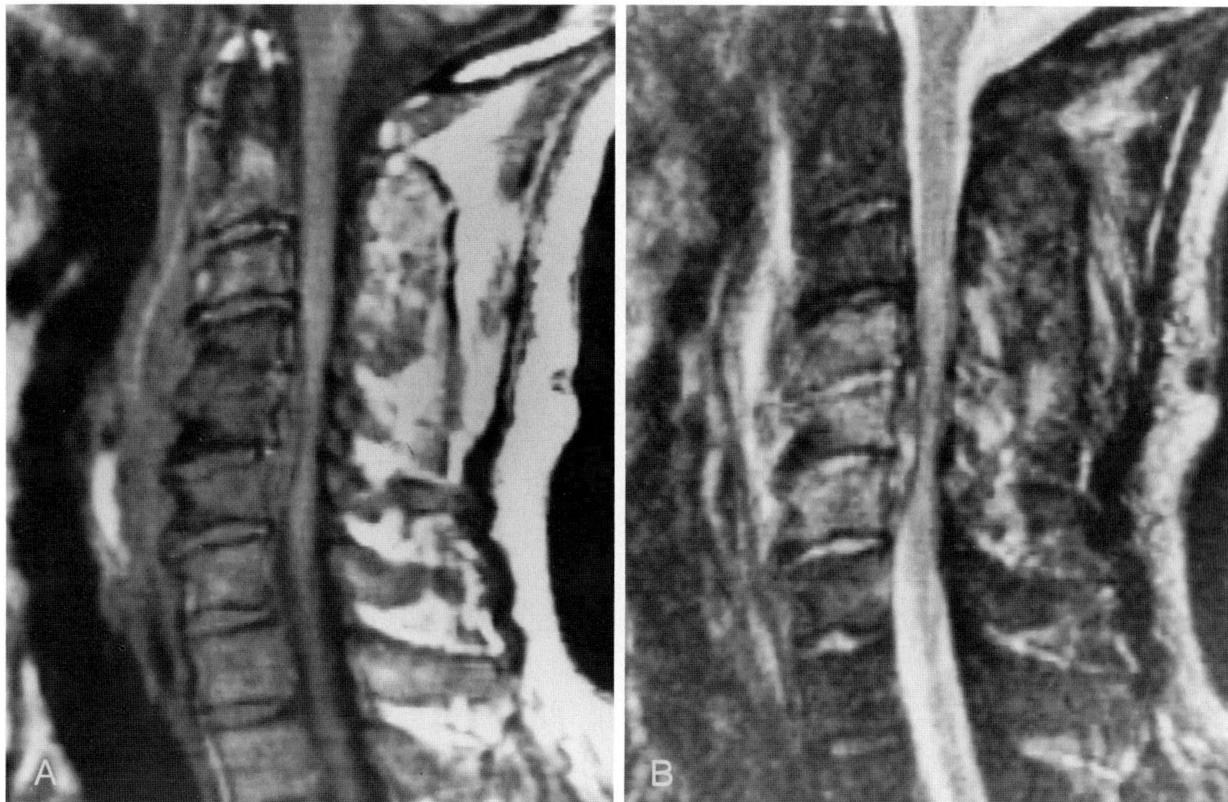

Figure 7.12 MRI of osteomyelitis, discitis, and epidural abscess. **A,** this sagittal T1-weighted spin echo image of a 42-year-old man with Staph. sepsis reveals decreased bone marrow signal in C4, C5, and C6 due to increase edema and replaced fat. There is bulging of the epidural tissues dorsally at these levels due to abscess with cord compression. The precervical tissue are distended by edema. **B,** this T2-weighted spin echo sagittal image of the same patient now shows increased signal in the vertebral bodies and mid-cervical intervertebral discs due to edema. Precervical edema shows increased signal, and there is increased signal due to fluid in the epidural abscess.

completely or partially extradural. On T1-weighted MRI, meningiomas appear as small soft tissue masses that are typically isointense with the spinal cord and displace it. On T2-weighted sequences they are isointense or slightly hyperintense with the spinal cord and are contrasted by high intensity CSF. Gadolinium greatly increases the conspicuity of meningiomas on T1-weighted sequences.

Schwannomas are composed of Schwann cells of peripheral sensory nerves, while neurofibromas are composed of Schwann cells and fibroblasts and occur multiply in patients with neurofibromatosis (41). Schwannomas occur in adults between 20 and 50 and are most frequent in the thoracic region. These tumors are typically completely intradural, but in up to 20% of patients may be partially or completely extradural in location (41). On T1-weighted sequences these tumors are relatively isointense with the spinal cord and are surrounded by lower intensity CSF (Fig. 7.16). On T2-weighted sequences they possess a higher signal then surrounding spinal and paraspinal soft tissues (47). Gadolinium also improves detection of lesions on T1-weighted sequences.

A number of tumors may metastasize to the intradural, extramedullary space including primary CNS tumors such as ependymoma, blioblastoma, and medulloblastoma, pineal tumors, and choriod plexus papillomas. Extra-CNS tumors such as breast or lung carcinoma and lymphoma, among others, also are potential sources of intradural lesions. Again, in general, gadolinium contrast agents increase the conspicuity of these lesions on T1-weighted sequences. Intradural, extramedullary lesions can cause syringomyelic cavitation within the cord secondary to obstruction of normal CSF flow dynamics (48).

Intramedullary Tumors

MRI is the procedure of choice in evaluating patients suspected of having intramedullary tumors, because of the ability to image the parenchyma directly, rather than on relying on cord expansion along. Ependymoma and astrocytoma constitute about 90% of intrinsic spinal cord tumors. Ependymomas are more typical in adults and usually occur in the conus region, but a significant number are

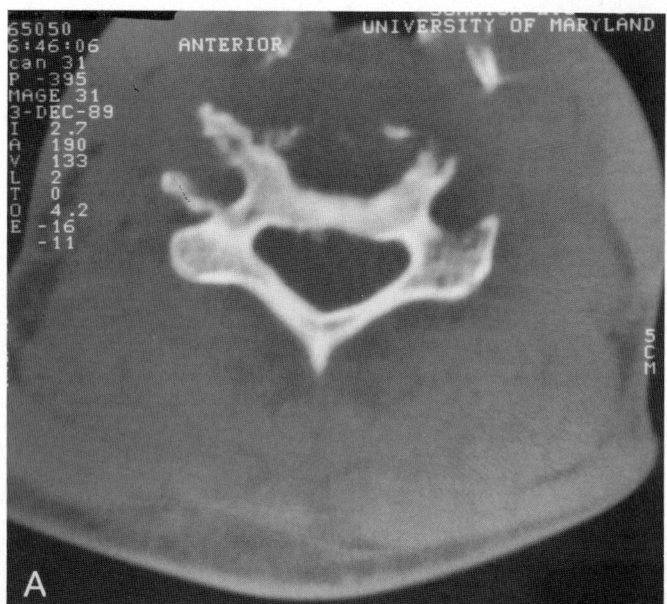

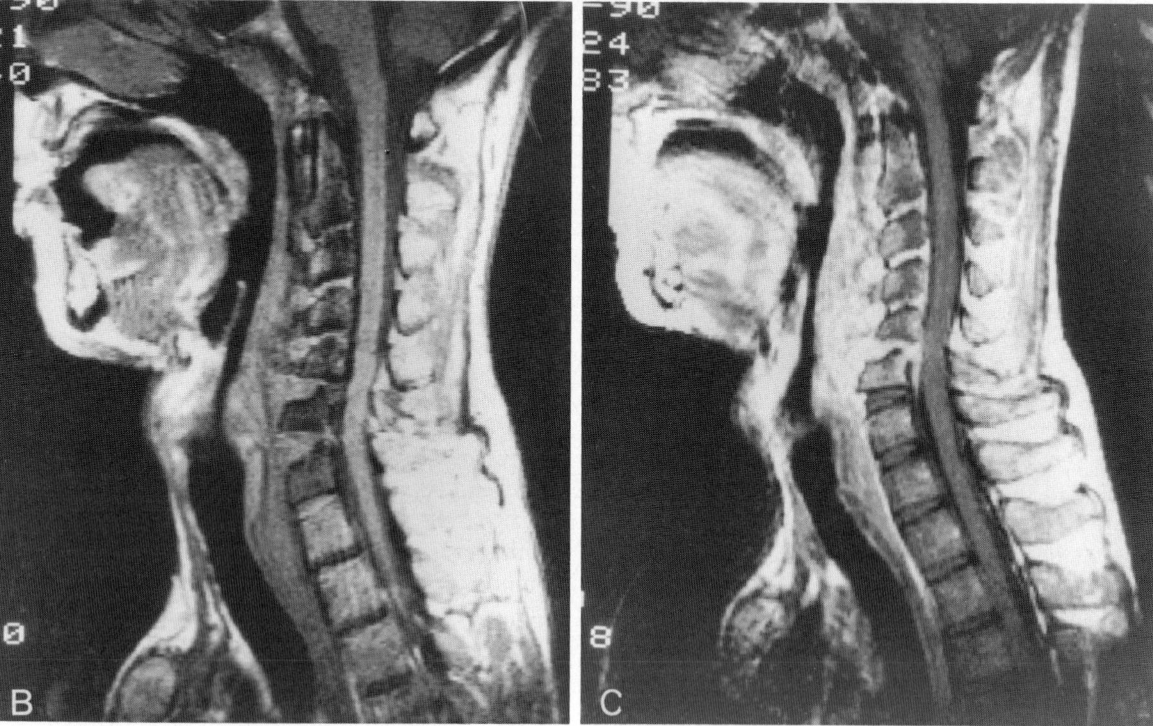

Figure 7.13. MRI of diffuse cervical osteomyelitis, discitis, and epidural abscess formation. **A,** CT image of the C5 level in patient with history of IV drug abuse using cervical injections complaining of neck pain, dysphagia, and fever shows destruction of the anterior aspect of the vertebral body and precervical soft tissue swelling. **B,** this sagittal T1-weighted MR image reveals multiple areas of decreased signal from C2 through C7 with destruction of the anterior superior aspects of C4, C5, and C6. There is marked precervical edema. Loss of bone marrow fat signal is due to infiltration with edema. **C,** this sagittal T2-weighted image shows increased signal in the vertebral bodies and intervertebral discs throughout the cervical region. There is marked precervical swelling partially compressing the airway. Also, there is effacement of the anterior cervical subarachnoid space. Percutaneous biopsy showed Staphylococcus infection that responded to long-term antibiotics.

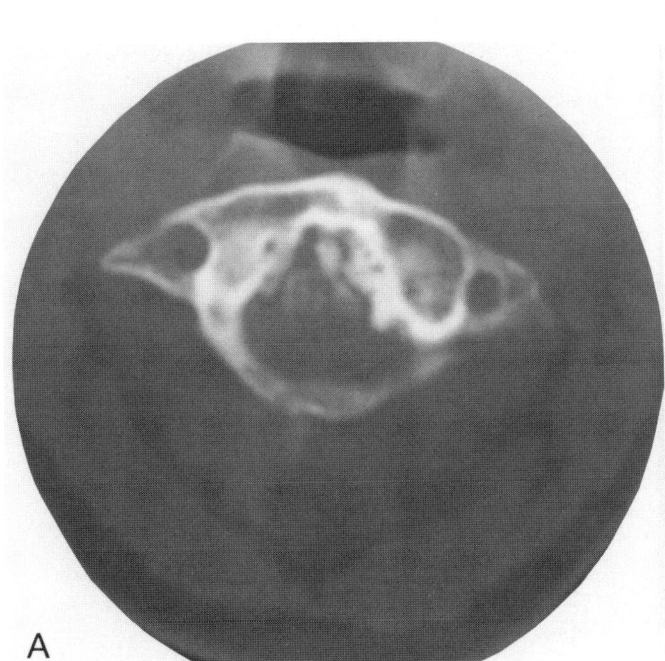

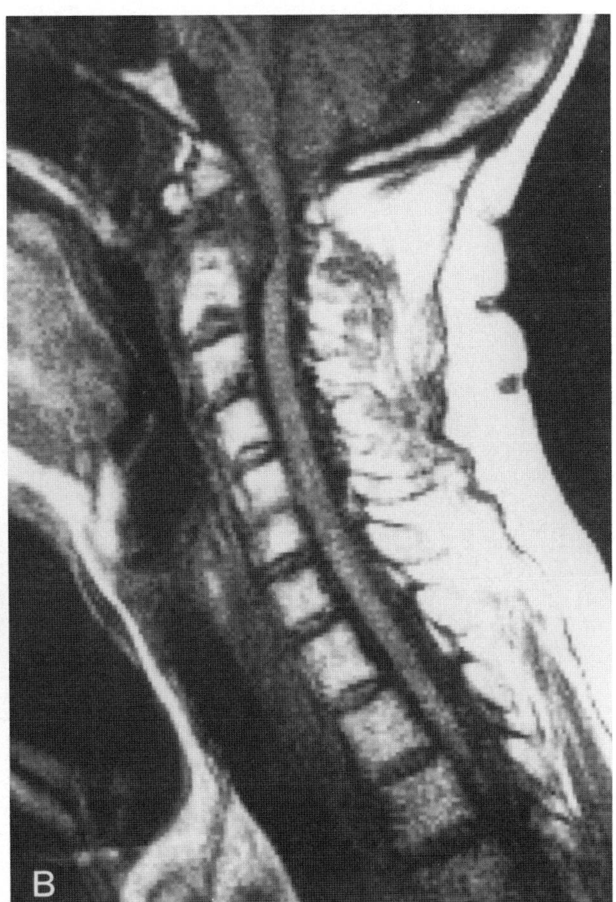

Figure 7.14. CT and MRI of cervical rheumatoid arthritis. **A,** CT scan through upper cervical spine in elderly women who developed cervical myelopathy after trauma reveals bony fragments and sclerosis involving the apical portion of the odontoid process. These findings are strongly suggestive of rheumatoid disease. **B,** T1-weighted mid-sagittal image reveals soft tissue mass indenting anterior cord at the level of the odontoid process. This is inflammatory pannus caused by rheumatoid disease. (From: Mirvis SE, Wolf A. Emerging MRI role: assessing cervical spine trauma. MRI Decisions 1990;4:21–31.)

also seen in the cervical spine (49). Astrocytomas are more common in the cevicothoracic region and are more frequent in children. On T1-weighted MR images both tumors lead to fusiform enlargement of the cord over one or more segments and demonstrate a slight decreased signal relative to the normal cord. On T2-weighted sequences both tumors show extensive areas of increased signal representing both neoplastic issue and edema. Cystic cavitation occurs in 38% of astrocytomas (Fig. 7.17) and 46% of ependymomas (Fig. 7.18) (50). Smooth contour cysts may extend rostral and/or caudal to the tumor, are typically non-neoplastic with gliotic linings, and contain fluid similar to CSF signal intensity (Figs. 7.17–7.19). These cysts are noncommunicating and contain fluid with an elevated protein content. MRI readily differentiates between the solid and cystic components of tumor better than myelography or CT (49). MRI, particularly with gadolinium enhancement, is more advantageous than CT in selecting the most appropriate biopsy site(s). Cysts developing within neoplastic masses are lined by abnormal glia and are filled with xanthochromic fluid or blood displaying different signal characteistics than CSF.

Hemangioblastoma is a rare spinal cord tumor that has a predilection for the cervicothoracic and thoracolumbar junctions (50). The tumors may be isolated or multiple and are usually associated with posterior fossa tumors occurring with von Hipple-Lindau disease. These tumors present as intramedullary cysts containing a vascular nidus. On T1-weighted images the cystic component has a low signal but a high signal on T2-weighted sequences (Fig. 7.19). The soft tissue nidus enhances markedly on T1-weighted images with gadolinium. Serpiginous "flow voids" related to enlarged feeding vessels may be seen in proximity to the vascular nidus (Fig. 7.19).

Metastatic disease may produce intramedullary involvement either secondary to leptomeningeal seeding as with glioma or medulloblastoma or via a hematogenous route such as with melanoma, adenocarcinoma, or lymphoma.

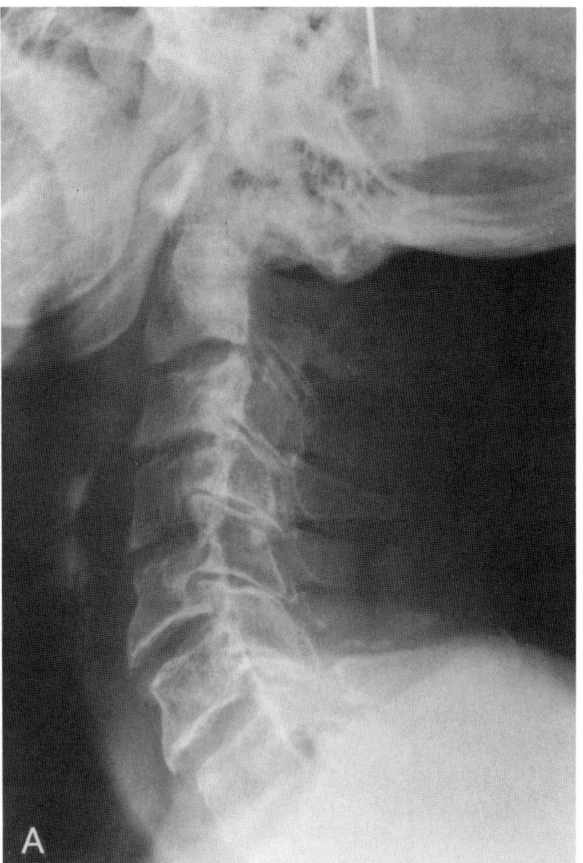

Figure 7.15. MRI of spinal metastatic disease. **A,** lateral cervical radiograph in elderly man with known metastatic lung carcinoma is essentially unremarkable. **B,** this sagittal T1-weighted MR image shows multiple foci of replaced bone marrow involving C2, C3, C4, and C7. Loss of signal involves both the vertebral bodies and posterior elements. Also note loss of marrow signal at T5 level indicating metastasis. **C,** T1-weighted axial image through the C3 level shows marked bony destruction (*arrows*) that was not appreciated radiographically. Tumor is encroaching upon the right thecal space (*arrowhead*).

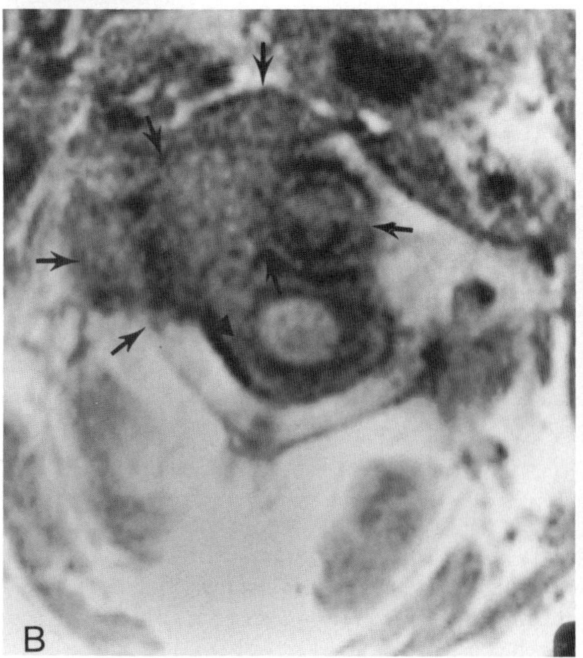

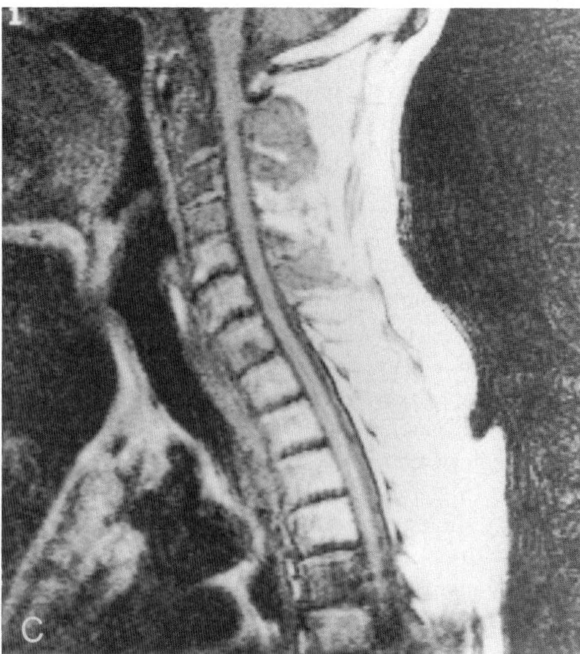

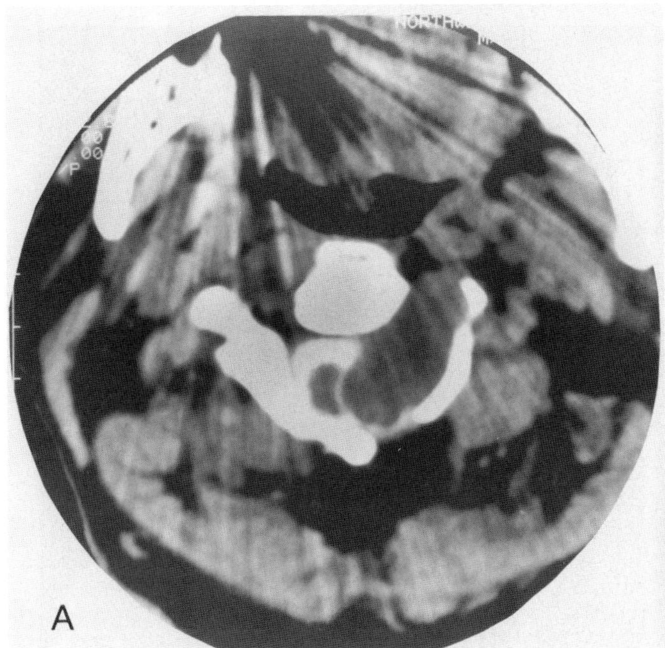

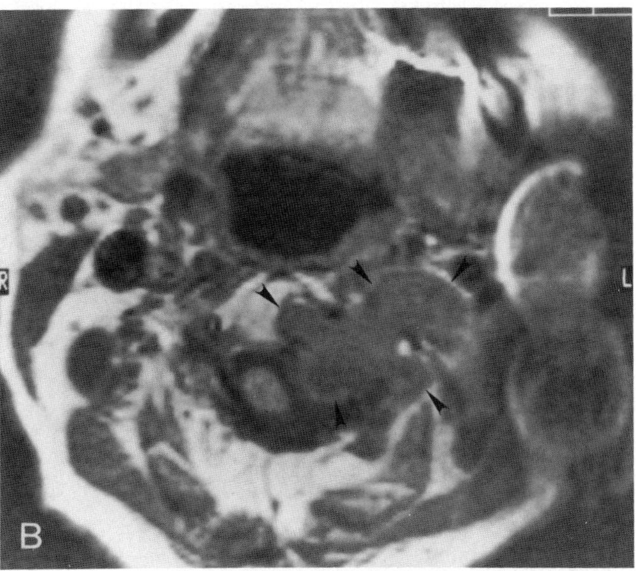

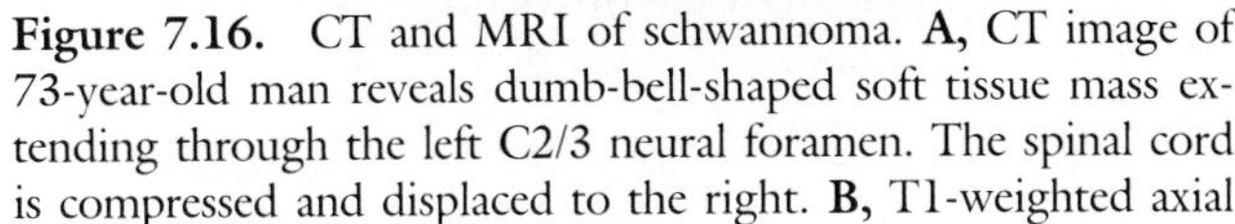
Figure 7.16. CT and MRI of schwannoma. **A,** CT image of 73-year-old man reveals dumb-bell-shaped soft tissue mass extending through the left C2/3 neural foramen. The spinal cord is compressed and displaced to the right. **B,** T1-weighted axial spin-echo image shows intermediate signal intensity mass (*arrowheads*) with intra- and extradural extension displacing spinal cord to the right and invading vertebral body. Neural foramen is significantly widened by surgically proven schwannoma.

On T1-weighted MRI the cord appears enlarged with metastases having a lower signal intensity than the normal cord. Tumor enhances to a greater extent than the normal cord on T1-weighted studies with gadolinium, and metastatic foci are increased in signal on T2-weighted images relative to the normal cord. Metastatic lesions may be confused with post-irradiation myelitis that develops in 2–3% of patients. Radiation myelitis occurs after 3300 rads over greater than 10 cm of cord or 4300 rads over less than 10 cm of cord and presents 6–12 months after treatment with a gradual onset of myelopathy at or below the treatment level (51). Tissue diagnosis may, on occasion, be required to differentiate between residual tumor and radiation necrosis.

Other inflammatory lesions, such as multiple sclerosis and transverse myelitis can present as focal areas of increase signal in the cord on T2-weighted sequences. However, these can be reliably differentiated from tumors on the basis of lack of significant cord expansion and relative lack of enhancement following Gd-DTPA administration. Acute multiple sclerosis plaques and regions of transverse myelitis will often enhance with Gd-DTPA, but can usually on clinical grounds be distinguished from tumors. In some cases, follow-up studies maybe required.

Postoperative Evaluation with MRI

Anterior decompression with bone graft fusion is most commonly performed for symptomatic single level intervertebral disk herniation, while multilevel laminectomy is required for multilevel spinal stenosis due to herniated disc and/or posterior osteophtyes. MRI is valuable to demonstrate the position of an anterior graft and the degree of restoration of canal patency (Figs. 7.20 and 7.21). The graft signal is determined by the acquisition site, the relative amount of cortical and cancellous bone, the state of the marrow, and trauma and edema related to harvesting (31). There are no definitive MRI findings to indicate graft fusion or stability. A homogeneous high signal from vertebral bodies and graft with no visible disc space usually indicates fusion, but the lack of this appearance does not indicate nonunion (31). The extent of spinal canal decompression and dorsal migration of the spinal cord following multilevel laminectomy can also be well assessed with MRI (Fig. 7.22). As discussed below, MRI can be used to assess posterior fusion, but is subject to significant artifact arising from stainless steel wire. This artifact is substantially decreased using titantium internal fixation plates and wires (15).

Following discectomy or chymopapain injection signal alterations similar to discitis occur in that the vertebral endplates show low signal on T1 and high signal on T2-weighted images. However, unlike discitis, the disc space signal remains decreased on both T1- and T2-weighted sequences. The signal alterations in the adjacent vertebral endplates may reflect ischemia or a sterile inflammatory process (49).

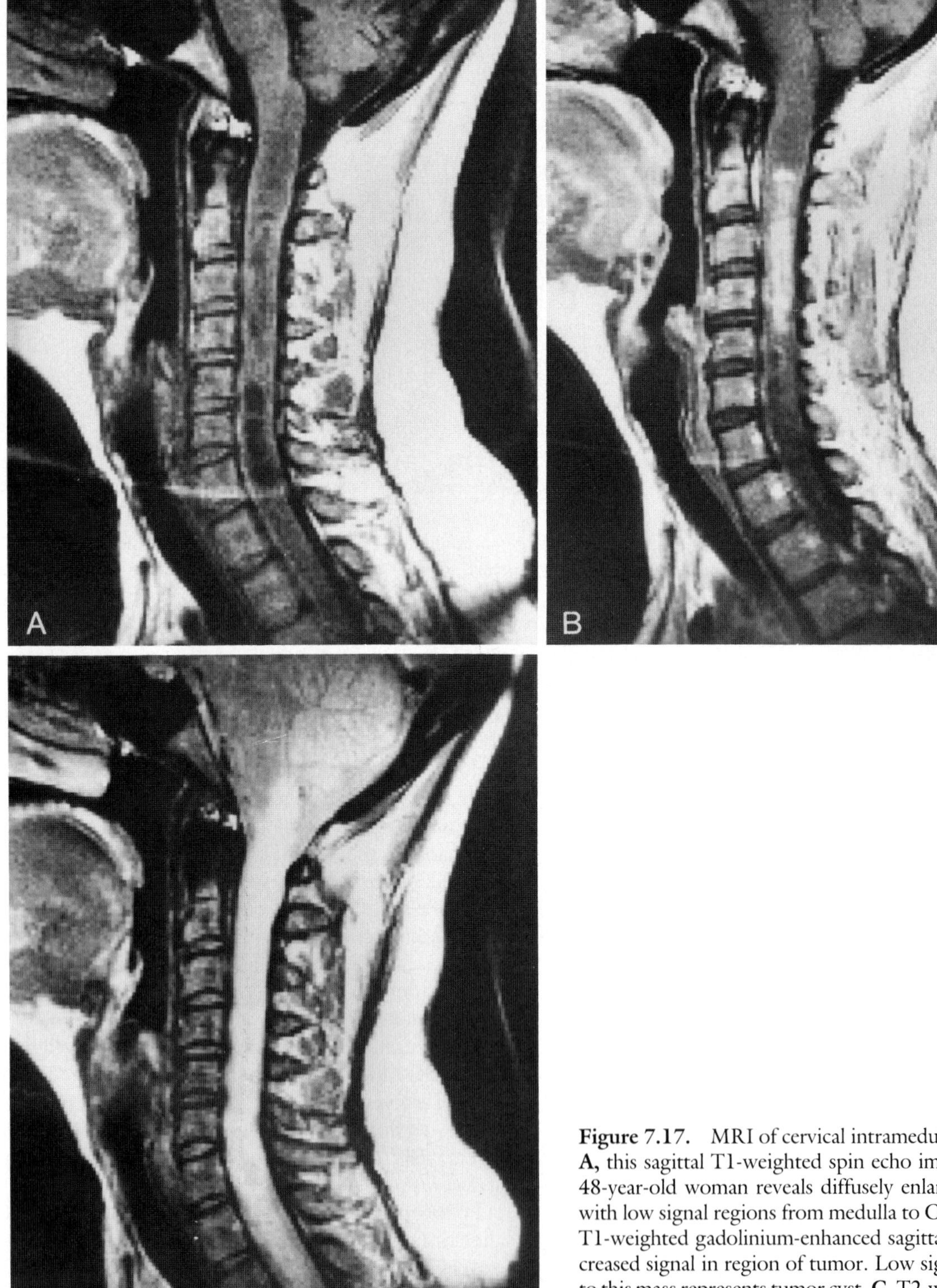

Figure 7.17. MRI of cervical intramedullary astrocytoma. **A,** this sagittal T1-weighted spin echo image obtained in a 48-year-old woman reveals diffusely enlarged cervical cord with low signal regions from medulla to C7/T1 level. **B,** this T1-weighted gadolinium-enhanced sagittal study shows increased signal in region of tumor. Low signal region caudal to this mass represents tumor cyst. **C,** T2-weighted spin echo sequence shows extensive increase in cord signal from medulla to T2 level due to edema.

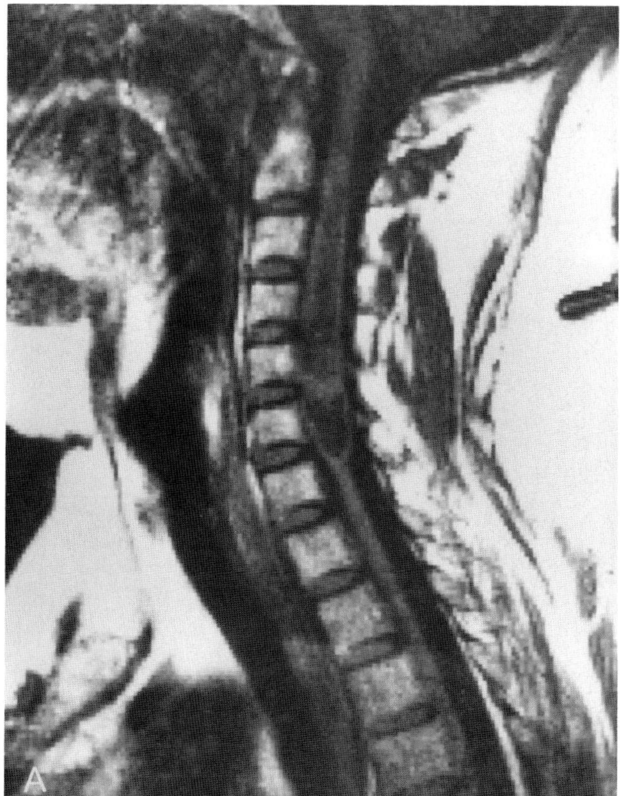

Figure 7.18. MRI of cervical ependymoma. **A,** this sagittal T1-weighted spin echo image obtained in a 52-year-old man shows marked cervical cord distension from C2 to C6 with low signal regions. **B,** this T1-weighted gadolinium-enhanced spin echo sequence shows increased signal in area of tumor. Tumor cysts extend rostrally and caudally from this mass.

MRI of Traumatic Cervical Pathology

Acute Injury

MRI has been utilized only relatively recently for the examination of patients with acute injury resulting from cervical spine trauma (9, 12, 13, 52). Initial studies using MRI for this application have demonstrated several advantages over plain CT or CT with intrathecal contrast including: *a*) the capacity to visualize the cervical soft tissues with greater contrast discrimination, *b*) the ability to directly image ligamentous injuries and acutely or chronically herniated intervertebral discs, *c*) the capacity to directly image the spinal canal in any orientation desired to enhance lesion detection, *d*) the ability to create "myelographic-equivalent" images using T2-weighted signal acquisition sequences to better evaluate the extent of spinal canal compromise from bone fragments, osteophytes, herniated disc material, and/or epidural hematoma, and *e*) the unique capability to directly image damage to the spinal cord parenchyma including edema, hemorrhage, myelomalacia, laceration, and synrix formation. In addition, MRI may provide unique prognostic information concerning potential for neurologic recovery. Application of MRI in acute cervical spine trauma eliminates many of the technical problems inherent in the use of CT-myelography. CT image quality is often compromised in the lower cervical region, especially in large or obese patients. Instilled intrathecal contrast may layer posteriorly in the supine patient and fail to adequately outline the extent of the ventral subarachnoid space. Complete blockage of the upper cervical canal prevents flow of contrast into the lower canal necessitating lumbar contrast instillation — dangerous in patients with mechanically unstable cervical spine injuries. Administration of intrathecal contrast into the upper cervical spine requires a C1–C2 puncture, which may be difficult to perform in an uncooperative patient and can lead to iatrogenic complications (53, 54). MRI can evaluate the entire cervical spine directly, while CT would require an excessive number of contiguous or overlapping axial images to cover the entire cervical region.

Some technical limitations currently must be faced when performing MRI in critically ill patients and/or those with potentially unstable cervical spine injuries. These patients may require extensive physiologic support and monitoring equipment including pulmonary catheter pressure measurements, pulse oximetry, finely regulated intravenous in-

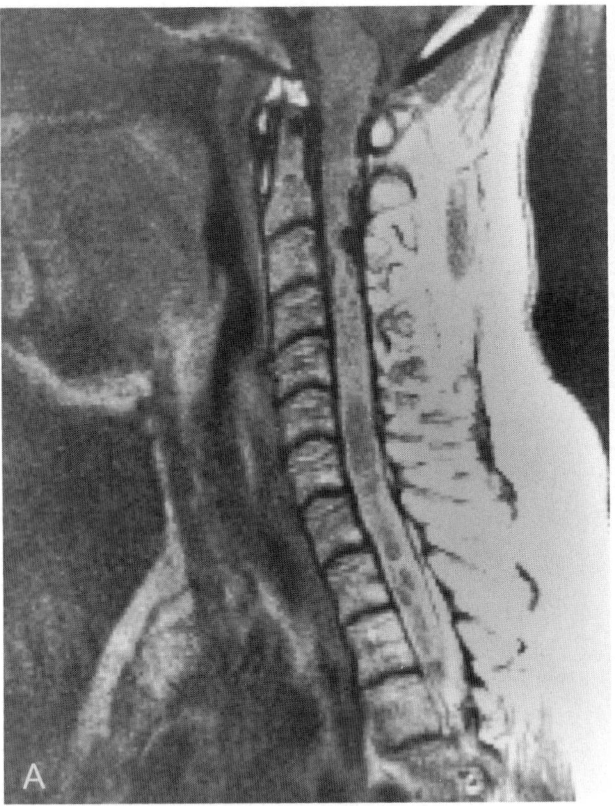

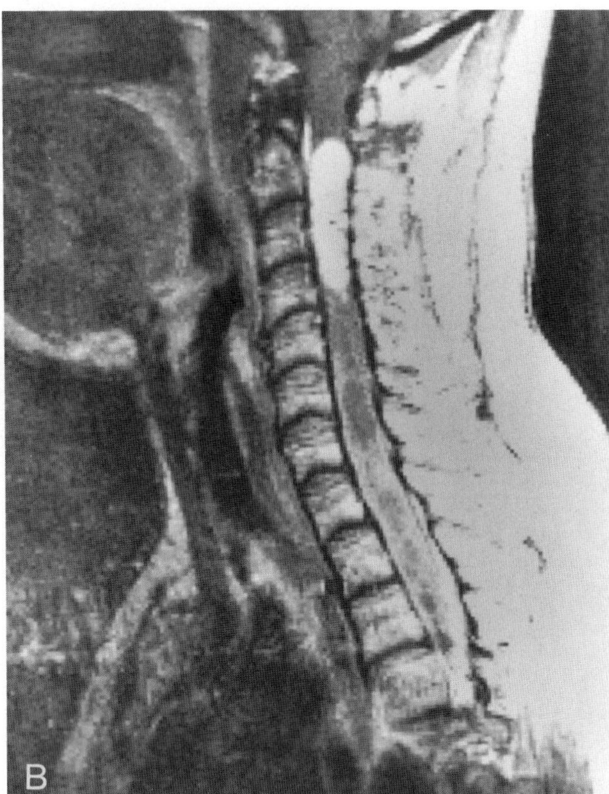

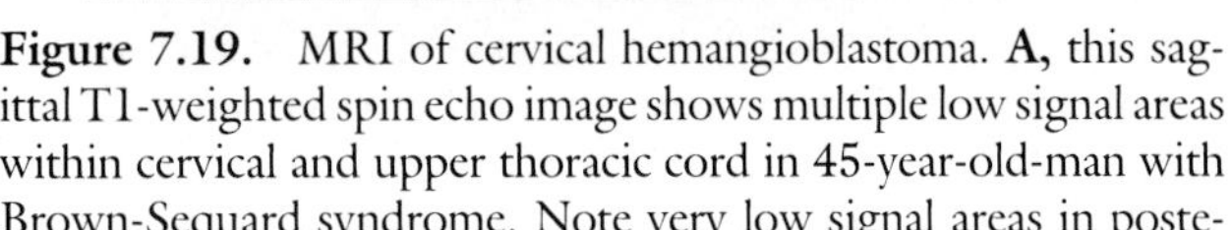
Figure 7.19. MRI of cervical hemangioblastoma. **A,** this sagittal T1-weighted spin echo image shows multiple low signal areas within cervical and upper thoracic cord in 45-year-old-man with Brown-Sequard syndrome. Note very low signal areas in posterior aspect of cord at C2/C3 level suggestive of flow-void in dilated vessels. **B,** this sagittal T1-weighted gadolinium-enhanced image shows tumor mass with caudal tumor cysts.

fusions such as vasopressors, and respiratory support. These devices may interfere with high quality image acquisition and are not guaranteed to function properly in the magnetic fringe field in close proximity to the magnet. When required, we have found that ventilatory support can be provided in the MR suite using a Siemens SV-900 C servo ventilator (Siemens-Elema, Iselin, NJ) placed at least 1.2 m from the magnet (14). A 12-ft (11m), low compliance pediatric circuit connects the ventilator to the patient's endotracheal or tracheostomy tube. This system provides all standard modes of respiratory support without detectible deterioration in image quality.

MR imaging times are relatively long as compared to CT, and patient motion must be restricted, which may be difficult for patients in severe pain or in those with impaired cognitive function. It is anticipated that application of ultra-fast imaging sequences, improved motion suppression techniques, and improved surface coil designs will all contribute to higher quality cervical spine MRI examinations in considerably shorter imaging times (16–18) than is generally available currently.

Some patients require cervical immobilization with or without maintained traction. In our center, most patients are immobilized in a rigid cervical Philadelphia collar (Philadelphia Collar Co, Westville, NJ) with plastic fasteners for the MRI examination. Clayman et al. have studied a variety of cervical spine braces (halo fixation) for MR compatibility (55). They noted that orthoses which contain electrically conductive loops were unsatisfactory, since the fluctuating magnetic field created by gradient coils induce "eddy" current within these conductive loops which in turn produced local magnetic field inhomogeneity causing alteration in the frequencies and phases of precessing protons and signal loss. They found that aluminum or graphite carbon composite components interconnected with plastic ball and socket joints were most successful at eliminating artifact. Two cervical immobilization devices which permitted acceptable MR image quality included a PMT halo cervical orthoses (PMT Corporation, Chanhassen, MN) and an MR-compatible Bremer halo system (Bremer Medical Corporation, Jacksonville, FL). Alternatively, appropriately placed splits in a nonferromagnetic halo device would also serve to eliminate eddy current induction (55).

In some patients cervical traction immobilization is required to maintain adequate reduction during imaging. If necessary, in-line cervical traction can be achieved via either

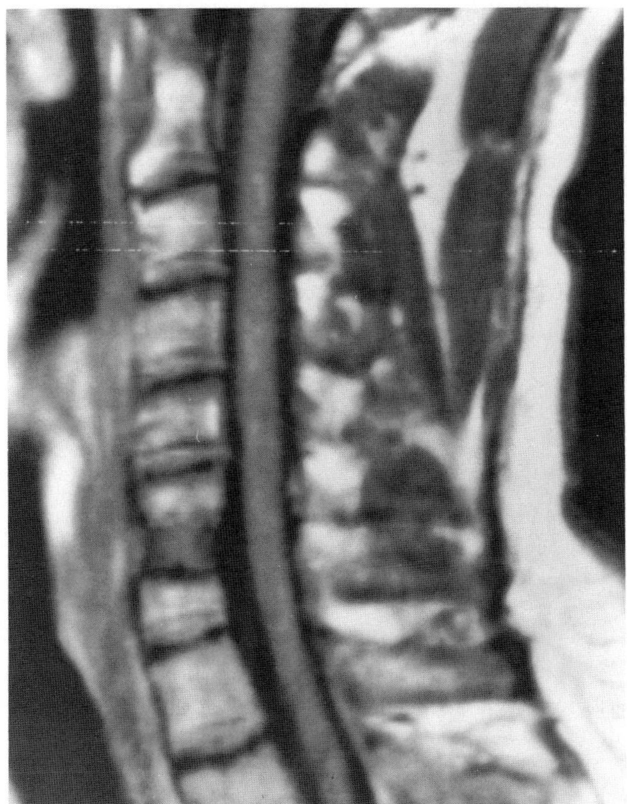

Figure 7.20. MRI of anterior decompression and bone graft fusion. This sagittal T1-weighted image obtained in 42-year-old-man after anterior decompression of herniated nucleus pulposis shows intermediate signal bone plug and confirms successful decompression of anterior thecal space.

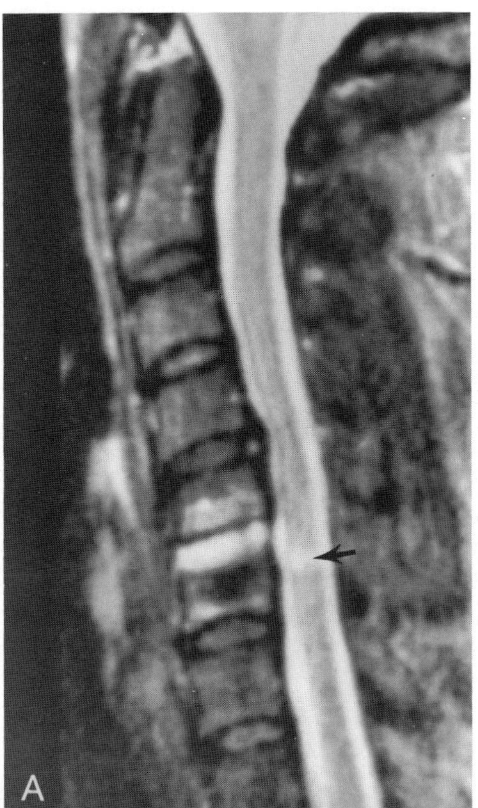

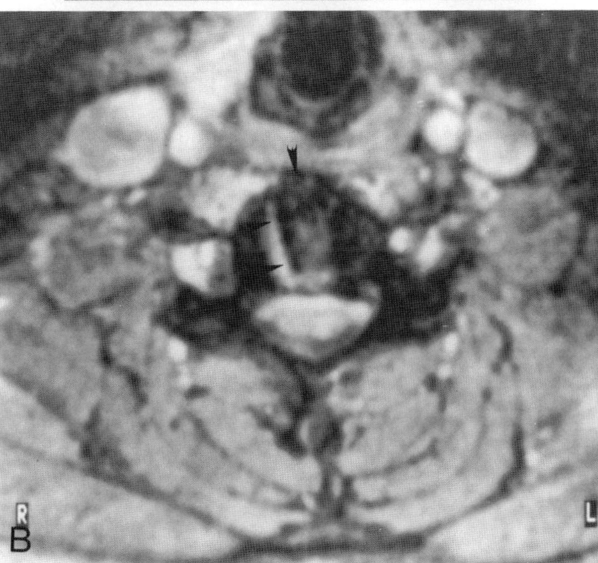

Figure 7.21. MRI of anterior bone graft fusion. **A,** this T2-weighted sagittal image was acquired in 43-year-old woman after discectomy at the C5/6 level. Bone graft at C5/6 shows increased signal probably due to edema. A posterior osteophyte indents the cord at the C4/5 level. The patient had developed urinary incontinence after surgery, and a focal area of contusion is observed in the cord just below the C5/6 interspace (*arrow*). **B,** this axial T2-weighted gradient echo image shows bone plug placement (*arrowheads*) with surrounding edema. The spinal canal appears decompressed, but increased signal in the cord indicates edema (contusion).

MRI-compatible graphite traction tongs and a series of nonferrous pulleys and water bags (56) or by using a Sokhoff board and plastic traction weights. The authors have performed some cervical MRI examinations using a commercially available nonferrous traction-immobilizer (TACIT device, Minto Research and Development, Redding, CA). However, this device places the cervical spine at a greater distance from the surface coil receiver, resulting in a decrease in the signal to noise ratio in the anterior cervical region compromising image quality. The ideal cervical immobilizer would combine MR-compatibility and low electron density to permit artifact-free CT imaging as well.

Acute Cervical Spine Pathology: Indications for MRI

MRI is indicated in the evaluation of patients sustaining neurologic deficits after cervical spine injury when permitted by the patient's overall clinical status. Typically, patients with acute cervical spine injury will initially receive cervical radiographs to evaluate for the presence of fractures and/or cervical dislocation. In many situations, cer-

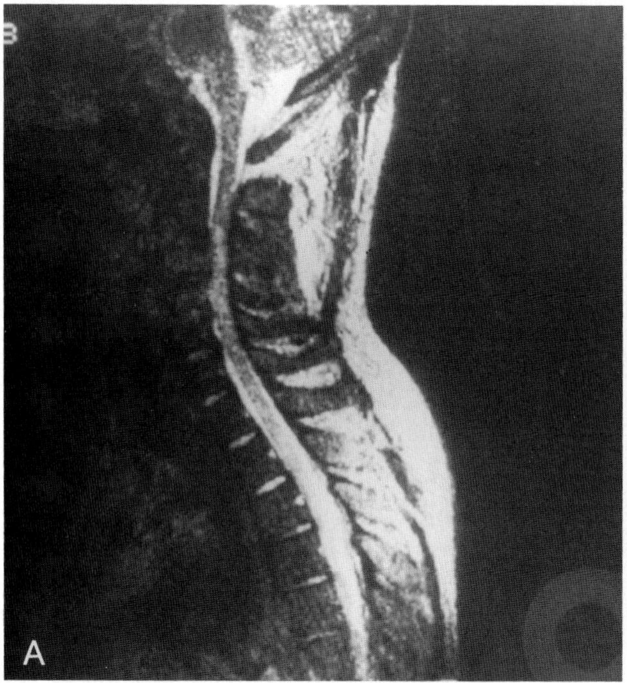

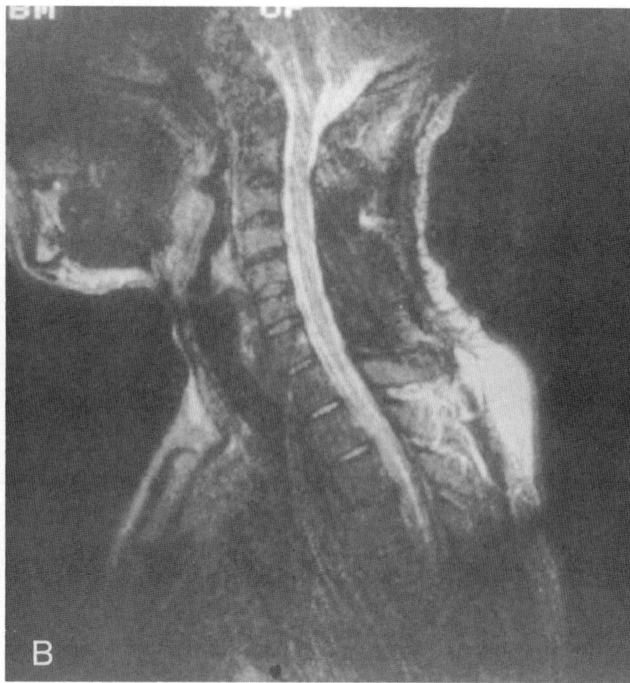

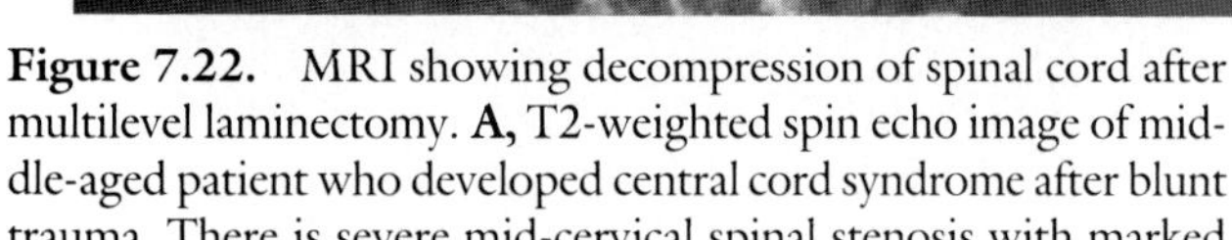

Figure 7.22. MRI showing decompression of spinal cord after multilevel laminectomy. **A,** T2-weighted spin echo image of middle-aged patient who developed central cord syndrome after blunt trauma. There is severe mid-cervical spinal stenosis with marked cord compression. **B,** Sagittal T2-weighted image performed after C2 through C7 laminectomy reveals excellent decompression of the spinal canal with restoration of the subarachnoid space.

Table 7.2. Acute Pathology Detected by Cervical MRI

Spinal cord contusion (predominantly nonhemorrhagic)
Spinal cord hematoma (predominantly hemorrhagic contusion)
Spinal cord laceration/transection
Spinal stenosis (congenital and acquired)
Ligament strain or interruption
Intervertebral disk disruption/herniation
Epidural hematoma
Fractures (particularly vertebral body)
Malalignment of vertebral bodies, facets
Paracervial soft tissue edema, hemorrhage
Cervical arterial disruption

vical CT may also be utilized to better define anatomic details of osseous injury that may not be easily diagnosed by plain radiographs. In most situations, information derived from radiographs and CT is sufficient to plan appropriate management, surgical or nonsurgical. In our center, MRI is performed in nearly all patients with *incomplete* neurologic deficits related to cervical spinal cord injury if the patient is hemodynamically stable and has no contraindication to MRI examination. Imaging is performed only after realignment of the spine has been effected by traction. MRI can best assess the patency of the thecal sac and detect the presence, location, and nature of any lesions compressing the spinal cord (see below) after reduction. Patients with cervical cord deficits after trauma, but with no injury detected by radiography or CT, should also be evaluated by MRI. In patients with cervical radiculopathy after trauma, MRI is used to detect the presence of nerve root compression within the intervertebral neural foramina or nerve root avulsion. MRI is also be performed in patients who manifest delayed progression of an initially stable neurologic deficit as well as those whose osseous injury does not correspond to the neurologic deficit. We do not perform MRI in patients who have cervical spine injury but who are neurologically intact.

MRI Appearance of Acute Cervical Spine Injury

Table 7.2 summarizes the types of acute cervical spine injuries that may be detected by MRI. Table 7.3 reviews the typical expected imaging characteristics of spinal cord hemorrhage on both T1- and T2-weighted sequences in the acute, subacute, and chronic phase after injury.

Cord contusions, that are predominantly nonhemorrhagic, appear isointense or hypointense to normal spinal cord parenchyma on T1-weighted spin echo sequences and hyperintense on balanced and T2-weighted sequences (Figs. 7.23 and 7.24). When significant hemorrhage is present within a contusion, its appearance on MRI depends largely on the chemical state of the hemoglobin molecule and thus

Table 7.3. Imaging Characteristics of Spinal Cord Hemorrhage

Time to initial imaging after trauma	T2-weighted signal	T1-weighted signal	Reason for signal intensity change
Acute hemorrhage: <24 hr	Decreased	Isointense or hypointense	Local heterogeneity of magnetic susceptibility; preferential T2 shortening due to intracellular deoxyhemoglobin
Subacute hemorrhage: >4 hr to 3–4 wk	Increased (lags T1 increase)	Increased	Paramagnetic effect of extracellular methemoglobin preferential T1 shortening
Chronic hemorrhage: >3–4 wk	Increased	Decreased	Myelomalacia or posttraumatic cyst; cystic regions often mimic CSF intensity patterns (predominantly free water).

CSF = Cerebrospinal fluid.
From Mirvis SE, Wolf A. MRI Decisions. PW Communications International 1990;4:23.

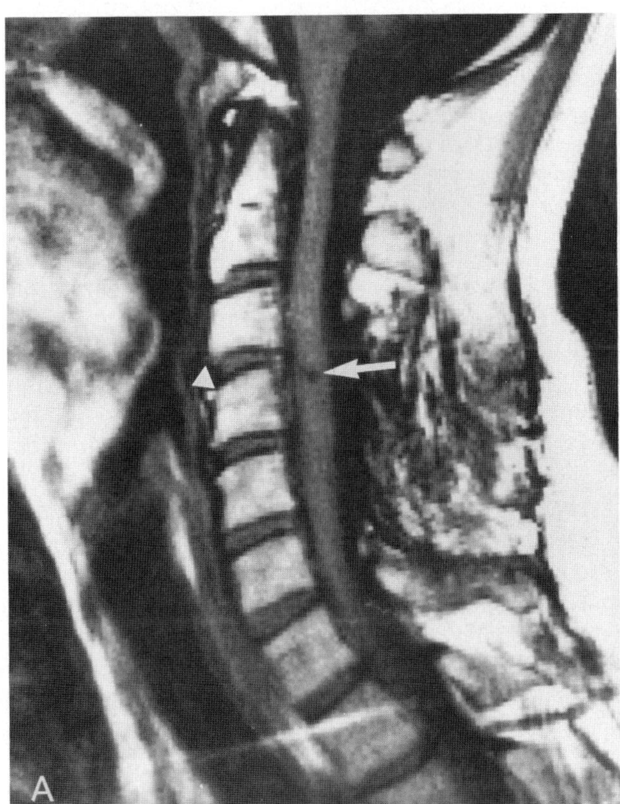

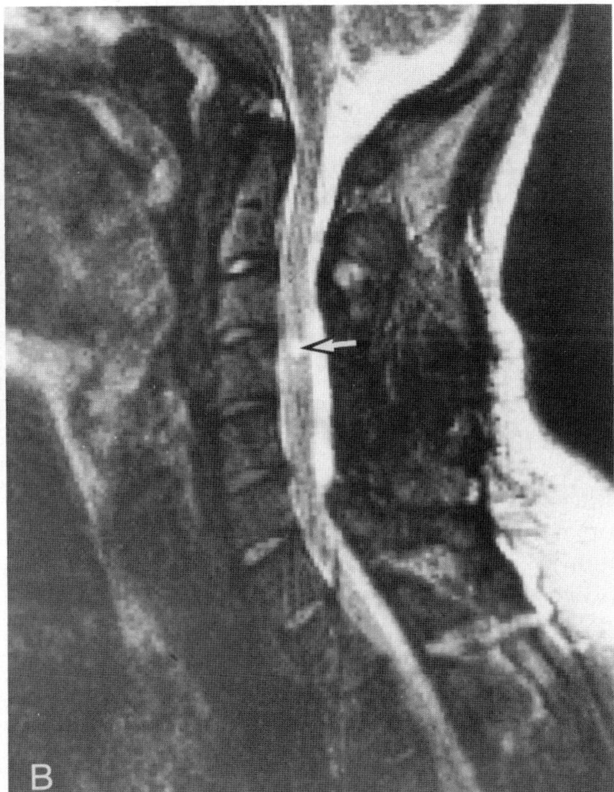

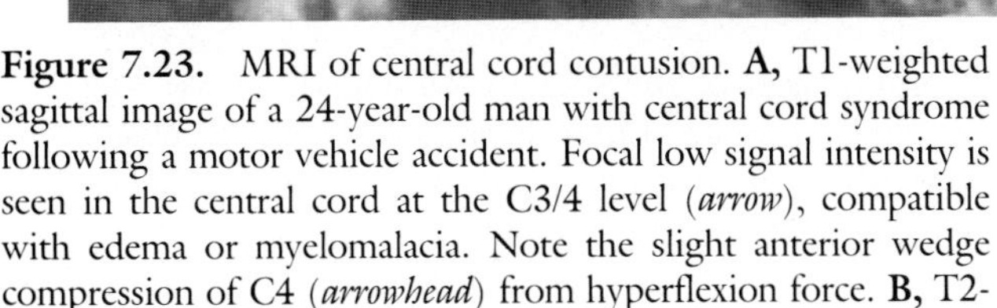

Figure 7.23. MRI of central cord contusion. **A,** T1-weighted sagittal image of a 24-year-old man with central cord syndrome following a motor vehicle accident. Focal low signal intensity is seen in the central cord at the C3/4 level (*arrow*), compatible with edema or myelomalacia. Note the slight anterior wedge compression of C4 (*arrowhead*) from hyperflexion force. **B,** T2-weighted sagittal image reveals focal increased signal (*arrow*) at C3/4, compatible with cord edema at this level. A decompressive laminectomy has been performed from C3 to C5. (From: Mirvis SE, Wolf A. Emerging MRI role: assessing cervical spine trauma. MRI Decisions 1990;4:21–31.)

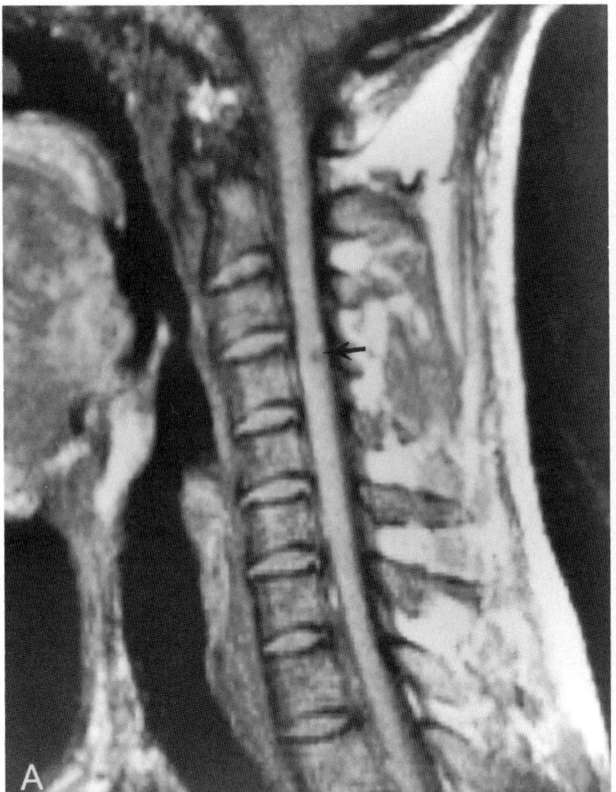

Figure 7.24. MRI of spinal cord contusion. **A**, this sagittal T1-weighted spin echo image shows a focal low signal area (*arrow*) in the dorsal cord at the C3/4 level in a young man with quadriplegia following a significant fall. **B**, the corresponding gradient echo T2-weighted image shows extent of edema within the cord as high signal. Posterior osteophyte at this level probable was point of impact against the cord.

on the time since injury (Table 7.2) (57). Acute hematomas appear as areas of low signal intensity on T2-weighted spin echo images (Figs. 7.25–7.27). This effect is attributed to loss of phase coherence caused by local field inhomogeneity created by the magnetic susceptibility of deoxyhemoglobin (57, 58). The persistence of intracellular deoxyhemoglobin within the cord over time may be due to the ischemic environment within the damaged cord (57). However, hematomas become hyperintense in the subacute period on both T1- and T2-weighted sequences, owing to the T1-shortening effects of paramagnetic extracellular methemoglobin (57) (Figs. 7.25–7.27). Regions of spinal cord contusion often display a spindle-shaped appearance centered at the point of cord impact with edema progressing cephalad and caudal from this point (Figs. 7.25–7.27).

In our experience to date, we have found sagittal images to be superior to axial images in the detection of acute spinal cord contusions. In addition, we have noted that T2-weighted spin echo images are more sensitive at contusion detection than are gradient echo images with small flip angles (T2-weighted).

Eventually, areas of severe contusion and/or hematoma formation progress to regions of myelomalacia or macrocyst formation that display low signal intensity on T1-weighted and high signal intensity on T2-weighted sequences (Fig. 7.28).

Traumatic lacerations of the spinal cord are uncommon but have been described as a complication of birth trauma, i.e., hypertraction on the spine and as a result of trauma, typically hyperdistraction. On CT, lacerations may be detected by complete transection of the spinal cord or as areas of cord parenchyma which fill with myelographic contrast immediately after contrast instillation. By MRI, cord lacerations are demonstrated as defects in the cord parenchyma of CSF signal intensity that extend to the subarachnoid space. As expected such injuries typically result in complete neurologic deficits. Hyperdistraction force may also lead to cord contusion without laceration.

Epidural Pathology

Compression of the spinal cord and thecal sac following trauma may arise from dislocated vertebrae, displaced bone fragments, acutely herniated discs, large osteophytes, ossification of the posterior longitudinal ligament (OPLL) and epidural hematomas (Figs. 7.10, 7.14, 7.29–7.31) among other entities. Although not confirmed statistically, it is our impression that the presence of preexisting cervical spinal stenosis increases the likelihood of neurologic injury from a given cervical spine stress due to the reduced potential for spinal cord movement away from impacting hard and soft tissues, as is observed in elderly males (59).

Epidural hematomas may develop acutely after trauma, in a delayed fashion, or after open or closed reduction of the spinal column. Again the appearance of the epidural hemorrhage depends on the age of the blood. Acutely, hematoma will appear of low signal of T2-weighted sequences due to intracellular deoxyhemoglobin, but will display progressive increased signal on T1-weighted images as extracellular methemoglobin content increases (Fig. 7.32). The presence of a cervical spinal cord deficit without obvious bony injury or delayed neurologic deterioration should suggest the presence of an epidural hematoma among other entities.

Acute intervertebral disc herniation may accompany fracture-dislocations of the cervical spine or may occur as an isolated lesion (Fig. 7.30). If the disc impacts the spinal cord, then focal injury may result producing either a transient deficit cord concussion (60), Brown-Sequard syndrome, or an anterior or central cord deficit. Demonstration of single level acute intervertebral disc herniation is crucial in surgical planning, since an anterior discectomy and fusion is indicated to appropriately decompress the spinal cord. Acute disc herniation is usually evident from T1-weighted sagittal studies but is best appreciated on gradient echo T2-weighted studies due to suppression of bone marrow signal. The advantages of MRI over CT without intrathecal contrast in detecting acute traumatic disc herniation were shown in the study of Flanders et al. (12) in which 40% of acute disc herniations detected by MRI were missed on noncontrast CT. In our experience, isolated acute intervertebral disk herniations producing neurologic deficits are very uncommon and account for <1% of neurologic deficits seen at our institution annually (61).

Large posterior osteophytes associated with or without spinal stenosis may provide an impact point for the cervical spinal cord during hyperflexion deformation. As the spinal column and cord bend suddenly forward the anterior cord impacts against the protruding osteophyte producing an anterior or central cord deficit (Fig. 7.29). In our expe-

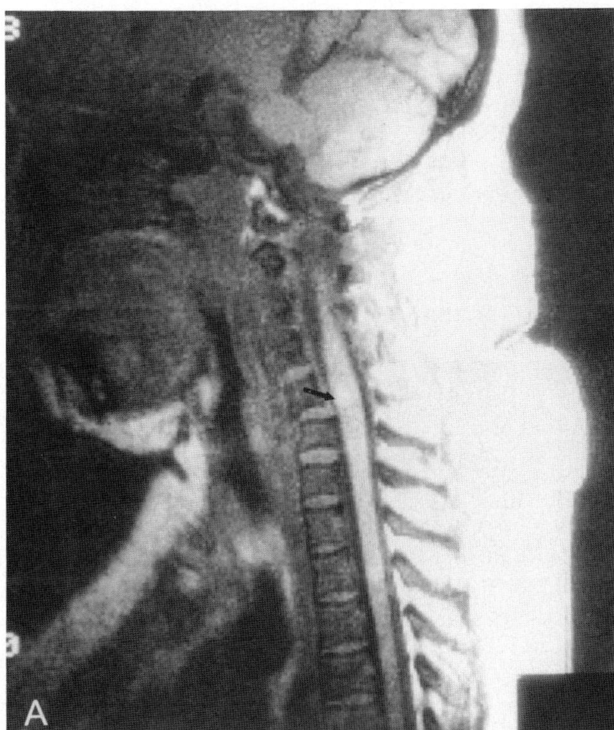

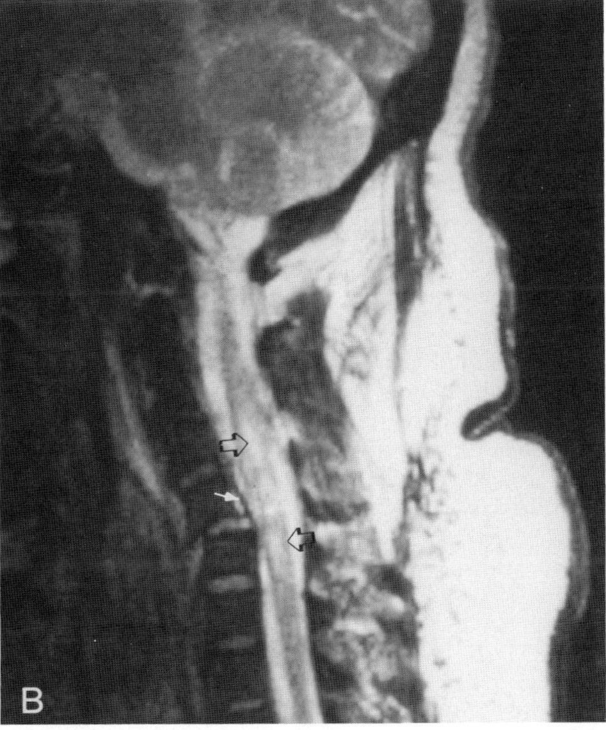

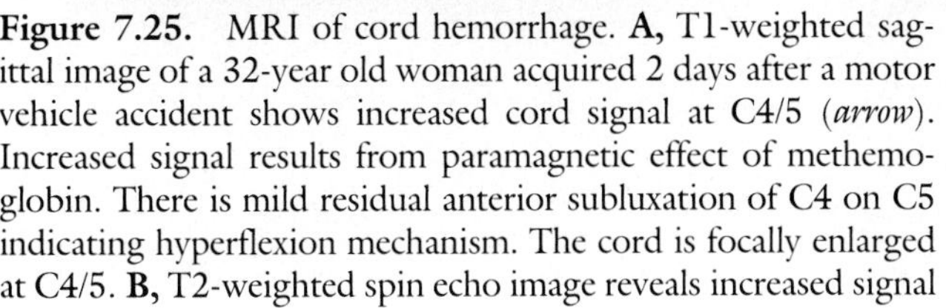

Figure 7.25. MRI of cord hemorrhage. **A,** T1-weighted sagittal image of a 32-year old woman acquired 2 days after a motor vehicle accident shows increased cord signal at C4/5 (*arrow*). Increased signal results from paramagnetic effect of methemoglobin. There is mild residual anterior subluxation of C4 on C5 indicating hyperflexion mechanism. The cord is focally enlarged at C4/5. **B,** T2-weighted spin echo image reveals increased signal extending cephalad and caudad from C4/5 (*open arrows*) in a spindle-shaped pattern indicating edema extending from the primary impact site. The posterior longitudinal ligament is stripped from the C4 vertebral body (*white arrow*). (From Young JWR, Mirvis SE. Cervical spine trauma. In: Mirvis SE, Young JWR, eds. Imaging in trauma and critical care. Baltimore: Williams & Wilkins, 1992.)

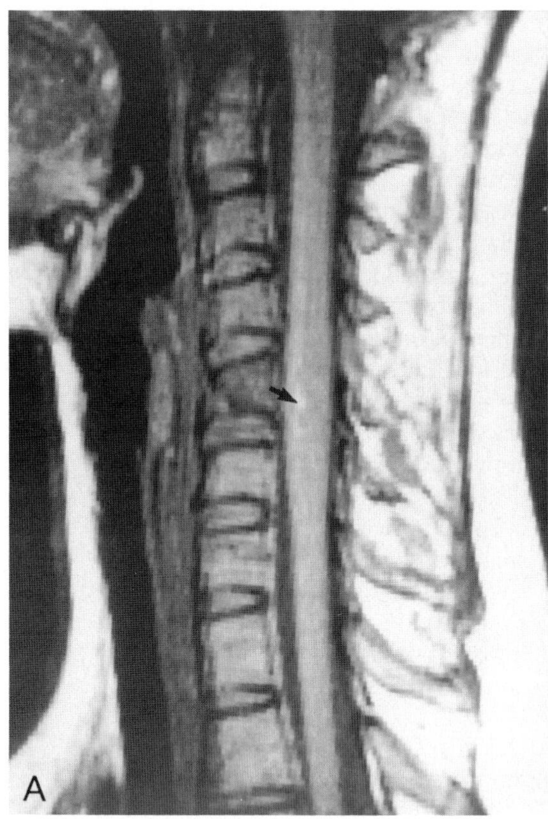

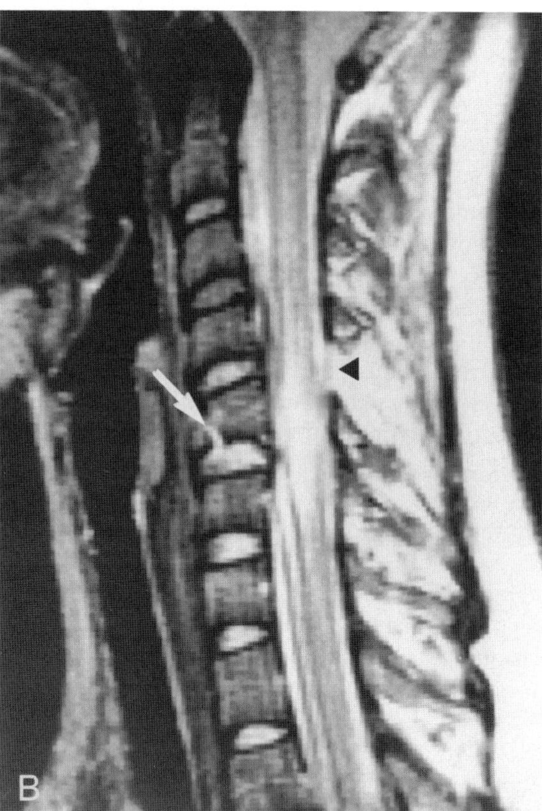

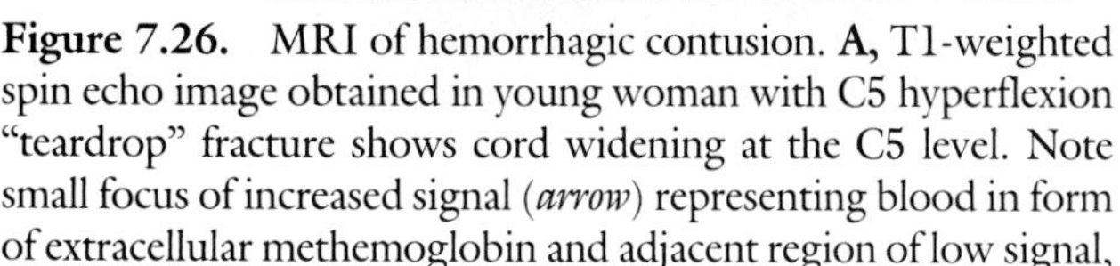
Figure 7.26. MRI of hemorrhagic contusion. **A,** T1-weighted spin echo image obtained in young woman with C5 hyperflexion "teardrop" fracture shows cord widening at the C5 level. Note small focus of increased signal (*arrow*) representing blood in form of extracellular methemoglobin and adjacent region of low signal, probably representing acute hemorrhage (deoxyhemoglobin). **B,** T2-weighted spin echo image shows diffuse increased signal extending above and below level of impact in spindle shape. Fracture of C5 (*arrow*) is easily observed as is flaring of C4 and C5 posterior osseous elements (*arrowhead*) and ligaments.

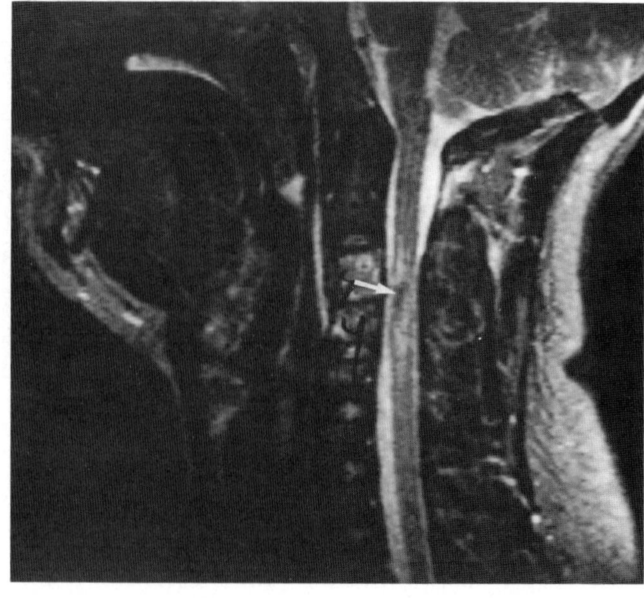

Figure 7.27. MRI of spinal cord hemorrhage. This T2-weighted spin echo image shows area of low signal in the cord at C3/4 (*white arrow*). This low signal represents acute hemorrhage caused by "magnetic susceptibility" effects of intracellular deoxyhemoglobin, which enhances T2 relaxation and decreases signal strength on T2-weighted sequences. Higher signal edema is seen above and below the hemorrhage.

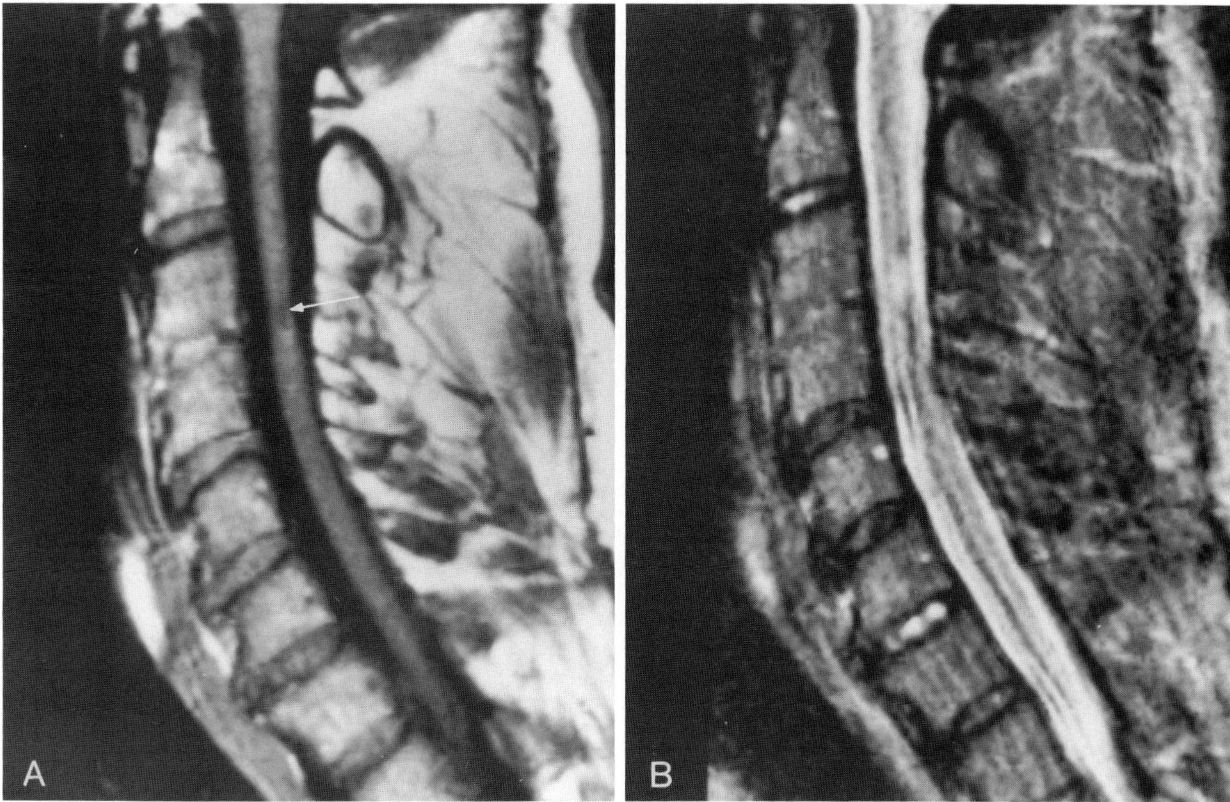

Figure 7.28. MRI of posttraumatic myelomalacia. **A,** this sagittal T1-weighted image of a 45-year-old man obtained several weeks after a fall that resulted in quadriplegia shows low cord signal at C3/4 (*arrow*) compatible with myelomalacia and focal cord atrophy. **B,** T2-weighted image is compromised by motion but shows area of increased signal at C3/4 represent increased fluid in region of gliosis (myelomalacia). MRI can not easily distinguish microcystic from macrocystic changes within the cord.

rience, the contusion produced occurs slightly below the level of the "critical" osteophyte due to the cephalad distraction of the cord at the time forced hyperflexion.

Displaced fracture fragments may produce persistent compression of the spinal cord following radiologically adequate reduction of vertebral body alignment. Identification of such bony fragments by CT is possible, but the extent of compression of the thecal sac and spinal cord is best defined by CT with intrathecal contrast (Fig. 7.31). MRI demonstrates such bone fragments quite well and can simultaneously demonstrate the extent of spinal cord compression, while avoiding the need for intrathecal contrast.

Injury in Support Tissues of the Cervical Spine

Vertebral fractures and/or dislocations are usually well assessed by radiography and selective use of CT with appropriate reformatted images. MRI, in our experience, usually detects fractures involving the vertebral bodies and may on occasion be useful to detect certain fractures (nondisplaced, horizontally-oriented fractures) to which radiography and CT are not sensitive. By T1-weighted MRI sequences, fractures appear as disruptions of the low signal cortical margin(s) and low signal intensity through the normally high signal of fatty marrow (Figs. 7.27, 7.30, 7.33–7.35). On T2-weighted images, the bone marrow is visualized as low signal while fractures are relatively intense due to edema and hemorrhage (Figs. 7.27, 7.30, 7.33–7.35). MRI has not, in our experience to date, been reliable in imaging many fractures of the posterior spinal column and should not be relied upon for that purpose, as the presence of combined anterior and posterior column disruption may alter the form of stabilization required. In the study by Flanders et al., MRI detected 25% of posterior vertebral fractures compared to 71% for CT (12).

Generally, ligament injuries of the cervical spinal column are **inferred** from the mechanism of injury and the direction and degree of vertebral body malalignment. In many cases, however, when patients are placed in cervical immobilization in the field, alignment may be restored and the mechanism of injury may be difficult to determine. This is especially true for hyperextension injuries without fracture that may be reduced to a normal or near normal appearance by cervical immobilization.

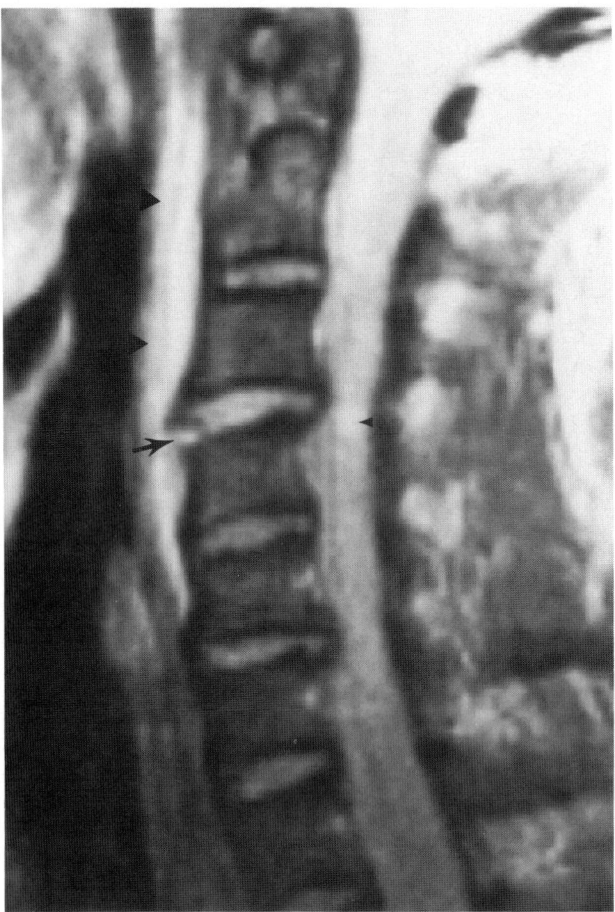

Figure 7.29. Posterior osteophyte leading to cord contusion. This spin echo (proton) image shows C3/4 osteophyte indenting anterior thecal space. There is a small anterior avulsion fracture of C4 (*arrow*) and edema in the precervical soft tissues (*arrowheads*) indicating hyperextension mechanism. A focal cord contusion (*small arrowhead*) is observed at the point of impact of the cord against the osteophyte. (From: Young JWR, Mirvis SE. Cervical spine trauma. In: Mirvis SE, Young JWR, eds. Imaging in trauma and critical care. Baltimore: Williams & Wilkins, 1992.)

MRI demonstates ligaments as regions of low signal intensity due to a paucity of mobile hydrogen. As has been well demonstrated in other body regions, injured (sprained) ligaments may manifest increased signal on T2-weighted sequences due to edema. Disrupted ligaments will demonstrate a discontinuity in the normal continuous low signal intensity of the ligament. Avulsion or "stripping" of the anterior and posterior longitudinal ligament from the vertebral body is well visualized by MRI and may be helpful in confirming the mechanism of the injuring force (Figs. 7.35 and 7.36). In addition, disruption of the low signal annulus fibrosis can be identified by MRI. The precise sensitivity and specificity of MRI for detection of ligament and annulus fibrosus injuries of the cervical spine is, to our knowledge, unknown.

Cervical vascular injury may accompany blunt force injury to the neck as a result of overstretching of the vessel, excessive torsion, direct impact, or by fracture fragment laceration (52, 62). In the assessment of the cervical spine by MRI the four major cervical cerebral arteries should be inspected for the presence of a flow void (spin echo) or increased signal (gradient echo). Absence of the expected signal may indicate vessel injury.

Correlation of MRI Appearance with Prognosis

Initial limited studies at the University of Maryland (9) and the University of Texas at Houston (7) suggested that the use of MRI in the acute period may provide information regarding the potential for recovery of neurologic function. In these two studies, patients who had spinal cord lesions with hemorrhage demonstrable on MRI showed significantly more limited recovery than those whose lesions were predominantly edematous or in patients in whom no lesion was identified in the spinal cord despite initial neurologic deficits.

In a more recent study, Flanders et al. (12) retrospectively compared the acute MRI cervical spine examination with neurologic outcome in 78 patients with acute cervical spine injury. In this series, intramedullary hemorrhage was always predictive of a *complete* lesion, and 91% of patients with complete deficits had intramedullary hemorrhage. The presence of intramedullary hemorrhage was five times more likely to be present with compressive injuries to the cervical cord.

Alternatively, patients with increased signal on T-2 weighted spin echo images due to extracellular edema or noncoalescent petechial hemorrhage had a relatively favorable prognosis. In this study, cord edema was detected as early as 4 hours after trauma and was maximal by 72 hours after injury. The clinical level of impairment was imprecisely related to the level of edema, but the extent of edema did correlate with the extent of neurologic injury. These authors also found that T2-weighted spin echo images were more sensitive to detect cord edema than gradient echo sequences.

Interestingly, in this series, the extent of bony and soft tissue injury, preexisting spondylosis, and disk herniation did not correlate with the severity of neurologic deficit. Hackney (63) suggests that patient selection and referral patterns may be in part responsible for this finding. Hackney suggests that similar injuries would be expected to produce both a range of functional deficits and MR findings, but still acknowledges the relatively poor neurologic outcome implied by acute cord hemorrhage.

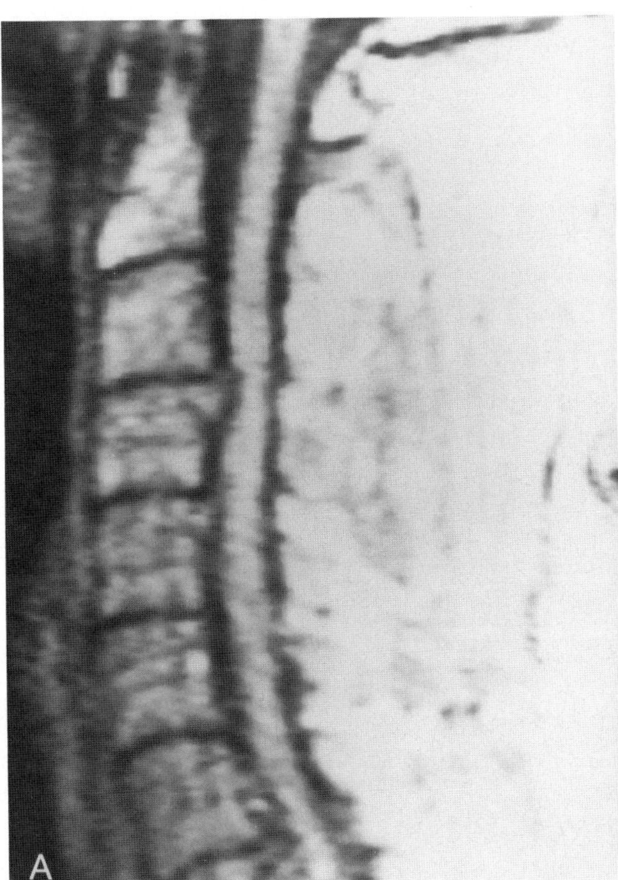

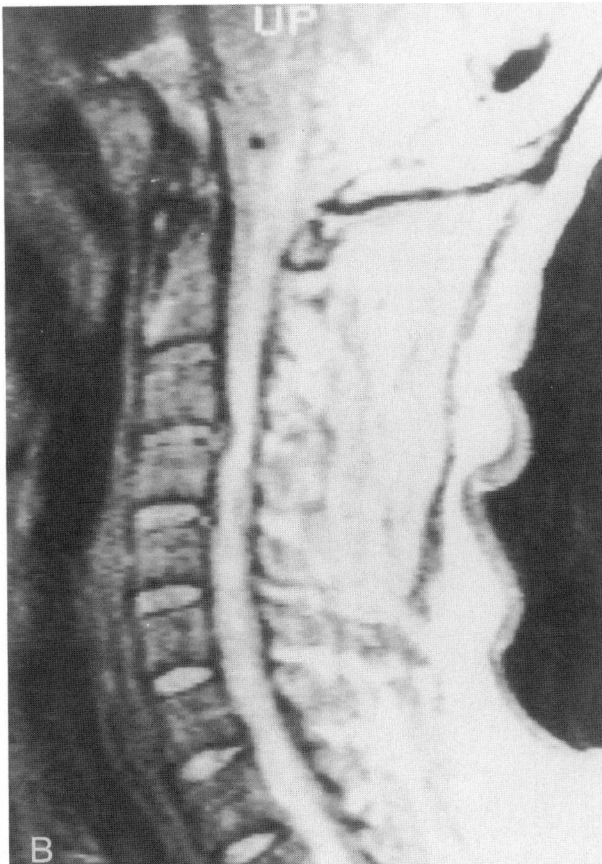

Figure 7.30. Herniated intervertebral disk material leading to cord contusion. **A,** this T1-weighted spin echo image shows marked herniation of disk material compressing the cord at C3/4. **B,** the corresponding spin echo proton image shows increased signal in the cord at this level corresponding to edema. The patient had an acute anterior cord syndrome.

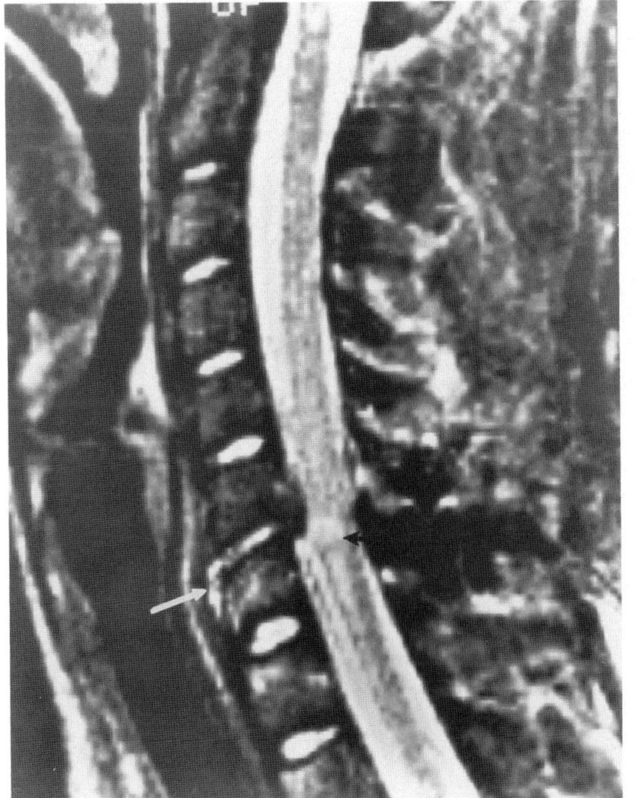

Figure 7.31. Retropulsed bone fragment leading to cord contusion. This T2-weighted spin echo image reveals a bone fragment arising from C6 compressing the cord and producing a contusion (*black arrow*). The intervertebral disc is herniated anteriorly (*white arrow*). The patient has been internally fixed posteriorly at C6/C7 using titanium wire that produces minimal artifact. (From: Mirvis SE, Geisler FH, Joslyn JN, Zrebeet H. Use of titanium wire in cervical spine fixation as a means to reduce MR artifacts. AJNR 1988;9:1229–1231.)

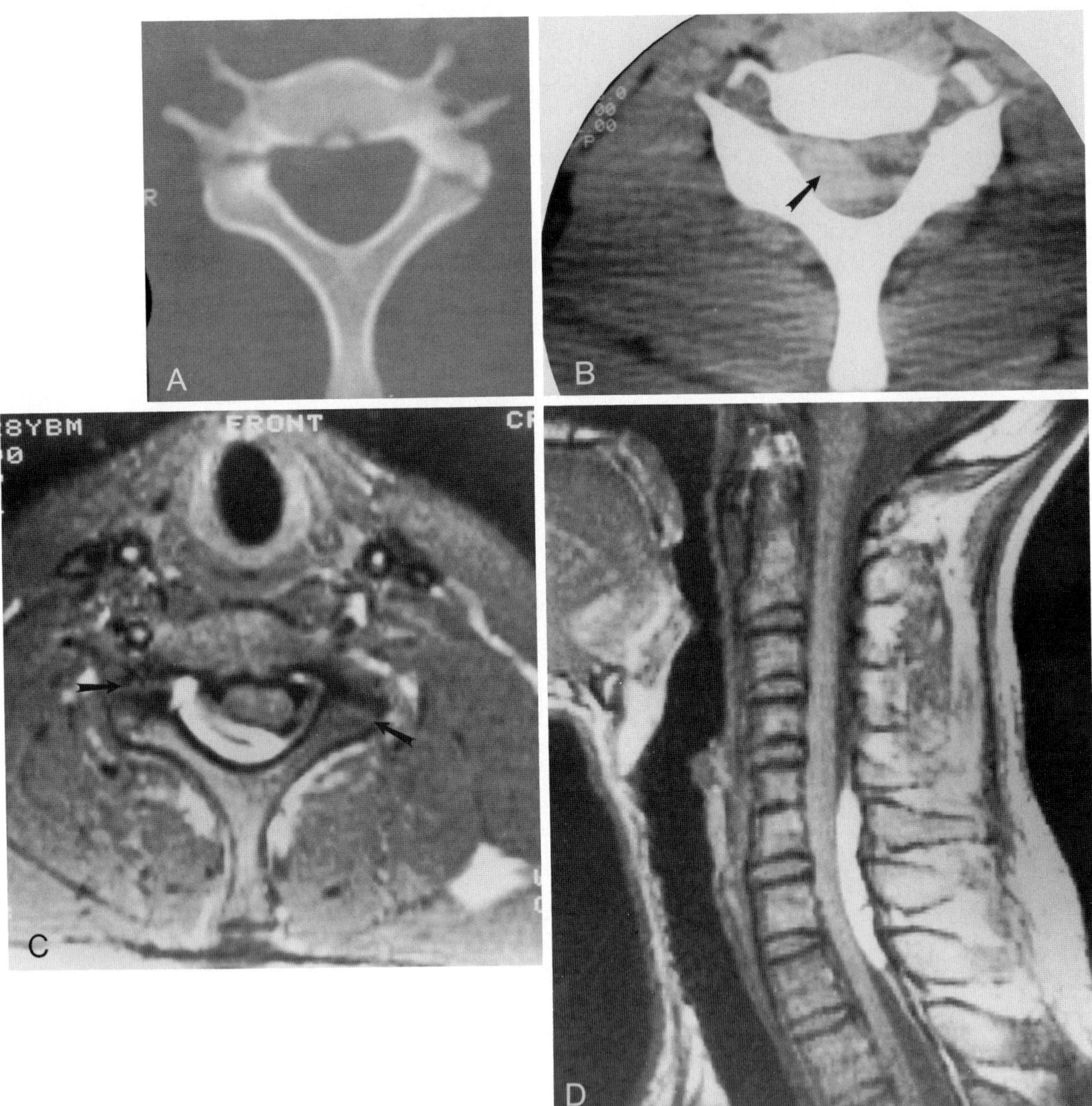

Figure 7.32. CT and MRI of acute posttraumatic epidural hematoma. **A,** axial CT image at C6 level (photographed in bone windows) of young man with neck pain after motorcycle accident shows fractures through both pedicles. **B,** CT image at C6 level obtained after onset of progressive quadriparesis shows high density hematoma (*arrow*) compressing the cord to the left. **C,** this T1-weighted spin echo image shows high signal hematoma (due to extracellular methemoglobin) compressing cord. Fractures through the pedicles are noted (*arrows*). **D,** this sagittal T1-weighted image shows extent of substantially posterior epidural collection from C5 to T1. The hematoma was surgically evacuated with restoration of normal neurologic function.

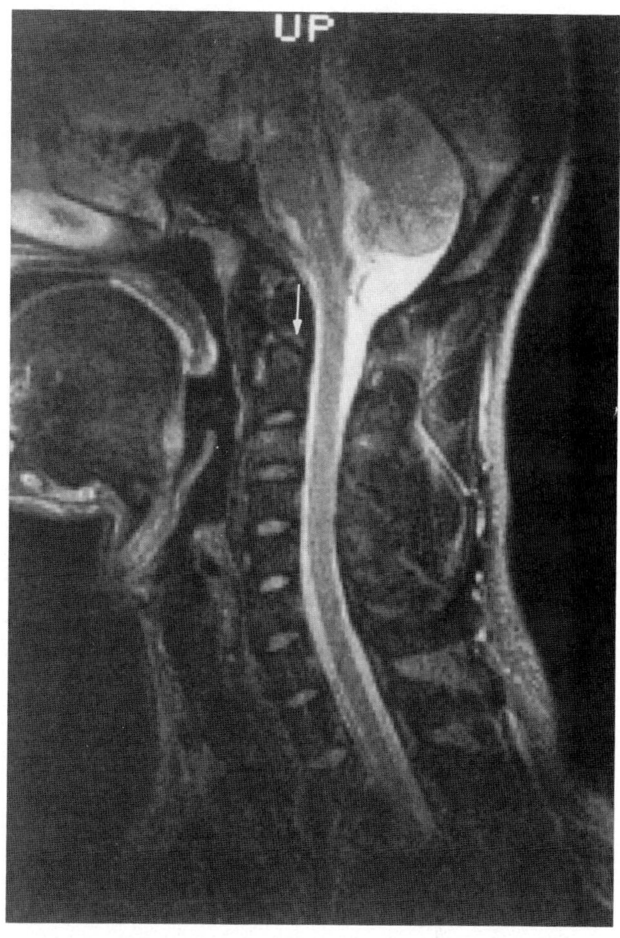

Figure 7.33. MRI of C2 fracture. This T2-weighted spin echo image obtained in a neurologically intact 24-year-old man with upper cervical pain (but no evidence of injury on radiography or CT) shows oblique, nondisplaced C2 fracture as line of increased signal in bone marrow (*arrow*). (From: Mirvis SE, Wolf A. Emerging MRI role: assessing cervical spine trauma. MRI Decisions 1990;4:21–31.)

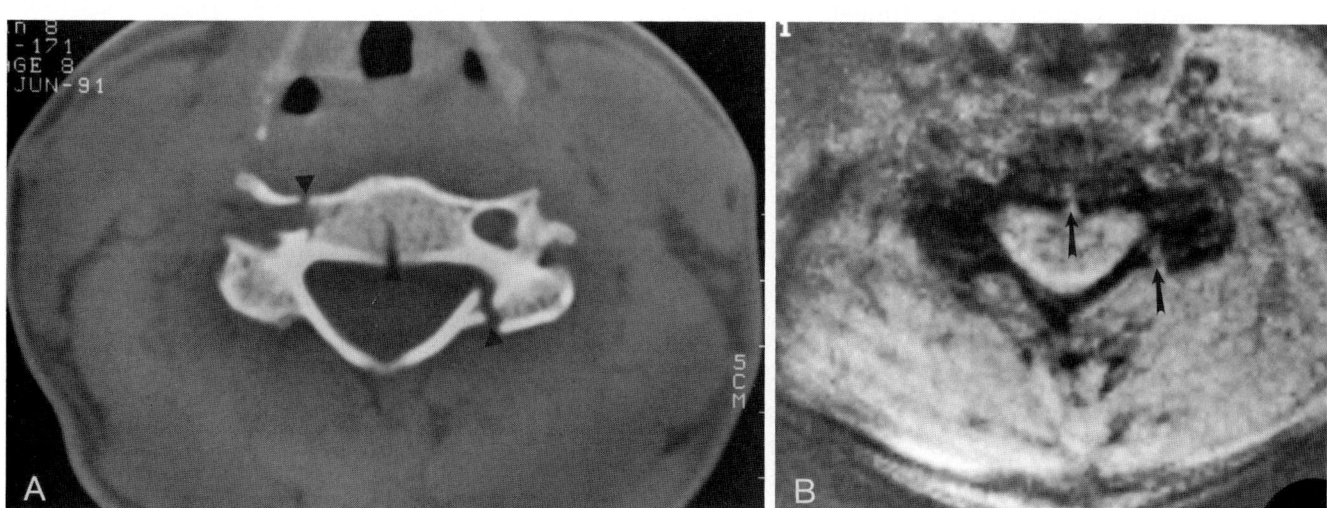

Figure 7.34. CT and MRI of cervical fractures. **A,** this axial CT image through C5 shows several fractures. **B,** gradient echo image clearly shows two fractures through left lamina and body (*arrows*), but does not detect right transverse process fracture due to lower spatial resolution.

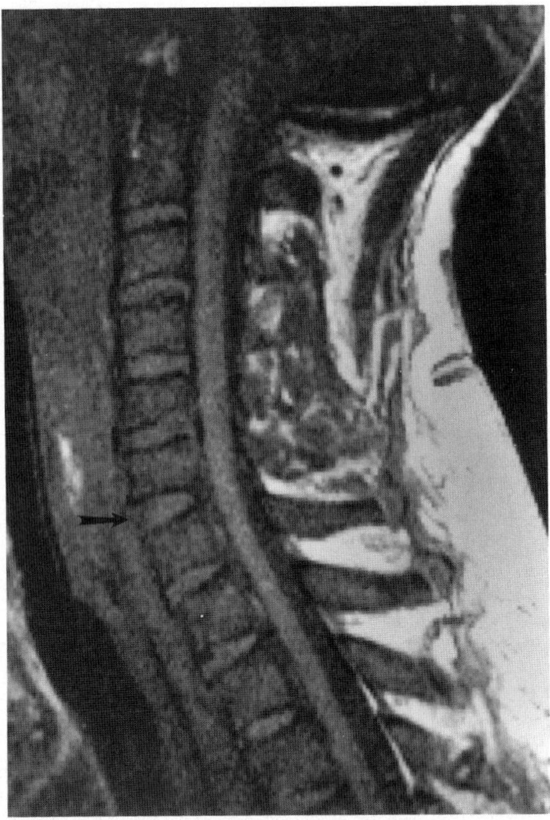

Figure 7.35. MRI of ligament injury. This T1-weighted spin echo image obtained after cervical trauma shows widening of the C6/7 anterior intervertebral space and loss of the expected low signal anterior longitudinal ligament and annulus fibrosis (*arrow*) indicating hyperextension disruption.

Chronic Cervical Spine Injury: MRI Evaluation

The chronically injured spinal cord may manifest a variety of MRI findings, depending upon the specific pathology present. Yamashita et al. (10) evaluated the MRI appearance of the spinal cord in 76 patients with chronic myelopathy secondary to cord injury. These authors identified five patterns in chronic injury based on the T1-weighted and T2-weighted appearance of the spine. Patients with normal T1 and T2 appearances had slight injury and an excellent prognosis (N/N). Patients with normal T1 but increased T2 signal had mild neurologic impairment and associated residual cord compression in 83% of 18 patients (N/Hi). Patients with decreased signal on T1 and increased signal on T2-weighted sequences (Lo/Hi) had the worst prognosis and most likely represent patients with macrocysts or syrinx formation (Figs. 7.37 and 7.38). Patients with a long history of myelopathy and/or cord atrophy also had poor longterm prognoses. In our experience as well, the presence of underlying cord atrophy is a poor prognostic factor after acute spinal cord injury.

Posttraumatic progressive myelopathy affects from 0.01 to 3.2% of patients with severe spial cord injury (10) and may be secondary to intramedullary cyst (syrinx), subarachnoid cysts, residual herniated disc or compressive bone fragment, and scarring (tethering). Patients with simple spinal cord contusion (predominantly nonhemorrhagic) typically progress to a normal MRI appearance or to myelomalacia manifesting as increased signal region to T2-weighted images. Alternatively, patients with cord hematoma or ischemic necrosis are more likely to progress to macrocyst or syrinx formation (low T1-weighted, high T2-weighted) (Figs. 7.37 and 7.38). As emphasized by Quencer (63), the distinction among these entities is clinically relevant, as syrinx or cysts which communicate with the subarachnoid space may expand due to CSF pulsations and could benefit from shunting. Myelomalacia (gliosis, neuronal degeneration, microcyst formation) does not typically lead to progressive symptoms. Intramedullary cysts may communicate with the subarachnoid space and require shunting. Evaluation of the cyst using nonmotion compensated T2-weighted sequences to detect fluid movement (local signal void within cyst) or CINE MRI modes to assess the cyst in a dynamic fashion are helpful to determine the need for cyst shunting (64).

Quencer (64) has pointed out that cysts tend to have uniform low signal on T1-weighted images and maintain sharp borders with the adjacent normal cord, while myelomalacia presents a heterogeneous hypodensity on T1-weighted sequences and presents an indistinct interface with the adjacent cord parechyma. As noted above, there is no evidence of CSF flow within areas of myelomalacia. A large intramedullary cyst may mimic cord atrophy. An obstructing subarachnoid cyst compressing the cord will create increased CSF turbulence above the lesion and decreased CSF motion below the cyst.

Evaluation of the patient with spinal cord injury who has undergone posterior wire stablization with ferromagnetic stainless steel is significantly compromised by signal loss created by loss of field homogeneity around the wires. In an effort to reduce such artifact we evaluated the imaging effects fixation with braided titanium wire (allow Ti-6 A1-4V). Titanium has good tissue compatibility, biomedical, and mechanical properties. In our studies (15), MR artifacts from titanium were far less than those produced by stainless steel and permitted an undistorted image of the spinal cord and canal immediately adjacent to the surgical fixation. The braided titanium wires used in this study are stiffer than stainless steel and were therefore more difficult to install. We are currently using titanium plates and screws (Synthes Products, Switzerland) for anterior fixation of the cervical spine that preserves postoperative MR image quality without difficult surgical instillation.

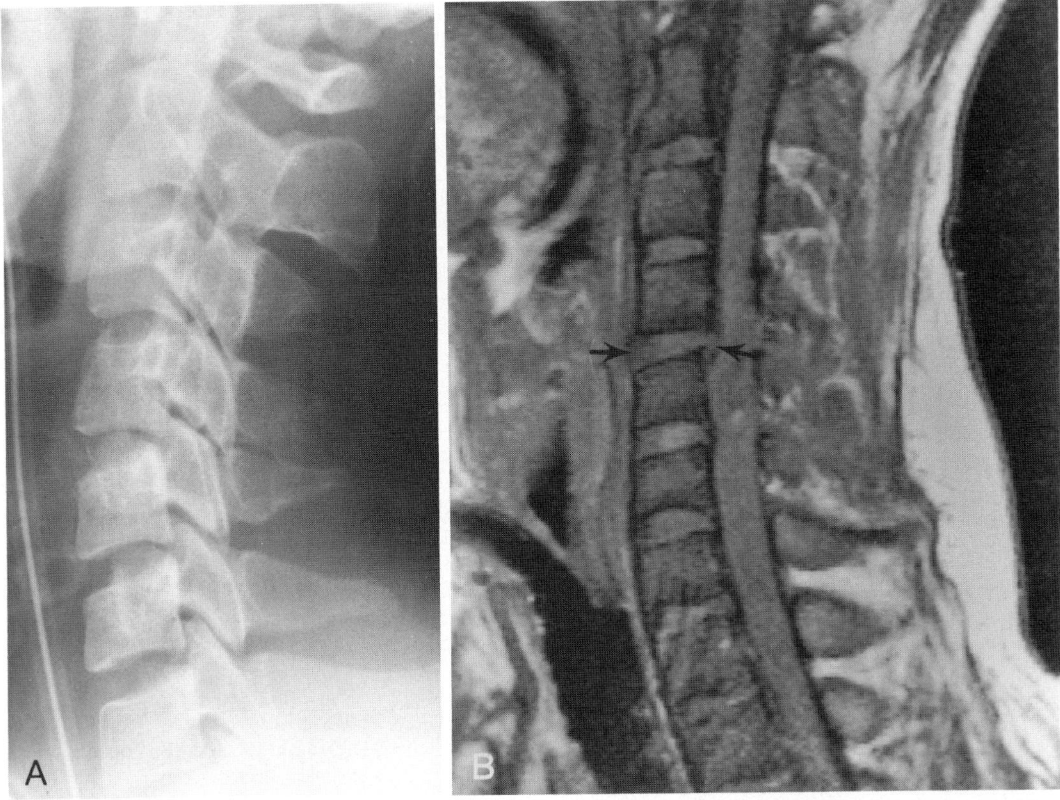

Figure 7.36. MRI of ligament disruption. **A,** lateral cervical radiograph obtained in 40-year-old man with quadriplegia after MVA shows slight widening of anterior disc space at C4/5 suggesting hyperextension force injury. The posterior osseous structures at C4 and C5 are compressed together. **B,** proton-weighted MRI shows loss of low signal for the anterior and posterior longitudinal ligaments (*arrows*) as well as interspinous ligaments. This much ligamentous disruption was not anticipated from plain radiographs and changed surgical management.

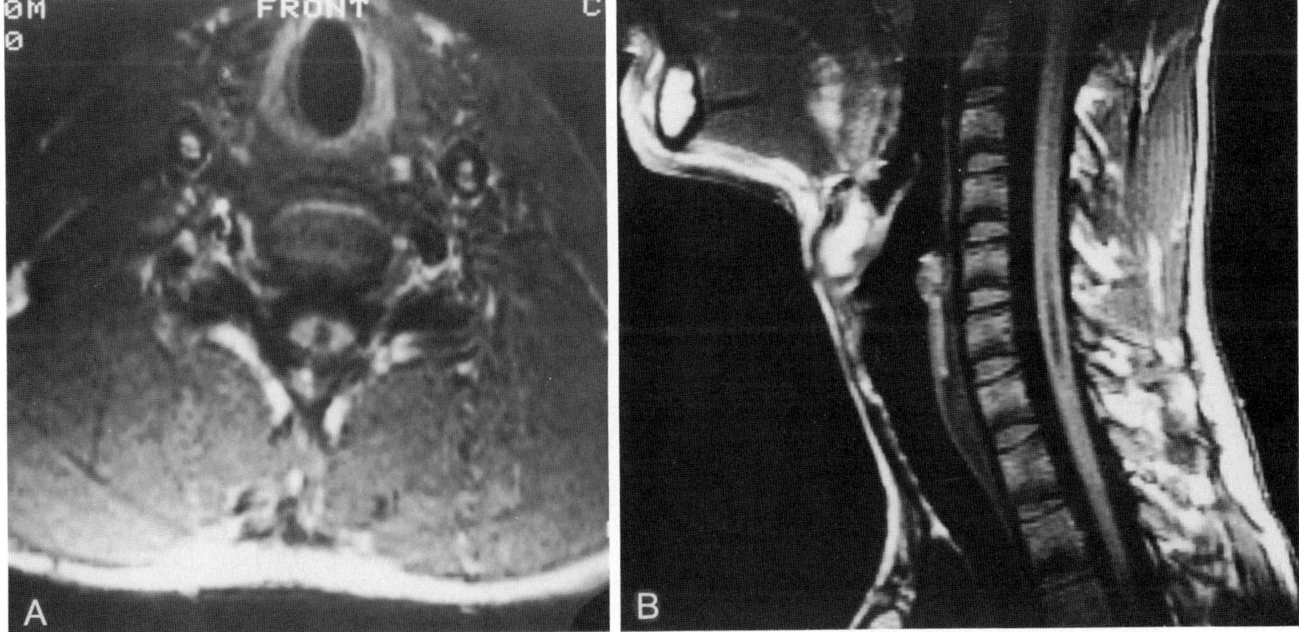

Figure 7.37. MRI of traumatic syrinx. **A,** axial T1-weighted and **B,** sagittal T1-weighted images show low signal syrinx in central cord from C5 to C7 several months after trauma. The patient did not have progressive symptoms.

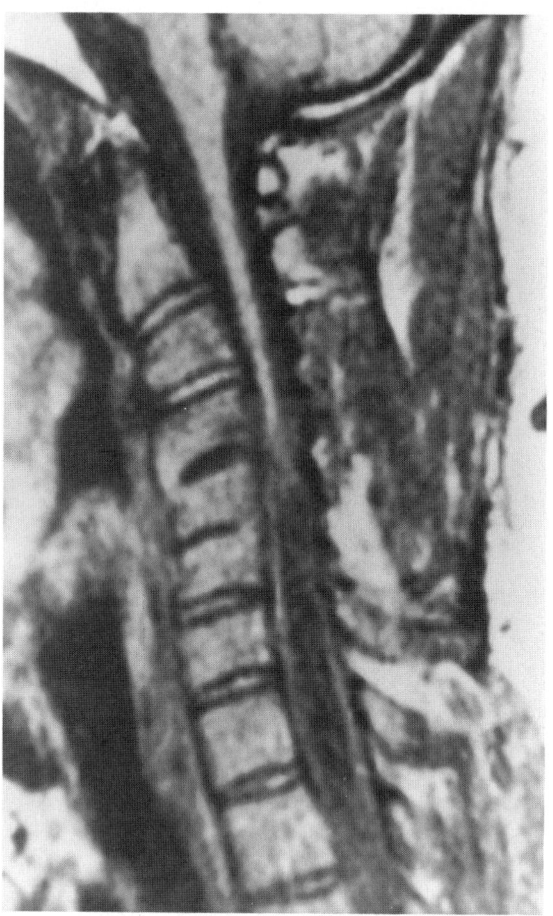

Figure 7.38. MRI of chronic posttraumatic syrinx. This T1-weighted sagittal shows marked cord atrophy at C3 and C4 level several months after injury leading to quadriplegia. A large low signal syrinx (cyst) extends caudally to the upper thoracic cord.

REFERENCES

1. Larsson EM, Holtas S, Brandi L. Comprison of myelography, CT myelography, and magnetic resonance imaging in cervical spondylosis and disk herniation. Pre- and post-operative findings. Acta Radiol 1989;30:233–239.

2. Karnaze MG, Gado MH, Sartor KJ, Hodges FJ. Comparison of MR and CT myelography in imaging the cervical and thoracic spine. AJR 1988;150:397–403.

3. Carmody RF, Yang PJ, Seeley GW, Geeger JF, Unger EC, Johnson JE. Spinal cord compression due to metastatic disease: diagnosis with MR imaging versus myelography. Radiology 1989;173:225–229.

4. Bates D, Ruggierri P. Imaging modalities for evaluation of the spine. In: Modic MT, ed. Imaging of the spine. Radiol Clin North Am 1991;29:675–690.

5. Lee SH, Coleman PE, Hahn FJ. Magnetic resonance imaging of degenerative disease of the spine. In Lee SH and Zimmerman RA, eds. Imaging in neuroradiology, Part II. Radiol Clin North Am 1988;26:949–964.

6. Zimmerman RA, Bilaniuk LT. Imaging of tumors of the spinal canal and cord. In: Lee SH, Zimmerman RA, eds. Imaging in neuroradiology, Part II. Radiol Clin North Am 1988;26:965–1008.

7. Kulkarni MV, McArdle CB, Kopanicky D. Acute spinal cord injury: MR imaging at 1.5 T. Radiology 1987;164:837–843.

8. McArdle CB, Wright JW, Provost WJ. MR imaging of the acutely injured patient with cervical traction. Radiology 1986;159:273–274.

9. Mirvis SE, Geisler FH, Jelinek JJ, Joslyn JN, Gellad FE. Acute cervical spine trauma: evaluation with 1.5 T MR imaging. Radiology 1988;166:807–816.

10. Yamashita Y, Takakashi M, Matsuno Y, Sakamoto Y, Organi T, Sakae T, Yoshizumi K, Kim EE. Chronic injuries of the spinal cord. Assessment with MR imaging. Radiology 1990;175:849–854.

11. Beers GJ, Raque GH, Wagner GG, et al. MR imaging in acute cervical spine trauma. J Comput Assist Tomogr 1988;12:755–761.

12. Flanders AE, Schaeffer DM, Doan HT, Mishkin MM, Gonzales CF, Northrup BE. Acute cervical spine trauma: correlation of MR imaging findings with degree of neurologic deficit. Radiology 1990;177:25–33.

13. Goldberg AL, Rothfus WE, Deeb ZZ. Impact of magnetic resonance on the diagnostic evaluation of acute cervicothoracic spinal trauma. Skeletal Radiol 1988;17:89–97.

14. Mirvis SE, Borg U, Belzberg H. MRI of ventilator-dependent patients: preliminary experience. AJR 1987;149:845–846.

15. Mirvis SE, Geisler F, Joslyn JN, Zrebeet H. Use of titanium wire in cervical spine fixation as a means to reduce MR artifacts. AJNR 1988;9:1229–1231.

16. Saini S, Stark DD, Rzedzian RR, Pykett IL, Rummeny E, Hahn PF, Wittenberg J, Ferrucci JT. Forty-millisecond MR imaging of the abdomen at 2.0 T. Radiology 1989;173:111–116.

17. Unger EC, Cohen MS, Gatenby RA. Single breath-holding scans of the abdomen using FISP and FLASH at 1.5 T. J Comput Assist Tomogr 1988;12:575–578.

18. Feinberg DA, Oshio K. GRASE (gradient- and spin-echo) MR imaging: a new fast clinical imaging technique. Radiology 1991;181:597–602.

19. Klein DS. Prevention of claustrophobia induced by MR imaging: use of alprazolam. AJR 1991;156:633.

20. Goldstein EJ, Burnett KR, Hansell JR, et al. Gadolinium DTPA (an NMR imaging contrast agent): chemical structure, paramagnetic properties and pharmacokinetics. Physiologic Chem, Phys Med NMR 1984;16:97–104.

21. Krestin GP, Neufang KFR, Friedmann G, Clauss W, Schuhmann-Giampieri G, Stoecki B. Functional dynamic MR imaging and pharmacakinetics of Gd-DTPA in patients with renal failure. Presented at Radiologic Society of North America meeting, Chicago, IL 1989.

22. Yu S. Haughton VM, Rosenbaum AE. Magnetic resonance imaging and anatomy of the spine. In: Modic MT, ed. Imaging of the spine. Radiol Clin North Am 1991;29:691–710.

23. Czervionke LF, Daniels DL. Cervical spine anatomy and pathologic processes: applications on new MR imaging techniques. In Lee SH, Zimmerman RA, eds. Imaging in neuroradiology, Part II. Radiol Clin North Am 1988,26:921–947.

24. Jahnke RW, Hart BL. Cervical stenosis, spondylosis, and herniated disc disease. In: Modic MT, ed. Imaging of the spine. Radiol Clin North Am 1991;29:777–792.

25. Youssem DM, Atlas SW, Goldberg HI, Grossman RI. Degenerative narrowing of the cervical spine neural foramina: evaluation with high-resolution 3DFT gradient-echo MR imaging. AJNR 1991:12:229–236.

26. Matsuda Y, Miyazaki K, Tada K, et al. Increased MR signal intensity due to cervical myelopathy: analysis of 29 surgical cases. J Neurosurg 1991;74:887–892.

27. Smith AS, Blaser SI. Infectious and inflammatory processes of the spine. In: Modic MT ed. Imaging of the spine. Radio Clin North Am 1991;29:777–792.

28. Modic MT, Pflanze W. Feiglin D, et al. Magnetic resonance imaging of musculoskeletal infections. Radiol Clin North Am 1986;24:247–258.

29. Modic MT, Pavlicek W, Weinstein MA. Magnetic resonance imaging of interveretebral disk disease: clinical and pulse sequence considerations. Radiology 1984;152:103–111.

30. Chandnani VP, Beltran J, Morris CS, et al. Acute experimental osteomyelitis and abscesses: detection with MR imaging versus CT. Radiology 1990;174:233–236.

31. Ross JS. Magnetic resonance assessment of the postoperative spine: degenerative disc disease. In: Modic MT, ed. Imaging of the spine. Radiol Clin North Am 1991;29:793–808.

32. Modic MT, Feiglin DH, Piraino DW, et al. Vertebral osteomyelitis: assessment using MR. Radiology 1985;157:157–166.

33. Hlavin ML, Kaminski HJ, Ross JS, Ganz E. Spinal epidural abscess: a ten-year perspective. Neurosurgery 1990;27:177–184.

34. Whelan MA, Schonfeld S, Post JD, et al. Computed tomography of non-tuberculous spinal infection. J Comput Assist Tomogr 1985;9:280–287.

35. Post MJ, Quencer RM, Montalvo BM, Katz BH, Eismont FJ, Green BA. Spinal infection: evaluation with MR imaging and intraoperative US. Radiology 1988;169:765–771.

36. Einig M, Higer HP, Meairs S, Faust-Tinnefeldt G, Kapp H. Magnetic resonance imaging of the craniocervical junction in rheumatoid arthritis: value, limitations, indications. Skeletal Radiol 1990;19:341–346.

37. Semble EL, Elster AD, Loeser RF, Laster DW, Challa VR, Pisko EJ. Magnetic resonance imaging of the craniocervical junction in rheumatoid arthritis. J Rheumatol 1988;15:1367–1375.

38. Glew D, Watt I, Dieppe PA, Goddard PR. MRI of the cervical spine: rheumatoid arthritis compared with cervical spondylosis. Clin Radiol 1991;44:71–76.

39. Dvorak J, Grob D, Baumgartner H, Gschwebd N, Grauer W, Larason S. Functional evaluation of the spinal cord by magnetic resonance imaging in patients with rheumatoid arthritis and instability of the upper cervical spine. Spine 1989;14:1057–1064.

40. Hollis PM, Malis LI, Zappulla RA. Neurologic deterioration after lumbar puncture below complete spinal subarachnoid block. J Neurosurg 1986;64:253–256.

41. Masark TJ. Neoplastic disease of the spine. In: Modic MT, ed. Imaging of the spine. Radiol Clin North Am 1991;29:829–845.

42. Sze G, Vichanco LS, Brant-Zawadski MN, et al. Chordomas: MR imaging. Radiology 1988;166:187–191.

43. Ross JS, Masaryk TJ, Modic MT, Carter JR, Mapstone T, Dengel FH. Vertebral hemangiomas: MR imaging. Radiology 1987;165:165–169.

44. Zimmer WD, Berquist TH, Sim FH, et al. Magnetic resonance imaging of aneurysmal bone cysts. Mayo Clin Proc 1984;59:633–636.

45. Sze G, Krol G, Zimmerman RD, Deck MDF. Malignant extradural spinal tumors: MR imaging with Gd-DTPA. Radiology 1988;167:217–223.

46. Smoker WRK, Godersky JC, Knutzon RK, Keyes WD, Norman D, Bergman W. The role of MR imaging in evaluating metastatic spinal disease. AJR 1987;149:1241–1248.

47. Burk DL, Brunberg JA, Kanal E, Latchaw RE, Wolf GL. Spinal and paraspinal neurofibromatosis: distinction from benign tumors using imaging techniques. AJR 1987;149:1059–1064.

48. Quencer RM, El Gammel T, Cohen G. Syringomyelia associated with intradural extramedullary masses of the spinal canal. AJNR 1986;7:143–148.

49. Norman D. The spine. In: Brant-Zawadski M, Norman D, eds. Magnetic resonance imaging of the central nervous system. New York: Raven Press, 1987, 289–328.

50. Sloof JL, Kernohan JW, MacCarty CS. Primary intramedullary tumors of the spinal cord and filum terminale. Philadelphia: WB Saunders, 1964.

51. Palmer JJ. Radiation myelopathy. Brain 1972;95:109–122.

52. Tarr RW, Drolshagen LF, Kerner TC. MR imaging of recent spinal trauma. J Comput Assist Tomogr 1987;11:412–419.

53. Alba AA, Rothfus WE, Maroon JC. Delayed spinal subarachnoid hematoma. Rare complication of C1-C2 cervical myelography. AJNR 1986;7:526–529.

54. Muller-Vahl H, Vogelsang H. Spinal cord injury caused by a lateral C1-2 puncture for cervical myelography. Eur J Radiol 1986;6:160–163.

55. Clayman DA, Murakami ME, Vines FS. Compatibility of cervical spine braces with MR imaging: A study of nine potential nonferous devices. AJNR 1990;11:385–390.

56. McArdle CB, Wright JW, Prevost WJ, Dornfest DJ, Amparo EG. MR imaging of the acutely injured patient with cervical traction. Radiology 1986;159:273–274.

57. Hackney DB, Asato R, Joseph P. Hemorrhage and edema in acute cervical spinal cord compression: demonstration by MR imaging. Radiology 1986;161:387–390.

58. Gomori JM, Grossman RI, Goldberg HI. Intracranial hematomas: imaging by high-field MR. Radiology 1985;157:87–93.

59. Cheng C, Wolf AL, Mirvis SE, Bellis E, Salcman M. Body surfing accidents resulting in cervical spine injury. Presented at the American Association of Neurologic Surgeons Annual Meeting. Washington, D.C., 1989.

60. Quencer RM. The injured spinal cord. Evaluation with MR and intraoperative sonography. Radiol Clin N Am 1988;26:1025–1045.

61. Ragheb J, Wolf Al, Mirvis SE, Robinson WL. CT myelography in acute spinal cord injury: is it necessary? Presented at the American Association of Neurologic Surgeons Meeting, Captiva Island, FL, 1990.

62. Katirji MB, Reinmuth OM, Latchaw RE. Stroke due to vertebral artery injury. Arch Neurol 1985;42:242–248.

63. Hackney DB. Denominators of spinal cord injury. Radiology 1990;177:18–20.

64. Quencer RM, Morse BMM, Green BA, Eismont FJ, Brost P. Intraoperative spinal sonography: adjunct to metrizamide CT in the assessment and surgical decompression of posttraumatic spinal cord cysts. AJNR 1984;5:71–79.

8

Angiography and Embolization of Cervical Spine Tumors

In Sup Choi and Graham Lee

Introduction

Selective angiography of the spinal cord and spine was first described by R. Djindjian and G. DiChiro in 1964 (1, 12), but initial clinical applications of spinal angiography were limited to spinal cord vascular lesions.

The development of a more aggressive and curative approach toward tumors of the spinal column, including metastasis (2, 3, 4) has increased the necessity of spinal angiography. Prior to surgical intervention, it is important to know the vascularity of the tumor and the location of radiculomedullary arteries in order to avoid unexpected excessive bleeding or clipping of unrecognized spinal arteries at the time of resection.

Since the first description of transfemoral embolization of spinal lesions by R. Djindjian in 1971 (5), a new era of endovascular treatment has developed. The techniques of superselective catheterization has rapidly improved with the development of new catheter systems and embolic materials. Endovascular embolization has become an important preoperative or palliative treatment for vascular neoplasms. Devascularizing vascular tumors may enable surgical resection to be performed without excessive blood loss and morbidity (6, 7). Some tumors initially considered unresectable may become resectable by decreasing their actual size and vascularity (8). Embolization by itself can provide symptomatic relief of pain (9, 10) and may relieve spinal cord compression in some cases (11).

Vascular Anatomy of the Spine

Since the introduction of selective spinal angiography, a number of articles have described angiographic anatomy of the spinal arteries and radiculomedullary branches (12). Less attention has been paid to the vascular supply of the vertebral bodies.

Each vertebra develops from a metamere which gives rise to its own segment of nervous, vascular, musculoskeletal, and cutaneous system. Therefore, the basic vascular supply to each vertebra is essentially the same regardless of its level.

Arterial supply of the spine can be divided simply into 4 territories (Fig. 8.1):

1. Anterolateral supply;
2. Anterior spinal canal supply;
3. Posterior spinal canal supply;
4. Posterior supply.

1. *Anterolateral supply:* These are fine perforating branches which enter the anterior and lateral surface and supply the anterolateral portion of the vertebral body. In the cervical region, they arise from the vertebral and ascending cervical arteries bilaterally.

2. *Anterior spinal canal supply:* This arterial arcade supplies the posterior surface of the vertebral body. In the cervical region, branches originate directly from the vertebral artery and give ascending and descending branches which form longitudinal anastomoses with corresponding branches of the adjacent levels. Terminal branches anastomose with the contralateral anterior spinal canal branches. These anastomoses represent a classical ladder pattern of H-shaped arterial arcade at the posterior surface of the vertebral bodies.

3. *Posterior spinal canal supply:* In the cervical region, small caliber posterior spinal canal branches originate from the vertebral artery and enter the spinal canal posterior to the nerve root. They pass through the posterior epidural space and anastomose with the contralateral arteries at the midline. The laminae of the spine obtain their blood supply from prominent midline branches which penetrate the base and run posteriorly to the tips of the spinous processes.

4. *Posterior supply:* The dorsal spinal artery passes posteriorly along the outer surface of the laminae and forms an open meshed plexus close to the spinous processes. Many fine arteries penetrate the laminae and spinous processes from the outer surface. Near the base of the spinous

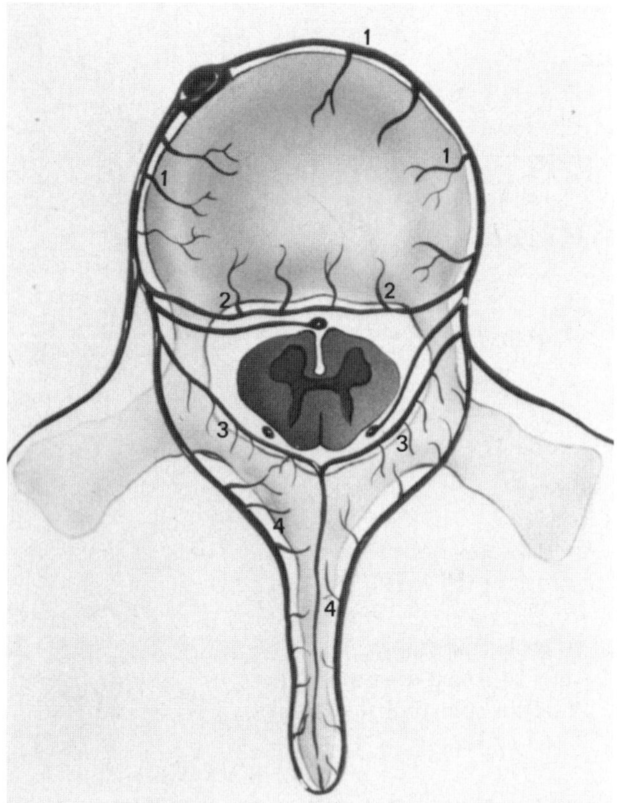

Figure 8.1. Vascular supply of the spine. 1. Anterolateral supply. 2. Anterior spinal canal supply. 3. Posterior spinal canal supply. 4. Posterior supply.

Table 8.1. Vascular Tumors of Spinal Column

Benign:
Hemangiomas
Aneurysmal bone cyst
Osteochondroma
Osteoid osteoma, osteoblastoma
Chondromas
Malignant:
Giant cell tumors
Osteogenic sarcoma
Chondrosarcoma
Malignant tumors of hematopoietic origin lymphomas, multiple myeloma
Hemangiopericytoma
Chordoma
Metastatic tumors, e.g., kidney, thyroid

process there is a longitudinal anastomosis with ipsilateral branches.

SPINAL ANGIOGRAPHY

Indications

Spinal angiography in most instances is performed as a preoperative or prebiopsy evaluation; however, it is often requested after an attempt to remove a tumor has been unsuccessful because of excessive bleeding. Noninvasive diagnostic imaging with CT and MRI define the location and extent of spinal tumors, but accurate determination of the vascularity of tumors is still difficult. Table 8.1 lists hypervascular tumors of the spinal column. The indications for spinal angiography largely depend upon the nature and extent of the lesion, the planned surgical approach (7), whether it is anterior or posterior, and how aggressive the removal of the lesion will be. If simple decompression laminectomy is planned for a vertebral tumor, it may not be necessary to perform spinal angiography even for a known vascular tumor. Evaluation by spinal angiography is useful for the following lesions:

1. Tumors of the lower cervical spine where the anterior spinal artery frequently originates;
2. Tumors with moderate or marked enhancement on contrast enhanced CT scan or with signal void areas or MRI suggestive of high blood flow;
3. Tumors of known vascular nature;
4. Tumors to be treated by embolization or chemoembolization.

Angiographic Protocol

Global injection of the aorta or subclavian artery will answer whether a tumor is highly vascular or not, but will miss certain tumors with a low or moderate vascularity and will not demonstrate dangerous anastomoses. We prefer selective catheterization of all possible feeding arteries to delineate the exact extent of tumor and for visualization of spinal arteries and anastomoses. At the same time, embolization can be done. The following list includes possible arterial supplies to tumors:

1. Upper cervical region (C1–C4);
   Vertebral artery;
   Occipital artery;
   Ascending pharyngeal artery;
   Thyrocervical trunk (ascending cervical artery);
   costocervical trunk (deep cervical artery).
2. Lower cervical region (C5–C7);
   Vertebral artery;
   Thyrocervical trunk (ascending cervical artery);
   Costocervical trunk (deep cervical artery);
   Supreme intercostal artery.

Most symptomatic vertebral tumors are not confined to the spine itself. For example, benign hemangiomas often have an extraspinal component which is seen at the time of surgery. As the tumor grows into the adjacent vertebra or extends into the paraspinal space, new vascular supplies are recruited. Utilizing a systematic approach as outlined in the above protocol, all possible arterial supplies can be thoroughly evaluated, and the presence of a spinal artery can be documented. If embolization is attempted it is important to know the anastomoses surrounding the lesion

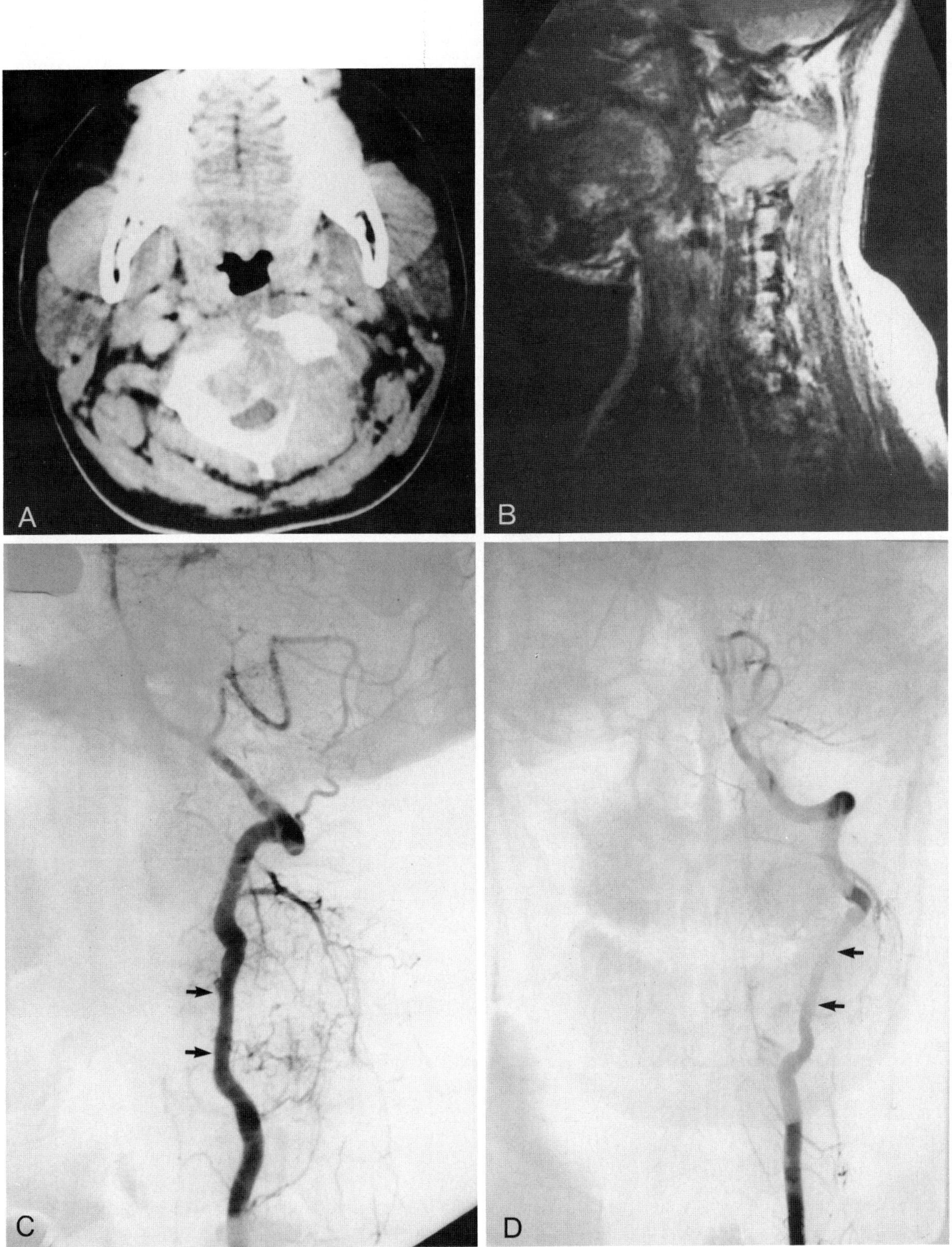

Figure 8.2. 17-year-old male with chordoma of C2 and C3 vertebrae. **A.** Axial CT scan at C2 level. Tumor mass destroying the vertebral body and narrowing the spinal canal. **B.** MRI of cervical spine. Paravertebral spread of tumor of C2 and C3. **C, D.** Left vertebral angiogram shows narrowing and anterior displacement of the vertebral artery at C2 and C3 (*arrows*) with fine neovascularity and vessel displacement by the mass. The right vertebral artery showed similar supply to the tumor.

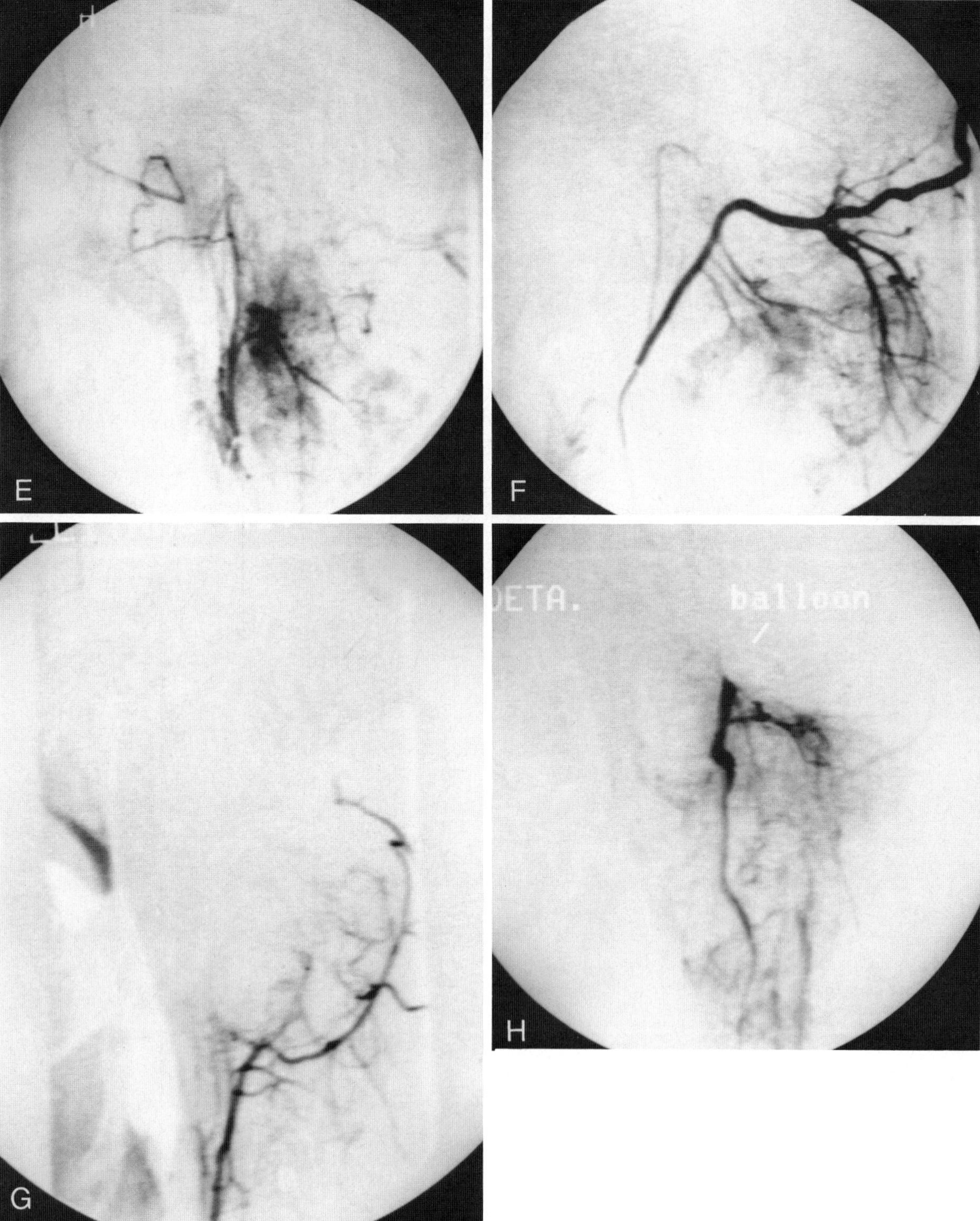

Figure 8.2. **E.** Left ascending pharyngeal arteriogram. Hypervascular tumor stain at C2 and C3 supplied by the spinomuscular branch. Then right ascending pharyngeal artery demonstrated similar supply. **F.** Left occipital arteriogram: Hypervascular tumor stain supplied by the C2 and C3 branches. **G.** Left ascending cervical arteriogram demonstrating supply to the inferior portion of the tumor. **H.** The left vertebral artery was occluded at the C1 level utilizing a detachable balloon. Complete occlusion of the vertebral artery and tumor hypervascularity are demonstrated. Embolization of the left occipital, ascending pharyngeal, and ascending cervical arteries was performed with PVA particles and ethanol. The right ascending pharyngeal and occipital arteries were embolized with PVA particles and ethanol.

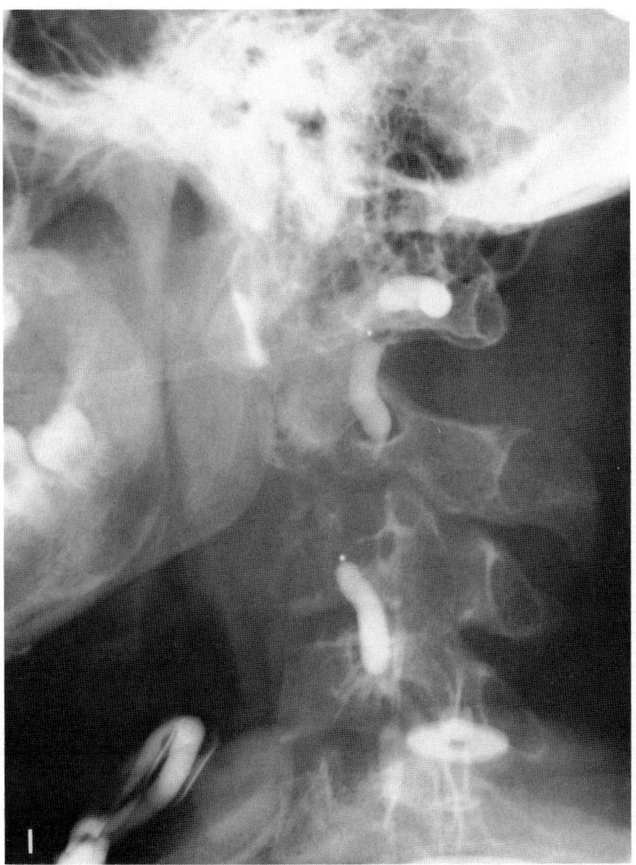

Figure 8.2. **I.** Postembolization film demonstrates the position of three balloons detached in the left vertebral artery.

in order to prevent inadvertent embolization of a spinal artery.

Spinal Cord Monitoring

Somatosensory evoked potentials (SEPs) have been effective in functional monitoring of the spinal cord (13). SEP monitoring during spinal angiography and embolization can reduce the complication rate (previously as high as 10–15%) (14) to less than 1%. This technique is very sensitive and effective in recognizing the spinal arteries, especially the anterior spinal artery (15). When contrast material is injected into the anterior spinal artery, the SEPs immediately decrease in amplitude and, at times, increase in latency (16). Clinical experience has shown that the presence of the anterior spinal artery can be recognized by SEP changes in over 80% of cases prior to angiographic confirmation.

It is also useful to monitor the actual embolizations. SEPs fluctuate due to different factors and conditions (depth of anesthesia, anesthetic agent, level of consciousness, etc.) but may provide an important warning signal during injection of embolic material. In cases where there is a decrease in amplitude of SEPs, embolization will be stopped until it recovers to baseline. SEP is also an excellent physiological indicator for a provocative test.

Provocative Test

In many instances, the anterior or posterior spinal artery can be readily recognized in conventional or digital subtraction angiography. But occasionally it may not be possible to document the presence of the spinal artery due to patient motion, subtraction artifact, or confusion with long anastomotic vessels of the spinal canal. If there is any doubt, a provocative test may be performed utilizing sodium amytal amobarbital (sodium), a short-acting barbiturate; 50–75 mg of sodium amytal (25 mg/cc dilution) is injected in the artery to be embolized. Neurological status is monitored clinically and electrophysiologically. If this test is positive, embolization will be aborted. Injection of xylocaine has also been used as a provocative test for the spinal cord, but experience with it is limited. Xylocaine is, however, used for provocative testing of the peripheral nerves including cranial nerves.

Angiographic Findings

In general the angiographic findings of spinal tumors are not specific except for a few benign lesions such as vertebral hemangiomas and osteoid osteomas. Voegeli and Fuchs (17) stated that arteriography in bone tumors increases the accuracy of the histological diagnosis by 20%. Analysis of the angiogram should be based on the differentiation between benign and malignant neoplasms (Fig. 8.2 and Fig. 8.3). The identification of typical vascular patterns may help to differentiate certain benign tumors.

Benign Tumors

Hemangioma

This is the most common benign vascular tumor in the spine, mostly in the thoracic and lumbar regions. On conventional radiography, the typical finding is a striated appearance of the vertebral body with thick trabeculations. Hemangiomas are usually asymptomatic and are found incidentally. Rarely they may present with backache, segmental pain, and spinal cord compression (17). Sudden paraplegia may occur due to compression fracture of the affected vertebra (18). The angiographic appearances are characteristic with a normal caliber of the feeding artery (19) and irregular opacification of the vertebral body with small pockets of contrast pooling. These contrast pools are of various size, without AV shunting and persist into the late venous phase. The draining veins are not dilated. Occasionally, atypical irregular vascular pools and stains may be seen, suggestive of a malignant lesion. The lack of AV shunting and a normal caliber filling artery favor a nonmalignant tumor. In the early stages, the tumor is confined

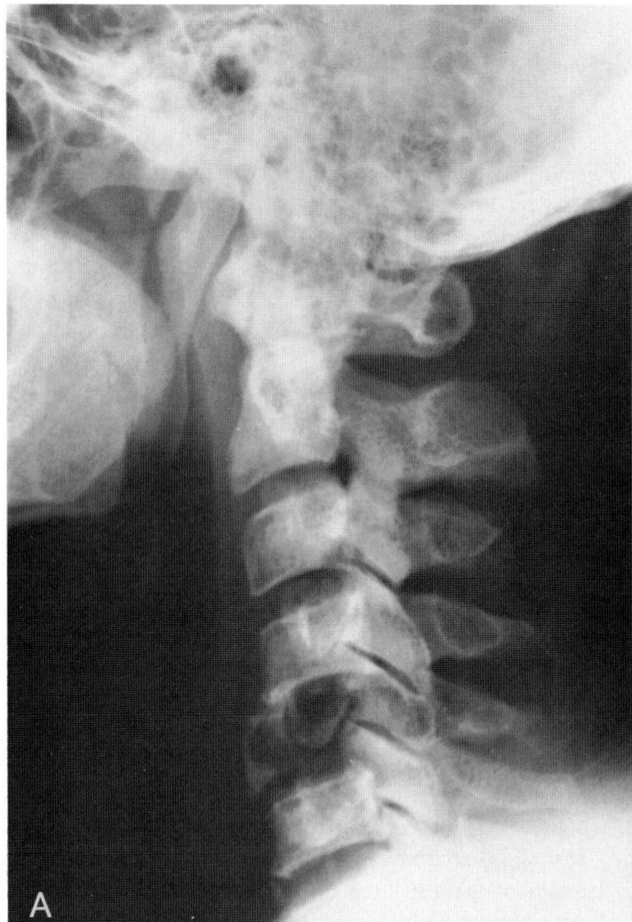

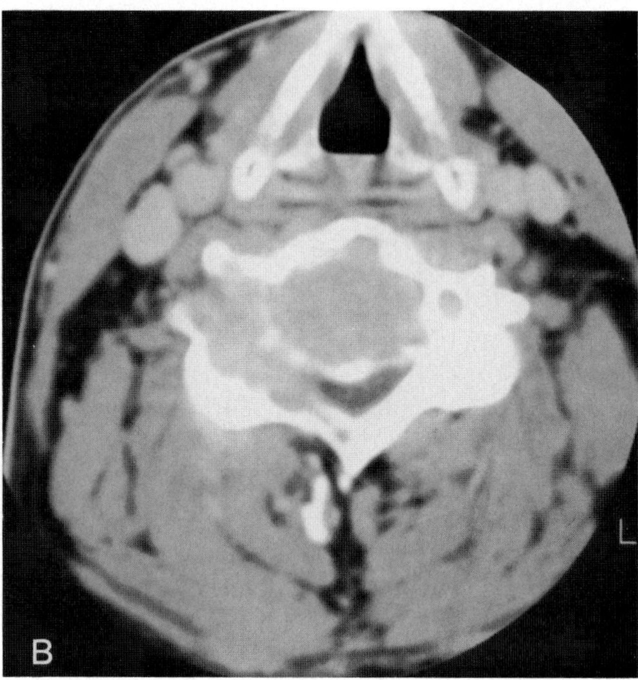

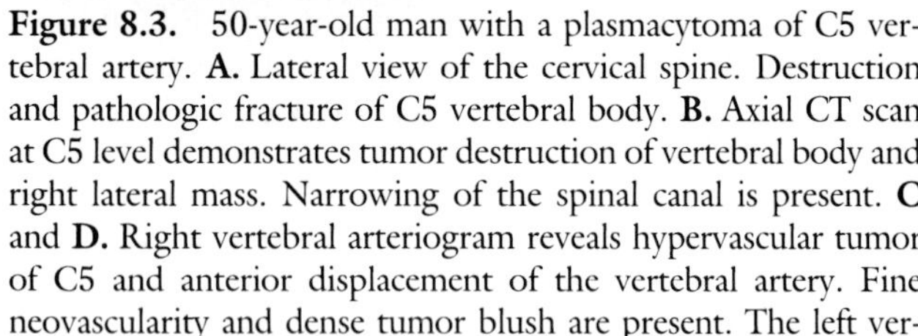

Figure 8.3. 50-year-old man with a plasmacytoma of C5 vertebral artery. **A.** Lateral view of the cervical spine. Destruction and pathologic fracture of C5 vertebral body. **B.** Axial CT scan at C5 level demonstrates tumor destruction of vertebral body and right lateral mass. Narrowing of the spinal canal is present. **C** and **D.** Right vertebral arteriogram reveals hypervascular tumor of C5 and anterior displacement of the vertebral artery. Fine neovascularity and dense tumor blush are present. The left vertebral artery provided minimal supply to the tumor. **E.** Right ascending cervical arteriogram demonstrating supply to the tumor. Note the artery of the cervical enlargement supplying the spinal cord (*small arrows*); therefore, this pedicle could not be embolized. **F.** A detachable balloon was placed at the C3 level to prevent inadvertent embolization of the vertebrobasilar system. Embolization of the right vertebral artery was then performed utilizing PVA particles.

to the vertebral body. However, most symptomatic lesions have paraspinal or epidural extension which is easily recognized on CT scan. There may be multiple hemangiomas in the spine or associated hemangiomas elsewhere in the body.

Aneurysmal Bone Cyst

The typical radiographic appearance of these lesions is a ballooned-out subperiosteal shell of bone with eccentric destruction of underlying cortex and cancellous bone (20). Paraspinal extension is common. The feeding arteries are usually enlarged with the cystic area opacified by contrast in the late arterial phase. This is often patchy and persists into the venous phase. This patchy opacification could be due to washout by unopacified blood through the cystic area (21). There is some degree of AV shunting, but it is not as intense as in malignant tumors.

Giant Cell Tumors

Giant cell tumors are rare in the cervical spine and are highly vascular with enlarged feeding arteries. Multiple dilated feeders can be seen on the surface entering the tumor. A dense irregular tumor stain with AV shunting is common, and the center of the tumor may show lack of stain. Differentiating this tumor from an aneurysmal bone cyst or a hypervascular malignant tumor may be difficult (22).

Other Vascular Benign Tumors

For benign tumors, conventional radiology and the CT scan are more useful for specific diagnosis than angiograms. Osteoid osteoma, osteochondroma, chondroma, or osteoblastoma frequently show a hypervascular tumor stain without AV shunting or dilated feeding arteries (23).

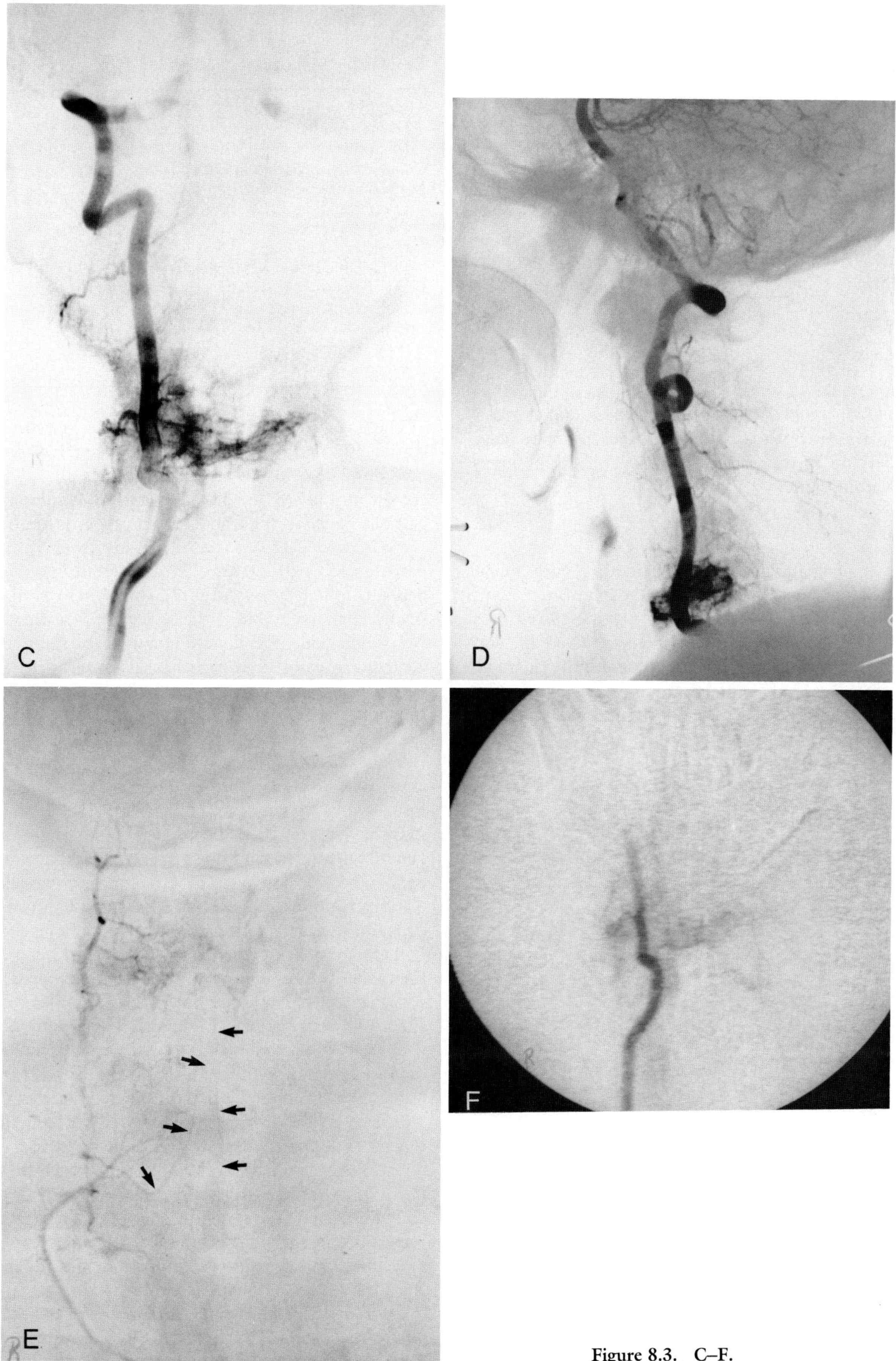

Figure 8.3. C–F.

MALIGNANT TUMORS

The differential diagnosis between malignant tumors is difficult and not practical, and only typical angiographic findings of malignancy will be discussed (24).

Feeding Arteries

The feeding arteries are usually dilated, and small osseous branches are recognizable. These may increase in number. The caliber is somewhat irregular, and abrupt angulations can be seen.

Vascularity

Vascularity may vary from lesion to lesion. Compared to benign lesions, tumor stains are seen earlier, and irregular vascular lakes are often seen. The tumor vessels are irregular in caliber and have a distorted course with abrupt angulation within the tumor.

Venous Drainage

Venous drainage often shows AV shunting. Early filling of the epidural or paravertebral venous plexuses is common. The draining veins may or may not be dilated.

Malignant lesions often extend to adjacent vertebra and recruit a new vascular supply. To recognize the extent of the lesion, the margins of the tumor must be identified by studying all possible collateral circulations and demonstrating normal surrounding tissues.

EMBOLIZATION

Since the introduction of selective spinal angiography and the development of selective endovascular embolization (5, 13), many reports have confirmed the value of embolization of vascular tumors of the spine (19). Embolization can reduce mass effect, relieve spinal block (11), and improve symptoms (9). Although embolization is not a curative treatment for spinal tumors, it can palliate symptoms, mainly intolerable pain, and possibly retard tumor growth. When surgical intervention is indicated, preoperative embolization may enable the tumor to be totally resected (8). Moreover, tumors which were considered unresectable may become resectable after embolization.

In order to maximize the effects of embolization, several factors must be considered.

a. The anatomy and flow characteristics in a given tumor;
b. The size and physical characteristics of the catheter system to be used;
c. The position of the catheter tip;
d. The physical, chemical, and biological characteristics of the embolic material;
e. The goal of embolization: preoperative, prebiopsy, or palliative;
f. The type of lesion, benign or malignant.

Table 8.2. Embolic Agents

Absorbable solid particles
Gelatin sponge and/or powder (Gelfoam TM)
Microfibrillar collagen (Avatine TM) (Angiostat TM)
Glutaraldehyde cross-linked collagen (GAX)
Nonabsorbable solids
Lyophilized dura (Lyodura)
Polyvinyl alcohol foam (PVA, Ivalon TM)
Metallic coils
Detachable balloons: latex, silicone
Fluids
Isobutyl-2-cyanoacrylate (IBCA)
N-butyl-cyanoacrylate (NBCA)
95% ethanol
Ethanol in various concentrations

These factors will determine the proper selection of the embolic agent so that the best and safest results can be accomplished. Various embolic materials are available as shown in Table 8.2. The following are commonly used embolic materials for embolization of spinal tumors.

a) *Gelfoam:* Gelfoam is available in powder form with particle sizes of 40–60 μm. These penetrate into the tumor bed producing perivascular necrosis. These particles are smaller than the caliber of the dangerous anastomoses and AV shunts and generally are not used for spinal tumors. Gelfoam strips or large particles have been used (18) but do not penetrate into the tumor bed, resulting in an effect similar to surgical ligation of a main feeding artery. The tumor bed will be resupplied by collateral circulation.

b) *Polyvinyl alcohol foam (PVA) (25, 26):* PVA is a nonabsorbable biocompatible sponge material. A particulated form is used varying in size from 149–1000 μm (149–250, 250–590, 590–1000 μm). These particles are suspended in contrast and injected through conventional or coaxial catheter systems to penetrate into the vascular bed. Various concentrations of PVA suspensions can be used depending upon flow rate and vascularity of a given tumor. If there are dangerous anastomoses, particles larger than the caliber of anastomotic vessels may be required to prevent inadvertent embolization. This is an excellent embolic agent for preoperative devascularization of tumors.

c) *Metallic coils:* These are short pieces of stainless steel or platinum guidewire to which dacron thread is attached to promote thrombosis. They are pushed or injected through a catheter to the artery at the catheter tip. If used alone this gives the same effect as surgical ligation of a feeding artery, but it is usually combined with particle embolization. Following injection of particles (PVA or Gelfoam), coils can occlude the trunk of the feeding artery and maximize the effect of particle embolization. Coils can be used to occlude branches supplying normal tissues or dangerous anastomoses prior to particle embolization.

d) *Isobutyl-2-cyanoacrylate (IBCA) or n-butyl-cyanoacrylate (NBCA):* These are low viscosity liquids which polymerize rapidly when in contact with ions and changes in

Ph. Polymerization time can be delayed by adding retardants (pantopaque or acetic acid) so that the distal tumor bed can be reached (27). Tantalum powder is added to increase radiopacity. Cyanoacrylates have tissue adhesive properties and cause an inflammatory reaction of the vascular walls. The *n*-butyl derivative is preferable to IBCA due to its lower tensile strength. They are useful for recurrent or unresectable tumors as well as tumors with fast AV shunting. Cyanoacrylates are not widely used due to difficulty in handling the agents and the amount of experience needed for proper use. Furthermore, there is controversy related to their potential carcinogenicity.

e) *Ethyl alcohol:* Ethanol has a potent sclerosing effect in endothelium which makes it an effective embolic material. When ethyl alcohol is injected intravascularly, it causes intimal damage and sludging of cellular blood elements which then produces mechanical emboli.

The long-term effect of intraarterial ethanol infusion has been studied. For up to 91 days, there was complete vascular occlusion and permanent infarction without evidence of recanalization (28). The flow characteristics, availability, and effectiveness as a long-term occlusive agent make ethanol the best embolic agent for vascular tumors. However, if inadvertently perfused into the normal tissue, serious complications can occur from necrosis of neural or visceral tissue (23). Ethanol can cause extensive skin necrosis by perfusing cutaneous branches. Therefore, we limit the use of ethanol to embolization of malignant tumors.

Ninety-five percent ethyl alcohol is opacified by metrizamide powder, which enables it to be seen under fluoroscopy. It is injected only when superselective catheterization of the tumor feeding pedicle is accomplished; 2–3 cc of opacified ethanol is injected slowly each time. Because of the low viscosity it can be easily refluxed to the normal territory. Therefore at the end stages of embolization, smaller amounts (0.5–1 cc) should be injected at a slower rate. For larger and highly vascular lesions, ethanol can be diluted and mixed with PVA particles. The PVA provides mechanical blocking and increases stasis of the ethanol. Significant tumor necrosis can be achieved with ethanol embolization, not only as a preoperative measure but as a palliative treatment.

f) *Detachable balloons:* Silicone or latex balloons are utilized for occluding large vessels such as the vertebral artery. They are filled with contrast material or a solidifying agent such as hydroxyethyl methacrylate (HEMA) or silicone. Contrast-filled balloons may deflate over a few weeks or months, but the vessel remains permanently occluded. Occlusion of the vertebral artery may be performed preoperatively when adequate surgical removal of the tumor will require sacrifice of the vertebral artery. Occlusion of the vertebral artery may also be required to facilitate thorough embolization of tumors receiving significant blood supply from vertebral artery branches, or from other cervical arteries with dangerous anastomoses with the vertebral artery. Occlusion of the vertebral artery in this instance enables devascularization of the tumor to be performed without the risk of emboli migrating into the vertebrobasilar system.

Several other embolic materials have been used clinically, such as particles of Bovine dura mater.

Direct retrograde injection of methyl methacrylate into a hemangioma of vertebral body has been reported (30). Following transarterial embolization, laminectomy was performed and methyl methacrylate was injected through a cannula positioned in the pedicles. The authors claimed that polymerized acrylate supports a weakened vertebral body so that no further stabilization is necessary. Long-term follow up has not been reported.

CHEMOEMBOLIZATION

The term chemoembolization was first introduced by Kato and Nemoto in 1978 (31). In order to increase the topical release of an active anticancerous agent in high concentrations, they prepared mitomycin C microcapsules with particle size of 224.6 +/− 45.9 μm and injected these particles through the angiographic catheter to the target organ. The microcapsules produced local ischemia, and the sustained release of mitomycin-C from the capsule increases the duration of contact between the drug and target cells.

Courtheoux et al. reported their experience of chemoembolization of spine metastases in 1985 (32). Mitomycin C microcapsules or Adriamycin mixed with dura mater was used. Improvement of clinical symptoms, pain, and neurological deficits were noticed in 58 months follow up.

Early results of chemoembolization indicate it can be an excellent palliative treatment for unresectable metastases. Further clinical and pharmacological studies are needed in conjunction with comparative studies with other cytotoxic embolic agents such as ethyl alcohol.

REFERENCES

1. Djindjian R, Merland JJ. Angiography of spinal column and spinal cord tumors. Stuttgart: Georg Thieme Verlag, 1981.

2. Fielding W, Pyle R, Fietti V. Anterior cervical vertebral body resection and bone-grafting for benign and malignant tumors. J Bone Joint Surg 1979;61-A:251–253.

3. Gilbert R, Kim J, Posner J. Epidural spinal cord compression from metastatic tumor: diagnosis and treatment. Ann Neurol 1978;3:40–51.

4. Marshall L, Langfitt T. Combined therapy for metastatic extra-[l]dural tumors of the spine. Cancer 1977;40:2067–2070.

5. Djindjian R, Cophignon J, Rey A, et al. Superselective arteriographic embolizations by the femoral route in neuroradiology, study of 50 cases: embolizations in vertebromedullary pathology. Neuroradiology 1973;6:132–142.

6. Slatkin N, Posner J. Management of spinal epidural metastases. Clin Neurosurg 1984;30:698–716.

7. Sundaresan N, Galicich J, Lane J, et al. Treatment of neoplastic epidural cord compression by vertebral body resection and stabilization. J Neurosurg 1985;63:676–684.

8. Sundaresan N, Scher H, DiGiacinto G, et al. Surgical treatment

of spinal cord compression in kidney cancer. J Clin Oncol 1986;4:1851–1856.

9. Nickolisen R, Fallon B. Locally recurrent hypernephroma treated by radiation therapy and embolization. Cancer 1985;56:1049–1051.

10. Treves R, Legoff J, Doyon D, et al. L'embolisation therapeutique ou embolisation palliative a visee antalgique des metastases osseuses d'origine renale. Rev Rhum 1984;51:1–5.

11. Gross C, Hodge C, Binet E, et al. Relief of spinal block during embolization and vertebral resection. Spine 1984;9:97–101.

12. Crock HV, Yoshizawa H. Origins of arteries supplying the vertebral column, in: The blood supply of the vertebral column and spinal cord in man. New York: Springer-Verlag 1977:1–21.

13. Hacke W. Neuromonitoring. Neurology 1985;232:125–133.

14. Doppman JL, DiChiro G. Risks and complications. In: Selective angiography of the spinal cord. Missouri: Warren H. Green, Inc., 1969:51–58.

15. Berenstein A, Young W, Ransohoff J, et al. Somatosensory evoked potentials during spinal angiography and therapeutic transvascular embolization. J Neurosurg 1984;60:777–785.

16. Young W, Berenstein A. Somatosensory evoked potential monitoring of intraoperable procedures: In: Schramm J, Jones SJ eds. Spinal cord monitoring. Heidelberg: Springer-Verlag Berlin, 1985:197–203.

17. Voegeli E, Fuchs W. Arteriography in bone tumors. Br J Radiol 1976;49:407–415.

18. Graham J, Yang W. Vertebral hemangioma with compression fracture and paraparesis treated with preoperative embolization and vertebral resection. Spine 1984;9:97–101.

19. Esparza J, Castro S, Portillo J, et al. Vertebral hemangiomas: spinal angiography and preoperative embolization. Surg Neurol 1978;10:171–173.

20. MacCarty C, Dahlin D, Doyle J, et al. Aneurysmal bone cysts of the neural axis. J Neurosurg 1961;18:671–6677.

21. Lindbon A, Soderberg G, Spjut H, et al. Angiography of aneurysmal bone cyst. Acta Radiol 1961;55:12–16.

22. Laurin S. Angiography in giant cell tumors. Radiology 1977;17:118–123.

23. MacLellan D, Wilson F. Osteoid osteoma of the spine. J Bone Joint Surg 1967;49-A:111–121.

24. Baylock R, Kempe L. Chondrosarcoma of the cervical spine. J Neurosurg 1976;44:500–503.

25. Tadavarthy SM, Moller JH. Polyvinyl alcohol (Ivalon): a new embolic material. Am J Roentgenol 1974;125:609–616.

26. Berenstein A, Graeb D. Convenient preparation of ready to use particles in polyvinyl alcohol foam suspensions for embolization. Radiology 1982;145:38–46.

27. Cromwell KD, Kerber CW. Modification of cyanoacrylate for therapeutic embolization: preliminary experience. Am J Roentgenol 1979;132:779–801.

28. Latchaw RF, Pearlman RL, Schaitkin BM, et al. Intra-arterial ethanol as a long term occlusive agent in renal hepatic and gastrosplenic arteries of pigs. Cardiovasc Intervent Radiol 1985;8:24–30.

29. Malligan BD, Espimosa GA. Bowel infarctions: complications of ethanol ablation of a renal tumor. Cardiovasc Intervent Radiol 1983;6:55–57.

30. Nicola N, Ling E. Vertebral hemangioma: retrograde embolization stabilization with methyl methacrylate. Surg Neurol 1987;27:481–486.

31. Kato T, Nemoto R. Microencapsulation of mitomycin C for intra-arterial infusion chemotherapy. Proc Japan Acad 1978;54-B:413–417.

32. Courtheoux P, Alachkar F, Casasco A, et al. Chimioembolization des metastases du rachis lombaire. J Neuroradiol 1985;12:151–162.

9

INTRAOPERATIVE ULTRASOUND IMAGING OF THE CERVICAL SPINE

William F. Chandler and Jonathan M. Rubin

The use of real-time ultrasound sector scanning for imaging the spinal cord during neurosurgical and orthopedic procedures has proven to be extremely helpful and adds significantly to the safety of the patient (13). Although ultrasound imaging was first recognized to be useful for localization during intracranial procedures as early as 1979 (2, 8, 16, 20), it was not until 1982 that the first report appeared documenting the intraoperative imaging of the spinal cord with ultrasound (4, 6, 7, 14, 18). Once the bony lamina have been removed over the area of interest, ultrasound is an ideal method for imaging the spinal cord and its surrounding structures. Since the dura is not an impediment to ultrasound waves, the spinal cord, subarachnoid spaces, and adjacent bone and disc spaces can all be "seen" in real-time on a television screen. The normal pulsations of the spinal cord can easily be observed. Since ultrasound waves are completely safe and the imaging is instantaneous, this method can be repeated as often as needed during a procedure. Imaging with ultrasound takes only a few minutes and in most situations actually saves operating time because the pathology can be localized and evaluated prior to even opening the dura.

Although modern static imaging techniques such as magnetic resonance imaging (MRI) and computed tomography (CT) scanning have improved dramatically, they still do not provide the surgeon with feedback during the operation. The intraoperative use of ultrasound imaging has the one unique and important quality that it provides continuous and real-time imaging information. It also provides in most instances an even more detailed image of the internal structure of the spinal cord than does the MRI. It will show the "new" position of the cord relative to a tumor or bony spur once the laminectomy has been completed. Ultrasound will demonstrate if the normal motion of the spinal cord has been restored by a particular procedure.

TECHNIQUES AND EQUIPMENT

The spinal canal is imaged with ultrasound during surgery by simply filling the wound with saline after the laminectomy has been completed and immersing the tip of the transducer in the saline. It is necessary for the patient to be in a prone position for this technique to be practical. Figure 9.1 shows this relationship between the transducer and the spinal canal. All ultrasound devices create an image in a particular plane, much as we are accustomed to viewing a specific "cut" with CT or MRI imaging. Since the surgeon is viewing the canal in real-time, the transducer is simply rotated 90° to switch from a longitudinal to a cross-sectional image of the cord. The transducer is moved from side to side or cephalad to caudad to view all aspects of the exposure. It is best to do this in a systematic fashion so as not to miss any area of the field. It is important to use an ultrasound transducer with a 7.5 MHz frequency, since the 3.5 or 5 MHz transducers that work well on the brain will not image the spinal cord.

Although this imaging technique can be managed by a

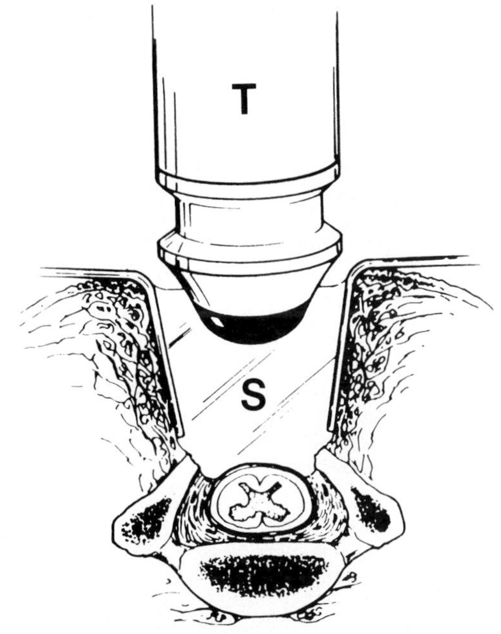

Figure 9.1. The ultrasound transducer (*T*) is shown immersed in the saline (*S*) filled wound during a laminectomy. A cross-sectional representation of the spinal canal and cord is shown at the bottom of the drawing.

surgeon alone, it is ideal to work along with an experienced radiologist trained in ultrasonography. This is particularly true when first starting out with this technique, since the ultrasound images created in real-time are quite foreign to most surgeons. Practice with maneuvering the transducer can be obtained in a beaker of water with objects placed in the bottom.

Ultrasound imaging of a normal cervical spinal cord is seen in Figure 9.2. At the top of each picture is a curvilinear white area that is not a true object but only the near field artifact just beneath the transducer head. This is why the standoff of saline between the transducer and the dura is necessary. The first layer beneath the near field artifact to be seen is the dura, which is very echogenic. Beneath that the nonechogenic subarachnoid space is seen, and then the spinal cord is imaged with both its anterior and posterior aspects being well delineated. A white echogenic line is routinely seen within the normal cord just anterior to its true center. We have called this the central canal, but in fact this may just be echoes emanating from the anterior median fissue of the cord. This has proven to be a useful landmark, since it tends to disappear with any significant intramedullary pathology. Anterior to the cord the subarachnoid space is once again seen well and anterior to that, the posterior aspects of the vertebral bodies and disc spaces are visualized. All of these structures can be identified in either the sagittal or transverse planes.

It should be mentioned that it is possible to visualize the spinal cord with ultrasound from the anterior approach if a complete corpectomy has been performed at one level. Although this is not used often, we have had occasion to use this technique in selected trauma cases, and it was sufficient to ascertain that the cord was not compressed and that a hematoma was not present.

In addition to the standard gray-scale sector scanning which is so helpful for localization and anatomical evaluation, another technique has recently become available for the specific identification and localization of small vascular anomalies. This system is called Color-Flow Doppler imaging and provides the ability to assign a different color to blood which is flowing either towards or away from the transducer (1). This allows even a small vascular malformation to stand out very colorfully against the gray-scale background of the normal spinal cord.

CERVICAL SPINE LESIONS

Tumors

Tumors within the cervical spinal canal are ideal for localization and characterization with intraoperative ultrasound imaging. This is true whether the tumors are intramedullary, extramedullary, or even extradural. We have had the opportunity to image a large variety of cervical tumors and have not yet failed to readily identify the neoplasm.

Ultrasound is particularly helpful in the intraoperative evaluation of intramedullary tumors such as astrocytomas and ependymomas (12). Before the dura is opened the overall extent of the tumor is visualized and specific areas of interest such as cysts or calcified regions can be localized. This imaging guides the opening of the dura and often directs the surgeon to a particular location to start the

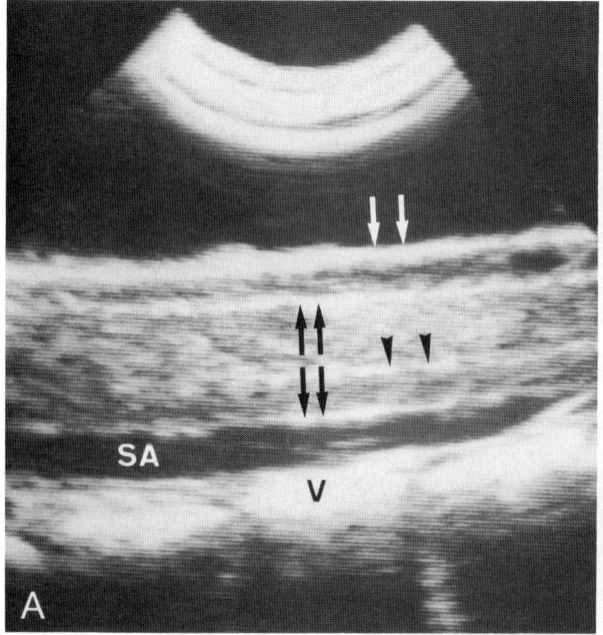

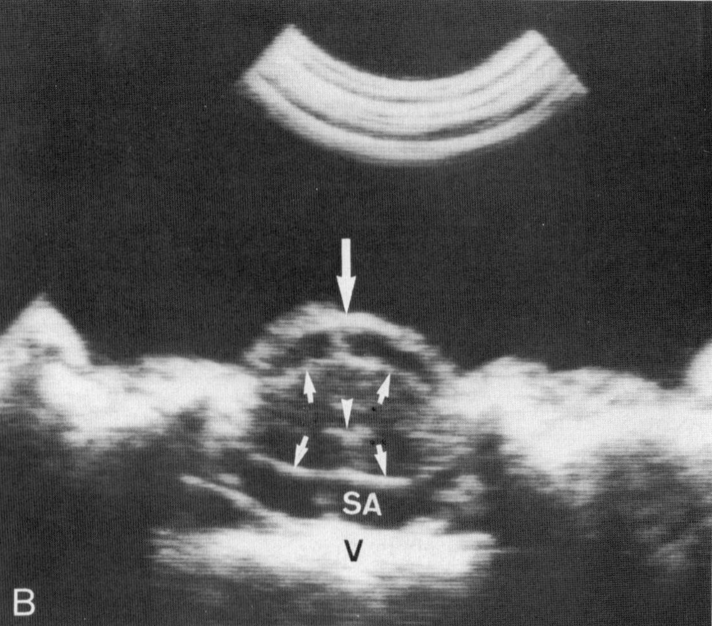

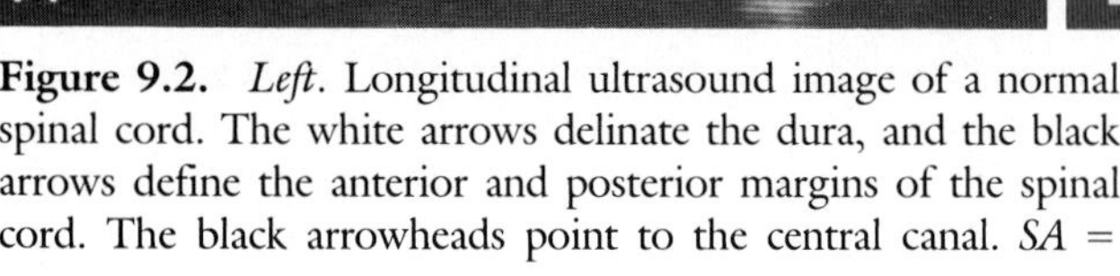
Figure 9.2. *Left.* Longitudinal ultrasound image of a normal spinal cord. The white arrows delinate the dura, and the black arrows define the anterior and posterior margins of the spinal cord. The black arrowheads point to the central canal. *SA* = subarachnoid space and *V* = vertebral body. *Right.* Cross-sectional ultrasound image of spinal cord. The large white arrow points to the dura, and the small white arrows define the spinal cord. The arrowhead points to the central canal.

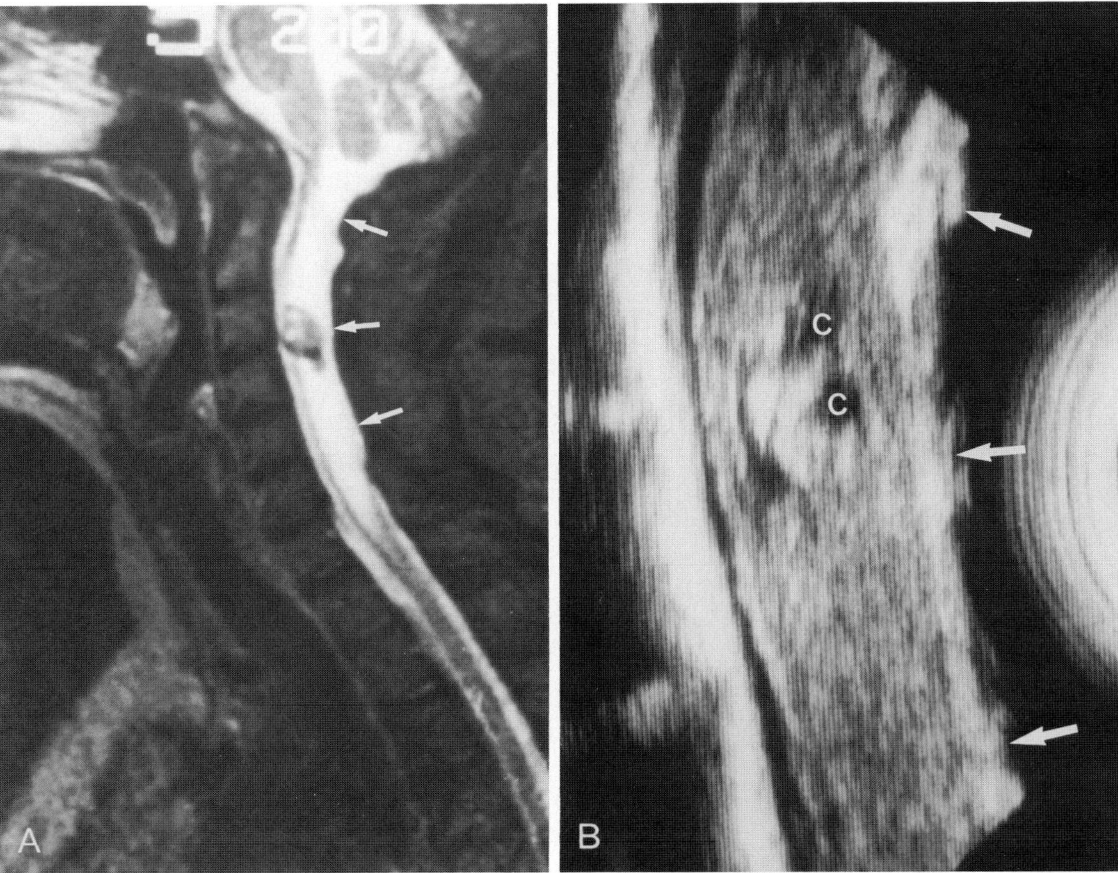

Figure 9.3. *Left.* Sagittal magnetic resonance image showing an intrinsic astrocytoma of the cervical spinal cord (all *arrows*) with a probable cystic area (at middle *arrow*). *Right.* Ultrasound image of the same area (*arrows*) showing the diffuse tumor and the cystic areas (*C*'s).

myelotomy and exploration. In cystic tumors such as astrocytomas or hemangiomas, ultrasound will identify the specific mural nodule of tumor (17). With intramedullary tumors the "central canal" will virtually always be absent to ultrasound imaging. This is helpful in determining the length of tumors. Edema proximal or distal to the tumor will also cause widening of the cord and loss of the central canal, thus creating some confusion in determining the absolute limits of the tumor. In most cases the tumor border is quite well defined and the edema is less echogenic. Figure 9.3 is an excellent example of how a low grade astrocytoma of the cervical cord was imaged with ultrasound. In this case the relatively small cystic portion of the tumor was localized and a myelotomy performed over the area of maximum tumor involvement. This provided the approach to the tumor with the least possibility of injury to the surrounding spinal cord.

Extramedullary intradural lesions such as meningiomas and neuromas can also be easily localized with ultrasound. Although precise localization of a lesion posterior to the cord may not be critical, if the lesion is primarily anterior then accurate localization becomes imperative to minimize cord retraction. Even with posteriorly located lesions ultrasound helps in directing the dural opening. Figure 9.4 is an example of a meningioma that was located anterior to the cord in the cervical region. Ultrasound localized the lesion and provided the surgeon with direction as to the side that was optimal for approaching the tumor. Figure 9.5 is an unusual neurenteric cyst that eroded the vertebral body but was located intradurally, causing distortion and compression of the spinal cord. Again, the ultrasound imaging directed the surgeon to the appropriate side for tumor resection. In each of these examples, postresection imaging ascertained that the tumor removal was complete and that the cord was no longer distorted.

Extradural tumors such as lymphomas, myelomas, or metastases can also be imaged lying anterior or lateral to the dura. Bone erosion may be identified, but bone invasion is not seen with ultrasound. Imaging of these extradural lesions is also helpful in assessing the degree of cord decompression after laminectomy and partial tumor removal.

Cysts and Syringomyelia

Ultrasound imaging is an excellent method for delineating and characterizing any type of cyst or syrinx within the cervical spinal cord. Ultrasound is capable in most instances of differentiating cystic regions from solid abnormalities, no matter what the protein content of the cyst (11). Cystic areas that are difficult or impossible to characterize with CT or MRI scanning are readily identified with ultrasound. Syrinx cavities within the cord can be accurately localized and any small septae identified and evaluated. In some instances, what appears on CT or MRI scanning to be a single syrinx turns out be a collection of small cystic areas within a given cross-section of the cord. We have had several examples where at the time of surgery the "syrinx" was either so small or composed of multiple channels that placement of a catheter was not even attempted.

Figure 9.6 is an example of a sizable cervical syrinx. The multilobulated configuration of the syrinx is much better appreciated on the ultrasound imaging than on the MRI.

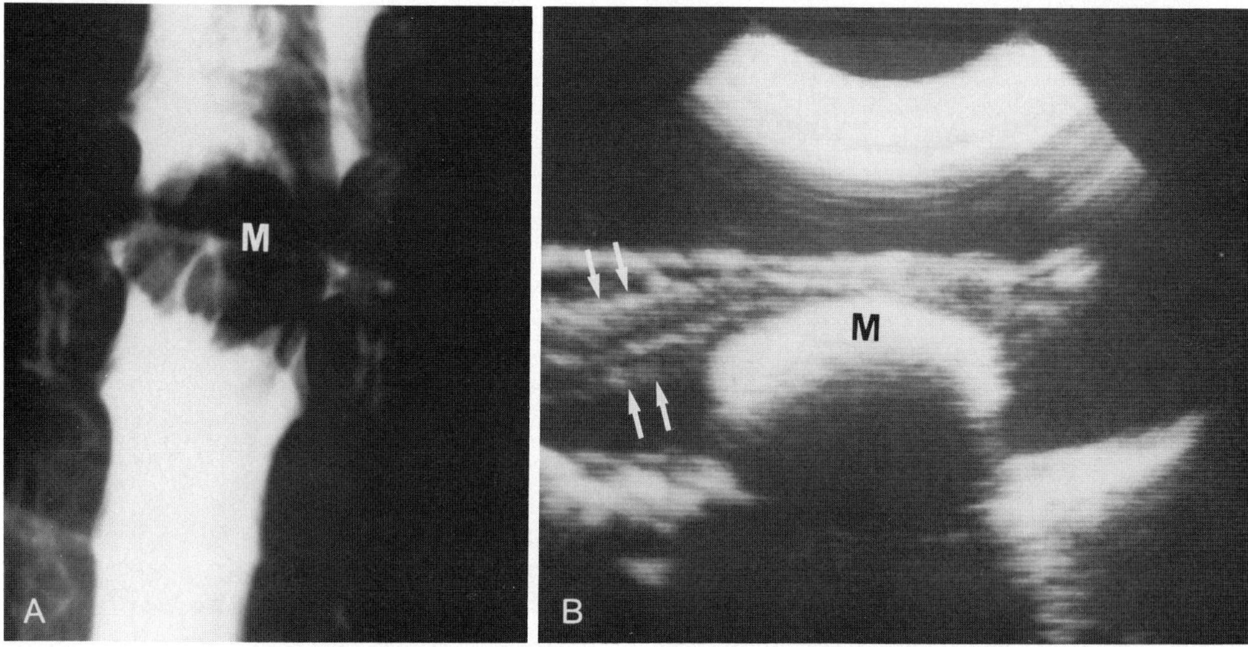

Figure 9.4. *Left*. Myelogram demonstrating a filling defect (*M*) caused by a meningioma. *Right*. Ultrasound imaging shows the meningioma (*M*) anterior to the spinal cord and the cord (between *arrows*) draped over the tumor.

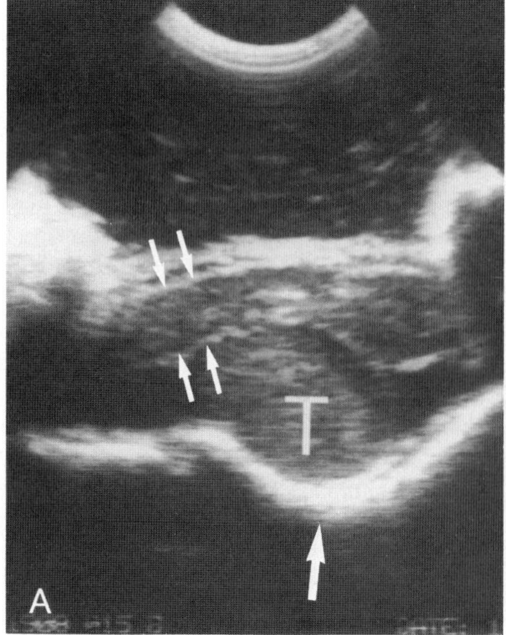

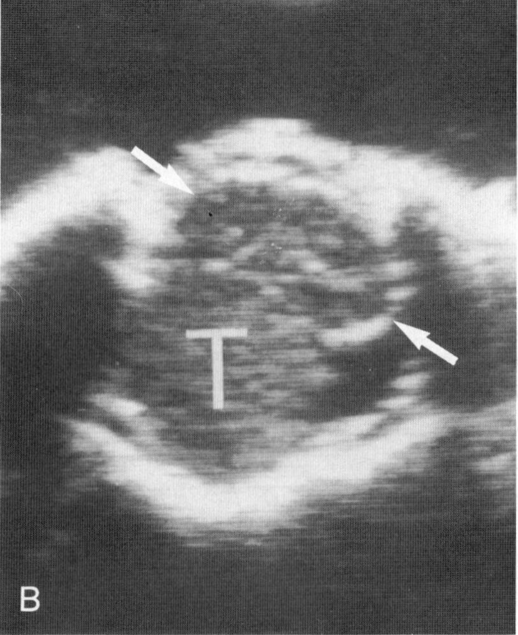

Figure 9.5. *Left*. Intraoperative ultrasound image (longitudinal) showing a neurenteric cyst (*T*) with the spinal cord (between *arrows*) draped posteriorly. The single arrow points to the vertebral body erosion. *Right*. Cross-sectional view demonstrating the spinal cord (between *arrows*) being displaced by the tumor (*T*).

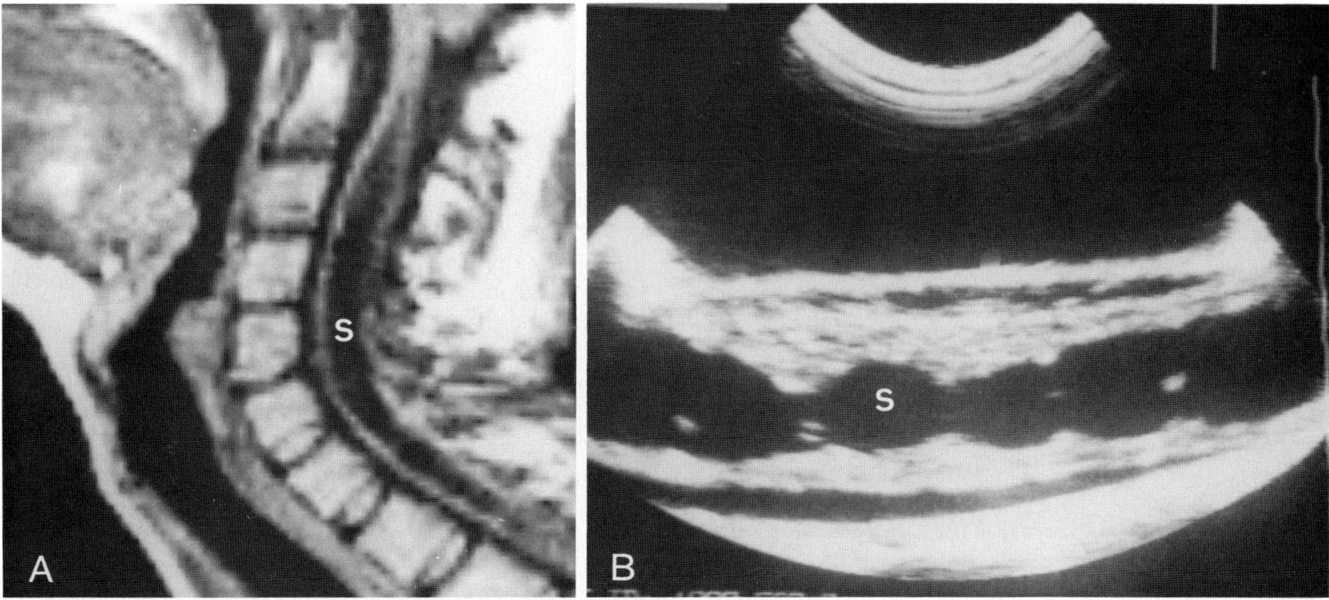

Figure 9.6. *Left*. Magnetic resonance image demonstrating a syrinx (*S*) of the cervical spinal cord. *Right*. The ultrasound image shows the syrinx (*S*) to have multiple septae and a beaded appearance.

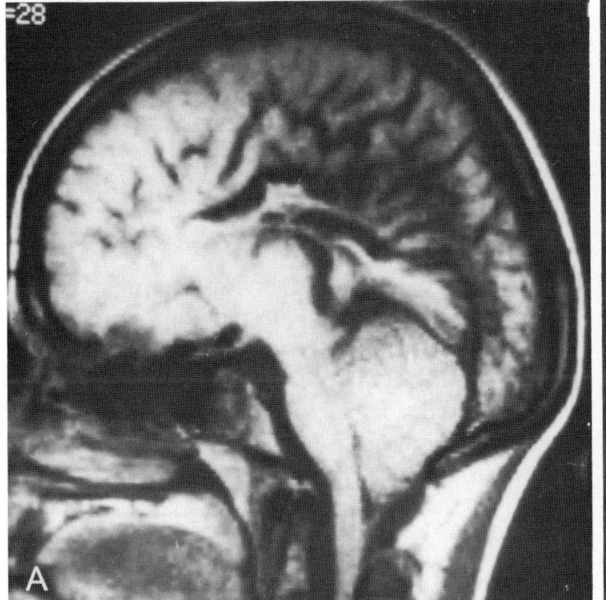

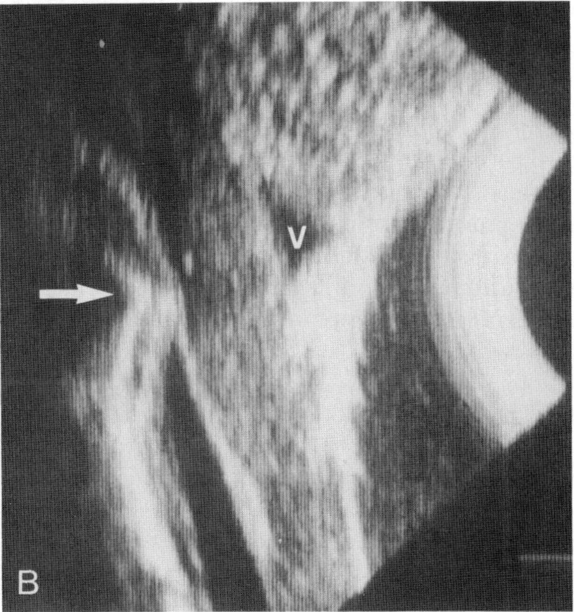

Figure 9.7. *Left*. Magnetic resonance image of a patient with an Arnold-Chiari malformation. *Right*. Ultrasound image of the posterior fossa showing the fourth ventricle (*V*) nearly below the foramen magnum (*arrow*).

Another useful aspect of ultrasound imaging in the treatment of syringomyelia is that the cord can be reimaged once the drainage tube has been placed. This will provide evidence for whether the entire syrinx has been drained or if an additional catheter is needed or the first catheter need be advanced.

Arnold-Chiari Malformation

In patients with Arnold-Chiari malformations the relationship of the cerebellar tonsils to the foramen magnum can be evaluated with intraoperative ultrasound, as well as the ability to look for associated anomalies within the upper cervical spinal cord (3, 19). Often a syrinx will be present in association with this malformation and may be connected to the low-lying fourth ventricle by only a thin tract. Ultrasound will clearly demonstrate these anatomic variations and help the surgeon to decide if the syrinx needs to be shunted as well as the cervical-medullary region decompressed.

Figure 9.7 is the ultrasound image of an Arnold-Chiari Malformation in a child demonstrating the very caudal

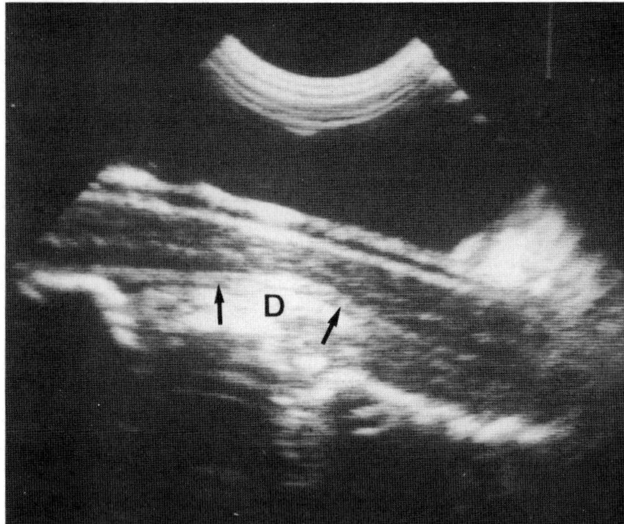

Figure 9.8. Ultrasound image of a centrally herniated cervical disc (*D*). The spinal cord (*arrows*) is draped over the disc fragment.

location of the fourth ventricle. In this case no syrinx was identified, and a simple decompression was performed.

Disc Disease and Spondylosis

Although most small herniated cervical discs are well characterized preoperatively and an anterior or posterior approach planned according to the location of the disc and the personal preference of the surgeon, there are still occasions when a large centrally herniated disc cannot be completely differentiated from a tumor. In these situations a laminectomy is usually carried out to identify and remove the compressive lesion. We have found that transdural imaging with ultrasound is very helpful prior to opening the dura to further assess the location of the lesion and its precise anatomical relationship to the anterior dura and the spinal cord.

Figure 9.8 is an example of a large centrally herniated disc that was believed by preoperative myelography and CT scanning to be a tumor displacing the spinal cord. The intraoperative ultrasound clearly demonstrated that the lesion was anterior to the dural sac and thus most likely a large disc fragment. Cross sectional images showed that the mass was slightly more to one side, and the disc was removed quite readily via an extradural dissection on that side. Without the ultrasound imaging, the dura would likely have been opened and the subarachnoid spaces explored.

Intraoperative ultrasound can also image the relationship of the spinal cord to any osteophytic spurring that might cause cord impingement. This is of course performed after the decompressive laminectomy so that the cord is being evaluated in its "new" position, which differs from that seen on the preoperative imaging studies. Since the ultrasound imaging is in real-time, it provides the unique opportunity to observe the actual movement of the spinal

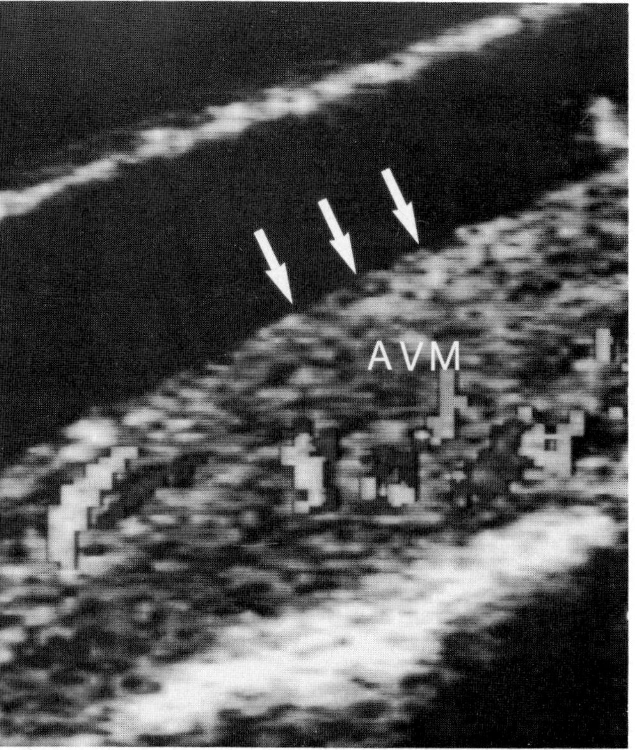

Figure 9.9. Color-Flow Doppler image of a small arteriovenous malformation of the cervical spinal cord. The arrows delineate the posterior aspect of the spinal cord, and the vascular malformation is shown as the area of mixed red and blue signals beneath the letters "*AVM*."

cord (5). In most cases of cervical stenosis related to diffuse spondylitic changes, the normal spinal cord pulsations return after decompressive laminectomy. If the cord is seen to be significantly displaced by a single bony ridge and cord pulsations remain absent below the ridge, additional anterior decompression could be considered if the patient does not improve clinically.

Trauma

Ultrasound imaging has become established as a very helpful way to assess the spinal canal and cord in operations for spine decompression related to trauma, often associated with spine stabilization procedures (9, 10). This is especially useful in the thoracic and thoraco-lumbar areas, but is occasionally useful in the cervical region. We have used this technique through very limited cervical laminectomies to be certain that an anterior disc fragment was not present. In one instance, we have used the ultrasound to image the spinal cord via the anterior approach through a corpectomy used for decompression and fusion. In this situation the imaging very clearly showed that the cord was decompressed and that there was no hematoma or bone fragment displacing the cord.

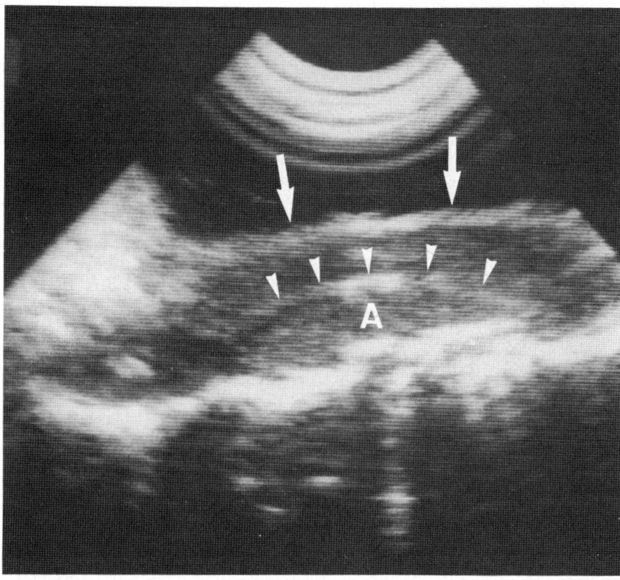

Figure 9.10. Longitudinal ultrasound image of the cervical spinal canal with an epidural abscess (*A*) lying anterior to the spinal cord. The large arrows delineate the posterior aspect of the cord, and the arrowheads show the limits of the abscess.

Vascular

Although vascular malformations of the spinal cord may well be imaged with conventional gray-scale sector scanning ultrasound (15), we have found recently that the use of Color-Flow Doppler ultrasound imaging adds significantly to the resolution of vascular anomalies (1). Color-Flow Doppler technology provides the ability for the imaging device to differentiate flowing blood from all other types of stationary tissue. Thus it is possible to recognize even a small collection of vessels within normal tissue or even within an abnormal area such as a hematoma. This technique adds one of two colors to blood which is flowing towards the transducer and a second color to blood which is flowing away from the transducer. Thus a collection of abnormal vessels will have a mixture of colors, and normal vessels will have only one color.

Figure 9.9 is an example of a small arteriovenous malformation involving the cervical spinal cord. The abnormal blood vessels stand out very clearly against the gray-scale image of the spinal cord.

Infections

Epidural abscesses which lie anterior to the spinal cord may be quite localized and difficult to diagnose definitively preoperatively and to find during surgery. Since intraoperative ultrasound has the ability to image the anterior dura, it can accurately localize the extent and thickness of an epidural abscess. Figure 9.10 demonstrates a cervical epidural abscess in a patient who was operated upon emergently late at night for a progressive quadraparesis with preoperative studies showing only a compressive lesion. With the accurate localization of this anterior epidural lesion, the dura was gently retracted medially, and the abscess was drained.

REFERENCES

1. Black KL, Rubin JM, Chandler WF, McGillicuddy JE. Intraoperative color flow Doppler imaging of AVM's and aneurysms. J Neurosurg 1988;68:635–639.

2. Chandler WF, Knake JE, McGillicuddy JE, Lillehei KO, Silver TM. Intraoperative use of real-time ultrasonography in neurosurgery. J Neurosug 1982;57:157–163.

3. DiPietro MA, Venes JL, Rubin JM. Arnold-Chiari II malformation: intraoperative real-time ultrasound evaluation. Radiology 1987;164:799–804.

4. Dohrmann GJ, Rubin JM. Intraoperative ultrasound imaging of the spinal cord: syringomyelia, cysts, and tumors—a preliminary report. Surg Neurol 1982;18:395–399.

5. Jokich PW, Rubin JM, Dohrmann GJ. Intraoperative ultrasonic evaluation of spinal cord motion. J Neurosurg 1984;60:707–711.

6. Knake JE, Chandler WF, McGillicuddy JE, Gabrielsen TO, Latack JT, Gebarski SS, Yang PJ. Intraoperative sonography of intraspinal tumors: initial experience. AJNR 1983;4:1199–1201.

7. Knake JE, Gabrielsen TO, Chandler WF, Latack JT, Gebarski SS, Yang PJ. Real-time sonography during spinal surgery. Radiology 1984;151:461–465.

8. Masuzawa H. Intraoperative ultrasonography of the brain. Jpn J Med Ultrasonics 1980;7:277–279.

9. McGahan JP, Benson D, Chehrazi B, Walter JP, Wagner FC. Intraoperative sonographic monitoring of reduction of thoracolumbar burst fractures. Am J Radiol 1985;145:1229–1232.

10. Montalvo BM, Quencer RM, Green BA, et al. Intraoperative sonography in spinal trauma. Radiology 1984;153:125–134.

11. Platt JM, Rubin JM Bowerman RA, DiPietro MA, Chandler WF. Intraoperative sonographic characterization of a cystic intramedullary spinal cord lesion appearing as solid. Am J Neuroradiol 1988;9:614.

12. Platt JM, Rubin JM, Chandler WF, Bowerman RA, DiPietro MA. Intraoperative spinal sonography in the evaluation of intramedullary tumors. J Ultrasound Med 1988;7:317–325.

13. Rubin JM, Chandler WF. Ultrasound in Neurosurgery. New York: Raven Press, 1989.

14. Rubin JM, Dohrmann GJ. Work in progress: intraoperative ultrasonography of the spine. Radiology 1983;146:173–175.

15. Rubin JM, Knake JE. Intraoperative sonography of a spinal cord arteriovenous malformation. Am J Neuroradiol 1987;8:730–731.

16. Rubin JM, Mirfakhraee M, Duda EE, Dohrmann GJ, Brown F. Intraoperative ultrasound examination of the brain. Radiology 1980;137:831–832.

17. Sanders WP, Ausman JI, Dujovny M, et al. Ultrasonic features of two cases of spinal cord hemangioblastoma. Surg Neurol 1986;26:453–456.

18. Theodotou BC, Powers SK. Use of intraoperative ultrasound in decision making during spinal operations. Neurosurgery 1986;19:205–211.

19. Venes JL, Black KL, Latack JT. Preoperative evaluation and surgical management of the Arnold-Chiari II malformation. J Neurosurg 1986;64:363–370.

20. Voorhies RM, Patterson RH. Preliminary experience with intraoperative ultrasonographic localization of brain tumors. Radiol Nucl Med 1980;10:8–9.

10

Radiographic Evaluation of Athletic Injuries to the Cervical Spine

Joseph S. Torg, Helene Pavlov, and Steven G. Glasgow

Cervical Spine

Athletic injuries to the cervical spine may involve the bony vertebrae, intervertebral discs, ligamentous supporting structures, the spinal cord, roots, and peripheral nerves, or any combination of these structures. The panorama of injuries observed runs the spectrum from the "cervical sprain syndrome" to fracture-dislocations with permanent quadriplegia. Fortunately, severe injuries with neural involvement occur infrequently. However, those responsible for the emergency and subsequent care of the athlete with a cervical spine injury should possess a basic understanding of the variety of problems that can occur.

The various athletic injuries to the cervical spine and related structures are:

1. Nerve root-brachial plexus neurapraxia;
2. Stable cervical sprain;
3. Muscular strain;
4. Nerve root-brachial plexus axonotmesis;
5. Cervical cord neurapraxia with transient quadriplegia;
6. Intervertebral disc injury (narrowing-herniation) without neurologic deficit;
7. Stable cervical fractures without neurologic deficit;
8. Subluxations without neurologic deficit;
9. Unstable fractures without neurologic deficit;
10. Dislocations without neurologic deficit;
11. Intervertebral disc herniation with neurologic deficit;
12. Unstable fracture with neurologic deficit;
13. Dislocation with neurologic deficit;
14. Quadriplegia;
15. Death.

Consideration of current diagnostic, management, and rehabilitation principles are presented in other appropriate chapters. The purpose of this chapter is to define several specific areas pertaining to cervical spine injury resulting from recreational and competitive athletic activities. These areas are:

1. On-field management;
2. Cervical cord neurapraxia;
3. Axial loading injuries to the middle cervical spine segment;
4. The axial load tear-drop fracture: the isolated and three-part, two-plane fractures;
5. Prevention of cervical injuries;
6. Criteria for return to contact activities following injury.

Although all athletic injuries require careful attention, the evaluation and management of injuries to the cervical spine should proceed with particular consideration. The actual or potential involvement of the nervous system creates a high-risk situation in which the margin for error is low. A proper diagnosis is imperative, but the clinical picture is not always representative of the seriousness of the injury at hand. An intracranial hemorrhage may initially present with minimal symptoms, yet follow a precipitous downhill course, whereas a less severe injury, such as neurapraxia of the brachial plexus that is associated with alarming paresthesias and paralysis, will resolve swiftly and allow for quick return to activity. Although the more severe injuries are rather infrequent, this low incidence coincidentally results in little, if any, management experience for the on-site medical staff.

There are several principles that should be considered by individuals responsible for on-the-field management of athletes who may sustain injuries to the head and neck.

(1) The team physician or trainer should be designated as the person responsible for supervising on-the-field management of the potentially serious injury. This person is the "captain" of the medical team.
(2) Prior planning must ensure the availability of all necessary emergency equipment at the site of potential injury. At a minimum, this should include a spineboard, stretcher, and equipment necessary for the initiation and maintenance of cardiopulmonary resuscitation (CPR).
(3) Prior planning must ensure the availability of a properly equipped ambulance, as well as a hospital equipped and staffed to handle emergency neurologic problems.
(4) Prior planning must ensure immediate availability of a telephone for communicating with the hospital

emergency room, ambulance, and responsible individuals in case of an emergency.

Managing the unconscious or spine-injured athlete is a process that should not be done hastily or haphazardly. Being prepared to handle this situation is the best way to prevent actions that could convert a repairable injury into a catastrophe. Be sure that all the necessary equipment is readily accessible, in good operating condition, and that all assisting personnel have been trained to use it properly. On-the-job training in an emergency situation is inefficient at the least. Everyone should know what must be done beforehand, so that on a signal the game plan can be put into effect.

A means of transporting the athlete must be immediately available in a high-risk sport such as football and must be "on-call" in other sports. The medical facility must be alerted to the athlete's condition and estimated time of arrival so that adequate preparation can be made.

Having the proper equipment is an absolute must. A spineboard is essential and is the best means of supporting the body in a rigid position. It is somewhat like a full body splint. By splinting the body, the risk of aggravating a spinal cord injury, which must always be suspected in the unconscious athlete, is reduced. In football, bolt cutters and a sharp knife or scalpel are also essential if it becomes necessary to remove the face mask. A telephone must be available to call for assistance and to notify the medical facility. Oxygen should be available and is usually carried by ambulance and rescue squads, although it is rarely required in an athletic setting. Rigid cervical collars and other external immobilization devices can be helpful if properly used. However, manual stabilization of the head and neck is recommended even if other means are available.

Properly trained personnel must know, first of all, who is in charge. Everyone should know how to perform CPR and how to move and transport the athlete. They should know where emergency equipment is located, how to use it, and the procedure for activating the emergency support system. Individuals should be assigned specific tasks beforehand, if possible, so that duplication of effort is eliminated. Being well prepared helps to alleviate indecisiveness and second-guessing.

Prevention of further injury is the single most important objective. Do not take any action that could possibly cause further damage. The first step should be to immobilize the head and neck by supporting them in a stable position (Fig. 10.1 A & B). Then, in the following order, check for breathing, pulse, and level of consciousness.

If the victim is breathing, simply remove the mouth guard, if present, and maintain the airway. It is necessary to remove the face mask only if the respiratory situation is threatened or unstable or if the athlete remains unconscious for a prolonged period. Leave the chin strap on.

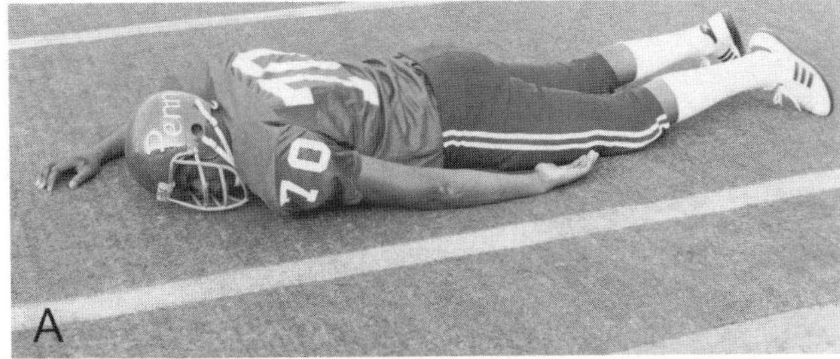

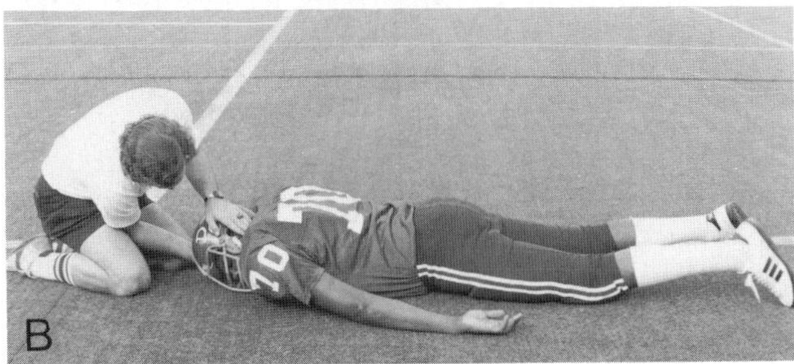

Figure 10.1. **A**, Athlete with suspected cervical spine injury may or may not be unconscious. However, all who are unconscious should be managed as though they had a significant neck injury. (With permission, from Torg JS, ed. Athletic injuries to the head, neck and face. Philadelphia: Lea & Febiger, 1982.) **B**, Immediate manual immobilization of the head and neck unit. First, check for breathing. (With permission, from Torg JS, ed. Athletic injuries to the head, neck and face. Philadelphia: Lea & Febiger, 1982.)

Once it is established that the athlete is breathing and has a pulse, evaluate the neurologic status. The level of consciousness, response to pain, pupillary response, and unusual posturing, flaccidity, rigidity, or weakness should be noted.

At this point, simply maintain the situation until transportation is available, or until the athlete regains consciousness. If the athlete is face down when the ambulance arrives, change his position to face up by logrolling him onto a spineboard. Make no attempt to move him except to transport him or to perform CPR if it becomes necessary.

If the athlete is not breathing or stops breathing, the airway must be established. If he is face down, he must be brought to a face-up position. The safest and easiest way to accomplish this is to logroll the athlete into a face-up position. In an ideal situation the medical-support team is made up of five members: the leader, who controls the head and gives the commands only; three members to roll; and another to help lift and carry when it becomes necessary. If time permits and the spineboard is on the scene, the athlete should be rolled directly onto it. However, breathing and circulation are much more important at this point.

With all medical-support team members in position, the

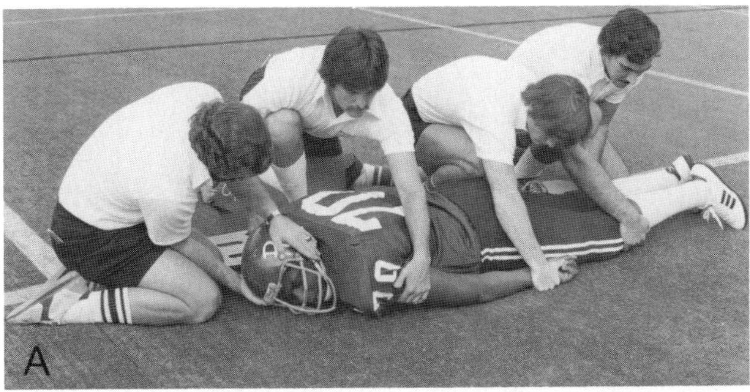

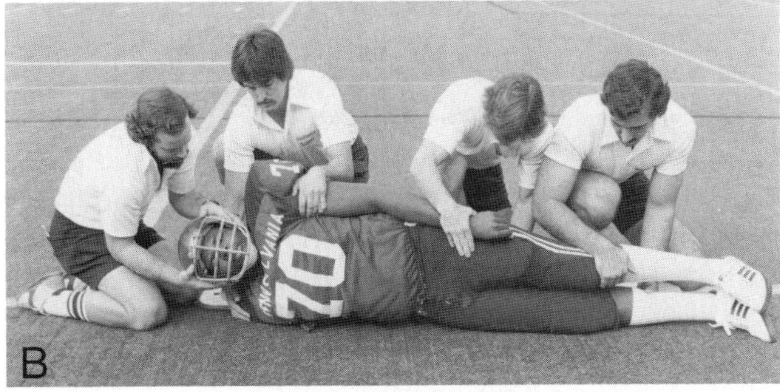

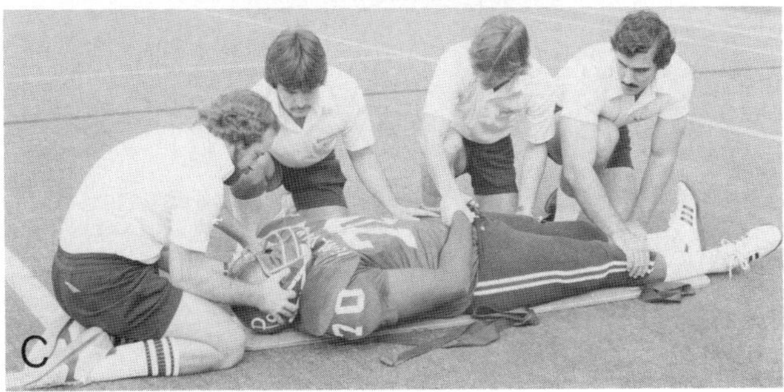

Figure 10.2. **A**, Logroll to a spineboard. This maneuver requires four individuals: the leader to immobilize the head and neck and to command the medical-support team. The remaining three individuals are positioned at the shoulders, hips, and lower legs. (With permission, from Torg JS, ed. Athletic injuries to the head, neck and face. Philadelphia: Lea & Febiger, 1982.) **B**, logroll. The leader uses the cross-arm technique to immobilize the head. This technique allows the leader's arms to "unwind" as the three assistants roll the athlete onto the spineboard. (With permission, from Torg JS, ed. Athletic injuries to the head, neck and face. Philadelphia: Lea & Febiger, 1982.) **C**, logroll. The three assistants maintain body alignment during the roll. (With permission, from Torg JS, ed. Athletic injuries to the head, neck and face. Philadelphia: Lea & Febiger, 1982.)

athlete is rolled toward the assistants—one at the shoulders, one at the hips, and one at the knees. They must maintain the body in line with the head and spine during the roll. The leader maintains immobilization of the head by applying slight traction and by using the crossed-arm technique. This technique allows the arms to unwind during the roll (Fig. 10.2 A to C).

The face mask must be removed from the helmet before rescue breathing can be initiated. The type of mask that is attached to the helmet determines the method of removal. Bolt cutters are used with the older single- and double-bar masks. The newer masks that are attached with plastic loops should be removed by cutting the loops with a sharp knife or scalpel. Remove the entire mask so that it does not interfere with further rescue efforts (Fig. 10.3 A to C).

Once the mask has been removed, initiate rescue breathing following the current standards of the American Heart Association.

Once the athlete has been moved to a face-up position, quickly evaluate breathing and pulse. If there is still no breathing or if breathing has stopped, the airway must be established.

"The jawthrust technique is the safest first approach to opening the airway of a victim who has a suspected neck injury, because in most cases it can be accomplished by the rescuer grasping the angles of the victim's lower jaw and lifting with both hands, one on each side, displacing the mandible forward while tilting the head backward. The rescuer's elbows should rest on the surface on which the victim is lying" (1a) (Fig. 10.4).

If the jaw thrust is not adequate, the head tilt-jaw lift should be substituted. Care must be exercised not to overextend the neck.

"The fingers of one hand are placed under the lower jaw on the bony part near the chin and lifted to bring the chin forward, supporting the jaw and helping to tilt the head back. The fingers must not compress the soft tissue under the chin, which might obstruct the airway. The other hand presses on the victim's forehead to tilt the head back" (1a) (Fig. 10.5).

The transportation team should be familiar with handling a victim with a cervical spine injury, and they should be receptive to taking orders from the team physician or trainer. It is extremely important not to lose control of the care of the athlete; therefore, be familiar with the transportation crew that is used. In an athletic situation, prior arrangements with an ambulance service should be made.

Lifting and carrying the athlete requires five individuals; four to lift, and the leader to maintain immobilization of the head. The leader initiates all actions with clear, loud verbal commands (Fig. 10.6 A and B).

The same guidelines apply to the choice of a medical facility as to the choice of an ambulance: be sure it is equipped and staffed to handle an emergency head or neck injury. There should be a neurosurgeon and an orthopedic surgeon to meet the athlete upon arrival. Roentgenographic facilities should be standing by.

Once the athlete is in a medical facility and permanent immobilization measures are instituted, the helmet is removed. The chin strap may now be unfastened and discarded. The athlete's head is supported at the occiput by one person while the leader spreads the earflaps and pulls the helmet off in a straight line with the spine (Fig. 10.7 A and B).

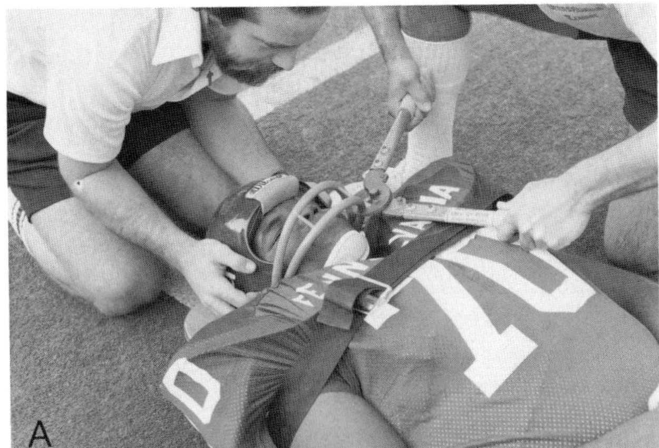

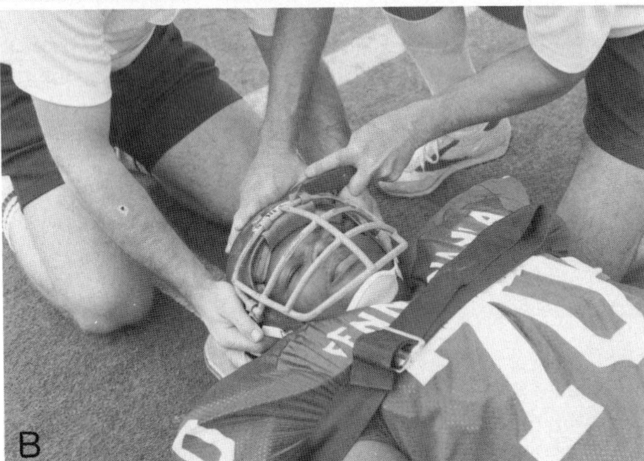

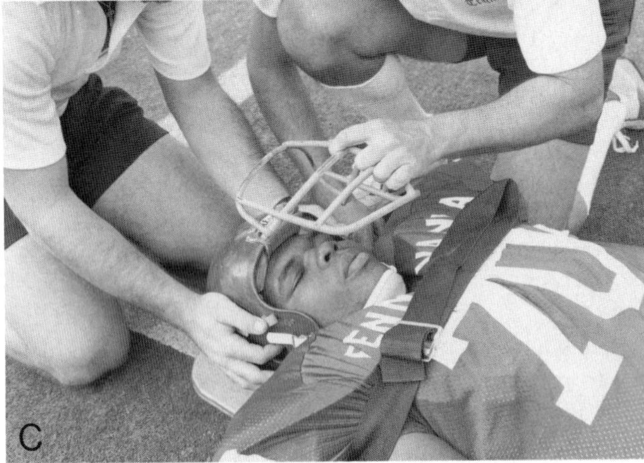

Figure 10.3. **A**, Remove double and single masks with bolt cutters. Head and helmet must be securely immobilized. (With permission, from Torg JS, ed. Athletic injuries to the head, neck and face. Philadelphia: Lea & Febiger, 1982.) **B**, remove "cage"-type masks by cutting the plastic loops with a utility knife. Make the cut on the side of the loop away from the face. (With permission, from Torg JS, ed. Athletic injuries to the head, neck and face. Philadelphia: Lea & Febiger, 1982.) **C**, remove the entire mask from the helmet so it does not interfere with further resuscitation efforts. (With permission, from Torg JS, ed. Athletic injuries to the head, neck and face. Philadelphia: Lea & Febiger, 1982.)

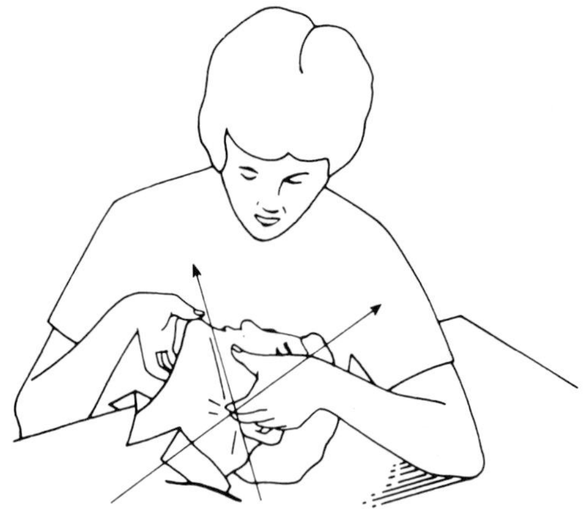

Figure 10.4. Jaw-thrust maneuver for opening the airway of a victim with a suspected cervical spine injury. From: Health care provider's manual for basic life support. Dallas, TX: American Heart Association, 1988.

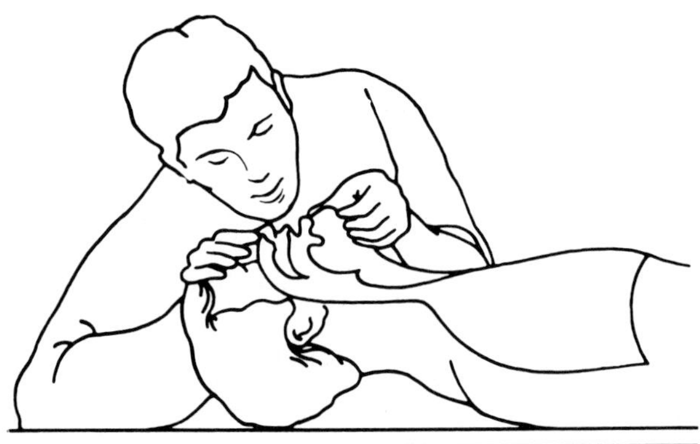

Figure 10.5. Head tilt-jaw lift maneuver for opening the airway. Used if jaw thrust is inadequate or if a helmet is being worn. From: Health care provider's manual for basic life support. Dallas TX: American Heart Association, 1988.

Cervical Spinal Stenosis with Cord Neurapraxia and Transient Quadriplegia

Characteristically, the clinical picture of cervical spinal cord neurapraxia with transient quadriplegia involves an athlete who sustains an acute transient neurologic episode of cervical cord origin with sensory changes that may be associated with motor paresis involving both arms, both legs, or all four extremities after forced hyperextension, hyperflexion, or axial loading of the cervical spine (1).

Sensory changes include burning pain, numbness, tingling, or loss of sensation; motor changes consist of weakness or complete paralysis. The episodes are transient, and complete recovery usually occurs in 10–15 minutes, although in some cases gradual resolution does not occur for 36–48 hours. Except for burning paresthesia, neck pain is not present at the time of injury. There is complete return of motor function and full, pain-free cervical motion. Rou-

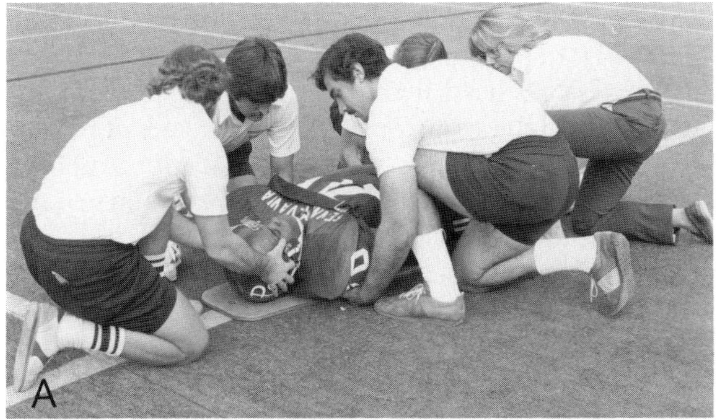

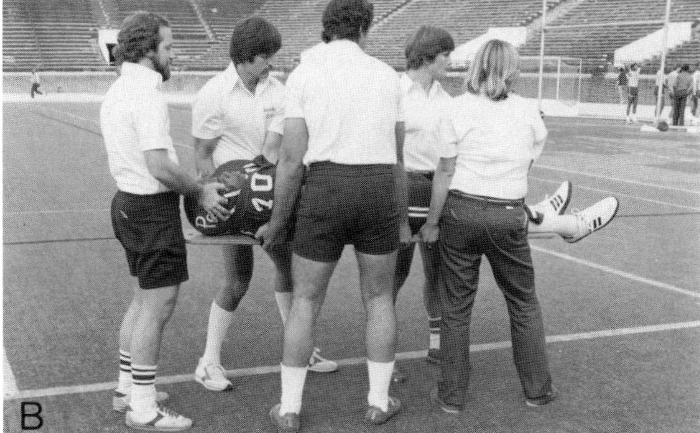

Figure 10.6. **A**, Four members of the medical support team lift the athlete on the command of the leader. (With permission, from Torg JS, ed. Athletic injuries to the head, neck and face. Philadelphia: Lea & Febiger, 1982.) **B**, the leader maintains the manual immobilization of the head. The spineboard is not recommended as a stretcher. An additional stretcher should be used for transporting over long distances. (With permission, from Torg JS, ed. Athletic injuries to the head, neck and face. Philadelphia: Lea & Febiger, 1982.)

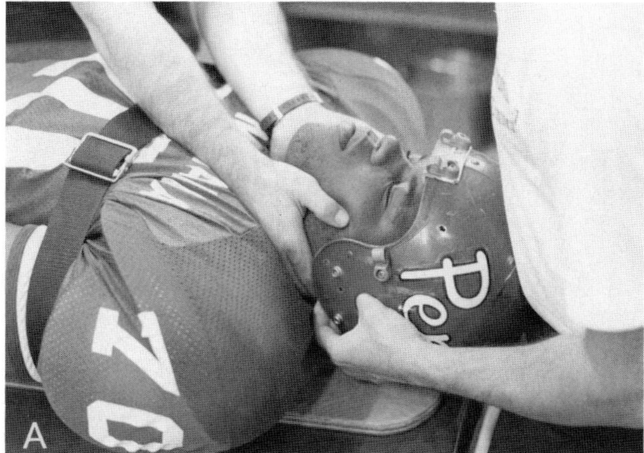

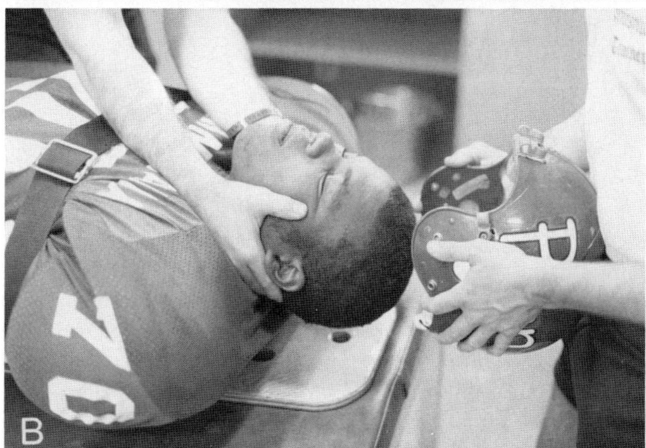

Figure 10.7. **A**, The helmet should be removed only whenever permanent immobilization can be instituted. The helmet may be removed by detaching the chin strap, spreading the earflaps, and gently pulling the helmet off in a straight line with the cervical spine. (With permission, from Torg JS, ed. Athletic injuries to the head, neck and face. Philadelphia: Lea & Febiger, 1982.) **B**, the head must be supported under the occiput during and after removing the helmet. (With permission, from Torg JS, ed. Athletic injuries to the head, neck and face. Philadelphia: Lea & Febiger, 1982.)

tine x-ray films of the cervical spine show no evidence of fracture or dislocation. However, a demonstrable degree of cervical spinal stenosis is present (1).

DETERMINATION OF SPINAL STENOSIS: METHOD OF MEASUREMENT

In order to identify cervical stenosis, a method of measurement is needed. The standard method, the one most commonly employed for determining the sagittal diameter of the spinal canal, involves measuring the distance between the middle of the posterior surface of the vertebral body and the nearest point on the spinolaminar line. Using this technique, Boijsen reported that the average sagittal diameter of the spinal canal from the 4th to the 6th cervical vertebra in 200 healthy individuals was 18.5 mm (range, 14.2 to 23 mm) (2). The target distance he used was 1.4 m. Kessler noted that values of less than 14 mm are uncommon and fall below the standard deviation for any cervical segment (3). Other measurements reported in the literature vary greatly. It is the variations in the landmarks and the methods used to determine the sagittal distance, as well as the use of different target distances for roentgenography, that have resulted in inconsistencies in the so-called normal values. Therefore, the standard method of measurement for spinal stenosis is a questionable one.

THE RATIO METHOD

An alternative way to determine the sagittal diameter of the spinal canal was devised by Pavlov and is called the ratio method (4). It compares the standard method of measurement of the canal with the anteroposterior width of the vertebral body at the midpoint of the corresponding vertebral body (Fig.10.8). The actual measurement of the sagittal diameter in millimeters, as determined by the conventional method, is misleading, both as reported in the literature and in actual practice; this is because of variations

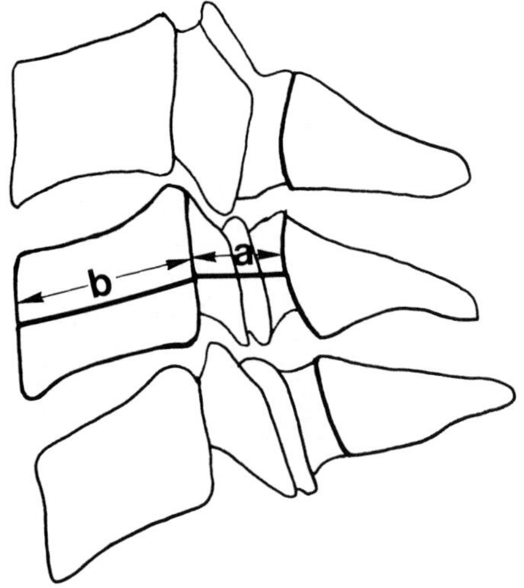

$$\text{ratio} = \frac{a}{b}$$

Figure 10.8. The ratio of the spinal canal to the vertebral body is the distance from the midpoint of the posterior aspect of the vertebral body to the nearest point on the corresponding spinolaminar line (*a*) divided by the anteroposterior width of the vertebral body (*b*). (With permission, from Torg et al. Neurapraxia of the cervical spinal cord with transient quadriplegia. J Bone Joint Surg 1986;68A(9):1354–1370.)

in the target distances used for roentgenography and in the landmarks used for obtaining the measurement. Using the standard method, the actual measurement of the canal in our observations has occasionally been within the acceptable normal range. The ratio method compensates for variations in roentgenographic technique because the sagittal diameter of both the canal and the vertebral body is affected similarly by magnification factors. The ratio method is independent of variations in technique, and the results are statistically significant. Using the ratio method of determining the dimension of the canal, a ratio of the spinal canal to the vertebral body of less than 0.80 is indicative of significant cervical stenosis (1). We believe that the ratio of the anteroposterior diameter of the spinal canal to that of the vertebral body is a more reliable way to determine cervical stenosis (Fig. 10.9 A & B).

On the basis of these observations, it may be concluded that the identified factor that explains the described neurologic picture of cervical spinal cord neurapraxia is diminution of the anteroposterior diameter of the spinal canal, either as an isolated observation or in association with intervertebral disk herniation, degenerative changes, posttraumatic instability, or congenital anomalies. In instances of developmental cervical stenosis, forced hyperflexion, or hyperextension of the cervical spine, a further decrease in the caliber of an already stenotic canal occurs, as explained by the pincer mechanism of Penning (see Fig. 10.10). In patients whose stenosis is associated with osteophytes or a herniated disc, direct pressure can occur, again with the spine forced in the extremes of flexion and extension. It is further postulated that with an abrupt but brief decrease in the anteroposterior diameter of the spinal canal, the cervical cord is mechanically compressed, causing transient interruption of either its motor or its sensory function, or both, distal to the lesion. The neurologic aberration that results is transient and completely reversible.

A review of the literature revealed that few reported cases of transient quadriplegia occurred in athletes. Attempts to establish the incidence indicate that the problem is more prevalent than expected. Specifically, in the population of 39,377 exposed participants, the reported incidence of transient paresthesia in all four extremities was six per 10,000, whereas the reported incidence of paresthesia associated with transient quadriplegia was 1.3 per 10,000 in the one football season surveyed. From these data, it may be concluded that the prevalence of this problem is relatively high and that an awareness of the etiology, manifestations, and appropriate principles of management is warranted.

Characteristically, after an episode of cervical spinal cord neurapraxia with or without transient quadriplegia, the first question raised concerns the advisability of restricting activity. In an attempt to address this problem, 117 young athletes have been interviewed who sustained cervical spine injuries associated with complete permanent quadriplegia while playing football between the years of 1971 and 1984. None of these patients recalled a prodromal experience of transient motor paresis. Conversely, none of the patients in this series who had experienced transient neurologic episodes subsequently sustained an injury that resulted in permanent neurologic injury. On the basis of these data, it is concluded that a young patient who has had an episode of cervical spinal cord neurapraxia with or without quadriplegia is not predisposed to permanent neurologic injury because of it.

With regard to restrictions in activity, no definite recurrence patterns have been identified to establish firm principles in this area. However, athletes who have this syndrome associated with demonstrable cervical spinal instability or acute or chronic degenerative changes should not be allowed further participation in contact sports. Athletes with developmental spinal stenosis or spinal stenosis associated with congenital abnormalities should be treated on an individual basis. Of the six youngsters with obvious cervical stenosis who returned to football, three had a second episode and withdrew from the activity, and three returned without any problem at 2-year follow-up. The data clearly indicate that individuals with developmental spinal stenosis are not predisposed to more

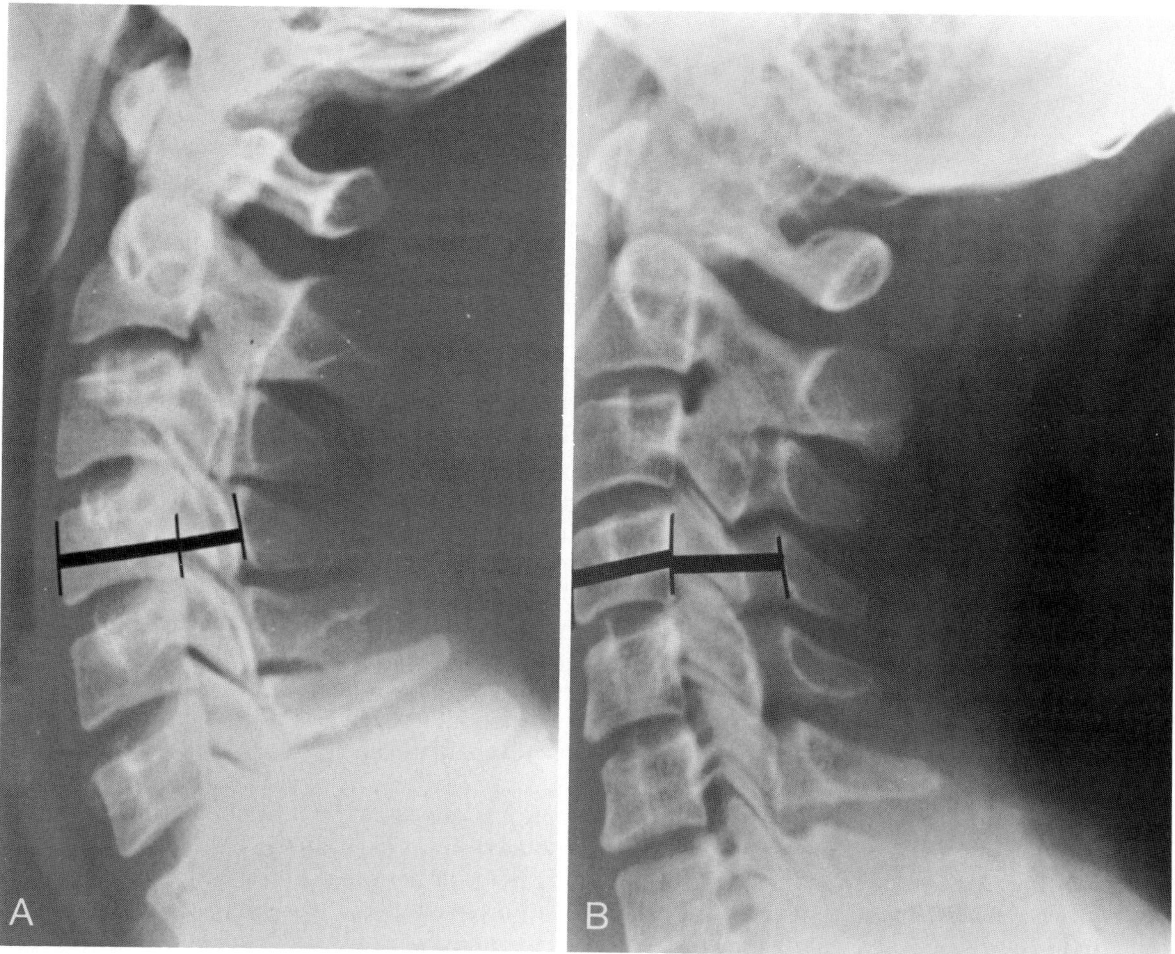

Figure 10.9. **A** & **B**, A comparison between the ratio of the spinal canal to the vertebral body of a stenotic patient versus that of a control subject is demonstrated on lateral roentgenograms of the cervical spine. The ratio is approximately 1:2 (0.50) in the stenotic patient (**A**) compared with 1:1 (1.00) in the control subject (**B**). (With permission from Torg et al. Neurapraxia of the cervical spinal cord with transient quadriplegia. J Bone Joint Surg. 1986;68A(9):1354–1370.)

severe injuries with associated permanent neurologic sequelae (1).

Axial Loading Injuries to the Middle Cervical Spine Segment

Injuries to the cervical spine at the C3–C4 level involving the bony elements, intervertebral discs, and ligamentous structures are rare. We have reported 25 cases of traumatic C3–C4 injuries sustained by young athletes and documented by the National Football Head and Neck Injury Registry (5). Analysis of this material revealed that the response of energy inputs at the C3–C4 level differ from those involving the upper (C1–C2) and lower (C4–C5–C6–C7) cervical segments. Specifically, the C3–C4 lesions appear unique with regard to the infrequency of bony fracture, difficulty in effecting and maintaining reduction and a more favorable recovery following early aggressive treatment. In the majority of instances, injury at this level results from axial loading of the cervical spine. Distribution of lesions into specific categories was as follows: 1) acute intervertebral disc herniation; 2) anterior subluxation C3 on C4; 3) unilateral facet dislocation; 4) bilateral facet dislocation; and 5) vertebral body fracture.

Review of these 25 cases suggests that traumatic lesions of the cervical spine in general can be classified as either involving: 1) upper (C1–C2); 2) middle (C3–C4); or 3) lower (C4–C7) segments. This is based on the observations in this series that C3–C4 lesions: 1) generally do not involve fracture of the bony elements; 2) acute intervertebral disc herniations are frequently associated with transient quadriplegia; 3) reduction of anterior subluxation of C3 on C4 is difficult to maintain; 4) reduction of unilateral facet dislocation is difficult to obtain by skeletal traction and is best managed by closed manipulation and reduction under general anesthesia (Fig. 10.11 A to C); and 5) reduction of bilateral facet dislocation is difficult to

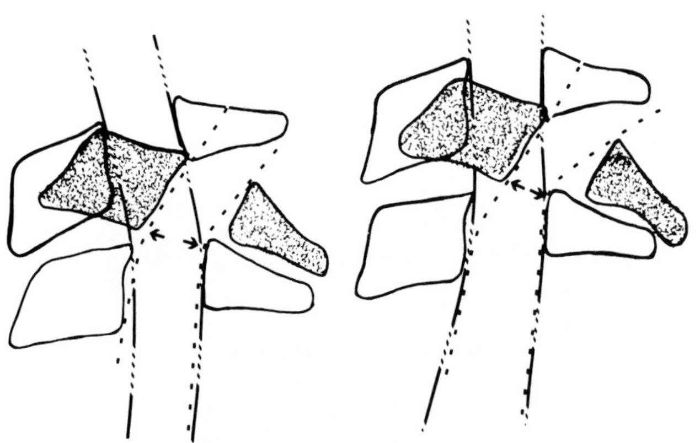

Figure 10.10. The pincers mechanism, as described by Penning, occurs when the distance between the posteroinferior margin of the superior vertebral body and the anterosuperior aspect of the spinolaminar line of the subjacent vertebra decreases with hyperextension, with compression of the cord occurring. With hyperflexion, the anterosuperior aspect of the spinolaminar line of the superior vertebra and the posterosuperior margin of the inferior vertebra would be the "pincers."

obtain by skeletal traction and is best managed by open methods (Fig. 10.12 A & B).

The more favorable results of immediate reduction of both unilateral and bilateral facet dislocations deserve emphasis. In two cases of unilateral facet dislocation reduced within 3 hours of the injury and subsequently fused anteriorly, significant neurologic recovery occurred. The other four cases, two who underwent an open reduction and laminectomy and two treated closed with skeletal traction remained quadriplegic.

In the four instances of bilateral facet dislocation where reduction was achieved by either closed or open methods, although there was no neurologic recovery, all four survived their injuries. However, the three youngsters who were not successfully reduced died.

THE AXIAL LOAD TEAR-DROP FRACTURE: THE ISOLATED FRACTURE AND THE THREE-PART—TWO-PLANE FRACTURE OF THE CERVICAL SPINE

A triangular fracture fragment at the anteroinferior corner of a cervical vertebral body is frequently referred to as a "tear-drop" fracture. This anteroinferior corner fracture fragment actually is an integral part of two specific cervical vertebral body compression fractures that occur in the lower cervical spine. One fracture pattern is an isolated anteroinferior fracture (Fig. 10.13 A & B), and the other, more common fracture pattern is a three-part—two-plane fracture (6). The three-part—two-plane fracture consists of the anteroinferior corner fracture fragment combined with a sagittal vertebral body fracture and fractures of the posterior neural arch (Fig. 10.14). These two fracture patterns have distant neurologic sequelae. In the medical literature, however, cervical spine fractures with an anteroinferior triangular fracture are often grouped together and referred to as a "flexion tear-drop" and/or a "burst" fractures. Analysis of 55 such injuries reveals that these commonly used terms are an incomplete description of the bony pathology and an inaccurate explanation of the mechanism of injury.

Schneider and Kahn were the first to describe the anteroinferior or "tear-drop" vertebral body fracture and to evaluate the neurologic consequence (7). In their original description, Schneider and Kahn enumerated the fracture findings, emphasizing the anteroinferior corner fracture fragment, posterior displacement of the fractured vertebral body into the spinal canal, and disc space narrowing. All of these observations were made from lateral roentgenograms. Descriptions of the roentgen findings from the anteroposterior view were not reported, and the possibility of a sagittal vertebral body fracture or posterior arch fracture was not mentioned. Essentially, their explanation of the tear-drop fracture was determined solely on the lateral roentgenogram. Because findings from the anteroposterior view were not presented, Schneider and Kahn did not distinguish between an isolated anteroinferior corner cervical vertebral body fracture and those associated with the sagittal fracture. They concluded that the "tear-drop" fracture was caused by "acute flexion" of the cervical spine and resulted in severe neurologic deficits. Subsequently, the terms "acute flexion" and "tear-drop" have been recognized and accepted as the descriptive label for vertebral body fractures with an anteroinferior corner fracture fragment. Similar injuries have also been described as "burst" or "compression" fractures, while other authors use the terms "flexion tear-drop" and "burst" interchangeably.

Inherent in the descriptive terminology of these injuries is confusion regarding the mechanism of injury. These fractures have been attributed to flexion, hyperflexion, or hyperflexion with compression, axial loading, hyperextension (presumably an avulsion of the anterior longitudinal ligament), and a combination of hyperextension and hyperflexion. Woodford reported that the sagittal fracture occurs in "burst fractures" caused by an axial force but not with "flexion tear-drop fractures" and stated that the two fractures can be differentiated based on the mechanism of injury (8). Allen, et al., claim that "vertical compression" fractures with an anterior fracture fragment can be differentiated from anteroinferior corner fractures caused by "compression flexion" (9).

Because of the inconsistency in regard to both terminology and mechanism of injury, the neurologic sequelae associated with the different fracture patterns has not been clarified. Richmond and Freedman reviewed 17 cases of cervical vertebral body fractures with an associated sagittal fracture in quadriplegic patients and concluded that the sagittal fracture indicated "severe trauma" (10). Lee reported that forceful flexion produces the anteroinferior

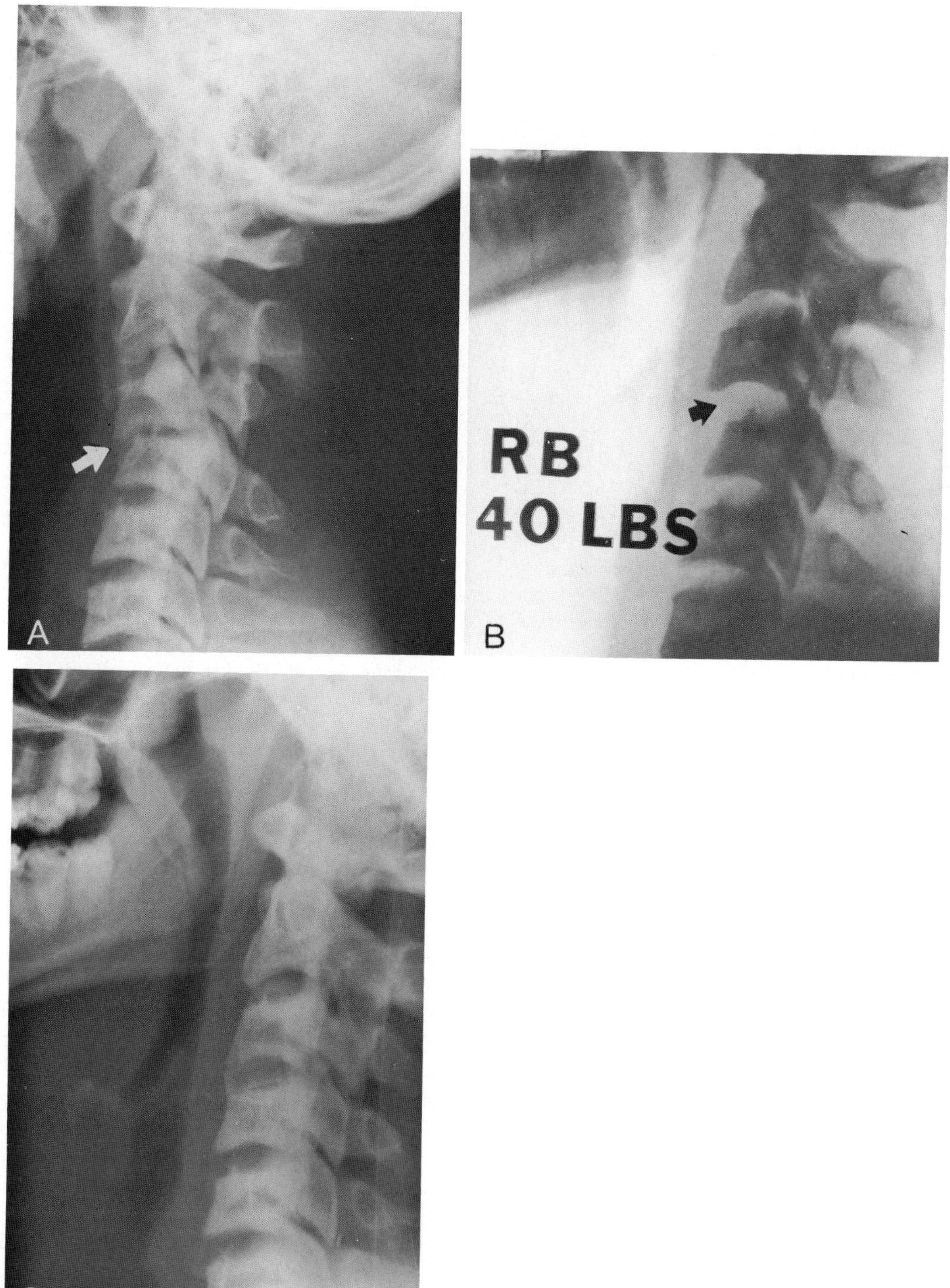

Figure 10.11. **A**, Lateral cervical spine roentgenogram demonstrates a unilateral facet dislocation of the third cervical vertebrae, in addition to anterior displacement and angulation of C3 on C4. Of note, the spinous process of C3 has rotated from its normal relationship with those of the second and third cervical vertebrae and is not seen on the lateral roentgenogram. Also, the dislocated left articular process of C3 (*arrowhead*) is clearly visible on the AP view. **B**, 18 kg of skull caliper traction distracted the interspace but was unable to disengage the locked facet. Closed manipulative reduction performed under nasotracheal general anesthesia resulted in successful reduction of the facet dislocation. A myelogram performed the day following the injury demonstrated a complete block to the flow of panopaque at the C3–C4 level. **C**, lateral roentgenograms immediately following anterior C3–C4 discectomy and interbody fusion. (With permission, from Torg, JS, Sennett B, Vegso JJ, et al. Axial load injuries to the middle cervical spine segment. Am J Sports Med 1991;19:6–20.)

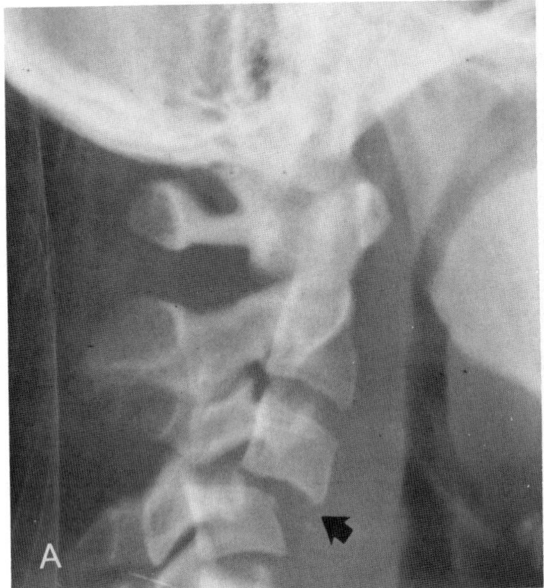

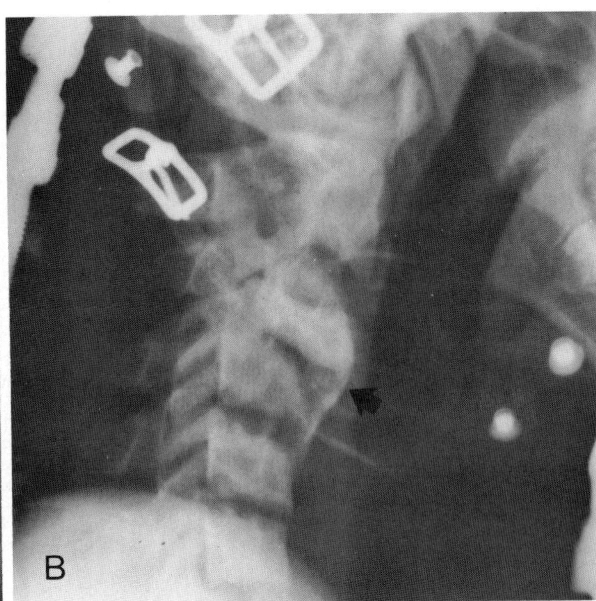

Figure 10.12. **A**, Lateral roentgenograms of the cervical spine obtained shortly after the patient's injury demonstrates a bilateral facet dislocation at C3–C4. In addition to marked anterior translation of C3, there is associated anterior angulation as well as increased distance between the spinous processes of C3 and C4; 11.2 kg of traction mediated through Crutchfield Tongs improved the alignment, however, failed to disengage the locked facet. **B**, lateral roentgenograms of the cervical spine obtained 3 months following injury demonstrates persistence of the bilateral facet dislocation. The lesion has gone on to an autofusion at C3–C4. Of interest is ossification that has occurred anteriorly within the confines of the anterior longitudinal ligament. (With permission, from Torg, JS, Sennett B, Vegso JJ, et al. Axial load injuries to the middle cervical spine segment. Am J Sports Med 1991;19: 6–20.

corner triangular fracture and strong axial load compression produces the sagittal fracture (11, 12). Lee, et al., observed the sagittal fracture in association with a teardrop fracture in 51 cases and reported that 94% had permanent neurologic deficits; 38 of the 51 were quadriplegic (11). In another study, Lee reported that 41 (61%) of 61 patients with an anterior triangular fracture fragment without a facet locking had an associated sagittal fracture of the vertebral body (12). Of this group of 61, 53 (87%) sustained a permanent neurologic injury, of which the majority were quadriplegic. Unfortunately, no mention of the neurologic status of the patients having only the isolated anteroinferior corner fracture was indicated in either of these studies.

Analysis of 55 fractures has indicated that, in most instances, the prevalent descriptive terms for these fractures inaccurately and/or incompletely describe both the bony pathology and the mechanism of injury (6). While our report was based on the injury pattern occurring in football, a similar fracture pattern associated with quadriplegia has also been reported in rugby (13, 14), ice hockey (15, 16), trampolining (17, 18, 19, 20), parachuting (21), and water sports (22, 23, 24, 25, 26).

Review of the 55 cases presented in this report establishes a distinction between the isolated anteroinferior corner and the three-part—two-plane fracture pattern. The three-part—two-plane fracture defines a cervical vertebral body compression fracture consisting of 1) an anteroinferior corner fracture fragment; 2) a sagittal vertebral body fracture; and 3) various injuries to the intervertebral disc, the facet joints, the posterior neural arch, and the posterior ligamentous structures (Fig. 10.15 A to C). This particular fracture pattern has not been included in common classifications.

Many reports regarding fractures of the lower cervical spine have relied solely on the lateral roentgenograms. However, in order to delineate the full extent of the injury associated with the anteroinferior fracture fragment, a minimum of two roentgenograms (an AP and a lateral projection) are required. On the lateral view, in addition to the anteroinferior corner vertebral body fracture fragment, it is essential to determine: 1) retropulsion and/or angulation of the posterior body fragment; 2) intervertebral disc space narrowing; and 3) loss of parallelism of the interfacetal joints and fanning of the intraspinous processes indicating a tear or rupture of the posterior ligamentous complex.

On the AP view, it is essential to determine: 1) the sagittal fracture of the vertebral body; 2) widening of the interpediculate distance; and 3) asymmetry of the lateral borders indicating a posterior neural arch fracture. Care must be taken not to confuse the air in the larynx (formed as the tracheal air column narrows to a slit as it projects over the vertebral bodies of C3, C4, or C5) with a sagittal

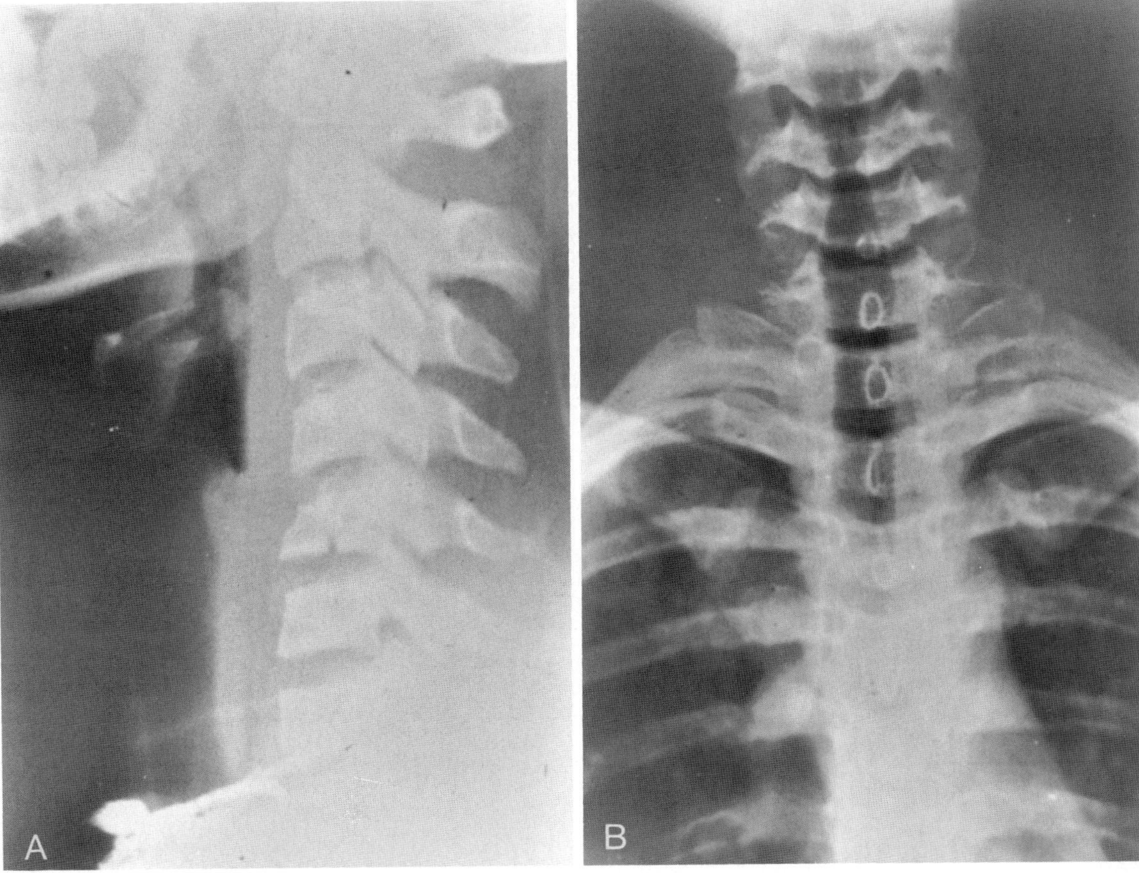

Figure 10.13. **A & B**, An isolated anteroinferior "tear-drop" fracture of C6 is demonstrated on the lateral roentgenogram. A sagittal component is not seen on the anterior-posterior view. (With permission, from Torg JS, O'Neill MJ, Pavlov H. The axial load teardrop fracture. Am J Sports Med, 1991;19:355–364.)

fracture. Anteroposterior tomograms or a CT examination may be necessary to exclude or confirm the presence of a sagittal fracture and/or posterior neural arch injuries. Lee reported that CT and polytomography were necessary to document the presence of a sagittal fracture and the fractures of the posterior arch (11). In his series, posterior arch fractures were present in association with six or seven isolated sagittal vertebral body fractures and in 36 of 51 tear-drop fractures associated with a sagittal vertebral body fracture. Of these 42 posterior arch fractures, only 13 were evident on the routine plain films. Posterior arch fractures are an expected occurrence with a sagittal fracture, as it is unlikely for a rigid ring structure to fracture in only one site.

Fracture Pattern and Associated Neurologic Sequelae

The isolated anteroinferior corner fracture pattern and the three-part—two-plane fracture pattern have vastly different neurologic sequelae. Of the 31 patients in our series with a documented three-part—two-plane injury, 27 (87%) were quadriplegic. In the remaining 4 cases, all had initial neurologic symptoms of paresthesias or paresis, including one case of central cord syndrome, all of which eventually resolved.

Of the six patients with an isolated anteroinferior corner fracture fragment without an associated sagittal fracture, five of these six (83%) had no serious neurologic sequelae. The one remaining patient had fractures to the posterior elements of the subadjacent vertebra and was quadriplegic.

An anteroinferior corner fracture without a sagittal fracture has a less detrimental pattern. This finding has been substantiated by other studies in which the sagittal fracture accompanying an anteroinferior corner fracture fragment has been reported associated with severe cord injury and/or quadriplegia. King noted a correlation between the sagittal fracture associated with an anteroinferior corner fracture and cord damage, while patients with an isolated anteroinferior corner fracture did not have cord damage. In a review of 45 patients with an anterior corner tear-drop fragment, Kim reported that five of six patients with intact neurologic status did not have an associated sagittal fracture compared with 38 of 39 patients with neurologic deficits who had an associated sagittal fracture (27).

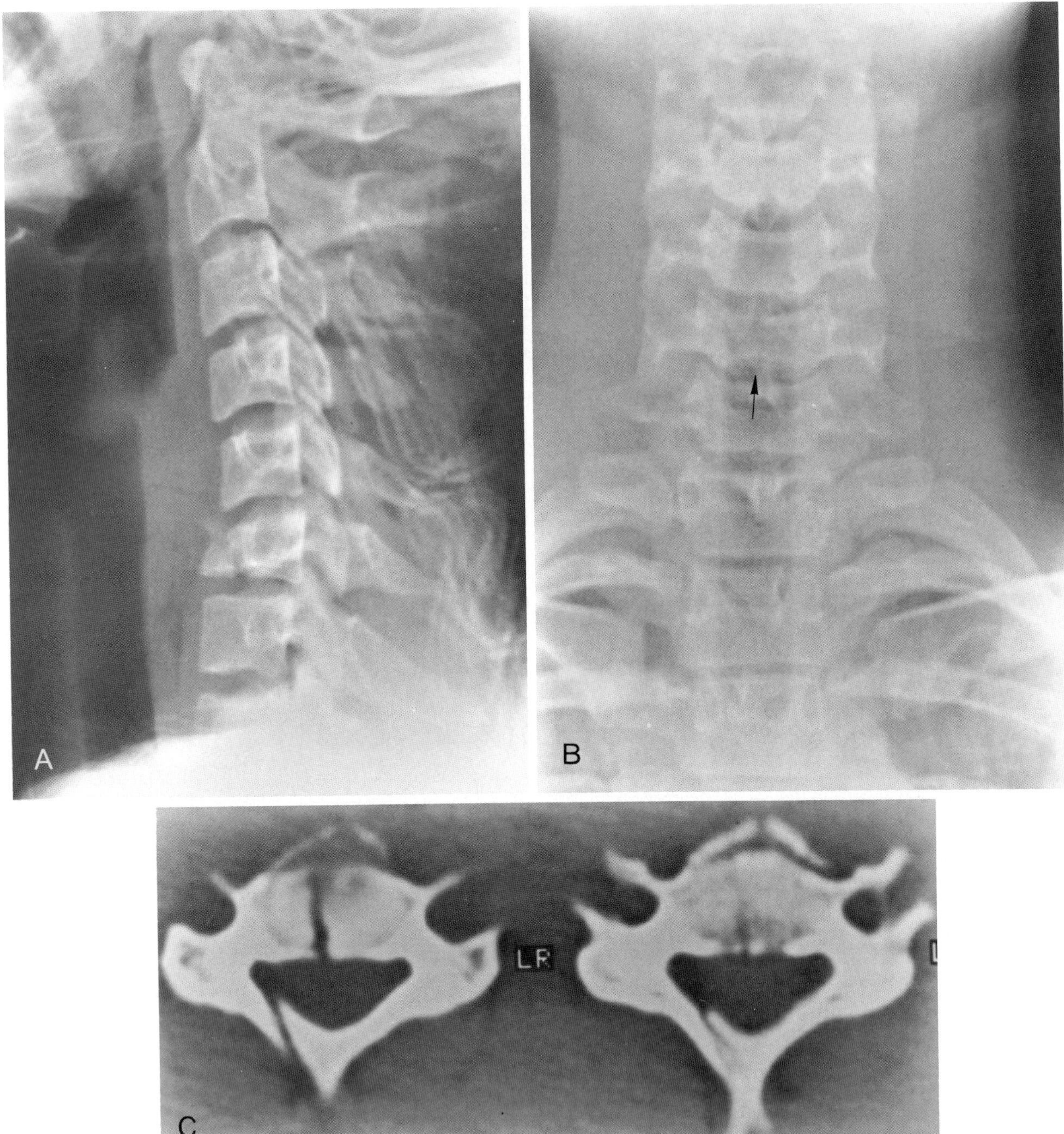

Figure 10.14. **A**, A three-part, two plane fracture of C6. Lateral view demonstrates prevertebral soft tissue swelling and an anteroinferior fracture fragment of C6 involving the entire vertebral body height (VBH) and ⅓ the vertebral body width (VBW). There is approximately 1 mm of posterior displacement of the inferior aspect of the posterior vertebral body. The C6–C7 intervertebral disc space is minimally narrowed posteriorly with associated capsular disruption and "fanning." **B**, frontal view demonstrates a faint, linear radiolucency through the C6 vertebral body indicating a sagittal vertebral body fracture (*arrow*). There is mild lateral mass displacement. **C**, CT examination demonstrates the sagittal fracture extending completely through the vertebral body with disruption of the lamina on the right. (With permission, from Torg JS, O'Neill MJ, Pavlov H. The axial load teardrop fracture. Am J Sports Med, 1991;19:355–364.)

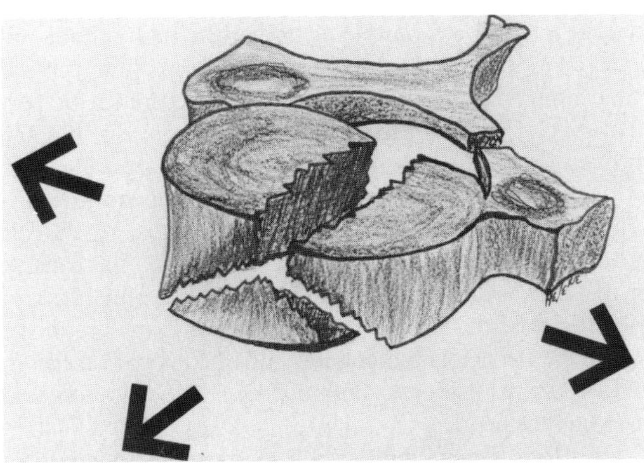

Figure 10.15. Diagrammatic representation of the three-part, two plane vertebral body compression fracture demonstrates the anteroinferior "tear-drop" as well as the sagittal vertebral body fractures and associated fracture through the lamina. (With permission from Torg JS, O'Neill MJ, Pavlov H. The axial load teardrop fracture. Am J Sports Med, 1991;19:355–364.)

MECHANISM OF INJURY

The most popular description of the mechanism responsible for fracture/dislocation of the cervical spine has been accidental forced hyperflexion. The reports describe the subject as an unsuspecting victim of some untoward circumstance, i.e., an accidental fall, a dive into shallow water, an unexpected blow to the head, or in the case of an athlete, a poorly executed physical act in which the cervical spine is unwittingly forced into the extreme of motion with resulting injury. This hyperflexion mechanism was established by Schneider and Kahn as the force responsible for the "acute flexion tear-drop" fracture (7). There are two major factors to differentiate the isolated anteroinferior corner fracture and the three-part—two-plane fracture described in this report from the classical hyperflexion (or hyperextension) injuries. First, the circumstances surrounding the event are usually not accidental. Injury reports and cinematographic analysis have clearly demonstrated that, in most instances, the subject was executing a maneuver in which the head was used as a battering ram, the initial point of contact being made with the top or crown of the helmet in an impact situation (28, 29). Second, the principle mechanism of injury is not cervical spine hyperflexion or hyperextension, but instead, axial loading. The vast majority of injuries occurred as the athlete struck another player or object, attempted a tackle, or performed a block with the crown of his helmet and his neck slightly flexed, reducing the cervical lordosis to a straight line. When the cervical spine is straight, it becomes a segmented column. Loading of this segmented column occurs when impact is exerted to the vertex of the head along the vertical axis of the straightened spine. In this situation, the forces are transmitted along the vertical axis of the cervical spine, obviating the impact-absorbing capacities of the discs, joints, and paravertebral muscles such that injury occurs to the bones, discs, and ligamentous structures. When the maximum axial compressive deformation is reached, cervical spine flexion and/or rotation occurs with fracture, subluxation, or unilateral or bilateral facet dislocation. An excessive axial load is one force that could theoretically produce the components of both the isolated anteroinferior corner of the three-part—two-plane cervical vertebral body fractures (30).

Multiple authors have supported axial compression as the mechanism responsible for the anteroinferior corner fracture pattern. Furthermore, other reports have suggested that a pure hyperflexion force cannot produce significant cervical spine fractures or dislocations. The axial loading mechanism of cervical spine injuries has been presented in previous published studies based on data from the National Head and Neck Injury Registry. These studies have demonstrated a causal relationship between axial loading and serious cervical spine injury based on injury reports, cinematographic analysis, and biomechanical models.

The mechanism of axial loading is supported by several biomechanical studies. Mertz, et al., Hodgson and Thomas, and Sances have measured stresses and strains within the cervical spine when axial impulses are applied to helmeted cadaver head-spine-trunk specimens and demonstrated that fractures of the lower cervical spine occur when the impulse is applied to the crown of the helmet. Hodgson and Thomas have determined that a direct vertex impact imparts a larger force to the cervical vertebrae than forces applied farther forward on the skull (32). Gosch, et al., have investigated three different injury modes: hyperflexion, hyperextension, and axial compression in their experiment involving anesthetized monkeys, and they conclude that axial compression produces cervical spine fractures and dislocations (33). Maiman, et al. (34), Roaf (35, 36), and White and Panjabi (37) have demonstrated vertebral body fractures in the lower cervical spine due to the axial loading of isolated spinal units. Roaf believes it is the failure of the vertebral body-intervertebral disc complex that accounts for the vertical fractures of the vertebral body occurring in burst fractures. He has shown that in the presence of an intact intervertebral disc, a compressive load initially causes endplate failure with herniation of the nucleus pulposus into the vertebral body followed by bony failure. White and Punjabe emphasize that axial loading is the major injury vector involved in the production of the tear-drop fracture in the cervical vertebrae.

Several clinical studies support these findings and emphasize that tackling with the head down is the major cause of serious cervical spine injuries occurring in rugby and tackle football. Based on these studies, it can be concluded that axial loading is the dominant mechanism of injury for the various cervical spine fractures and dislocations occurring in tackle football, including the two types discussed in this report.

The fracture pattern originally described by Schneider and Kahn as the "acute flexion tear-drop fracture" was made on the basis of an incomplete roentgenographic analysis of the problem. As the cases that we have reported demonstrate, two types of fractures exist which involve the anteroinferior corner of the vertebral body, either an isolated fracture or a three-part—two-plane injury in which there is a sagittal vertebral body fracture. Both lesions are primarily produced by an excessive axial load to the cervical spine. An axial load can theoretically and experimentally produce the fractures to both the anterior and posterior elements of the vertebral body as well as the posterior ligamentous disruption and posterior displacement of the vertebral body that are seen clinically. Hyperflexion or hyperextension mechanisms fail to account for all the pathologic aspects of either the isolated anteroinferior corner fractures or the three-part—two-plane fracture (38, 39).

In summary, the following points must be emphasized:

1) The terms "flexion tear-drop," "acute flexion tear-drop," and "burst fracture," to describe a comminuted fracture of the cervical vertebral body are incomplete descriptive terms and inaccurately explain the mechanism of injury.
2) There are two fracture patterns associated with the anteroinferior corner fracture (tear-drop) fragment: a) the isolated fracture, which is usually not associated with permanent neurologic sequelae, and b) the three-part—two-plane fracture in which there is a sagittal vertebral body fracture and fractures of the posterior neural arch and which is usually associated with permanent neurologic sequelae, specifically quadriplegia.
3) Axial load is the mechanism of injury for both fracture patterns.
4) The predominant level of involvement is at C5 (74%), then C4 (16%), and C6 (10%).
5) In football, the majority (73%) of these fractures occur while attempting a tackle.
6) A complete radiologic examination including a lateral view to determine the extent of posterior displacement and angulation of the posterior vertebral body fragment and an AP view, with CT or tomography as necessary to determine the presence of a sagittal vertebral body and the integrity of the posterior neural arch is essential in evaluating patients following cervical spine trauma when either type of lesion is suspected.

PREVENTION

Data on cervical spine injuries resulting from participation in football have been compiled by a national registry since 1971 (28, 40, 41). Analysis of the epidemiologic data and cinematographic documentation clearly demonstrates that the majority of cervical fractures and dislocations were due to axial loading. On the basis of this observation, rule changes banning both deliberate "spearing" and the use of the top of the helmet as the initial point of contact in making a tackle were implemented at the high school and college levels. Subsequently, a marked decrease in cervical spine injury rates has occurred. The occurrence of permanent cervical quadriplegia decreased from 34 in 1976 to five in the 1984 season (Fig. 10.16).

Identifying the cause and prevention of cervical quadriplegia resulting from football involves four areas: (1) the role of the helmet-face mask protective system; (2) the concept of the axial loading mechanism of injury; (3) the effect of the 1976 rule changes banning spearing and the use of the top of the helmet as the initial point of contact in tackling; and (4) the necessity for continued research, education, and rules enforcement.

The protective capabilities provided by the modern football helmet have resulted in the advent of playing techniques that have placed the cervical spine at risk of injury with associated catastrophic neurological sequelae. Available cinematographic and epidemiologic data clearly indicate that cervical spine injuries associated with quadriplegia occurring as a result of football are not hyperflexion accidents. Instead, they are due to purposeful axial loading of the cervical spine as a result of spearing and head-first playing techniques (Fig. 10.17). As an etiological factor, the present-day helmet-face mask system is secondary, contributing to these injuries because of its protective capabilities that have permitted the head to be used as a battering ram, thus exposing the cervical spine to injury.

Classically, the role of hyperflexion has been emphasized in cervical spine trauma whether the injury was due to a diving accident, trampolining, rugby, or American football. Epidemiologic and cinematographic analyses have established that most cases of cervical spine quadriplegia that occur in football have resulted from axial loading. Rather than an accident, an untoward event, techniques are deliberately used that place the cervical spine at risk of catastrophic injury. Recent laboratory observations also indicate that athletically induced cervical spine trauma results from axial loading (31, 35, 36, 38).

In the course of a collision activity, such as tackle football, most energy inputs to the cervical spine are effectively dissipated by the energy-absorbing capabilities of the cervical musculature through controlled lateral bending, flexion, or extension motion. However, the bones, discs, and ligamentous structures can be injured when contact occurs on the top of the helmet with the head, neck, and trunk positioned in such a way that forces are transmitted along the longitudinal axis of the cervical spine.

With the neck in the anatomic position, the cervical spine is extended due to normal cervical lordosis (Fig. 10.18). When the neck is flexed to 30°, the cervical spine straightens (Fig. 10.19). In axial loading injuries, the neck is slightly flexed and normal cervical lordosis eliminated, thereby converting the spine into a straight segmented column. Assuming the head, neck, and trunk components to be in motion, rapid deceleration of the head occurs when it strikes

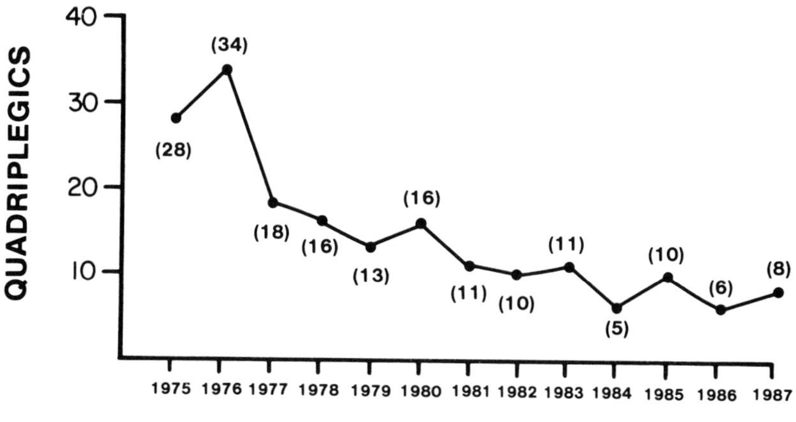

Figure 10.16. The yearly incidence of permanent cervical quadriplegia for all levels of participation (1975–1987) decreased dramatically in 1977 following the initiation of the rule changes prohibiting the use of head first tackling and blocking techniques. (With permission, from Torg JS, Vegso JJ, O'Neill MJ. The epidemiologic, pathologic, biomechanical and cinematographic analysis of football induced cervical spine trauma. Am J Sports Med 1990;18:56–57.)

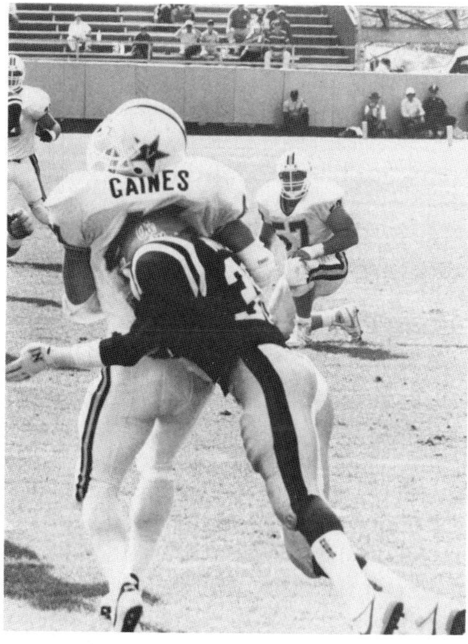

Figure 10.17. An intercollegiate defensive back making a head tackle which resulted in an axial loading injury to his cervical spine and quadriplegia. (With permission, from Torg JS, Vegso JJ, O'Neill MJ. The epidemiologic, pathologic, biomechnical and cinematographic analysis of football induced cervical spine trauma. Am J Sports Med 1990;18:56–57.)

another object, such as another player, trampoline bed, or lake bottom. This results in the cervical spine being compressed between the rapidly deaccelerated head and the force of the oncoming trunk. When the maximum vertical compression is reached, the straightened cervical spine fails in a flexion mode, and fracture, subluxation, or unilateral or bilateral facet dislocation can occur (Fig. 10.20 A to E).

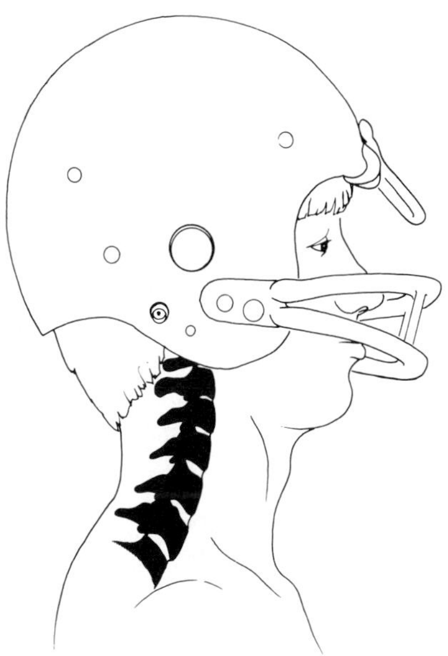

Figure 10.18. When the neck is in a normal, upright, anatomical position, the cervical spine is slightly extended because of the natural cervical lordosis. (With permission, from Torg JS, Vegso JJ, O'Neill MJ. The epidemiologic, pathologic, biomechanical and cinematographic analysis of football induced cervical spine trauma. Am J Sports Med 1990;18:56–57.)

Refutation of the "freak accident" concept with the more logical principle of cause and effect has been most rewarding in dealing with problems of football-induced cervical quadriplegia. Definition of the axial-loading mechanism in which a football player, usually a defensive back, makes a tackle by striking an opponent with the top of his helmet had been key in this process. Implementation of rules changes and coaching techniques in 1976 eliminating the use of the head as a battering ram have resulted in a dramatic reduction in the incidence of quadriplegia since 1976 (Fig.

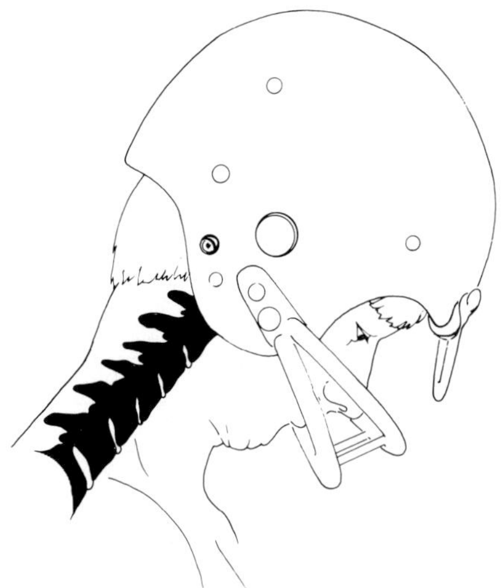

Figure 10.19. When the neck is flexed slightly, to approximately 30°, the cervical spine is straightened and converted into a segmented column. (With permission, from Torg JS, Vegso JJ, O'Neill MJ. The epidemiologic, pathologic, biomechanical and cinematographic analysis of football induced cervical spine trauma. Am J Sports Med 1990;18:56–57.)

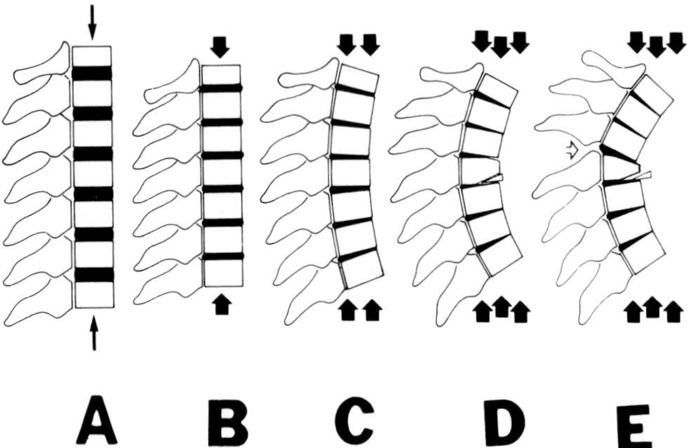

Figure 10.20. Axial loading of the cervical spine first results in compressive deformation of the intervertebral discs (**A** and **B**), followed by maximum compressive deformation, and then angular deformation and buckling occur. The spine fails in a flexion mode (**C**) with resulting fracture, subluxation, or dislocation. (**D** and **E**) Compressive deformation to failure with a resultant fracture, dislocation, or subluxation occurs in as little as 8.4 msec. (With permission, from Torg JS, Vegso JJ, O'Neill MJ. The epidemiologic, pathologic, biomechanical and cinematographic analysis of football induced cervical spine trauma. Am J Sports Med 1990;18:56–57.)

10.16). We believe that the majority of athletic injuries to the cervical spine associated with quadriplegia also occur as a result of axial loading.

Tator et al. (26) identified 38 acute spinal cord injuries due to diving accidents and observed that "in most cases the cervical spine was fractured and the spinal cord crushed. The top of the head struck the bottom of the lake or pool." Sher (42), reporting on vertex impact and cervical dislocation in rugby players, observed that, "when the racket is slightly flexed, the spine is straight. If significant force is applied to the vertex when the spine is straight, the force is transmitted down the long axis of the spine. When the force exceeds the energy-absorbing capacity of the structures involved, cervical spine flexion and dislocation will result." Tator and Edmonds (15, 16) have reported on the results of a national questionnaire survey by the Canadian Committee on the Prevention of Spinal Injuries due to Hockey which recorded 28 injuries involving the spinal cord, 17 of which resulted in complete paralysis. They noted that in this series, the most common mechanism involved was a check with the injured players striking the boards "with the top of their heads, while their necks were slightly flexed."

These reports in the recent literature that deal with the mechanism of injury involved in cervical spine injuries resulting from water sports (diving), gymnastics, rugby, and ice hockey support our thesis.

Criteria for Return to Contact Activities Following Cervical Spine Injury

Injury to the cervical spine and associated structures as a result of participation in competitive athletic and recreational activities is not uncommon. It appears that the frequency of these various injuries is inversely proportional to their severity. Whereas Albright has reported that 32% of college football recruits sustained "moderate" injuries while in high school, catastrophic injuries with associated quadriplegia occurs to less than 1/100,000 participants per season at the high school level (43). The variety of possible traumatic lesions to the cervical spine resulting from athletic trauma is considerable and the severity variable. The literature dealing with diagnosis and treatment of these problems is considerable. However, conspicuously absent is a comprehensive set of standards or guidelines for establishing criteria for permitting or prohibiting return to contact sports (boxing, football, ice hockey, lacrosse, rugby, wrestling) following injury to the cervical spinal structures. The explanation for this void appears to be twofold. First, the combination of a litigious society and the potential for great harm should things go wrong makes "no" the easiest, and perhaps most reasonable, advice. Second, and perhaps most important, with the exception of the matter of transient quadriplegia, is the lack of credible data pertaining to postinjury risk factors. Despite a lack of credible data, this chapter will attempt to establish guidelines to assist the clinician as well as the patient and his parents in the decisionmaking process.

Cervical spine conditions requiring a decision as to whether or not participation in contact activities is advisable and safe can be divided into two categories: 1) congenital or developmental; and 2) posttraumatic. Each condition has been determined to present either: 1) no contraindication; 2) relative contraindication or; 3) an absolute contraindication on the basis of a variety of parameters. Information compiled from over 1200 cervical spine injuries documented by the National Football Head and Neck Injury Registry has provided insight into whether various conditions may or may not predispose to more serious injury (40, 41). A review of the literature in several instances provides significant data for a limited number of specific conditions. Analysis of many conditions predicated on an understanding of recognized injury mechanisms has permitted categorization on the basis of "educated" conjecture. And lastly, much reliance has been placed on personal experience that must be regarded as anecdotal.

The structure and mechanics of the cervical spine enables it to perform three important functions. First, it supports the head as well as the variety of soft tissue structures of the neck. Second, by virtue of segmentation and configuration, it permits multiplanar motion of the head. Third, and most important, it serves as a protective conduit for the spinal cord and cervical nerve roots. A situation that would impede or prevent the performance of any of the three functions in a pain-free manner either immediately or in the future is unacceptable and contraindicated.

The following proposed criteria for return to contact activities in the presence of cervical spine abnormalities or following injury are intended only as guidelines. It is fully acknowledged that for the most part they are, at best, predicated on the antidotal, and no responsibility can be assumed for their implementation.

Critical to the application of these guidelines is the implementation of coaching and playing techniques that preclude the use of the head as the initial point of contact in a collision situation. Exposure of the cervical spine to axial loading is an invitation to disaster and relegates any and all safety standards as meaningless.

Criteria

CONGENITAL CONDITIONS

A) Odontoid anomalies—Hensinger has stated that "patients with congenital anomalies of the odontoid are leading a precarious existence. The concern is that a trivial insult superimposed on already weakened or compromised structure may be catastrophic" (44). This concern became a reality during the 1989 football season when an eighteen-year-old high school player was rendered a respiratory-dependent quadriplegic while making a head tackle that was vividly demonstrated on the game video. Postinjury roentgenograms revealed an os odontoidium with marked C1–C2 instability. Thus, the presence of odontoid agenesis, odontoid hypoplasia, or os odontoidium are all absolute contraindications to participation in contact activities.

B) Spina bifida occulta—a rare, incidental roentgenographic finding that presents no contraindication.

C) Atlantoccipital fusion—a rare condition characterized by partial, or complete congenital fusion of the bony ring of the atlas to the base of the occiput. The onset of signs and symptoms are referable to the posterior columns due to cord compression by the posterior lip of the foramen magnum, usually occurring in the third or fourth decade. They usually begin insidiously and progress slowly, but sudden onset or instant death have been reported. Atlantoccipital fusion as an isolated entity or coexisting with other abnormalities constitute an absolute contraindication to participation in contact activities.

D) Kipple-Feil anomaly is the eponym applied to congenital fusion of two or more cervical vertebrae. For purposes of this discussion, the variety of abnormalities can be divided into two groups: Type I—mass fusion of the cervical and upper thoracic vertebrae and; Type II—fusion of only one or two interspaces. To be noted, the variety of associated congenital problems have been identified to be associated with congenital fusion of the cervical vertebrae and include pulmonary, cardiovascular, and urogenital. Pizzutillo has pointed out that "children with congenital fusion of the cervical spine rarely develop neurologic problems or signs of instability" (45). However, he further states, "the literature reveals more than 90 cases of neurologic problems . . . that developed as a consequence of occipital cervical anomalies, late instability, disc disease, or degenerative joint disease" (45). These reports included cervical radiculopathy, spasticity, pain, quadriplegia and sudden death. Also, "more than two-thirds of the neurologically involved patients had single level fusion of the upper area, whereas many cervical patients with extension fusions of five to seven levels had no associated neurologic loss" (45). Despite this, the Type I lesion, a mass fusion, constitutes an absolute contraindication to participation in contact sports. As well, a Type II lesion with fusion of one or two interspaces with associated limited motion and/or associated occipitocervical anomalies, instability, disc disease, or degenerative changes also constitutes absolute contraindication to participation. On the other hand, Type II lesion involving fusion of one or two interspaces at C3 and below in an individual with full cervical range of motion and an absence of occipital cervical anomalies, instability, disc disease, or degenerative changes should present no contraindication.

DEVELOPMENTAL CONDITIONS

A) Developmental narrowing (stenosis) of the cervical spinal canal and its association with cervical cord neurapraxia and transient quadriplegia has been well defined (1). Defining narrowing or stenosis as a cervical segment with one or more vertebrae having a canal/body ratio of 0.8 or less is predicated on the fact that 92% of all reported clinical cases have fallen below this value at one or more levels. To be noted, 12% of asymptomatic controls also fell below the 0.8 level as did 48% of asymptomatic professional and 45% of asymptomatic college players. In the group of reported symptomatic players, there was in every instance complete neurologic return, and in those who continued with contact activities reoccurrence was not predictable.

Clearly, the presence of developmental narrowing of the cervical spinal canal does not predispose permanent neurologic injury. Eisman et al. have indicated, on the basis of experience of cervical fractures/dislocations resulting from automobile accidents, that the degree of neurologic impairment was inversely related to the anterior-posterior diameter of the canal (46). Due to the all or nothing pattern of axial load football spine injuries, this phenomenon has not been observed in athletic-related injuries.

The presence of a canal/vertebral body ratio of 0.8 or less is no contraindication to participation in contact activites in asymptomatic individuals. We further recommend against preparticipation screening roentgenograms in asymptomatic players. Such studies will not contribute to safety, are not cost effective, and will only contribute to the hysteria surrounding this issue.

In those individuals with a ratio of 0.8 or less who experience either motor and/or sensory manifestations of cervical cord neurapraxia there is a relative contraindication to return to contact activities. In these instances, each case must be determined on an individual basis depending on the understanding of the player and his parents and their willingness to accept any presumed theoretical risk.

Absolute contraindications to continued participation applies to those individuals who experience a documented episode of cervical cord neurapraxia associated with any of the following:

a. Ligamentous instability;
b. Intervertebral disc disease;
c. Degenerative changes;
d. MRI evidence of cord defects or swelling;
e. Symptoms or positive neurologic findings lasting more than 36 hours;
f. More than one reoccurrence.

B) "Spear Tackler's Spine" Analysis of material recently received by the National Football Head and Neck Injury Registry has allowed for the description of "Spear Tackler's Spine," an entity which consists of: 1) developmental narrowing; 2) reversal of normal cervical lordosis or kyphosis; and 3) subtle torticollis in an individual who employs spear tackling techniques (Fig. 10.21 A & B). Two cases with preinjury roentgenograms as well as video documentation of axial loading of the spine due to spear tackling resulted in a bilateral C3–C4 facet dislocation in the other, with both being rendered quadriplegic. Whether the straightened "segmented column" alignment of the spine or the head-first tackling technique, or a combination of the two predisposes those with "spear tackler's spine" to catastrophic injury is not clear. However, this combination of factors constitutes an absolute contraindication to further participation in contact sports.

TRAUMATIC CONDITIONS OF THE UPPER CERVICAL SPINE (C1–C2)

The anatomy and mechanics of C1–C2 segment of the cervical spine differ markedly from the middle or lower segments. Lesions with any degree of occipital or atlantoaxial instability portend a potentially grave prognosis. Thus, any injury involving the upper cervical segment that involves a fracture or ligamentous laxity is an absolute contraindication to further participation in contact activities. Healed, nondisplaced Jefferson fractures, healed type I and type II odontoid fractures, and healed lateral mass fractures of C2 constitute a relative contraindication providing the patient is pain free, has a full range of cervical motion, and no neurologic findings. Because of the uncertainty of the results of cervical fusion, the gracile configuration of C1, and the importance of the alar and transverse odontoid ligaments, fusion for instability of the upper segment constitutes an absolute contraindication regardless of how successful the fusion appears roentgenographically.

TRAUMATIC CONDITIONS OF THE MIDDLE AND LOWER CERVICAL SPINE

A) Ligamentous injuries. The criteria of White and Panjabi for defining clinical instability were intended to help establish indications for surgical stabilization (47). However, although the limits of displacement and angulation correlated with disruption of known structures, no one determinant was considered absolute. In view of the observations of Albright, et al. (43), that 10% (7/75) of the college freshman in his study demonstrated "abnormal motion," as well as on the basis of our own experience, it appears that in many instances some degree of "minor instability" exists in populations of both high school and college football players without apparent adverse effects. The question of course is: what are the upper limits of "minor" instability? Unfortunately, there is no available data to relate this to the clinical situation and from which to develop reliable standards. Clearly, however, where lateral roentgenograms demonstrate more than 3.5 mm of horizontal displacement of either one vertebra in relationship to another or more than 11° rotation than either adjacent vertebra, an absolute contraindication to further participation in contact activities exists. With regard to lesser degrees of displacement and rotation, further participation enters the realms of "trial by battle," and such situations can be considered a relative contraindication, depending on such factors as level of performance, physical

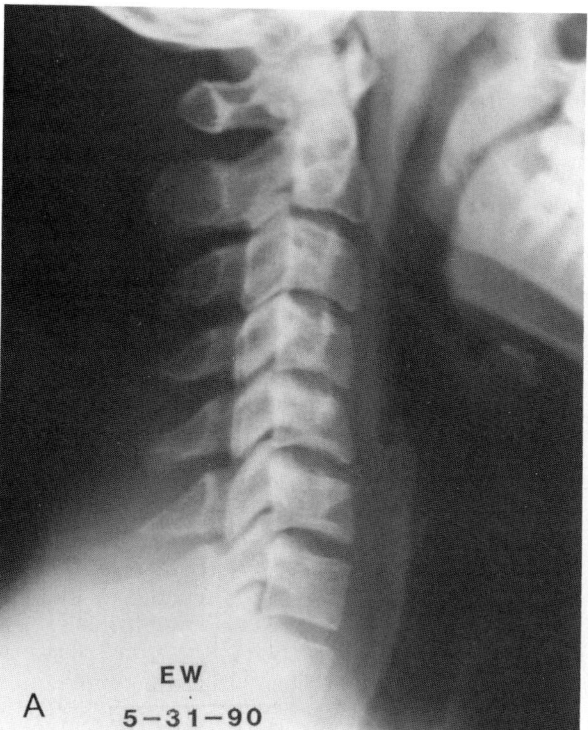

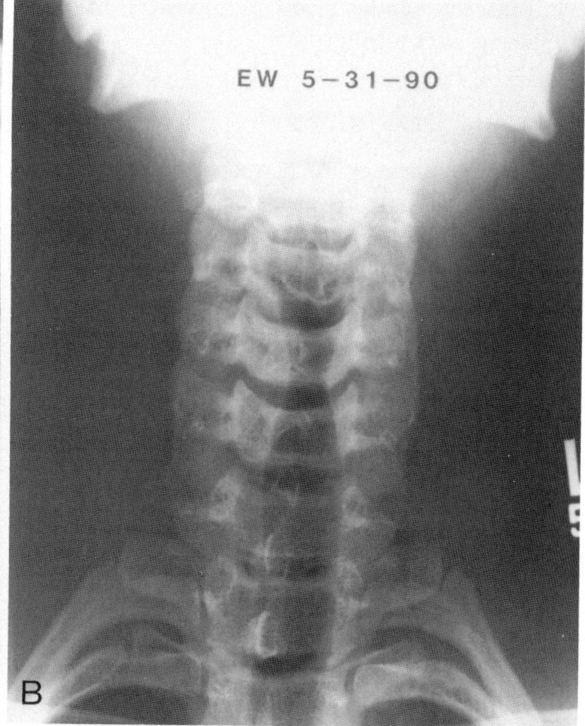

Figure 10.21. **A & B**, Roentgenographic characteristic of "spear tackler's spine" includes developmental narrowing, reversal of the normal cervical lordosis in the erect, neutral position on the lateral views, and suggestion of a wryneck attitude with tilt of the cervical spine to the left on the anteroposterior views. This particular 18-year-old high school football player's cervical CAT scan and MRI were normal. He was precluded from further participation in contact sports.

habitus, and position played (interior lineman vs. defensive back, etc.).

B) Fractures. An acute fracture of either the body or posterior elements with or without associated ligamentous laxity constitutes an absolute contraindication to participation.

The following healed, stable fractures in an asymptomatic patient who is neurologically normal and has a full range of cervical motion can be considered to be no contraindication to participation in contact activities:

1. Stable compression fractures of the vertebral body without a sagittal component on anterior/posterior roentgenogram and without involvement of either the ligamentous or posterior bony structures;
2. A healed stable endplate fracture without a sagittal component on anterior/posterior roentgenograms or involvement of the posterior or bony ligamentous structure;
3. Healed spinous process "clay shoveler" fractures.

Relative contraindications apply to the following healed stable fractures in individuals who are asymptomatic, neurologically normal, and have a full pain free range of cervical motion.

1. Stable displaced vertebral body compression fractures without a sagittal component on anterior/posterior roentgenograms. The propensity for these fractures to settle with increased deformity must be considered and carefully followed.
2. Healed stable fractures involving the elements of the posterior neural ring in individuals who are asymptomatic, neurologically normal, have a full pain free range of cervical motion. In evaluating radiographic and imaging studies to find the location and subsequent healing of posterior neural large fractures it is important to understand that, as pointed out by Steel (48), a rigid ring cannot break in one location. Thus, healing of paired fractures of the ring must be demonstrated.

Absolute contraindication to further participation in contact activities exists in the presence of the following fractures:

1) vertebral body fracture with a sagittal component;
2) fracture of the vertebral body with or without displacement with associated posterior arch fractures and/or ligamentous laxity;
3) comminuted fractures of the vertebral body with displacement into the spinal canal;
4) any healed fracture of either the vertebral body or posterior components with associated pain, neurologic findings, limitation of normal cervical motion;

5) healed displaced fractures involving the lateral masses with resulting facet incongruity.

INTERVERTEBRAL DISC INJURY

There is no contraindication to participation in contact activities in individuals with a healed anterior or lateral disc herniation treated conservatively, or those requiring an intervertebral discectomy and interbody fusion for a lateral or central herniation who have a solid fusion, are asymptomatic, neurologically negative, and have a full pain free range of motion.

A relative contraindication exists in those individuals with either conservatively or surgically treated disc disease with residual facet instability.

An absolute contraindication exists in the following situations:

1. Acute central disc;
2. Acute or chronic "hard disc" herniation with associated neurologic findings, pain, and/or significant limitation of cervical motion;
3. Acute or chronic "hard disc" herniation with associated symptoms of cord neurapraxia due to concomitant congenital narrowing "stenosis" of the cervical canal.

STATUS POST CERVICAL SPINE FUSION

A) A stable one-level anterior or posterior fusion in a patient who is asymptomatic, neurologically negative, pain free, and has a normal range of cervical motion presents no contraindication to continued participation in contact activities.

B) Individuals with a stable two or three level fusion who are asymptomatic, neurologically negative, and have a pain free full range of cervical motion present a relative contraindication. Because of the presumed increased stresses at the articulations of the adjacent uninvolved vertebra and the propensity for the development of degenerative changes at these levels, it appears to be the rare exception who should be permitted to continue contact activities.

C) In those individuals with more than a three level anterior or posterior fusion, an absolute contraindication exists concerning continued participation in contact activities.

REFERENCES

1a. American Heart Association. Health care provider's manual for basic life support. Dallas, TX: AHA, 1988.

1. Torg JS, Pavlov H, Genuario SE, Sennett B, Robie B, Jahre C. Neuropraxia of the cervical spinal cord with transient quadriplegia. J Bone Joint Surg 1986;68A:1354.

2. Boilsen E. The cervical spinal canal in intraspinal expansive processes. Acta Radiol 1954;42:101–115.

3. Kessler, JT. Congenital narrowing of the cervical spinal canal. J Neurol Neurosurg Psychiatry 1975;38:1218–1224.

4. Pavlov H, Torg JS, Robie B, Jahre C. Cervical spinal stenosis: determination with vertebral body ratio method. Radiology 1987;164:771–775.

5. Torg JS, Sennett B, Vegso JJ, Pavlov H. Axial load injuries to the middle cervical spine segment: an analysis and classification of 25 cases. Am J Sports Med 1991;19:6–20.

6. Torg JS, Pavlov H, O'Neill MJ, Nichols CE, Sennett B. The axial load teardrop fracture: the biomechanical, clinical and roentgenographic analysis. Am J Sports Med 1991;19:355–364.

7. Schneider RC, Kahn EA. Chronic neurologic sequelae of acute trauma to the spine and spinal cord. Part I. The significance of the acute-flexion or "tear-drop" fracture dislocation of the cervical spine. J Bone Joint Surg 1956;38A:985–997.

8. Woodford MJ. Radiography of the acute cervical spine. Radiography 1987;53:3–8.

9. Allen BL, Jr, Ferguson RL, Lehman TR, O'Brien RP. A mechanistic classification of closed, indirect fractures and dislocations of the lower cervical spine. Spine 1982;7:1–27.

10. Richman S, Friedman R. Vertical fracture of cervical vertebral bodies. Radiology 1954;62:536–542.

11. Lee C, Kim KS, Rogers LF. Sagittal fracture of the cervical vertebral body. Am J Roentgenol 1982;139:55–60.

12. Lee C, Kim KS, Rogers LF. Triangular cervical body fragments: diagnostic significance. Amer J Roentgenol 1982;138:1123–1132.

13. Carvell JE, Fuller DJ, Duthrie RB, Cockin J. Rugby football injuries to the cervical spine. Br Med J 1983;286:49–50.

14. Silver JR. Injuries of the spine sustained in rugby. Br Med J 1984;288:37–43.

15. Tator CH, Ekong CEU, Rowed DA, Schwartz ML, Edmonds VE, Cooper PW. Spinal injuries due to hockey. Can J Neurol Sci 1984;11:34–41.

16. Tator C, Edmonds VE. National survey of spinal injuries to hockey players. Can Med Assoc J 1984;130:875–880.

17. Frykman G, Hilding S. Hop pa stusmatta kan orska allvarliga skador. (Trampoline jumping can cause serious injury). Lakartidningen 1970;67:5862–5864.

18. Hammer A, Schwartzbach AL, Darre E, Osgaard O. Svaere neurologiske skader some folge af trampolinspring. (Severe neurologic damage resulting from trampolining.) Ugeskr Laeger 1981;143:2970–2974.

19. Steinbruck J, Paeslack V. Trampolinspringen—ein gefahrlicher sport? (Is trampolining a dangerous sport?) Munchener medizinischer Wochenschrift 1978;120:985–988.

20. Torg JS, Das M. Trampoline-related quadriplegia: review of the literature and reflections on the American Academy of Pediatrics' position statement. Pediatrics 1984;74:804–812.

21. Ciccone R, Richman R. The mechanism of injury and the distribution of three thousand fractures and dislocations caused by parachute jumping. J Bone Joint Surg 1948;30-A:77–100.

22. Mennen U. Survey of spinal injuries from diving: a study of patients in Pretoria and Cape Town. S Afr Med J 1981;59:788–790.

23. Coin CG, Pennink M, Ahmad WD, Keranen VJ. Diving-type injury of the cervical spine: contribution of computed tomography to management. J Comput Assist Tomogr 1979;3:362–372.

24. Albrand OW, Corkill G. Broken necks from diving accidents: a summer epidemic in young men. Am J Sports Med 1976;4:107–110.

25. Albrand Otmar W, Walter Janet. Underwater deceleration curves in relation to injuries from diving. Surg Neurol 1975;4:461–465.

26. Tator CH, Edmonds VE, New ML. Diving: frequent and potentially preventable cause of spinal cord injury. Can Med Assoc J 1981;124:1323–1324.

27. Kim KS, Chen HH, Russel EJ, Roger LF. Flexion teardrop fractures of the cervical spine: radiographic characteristics. Am J Roentgenol 1989;102:319–326.

28. Torg JS, Treux R, Jr, Quedenfeld TC, Burstein A, Spealman A, Nichols C, III. The national football head and neck injury registry—report and conclusions 1978. J Am Med Assoc 1979;241:1477–1479.

29. Torg JS, Vegso JJ, Torg E. Cervical quadriplegia resulting from axial loading injuries: cinematographic, radiographic, kinetic and pathologic analysis. American Academy of Orthopaedic Surgeons Audio-Visual Library, 1987.

30. Burstein AH, Otis JC, Torg JS. Mechanisms and pathomechanics of athletic injuries to the cervical spine. In: Torg JS, ed. Athletic injuries to the head, neck and face. Philadelphia: Lea & Febiger, 1982:139–142.

31. Mertz HJ, Hodgson VR, Thomas LM, Nyquist GW. An assessment of compressive neck loads under injury-producing conditions. Physician Sports Med 1978;6:95–106.

32. Hodgson VR, Thomas LM. Mechanisms of cervical spine injury during impact to the protected head. Twenty-Fourth Stapp Car Crash Conference 1980:1542.

33. Gosch HH, Gooding E, Schneider RC. An experimental study of cervical spine and cord injuries. J Trauma 1972;12:570–575.

34. Maiman DJ, Sances A, Myklebust JB, et al. Compression injuries of the cervical spine: a biomechanical analysis. Neurosurgery 1983;13:254–260.

35. Roaf R. A study of the mechanics of spinal injuries. J Bone Joint Surg 1960;42-B:810–823.

36. Roaf R. International classification of spinal injuries. Paraplegia 1972;10:78–84.

37. White AA, III, Punjabi MM. Clinical biomechanics of the spine. Philadelphia: JB Lippincott, 1978.

38. Bauze RJ, Ardran GM. Experimental production of forward dislocation in the human cervical spine. J Bone Joint Surg 1978;60-B:239–245.

39. Holdsworth F. Fractures, dislocations, and fracture-dislocations of the spine. J Bone Joint Surg 1970;52-A:1534–1551.

40. Torg JS, Vegso JJ, Sennett B. The national football head and neck injury registry; 14 year report on cervical quadriplegia, 1971 through 1985. JAMA 1985;254:3439–3443.

41. Torg JS, Vegso JJ, O'Neill J. The epidemiologic, pathologic, biomechanical and cinematographic analysis of football-induced cervical spine trauma. Am J Sports Med 1990;18:50–57.

42. Scher AT. Vertex impact and cervical dislocation in rugby players. S Afr Med J 1981;59:227–228.

43. Albright JP, Moses JM, Feldich HG, et al. Non-fatal cervical spine injuries in interscholastic football. JAMA 1976;236:1243–1245.

44. Hensinger RN. Congenital anomalies of the odontoid: the cervical spine. 2nd. ed. The Cervical Spine Research Society Editorial Committee: Philadelphia: JB Lippincott, 1989:248–257.

45. Pizzutillo PD. Klippel-Feil syndrome; the cervical spine, 2nd ed. The Cervical Spine Research Society Editorial Committee: Philadelphia: JB Lippincott, 1987:258–271.

46. Eismont FJ, Clifford S, Goldberg M, et al. Cervical sagittal spinal canal size in spine injuries. Spine 1984;9:663–666.

47. White AA, Johnson RM, Panjobi MM, et al. Biomechanical analysis of clinical stability in the cervical spine. Clin Orthop 1975;109:85–86.

48. Steel HH. Personal communication.

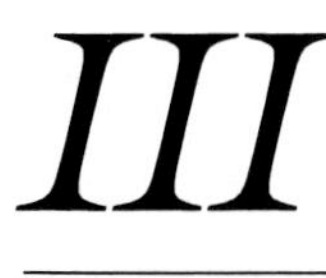

Nonsurgical Management of Cervical Spine Conditions

11

Medical Management of Cervical Spine Disease

Charles L. Christian

Cervical spine disease is common. Its long-term management requires an appreciation of its origins as well as of the therapeutic modalities available to the practitioner. This chapter includes a brief review of anatomy and the pathology of certain forms of arthritides followed by a discussion of the medical management of cervical spine complaints.

Anatomy of the Cervical Spine

The anatomy of the cervical spine is presented in more detail elsewhere in this book. As arthritis is a process primarily of joints, we will review those areas relative to articular structures which frequently are the sites of disease. The bodies of the vertebrae themselves are separated by intervertebral discs which contain glycosaminoglycans and type I collagen in the nucleus pulposus and type II collagen in the annulus fibrosus. The anterior and posterior longitudinal ligaments stabilize these structures. Luschka in 1858 described the presence of synovial spaces lateral to the cervical intervertebral discs. Whether such structures are normal anatomic entities or potential spaces which develop with age has remained controversial (1, 2). The anatomy posterolateral to the canal is stabilized by an interlacing continuity of ligaments — capsular, flavum, interspinous, and supraspinous. The true synovial joints of the cervical spine include the 14 apophyseal (interlaminar) joints which are the approximation of the inferior and superior articular processes and are embedded within the capsular ligaments. Additionally, there are two atlantoaxial synovial bursae separating the odontoid process from the anterior arch of the atlas and, posteriorly, from the transverse ligament.

Functionally, the anatomy of these parts provides support (body of vertebrae), protection of the spinal cord (vertebral arches), movement by acting as levers for muscle attachment (spinous and transverse processes), and limitation of movement (ligaments and apophyseal joints), especially anterior slipping. The anatomical alterations produced by varied expression of inflammation and from both destructive and hypertrophic lesions of bone and periarticular tissues result in the signs and symptoms of cervical spine disease.

Types of Arthritis Affecting the Cervical Spine

Osteoarthritis (Degenerative Joint Disease)

It is generally accepted that nearly 100% of individuals will develop osteoarthritis (OA) by late adulthood. Fortunately, the process is usually slowly progressive and often is asymptomatic. However, many individuals for unknown reasons have a more rapid development of both disease and symptoms. Characteristically, OA involves the weight-bearing diarthrodial joints. The cause is unknown, and only recently has a better understanding of the process been elucidated. The two salient features are damage to articular cartilage and subchondral bone remodelling. At some point, consequent to uncertain alterations, focal and erosive lesions appear at the surface of the hyaline cartilage. Chondrocyte proliferation occurs, and there is increased synthesis of type II collagen and prostaglandins. Alterations in proteoglycan content, subunit size, and aggregates occur (3). Increase in water content accompanies the disintegration (4). Increased density, microinfarction, and remodelling of the subchondral bone with a range of hypertrophy or atrophy eventuates. Classic osteophytes result. The degree of inflammatory cell infiltrate is variable, and it remains controversial as to whether inflammation plays a significant role in the destructive process or is an incidental response to tissue injury (5, 6). The cells are mixed mononuclear and appear more commonly at the cartilage juncture areas. The degree of inflammation is typically far less severe than in the other forms of chronic joint destruction such as rheumatoid arthritis. Pannus formation when it occurs is likewise reminiscent of that in rheumatoid, except usually not of same extent (7). The distribution of OA may be localized or general and in certain cases can be related to previous joint injury.

The process in the cervical spine is similar to that in

other distributions except that eburnation does not occur. In the cervical spine, the lower intervertebral disc spaces diminish with the bony hypertrophy. Osteophytes develop at the joints of Luschka and apophyseal joints. Hypertrophy of the longitudinal ligaments and ligamentum flavum is typical. The overall mechanical effects are reduced range of motion and impingement of neurovascular structures.

In the case of intervertebral disc disease, the most common manifestation is protrusion of the nucleus pulposus into the spinal canal and is predictably most frequent at the C5–C6 and C6–C7 level. This often appears acutely. The distribution (dorsomedial, dorsolateral, or intraforaminal) determines whether radicular and/or cord compression symptoms are present. Neck pain is common, and paresthesias, anesthesia, or motor deficits may appear along the distribution of the involved nerve roots. Interestingly, this acute consequence of OA occurs in a younger age group than that of other OA manifestations.

On the other hand, OA of the synovial joints more commonly involves those upper cervical segments which are also the most mobile (apophyseal and atlantoaxial joints), and symptoms usually appear at a later age. Limitation of range of motion is a classic feature, except forward flexion is usually preserved. Tenderness may be elicited by direct compression of the apophyseal joints. Occipital and frontal headache are common, especially in the morning.

Hypertrophy of the ligaments may result in cord impingement producing myelopathic symptoms. Bone remodeling, ligamentous hypertrophy, and intervertebral space narrowing leads to foraminal encroachment with resulting radiculopathies (8). Similar processes may cause vascular compromise especially of the vertebral arteries, but fortunately such events are uncommon.

Rheumatoid Arthritis

Rheumatoid arthritis (RA) is a systemic disease characterized by granulomatous inflammation. Joints, juxtaarticular tissues, serosae, and eyes are most commonly affected, but the spectrum of organ damage may be vast, particularly if vasculitis develops in the late stages. Classic RA is polyarticular and symmetrical. The cause is unknown, but it appears that the earliest changes involve synovial membranes. Via complex processes not completely understood, proliferation and inflammatory changes in synovium result in destructive lesions in cartilage, bone, and periarticular tissues. This leads to a wide variety of anatomical deformities characteristic of the disease. At times, functional ankylosis occurring as the joint becomes an inflammatory and/or fibrotic mass. Pain is caused not only by chemical mediators but also by mechanical disruption and impingement of neurovascular tissues. Swelling represents inflammation as well as synovial proliferation. The natural history and aggressiveness of this disease is quite variable, but in the majority of patients it is unrelenting. The presence of rheumatoid factor is statistically associated with more aggressive joint destruction and with nodule formation.

Cervical spine involvement in RA is common. Its frequency in general correlates with the duration and aggressiveness of extra-axial disease and thus with seropositivity. In the largest prospective studies, the incidence of cervical involvement in RA has been as high as 88% (2). As RA typically involves diarthrodial, movable joints, it is not surprising that manifestations in the cervical spine affect the upper, more mobile regions, especially the synovial-lined atlantoaxial and apophysial joints. Atlantoaxial pannus can lead to transverse ligament laxity, lateral body destruction, dens erosion, and even invasion of the cranial vault. As these prominent barriers are compromised, displacement occurs, especially anteriorly (9, 10). *Atlantoaxial subluxation* has been reported in 19%–42% of patients in radiographic surveys (2). Seropositivity and appendicular disease activity does correlate with subluxation, but perhaps less appreciated is how early in the disease this may occur (11). In a prospective radiographic study, over 80% of patients with subluxation developed evidence within the first 2 years of disease (12). In addition to anterior C1–C2 subluxation, rheumatoid destruction of the odontoid process at C-1 and C-2 further predisposes to *posterior dislocation* of the atlas (13). *Vertebrobasilar invagination and rotational* or *lateral dislocations* may result from partial or complete collapse of the lateral mass of the atlas, axis, or occiput erosion (14). Fortunately, these are far less common occurrences. Both ligamentous laxity and apophyseal joint destruction contribute to *subaxial anterior dislocation*.

Intervertebral disc space narrowing occurs as a consequence of improper loading from anterior subluxation and/or direct rheumatoid infiltration (15). Lesions from the joints of Luschka have been noted to extend into both intervertebral discs and bodies of vertebrae. Resultant disc space narrowing without osteophytosis in the upper levels of the cervical spine are virtually pathognomonic of rheumatoid disease in contradistinction to osteoarthritis. Disc space collapse, by shortening the vertical length of the spine anteriorly, further accentuates the forces toward anterior subluxation.

Besides bony compromise of the canal and foramina via subluxation and disc space narrowing, ligamentous thickening can compress the cord or nerve roots as well, with manifestations referable to spinal stenosis or radiculopathy. Additionally, rheumatoid nodules arising in any location may alter contiguous structures and function (16). Pachymeningitis with dural nodules may impact the cord (17). In late stage disease, a small percent of individuals develop widespread granulomatous lesions or vasculitis which can affect multiple organ systems, including the spinal cord.

The Seronegative Spondyloarthritides

The seronegative spondyloarthritides are a group of disorders significantly different from rheumatoid arthritis. (See Table 11.1.) RA occurs more frequently in women than men (F:M > 2:1), has a global racial distribution, and characteristically involves appendicular joints symmetrically. Axial involvement of clinical consequence is essentially limited to the cervical spine. In contrast, there is a male predominance in the seronegative spondyloarthritides. Genetically, Caucasians are more frequently affected, especially those expressing HLA-B27, and a familial predisposition is not uncommon. A further important clinical distinction is that peripheral joint involvement in seronegative disease is typically asymmetric. Rheumatoid factor is absent (thus "seronegative"), and nodule formation does not occur.

In contrast to rhematoid arthritis where the primary pathologic lesion is synovial, the spondyloarthritides appear to involve the entheses, sites of insertion of ligaments, tendons, or capsule into bone. It is at these insertions that the inflammatory lesions of spondyloarthritis appear, particularly in the spine. Appendicular arthritis frequently demonstrates both a combination of enthesopathy and synovitis. The spectrum of erosive disease, new bone formation, and ankylosis are typical radiologic features.

1) Ankylosing Spondylitis (AS) is the classic example of enthesopathy. Inflammation at the enthesiae leads to an osteitis and resorption of bone at the insertion of the annulus fibrosis into vertebral bodies. Squaring of the bodies, ossification of the annulus, and anterolateral and posterior bony bridging develop, the latter corresponding to the anterior and posterior longitudinal ligaments (18). Much less commonly, the spinal ligaments and their enthesiae involved. The apophyseal joints become involved with a frank synovitis not unlike that associated with RA, but ossification is the usual outcome. Peripheral arthritis occurs in 20%–25% of individuals. Approximately 50% of individuals with AS have cervical spine involvement (2). Unlike in RA, atlantoaxial subluxations are rare (2%), but they may occur early on due to ligamentous destruction (19). Pain is common, but limitation of neck range of motion is the prominent feature as ankylosis progresses. More worrisome, the formation of such a rigid unit predisposes the spine to through-and-through fracture from

Table 11.1. Comparison of Seronegative Spondylarthropathies and Rheumatoid Arthritis

	Ankylosing spondylitis	Reiter's syndrome	Psoriatic arthropathy	Intestinal arthropathy	Juvenile ankylosing spondylitis	Reactive arthropathy	Rheumatoid arthritis
Sex distribution	Male ≥ female	Male ≥ female	Female ≥ male	Female = male	Male ≥ female	Male = female	Female > male
Age at onset (yrs)	≥20	≥20	Any age	Any age	<15	Any age	Any age
Uveitis	+	++	+	+	++	+	++
Prostatitis	+	+	–	–	–	?	–
Peripheral joints	Lower limb, often	Lower limb, usually	Upper > lower limb	Lower > upper limb	Upper or lower limb	Lower > upper limb	Upper = lower
Rheumatoid nodules	<1%	<1%	<1%	<1%	<1%	<1%	>50%
Sacroiliitis	Always	Often	Often	Often	Always	Often	Rare
Plantar spurs	Common	Common	Common	?	?	?	Rare
Rheumatoid factor	<5%	<5%	<5%	<5%	<10%	<5%	>80%
HLA-B27 positive	90%	90%	20% (50% with sacroiliitis)	5% (50% with sacroiliitis)	90%	90%	Normal popul distribution
Enthesopathy	+	+	+	?+	+	?	Synovitis
Familial aggregation	+	+	+	+	+	+	±
Onset	Gradual	Sudden	Variable	Peripherally: sudden; axial: gradual	Variable, often knees first	Sudden	Sudden or gradual
Urethritis	–	+	–	–	–	+	–
Conjunctivitis	+	+++	+	+	+	+	++
Skin involvement	–	+	+++	–	–	–	+
Mucous membrane involvement	–	++	–	+	–	–	±
Spine involvement	+++	+	+	+	+	+	++
Symmetry	+	–	–	+	±	±	++
Self-limiting	–	±	±	±	±	±	–
Remissions, relapses	–	±	±	±	±	±	±

*Modified from Calin A. Spondylarthritis. Medicine. Sci Am 1982;3(6):15.

even seemingly minor trauma (20). Fractures typically occur at the C5–C7 level, usually after simple falls. Fatality rates as high as 50% have been reported (21).

2) Reiter's Disease and Reactive Arthritis — Reiter originally described the triad of arthritis, conjunctivitis, and urethritis following a postdysenteric syndrome. We now recognize a spectrum of "reactive arthritis" subsequent to infection, especially with Gram-negative enteric pathogens (i.e., *Salmonella*, *Shigella*, *Yersinia*, and *Campylobacter*) or sexually transmitted agents (*Chlamydia* and *Mycoplasma*). Individuals possessing HLA-B27 are particularly predisposed to development of these syndromes (22). Other frequent manifestations include cervicitis, keratoderma blennorrhagia, circinate balanitis, nail lesions, and stomatitis. The nonarticular involvement is variable, and incomplete expression of the classic triad of Reiter is common (23). A significant number of patients with otherwise typical reactive arthritis lack a history of antecedent infection. Once thought to have an overwhelming male predominance, the incidence in women in some studies has approached that in men. This is in part due to the less symptomatic character of genitourinary infection in women or the characterization of dysuric syndromes and cervicitis as "nonspecific."

Distinguishing early AS from Reiter's may be difficult, but there are notable differences. In contrast to Reiter's disease, skin and mucosal lesions are rare in AS. Further, sacroiliitis is universal in AS, while appearing in only 20% of patients with Reiters disease. Peripheral joint disease is comparatively more common in reactive arthritis. Spine lesions in AS are typically symmetric and ascending. Skip, asymmetric lesions are more frequent in the reactive arthritides. Therefore, the extent of ankylosis, limitation in range of motion, and frequency of serious fractures are much less. The course of reactive arthritis is highly variable; complete remission after several weeks or more is common, while others have remittant/recurrent or chronic progressive patterns.

3) Psoriatic Arthropathy — The musculoskeletal manifestations of psoriasis are quite variable (24). To some extent it represents coincidence of common diseases, but there is a highly significant increased frequency of inflammatory arthropathy of peripheral and axial joints. Both synovitis and enthesopathy occur. Distal interphalangeal joint involvement is more common than in Reiters, and there is a comparative predilection for the upper extremities. Asymmetric disease is typical and dactylitis ("sausage digits") are common, a feature shared with Reiter's disease. Some patients develop a particularly aggressive form known as "arthritis mutilans" with telescoping and "pencil-in-cup" deformities of the digits. Another group develops symmetric polyarthritis essentially indistinguishable from RA. In such subjects, the presence or absence of rheumatoid factor is often used in arbitrarily distinguishing RA from psoriatic arthropathy.

Spine disease occurs in as many as 25% of patients with psoriatic arthropathy (25, 26). Spondylitis is more common in HLA-B27 individuals, but axial disease is not as closely associated (<50%) with this genetic factor as it is in AS or Reiters. Syndesmophyte formation is particularly more frequent in psoriatic arthritis, but it tends to be asymmetrical and "nonmarginal" in location, and there is a predilection for the cervical spine. Though the extent of bridging seen with AS is rare, a subset of patients develop a picture of ascending spondylitis of the classic ankylosing type.

4) Enteropathic Arthropathy — Peripheral joint arthritis occurs in 10–20% of patients with inflammatory bowel disease, being more common in Crohn's disease than in ulcerative colitis. The appendicular arthritis typically appears in patients who have established gut disease and other extraintestinal manifestations. By contrast, spondylitis may precede the onset of gut symptoms by years, especially in ulcerative colitis. In both Crohn's disease and ulcerative colitis, sacroiliitis and other manifestations of ankylosing spondylitis occur in up to 10% of subjects. AS has been found in approximately 5% of patients with Whipple's disease.

5) Juvenile Spondyloarthropathies — All of the preceding forms of arthritis may occur in children. There is a stronger male predominance for spondylopathy in juvenile arthritis. As in adults, the association of HLA-B27 corresponds with development of axial disease. Pauciarticular peripheral joint disease may precede symptomatic spine involvement by years. Reiter's disease and enteropathic arthropathy may be particular difficult to diagnose as abdominal pain, diarrhea, dysuria, and conjunctivitis are relatively frequent pediatric problems. As well, the arthropathy of psoriasis may precede the skin manifestations by years. Involvement of the apophyseal joints of the cervical spine occurs in as many as 50% of children with juvenile polyarthritis. Atlantoaxial subluxation is most typically found. Bony fusion, especially at the C2–C3 level occurs with concomitant growth retardation of the vertebral bodies and narrowing of the disc space.

Other Arthroses

Diffuse Idiopathic Skeletal Hyperostosis (DISH), also known as Forrestier's disease, is a common disorder of advancing age, especially in men. The primary feature is the ossification of ligaments and enthesiae. Particularly the anterolateral spinal ligaments are affected, leading to bony bridging. The extent of involvement is variable and may lead to decreased mobility, but symptoms are usually less than what one would expect from radiographic findings. Disease in the cervical spine is most typical at the C4–C6 level. Hoarseness, dysphagia, a foreign body sensation in the pharynx, and fractures with minimal trauma have been reported as a consequence of DISH. Rarely, posterior longitudinal ligament disease produces spinal stenosis. Extraspinal ossifications also occur. An association with diabetes mellitis has been noted. Unlike the other spondyloarthropathies, there is no association with HLA-B27.

Cervical spine involvement is a rare manifestation of gout, although destruction of the atlas or odontoid and spinal compression have been reported. Sarcoidosis may particularly affect vertebral bone and discs. Calcium pyrophosphate deposition (CPPD) in the intervertebral discs increases with age, but the significance of this finding is uncertain. CPPD-associated ligamentum flavum hypertrophy has been reported to produce spinal compression.

THE MEDICAL MANAGEMENT OF ARTHRITIS OF THE CERVICAL SPINE

General Principles

The goals of therapy in cervical spine arthritis are to relieve pain and to improve function. A program of care should be approached with knowledge of the pathology as well as an appreciation that the majority of these diseases are chronic and that exacerbations and remissions are common. At all times, the clinician must be aware of the potential for neurovascular compromise which may warrant immediate surgical intervention. Additionally, the recent experience with the use of high-dose methylprednisolone in acute spinal cord injury suggests that such therapy may be important when acute myelopathy complicates cervical level arthropathies (27).

EDUCATION

To begin, patients should become acquainted with the nature of their disease. An awareness of anatomy and pathology sets the stage for understanding the modalities to alleviate the symptoms, improves compliance, and guards against the sense of futility which is always problematic in chronic or recurrent debility. A model of the cervical spine is particularly helpful in demonstrating and answering questions. During the discussion, choice of words is extremely important. "Degenerative" probably more than "arthritis" raises the specter of the wheelchair-bound invalid. This is particularly true for the younger adult or anyone who has yet to experience other chronic disease manifestations. Patients with longstanding peripheral joint disease are usually better able to incorporate cervical spine involvement within the framework of existing disease. Though during acutely painful presentations immediate comfort is the most pressing issue, early on, the concept of potential chronicity needs to be introduced. This should be done always with the assurance that care can be given and that the patient has a significant role to play in therapy.

A thorough examination of work and lifestyle habits often reveals points of practical alteration which may prevent exacerbation of symptoms. For example, the arrangement of desks and computer consoles, the proper elevation of keyboards or viewing screens, the use of swivel rather than stationary chairs, the use of book or paper holders — all may be important variables, reasonably altered. Reading in bed and watching television while lying on a sofa should be discouraged. Patients engaged in high impact aerobics or sports that require extremes of neck range of motion should explore alternative forms of exercise. Modes of transport which are particularly agitating (e.g., buses, subways) or prolonged travel without sufficient recess are to be avoided. Carrying groceries, ladened brief cases, shoulder bags, or luggage should be minimized or eliminated. Home health agencies may assist with marketing and more difficult house chores. The patient should be encouraged to buy a cervical pillow or use only one small pillow at bedtime.

Understanding the proper use of medications is paramount. In today's anti-drug environment, patients will avoid analgesics sufficient to alleviate exacerbations with subsequent increased pain and frustration. Often, they will decrease the dose of antiinflammatory medications, thus never achieving the intended effect. Education as to the role of medication, anticipating and explaining side-effects, and counseling as to toxicity are vital for safety and compliance. Two particular fears of patients are that they may become addicted or that the drugs will lose their efficacy with use. Dealing with these concerns forthrightly can strengthen the therapeutic relationship.

A propensity to falling, a common cause of morbidity and mortality in the elderly, is further aggravated in the patient with cervical spine disease. Limited neck range of motion interferes with visual cues, station, balance, and coordination. Installing adequate lighting, nailing down rugs, and eliminating other floor hazards such as thresholds or exposed electrical cords are practical home safety measures. Visiting home nurses can further investigate and reinforce instruction. Non-slip, broad-based footwear need not be expensive; running shoes are now fashionable. Canes, if used properly, are good ambulatory adjuncts. Maximization of visual acuity requires regular ophthalmologic care.

Lastly, an awareness of how chronic pain itself leads to its own set of problems can fortify the patient to better deal with disease. Understanding stress and the need for restful sleep may enable the patient to make alterations in lifestyle which reduce dependence on medication and decrease depression. With each encounter, the physician should reassess the patient's understanding of the modalities of therapy, review previous instruction and analyze lifestyle changes. Important points should be reemphasized and instructions written on prescription pads for the patient to later review. By this means, patients begin to appreciate that simple measures are worth more than chatter.

DRUGS AND THEIR USE

Pharmacologic intervention should be tailored to basic mechanisms of insult. Analgesics, nonsteroidal antiinflammatory drugs (NSAIDs), steroids, disease "remittive" agents, muscle relaxants, neuroleptic medications, and hypnotics ameliorate different levels of disease. They may be used separately or in combination but always with full knowledge of potential adverse effects.

1) Analgesics — Mild pain will often respond to acetaminophen. Analgesic doses of salicylates or NSAIDs are likewise useful but with potentially greater side-effects. Acetaminophen with codeine, hydrocodone, and oxycodone provide stepwise stronger opiate relief, but with concomitant constipation and depression of mental alertness. For extreme pain (e.g., acute disc herniation, torticollis) it is usually best to maximize analgesia at the beginning of therapy rather than progressively increase the potency of medications. Likewise, it is important for the patient to realize that early analgesic use (or other therapeutic modalities as well) may obviate the need for both stronger and more longterm measures later. "Toughing out" a flare rarely works. Increasing water intake and bulk in the diet and employing stool softeners can ameliorate constipation. Opiates may be too potent for use in the elderly without close supervision. They should be gingerly applied when necessary, aware of the increased potential of falling and overdose. In extreme circumstances, hospitalization may be warranted to gain control.

2) Aspirin and Nonsteroidal Antiinflammatory Drugs — Salicylates and NSAIDs at low to moderate doses are effective analgesics. As analgesics, their use should be weighed against their special toxicity profiles — gastrointestinal and renal in particular. At higher doses, the antiinflammatory potential of these agents is achieved. Therefore in diseases with inflammatory components, they may be the mainstay of therapy. Too often, however, these medications are improperly used. To attain their antiinflammatory effect, some preparations require regular use for at least 10–14 days. It is important to educate the patient that intermittent use of these medications may therefore fail to achieve the desired result while still exposing the patient to adverse effects. For patients requiring sustained NSAID therapy, regular monitoring of hemograms, urinalyses, renal and liver function, and stool heme may be indicated. Ulcer prevention or treatment by H2 blockers, sucralfate, or misoprostol are indicated for patients experiencing gastrointestinal intolerance to NSAID therapy.

3) Other Pharmaceuticals — Neuroleptic agents are increasingly used in patients with inflammatory diseases, especially to treat chronic pain, neuropathy, and sleep disturbance. The tricyclic antidepressants (imipramine, amitryptyline, and doxepin) anecdotally decrease pain in patients with rheumatoid arthritis. These same compounds as well as phenytoin and carbamazepine are extensively used for treatment of neuropathic pain with variable success. In this regard we have found them effective in treating nerve root compressive symptoms and reflex sympathetic dystrophy. The dose required of tricyclic agents is usually much less (<50 mg/day) than antidepressant dosing. They are particularly helpful if given in the evening hours where they may prolong the time of uninterrupted sleep. They further provide an advantage to benzodiazepines, particularly in the elderly, where mental alertness and memory are of particular concern.

Muscle relaxants (cyclobenzaprine, methocarbamol, diazepam) are useful adjuncts in the acute setting of neck pain where paraspinal muscle spasm is apparent. As single agents or in chronic application, they are less efficacious. Associated with potentially significant side effects (depressed mental status, incoordination, increased intraocular pressure), their use should be restricted, especially in the elderly.

PHYSICAL AND MECHANICAL MODALITIES

Cervical collars have roles in the management of pain associated with cervical spine disease. Soft collars do not immobilize, but they provide tactile cues to reinforce decreased movement, and they have the advantage of easy transport. Anterior subluxation continues to occur with the use of soft collars in patients with rheumatoid arthritis; however, this does not negate their usefulness in decreasing pain. Hard collars, on the other hand, provide some immobilization, but they require custom fitting and adjustment, and they may aggravate subluxation anteriorly (28).

Physical therapy is discussed in detail elsewhere in this text. Upper extremity range of motion within the limits of comfort will minimize the complications of atrophy, contracture, and reflex sympathetic dystrophy. Heat applications are easily administered at home and office. Traction requires assurance that the equipment is safe and user friendly, and ideally the physical therapist should visit the patient's home setting to assure proper use. Transcutaneous electrical nerve stimulation (TENS) appears to be helpful for some patients with radiculopathy, but there is continuing controversy regarding the role and efficacy of such devices.

Considerations Relative to Specific Types of Arthritis

OSTEOARTHRITIS

Since inflammation is not primary in OA of the spine, the therapeutic approach should emphasize physical modalities and analgesics. Physical therapy, heat, and collars are particularly effective, often obviating drug use. TENS and a tricyclic antidepressant may ameliorate radicular symptoms. Home traction provides relief for many. Acetaminophen is adequate for the majority of patients, and supplementation with NSAIDs is usually sufficient during flares. Opiates should be avoided or used for brief periods only. Steroids, especially for acute impingement and radicular syndromes may be helpful in the short term and they may be better tolerated than opiates or NSAIDs in the elderly. Systemic steroid therapy should rarely be used for more than 10 days.

Rheumatoid Arthritis

In contrast to OA, physical therapy techniques have more restricted roles in the management of cervical spine problems in RA. Due to the propensity for subluxation and cord compression, protection of the neurovascular tissues often necessitates decreased range of motion and restricts the use of traction. Education is important in this regard. Patients must understand the importance of informing health care personnel of their cervical spine disease so that caution will prevent inappropriate manipulation. This is particularly important during the perioperative period. Wearing a soft collar in the operating theater and recovery room is as much a constant reminder to medical personnel as it is in the nonhospital setting.

NSAIDs are the mainstay of therapy, sustained at high doses for antiinflammatory efficacy. As in other diseases, the use of steroids should be limited to those severe situations where inflammation is paramount and debility extreme. The goal is to mobilize the patient until other agents achieve control. Steroids are of particular concern in rheumatoid arthritis where bone destruction occurs as part of the disease process. Even low doses (5 mg/day) appear to accelerate osteoporosis. Prospective studies have shown that atlantoaxial subluxation is more frequent and to greater degree in individuals treated with corticosteroids (29). One may argue that this only reflects the subset of individuals with fulminant disease requiring corticosteroid therapy, but it should give cause for further pause before therapy is instituted.

DMARDs (acronym for Disease Modifying Antirheumatic Drug) refers to a group of medications that have proven, but not predictable, roles in decreasing activity of RA. They include injectable and oral gold, penicillamine, azathioprine, sulfasalazine, and methotrexate. It remains controversial as to whether any DMARD clearly halts or significantly delays joint and bone destruction. Frequently, the disease process escapes the control achieved, or the patient develops intolerable adverse effects. Another feature of these medications, except for methotrexate, is that several weeks or more are usually required before one sees signs of efficacy. Some rheumatologists now argue that the classic stepwise trial of these slow-acting agents allows irreversible joint destruction to occur in the early stages of disease. They propose that the application of methotrexate or combination chemotherapy within the first few months of onset may diminish the long-term destruction by arresting the disease during early stages. This "reversal of the pyramid" is attractive vis-a-vis the cervical spine where it is evident that the most common and problematic lesions (anterior subluxations) usually appear within the first 2 years of disease. The problem is that data from clinical trials with this approach are not yet available. The classic stepwise approach is based in part on an awareness of the incremental toxicity of the agents used. At this time it is our bias that, until clinical studies suggest otherwise, introduction of disease "remittive" drugs should be based on their known ability to decrease pain and to improve function.

Seronegative Spondyloarthropathies

The primary goals of therapy in these diseases are to maintain posture and preserve motion. This is particularly true in the ankylosing patterns of disease. In this regard, patient education should emphasize adapting physical modalities of therapy to lifestyle and maintaining both nonimpact and range of motion exercise regimens. Occupational therapy may train the patient in the use of assistive devices to accommodate for the loss of neck motion. NSAIDs significantly reduce pain and stiffness augmenting the results of physical therapy. Typically, these drugs are employed chronically and in high dose. Months of use may be required before a gradual reduction in dose can be attempted. For unknown reasons, indomethacin and phenylbutazone are notable for their particular efficacy in spondylitis. As with all NSAIDs, however, an empiric trial of a different drug is indicated when another achieves less than desirable results. Again, one may require a number of weeks to ascertain the full benefit of any agent.

"Disease-modifying" chemotherapy of the spondyloarthropathies is less clear. In ankylosing spondylitis, three placebo-controlled, double-blind studies have suggested the effectiveness of sulfasalazine (30, 31, 32). In addition to ameliorating peripheral joint disease, there was decreased spine pain and increased chest expansion. As well, more subjects were able to discontinue NSAID use. In view of these findings, sulfasalazine has been employed in poorly controlled trials in Reiter's disease and psoriatic arthropathy (33, 34). The results suggested that it may likewise be effective in these diseases, but the amelioration of axial disease was less clear. The activity of peripheral joint involvement in psoriatic arthritis frequently parallels that of skin disease. Methotrexate predictably improves the skin condition and appendicular arthropathy, but its role for treatment of spine involvement is less well established. Similarly parenteral gold therapy has significant efficacy in controlling the peripheral joint manifestations of patients with the RA-like pattern of psoriatic arthritis. Until further studies are available, it seems reasonable to begin therapy with sulfasalazine in patients with spondyloarthropathies who have not benefited from several months of NSAID use.

INDICATIONS FOR SURGERY

Any suspicion of spinal stenosis, cord compression, or vascular compromise demands immediate assessment by radiographic, neurologic, and surgical consultants. In osteoarthritis, the clinical setting and presentation in most cases provide adequate information to establish a diagnosis and initiate therapy. As a general rule, pain which does not abate and allow reduction in analgesia within 7–10 days requires radiographic examination and appropriate laboratory or electrophysiologic evaluation. Acute disc herniation with motor deficit should prompt immediate surgical consultation, and the persistence of such deficits or truly intractable severe pain may warrant surgical intervention. These patients respond well to disc excision and spine fusion. Severe disability may occur within days in some if surgery is delayed. Likewise, the patient with chronic myelopathic signs or intractable pain may benefit from posterior fusion to prevent progressive deterioration. However, as Bland cautions, the anteroposterior diameter of the spinal canal may be already significantly narrowed in patients with longstanding hypertrophy and fibrosis (35). Even the minor trauma of surgery may cause acute myelopathy in these patients. For this reason, pain alone in the older patient with extensive degenerative disease is seldom an indication for operative intervention.

The patient with RA poses a more difficult problem. Radiographic findings too often do not correlate with clinical symptoms. Severe occipital headache or neck pain suggests significant atlantoaxial subluxation. Paresis, tonic-clonic movements, or alterations in urinary function are classical indications of cord compromise (36). Urinary frequency, however, may be inappropriately attributed to infection or prostatic hypertrophy. Subtle alterations in gait or complaints of pain and weakness may be misinterpreted as manifestations of peripheral arthritis or peripheral neuropathy. Isolated stocking-glove sensory loss has been reported. Proprioceptive disturbance is particularly difficult to define, especially early, by physical examination alone. Suspicion demands clarification by imaging and electrophysiologic studies (37). Neurological manifestations of vertebrobasilar vascular compromise, though infrequent, are significant complications of RA spine involvement (38). Therefore, stroke in the vertebrobasilar distribution, syncope, or sudden unexplained collapse without loss of consciousness demand investigation and intervention if a lesion amenable to surgical approach is found. Though cervical spine destruction begins early in disease, years usually pass before operative intervention is necessary (39). Wound healing and fixation of implant materials are less than optimal in patients with rheumatoid disease (40, 41, 42). This observation along with the advanced longstanding systemic disease of most patients may account for the relatively high postoperative mortality and poor surgical result of some series (43). In the hands of surgeons experienced in the management of cervical spine complications, timely intervention can arrest and sometimes reverse neurological complications.

Demonstration of upper cervical subluxation in the spondyloarthritides with resultant neurovascular compromise is infrequent but should prompt surgical intervention when signs appear as discussed above. Internal fixation of fracture in AS is indicated where instability is possible. Otherwise, based on our present level of knowledge there is good reason to avoid intervention in most cases of spondylitis.

ACKNOWLEDGMENT

We wish to acknowledge our debt to Dr. John Bland who, more than any other individual, has both expanded our knowledge of cervical spine disease and influenced our patient care and this writing.

REFERENCES

1. Bland JH. Luschka's joint? A cleft in the annulus fibrosis; not a joint at all. [Abstract]. Arthritis Rheum 1990;33(5)Supplement:R37.

2. Mohr W. Pathogenesis and morphology of degenerative and inflammatory changes in the cervical spine. Eur League Against Arth Bull 1987;2:49–58.

3. Kresina TF, Malemud CJ, Moskowitz RW. Analysis of osteoarthritic cartilage using monoclonal antibodies reactive with rabbit proteoglycan. Arthritis Rheum 1986;29:863–871.

4. Maroudas A, Venn M. Chemical composition and swelling of normal and osteoarthritic femoral head cartilage. II. Swelling. Ann Rheum Dis 1977;36:399–406.

5. Gardner DL. The nature and causes of osteoarthritis. Br Med J 1983;286:418–424.

6. Glynn LE. Primary lesion in osteoarthritis. Lancet 1977;1:574–575.

7. Goldenberg DL, Egan MS, Cohen AS. Inflammatory synovitis in degenerative joint disease. J Rheumatol 1982;9:204–209.

8. Beamer YB, Garner JT, Shelden CH. Hypertrophied ligamentum flavum. Clinical and surgical significance. Arch Surg 1973;106:289–292.

9. Bland JH. Rheumatoid artritis of the cervical spine. J Rheumatol 1974;1:319–341.

10. Konttinen YT, Bergroth V, Santavirta S, Sandelin J. Inflammatory involvement of cervical spine ligaments in rheumatoid arthritis patients with atlantoaxial subluxation. J Rheumatol 1987;14:532–534.

11. Eulderink F, Meijers KA. Pathology of the cervical spine in rheumatoid arthritis: a controlled study of 44 spines. J Pathol 1976;120(2):91–108.

12. Winfield J, Cooke D, Brook AS, Corbett M. A prospective study of the radiological changes in the cervical spine in early rheumatoid disease. Ann Rheum Dis 1981;40(2):109–114.

13. Santavirta S, Sandelin J, Slatis P. Posterior atlantoaxial subluxation in rheumatoid arthritis. Acta Orthop Scand 1985;56:298–301.

14. Menezes AH, Vangilder JC, Clark CR, el-Khoury G. Odontoid

upward migration in rheumatoid arthritis. An analysis of 45 patients with "cranial settling." J Neurosurg 1985;63(4):500–509.

15. Martel W. Pathogenesis of cervical discovertebral destruction in rheumatoid arthritis. Arthritis Rheum 1977;20(6):1217–1225.

16. Pettersson H, Larsson EM, Holtas S, Cronqvist S, et al. MR imaging of the cervical spine in rheumatoid arthritis. AJNR 1988;9(3):573–577.

17. Gutmann L, Hable K. Rheumatoid pachymeningitis. Neurology 1963;13:901–905.

18. Calin A. Ankylosing spondylitis. In: Kelly WN, Harris ED, Ruddy S, Sledge CB, eds. Textbook of rheumatology. Philadelphia: W B Saunders, 1989:1021–1037.

19. Sorin S, Askari A, Moskowitz RW. Atlantoaxial subluxation as a complication of early ankylosing spondylitis. Two case reports and a review of the literature. Arthritis Rheum 1979;22(3):273–276.

20. Hunter T, Dubo H. Spinal fractures complicating ankylosing spondylitis. A long-term follow-up study. Arthritis Rheum 1983;26(6):751–759.

21. Hunter T, Dubo H. Spinal fractures complicating ankylosing spondylitis. Int Med 1978;88(4):546–549.

22. Espinoza LR, Aguilar JL, Gutierrez F. Infections in the seronegative spondyloarthropathies. Curr Opin Rheum 1989;1(2):151–158.

23. Arnett F, McClusky OE, Schacter BZ, et al. Incomplete Reiter's syndrome: discriminating features and HL-A W27. Ann Int Med 1976;84:8–12.

24. Michet CJ, Conn DL. Psoriatic arthritis. In: Kelly WN, Harris ED, Ruddy S, Sledge CB, eds. Textbook of rheumatology. Philadelphia: W B Saunders, 1989:1053–1063.

25. Green L, Meyers OL, Gordon W, Briggs B. Arthritis in psoriasis. Ann Rheum Dis 1982;40:366–369.

26. Lambert JR, Wright V. Psoriatic spondylitis: A clinical and radiological description of the spine in psoriatic arthritis. Q J Med 1977;46:411–425.

27. Bracken MB, et al. A randomized, controlled trial of methylprednisolone or naloxone in the treatment of acute spinal cord injury. Results of the second national acute spinal cord injury study. N Engl J Med 1990;322(20):1405–1411.

28. Althoff B, Goldie IF. Cervical collars in rheumatoid atlantoaxial subluxation: a radiographic comparison. Ann Rheum Dis 1980;39(5):485–489.

29. Rasker JJ, Cosh JA. Radiological study of cervical spine and hand in patients with rheumatoid arthritis of 15 years' duration: an assessment of the effects of corticosteroid treatment. Ann Rheum Dis 1978;37(6):529–535.

30. Dougados M, Boumier P, Amor B. Sulphasalazine in ankylosing spondylitis: a double blind controlled study in 60 patients. Br Med J [Clin Res] 1986;293:911–914.

31. Feltelius N, Hallgren R. Sulfasalazine in ankylosing spondylitis. Ann Rheum Dis 1986;45:396–399.

32. Nissila M, Lehtinen K, Leirisalo-Repo M, Luukkainen R, Mutru O, Yli-Kerttula U. Sulfasalazine in the treatment of ankylosing spondylitis—a 26-week, placebo-controlled clinical trial. Arthritis Rheum 1988;31:1111–1116.

33. Farr M, Kitas GD, Waterhouse L, Jubb R, Felix-Davies D, Bacon PA. Treatment of psoriatic arthritis with sulphasalazine: a one year open study. Clin Rheumatol 1988;7:372–377.

34. Trnavsky K, Peliskova Z, Vacha J. Sulphasalazine in the treatment of reactive arthritis. Scand J Rheumalol 1988;67(suppl):76–79.

35. Bland JH. Disorders of the cervical spine. Diagnosis and medical management. Philadelphia: W B Saunders, 1987.

36. Marks JS, Sharp J. Rheumatoid cervical myelopathy. Q J Med 1981;50(199):307–319.

37. Toolanen G, Knibestol M, Larsson SE, Landman K. Somatosensory evoked potentials (SSEPs) in rheumatoid cervical subluxation. Scand J Rheumatol 1987;16(1):17–25.

38. Lipson SJ. Rheumatoid arthritis of the cervical spine. Clin Orthop 1984;182:143–149.

39. Wolfe BK, Okeeffe D, Mitchell DM, Tchang SP. Rheumatoid arthritis of the cervical spine: early and progressive radiographic features. Radiology 1987;165(1):145–148.

40. Glynn MK, Sheehan JM. Fusion of the cervical spine for instability. Clin Orthop 1983;179:97–101.

41. Fehring TK, Brooks AL. Upper cervical instability in rheumatoid arthritis. Clin Orthop 1987;221:137–148.

42. Bryan WJ, Inglis AE, Sculco TP, Ranawat CS. Methylmethacrylate stabilization for enhancement of posterior cervical arthrodesis in rheumatoid arthritis. J Bone Joint Surg 1982;64(7):1045–1050.

43. Zoma A, Sturrock RD, Fisher WD, Freeman PA, Hamblen DL. Surgical stabilization of the rheumatoid cervical spine. A review of indications and results. J Bone Joint Surg [Br] 1987;69(1):8–12.

12

NONOPERATIVE MANAGEMENT OF CERVICAL DISC DISEASE

Scott D. Boden and Sam W. Wiesel

All patients with neck pain, excluding those with fractures, dislocations, or cervical myelopathy should be given an initial period of conservative therapy. There are many noninvasive treatment modalities available; unfortunately, most of them are based on empiricism and tradition. While there are few prospective, randomized, double-blind studies for conservative treatment of lumbar disc disease, even less scientifically valid data exist for cervical disc disease (1). Each treatment in popular use today is surrounded by conflicting claims for its indication and efficacy.

The goals of noninvasive treatment of cervical disc disease are to return the patient to normal activity rapidly with the least diagnostic and therapeutic expense and, most of all, to do no harm. The purpose of this chapter is to outline one strategy for conservative management of cervical disc disease. The treatment protocol presented here has been empirically developed by the authors; other temporal sequences of the various treatment modalities may also be effective. Finally, several of the more common therapeutic modalities will be described along with the available scientific evidence for and against their use.

NONOPERATIVE TREATMENT PROTOCOL

After a cervical myelopathy has been ruled out, the remainder of neck pain patients, which constitute an overwhelming majority, should be started on a course of conservative (nonoperative) management. Initially, a specific diagnosis, whether it be a herniated disc or neck strain, is not required, as the entire group is treated in the same fashion, unless there is neurological defect.

Immobilization is the mainstay of therapy in both acute episodes and exacerbations in patients with chronic cervical disc disease (2). A soft felt collar should fit properly and will usually provide comfort for the patient. The collar should initially be worn continuously, day and night. The patient must understand that the neck is especially unprotected from awkward positions and movements during sleep and that the collar is very important. The other major component of the initial treatment program is drug therapy. Antiinflammatory drugs, analgesics, and muscle relaxants will usually improve patient comfort and should supplement immobilization. Medication is not a substitute for proper immobilization.

Most patients will respond to this approach of immobilization and pharmacotherapy in the first 10 days. The patients that do improve should be encouraged to gradually increase their activities and begin a program of exercises directed at strengthening the paravertebral musculature, rather than at increasing the range of motion. The soft collar is then weaned over the subsequent 2–3 weeks. The unimproved group of patients should continue with immobilization and antiinflammatory medication.

If there is not a significant improvement in symptoms at 3–4 weeks, a local injection into the area of maximum tenderness in the paravertebral musculature and trapezii should be considered. Marked relief of symptoms is often achieved dramatically by infiltration of these trigger points with a combination of 3–5 ml of lidocaine (Xylocaine) and 10 mg of a corticosteroid preparation. If the trigger point injection is not successful at 4–5 weeks since the onset of symptoms, a trial of cervical traction may be instituted. A home traction device with minimal weights is preferred.

The patient should be treated conservatively for up to 6 weeks. The majority of cervical spine patients will get better. If the initial conservative treatment regimen fails, symptomatic patients may be separated into two groups. The first group is comprised of patients with neck pain as a predominant complaint, with or without interscapular radiation. The second group consists of those who complain primarily of arm pain (brachalgia).

If no symptomatic improvement in neck pain is achieved after 6 weeks of conservative therapy, further studies including lateral flexion-extension x-rays, a bone scan, and a medical evaluation must be obtained to assess the cervical spine for instability, arthritis, tumor, and infection. X-rays before this point are not always helpful because of the lack of significant differences between symptomatic and asymptomatic patients (3, 4). A thorough medical examination may also reveal problems missed in the early stages of neck pain evaluation. If the above workup is negative, the patient should have a complete psychosocial evaluation and receive treatment when appropriate for depression or substance dependence, frequently seen in association with neck pain.

If the psychosocial evaluation proves normal, the patient is considered to have chronic neck pain. These patients require encouragement, patience, and education. They especially need to be detoxified from narcotic drugs and placed on an exercise regimen. Many will respond to antidepressant drugs such as amitryptyline (Elavil). Regardless, these patients need to be periodically reevaluated to avoid missing any new problems.

Occasionally, it is difficult to distinguish those patients who have a true neck problem from those individuals using their neck as an excuse to stay out of work and collect compensation or because of pending litigation. The outcome of treatment of cervical disc disease has been shown to be adversely affected by litigation (5). Frequently with hyperextension neck injuries, there are no objective findings to substantiate the subjective complaints. The best solution to this dilemma in the compensation setting is to recommend an independent medical examination early in the treatment course.

The patients with predominantly arm pain (brachalgia) may have symptoms due to mechanical pressure from a herniated disc and secondary inflammation of the involved nerve roots (6). Extrinsic pressure on the vascular structures or peripheral nerves is the most likely imitator of brachalgia and must be ruled out. Pathology in the chest and shoulder must also be considered. Otherwise, if there is unequivocal evidence of nerve root compression (neurologic deficit, positive EMG, and positive myelogram or MRI) consistent with the physical findings, surgical decompression should be considered. Some studies suggest that patients with radicular symptoms seem to do better with surgery (7). Although conservative management of patients with radicular symptoms has shown that this problem rarely progresses to cervical myelopathy, persistent symptoms are common (8).

NONOPERATIVE TREATMENT MODALITIES

As stated earlier, most patients with pain from cervical disc disease will achieve some relief from a conscientious program of conservative care. The multitude of treatment modalities are based on empiricism and tradition. The following section will discuss the rationale behind the use of some of the more common therapeutic measures.

Immobilization

The cornerstone of conservative therapy is immobilization of the cervical spine (9). The goal of immobilization is to rest the neck to facilitate healing of torn and/or attenuated soft tissues. In patients with an exacerbation of chronic symptoms, the purpose of immobilization is to reduce any inflammation in the supporting soft tissues and around the nerve roots.

Immobilization can be best achieved by use of a soft cervical collar that holds the head in a neutral or slightly flexed position. The collar must fit properly; if the neck is held in hyperextension the patient is often uncomfortable and will not derive any benefit from its use. Acutely, the collar should be worn 24 hours a day, until the pain subsides. The amount of immobilization required varies for each patient and should be guided by improvement of symptoms. Once acute symptoms have improved, the ideal long-term immobilization is strong paracervical musculature. Therefore, excessive external immobilization which will cause atrophy of the muscles should be avoided.

In addition to the soft collar, other devices such as plastic collars and metal braces are available to achieve immobilization. In the authors' experience, these are more burdensome to the patient than soft collars and may be less effective in the relief of pain. Furthermore, when the rigid devices are used for a prolonged period of time, they may lead to marked soft tissue atrophy and stiffness, which are not generally found with use of the soft collar.

Another component of immobilization is bedrest for limited periods of time. The benefits are not only the relief of axial compressive forces on the cervical spine, but confinement to bed also limits other daily activities which would exacerbate the problem. Bedrest with cervical support is a viable option for extremely severe pain or for patients who would not otherwise comply with limitation of physical activities.

Drug Therapy

Antiinflammatory medications are used because it is felt that inflammation in the soft tissues is a major contributor to pain production in the cervical spine. This is especially true for those patients with symptoms secondary to cervical disc herniation. The resulting arm pain is due not only to mechanical pressure from the ruptured disc but also to inflammation around the involved nerve roots.

None of the vast spectrum of antiinflammatory drugs has been proven superior. Accordingly, the usual treatment plan is to begin the patient on adequate doses of aspirin, which is effective and inexpensive. If the response is not satisfactory, other agents such as naproxen, ibuprofen, or indomethacin are tried. It should be stressed that antiinflammatory agents are utilized in conjunction with immobilization; they do not replace adequate rest.

Analgesic medication is also very important during the acute phase of an episode of neck pain. Most patients respond to the equivalent of 30–60 mg of codeine every 4–6 hours. If stronger analgesia is required, the patient should be monitored very closely and admitted to the hospital for observation. Patients with peptic ulcer disease should not be treated with conventional antiinflammatories. Some salicylates are now available with a pH-sensitive coating which prevents digestion in the stomach and duodenum.

Muscle relaxants are another useful class of medication in the conservative treatment of cervical disc disease. Painful muscle spasm may frequently be a significant contributor to pain following injury to any of the tissues in the cervical spine. Spasm leads to ischemia which causes a further increase in pain. A muscle relaxant can frequently break the muscle spasm-pain cycle and allow an increased range of motion in the cervical spine. Methocarbanol or carisoprodol in adequate doses are the drugs commonly utilized. Valium is not recommended for use in these patients as a muscle relaxant because it is also a psychologic depressant, and many neck pain patients may already have some degree of clinical depression.

Traction

Although cervical traction has been used for many years, current opinions regarding its effectiveness are variable. While some studies have suggested that traction is a valuable clinical therapy (10, 11), others have concluded that it is either ineffective or potentially harmful in an acutely injured cervical spine (12, 13). Certainly, traction should never be prescribed unless x-rays have been reviewed for fracture, tumor, and infection. Traction is still an empirical form of therapy and should be employed only when more conservative treatment is not effective.

Cervical traction is contraindicated in several situations. Malignancy, cord compression, infection, osteoporosis, and rheumatoid arthritis. It is also commonly believed that when there is a sequestered herniated disc present either in the midline or laterally, traction should not be considered.

Cervical traction may be administered in several ways: mechanical or manual, continuous or intermittent, and sitting or supine. Many feel that manual traction is preferable, due to the interaction between the therapist and patient and the potential for individually varying the traction. We prefer a home traction device with minimal weights (5–10 pounds) pulling in slight flexion. Since there is evidence that at least 25 pounds are necessary to actually distract the cervical vertebrae, the major benefit of low weight traction is probably from the immobilization (14). There is no uniform idea as to how traction actually works, and there is no valid scientific evidence available that traction in and of itself is effective.

Trigger Point Injection

Many patients complain of very localized tender points in the paravertebral area. The objective of a trigger point injection is to decrease the inflammation in a specific anatomic area. The more localized the trigger point, the more effective this form of therapy. Injections may be repeated at intervals of 1–3 weeks. There have been no true randomized clinical trials to study the efficacy of this modality in the cervical spine, but the injections empirically seem to work quite well for both neck pain and brachalgia in some patients.

Epidural Steroids

A large component of cervical radiculopathy is often due to secondary inflammation of the involved nerve root. Reduction of the edema and the local inflammatory response should theoretically help to relieve symptoms. Cervical epidural injections of a local anesthetic and steroid may provide some pain relief. This procedure, however, requires experience, technical competence, and is not without complications. While some have had success with this technique, we do not utilize cervical epidural injections.

Exercises

After a patient's acute symptoms have resolved and there is no significant pain or spasm, an exercise regimen is recommended. The exercises should be directed at strengthening the paravertebral musculature rather than at increasing the range of motion. Motion will generally return with the disappearance of pain.

The authors suggest isometric exercises be performed once each day with increasing repetitions. It should be appreciated that there are no scientific studies which demonstrate that isometric or any type of exercises will reduce the frequency or duration of recurrent neck pain episodes. Empirically, exercise regimens do appear to have a positive psychologic effect and give the patient an active part in the treatment program.

Other Modalities

Manipulation of the cervical spine should be approached very carefully. There is no real scientific evidence that manipulation is effective in the treatment of acute or chronic neck problems. There have been a number of tragic complications associated with the use of cervical manipulation (15). It is the authors' feeling that the hazards are too great to warrant its use and that manipulation at this time has no place in the treatment of cervical spine disorders.

Other unproven modalities are safer and may achieve relief in some patients. Moist heat, transcutaneous electrical nerve stimulation (TENS), and ultrasound may be effective. Scientific data supporting these modalities are scant; however, they are safe, relatively inexpensive, and worthy of a brief trial in refractory patients. In addition, patient education about sleeping with the neck in a neutral position, avoiding automobile travel during the acute injury phase, and customizing work areas to avoid extreme neck flexion, extension, or rotation is worthwhile.

SUMMARY

Unlike acute lumbar disc disease, which is usually self-limiting, at least one third of the cervical disc disease patients have persistent pain (16). The role for conservative therapy in this disease is strengthened by some studies which suggest that operative intervention may not provide any long-term advantages over nonoperative management (5, 7). However, much of the evidence for the conservative treatment modalities is empiric, and there are no data to suggest that any of the conservative modalities influence the natural history of cervical disc disease other than alleviating acute symptoms (16).

The authors maintain that all patients with an exacerbation of cervical disc disease should have up to 6 weeks of conservative therapy in the absence of myelopathy. The specific temporal sequence for use of the various conservative modalities may be variable. A conscientious program of a soft cervical collar and antiinflammatory medications is recommended, occasionally followed by trigger point injections or home traction if necessary. This regimen has empirically been effective in treating the vast majority of patients with exacerbations of cervical disc disease.

REFERENCES

1. Bloch R. Methodology in clinical back pain trials. Spine 1987;12:430–432.

2. DePalma AF, Rothman RH. The intervertebral disc. Philadelphia: W B Saunders, 1970.

3. Friedenberg ZB, Miller WT. Degenerative disease of the cervical spine. J Bone Joint Surg 1963;45-A:1171–1178.

4. Gore DR, Sepic SB, Gardner GM. Roentgenographic findings of the cervical spine in asymptomatic people. Spine 1986;11:521–524.

5. Dillin W, Booth R, Cuckler J, et al. Cervical radiculopathy: a review. Spine 1986;11:988–991.

6. Rothman RH, Marvel JP. The acute cervical disc. Clin Orthop 1975;129:59–68.

7. DePalma AF, Rothman RH, Levitt RL, et al. The natural history of severe cervical disc degeneration. Acta Orthop Scand 1972;43:392–396.

8. Lees F, Turner JW. Natural history and prognosis of cervical spondylosis. Br Med J 1963;2:1607–1610.

9. Rothman RH, Simeone F. The Spine. 2nd ed. Philadelphia: W B Saunders, 1982.

10. Harris W. Cervical traction: review of the literature and treatment guidelines. Phys Ther 1977;57:8.

11. Zhongda L. A study of the effect of manipulative treatment on 158 cases of cervical syndrome. J Tradit Chin Med 1987;7:205–208.

12. British Association of Physical Medicine. Pain in the neck and arm: a multicentre trial of the effects of physiotherapy. Br Med J 1966;1:253.

13. Greenfield J, Ilfeld FW. Acute cervical strain. Clin Orthop 1977;122:196–200.

14. Rath WW. Cervical traction, a clinical perspective. Orthop Rev 1984;13:430–449.

15. Livingston MCP. Spinal manipulation causing injury (a three-year study). Clin Orthop 1971;81:82–86.

16. Gore DR, Sepic SB, Gardner GM, et al. Neck pain: a long-term follow-up of 205 patients. Spine 1987;12:1–5.

13

Epidural Injections of Steroids in the Management of Cervical Pain

Jeffrey Y. F. Ngeow

Since its introduction about 30 years ago, injection of steroids into the lumbar epidural space for treatment of low back pain and sciatica has become a widely accepted practice.

By contrast, the use of this method of therapy for pain in the neck and cervical radiculopathy has not achieved similar recognition. Lack of familiarity with this technique probably accounts for its infrequent use. However, recent reports do indicate a growing interest and popularity in the use of cervical epidural steroids as an acceptable method for controlling pain in the cervical spine (1).

Despite considerable experience in its use, the efficacy of lumbar epidural steroid injection has not been firmly established. Published reports gave improvement rates that ranged from 90% (2) to no more effective than local anesthetic placebo (3). The disparity of the outcomes have been attributed to differences in patient population, injection techniques, and the varying periods of follow-up (4).

Similar caveat will be applicable when evaluating results of cervical epidural steroid injections. Nonetheless, reports of several series of patients treated with cervical epidural steroid injections using the patients' own assessments as the criterion of improvement showed favorable response rates ranging from 68–88% (5). This is comparable to that obtained from lumbar epidural steroid injections.

Indications for Epidural Steroids

Epidural steroid injections have been used in patients with degenerative cervical spondylosis, radiculopathy with or without demonstrable disc herniation, post-laminectomy syndromes, spinal stenosis, and neck pain with nonspecific dermatomal involvements.

The data from several published series suggest that patients with dermatomal specific radiculopathies have the best results following steroid injections (1, 7, 8). Those with radiographic evidence of spondylosis may also benefit from the therapy, whereas nonspecific neck pain profits the least (9). However, this is not to say that other groups of patients will not be helped by this technique. Catchlove (10) has employed local anesthetic injections alone as part of a multimodality approach to neck and occipital pains of muscular and posttraumatic origin and found it to be effective.

Radiographic evidence of cervical degenerative changes have been emphasized as a prognostic feature in the prediction of outcome of epidural steroid injections. However, some patients who do not have radiographically demonstrable degenerative disc disease when first seen, will eventually develop anterior or posterior osteophytes. This occurs particularly in patients who initially present with severe pain which persists despite a variety of conservative treatments (11). Following existing guidelines, this group of patients may not be considered for or receive an adequate trial of epidural steroid injections, when, in fact, they actually belong to the group that will show a favorable response.

In one series of patients there is evidence to suggest that following routine use of cervical epidural steroid injections on those with demonstrable neurologic deficit accompanying their cervical pain, the incidence of surgical intervention is decreased. This relationship, however, does not hold true for lumbar pathology (12).

The use of epidural steroid is based upon the assumption that there is inflammatory change in the nerves in the epidural space which causes the pain. This condition is more likely to exist in patients with acute or subacute symptoms. When the complaint has been chronic or persists after surgical intervention, it is more likely due to perineural fibrosis. In these cases, steroid injection is less likely to provide any benefit.

The situation is somewhat different in the patient who has been stable after a previous operation, a spinal fusion, for example, and who then develops an episode of acute exacerbation. Such episodes may indicate an acute inflammatory process, particularly if an edematous nerve root can be seen on magnetic resonance imaging. It is reasonable to offer such a patient an injection of epidural steroid to see if it can bring about a rapid remission.

TECHNIQUE

Patient Preparation

Preliminary evaluation of the patient should include an adequate history and examination. Anticoagulant medications should be withheld beforehand, and those with a history of peptic ulceration should be prepared with the appropriate medications. Limitations of head and neck movements should be noted, and diagnostic studies such as EMGs, CT scans, and MRIs should be reviewed to assist in selecting the best interspace for the injection.

Selection of Injection Site

The prominent C7 spine renders itself to ready identification. Many practitioners have chosen this landmark and inject the C6–7 or C7–T1 interspace. The diameter of the spinal cord at C7–T1 is reduced compared to the levels above it. Conversely, the epidural space here is wider, that is, 3–4 mm compared to 2 mm at C4, making its identification easier. There is a disadvantage, however, of using the lower cervical spaces. Larger volume of a carrier solution will be required to spread the steroid over the targeted nerve root if it lies higher up. This will inevitably result in partial loss of the medication to unaffected areas. An alternative will be to insert an epidural catheter through a large bore needle so that the catheter tip lies next to the targeted nerve root. This will require delicate manipulations, since advancing a catheter in the narrow cervical epidural space is apt to cause painful paresthesia, resulting in sudden patient movements. I prefer to use a 22-gauge short beveled spinal needle at the desired interspace if it is below C4. Above the C4 level, identification of landmarks can be difficult. Injection at those levels is not recommended unless guided by an imaging device.

Positioning

The patient may be positioned sitting upright, lying prone, or in lateral decubitus with the affected side down. In the sitting position, the patient should be placed on a low stationary sitting stool. The body leans slightly forward with both feet on the floor and the forehead resting comfortably on a firm support. The height of the support should be adjusted to achieve full flexion of the neck without discomfort. The arms should rest on the knees to relax the shoulder and neck muscles (Fig. 13.1). The operator stands behind the patient so that he can view the needle from all directions.

When working with imaging equipments, the prone position may have to be adopted. In this situation, the patient's chest is supported by a thick cushion while the forehead rests on a thin pillow to maintain neck flexion. Since the operator will need to stand on the patient's side, it is harder to judge the direction of the needle and to maintain its midline course. This difficulty is reduced by having the patient lie on the side, but sudden movement of the head is much less preventable in the lateral position.

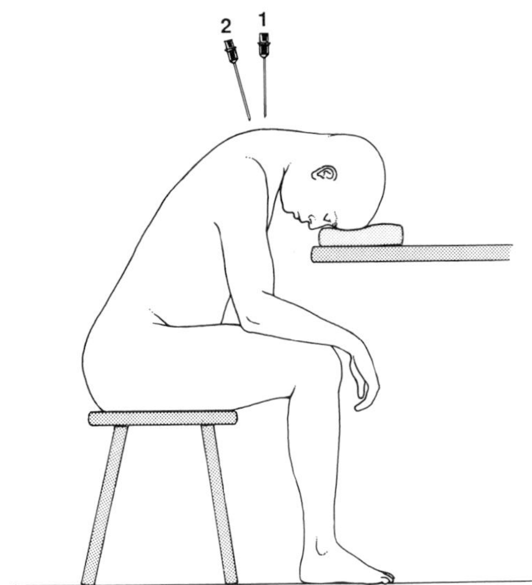

Figure 13.1. Patient position for cervical epidural injection as described in the text. Note: needle position **1** for C6/7 interspace injection is virtually vertical, and needle position **2** for C7/T1 interspace injection is about 15° to the vertical.

The Injection

Under sterile precautions, the skin of the chosen interspace is locally anesthetized using a fine gauge needle. The spinal needle is now inserted in the midline to a depth of 2 cm so that it is embedded in the interspinous ligament. The stylet is withdrawn, and the resistance is tested with a lubricated glass syringe filled with 1 or 2 ml of normal saline. Above C6 level, both the interspinous ligament and the ligamentum flavum are broad and thin (13). The feel of resistance is less than that at the lumbar levels, but it must be tested each time before the needle is advanced. In my experience, the use of a "hanging drop" to look for negative pressure of the epidural space is not always reliable with a 22-gauge needle. When loss of resistance is detected, careful aspiration is done to look for CSF or blood flowback. If either blood or CSF is aspirated, the needle should be withdrawn and the patient asked to return on a subsequent day for another attempt.

Following negative aspiration a test dose of 1 ml 0.5% lidocaine is injected. If numbness or weakness of the dermatome involved occurs there is probably a dural puncture, and the procedure should be postponed. Otherwise, a mixture of Triamcinolone Acetonide (Kenalog)® at 1 mg/kg and 2% lidocaine 2 ml is injected. A gradual warming and slight sensation of numbness indicates correct needle placement.

If higher spread is desired from a low cervical injection, the volume of local anesthetic can be increased to 4 ml.

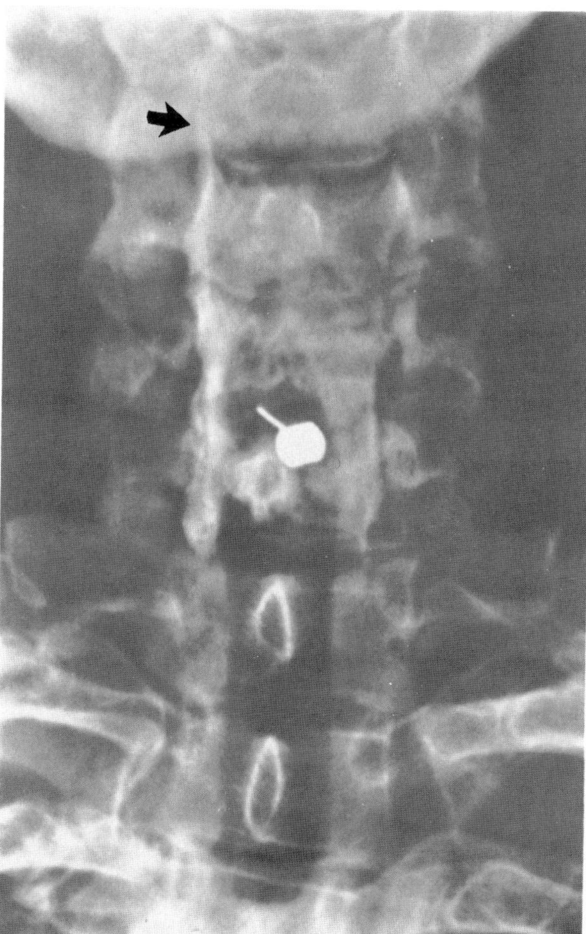

Figure 13.2. PA view of the cervical spine with patient lying prone. Note spinal needle at the C6/7 interspace. Injected dye (Omnipaque 180, 4 ml) showed a characteristic hazy distribution in the epidural space, reaching up to C4 (*arrow*).

When mixed with the steroid, the final volume will be about 6 ml, which is adequate for a spread up to C2 (Figs. 13.2, 13.3). Larger volume will simply force the injectate into the thoracic epidural space and out the transverse foramena. Since the potential epidural space stops at the foramen magnum and is essentially nonexistent dorsally above C3 (13), spreading above C2 cannot always be achieved, even with larger volumes (14). If methylprednisolone is used, the patient should lie with the affected side down after withdrawal of the needle, to encourage the medication to settle on that side.

Complications

Direct trauma to the spinal cord and epidural hematoma are potentially the most serious complications. Fortunately these are extremely rare and have not been reported following cervical epidural steroid injections. Accidental subarachnoid injections of even small volumes of local anesthetic solution at this level will result in total spinal blockade, and the patient will require the usual support until the anesthesia recedes. Intraarterial injection into the vertebral artery is also a possibility, and this will be manifested by CNS toxicity. Immediate complaints of tinnitus or facial or tongue numbness forewarns an imminent grand mal seizure from an intraarterial leak of local anesthetic.

These events, though life-threatening, do not leave permanent deficits if promptly and appropriately treated. For this reason the procedure should only be done where resuscitation facilities are immediately available. Also because of these potential complications, injection into surgical scar is best avoided, since the epidural space under the scar is likely to be obliterated by fibrosis. If steroids are to be given to previously operated patients it should be injected at neighboring interspaces. Clearly, in this case one is less certain if the medication will reach the desired area (4).

Subdural extraarachnoid injection of medications can happen and has been documented (15). In this situation a small volume of injectate may spread over a wide segment of the subdural space. Unexpectedly high anesthetic blockade level which is of a slow onset, should alert one to this happening. Therefore, all patients should be observed for at least 30 minutes following an "uneventful" epidural injection.

Dural puncture with large bore needles has been reported (12) and did not cause any sequelae. One would expect postural headache to occur far less frequently from dural punctures in the neck, since the CSF pressure here would be relatively low in the upright position.

Systemic absorption of steroids may cause depressed plasma cortisol levels lasting usually 2 weeks (16). Guidelines of not more than 3 mg/kg have been recommended to avoid suppression of the pituitary-adrenal axis. However, idiosyncratic response to a single injection resulting in Cushing's syndrome has been reported (17).

Other minor complications that have been reported include nausea, vomiting, dizziness, and hypotension as well as transient increase in pain and stiffness of the neck lasting 24 hours (9). Depression of respiration or heart rate from phrenic nerve and cardiac sympathetic nerve blockade undoubtedly may occur, but, interestingly, have not been reported to be a problem even in the operating room where much larger volumes of local anesthetic agents are used (18).

Conclusion

Cervical epidural steroid injection is a reasonably simple and safe method for treating cervical radiculopathy and neck pain. Shulman (7) has shown that patients who have the best initial pain relief from this treatment will also have the longest period of remission. For these patients repeated injections are unnecessary. On the other extreme, patients who have no benefit from the first properly placed epidural steroid injection for a single disc herniation or monoradiculopathy is unlikely to respond to multiple injections

Figure 13.3. Lateral view of the same patient. The needle (*dark arrow*) is partially obscured by the shoulders. Dye can be seen reaching to C4 dorsally and C2 ventrally (*light arrows*).

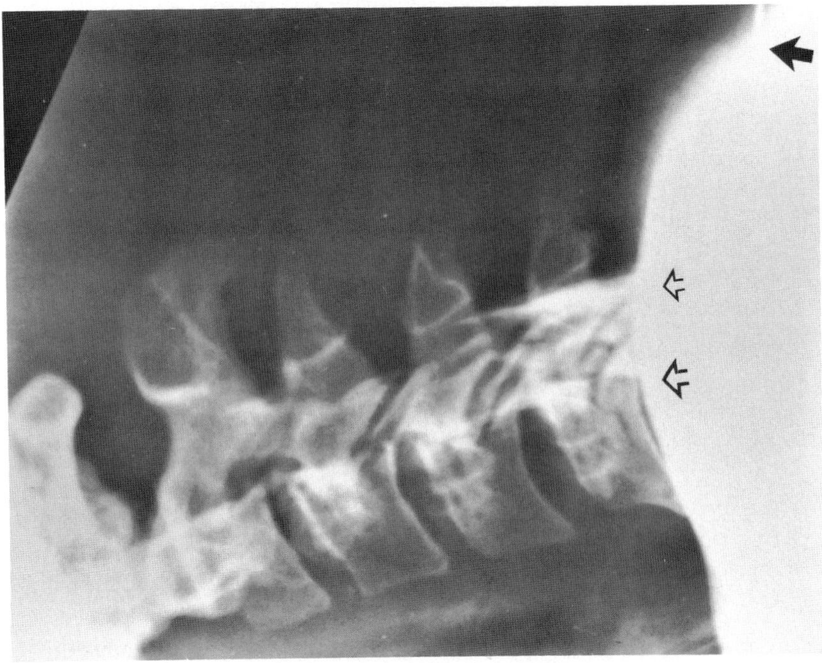

either. When there is partial relief from the first injection or when multiple level pathology is present, such as in spinal stenosis, a second injection at the same level or in a different level to achieve further symptom reduction is justifiable. With multiple injections the consequence of steroid overdose is likely to obscure its benefit.

The successful use of epidural steroid injections to treat reflect sympathetic dystrophy which has failed to respond to standard therapies (19) points to the fact that steroids may work via mechanisms that are as yet unclear to us. Judicious use of this treatment modality may considerably expand our armamentarium to deal with other chronic pain syndromes.

REFERENCES

1. Rowlingson JC, Kirschenbaum LP. Epidural analgesic techniques in the management of cervical pain. Anesth Analg 1986;65:938–942.

2. Heyse-Moore G. A rational approach to the use of epidural medication in the treatment of sciatic pain. Acta Orthop Scand 1978;49:366–370.

3. Cuckler JM, Bernini PA, Wiesel SW, et al. The use of epidural steroids in the treatment of lumbar radicular pain. J Bone Joint Surg 1985;67A(1):63–66.

4. Sharrock NE. Nerve blocks, the use of epidural steroids. In: The lumbar spine. Camins MB, O'Leary PF, eds. New York: Raven Press, 1987.

5. Cicala RS, Williams CH. Cervical epidural injections for the treatment of neck pain. A review. Pain Man 1989;2:141–148.

6. Kepes ER, Duncalf D. Treatment of backache with spinal injections of local anesthetics, spinal and systemic steroids. A review. Pain 1985;22:33–47.

7. Shulman M. Treatment of neck pain with cervical epidural steroid injection. Reg. Anaesth. 1986;11:92–94.

8. Wilson SP, Iacobo RS, Rocco AG, Ferrante FM. Pathophysiology of cervical radiculopathy as a predictor of efficacy of epidural steroid injection. Anesthesiology 1989;79(3):A733.

9. Cicala RS, Thoni K, Angel JJ. Long-term results of cervical epidural steroid injections. Clin J Pain 1989;5:143–145.

10. Catchlove RFH, Braha R. The use of cervical epidural nerve blocks in the management of chronic head and neck pain. Can Anaesth Soc J 1984;31:188–191.

11. Gore D, Sepic S, Gardner GM, Murray MP. Neck pain: a long term follow up of 205 patients. Spine 1987;12(1):1–5.

12. Pawl RP, Anderson W, Shulman M. Effect of epidural steroids in the cervical and lumbar region on surgical intervention for diskogenic spondylosis. In: Fields H, ed. Advances in pain research and therapy. Vol. 9. New York: Raven Press, 1985:791–798.

13. Cheng PA. The anatomical and clinical aspects of epidural anesthesia, Part I. Anesth Analg 1963;42:398–406.

14. Jacobs S, McCormick CC. Some observations of the spread of solution in the cervical epidural space using metrizamide. Anaesth Intensive Care 1979;7:350–352.

15. Mehta M, Maher R. Injection into the extraarachnoid subdural space. Experience in the treatment of intractable cervical pain and in the conduct of extradural (epidural) analgesia. Anaesthesia 1977;32:760–766.

16. Burn JMB, Langdon L. Duration of action of epidural methylprednisolone. Am J Phys Med 1974;53:29–34.

17. Tuel SM, Meythaler JM, Cross LL. Cushing's syndrome from epidural methylprednisolone. Pain 1990;40:81–84.

18. Takasaki M, Takahashi T. Respiratory function during cervical and thoracic extradural analgesia in patients with normal lungs. Br J Anaesth 1980;52:1271–1276.

19. Dirksen R, Rutgers MJ, Coolen JMW. Cervical epidural steroids in reflex sympathetic dystrophy. Anesthesiology 1987;66:71–73.

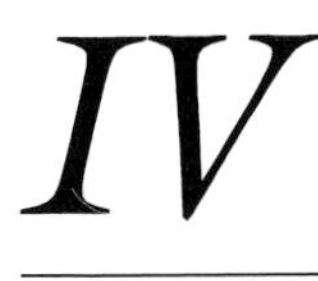

Congenital Developmental and Acquired Diseases

14

TORTICOLLIS—NEWBORN, INFANT, AND CHILD

Stephen W. Burke

Torticollis must be considered a symptom or sign, rather than a pathologic diagnosis. Common usage of the term generally denotes "congenital muscular torticollis," but clearly there exist multiple etiologies, both congenital and acquired, each having a different natural history, prognosis, and method of treatment.

CONGENITAL TORTICOLLIS

Muscular

Congenital muscular torticollis is the most common form of torticollis, occurring in perhaps 4 per 1000 live births.

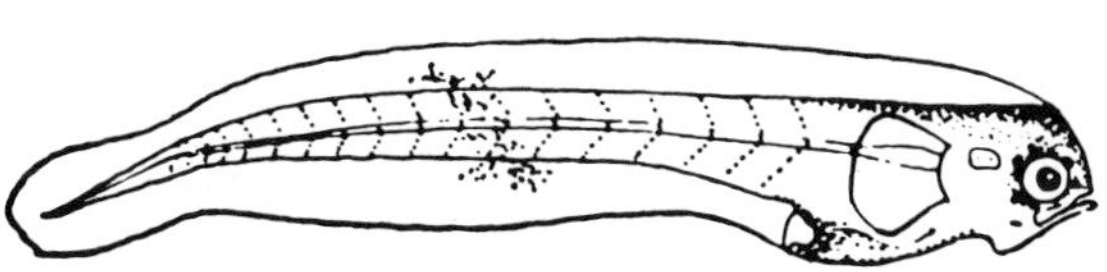

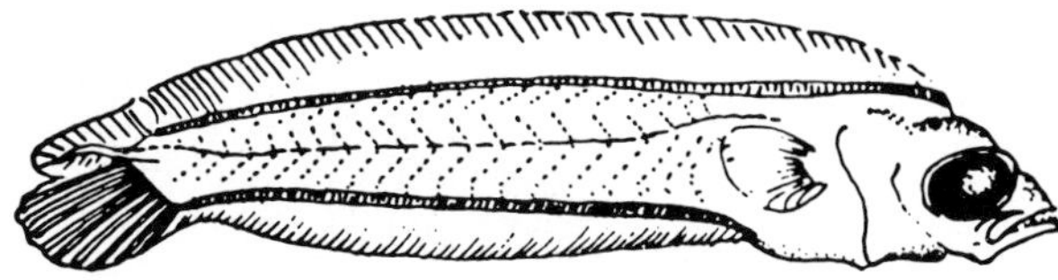

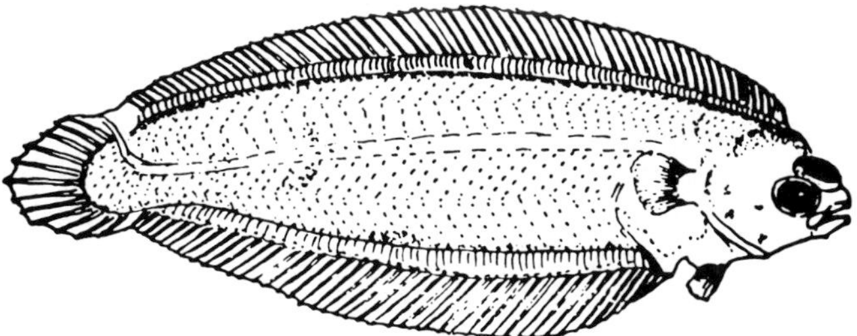

Figure 14.1. Ocular migration seen in *Bothidae* (flukes and flounders). Similar, though less marked, changes can occur in untreated torticollis. (Reproduced from McClane's new standard fishing encyclopedia. New York: Holt, Rinehart and Winston, 1974.)

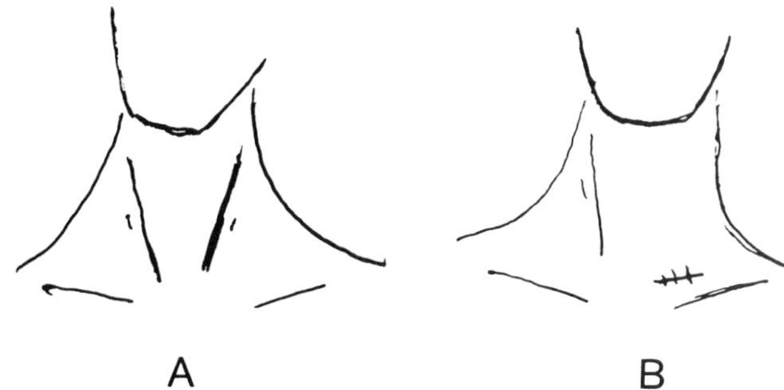

Figure 14.2. The sternocleidomastoid borders form an inverted triangle. With a distal release this is lost.

Male to female and right to left ratios appear approximately equal with some significant variations among the published series (1, 2, 11, 15, 17, 19). Of the various associations, the ones of some importance are those of breech presentation (5- to 8-fold increase) (1, 8), and congenital dysplasia and dislocation of the hip (7–20 percent of patients with torticollis) (9, 17).

Etiology

There is little disagreement that the sternocleidomastoid is the offending muscle, with cicatricial contracture and loss of pliability leading to the clinical picture seen. Some difference of opinion exist, however, as to the cause of the sternocleidomastoid scarring. Theories of etiology include: trauma, infection, ischemia, and neurogenic problems (8, 10, 13).

Birth trauma is an attractive hypothesis, but the lack of hemosiderin deposition in the tissues (which should be seen if there were a traumatic, hemorrhagic event) and the presence of sternocleidomastoid scarring in Cesarean (presumably atraumatic) births tend to discount this as a cause.

Infection may play a role in some rare acquired torticollis cases, but there is no bacterial or clinical evidence to suggest that this is of significance in the congenital form.

The vascular supply of the sternocleidomastoid has been extensively studied with regard to congenital torticollis in both humans and experimental animals. It appears that ischemia of the sternocleidomastoid, most probably sec-

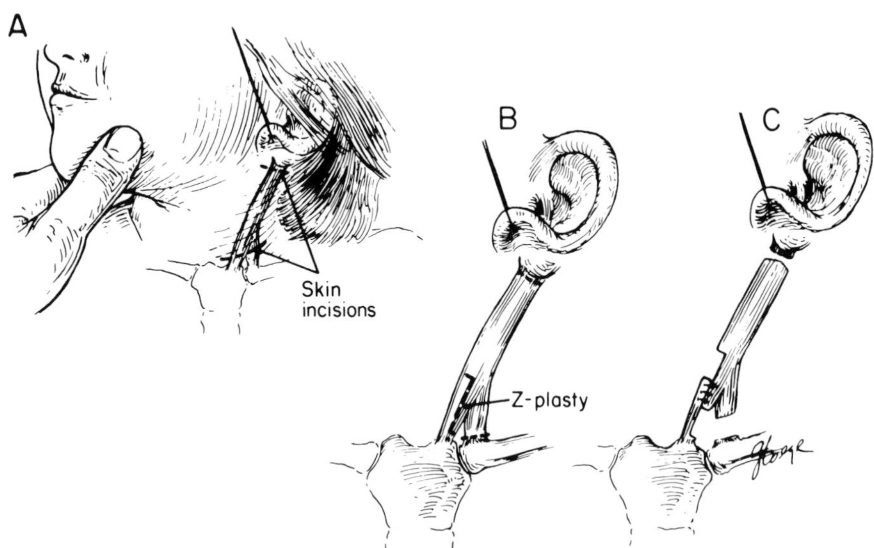

Figure 14.3. Technique of bypolar sternocleidomastoid lengthening. (Reproduced with permission from Ferkel RD, Westin GW, Dawson EG, Oppenheim WL. Muscular torticollis: a modified surgical approach. J Bone Joint Surg 1983;65-A:895.)

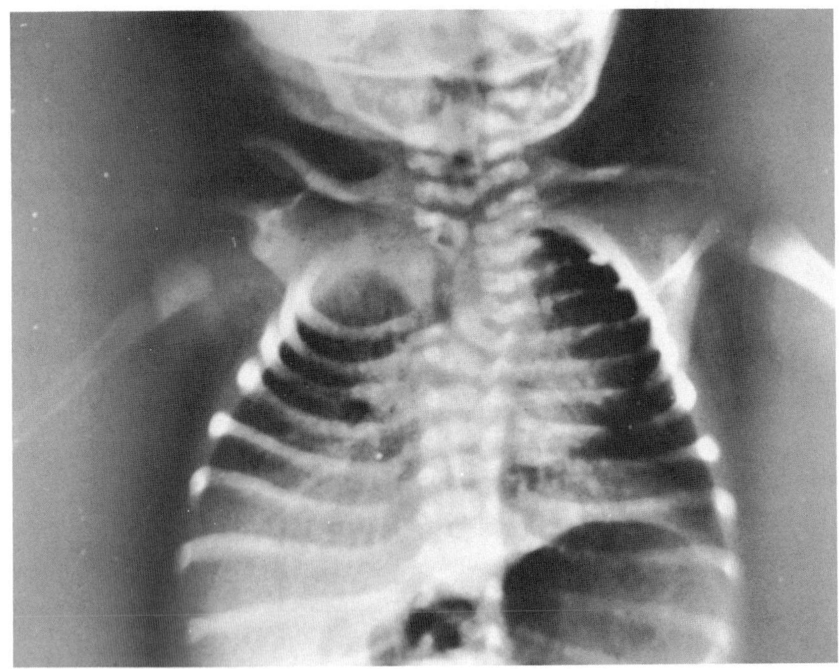

Figure 14.4. Radiograph of a newborn with severe torticollis. Note the congenital vertebral anomalies causing this.

ondary to venous obstruction due to position of the neck, is the cause of congenital muscular torticollis.

Sarnat and Morrissey (24) biopsied the sternocleidomastoid of 9 children with congenital muscular torticollis; their findings suggest the possibility of an entrapment neuropathy of the spinal accessory nerve superimposed upon the fibrosis of the sternocleidomastoid as a cause for perpetuation and worsening of the deformity.

Presentation and Natural History

Physical findings in congenital muscular torticollis depend upon the age at presentation. In the newborn, findings include sternocleidomastoid "tumor," plagiocephaly, and limited cervical spine motion.

The "tumor," actually the fibrotic sternocleidomastoid, is usually located in the mid substance of the sternocleidomastoid. It is present in 15–20 percent of cases, though it can easily be overlooked; the "tumor" generally resolves by early infancy (15).

Plagiocephaly refers to the flattening or asymmetry of one portion of the skull. While most noticeable in the frontal region, with careful inspection, there is generally found to be opposite flattening posteriorly. In the neonatal period, plagiocephaly is due to in utero molding; subse-

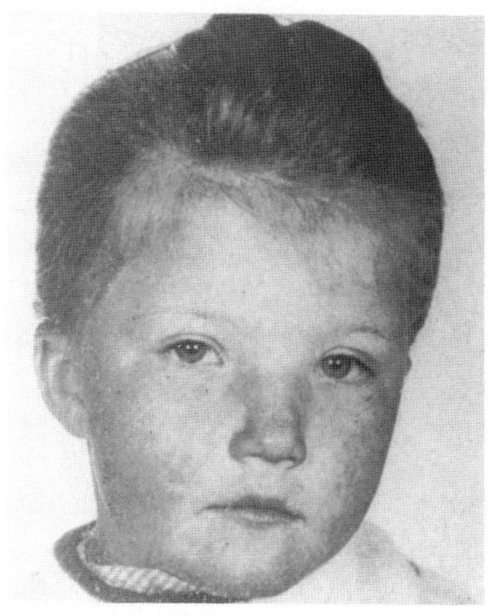

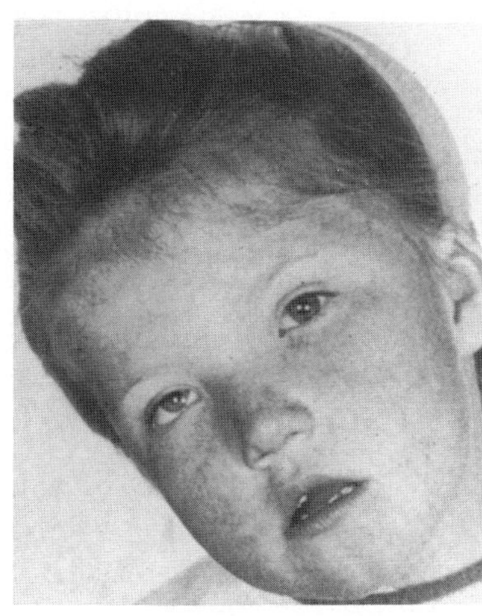

Figure 14.5. Bielschowsky phenomenon. Tilting of the head is done to maintain conjugate gaze. With righting the head, the paretic muscle is unable to adjust the eye, and divergent gaze results. (Reproduced from Duke-Elder S. System of ophthalmology: MO: CV Mosby, 1973:669.)

quently, persistent plagiocephaly may be due to sleeping or lying in one position—prone or supine, with pressure applied to one portion of the skull, due to limited cervical spine motion.

The sternocleidomastoid muscle acts to flex and laterally rotate (to the opposite side) the head, as well as laterally flex the head to the same side. Unilateral contracture thus results in the characteristic "cock-robin" position with the head tilted toward, and the chin rotated away from, the contracture.

With advancing age and cervical spine growth, the deformity slowly worsens. With persistent malposition of the skull, impressive facial asymmetry may develop, analogous to the ocular migration seen in fish of the family, *Bothidae* (Figure 14.1). Occasionally, one may see sufficient facial deformity and ocular asymmetry that a scoliosis develops as a compensating mechanism.

By adulthood, untreated congenital muscular torticollis may result in significant degenerative arthritis of the cervical spine as a result of asymmetric loading of the facet joints.

Treatment

Congenital muscular torticollis has significant functional as well as cosmetic sequelae; therefore, treatment is indicated in virtually all cases.

In the first year of life, conservative treatment in the form of stretching exercises has an excellent probability of resulting in a cure.

The sternocleidomastoid rotates the head and chin away from itself and laterally tilts the head toward itself in order to stretch the sternocleidomastoid; these positions must be reversed. It is the author's feeling that it is easier to perform this as two separate exercises, both done with the infant supine with the head off the edge of the bed or dressing table.

First, the chin is rotated toward the contracture as far as gently possible and held in this position for a count of 10, then released. The ear opposite the contracture is brought as close as possible to its corresponding shoulder and held for a count of 10. These are each repeated a total of 20 times throughout the day.

Infants dislike these exercises intensely. It is difficult for a parent to perform these without constant reinforcement and encouragement. Therefore, frequent physician follow-up visits as well as the enlistment of a therapist to follow the child and parents closely, seem to improve the results.

The exercises are continued until there is a full range of both rotation and lateral flexion, and the infant holds his or her head in the neutral position. Rotation improves most quickly, soon followed by lateral flexion. Active positioning of the head in the neutral position may take some time.

In this age group, it appears that restoration of full range of motion is promptly followed by a relatively rapid improvement of any plagiocephaly present.

After 1 year of age, conservative treatment is generally ineffective, and surgical correction is necessary.

Correction can be accomplished by a number of operative methods including tenotomy (either proximal or distal), Z-lengthening, or excision of all or part of the sternocleidomastoid.

Distal tenotomy is the most widely used surgical technique; its major drawback is that there is loss of the subcutaneous prominence of the sternal head (termed "loss of the sternocleidomastoid column"), which may be a significant cosmetic problem (Fig. 14.2). For this reason the bipolar release as described by Ferkel, et al. (5) has certain distinct advantages and is the author's procedure of choice.

Surgery is performed with a rolled towel under the shoulders. The head should be sufficiently mobile that the anesthetist is able to rotate the head allowing for intraoperative range of motion evaluation. The proximal incision is placed at the tip of the mastoid process, avoiding the spinal accessory nerve which enters the sternocleido-

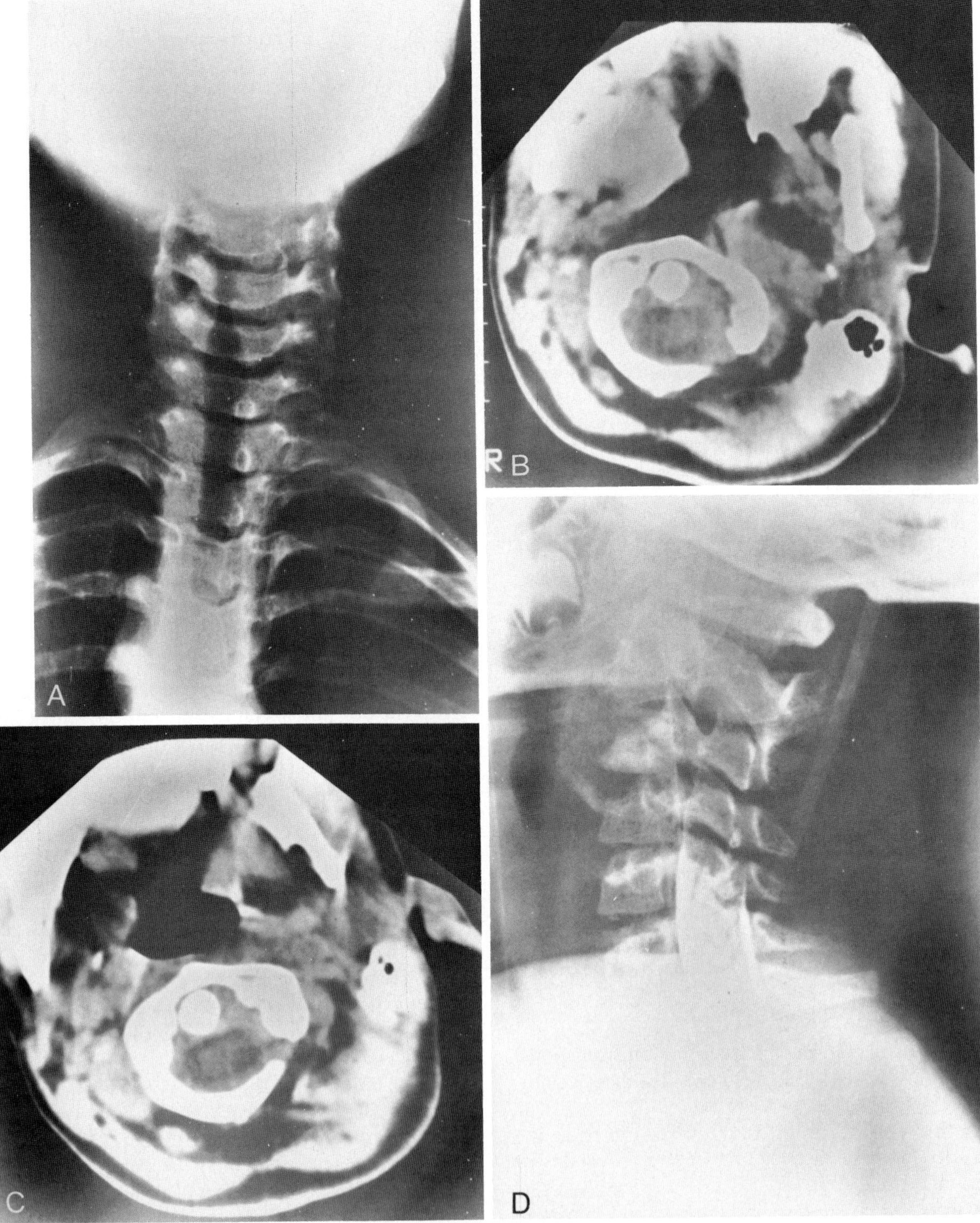

Figure 14.6. **A,** plain radiograph of an 8-year-old female who presented with a 6-month history of a painful torticollis. **B,C,** CT scans with head rotated left and right show some motion between C1 and C2. **D,** myelogram shows a complete block from what proved to be a cervical chordoma. The child subsequently succumbed to her disease.

mastoid in its proximal portion. The distal incision should be placed in the base of the neck rather than over the clavicle to avoid hypertrophic scarring. Identification and isolation of the sternocleidomastoid in both wounds is helped by performing this before tenotomy or lengthening. The proximal portion is tenotomized at its origin on the mastoid process, and the distal portion is Z-lengthened as illustrated (Fig. 14.3).

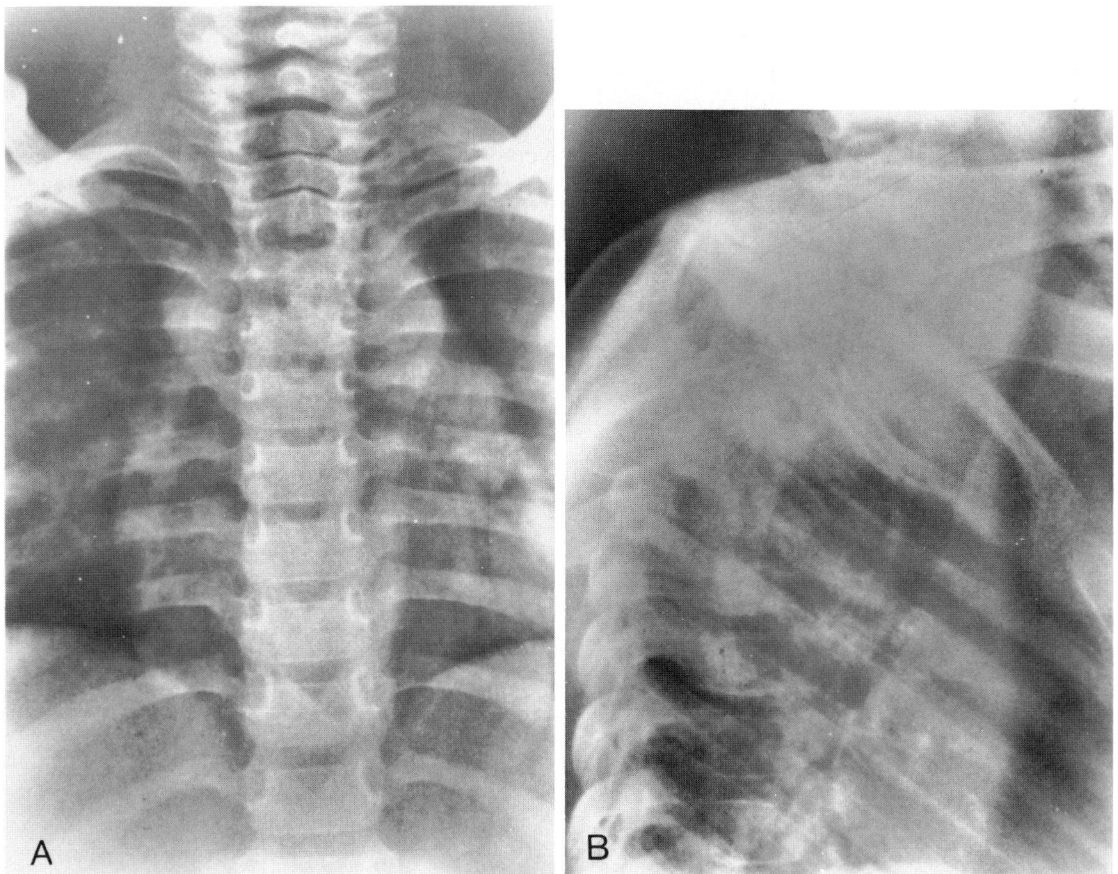

Figure 14.7. A 2-year-old female presented with a painful torticollis. **A,** AP radiograph. Note the large paraspinal mass. **B,** Lateral radiograph. Note destruction of the body of T3. *Mycobacterium Tuberculosis* was grown from the lesion.

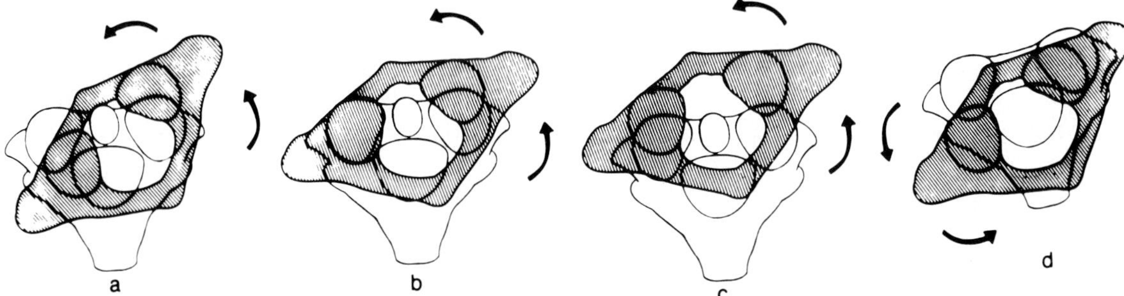

Figure 14.8. Drawings showing the four types of rotatory fixation. **a,** Type I—rotatory fixation with no anterior displacement and the odontoid acting as the pivot; **b,** Type II—rotatory fixation with anterior displacement of 3–5 mm, one lateral articular process acting as the pivot; **c,** Type III—rotatory fixation with anterior displacement of more than 5 mm; and **d,** Type IV—rotatory fixation with posterior displacement. (Reproduced with permission from Fielding JW, Hawkins RJ. Atlanto-axial rotatory fixation (fixed rotatory subluxation of the atlanto-axial joint). J Bone Joint Surg 1977;59-A:705–708.)

Postoperatively, the patient is nursed in halter traction until comfortable, usually 2 to 3 days, then allowed up in a Philadelphia collar. Critical to the success of the procedure is a vigorous, conscientious postoperative range of motion program. This is begun at the time the patient is allowed out of bed. The patient remains in the hospital until a virtually full range of motion is achievable. The exercises are continued at home wearing the collar, otherwise full-time for 8 to 12 weeks.

Surgery is generally well-tolerated, but there is a significant residual cosmetic deformity in up to one-third of patients (1, 5, 11, 12, 16, 19) due to residual facial asymmetry, limited motion, head tilt, or cosmetically unacceptable scarring. Suboptimal results are generally related

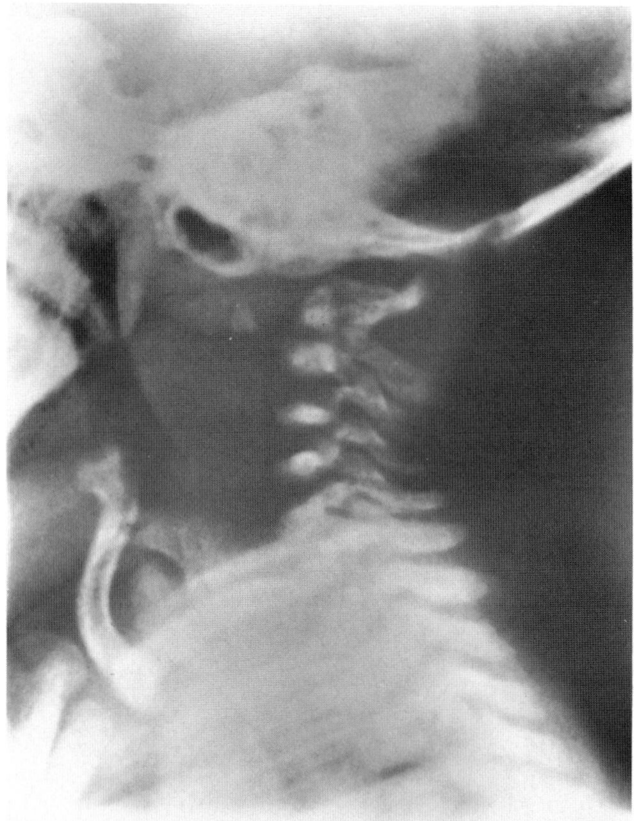

Figure 14.9. Grisel's syndrome. Note the massive retropharyngel swelling coupled with atlanto-axial subluxation.

to the severity of the deformity, the duration of the disease, and the age of the patient at operation.

BONY TORTICOLLIS

Congenital cervical spine deformity may be the cause of an infantile torticollis (4, 20). The presentation may be identical to that of congenital muscular torticollis with a painless head tilt.

Several features serve to distinguish bony from muscular torticollis, however. First, features suggestive of Klippel-Feil (low hairline, webbed neck, cervical synostosis) are present. Secondly, there is frequently a disparity between the lateral flexion deformity (frequently significant) and the rotational deformity (frequently relatively mild), whereas in congenital muscular torticollis these are generally of similar magnitude. Finally, there is relatively frequent coexistence of other major congenital abnormalities, orthopaedic and otherwise. In congenital muscular torticollis, on the other hand, with the exception of congenital dysplasia of the hip (CDH), congenital malformations are no more common than in the general population. While these may or may not be present, the sine qua non remains x-ray demonstration of a bony abnormality. Routine radiographic examination of all torticollis patients is therefore warranted (Fig. 14.4).

Similar to congenital spine deformity in other areas, cervical spine bony abnormalities are associated with abnormalities of other major organ systems: genitourinary tract (15–25%), cardiac system (10%), and central nervous system (10–20%). Careful investigation of these organ systems should follow the diagnosis of congenital cervical spine bony abnormalities.

The natural history of the deformity is variable in terms of its progression. Conservative treatment has very little role. Early spine fusion coupled with preoperative halo traction alignment may be indicated for progressive deformity (4, 20).

Plagiocephaly can be a difficult problem in this form of torticollis. Water pillows and custom molded helmets have been used in other situations with some success but have not been particularly helpful in this context.

OCULAR TORTICOLLIS

Ocular torticollis is perhaps the rarest of the etiologies of congenital wry neck. It is, in fact, the result of an incomitant strabismus—a "dissociation of ocular movements wherein the deviation is irregular varying in an incoordinate manner in different direction of gaze" generally involving the superior oblique muscle associated with overactivity of the ipsolateral inferior oblique muscle (3, 14). It is listed as congenital because its presence can virtually be accepted as evidence that the ocular palsy is of congenital or early infantile origin (14).

The attitude of the head is adopted to avoid diplopia and maintain binocular vision. Typically, the neck deformity is functional, and the head can be passively straightened (at the cost of developing diplopia). This is the basis of the Bielschowsky phenomenon, wherein returning the head to the straight position results in a visible divergence of gaze (Fig. 14.5).

Differentiating ocular from orthopaedic torticollis is generally not difficult if looked for. Ocular torticollis patients have a full range of motion of the cervical spine, little plagiocephaly (with the eyes closed there is no fixed contracture, therefore no molding), and a lack of symmetric ocular movements.

Treatment of ocular torticollis is directed at balancing the extraocular muscles to give balanced conjugate gaze. Successful treatment of this generally results in rapid resolution of the torticollis.

ACQUIRED TORTICOLLIS

Torticollis with its onset after the neonatal period has a number of different etiologies. While transitory torticollis ("crick in the neck") is reasonably common, persistent acquired torticollis lasting more than a few days is uncommon and should prompt a workup to determine its etiology.

The etiologic considerations in acquired torticollis are primarily irritative- or instability-related. Irritative processes can be considered neurologic, orthopaedic, or gastrointestinal.

Neurologic problems leading to torticollis are primarily tumors involving either the posterior fossa or cervical cord. A high index of suspicion and a careful neurologic examination are the keys to diagnosis. MRI in suspected cases is warranted (Fig. 14.6).

Orthopaedic causes include a variety of tumors and infections of the upper ribs or cervical or cervical-thoracic spine (23, 25, 26). Plain x-rays are frequently negative; laboratory studies (CBC, sedimentation rate) and bone scan are helpful in securing the diagnosis. (Fig. 14.7).

Gastrointestinal problems in the form of gastroesophagela reflux may cause acquired torticollis; this has been termed Sandifer syndrome (22). The physiologic basis for this is not understood, but it nevertheless exists. The torticollis may be on either side and may be intermittent. Neck symptoms are generally lacking, but a history of postprandial vomiting or colic may be elicited. The diagnosis of reflux is most easily confirmed by esophageal pH probe studies.

The literature suggests that surgical correction of the reflux (by Nissen fundoplication) is necessary for a cure; the author's personal experience is that medical management in the form of proper positioning after feeding, coupled with the use of antacids and gastric motility enhancers is frequently effective. Control of the reflux should lead to prompt resolution of the torticollis.

Instability

Acquired torticollis in the absence of a defined cause has been termed atlanto-axial rotatory subluxation (6) and can be considered a spectrum of instability (Fig. 14.8). The cause of this instability may be inflammatory or traumatic.

Nasopharyngeal inflammation leading to atlanto-axial instability has been termed Grisel's syndrome (10, 18, 27). The mechanism is felt to be a local hyperemia and edema of the supporting ligaments of the atlanto-axial articulation (Fig. 14.9).

A history of trauma is given by many patients with atlanto-axial rotatory subluxation, but distinct bony injury is rarely seen. Presumably the trauma is sufficient to create a sprain of the atlanto-axial joint that then leads to the fixed malalignment.

Clinically the patient complains of stiffness and, occasionally, pain. The head is held in a tilted, rotated "cock robin" position. Attempts to manipulate the head into a corrected or over-corrected position are unsuccessful. Plain radiographs may suggest a diagnosis by asymmetry of the size of the lateral masses of the atlas and narrowing of the joint on one side as well as eccentricity of the dens and rotation of the spinous process of the atlas (6), but confirmation of the diagnosis is most easily accomplished by sequential CT scans of the atlanto-axial joint in maximum rotation to the right and to the left (7).

Treatment principles have been recommended by Phillips and Hensinger (21). Acute torticollis of less than 1 week duration should be managed by symptomatic treatment (analgesics, muscle relaxants, soft collar) and follow-up.

Acute torticollis lasting over 1 week should be worked up by CT scan. If atlanto-axial rotatory subluxation is diagnosed, the patient should be admitted to the hospital and placed in cervical halter traction until full range of motion is restored. A collar is then worn, generally for about 6 weeks. For patients with symptoms of more than a month's duration, the same treatment protocol is undertaken, but the likelihood of failure or recurrence is quite high.

For refractory or recurrent cases, atlanto-axial fusion is recommended. Due to the tendency of the deformity to recur even with internal fixation with wires, halo immobilization should be considered to maintain head alignment until the fusion is solid.

REFERENCES

1. Canale ST, Griffin DW, Hubbard CN. Congenital muscular torticollis. J Bone Joint Surg 1982;64-A:810–816.

2. Coventry MB, Harris LE. Congenital muscular torticollis in infancy. J Bone Joint Surg 1959;41-A:815–822.

3. Duke-Elder S, Wybar K. Ocular motility and strabismus. Chapter X: Incomitant strabismus. CV Mosby, 1973.

4. Dubousset MD. Torticollis in children caused by congenital anomalies of the atlas. J Bone Joint Surg 1986;68-A:178–188.

5. Ferkel RD, Westin GW, Dawson EG, Oppenheim WL. Muscular torticollis. J Bone Joint Surg 1983;65-A:894–900.

6. Fielding JW, Hawkins RJ. Atlanto-axial rotary fixation. J Bone Joint Surg 1977;59-A:37–44.

7. Fielding JW, Stillwell WT, Chynn KY, Spyropoulos EC. Use of computed tomography for the diagnosis of atlanto-axial rotatory fixation. J Bone Joint Surg 1978;60-A:1102–1104.

8. Hulbert KF. Congenital torticollis. J Bone Joint Surg 1950;32-B:50–59.

9. Hummer CD, MacEwen GD. The coexistence of torticollis and congenital dysplasia of the hip. J Bone Joint Surg 1972;54-A:1255–1256.

10. Hunter, GA. Non-traumatic displacement of the atlanto-axial joint. J Bone Joint Surg 1968;50-B:45–51.

11. Ippolito E, Tudisco C, Massobrio M. Long-term results of open sternocleidomastoid tenotomy for idiopathic muscular torticollis. J Bone Joint Surg 1985;67-A:30–38.

12. Lee EH, Kang YK, Bose K. Surgical correction of muscular torticollis in the older child. J Pediatr Orthop 1986;6:585–589.

13. Lidge RT, Bechtol RC, Lambert CN. Congenital muscular torticollis. J Bone Joint Surg 1957;39-A:1165–1182.

14. Liebman SD, Gellis SS. The pediatrician's ophthalmology. Chapter 9. Neuro-ophthalmology in children. CV Mosby, 1966.

15. Ling DM, Low YS. Sternomastoid tumor and muscular torticollis. Clin Orthop 1972;86:144–150.

16. Ling CM. The influence of age on the results of open sternomastoid tenotomy in muscular torticollis. Clin Orthop 1976;116:142–148.

17. MacConald D. Sternomastoid tumour and muscular torticollis. J Bone Joint Surg 1969;51-B:432–443.

18. Mathern GW, Batzdorf U. Grisel's syndrome. Clin Orthop 1989;244:131–146.

19. Morrison DL, MacEwen GD. Congenital muscular torticollis: observations regarding clinical findings, associated conditions, and results of treatment. J Pediatr Orthop 1982;2:500–505.

20. Nicholson JT, Sherk HH. Anomalies of the occipitocervical articulation. J Bone Joint Surg 1968;50-A:295–304.

21. Phillips WA, Hensinger RN. The management of rotatory atlantoaxial subluxation of children. J Bone Joint Surg 1989;71-A:664–668.

22. Ramenofsky ML, Buyse M, Goldberg MJ, Leape LL. Gastroesophageal reflux and torticollis. J Bone Joint Surg 1978;60-A:1140–1141.

23. Robb JE, Southgate GW. An unusual case of torticollis. J Pediatr Orthop 1986;6:469.

24. Sarnat HB, Morrissey RT. Idiopathic torticollis: sternocleidomastoid myopathy and accessory neuropathy. Muscle Nerve 1981; Sept/Oct:374–379.

25. Sovio OM, Beauchamp, RD, Morton KS, Baldwin VJ. Osteoblastoma in the very young: report of two cases. J Pediatr Orthop 1988;8:342–344.

26. Steinberg GG. Osteomyelitis of the rib presenting as painful torticollis. J Bone Joint Surg 1979;61-A:614–615.

27. Wilson BC, Jarvis Bl, Haydon RC. Nontraumatic subluxation of the atlantoaxial joint: Grisel's syndrome. Ann Otol Rhinol Laryngol 1987;96:705–708.

15

Torticollis in Adults

Robert E. Barrett

Torticollis, as the term describes, is a twisting of the neck. Torticollis, as a disease state, is perhaps the most common manifestation of a group of neurologic disorders that go under the name of torsion dystonia. Dystonia musculorum deformans was the term initially used by Oppenheim (1) in 1911 to describe the multifocal abnormal increase in tone and development of abnormal postures in a family with three affected siblings. This family had previously been described by Schwalbe (2) in 1908, and the descriptive label he had applied was "chronic cramp syndrome with hysterical symptoms." Schwalbe held the belief, because of his psychiatric training, that the symptoms were psychological in origin. Oppenheim, however, was convinced appropriately that the abnormal twistings were of an organic origin.

The term "Torticollis spasmodique" was first used in 1901 by Destorac (3) to describe the twisting neck and pelvic movements in a 17-year-old girl. He emphasized that these movements were aggravated or magnified during activity and were often reduced or disappeared when recumbent or at rest and could be modified by certain positional maneuvers.

Dystonia is a hyperkinetic movement disorder characterized by twisting, involuntary movements which can affect any groups of muscles in the body. Herz (4, 5) originally defined dystonic movements as "slow, long sustained turning movements of the head and trunk and rotations of the upper or lower extremities." Subsequent descriptions of dystonia by Denny-Brown (6) indicated that the body part involved assumed a "fixed or relatively fixed attitude." Even in the earlier descriptions by Oppenheim (1) it was noted that in addition to the twisting and turning postures assumed, there were tremor-like movements, especially seen in the process of attempting to overcome the abnormal postures and the spasmodic contractions of the muscles involved. When dystonia affects the muscles of the neck and shoulders, the clinical picture of spasmodic torticollis is produced. While the most common manifestation is the appearance of abnormal neck posture of axial rotation, there may be included a degree of retrocollis or antecollis, or these abnormal postures may be the only features of the dystonic syndrome without the axial rotation.

The Clinical Picture of Spasmodic Torticollis

As in all classification systems, focal or segmental dystonia involving the head and neck region can be classified according to clinical characteristics, severity, and etiology. The vast majority of torticollis would fit under the classification of primary idiopathic torsion dystonia of focal type. This can occur on an inherited basis; however, it is usually unassociated with a family history. The onset is usually in the 3rd or 4th decade of life; however, it can have its onset in the 2nd decade or as late as the 6th decade of life. The occurrence is equal in both sexes. There can be great variability in the clinical manifestations. The onset usually commences with a sensation of pain in the neck, associated with a feeling of increased tone and an inability to maintain the head in a free posture. Head tremor is an early manifestation produced by an attempt to keep the head straight. With varying rapidity the head may assume a variety of different postures, the most common of which is that of the head turned to one side with the chin pointed upward or downward. There is often an upward movement and forward thrust of the shoulder on the side to which the chin is turned. There is downward and posterior movement of the opposite shoulder. Sometimes the occiput is tilted toward the side opposite which the chin is turned. While in some patients the head deviation produced by cervical dystonia is constant, the large majority demonstrate "spasmodic" contractions of the muscles in the neck, resulting in a jerky movement of the head in the direction produced by the most active muscles. These rhythmic contractions of the muscles in the neck can be misinterpreted as essential tremor of the head; however, it should be pointed out that about 30% of all patients with cervical spasmodic torticollis will manifest essential tremor of the hands, best demonstrated with the hands outstretched or on intention, sustention (7). (There is also a high incidence of essential familial tremor in other family members of individuals with spasmodic torticollis.)

It must not be assumed that the abnormal posture of the neck is due only to dystonic contractions of the muscles which produce the abnormal posture. There is electromyographic evidence to support abnormal tonic input to antagonistic muscle groups involved in neck turning (8).

The distinction between the essential tremor characteristics and the tremor of the dystonic muscle contraction can be made by attempting resistance against forced correction of the abnormal posture. By this maneuver in spasmodic torticollis the tremor increases; however, in essential tremor the tremor becomes reduced or completely relieved (7).

Spontaneous and lasting remissions have been described in individuals suffering from spasmodic torticollis in up to 23% of patients (9). Such remission is most frequently experienced during the first 3 years after the onset of symptoms. It is more likely to occur in individuals with jerky dystonia or dystonia that disappears when recumbent than in those with constant persistent neck deviation. In the majority of individuals with cervical dystonia, the disorder is a lifelong disability. In about 15–20% of individuals there is a progression to segmental or generalized dystonia (7).

One of the striking characteristics of spasmodic torticollis is the use of postural tricks to assist in control of the abnormal head posture. This is usually accomplished by placing the thumb or the knuckles against the chin as if to supply support. Occasionally the trick is to place the palm of the hand over the occiput on the side opposite to the direction of head turning. Another maneuver not infrequently seen is to drape the arm over the vertex of the head. These movements seems to help control not only the dystonic tremor, but also the head posture. Early in the course of disorder, it is common for the abnormal posture of the head to disappear when a patient is in a recumbent position. Sometimes this freedom from dystonic posturing persists throughout life; however, it is more common for the abnormal neck posture to evolve so that the recumbent position no longer gives relief.

In about one-third of patients with spasmodic torticollis, there is disabling pain which has been thought to be due to intense muscle spasms. While ischemic phenomena in the muscles of the neck can be used to explain the pain, it seems more likely that the pain is either due to nerve irritation in the cervical region produced by spasm or to twisting effects on the ligaments which bind the cervical spine in its delicate conformation. In the author's experience, it is not uncommon for pain to extend into the occipital region or into the upper arms. It is, however, uncommon for a radicular syndrome to be part of the clinical picture. Occasional ulnar neuropathic symptoms and clinical signs occur because of excessive use of elbow pressure on tables or chair arms to maintain the head posture. Rarely in the author's experience has an ulnar sensory or motor neuropathy been observed secondary to nerve root compromise at the level of the cervical foramina.

Usually with the passage of time and the administration of medications to relieve some of the painful dystonic spasms, the pain aspect of the disorder subsides. When pure antecollis or retrocollis occurs, there is usually an associated dystonic manifestation of other muscles including the muscles enervated by cranial nerve V. This is usually referred to as "oro-mandibular dystonia" (7). There is occasional retraction of the jaw, and less often it is deviated to one side by forceful contraction. When the dystonic movements of neck flexion are associated with blepharospasm and forceful facial grimacing, the disorder becomes known as Meige syndrome (7). With either neck flexion or hyperextension, there is occasional spasmodic dysphonia, in which instance the speech becomes constricted and difficult to understand. Occasionally the tongue is involved in these dystonic movements.

PATHOLOGY

The pathology underlying spasmodic torticollis is unknown. Neuropathological studies of brains from individuals with torticollis have in general been normal. A recent pathological study by Zweig and Hedreen (11) showed numerous neurofibrillary tangles and mild neuronal loss within the locus ceruleus of a patient with a 15-year history of dystonia musculorum deformans. A patient with a 35-year history of Meige syndrome had moderate to severe neuronal loss in several brainstem nuclei including the substantia nigra, locus ceruleus, raphe nuclei, and pedunculopontine nucleus. A similar examination of a 10-year-old boy with a 6-year history of dystonia musculorum deformans and a 50-year-old woman with a 3-year history of spasmodic torticollis did not disclose similar abnormalities. In general, it is the consensus that the pathologic substrate of spasmodic torticollis or dystonia musculorum deformans is unknown as was pointed out by Zeman and Dyken (12) in a review of the neuropathological material reported by Vogt (the original Oppenheim cases) and a careful study of brains from more recent cases.

PATHOPHYSIOLOGY OF TORSION DYSTONIA

Some studies have implicated the vestibular system, as evidenced by a small group of patients studied by Bronstein and Rudge (1986) (10) in which 70% demonstrated a directional preponderance of vestibular nystagmus opposite to the chin deviation. The authors suggested a "tonic imbalance of muscle activity both in the neck and the extraocular system."

One of the physiological hallmarks of dystonia is the dramatic cocontraction of agonist and antagonist muscles. There is often an overflow of muscle contractions to other muscles, more apparent during attempted voluntary movement of the affected part. In many individuals with focal or segmental dystonia, however, there is no EMG recordable involuntary muscle activity at rest. In generalized dystonia, involuntary muscle contractions persist even at rest. Electromyographic abnormalities have been classified by Rothwell, et al. (13) and include: *a*) continuous 30-second periods of activity terminated by short periods of silence, *b*) repetitive rhythmic spasms of 1 to 2 seconds each, separated by periods of relative EMG silence, and *c*) rapid irregular brief jerks, lasting only 100 ms and resembling myoclonus. Occasionally these jerky movements last up to 500 ms and are not associated with any recordable synchronous electroencephalographic event. Occasionally in dystonic patients the second phase of the H-reflex is abnormal; however, the mechanism underlying this is unknown. None of these physiologic abnormalities are specific for torsion dystonia; however, their findings in dystonic individuals suggests a neurological origin. There is no physiological tool that allows for diagnosis of torticollis as a neurogenic disease; however, most of the evidence would suggest that its origin is in a disturbance of brain function in the basal ganglia structures that, in general, control body movement. This is evidenced by the occurrence of dystonia in known diseases of central nervous system origin such as Parkinson's disease, Wilson's disease, Huntington's disease, progressive supranuclear palsy, Hallervorden-Spatz disease, etc. (7). In addition, centrally active drugs which block or modify dopamine receptors (the phenothiazines) may be associated with idiosyncratic dystonic reactions. There is, however, a body of observation that peripheral trauma can induce dystonic movements (14, 15). This suggests a possible peripheral influence in dystonia. The evidence suggests a latency between the onset of the abnormal involuntary movements and the peripheral injury ranging from 1 day to 36 months. In many individuals in whom trauma has been suggested, there have been noted possible predisposing factors including previous exposure to psychoactive drugs and family history of dystonia or essential tremor. These observations suggest that in certain susceptible individuals peripheral trauma, including head trauma, can induce focal segmental or generalized dystonia.

Animal experiments in which unilateral labyrinthectomy has resulted in permanent head torsion have implicated the vestibular system in torticollis (16). A lesion between the red nucleus and the interstitial nucleus of Cajal has been shown to cause tonic neck torsion in the monkey (17). The nucleus of Cajal receives projection systems from the contralateral vertical canal neurons. Lesions in the nucleus of Cajal have been reported to improve torticollis in humans (18). There is a high incidence of abnormalities in caloric testing in patients with spasmodic torticollis, and ocular counterrolling abnormalities have been investigated in individuals with this disorder as reported by Diamond, et al. (19), pointing to a vestibular dysfunction, probably central. A question remains whether the central vestibular imbalance is primary and causal or secondary to a chronically tipped head or asymmetric afferent impulses from the neck to the vestibular nuclei.

While idiopathic spasmodic torticollis on a sporadic basis is the most common manifestation of abnormal neck postures, there are other diseases which must be considered when abnormal neck posture is encountered. The variety of disease states that may manifest torsion dystonic features involving neck turning is extensive, and analysis of these is excessive for this chapter. Reference should be made to the compendium of Fahn, Marsden, and Calne (20). There are, however, certain of these that are important to note.

Intrinsic structural organic lesions in the posterior fossa such as arachnoid cysts under pressure or arteriovenous malformations may exhibit unusual tilted or rotated head postures. Syringomyelia, most often seen as a component of the Arnold-Chiari malformation, and intrinsic cervical cord tumors (ependymoma and hemangioglastoma) may manifest axial neck rotations. In these disease states, however, the torticollis is only a small part of the clinical picture, and careful neurological evaluation should serve to diagnose these conditions. More importantly, unusual head postures may be experienced with atlanto-axial dislocation or subluxation which may be either traumatic or nontraumatic (Grisel's syndrome) (21). The overriding distinction, however, is that the torticollis produced by these pathological substrates is not associated with the dystonic tremor so characteristic of spasmodic torticollis, and the antecedent history and anamnesis should lead to diagnosis.

Neck trauma must always be considered in evaluating torticollis, since occult traumatic lesions of the cervical spine usually involve the smaller posterior elements of the vertebrae. The chronic neck pain associated with these lesions is intermittent and variable in character and severity. The joints of Lushka laterally, the apophyseal joints posteriorly, and the intervertebral joint in front constitute a closed 5 point dynamic suspension system at each of the levels of the cervical spine from C2 down. Whenever one of these points is stressed, distorted, or malaligned there follows bilateral hypertrophic changes and disc deterioration of the remaining elements. This may result in rotation of the elements, cervical malalignment and subsequent muscle imbalance with slight neck rotation (22). In this situation the pain is the overriding clinical manifestation, and the severe torsion phenomena are not experienced.

The clinical picture of severe torsion spasms of the neck, often associated with facial grimacing resulting from the administration of phenothiazines is important to recognize. This is an idiosyncratic reaction and not a tardive response to prolonged phenothiazine administration. It responds acutely to the intravenous administration of Benadryl or other centrally active anticholinergic medications.

Therapy of Spasmodic Torticollis

One of the clear-cut observations in patients with spasmodic torticollis is that the pain and the severity of torsion are increased with stress, fatigue, and increasing exercise. Sleep and relaxation are always helpful. Behavioral modification therapy has been used extensively in the management of torticollis. Brierly (23) reported on using a Pavlovian approach with EMG and cutaneous shocks. While patients were attached to the training apparatus, they were often able to reduce the severity of the spasms. Sensory biofeedback, coupled with relaxation therapy, has been reported to produce clinical benefit (24). Unfortunately, many patients give up on this approach because of its expense and lack of extended carry-over beyond the training sessions. The lack of sustained success with the biofeedback approach makes it of little practical value, and patients are seldom referred for this approach unless they wish to avoid drug or injection therapy. Psychotherapy is generally of no benefit in treating torticollis except as an ancillary approach to reassure the patient of the organic nature of his disease. Often a psychiatric diagnosis has been applied, resulting in conflictual interactions with other family members.

The use of cervical collars in some occasions may reduce the intensity of cervical muscle spasm; however, in most patients, the introduction of a foreign body around the neck, producing further restriction of neck motion, results in an increase of muscle spasms. This seems paradoxical in view of the fact that sensory tricks such as earlier described, using the knuckles against the chin or the palm of the hand against the occipital region, can help in controlling the abnormal posture.

PHARMACOTHERAPY

The history of pharmacotherapy for spasmodic torticollis is filled with anecdotal reports of many different pharmacologic agents possessed of central effects producing variable clinical responses. These agents range from anticonvulsants including phenytoin and carbamazepine, barbiturates, muscle relaxants such as baclofen, dopamine agonist and antagonist, and drugs capable of reducing monoamine storage in brain such as reserpine and tetrabenazine (25). The most consistently effective drugs, however, have had central nervous system anticholinergic activity. Only during the past 15 years have well-controlled studies been performed using the anticholinergic medications. Early studies using low dosages of anticholinergics reported benefit, but not until the controlled double blind investigations of Burke, Fahn, and Marsden in 1986 (26) did it become clear that high dosage anticholinergic medication was singularly the most effective in the management of spasmodic torticollis. In general, these studies showed that approximately 50% of children with dystonia and 40% of adults with a variety of idiopathic dystonic manifestations obtained significant benefit from this class of drugs.

Adverse effects from anticholinergic drugs constitute the dose-limiting problem. The peripheral adverse effects, such as blurred vision and dry mouth, are fairly common but can frequently be accommodated if the clinical improvement is significant. Urinary retention can occasionally be a significant limiting factor. The central adverse effects include behavioral changes, lethargy, forgetfulness, confusion, memory impairment, and hallucinations. These side effects occur more commonly in adults than in children; however, they may be dose related, and their appearance does not necessarily dictate total cessation of the drug. Children and adults have been treated with doses of trihexyphenidyl up to 50 mg per day for periods of over 10 years without adverse effect. Of equal importance to the dosage level is continuation of a dose that is tolerated for a sufficient period of time, since the effect on the torticollis may not be manifest until the drug has been administered for periods of 2 months or longer. Greene, et al. (27) also showed that there was a statistically significant likelihood for improvement if medication was begun within 5 years of onset of the dystonia.

The mechanism by which anticholinergics are effective in modifying the symptoms of spasmodic torticollis is unknown. Also the mechanism involved in the relief of acute dystonic reactions due to phenothiazine drugs is also not understood. There is a striatal balance between cholinergic and dopaminergic mechanisms which when tilted acutely seems to result in peculiar dystonic symptoms.

Soon after the demonstration of high dose levodopa therapy for the amelioration of Parkinson's disease symptoms, this drug was tried on patients with dystonia. The initial responses were quite variable and inconsistent between investigators. Patients with diurnal fluctuations of dystonia were shown to obtain a dramatic response to low dosage levodopa or dopamine agonist therapy (28). There are some children with dystonia without diurnal fluctuations in whom low dosage levodopa therapy produces a significant improvement (29). There is no good indication that levodopa or dopamine agonists have any significant effect on spasmodic torticollis except in a rather small number of individuals. Lang (in 1987) (30) reviewed the literature on dopamine antagonist therapy in idiopathic dystonia. The frequency of response of these drugs varied widely, and for spasmodic torticollis the response rate was from 9–46%. The most commonly used drugs of this class have been the phenothiazines, haloperidol, pimozide, and tetrabenazine. The former three are dopamine receptor antagonists, and the last is a short-acting depleter of presynaptic monoamine stores. Occasionally a dopamine receptor blocker, an anticholinergic agent, and a dopamine depleter can be used together with greater clinical effect than any single drug (31).

Other drugs including benzodiazepines, carbamazepine, clonidine, lithium, baclofen, flexeril, robaxin, etc. have been used with marginal effectiveness.

Localized injections of *botulinus* toxin: the injection of *botulinus* toxin into eye muscles to correct strabismus was started in 1981 (32) and used for the treatment of blepharospasm in 1983 (33). *Botulinus* toxin acts presynaptically at nerve terminals in muscle to prevent calcium dependent release of acetylcholine. Injections of *botulinus* toxin locally produce the effect of chemical denervation. Three studies have been conducted so far reporting on the effectiveness of *botulinus* toxin in the treatment of spasmodic torticollis (34, 35, 36). All of these studies have demonstrated the frequent but variably sustained relief of muscle pain following injection of the toxin directly into the painful sites in torticollis patients. Injections are made at multiple sites using varying doses at many different points in the involved muscles. Up to 275 units of Botox are used over three injection periods. The average injection at any one period was approximately 80 units of Botox. In general, modification of the motor symptoms occurs in 3 to 4 days, reaching a peak at 7 days and having a duration of approximately 12 weeks. In the study conducted by Brin, et al. (35) many patients requested retreatment before the allotted time period because of the return of pain. It is apparent that this form of muscle paralysis therapy is an important adjunct to the treatment of spasmodic torticollis.

SURGICAL THERAPY

Brain Lesioning

A review of the history of brain surgical approaches for the relief of movement disorders is too extensive to be more than synopsized. Perhaps the most significant discovery was made by Cooper (37) in 1953 when, while performing a surgical leukotomy for treatment of Parkinson's disease, the anterior choroidal artery was cut, forcing ligation of this vessel. The patient sustained a dramatic relief of tremor and rigidity on the contralateral side. Further use of this anterior choroidal artery ligation approach carried a high mortality and pushed investigations toward the introduction of stereotaxic surgery with the injection of alcohol, followed by the use of freezing probes and subsequently controlled radio frequency lesioning, involving destruction of the ventral lateral nucleus of the thalamus. When applied to the group of dystonias, the general observations were that thalamotomy tended to be more successful for dystonia of the limbs, as compared to dystonia of the axial musculature. Patients with spasmodic torticollis required bilateral thalamotomies. Cooper (38) reported the surgical results of some 160 patients with this condition, 60% of whom were reported as improved, although 20% developed the most troublesome effect of bilateral thalamotomy, dysphonia. Others have reported a frequency of 56% of patients experiencing permanent dysphonia after bilateral thalamotomy (39). Bertrand (40), who has considerable experience in performing thalamotomies for patients with spasmodic torticollis, has indicated that peripheral denervation of the involved neck muscles is the preferred surgical approach.

Peripheral Surgery

The segmental innervation of the sternomastoid and trapezius muscles differ. The sternocleidomastoid is innervated primarily from the C1–C2 level of the cord, and the trapezius is innervated primarily from C2–C3–C4 segments (41). The corticospinal input to the two muscle groups may also differ. Marcus (42) has observed that trapezius function is lost in hemiplegic children while sternocleidomastoid function is retained.

The goal of surgery for spasmodic torticollis should be interruption of abnormal output of the motor system into those muscles producing the abnormal torsion posture. It is apparent from electrical studies that the abnormal motor output is not a unilateral phenomenon, nor are the muscles involved only the sternocleidomastoid, splenius capitis, and trapezius muscles. The standard rhizotomy procedure has been to section the anterior roots of C1–C3 bilaterally, including a contribution to C1 from the spinal accessory nerve. Several reports on this general procedure, modified after McKenzie (43) and Dandy (44), have indicated benefit in nearly 80% of patients. The results of such operations are frequently far from satisfactory, leading to major weakness in neck muscles and instability of the head, along with swallowing difficulty and subluxation of the cervical spine (45, 46). Studies by Freckmann, et al. (47) have shown a high variety of anatomic relationships in the cranial cervical region. They presented a series of 33 patients who underwent bilateral microsurgical lysis of the spinal accessory nerve roots and anastomoses between these nerve roots and the dorsal roots of the first and second cervical nerves. The clinical results were reported as markedly in five, good in 10, improved in 12, and unchanged or worse in five. As a result of their studies, they concluded that spasmodic torticollis is based on a pathology in the afferent component of head control, and not in the efferent part. Bertrand and Molina-Negro (48) have promoted surgical selective extraspinal peripheral denervation for the treatment of torticollis. They have also strongly opposed bilateral denervation, indicating that they believe the bilateral contractions of neck muscles seen on electromyography are due to compensatory contractions of antagonist muscles. These authors have evolved a mediolateral approach for exposure of the C1 and C2 rami and the posterior primary divisions of C3-C4-C5-C6 with selective denervation under light anesthesia. In their reported results, in 131 patients treated exclusively by selective denervation over a 10-year period, all or almost all the abnormal movements of spasmodic torticollis were suppressed in 115 (88%), while preserving posture and mobility (49). If these results are correct and can be duplicated by others, then this would be the preferred surgical approach, failing adequate response to pharmacotherapy.

CONCLUSIONS

Spasmodic torticollis is a focal dystonic movement disorder characterized by forceful muscle spasms, resulting in torsion neck postures. The clinical appearance of abnormal neck postures should be thoroughly investigated with a careful history, the performance of appropriate cervical spine x-rays and/or computerized scans, and the performance of a careful neurological examination to exclude the possibility of other diseases presenting with abnormal neck postures. Therapy should be dictated by the findings on these examinations.

Electromyographic studies and vestibular function studies should be performed where indicated. The appropriate therapy in idiopathic spasmodic torticollis in adults should start with pharmacotherapy, along with supportive psychotherapy. Surgical intervention should be through selective denervation only when pharmacotherapy fails.

REFERENCES

1. Oppenheim H. Uber eine eigenartige Krampfkrankheit des kinlichen und jugendlichen alters (dysphasia lordotica progressiva, dystonia musculorum deformans). Neurol Centrabl 1911;30:1090–1107.

2. Schwalbe W. Eine eigentumliche touische Krampfform mit hysterischen Symptomen. Berlin:Schade, 1908.

3. Destarae. Torticolis spasmodique et spasmes fonctionnels. Rev Neurol 1901;9:591–597.

4. Herz E. Dystonia. I. Historical review analysis of dystonic symptoms and physiologic mechanisms involved. Arch Neurol Psychiatry 1944a;51:305–318.

5. Herz E. Dystonia II. Clinical classification. Arch Neurol Psychiatry 1944b;51:319–355.

6. Denny-Brown D. The basal ganglia and their relation to disorders of movement. London: Oxford University Press, 1962:78.

7. Jankovic J, Fahn S. Dystonic syndromes. Parkinson's disease and movement disorders. Jankovic J, Tolosa E, Eds. Baltimore-Munich: Urban & Schwarzenberg, 1988:283–314.

8. Rothwell JC, Obeso JA. The anatomical and physiological basis of torsion dystonia. In: Marsden CD, Fahn S, eds. Movement disorders 2. London: Butterworths, 1987:313–331.

9. Friedman A, Fahn S. Spontaneous remissions in spasmodic torticollis. Neurology 1986;36:398–400.

10. Bronstein AM, Rudge P. Vestibular involvement in spasmodic torticollis. J Neurol. Neurosurg Psychiatry 1986;49:290–295.

11. Zweig RM, Hedreen JC. Pathology in brainstem regions of individuals with primary dystonia. Neurology 1988;38:701–706.

12. Zeman W, Dyken P. Dystonia musculorum deformans: clinical, genetic and pathoanatomic studies. Psychiatr Neurol Neurochir 1967;10:77–121.

13. Rothwell JC, Obeso JA, Day BL, Marsden CD. Pathophysiology of dystonias. In: Desmedt JE, ed. Motor control mechanisms in health and disease. New York: Raven Press, 1983:851–863.

14. Scherokovan B, Hussain F, Guetter A, et al. Peripheral dystonia. Arch Neurol 1986;43:830–832.

15. Schott GD. Induction of involuntary movements by peripheral trauma: an analogy with causalgia. Lancet 1986;2:712–716.

16. Patterson RM, Little SC. Spasmodic torticollis. J Nerv Ment Dis 1943;98:571–599.

17. Denny–Brown D. The midbrain and motor integration. Proc R Soc Med 1962;55:527–538.

18. Sano K, Sekino H, Tsukamoto Y, et al. Stimulation and destruction of the region of the interstitial nucleus in cases of torticollis and seesaw nystagmus. Confinia Neurol 1972;34:331–338.

19. Diamond SG, Markham CH, Balok RW. Ocular counterrolling abnormalities in spasmodic torticollis. Arch Neurol 1988;45:164–169.

20. Fahn S, Marsden CD, Calne DB. Classification and investigation of dystonia. In: Marsden CD, Fahn S, eds. Movement disorders 2. London: Butterworths, 1987:332–358.

21. Wilson B, Jarvis B, Haydon III R. Nontraumatic subluxation of the atlanto axial joint: Grisel's syndrome. Ann Otol Rhinol Laryngol 1987;96:705–708.

22. Abel MS. The radiology of chronic neck pain: sequelae of occult traumatic lesions. Crit Rev Diagn Imaging 1988;20:27–78.

23. Brierly H. The treatment of hysterical spasmodic torticollis by behaviour therapy. Behav Res Ther 1967;5:139.

24. Korein J, Bruduy J, Grynbaum B, et al. Sensory feedback therapy of spasmodic torticollis and dystonia: results in treatment of 55 patients. Adv Neurol 1976;14:375–402.

25. Fahn S, Marsden CD, In: Marsden CD, Fash S, eds. Movement disorders 2. London: Butterworths, 1987:359–382.

26. Burke RE, Fahn S, Marsden CD. Torsion dystonia: a double-blind, prospective trial of high-dosage trihexyphenidyl. Neurology 1986;36:160–164.

27. Greene P, Shale H, Fahn S. Analysis of open-label trials in torsion dystonia using high dosage of anticholinergies and other drugs. Mov Disord 1988;3:46–60.

28. Rondot PL, Ziegler M. Dystonia—L-Dopa responsive or juvenile Parkinsonism? J Neurol Trans 1983;19:273–281.

29. Nygaard TG, Duovisin RC, Marsden CD. Dopamine responsive dystonia. In: Fahn S, Marsden CD, Calne DB, eds. Dystonia: advances in neurology. New York: Raven Press, 1988:377–384.

30. Lang AE. Dopaminic agonists and antagonists in the treatment of idiopathic dystonia. In: Fahn S, Marsden CD, Calne DB, eds. Dystonia: advances in neurology. New York: Raven Press, 1988: 561–570.

31. Marsden CD, Marion MH, Quinn N. The treatment of severe dystonia in children and adults. J Neurol Neurosurg Psychiatry 1984;47:1166–1173.

32. Scott AB. Botulinum toxin injection of eye muscles to correct strabismus. Trans Am Ophthalmol Soc 1981;79:734–770.

33. Scott AB, Kennedy RA, Stubbs MA. Botulinum toxin injection as a treatment for blepharospasm. Arch Ophthalmol 1985;103:347–350.

34. Tsui JK, Eisen A, Mak E, Carruthers J, Scott AB, Calne DB. A pilot study on the use of *botulinum* toxin in spasmodic torticollis. Can J Neurol Sci 1985;12:314–316.

35. Brin MF, Fahn S, Mookowitz C, et al. Localized injections of *Botulinum* toxin for the treatment of focal dystonia and hemifacial spasm. Mov Disord 1987;2:237–254.

36. Jankovic J, Orman J. *Botulinum A* toxin for cranial-cervical dystonia: a double-blind, placebo-controlled study. Neurology 1987;37:616–623.

37. Cooper IS. Ligation of the anterior choroidal artery for involuntary movements of parkinsonism. Psychiatr Q 1953;27:317–319.

38. Cooper IS. Neurosurgical treatment of the dyskinesias. Clin Neurosurg 1977;24:367–390.

39. Andrew J, Fowler CJ, Harrison MJG. Stereataxic thalamatomy in 55 cases of dystonia. Brain 1983;106:981–1000.

40. Bertrand CM. Peripheral versus central surgical approach for the treatment of spasmodic torticollis. In: Marsden CD, Fahn S, eds. Movement disorders. London: Butterworths, 1982:315–318.

41. Jenny A, Smith J, Decker J. Motor organization of the spinal accessory nerve in the monkey. Brain Res 1988;111:352–356.

42. Marcus JC. The spinal accessory nerve in hemiplegia. Ann Neurol 1985;18:388.

43. McKenzie KG. Intrameningeal division of the spinal accessory and roots of the upper cervical nerves for the treatment of spasmodic torticollis. Surg Gynecol Obstet 1924;39:5–10.

44. Dandy WE. Operation for treatment of spasmodic torticollis. Arch Surg 1930;20:10–32.

45. Arseni C, Maretsis M. The surgical treatment of spasmodic torticollis. Neurochirurgia 1971;14:177–180.

46. Maccabe JJ. Surgical treatment of spasmodic torticollis. In Marsden CD, Fahn S, eds. Movement disorders. London: Butterworths, 1982:308–314.

47. Freckmann N, Hagenah R, Herrmann HD, Muller D. Bilateral microsurgical lysis of the spinal accessory nerve roots for treatment of spasmodic torticollis. Aeta Neurochirongica (Wein) 1986;83:47–53.

48. Bertrand CM, Molina-Negro P. Selective peripheral denervation in 111 cases of spasmodic torticollis: rationale and results. Adv Neurol 1988;50:637–643.

49. Bertrand CM, Molina-Negro P, Bouvier G, Goorczyca W. Observations and analysis of results in 131 cases of spasmodic torticollis after selective denervation. Appl Neurophysiol 1987;50:319–323.

16

Thoracic Outlet Syndrome

William R. Francis

The thoracic outlet syndrome is a poorly understood clinical condition which is often misdiagnosed and, consequently, ill-treated. Clinical interest and approaches to treatment have varied widely for the last 100 or more years.

It is by definition a constellation of symptoms involving the base of the neck and the upper extremities. These symptoms occur on the basis of neuro, venous, or arterial compression, with nerve compression far exceeding cases of vascular involvement almost eight to one. By consensus of opinion, it is caused by compression of the lower cervical-upper thoracic nerve roots, the subclavian artery, and the subclavian vein. This compression occurs between the clavicle and the first thoracic rib or between the clavicle and the scalenus complex as the arm is abducted and externally rotated (59, 95).

History

Historically, because of the lack of understanding of the etiology of this syndrome, various names have been attached or associated with the clinical entity we know as thoracic outlet compression syndrome. These include "scalenus anticus syndrome" (24), "costoclavicular syndrome" (10), "cervical rib syndrome," and "hyperabduction syndrome," as well as lesser known names for this syndrome as seen in Table 16.1. Peet in 1956 first noticed the similarity of presenting symptoms and referred to this entity collectively as thoracic outlet syndrome (63). It was Rob Standeven in 1958 who referred to this syndrome as thoracic outlet compression syndrome (68).

Table 16.1. Thoracic Outlet Syndrome: Various Synonyms

Shoulder-hand syndrome	First thoracic rib syndrome
Fractured clavicle syndrome	Humeral head syndrome
Pneumatic hammer syndrome	Rucksack paralysis
Effort vein thrombosis	Brachiocephalic syndrome
Pectoralis minor syndrome	Cervicothoracic outlet syndrome
Subcoracoid syndrome	Nocturnal paresthetic brachialgia
	Cervicobrachial neurovascular compression syndrome
	Syndrome of the scalenus medius band

Cervical thoracic abnormalities have been recognized for several hundred years. Cervical ribs were first known and described by early anatomists, including Gaylon and Versailles who described the presence of cervical ribs on morbid specimens (33). The French anatomist Hunauld in 1740 noted this anomaly in several of his specimens (33). Clinically, the first reports of pain, paresthesias, and weakness associated with cervical ribs were reported by Willshire (94) in 1860 and later by Gruber in 1869 (27). Coote in 1861 was the first to attempt the removal of the first rib for treatment of this condition (13). The syndrome received very little attention until 1905, when Murphy implicated compression of the subclavian artery between the scalenus anticus muscle and the cervical rib and successfully resected a cervical rib that had produced an aneurysm of the subclavian artery (54, 55). Following Murphy's interest, Keen wrote in 1907 an extensive review on the relationship of neurovascular compression to cervical ribs (37). Subsequent to this, Murphy again in 1910 removed a first thoracic rib for treatment of symptoms of thoracic outlet syndrome and was probably the first to perform this operation in the absence of a cervical rib (56).

The findings prompted Halsted in 1916 to begin his investigation of cervical ribs, noting that 35% of his patients presented with vascular symptoms (29). Halsted and others in the early 1900s significantly influenced the concept of the etiology of vascular compression in thoracic outlet syndrome, but soon contrary opinions were expressed (9, 59, 85). Stopford and Telford reported a compression of the brachial plexus as well as the subclavian artery by the first thoracic rib (85). A year later, Law was the first to recommend division of the banding elements for which he termed "advanticious ligaments," and the scalenus anticus muscle for relief of the symptoms (44). In 1927 Adson and Coffey wrote their famous article suggesting that the scalenus anticus muscle to be of paramount importance in this syndrome and therefore recommended scalenus anticus division as its sole treatment (4). This article was the first in which Adson described the maneuver to detect arterial compression in thoracic outlet syndrome (2–4).

In 1935 Ochsner, Gage, and DeBakey wrote an extensive article on arterial involvement by the scalenus anticus muscle and supported if not advocated that scalenotomy was sufficient as the only treatment for this syndrome (24, 62). The term scalenus anticus syndrome prevailed until 1958. Even though Stopford and Telford supported the importance of the first thoracic rib in this syndrome rather than either the cervical ribs or scalenus muscle, it was not well accepted until several years later (88) with the introduction of the term costoclavicular compression syndrome (10, 22, 84). Wright in 1945 described "hyperabduction syndrome," emphasizing the symptomatology of the syndrome while the arm was hyperabducted in either a stationary position or in the course of work-related activities (5, 35, 45, 87, 96).

Gradually, attention was shifted away from the importance of the scalenus anticus muscle in the mid 1950s (53) Lord in 1953 wrote on clavisectomy and division of the scalenus anticus muscle (48). In 1956, Lord and Stone reported good results with division of the pectoralis minor tendon (49). In the mid 1950s articles showing less than acceptable results with scalenus anticus division began to appear. Raaf, in 1955, expressed disfavor with anterior scalenotomy procedures, reporting less than 50% good results (64). Clagett, in his presidential address to the American Association of Thoracic Surgeons, reported a 60% failure rate versus the apparent good results of first rib resections (12). Shenkin and Somach in 1963 reported a success rate of less than 70% for simple scalenotomies (24, 66, 67, 80).

In contrast to these adverse reports in 1962, Falconer and Li reported good results in 11 patients following first rib resection (13, 21). Anecdotally, in 1945 LeVay had reported first rib resections with good results; however, his reports were far over-shadowed by the recommendation of Adson and Coffey in their report for simple scalenotomies (49, 65).

Primary venous obstruction with multiple intraluminal thrombi was elucidated by Nelson, Hess, and Lyman in 1963, and the term Paget-Schroetter syndrome was adopted (60). Drapanas and Curran later supported this work by pointing out the relationship of venous occlusion of the brachial and innominate veins at the region of the first thoracic rib, thereby supporting their evidence as contributing to compression in thoracic outlet syndrome (17).

The usefulness of arteriography in the diagnosis of arterial compression was revealed by Lang and Associates, Rosenberg, and Nelson and Jenson (40–43, 61, 76). Now the roles of arteriography and phlebography are being replaced almost entirely by noninvasive doppler techniques.

Roos in 1966 first called attention to the importance of

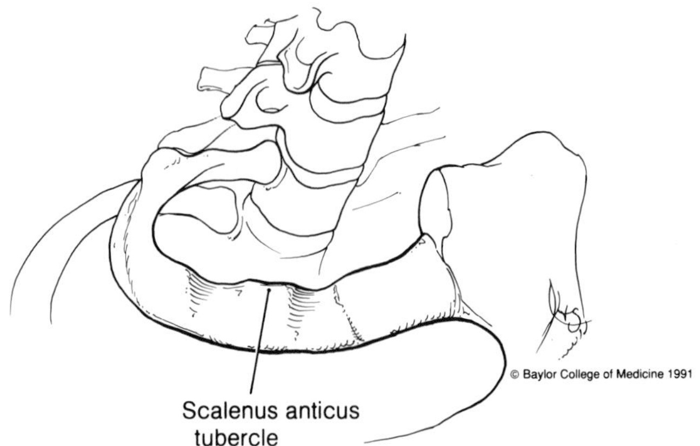

Figure 16.1. Right anterior oblique projection of the first thoracic rib reveals the location for the point of attachment of the scalenus anticus muscle and the groove for the neurovascular structures.

neurocompression as the primary etiology of the presenting symptoms in thoracic outlet syndrome (73). First rib resection for the treatment of thoracic outlet syndrome now became accepted, especially after Roos reported a 93% success rate with transaxillary approaches to first rib resection (73). Nelson and Jenson reported an anterior rib resection with division of the musculature around the first rib through a small anterior incision. This approach later proved to be inadequate for patients with cervical ribs for congenital abnormalities of the first rib and for retained or recurrent portions of the first rib following previous transaxillary surgery (61). Posterior rib resections were also performed but fell into disfavor owing to the potential for nerve injury and the difficult exposure with inadequate visualization of the thoracic outlet (12, 73). This was reported as early as 1961 by Rosati and Lord (235). The transaxillary approach for rib resection has received the most favorable results reported by Roos in several articles (70, 72–74) and McBurney and Howard (52). Both groups reported favorable results in excess of 90% of their cases. In 1968 Urschel and Associates compared first rib resection with scalenus anticus division and found an 80% to 23% favorable outcome ratio for first rib resections. Urschel also found that 150 patients undergoing simple scalenotomies or pectoralis major or minor incision and cervical rib resection only of 60% had recurrent symptoms and 40% required reoperation (91).

ANATOMY

An understanding of the anatomy of the region is essential in diagnosis and treatment of thoracic outlet compression syndrome. The first thoracic rib is C-shaped and flattens superiorly. On its middle, anterior portion are two transverse grooves separated by the scalenus anticus tubercle (Fig. 16.1). The scalenus anticus muscle attaches to the tubercle. Anterior to this is a subclavian vein, and posterior lies the subclavian artery and the lower trunks of the brachial plexus. Posterior to this structure is the scalenus medius muscle (7) (Fig. 16.2). At the point where the subclavian artery and brachial plexus cross the first thoracic rib, the clavicle immediately overrides the structures and produces a significant compressing effect when the arm is abducted and externally rotated (Fig. 16.3). Congenital rib malformations can also contribute to thoracic outlet compression, and a commonly seen variant of the first thoracic rib is when the normal C-shape of the rib is replaced by a foreshortened more appropriately labeled J-shaped rib with a fibrous band that attaches from the rib to the sternum as seen in Fig. 16.4.

Within the thoracic outlet itself lies the cupula of the lung shown in fig. 16.5 with the medial fibers of the scalenus anticus attached to the apical pleural fibers of this cupula (38).

Nerves that subtend the region of the thoracic outlet consist of the lower cervical root portions of the brachial plexus. The brachial plexus is formed by the anterior rami of the five spinal nerves including C5, C6, C7, C8, and T1 (Fig. 16.6). Anatomically, these rami combined to form the trunks which subsequently divide and reunite in combination to form posterior lateral and medial cords. The rami from C8 and T1 unite to form the lower trunk, which traverses the first rib behind the subclavian artery (Fig. 16.7), the course of this trunk takes a more circuitous route delving into the thoracic outlet and then up over the first rib to exist just posterior and inferior to the innominate artery consequently, the lower cervical and upper root

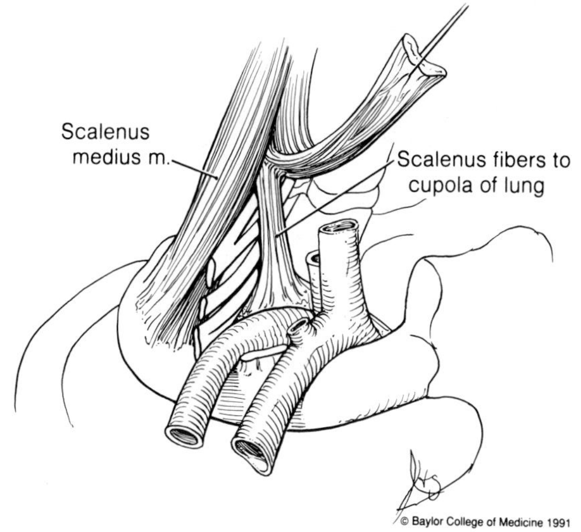

Figure 16.2. The neurovascular bundle is divided by the scalenus anticus muscle between the artery and vein. The scalenus medius muscle lies posterior to the neurovascular bundle.

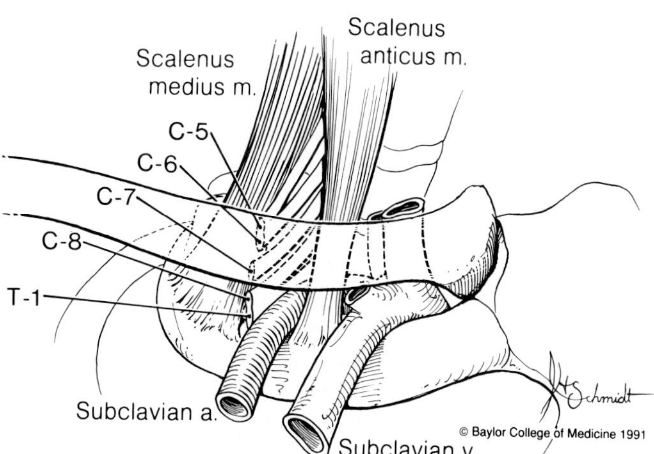

Figure 16.3. The neurovascular bundle and the clavicle cross the first thoracic rib approximately at the same point.

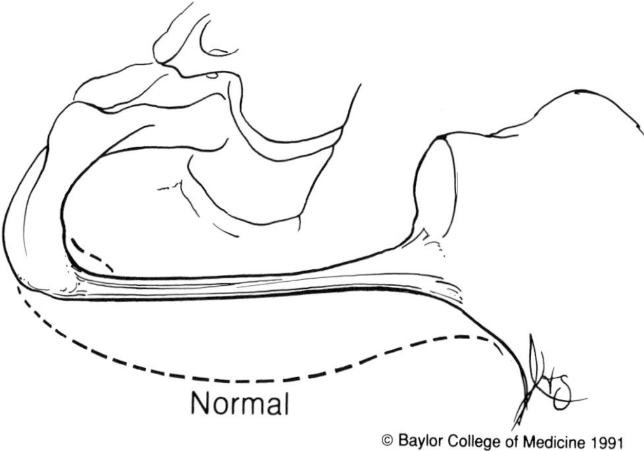

Figure 16.4. As the normal configuration of the rib is lost, and it becomes more J-shaped; the fibrous bands often contribute to the loss of mobility and hence increase the potential for thoracic outlet compression.

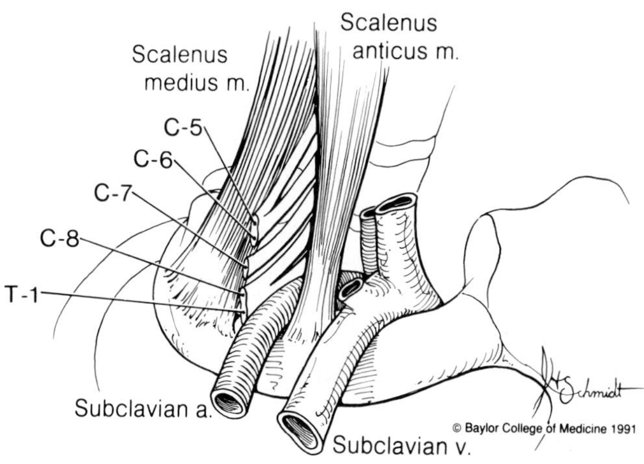

Figure 16.5. Medial fibers of the scalenus anterior muscle attach to the cupola of the lung. Between the fibers of the scalenus anticus and medius muscles traverse both the subclavian artery and the lower cervical roots as they join to become the brachial plexus.

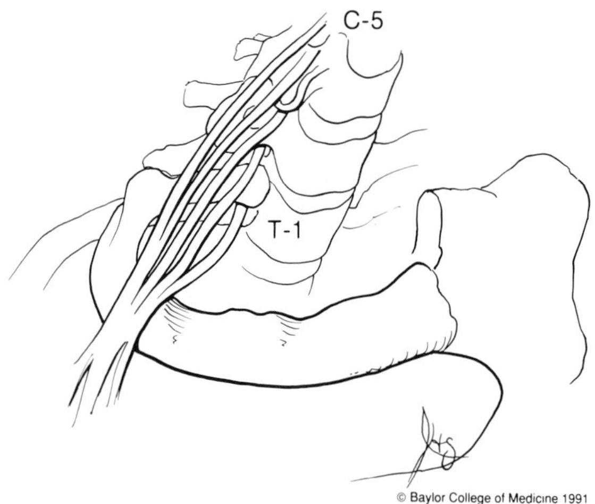

Figure 16.6. The brachial plexus is formed by the anterior rami of the lower cervical roots and the upper thoracic root, C-5 through T-1. The C-8 and T-1 roots are the most commonly involved.

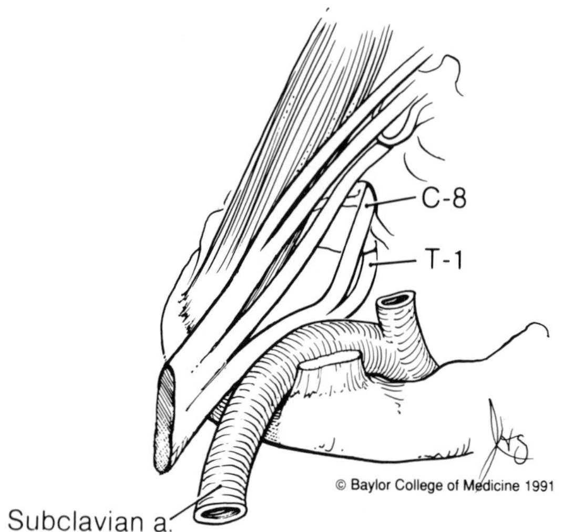

Figure 16.7. The lower trunk of the brachial plexus, formed by the C-8 and T-1 roots, traverses posterior to the subclavian artery and takes a more acute course over the first thoracic rib. These anatomic features are felt to be responsible for the predominance of lower cervical root symptoms as the initial presenting complaint.

symptoms are the most commonly seen as presenting complaints.

ETIOLOGY

While the etiology of thoracic outlet compression syndrome is not entirely understood, there are several consistent findings common with patient's exhibiting these symptoms.

The patient's habitus assumes one of two characteristic patterns. Patients are either muscular individuals with short, thickened necks often seen in athletes, or they tend to be esthenic individuals with very poor musculature, long, hypermobile necks, and low-riding shoulder girdles (89, 90) (Fig. 16.8). Patients with an increase in neck musculature have overdevelopment of the scalenus anticus muscle and the subclavian muscle; this produces an increasing compression of the neurovascular bundle (36). This differs from patients with long necks and low-riding shoulder girdles, who manifest compression by decreasing the space between the first thoracic rib and the clavicle. This condition is more commonly seen in middle-aged individuals where deterioration of muscle tone alone can cause the shoulder girdle to droop, producing the symptoms.

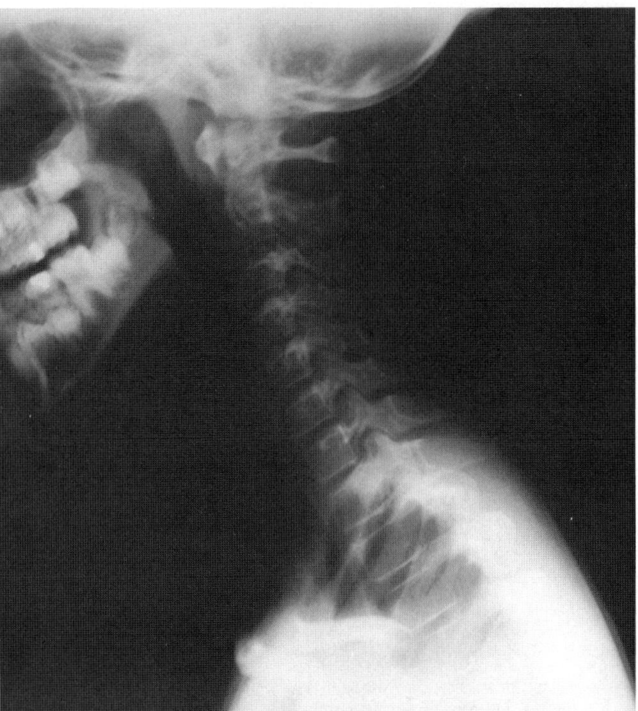

Figure 16.8. (LATERAL C-SPINE) A lateral radiograph of the C-spine may visualize the upper thoracic vertebrae distally as far as T4 or T5. The ability to see these vertebrae are indicative of the presence of low-riding shoulders.

Congenital anomalies, including cervical ribs or bifid clavicles, bony chondromas, fracture callouses, or exostosis of the first rib have been associated with thoracic outlet syndrome (59, 69, 72, 73, 77, 92). Cervical ribs are present in approximately 1% of the population; when present, they are bilateral in 80% of the cases (16, 78) (Fig. 16.9). Even though they are associated with C7, C8, and T1, less than 10% of all cervical ribs diagnosed become symptomatic (81, 132). Patients with other congenital anomalies of the cervicothoracic junction include elongated transverse processes of C7, the presence of eight cervical vertebrae or foreshortened first thoracic vertebrae, and the J-shaped first thoracic rib previously mentioned. These can all be susceptible to increasing symptomatology. In addition to the bony abnormalities, associated various fibrous bands can contribute to thoracic outlet symptoms. The most commonly occurring are those that originate from a cervical rib or elongated transverse process and transect the thoracic outlet attaching to various places on the first thoracic rib (59, 36). These variations compress the neurovascular bundle dramatically and are especially troublesome with arm elevation and rotation (36). Anatomic variations of the scalenus musculature are also known to contribute to compression of the neurovascular system (36, 46, 59). Roos initially divided the anatomical variance into five groupings (73, 74). However, more recently he has expanded his classification to nine (70, 95).

Type I is a short, cervical rib with a fibrous band passing under the first thoracic root (Fig. 16.10). Type II is a fibrous band arising from the elongated tip of the C7 transverse process which again transects the thoracic outlet to insert posterior to the scalenus anticus tubercle (Fig. 16.11). Type III is located slightly lower, passing from the neck of the first rib horizontally across the thoracic outlet and again under the first thoracic root of the plexus, and it attaches to the inner ridge of the first rib, often between the T1 trunk and the subclavian artery. This is the most common of all congenital abnormalities and is present in most patients who require operation for thoracic outlet compression syndrome (Fig. 16.12). Type IV is a fibral muscular band on the anterior edge of the middle scalene muscle, forming a fibral muscular laying under the plexus and subclavian artery and joining with the anterior scalene muscle. This band may cause irritation of all five roots contributing to the brachial plexus by elevating the plexus when the scalene contracts by exertion or spasm (Fig. 16.13). Type V is the scalenus minimum muscle, an anomalous ribbonlike muscle passing obliquely downward, parallel to the anterior scalene from C5 and C6 transverse process. It passes between the plexus and subclavian artery and at-

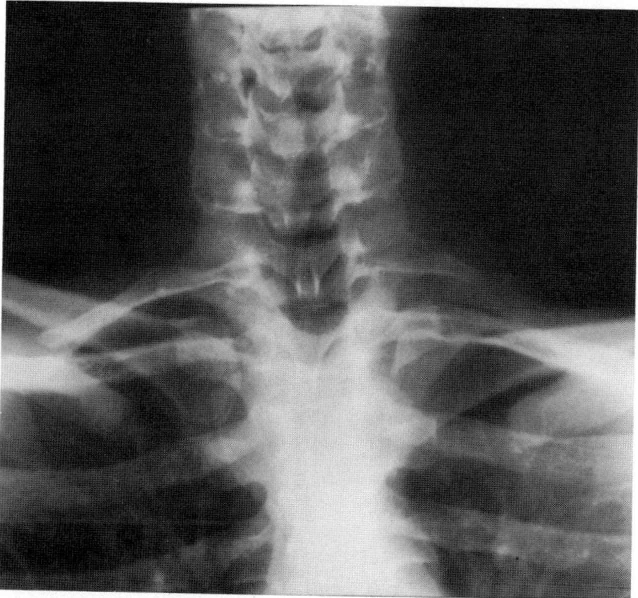

Figure 16.9. The presence of bilateral cervical ribs with a formed rib on the right and a rudimentary rib on the left.

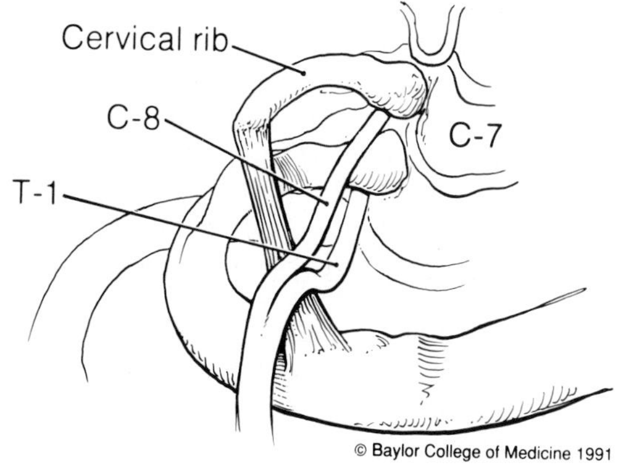

Figure 16.10. Type I variant.

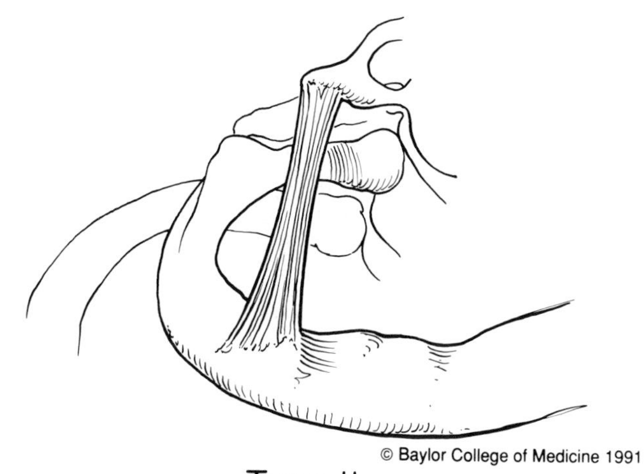

Figure 16.11. Type II variant.

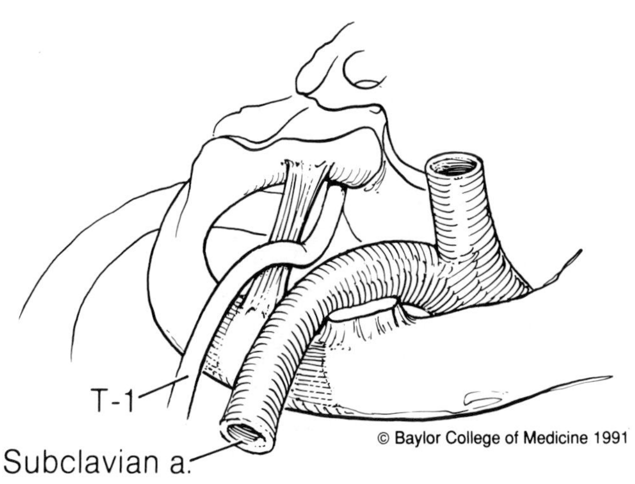

Figure 16.12. Type III variant.

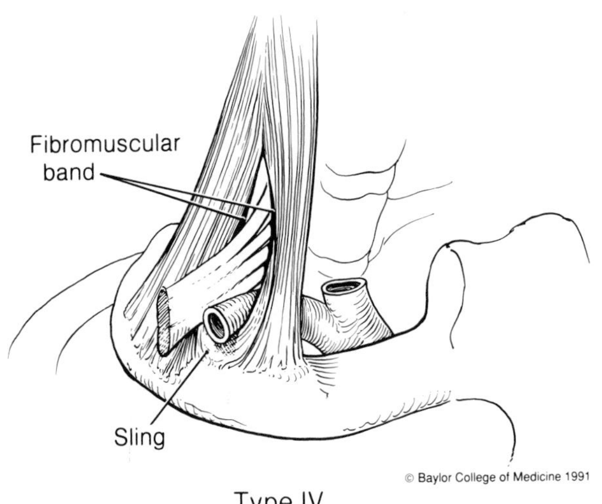

Figure 16.13. Type IV variant.

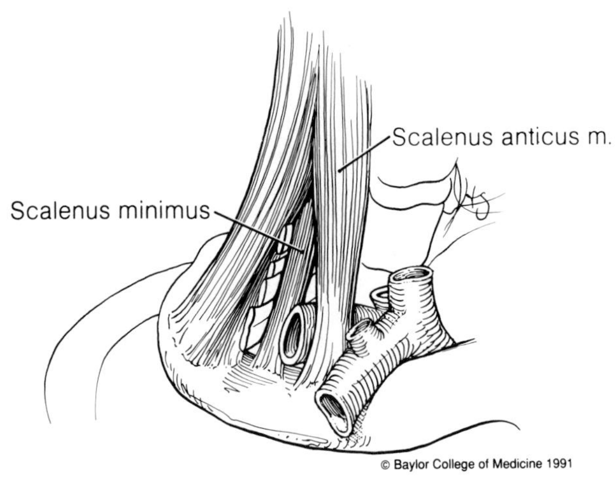

Figure 16.14. Type V variant.

taches on the inner edge of the first rib between the anterior and middle scalene (Fig. 16.14) (72). Type VI is a scalene minimus muscle that inserts posterior to the rib on the lung and on the pleura or Sibson's fascia and is not attached to the first rib. This is important because it may be taut even after rib resection (Fig. 16.15). Type VII is a fibrous band arising from the anterior scalene muscle and passes under the subclavian vein attaching to the posterior sternum (Fig. 16.16). This variation is felt to be primarily responsible for the proximal vein thrombosis of the subclavian vein termed the Pagett-Schrotter syndrome. Type VIII is similar to type VII but arises from the anterior surface of the scalenus medius muscle and passes under the brachial plexus artery and vein to insert on the posterior sternum (Fig. 16.17). Type IX is a taut web of fibers filling the entire thoracic outlet (Fig. 16.18). Trauma plays an important role in the etiology of this syndrome. Reports state that 35 to 50% of cases are precipitated by some traumatic episode, either a blow to the basilar region of the neck, a sharp, jerking motion, or a flexion extension injury commonly referred to as whiplash (72, 73, 95). In these types of injuries, neck pain develops almost immediately, while hand and arm pain may take several days or even weeks to develop (73, 95). Of particular recent interest is the concept expressed by Machleder and others that looked at sections of muscle fibers histologically with thoracic outlet syndrome and found there was a marked percentage of type 1 tonic contracting fiber predominance as well as type 1 fiber hypertrophy (50). This change clearly identified that the anterior scalene muscle was uniquely structured to sustain rather prolonged contractures.

INCIDENCE

The incidence of this syndrome is not well established. Females seem to predominate in a ratio between two to one and four to one, depending on the particular series

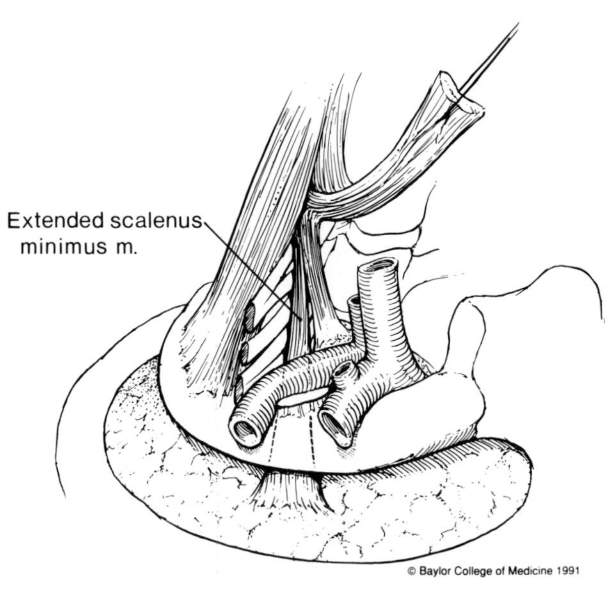

Figure 16.15. Type VI variant.

(72–74, 95). They tend to be morphologically more slender and esthenic, while the males tend to be well-developed and heavy in their musculature, especially in their neck and shoulder regions. The younger and middle-age groups are more commonly involved, with a mean age of approximately 35 years (12, 59, 61, 73, 82).

SIGNS AND SYMPTOMS

The symptoms of thoracic outlet syndrome vary according to specific structures that are compressed and their point of compression. The symptoms of neurocompression far exceed any vascular presenting symptoms. Neurologic symptoms are produced by compression of the brachial plexus; they consist of pain, paresthesias, and loss of strength in the fingers, hands, and upper extremities. Symptoms

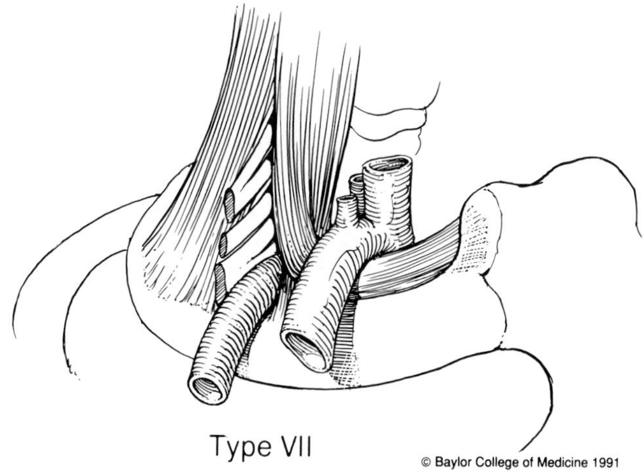

Figure 16.16. Type VII variant.

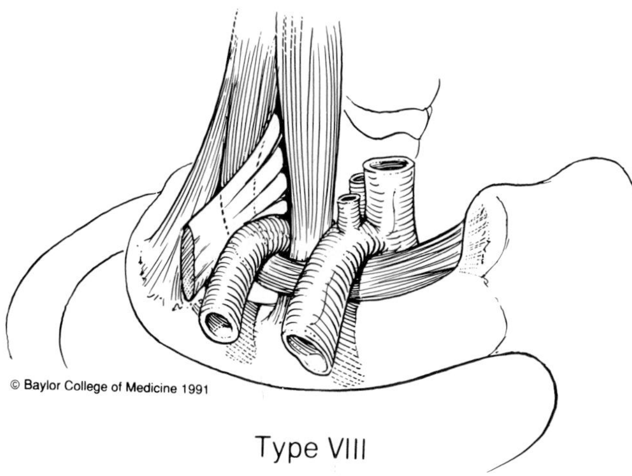

Figure 16.17. Type VIII variant.

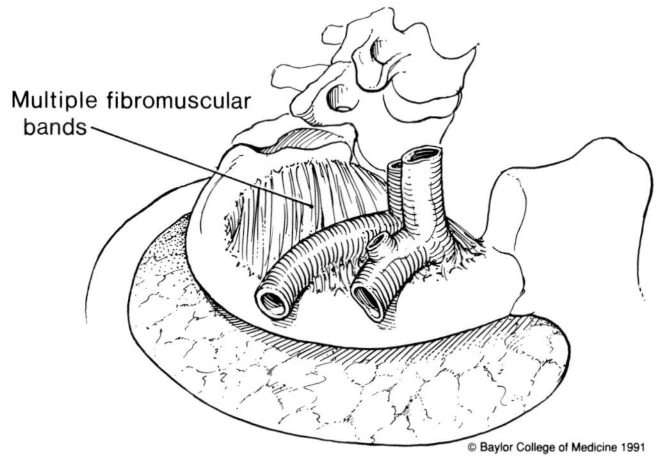

Figure 16.18. Type IX variant.

occur primarily along the ulnar distribution of the forearm and hand consisted with C7, C8, and T1 dermatomes. Symptoms may occur in the upper arm or in the shoulder girdle, but this event is unusual. Late manifestations include profound sensory deficits with a weakness and occasional muscular atrophy. To a lesser degree it is not unusual to find pain in the neck and shoulder region associated with headaches, anterior chest pain, and scapular pain. The intensity of this pain varies dramatically from a mild discomfort to almost incapacitating pain. Dysfunctional changes of the upper extremities can also occur such as dropping objects, especially small objects, impairment of handwriting, loss of dexterity, or the inability to comb the hair or manipulate objects above the level of the shoulder or overhead. Additional, complaints include headaches, usually originating in the posterior occipital region and radiating to the frontal area, frequently in the retro-occular area. Blurring of vision, difficulty in concentration, changes in personalities such as irritability and depression can be present (86). Other less common complaints include stiffness in the shoulder area, elbow pain, chest wall pain especially in women with particularly large, pendulous breasts (86). Generally, these neurologic symptoms are very subtle, often vague and intermittent in nature.

Arterial compression produces slightly different symptomatology. Classically this is the pain of ischemia described as a diffuse pain associate with numbness, fatigue, pallor, coolness, and sensitivity to cold with definite aggravation by elevation of the upper extremity. Other symptoms include claudication and weakness of the arm or hand, especially during activities. Elevation of the arms and hands or a patient's sleep position with the hands up around the face or above the head often produce these symptoms. In far advanced cases, vascular ulceration and gangrene of the finger tips can actually occur. Rarely, a unilateral type of Raynaud's phenomenon has been noted (39). Venous compression produces aching, swelling, and a blueish discoloration with an occasional unilateral enlargement of the upper extremity. Visually, one can see distended collateral veins around the shoulder area and anterior chest with often a cyanotic cast to the upper extremity that may actually disappear with elevation of the entire arm. Characteristically a typical story involves pain beginning gradually and intermittently then becoming progressively worse over a period of time. Characteristically it is described as an aching discomfort, beginning in the back of the neck and shoulders and gradually moving to the upper extremities. This discomfort traverses the arm and forearm into the hand, usually the ulnar three fingers, but occasionally the entire hand is involved. Pain can be associated with occasional numbness and tingling in the fingers occurring in a polyneural fashion. Patients frequently ignore these symptoms for a considerable length of time until the symptoms actually become somewhat refractory to conservative treatment.

In questioning individuals in the process of history taking, important events that can be derived from the history often contribute to the diagnosis of thoracic outlet. The first and most important is that it does involve the neck and upper extremities in a polyneural distribution with this distribution of pain and paresthesias almost always involving the C7, C8, and T1 roots. Only rarely do contributions occur from C5 and C6, giving radial side arm and hand paresthesias. Secondarily, the nature at which the symptoms occur, that is with fine motor movement or using the hands in an overhead fashion or at the level of the horizontal, is most informative.

PHYSICAL EXAMINATION

Observation and the general appearance of a patient is helpful in initially assessing the patient's likelihood of developing this syndrome. As previously mentioned, patients with long, esthenic necks with low-drooping shoulders as well as those with short, heavy muscular necks are prime candidates. Examination by observation of the hand and upper extremities may reveal swelling, discoloration, and intrinsic muscle atrophy.

Since only in the most severe cases do patients exhibit gross muscular weakness of the upper extremity, examination of the intrinsic muscles of the hand is often a subtle way to detect small changes in the lower cervical roots. An easy example is to ask a patient to grip a playing card between the interphalangeal joints with the fingers extended (36, 72, 81). Opposition of the thumb by flexing the thenar muscles is a good test for median nerve involvement. Less commonly involved muscular groups include the radial nerve as well as muscles about the elbow, specifically in flexion. Important examinationof the biceps, triceps, and radial wrist extensors should be done to differentiate those patients with possible cervical disc disease. Reflex activity is rarely affected in thoracic outlet syndrome. Therefore, absent reflexes or increase reflexes at the biceps, tricips, and brachial radialis may give indications of cervical disc disease or primary upper motor neuron disease.

Direct palpation or percussion over the brachial plexus can cause notable tenderness in the presence of acute thoracic outlet symptoms. This can be elicited by applying thumb pressure over the patient's brachial plexus in a supraclavicular fossa for 10 to 30 seconds. A positive test is indicated by gradually increasing pain and cephalad migration of the pain at the site of the neck to the base of the head or distally through the axilla to the interbrachium. Ordinarily, this test should not produce radiating symptoms unless thoracic outlet compression is present (73, 72). Asking the patient to flex the chin to the chest area and percussion over the cervical thoracic spinous processes often cause sharp, lancinating pains that can be associated with this syndrome.

The classic maneuver for establishing the presence of cervical disc disease is to have the patient extend and rotate the head from side to side. This can be done with or without axial compression. This maneuver rarely causes pain with thoracic outlet syndrome.

Upper extremity sensation may be difficult to test because of the polyneural presentation of these symptoms, but almost always it characteristically involves the ulnar border of the forearm and the ulnar two fingers of the affected hand.

Arterial compression must be evaluated in thoracic outlet compression. Radial and ulnar pulses are first palpated at the wrists with the hands in the resting or lap position. Next, while the radial pulse is being monitored, the arm is brought to 90° of abduction and external rotation. The position of the head toward the affected side is termed the Adson maneuver, whereas the head toward the opposite side is either the modified Adson maneuver or the Allen's test (72). With the arm in the position for the Adson maneuver the pulse is dampened in approximately 70% of the normal population. Therefore, the Adson test alone is highly unreliable for definitive diagnostic testing (72). In a retrospective review Adson's test was found to be positive in approximately 2% of patients with well documented thoracic outlet syndromes (72). The Allen test has a reasonable degree of accuracy and is used primarily as a secondary or supportive test for arterial compression (59, 36, 72, 73, 86).

According to Roos the most reliable test for thoracic outlet syndrome is the elevated arm stress test, termed the EAST test (Fig. 16.19). The patient elevates the arms 90° in abduction externally rotated position, with the shoulders and elbows braced back, similar to a military posture. The hands are opened and closed at moderate speed for 3 minutes. Normally a patient without thoracic outlet syndrome can do this with only minor forearm fatigue and minimal distress. Those with pronounced outlet syndrome will usually produce a gradual increase in pain, beginning in the back of the neck and shoulders and progressing down the arm across the forearms into the hands. Paresthesias develop in the lower arm, forearm, and fingers often causing the patients to be unable to complete the entire 3 minutes, therefore dropping the arms with profound weakness and marked distress in the neck and arms usually within 1 to 2 minutes. The symptoms are usually similar to the patient's own distress symptoms (72). Patients with carpal tunnel syndromes may develop numbness in the fingers due to compression of the median nerve, usually confined to the radial three fingers of the hand, however, the Tinel or Phalans tests are very adequate ways to help differentiate these findings. Patients having a double crush syndrome can be differentiated also by testing for carpal tunnel disease, especially with electrodiagnostic measures (95).

The blood pressure should be observed in both arms. Normally it is found to be 5 to 10 mm of mercury less in

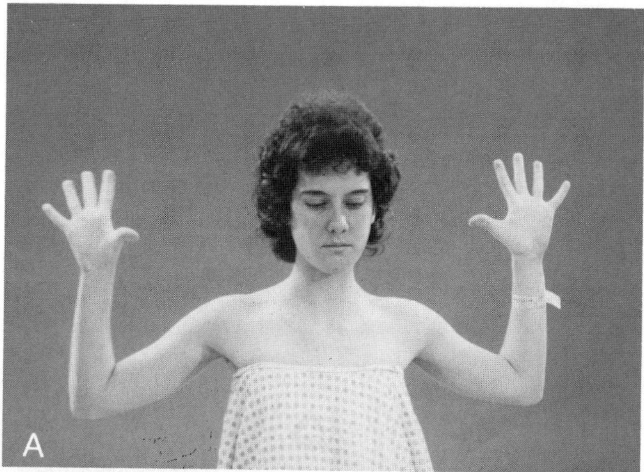

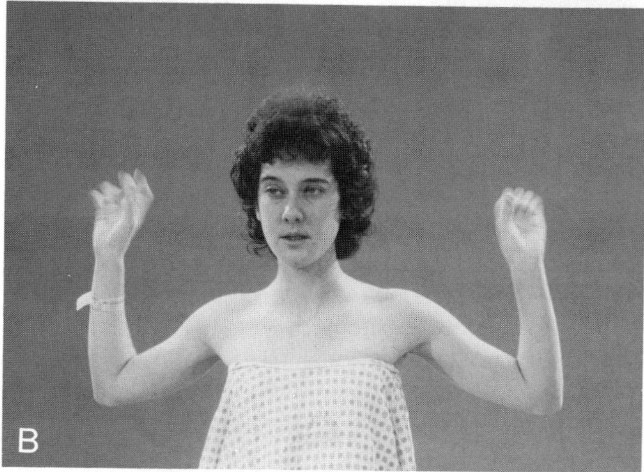

Figure 16.19. Patient performing the EAST maneuver, **A**. This has proven to be a very reliable clinical test of thoracic outlet syndrome. Note the painful expression on the patient's face, **B**.

the left arm. However, if the blood pressure should exceed a differential of 10 to 20 mm of mercury, a high level of suspicion for arterial abnormalities productive of these symptoms should be anticipated. Measurement of the blood pressure with the arm in the elevated abducted position to establish the costoclavicular compression is also quite helpful. Patients observing a loud bruit in the supraclavicular fossa, especially with the arms in the rest position, should have arteriography to rule out any substantial or difficult arterial abnormality or aberration.

Patients with venous obstruction are the most infrequent of all patient groups but are usually the most easily diagnosed. They tend to have a bluish tint to the hand, which is usually swollen unilaterally with severe venous congestion. Often this discoloration and swelling can be relieved with simple elevation of the extremity. Only in severe cases are cyanosis and mottling present.

Diagnostic and Objective Testing

There are few objective tests which clearly define or diagnostically indicate the presence of thoracic outlet syndrome. The diagnosis of thoracic outlet syndrome is primarily a clinical evaluation with supporting evidence occasionally obtained through objective diagnostic procedures.

A standard x-ray of the spine centered at C7 and T1 with a 10 to 15° upshoot is an important test in establishing the presence of cervical ribs or the presence of an eighth cervical vertebra. Likewise, abnormalities of the first thoracic rib including the J variant, anomalous insertions of the second rib, any bony exostosis or abnormalities of the clavicles, including previous fractures, or evidence of arthritis either in the sternoclavicular area or lower cervical areas can be detected. Complete cervical spine x-rays should also be obtained including AP, lateral, oblique, and flexion and extension lateral views to help rule-out the presence of congenital abnormalities of the spine, exostoses, and cervical spondylosis.

Cervical myelography is indicated to differentiate cervical disc disease from thoracic outlet syndromes and can be used in conjunction with computerized axial tomography of the cervical thoracic area to clearly examine both C-T abnormalities as well as supraclavicular soft tissue changes presence near the apex of the lung.

CT scanning of the apical lung region can often reveal abnormal soft tissue bandings as well as apical tumors within the lung itself that can produce symptoms similar to thoracic outlet syndrome.

While electrodiagnostic testing optimistically would give us the best indication of compression at the thoracic outlet it may also be dismally unrewarding. There have been several attempts at inductively implying the techniques of electromyography to diagnosing thoracic outlet syndrome, however. Jebsen describes a difficult technique of placing a stimulating electrode in the ulnar trunk of the brachial plexus and the receiving pole across the arm and hand; unfortunately the success of this operation is purely dependent on the interpretation of the examiner and the expert skills in placing the proximal electrode. Therefore, reproducibility of this test is often dubious. However, his work is supported by Urschel in 17 patients with thoracic outlet syndrome, in which all 17 conduction defects were established across the thoracic outlet and were relieved with excision of the thoracic rib. The conduction velocity times that were measured all returned to the normal range (34, 91). Unfortunately, this was subsequently challenged by the works of Wilburn and Letterman in 1984. Another analysis is the study of the F-wave analysis of the ulnar nerve and has been reported as showing varying accounts of some reproducibility (95). This is an inductive test, however, and is seen by all reports to have a wide range of variability. At best, this test in the hand of a skilled electromyographer can be considered a reasonable adjunctive electrodiagnostic test in the presence of other symptoms or other findings of thoracic outlet syndrome (25, 97). Entry of both potentials have also had some promising reports as electrodiagnostic trials: however, they are still somewhat speculative in this condition and are not generally acceptable as totally reliable (25, 97). Therefore, SSEP's and motor for both potentials MEP's are still in the investigative stage at best.

Arterial obstruction initially was studied by mercury strain gage plethysmography (59, 81). This was subsequently replaced by selective subclavian arteriography which continues to the present day; however, even this test, as sophisticated as it is, is progressively being replaced by the highly reliable byphasic doppler echoangiography. Since plethysmography was not reliable and angiography is certainly not without its own risks, it is not an innocuous procedure.

The popularity of noninvasive doppler studies is greatly enhanced. Invasive angiography is still required if doppler studies are inconclusive or if a question regarding particular anatomic extent of the vascular lesion cannot be established. The preferred method is still by femoral percutaneous introduction of the needle and selective angiography of the right and left subclavian arteries differentially (41, 46, 61). Some authors still feel that arteriography of the upper extremities should be done with both arms at the patient's side as well as in the abducted externally-rotated position with the shoulders braced, mimicking the condition which reproduces the symptoms (36, 59, 86). Because the lesions may be intermittent and purely positional, arteriography may not demonstrate the lesion even if it is present (74). Many patients with severe symptoms of thoracic outlet syndrome may have no arterial compression; therefore, a normal arteriogram would have no meaning in these cases (74). Additionally, patients without thoracic outlet syndromes can have subclavian artery compression in the arm in the elevated or shoulder braced position such that an abnormal arteriogram in these patients may produce a diagnostic and therapeutic dilemma (72, 74). The previously held concept of severe vascular compression as the major underlying etiology of thoracic outlet syndrome has been replaced by the concept of neural involvement as the major pathology, consequently, there seem to be fewer indications for arteriography. Certainly, the requirements of a positive arteriogram before advising surgery is no longer valid. Lastly, it is worth mentioning that arteriography is not an innocuous procedure, and its potential risks and complications can be severe. Arteriogram should be limited and is recommended in these particular instances (72): *a*) patients with arm complaints who are found to have weak pulses or pressure differentials of more than 20 mm of mercury as compared to the opposite asymptomatic side; *b*) patients suspected of plaque stenosis of the subclavian artery (e.g., loud bruit when the hands are held in the lap); *c*) patients suspected of possible subclavian aneurysm formation; or *d*) when the source of a peripheral embolus is sought.

Phlebography is recommended only in patients with obvious evidence of venous hypertension and stasis as the primary manifestation of the thoracic outlet syndrome. Phlebogram may help differentiate among compression of the axillary subclavian vein by the thoracic outlet structures, aneurysms, tumors, or thrombosis of the vein (36, 81).

DIFFERENTIAL DIAGNOSIS

Several conditions may simulate symptoms of the thoracic outlet compression syndrome. The most common are cervical disc disease, cervical neuritis or spondylitis and cervical spondylosis in general. Carpal tunnel syndrome is also quite commonly confused. Table 2 lists other less commonly seen diagnosis that may be confused with thoracic outlet syndrome (11, 19, 20, 36, 59, 69, 72, 82, 81, 86). Any neurologic symptom suggestive of reflex sympathetic dystrophy may also mimic thoracic outlet syndrome. This would include pallor and coldness of the hands or upper extremities, weakness and a pseudoparalysis. Occasionally, neuropathic changes in the hand or upper extremity can cause a dusky cyanotic appearance suggestive of venous obstruction but in reality represent sympathetic changes only.

Neck pain is common to both thoracic outlet syndrome and cervical disc disease. Extremity pain may be present in carpal tunnel syndrome even ascension of pain from the wrist to the level of the shoulder is not uncommon in some retrograde carpal tunnel syndromes.

Patients do complain of intense cramping of the forearm and hand are more likely to have symptoms of carpal tunnel disease especially in the presence of a positive Tinel or Phalan's test (29).

The relationship of trauma to thoracic outlet compression syndrome is important since there is a high correlation of patients with posttraumatic symptomatology. These patients are felt to be susceptible or have predisposing factors of developing thoracic outlet compression based on their cervical thoracic anatomy or general morphology. The symptoms of post-traumatic thoracic outlet syndrome are felt to be mediated through muscular spasm of the middle scalene muscles involving the brachial plexus.

TREATMENT

Initial treatment should always be non-operative. Rosati and Lord found that effective management was obtained with nonoperative treatment on initial clinic visits in 70% of cases (75). Urschel reported 40 to 50% of patients were helped by conservative measures (91).

Most non-operative treatment regimes are designed to instruct patients in the avoidance in positions or activities that precipitate their symptoms. Patients most likely to benefit from conservative treatment or those with mild symptoms, initial presentations exhibiting only occasional fatigue and numbness in the upper extremities. They are usually instructed to avoid hyperabduction maneuvers, excessive weight gain and any depression of the shoulder girdle such as carrying heavy objects. Physiotherapeutic measures are designed to increase the shoulder girdle and neck muscular tone in those esthenically build or hypotonic individuals. Sedentary patients are encouraged to proceed with an active physical therapy exercise program. These patients are usually more responsive to conservative treatment since normal muscle tone has been lost producing a drooping shoulder girdle and can with some degree of expectancy resolve with exercise alone. Most exercise programs can be done at home usually promoting general acceptance. Patients are educated as to the avoidance of sleep patterns that might cause precipitations of their symptoms. Reverse positioning exercises including isometrics for the trapezius, or levator muscles are emphasized. Adjunctive treatments can include non-steroidal anti-inflammatory medication and muscle relaxants as necessary. Non-operative treatment regimes should be pursued as long as effective means of pain relief can be established (31). Indications for operative intervention when conservative measures have failed are as follows (72). One, intolerable pain and sufficient loss of function or strength in the hand or upper extremities; two, lack or sleep or inability to maintain sleep patterns; three, unacceptable degree of personal inconvenience; four, personality changes from symptoms of thoracic outlet syndrome; five, significant arterial or venous symptoms; six, chronic use of strong analgesic medication; or seven, threatened job loss or poor performance as a result of thoracic outlet symptomatology.

The goal of surgical intervention is to decompress the thoracic outlet by removal of the first thoracic rib and the cervical rib if present. Various approaches have been employed, including posterior and anterior as well as supraclavicular, but the preferred approach today is the transaxillary approach reported to provide 90% good to excellent results with a minimum of complications (12, 13, 59, 73, 74). While morbidity is low there are potentially serious complications that can occur with transaxillary surgery (73–74). Hemorrhage from injury to the subclavian vein or artery or permanent neurological damage to the brachial plexus especially from T1 or C8 injuries are the most devastating complications. A neurologic injury could produce permanent ulnar sided neuropathies manifested by claw hand deformity, forearm atrophy and intrinsic atrophy. This can impair function and permanent numbness and pain can exist. Winging of the scapula can result from long thoracic nerve injuries. Fortunately, all of these complications are rare.

Vascular injuries are few in number even though the potential for injury is great. The incident of pneumothorax is small and in those pneumothoraxes that do occur, evacuation by suction catheter at the time of wound closure without indwelling suction test tube can usually be successfully managed. If chest tube thoracotomies are necessary they can usually be removed within 24 to 48 hours of surgery causing no long lasting sequelae. Some minor complications including intercostal brachial neuropathies producing axillary numbness and discomfort is usually temporary and does occur usually as a result of sectioning or traction on the intercostal brachial nerve. Likewise thoracodorsal traction injuries are long thoracic traction injuries can occur with retraction of the lower brachial plexus but again these usually resolve and don't produce substantial losses except in those cases of wing scapula which fortunately is ware.

TECHNIQUES OF SURGERY

The most satisfactory operation is carried out under general anesthesia with the patient rolled into a lateral position and taped at the hip level with the upper torso being reclined at an angle of 45 to 60 degrees. It is important to drape the arm free, having an assistant placed in a proper position to apply traction with a wrist lock type of hold when necessary (72). The incision is made low in the axilla approximately at the inferior border of the hairline with the arm abducted, this places the incision approximately over the third thoracic rib or just inferior to it (Fig. 16.20). The approach should be directed perpendicular to the skin and not in a slanted direction. Blunt dissection of the axilla should be used and is carried out to the external aspect of the rib cage, deep to the axillary fat pad, nodes and vessels. The intercostal brachial nerve is found in the mid field arising from the second intercostal space. This should be carefully dissected widely allowing retraction of the nerve to occur. Sectioning and ligating the nerve with its associated vascular bundle should not be performed in that a neuroma formation would be likely. Trauma to the nerve can cause numbness in the axilla and is fairly common but usually regresses quickly.

When the first rib is encountered after ligating small vessels, a light membrane of fascia will be noted. This forms a pocket or a culdesac at the lateral edge of the rib. It should be freed blunt dissection; fingertip dissection is then done along the first rib anteriorly thereby identifying the subclavian vein anterior to the vein subclavius muscle as it inserts on the inferior aspect of the clavicle. After the subclavian vein is identified immediately posterior to this structure is the scalenus anticus muscle. The subclavian artery is immediately posterior to the muscle and lies in direct proximity to the brachial plexus and the first thoracic root. The scalenus medium muscle is posterior to the plexus itself (Fig. 16.21).

As the axillar tunnel becomes deeper it is important to slowly and gently elevate the shoulder to elevate the shoulder to provide proper exposure for the operating surgeon. This should be relaxed periodically to release tension on the plexus and the vascular structures. With elevation of the shoulder girdle, the costoclavicular impingement anteriorly can easily be tested by placing a finger on each side of the scalenus anticus muscle on top of the rib. The pa-

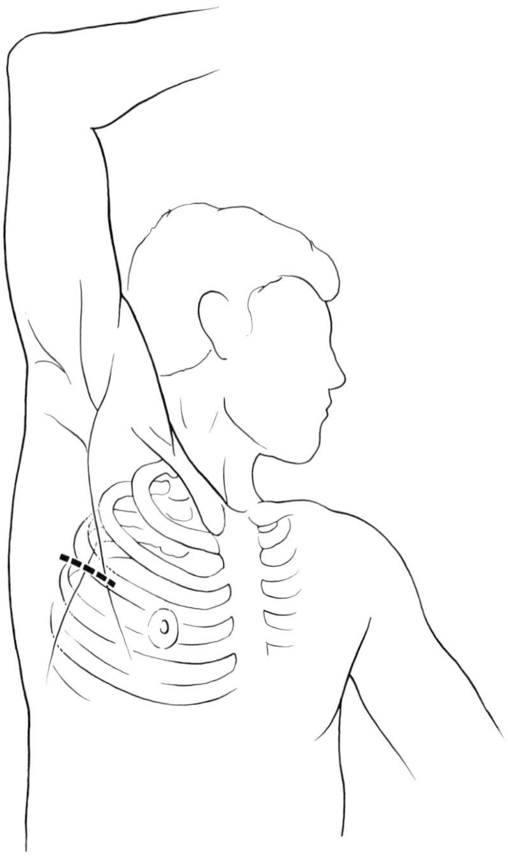

Figure 16.20. With the patient in a lateral decubitus position, a 3-in (8-cm) incision is made over the third rib in a curvilinear fashion between the latissimus dorsi and the pectoralis major muscles.

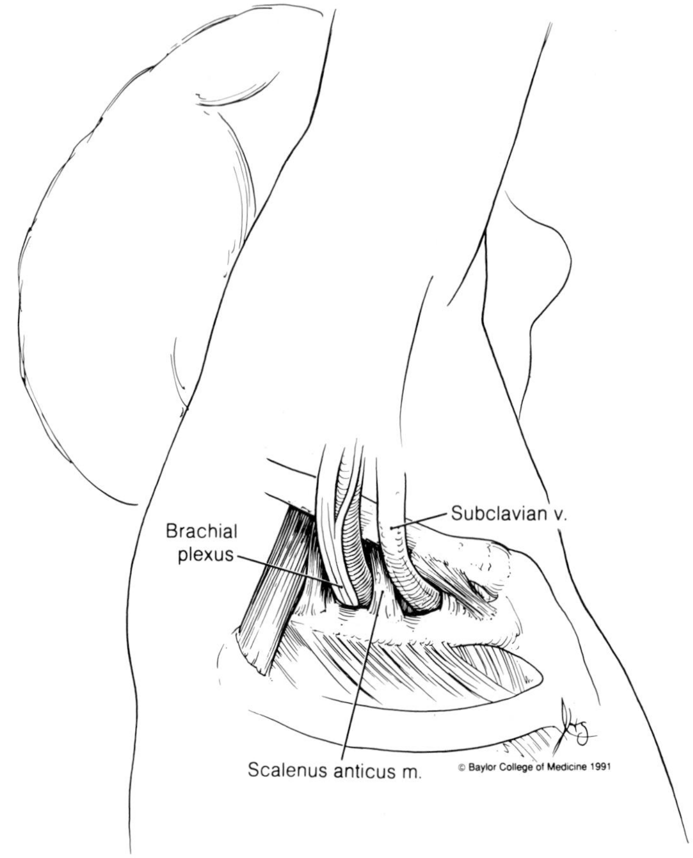

Figure 16.21. The appearance of the neurovascular bundle and the course and insertion of the scalene muscles are initially confusing because of the abducted arm. This coursing of the vessels and brachial plexus actually aids in exposure and removal of the first rib, minimizing neurovascular injury.

tient's shoulder is then relaxed or depressed in caudad fashion. With the shoulder depressed the patient's arm is placed in a position of 90 degrees of abduction and external rotation. Usually, the surgeon can feel a remarkably hard pinch with the patient that has profound thoracic outlet symptomatology. This closure of the costoclavicular space plays an important role in producing these symptoms.

Beginning anteriorly the subclavius tendon is felt on the first rib as a taught band under the head of the clavicle. Its origin is at the costochondral junction and can be divided with long scissors (Fig. 16.22). The subclavian vein lies immediate adjacent to the tendon, passing medial and posterior to it, and should be of course protected during the subclavius sectioning. The scalenus anticus muscle will then be encountered and isolated by a right angle clamp. Great care should be taken not to entrap the artery posterior and medial to the scalenus muscle. The muscle was then divided as shown in (Fig. 16.23). Medial fibers of the scalenus anticus muscle must then be divided by scissor dissection off the cupula of the lung. A scalpel should not be used in this area because of the danger of creating a pneumothorax (Fig. 16.24).

Following the removal of the scalenus anticus muscle,

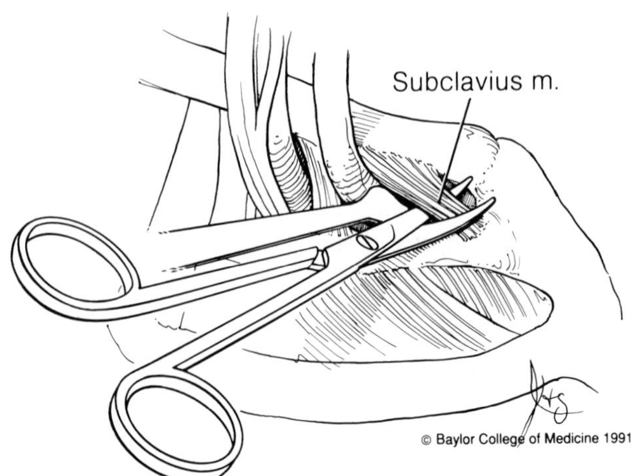

Figure 16.22. In dividing the origin of the subclavius tendon, great care should be taken because of the proximity of the subclavian vein. The tips of the scissors should be visualized to ensure the safety of the vein.

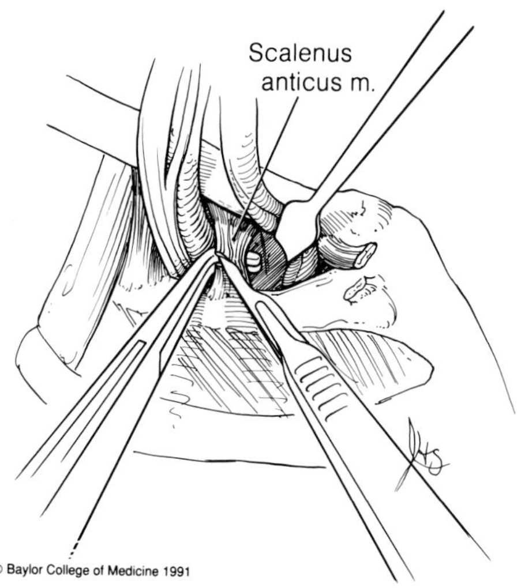

Figure 16.23. The scalenus anticus muscle is easily divided with a scalpel over a right angle clamp. The brachial plexus and the subclavian artery are protected by the clamp, but the vein should be retracted gently with a vein retractor.

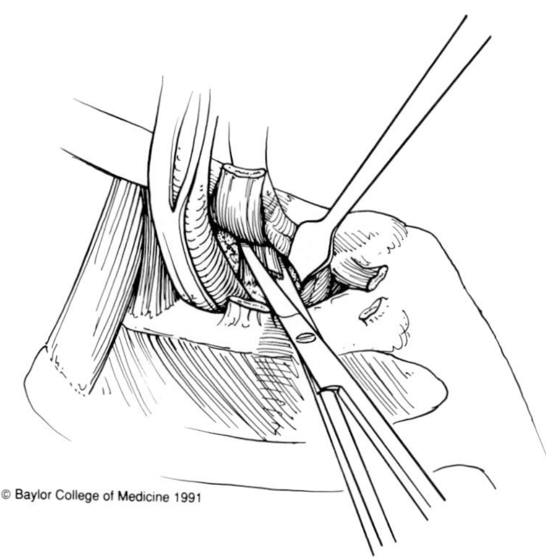

Figure 16.24. Following sectioning of the scalenus anticus muscle, the medial fibers should be transected with scissors, rather than a scalpel. The cupola of the lung is inferior to their attachment, and the danger of a pneumothorax is greater if a scalpel is used.

the subclavian artery is mobilized and the scalenus medius muscle is elevated from the first rib, using either periosteal elevator or extra periosteal dissection (Fig. 16.25). While most articles recommend extra periosteal dissection of this rib to prevent intramembranous reossification this is in a practical sense has not been encountered especially in adults. It is only rarely been reported as recurrence in children and probably a subperiosteal dissection is a safer more prudent manor of exposing the first thoracic rib. The first rib is then cleaned of all muscular attachments, including the intercostal muscle inferiorly. Extra periosteal dissection while desirable in order to prevent intramembranous reossifica-

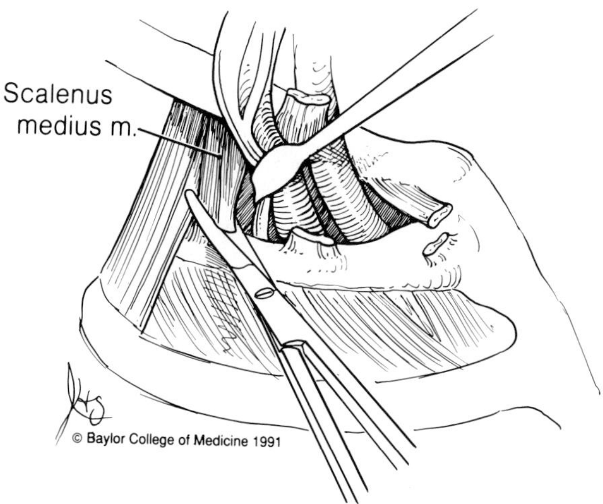

Figure 16.25. After mobilizing the brachial plexus and the subclavian artery and carefully and gently retracting them, the scalenus medius muscle is removed from the first rib to the transverse process of the vertebra. Frequent relaxation on the neurovascular retractor is necessary to ensure that no neuroproxia occurs. Following this resection, the rib is mobilized extraperiosteally from the costosternal junction to the tip of the transverse process. This maneuver helps to prevent entrapment of the neurovascular bundle should intramembranous callus formation occur.

tion and re-entrapment of thoracic structures is probably not necessary and certainly presents an increase in risk factor in damaging the thoracic outlet structures themselves. When dissection reaches the transverse process of the vertebrae posteriorly, the lower roots of the brachial plexus are elevated from the first thoracic rib and an angle rib cutter is introduced (Fig. 16.26). The rib is divided at the level of the transverse process. Care must be taken to ensure that the sharp edge of the rib does not perforate the pleural space on removal. The rib is then freed from the costochondral attachment and removed.

Congenital rib abnormalities or fibrous bandings that connect either congenital ribs or normal ribs with elongated process must be resected or released following removal of the first thoracic rib. Usually, this can be accomplished simply by extending the dissection cephalad. Cervical ribs less than two centimeters in length require no resection because they are too short and lie too far posterior and are usually not associated with fibrous banding to involve neurovascular structures. A congenital fibrous band arising from the tip of such a rib or a long C7 transverse process inserting on the scalene tubercle should however be removed not merely divided.

Prior to closure, the area should then be flooded with a saline solution and the lung placed under a val salva maneuver to examine for leaks within that have gone undetected. If a leak is present, a small chest tube suction catheter is placed in the hole itself or just over the third rib and brought out through a separate stab wound adjacent to the incision. This catheter can usually be re-

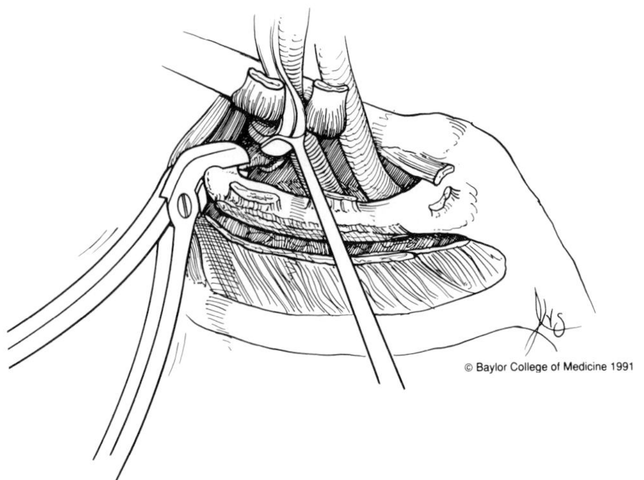

Figure 16.26. The rib is freed at the level of the transverse process with angled rib cutters. Care should be exercised to visualize the tips of the cutters. The neural structures should be retracted gently and relaxation should be frequent. The anterior division is done in a similar fashion, with care taken to protect the subclavian vein.

moved in the recovery room following an upright chest x-ray to determine if the free air has been evacuated from the chest. If no leak has been found, the wound can be closed with the area flooded with saline to prevent entrapment of air.

The arm is immobilized and the patient is cautioned not to use the arm particularly in elevation, but gentle pendulous or circumduction motion is allowed at the level of the shoulder with the elbow supported in a sling. Hand and elbow functions are encouraged during the postoperative period for a period of three to six weeks protection of the shoulder girdle by envelope sling alone.

VASCULAR ASPECTS OF THORACIC OUTLET SYNDROME

In the unusual cases of true arterial stenosis or occlusion caused by thoracic outlet syndrome or by venous obstruction necessitating thrombectomy, the vascular problems are handled similar to vascular injuries of like-type anywhere in the body (2 3, 6, 18). The operative approach is essentially the same but is normally combined with a supraclavicular approach to facilitate exposing the subclavian artery (46). The first rib is removed through the axillary approach initially with any congenital bands in the standard fashion. This opens up the axillar angle and somewhat facilitates the supraclavicular approach to the artery and vein. Since standard heparinization is performed prior to arterial cross clamping and then neutralized prior to wound closure, small fluid loculations can occur; therefore, a small penrose drain is recommended and brought out through the anterior tip of the supraclavicular incision. The supraclavicular fossa occasionally collects serous and lymphatic fluid postoperatively, and the drain provides easy egress for fluid control (8, 23, 79).

In rare cases of venous obstruction in thoracic outlet syndrome, especially one that occurs acutely, subclavian venous thrombectomy performed in the usual fashion is the preferred method (1). In the case of an acute thrombotic occlusion, the established choice of elevation and heparinization led to post phlebetic arm syndromes in 70 to 80% of patients reviewed (81). More recent reports suggest extraction of subclavian artery vein thrombosis through the brachial vein thrombectomy catheter described by Fogarty (51), similarly the use of human thrombolysing enzymes injected intravenously at the wrist or hand to digest acute thrombus has received favorable criticism (23).

RESULTS

Roos reported a remarkably good series. Of 566 patients evaluated for thoracic outlet syndrome 232 or 41% ultimately required surgery. There were 88.8% good or excellent results in this group with 11% being fair or poor. No patient has become worse as a result of the operative procedure (71, 72). This record compares quite favorably with reports of 60% failure rate with scalenotomies alone (80).

Taylor reported series of 256 patients with 351 operations performed. (Bilateral procedures in 93 patients). He reported 90% good to excellent results with minimal complications. Of the 90% of patients with good or excellent results all returned to full time employment and the level of activity enjoyed prior to the onset of thoracic outlet compression symptoms. There was a low percentage of poor results and no one was worse following surgery. It was also of particular note that 36% of his patients had bilateral procedures performed. Favorable results were reported in all 36 bilateral cases (86). McBurney and Howard reported success rates in excess of 90% utilizing the transaxillary approach (52). Urschel and Associates reported that 84% of their patients had first rib resections with a good result while only 23% had good results following scalenotomies alone (12). Wood, et al., in a more recent study showed that his first 100 consecutive patients utilizing the standards of diagnostic technique and surgical approaches of transaxillary resection reported greater than 90% of good results with no patients being worse following surgery.

In conclusion, thoracic outlet syndrome is an important clinical entity that because of the difficulty in diagnosis and understanding of the etiology of this syndrome is often misdiagnosed or simply overlooked by the examining physician. Attention and awareness of this condition and treatment or referral for treatment can greatly enhance expected return to normalcy or return to productivity of the compromised individual experiencing symptoms of compression thoracic outlet compression syndrome.

REFERENCES

1. Adams JT, DeWeese JA, Mahoney EB, Rob CC. Intermittent subclavian vein obstruction without thrombosis. Surgery, 1968;63:147.

2. Adson AW. Surgical treatment of cervical ribs. Tex Med 1933;28:739.

3. Adson AW. Surgical treatment of symptoms produced by cervical ribs and the scalenus anticus muscle. Surg Gynecol Obstet 1947;85:687.

4. Adson AW, Coffey JR. Cervical rib: a method of anterior approach for relief of symptoms by division of the scalenus anticus. Ann Surg 1927;85:839.

5. Beyer JA, Wright IS. The hyperabduction syndrome. With special reference to its relationship to Raynaud's Syndrome. Circulation 1951;4:161.

6. Bharucha EP, Dastur HM. Cranio-vertebral anomalies (a report on 40 cases). Brain 1964;87:469–480.

7. Bonney GLW. The Scalenus Medius Band. Read before the combined Canadian, British and American Orthopedic Associations, Vancouver, British Columbia, Canada, (June 1964).

8. Brannon EW, Wickstrom J. Surgical approaches to neurovascular compression syndromes of the neck. Clin Orthop 1967;51:65.

9. Brickner WM. Brachial plexus pressure by the normal first rib. Ann Surg 1927;85:858.

10. Brintnall ES, Hyndman OR, Van Allen MW. Costoclavicular compression associated with cervical rib. Ann Surg 1956;144:921.

11. Bucy PC, Oberhill HR. Pain in the shoulder and arm from neurological involvement. J.A.M.A. 1959;169:798.

12. Clagett OT. Presidential address: research and prosearch. J Thorac Cardiovasc Surg 1962;44:153.

13. Coote H. Pressure on the axillary vessels and nerve by an exostosis from a cervical rib: interference with the circulation of the arm, removal of the rib and exostosis; recovery. Med Times Gaz 1861;2:108.

14. Cunning AJ. Mural thrombosis of the subclavian artery and subsequent embolism in cervical rib. Q J Med 1964;33:133.

15. Dale WA. Thoracic outlet compression syndrome. Arch Surg 1982;117:1437.

16. Davis DB, King JC. Cervical rib in early life. Am J Dis Child 1938;56:744.

17. Drapanas T, Curran WL. Thrombectomy in the treatment of "Effort" thrombosis of the axillary and subclavian veins. J Trauma 1966;6:107.

18. Eastcott HHG. Reconstruction of the subclavian artery for complications of cervical rib and thoracic outlet syndrome. Lancet 1962;2:1243.

19. Edmonson RL. Neurovascular compression syndromes of the upper extremity. South Med J 1965;58:754.

20. Edwards EA. Anatomic and clinical comments on shoulder girdle syndromes. In: WF Barker, ed. Surgical Treatment of Peripheral Vascular Disease. New York: McGraw-Hill; 1962.

21. Falconer MA, Li FWP. Resection of the first rib in costoclavicular compression of the brachial plexus. Lancet 1962;1:59.

22. Falconer MA, Weddell G. Costoclavicular compression of the subclavian artery and vein. Relation to the scalenus anticus syndrome. Lancet 1943;2:539.

23. Ferguson JB, Burford TH, Roper CL. Neurovascular compression at the superior thoracic aperture: surgical management. Ann Surg 1947;167:573.

24. Gage M, Parnell H. Scalenus anticus syndrome. Am J Surg 1947;73:252.

25. Gilliatt RW, Willison RG, Dietz V, Williams JR. Pheripheral conduction in patients with cervical rib and band. Ann Neurol 1978;4:124.

26. Gilroy J, Meyer JS. Compression of the subclavian artery as a cause of ischemic brachial neuropathy. Brain 1963;86:733.

27. Gruber W. Uber die halsrippen des menschen mit vergleichenden and anatomischen bemerkungen. Mem Acad Imp Sci St Petersburg 1869;7:Ser 13.

28. Haggart GE. Value of conservative management in cervico-brachial pain. JAMA 1948;137:508.

29. Halsted WS. An experimental study of circumscribed dilation of an artery immediately distal to a partially occluding band, and its bearing on the dilation of the subclavian artery observed in certain cases of cervical rib. J Exp Med 1916;24:271.

30. Harvey W. Exercitatio anatomica de motu cordis et sanguinis in animalibus. (1627) Edition 5. Leake CD (TRANS) Charles C. Thomas, Springfield, IL: 1970:36.

31. Hill RM. Vascular anomalies of the upper limb associated with cervical ribs. Br J Surg 1939;27:100.

32. Holman E. The obscure physiology of poststenotic dilatation: its relation to the development of aneurysms. J Thorac Surg 1954;28:109.

33. Hunauld. Sur le nombre des Cotes, Moindre ou plus grande qu'a l'ordinaire. Hist Acad Roy Sci Mem Paris, 1740.

34. Jebsen RH. Motor conduction velocities in the median and ulnar nerves. Arch Phys Med 1967;48:185.

35. Jelsma F. The scalenus anticus syndrome—end result of 115 cases: report of 5 illustrative cases. Int Clin 1940;4:219.

36. Kelly TR. Thoracic outlet syndrome. Am Surg 1979;190:657.

37. Keen WW. The symptomatology, diagnosis and surgical treatment of cervical ribs. Am J Med Sci 1907;133:173.

38. Kirgis HD, Reed AF. Significant anatomic relations in the syndrome of the scalene muscles. Am Surg 1948;127:1182.

39. Kirtley JA, Riddell DG, Stoney WS. Cervico-thoracic sympathectomy in the treatment of neurovascular abnormalities of the upper extremity. Experience in 76 patients. Ann Surg 1967;165:869.

40. Lang EK. Arteriographic diagnosis of the thoracic outlet syndrome. Radiology 1965;84:296.

41. Lang EK. Neurovascular compression syndromes. Dis Chest 1966;50:572.

42. Lang EK. Roentgenographic diagnosis of the neurovascular compression syndromes. Radiology 1962;79:58.

43. Lang EK, Hann EC, Luros TJ. External-internal carotid artery anastomosis and its correlation to RISA circulation studies. Radiology 1964;83:632.

44. Law AA. Adventitious ligaments simulating cervical ribs. Ann Surg 1920;72:497.

45. Lawson FC, McKenzie KG. The scalenus minimus muscle. Can Med Ass J 1951;65:358.

46. LeVay AD. First rib resection for relief of subclavian artery compression. Lancet 1945;2:164.

47. Lindskog GE. ed Thoracic and cardiovascular surgery with related pathology. New York: Appleton-Century-Crofts, 1962.

48. Lord JW Jr. Surgical management of shoulder girdle syndromes. AMA Arch Surg 1953;66:69.

49. Lord JW, Stone PW. Pectoralis minor tenotomy and anterior scalenotomy with special reference to the hyperabduction syndrome and "effort thrombosis" of the subclavian vein. Circulation 1956;13:537.

50. Machleder HI, Moll F, Verity A. The anterior scalene muscle in thoracic outlet compression syndrome. Histochemical and morphometric studies. Arch Surg 1986;121:1141.

51. Mahorner H, Castleberry JW, Coleman WO. Attempts to restore function in major veins which are the site of massive thrombosis. Ann Surg 1957;146:510.

52. McBurney RP, Howard H. Resection of the first rib for thoracic outlet syndrome. A Surg 1966;32:165.

53. Moore J Jr. Scalenus anticus syndrome. South Med J 1966;59:954.

54. Murphy JB. Case of cervical rib with symptoms resembling subclavian aneurysm. Ann Surg 1905;41:399.

55. Murphy JB. The clinical significance of cervical ribs. Surg Gynecol Obstet 1906;3:514.

56. Murphy T. Brachial neuritis caused by pressure of the first rib. Aust Med J 1910;15:582.

57. Naffziger HC. The scalenus syndrome. Surg Gynecol Obstet 1906;3:514.

58. Naffziger HC, Grant WT. Neuritis of the brachial plexus me-

chanical in origin: the scalenus syndrome. Surg Gynecol Obstet 1938;67:722.

59. Nelson RM, Davis RW. Collective review: thoracic outlet compression syndrome. Ann Thorac Surg 1969;8:437.

60. Nelson RM, Hess WE, Lyman JH. Venous obstruction with hypertrophy of an upper extremity due to osteochondroma. Surgery 1963;54:871.

61. Nelson RM, Jenson CB. Plotocostotomy for thoracic outlet obstruction syndrome (abstract). Circulation 36 1967;(Suppl. 2):198.

62. Ochsner A, Gage M, DeBakey ME. Scalenus anticus (Naffziger) syndrome. Am J Surg 1935;28:669.

63. Peet RM, Hendricksen JD, Guderson TP, et al. Thoracic outlet syndrome. Evaluation of a therapeutic exercise program. Proc Mayo Clinic 1956;31:281.

64. Raaf J. Surgery for cervical rib and scalenus anticus syndrome. JAMA 1955;157:219.

65. Riddell DH. Thoracic outlet compression: The role of anterior scalenotomy. J Miss Med 1961;11:284.

66. Riddell DH. Thoracic outlet syndrome: thoracic and vascular aspects. Clin Orthop 1967;51:53.

67. Riddell DH, Kirtley JA, Moore JL, Goduco RS. Scalenus anticus syndrome symptoms: evaluation and surgical treatment. Surgery 1960;47:115.

68. Rob CG, Standeven A. Arterial occlusion complicating thoracic outlet compression syndrome. Br Med J 1958;2:709.

69. Rogers L. Upper limb pain due to lesions of the thoracic outlet, the scalenus syndrome cervical rib and costoclavicular compression. Br Med J 1949;2:956.

70. Roos DB. New concepts of thoracic outlet syndrome that explain etiology, symptoms, diagnosis and treatment. Vasc Surg 1979;13:313.

71. Roos DB. Personal communication, 1968.

72. Roos DB. Thoracic outlet and carpal tunnel syndromes. In: Rutherford ed. Vascular Surgery. Philadelphia: Saunders, 1977.

73. Roos Db. Tranaxillary approach for first rib resection to relieve thoracic outlet syndrome. Ann Surg 1966;163:354.

74. Roos DB, Owens JC. Thoracic outlet syndrome. Arch Surg (Chicago) 1966;93:71.

75. Rosati LM, Lord JW. Neurovascular compression syndromes of the shoulder girdle. Modern Surgical Monographs New York: Grune & Stratton, 1961:168.

76. Rosenberg JC. Arteriographic demonstration of compression syndromes of the thoracic outlet. South Med J 1966;59:400.

77. Sargent P. Lesions of the brachial plexus associated with rudimentary ribs. Brain 1921;44:95.

78. Sargent P. Some points in the surgery of cervical ribs. In discussion of cervical ribs. Proc Roy Soc Med 1913;6:117.

79. Schein CJ, Haimovici J, Young H. Arterial thrombosis associated with cervical ribs: surgical considerations. Report of a case and review of literature. Surgery 1956;40:428.

80. Shenkin HA, Somach FM. Scalenotomy in patients with and without cervical ribs. Arch Surg (Chicago) 1963;87:892.

81. Silver D. The thoracic outlet syndrome. Practice of Surgery New York: Harper & Row, Vol. II, 1968:1.

82. Silver D. Thoracic outlet syndrome. Miss Med 1980;77:189.

83. Spurling RG, Bradford FK. Scalenus neurocirculatory compression. Ann Surg 1938;107:708.

84. Stammers FAR. Pain in the upper limb from mechanisms in the costoclavicular space. Lancet 1950;1:603.

85. Stopford JSB, Telford ED. Compression of the lower trunk of the brachial plexus by a first dorsal rib with a note on the surgical treatment. Br J Surg 1919;7:168.

86. Taylor MF. Twelve years experience with thoracic outlet syndrome. J Fla Med Assn 66#10, PP1022–1024, (October 1979).

87. Telford ED, Mottershead S. Pressure at the cervico-brachial junction. J Bone Joint Surg (Brit.) 1948;30:249.

88. Telford ED, Stopford JSB. The vascular complications of the cervical rib. Br J Surg 1937;18:559.

89. Todd TW. The descent of the shoulder after birth; its significance in the production of pressure symptoms on the lowest brachial trunk. Anat Anz 1912;41:385.

90. Todd TW. Posture and the cervical rib syndrome. Ann Surg 1922;75:105.

91. Urschel HC Jr, Paulson DL, and McNamara JJ. Thoracic outlet syndrome. Ann Thorac Surg 1968;6:1.

92. White JC, Poppel MH, Adams R. Congenital malformations of the first thoracic rib. Cause of brachial neuralgia which simulates cervical rib syndrome. Surg Gynecol Obstet 1945;81:643.

93. Willshire WH. Supernumerary first rib, clinical records. Lancet 1860;2:633.

94. Wilborn AJ, Lederman RJ. Evidence for conduction delay in thoracic outlet syndrome is challenged. N Engl J Med 1984;310:1052.

95. Wood VE, Twito R, Verska JM. Thoracic outlet syndrome. The result of first rib resection in 100 patients. Ortho Clin North Am 1988;19(1):131.

96. Wright IS. Neurovascular syndrome by hyperabduction of the arms. Am Heart J 1945;29:1.

97. Yiannikas C, Walsh JC. Somatosensory evoked responses in the diagnosis of thoracic outlet syndrome. J Neurol Neurosurg Psychiatry 1983;46:234.

17

Congenital Anomalies of the Base of the Skull and the Atlanto-Axial Joint

T.S. Whitecloud III and Mark R. Brinker

Introduction

Congenital anomalies of the base of the skull and atlanto-axial joint are uncommon conditions which arise from abnormal fetal development. While these abnormalities most often remain clinically silent in childhood, onset of symptoms following minor trauma or progressive deformity with aging may lead to bony impingement on neural and vascular structures.

Assessment of congenital anomalies of the base of the skull and proximal cervical spine is difficult. Radiographic evaluation of the pediatric cervical spine is encumbered by the wide variation in normal growth and ossification. Fixed bony deformities and associated congenital anomalies make patient positioning difficult and further complicate radiographic evaluation in both the adult or pediatric patient. Early recognition and prompt appropriate treatment of congenital anomalies of the base of the skull and upper cervical spine are essential.

Basilar Impression

Basilar impression is a deformity of the bony structures in the region of the foramen magnum. The osseous components surrounding the foramen magnum appear to bear the impression of the upper cervical spine and are invaginated upward. The base of the skull is pushed upward which may result in compression of the proximal cervical cord and the contents of the posterior cranial fossa or in impairment of blood flow or cerebrospinal fluid. The tip of the odontoid process lies in a more superior attitude and may protrude through the foramen magnum dangerously close to the brainstem.

While basilar impression is a relatively rare condition, it is the most common congenital anomaly of the atlanto-occipital articulation (1). Primary basilar impression is a congenital malformation which may be associated with a variety of vertebral anomalies. The Klippel-Feil syndrome, occipitalization of the atlas, odontoid malformation, hypoplasia of the atlas, achondroplasia, and bifid posterior arch of C1 have all been associated with primary basilar impression (2–4). The Arnold-Chiari malformation, syringomyelia, and kyphoscoliosis have also been seen with basilar impression (1, 5). Secondary basilar impression is the result of softening of the bony structures which comprise the base of the skull. The deformity typically develops in adulthood secondary to trauma, severe osteoporosis, osteogenesis imperfecta, osteomalacia, renal osteodystrophy, rickets, and Paget's disease (2, 3 6–9).

Clinical Findings

The signs and symptoms of basilar impression are related to impingement of neurologic and vascular structures. The diagnosis is often difficult to make in that symptoms are common to a vast array of neurologic disorders. The clinical picture is further clouded by symptoms of associated cranial vertebral anomalies, vertebral artery anomalies, and neurologic conditions (5, 10–12). Motor weakness, spasticity, and sensory defects are not uncommon findings. DeBarros et al. (10) have reported that paresthesias and weakness of the extremities were the most common complaints in symptomatic patients with pure basilar impression. Headache in the distribution of the greater occipital nerve is a common complaint. Ataxia, dysarthria, dysphasia, nystagmus, and unusual breathing patterns have been described (1, 10, 13). DeBarros et al. (10, 14) reported sexual impotence as a common finding in patients with basilar impression. Taylor and Chakravorty (15) have reported confusion and altered states of consciousness. Neurologic findings in basilar impression have often been confused with multiple sclerosis, amyotrophic lateral sclerosis, spinal cord and posterior fossa tumors, syringomyelia, and polio.

While primary basilar impression is present at birth, symptoms often do not develop until the second or third decade (10, 16). Hensinger and MacEwen (2) have suggested that this may be due to progressive ligamentous laxity and instability with aging. Other authors have suggested that the brain may become less tolerant of com-

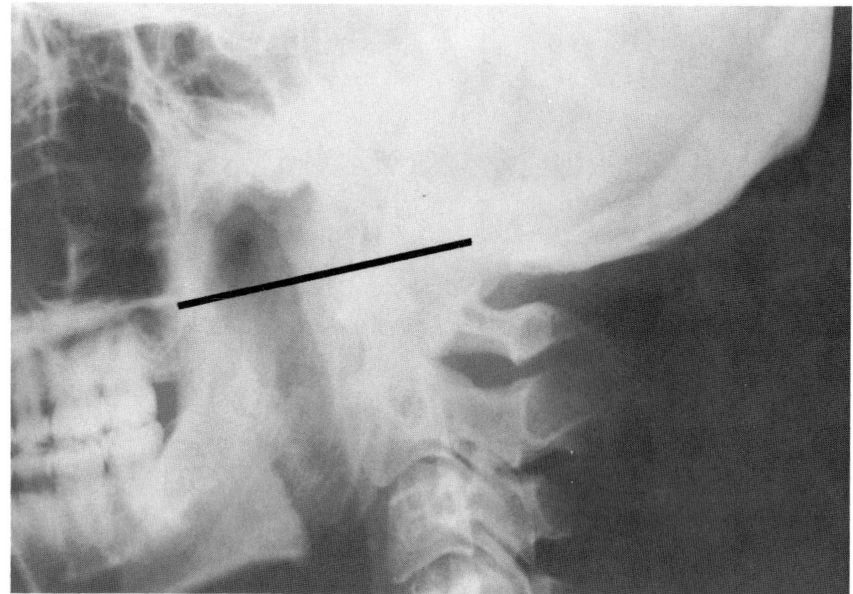

Figure 17.1. Lateral radiograph depicting Chamberlain's line which connects the dorsal edge of the hard palate with the posterior border of the foramen magnum.

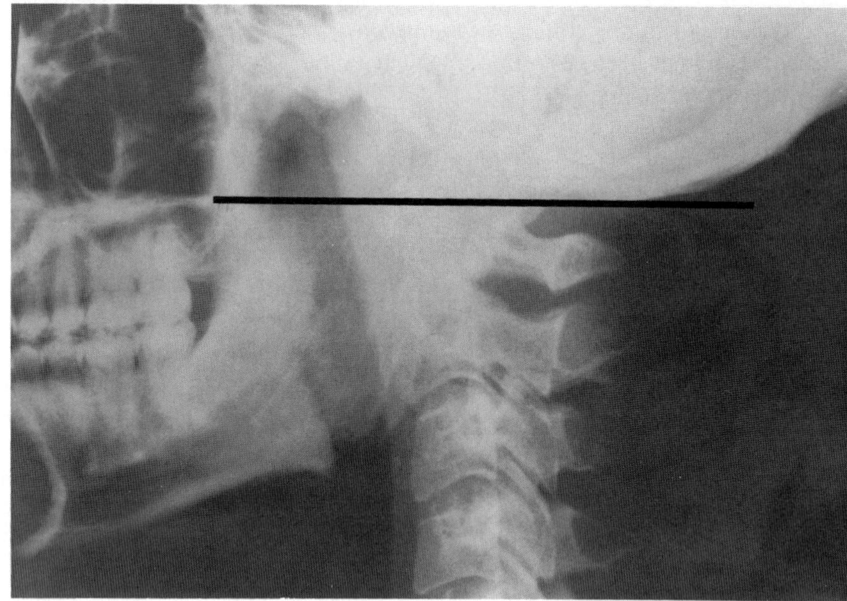

Figure 17.2. Lateral radiograph depicting McGregor's line which connects the posterior aspect of the hard palate with the most inferior aspect of the occiput.

pressive forces with aging (5, 16, 17). Additionally, temporary impingement of an aging sclerotic vertebral artery is more likely to lead to ischemic damage.

Radiographic Evaluation

Radiographic evaluation of basilar impression is difficult. A variety of radiographic criteria have been proposed in an attempt to simplify diagnosis. Chamberlain (16) felt that any projection of the odontoid process and body of C1 above a line connecting the posterior border of the foramen magnum and dorsal edge of the hard palate (Chamberlain's line) on a lateral radiograph constituted basilar impression (Fig. 17.1). McGregor (18) introduced a modification of Chamberlain's line because he felt the posterior edge of the foramen magnum was difficult to visualize on the lateral radiograph and was a moving reference point in advancing basilar impression. On the true lateral radiograph, McGregor's line connects the upper posterior edge of the hard palate and the most inferior point of the occipital curve (Fig. 17.2). McGregor suggested that the tip of the odontoid could project 4.5 mm above his line and be within the upper limit of normal. While Hinck et al. (9) have commented that McGregor's line represents the "most satisfactory available system for measurement" of basilar impression on lateral radiograph, results of their study suggest a wide range of normal odontoid projection and differences between men and women.

McRae and Barnum (19) base their line upon the opening of the foramen magnum (Fig. 17.3). The line is of value in assessing the position of the tip of the odontoid process relative to the opening of the foramen magnum.

Fischgold and Metzger (20) felt that McGregor's and Chamberlain's lines could be distorted by anatomical changes not involving the base of the skull (e.g., abnormally long or short odontoid process, high arch palate, abnormal structure of facial bones). The authors described the line connecting the two digastric grooves on anteroposterior laminograph as a method of assessing basilar impression. Hinck et al. (9) have commented that the digastric line is the best measurement for diagnosing basilar impression on anteroposterior radiograph. The normal distance from the digastric line to a line across the center of the atlanto-occipital joint is approximately 10 mm. In the presence of basilar impression this distance is reduced.

Various other measurements for assessing basilar impression have been described. Bull et al. (21) defined an angle formed by the intersection of a line along the plane of the hard palate and another line along the plane of the atlas (Fig. 17.4). Bull's angle is not normally greater than 13°, although abnormalities of the hard palate or excessive flexion or extension can lead to significant variation (9, 22). The basilar angle is defined at the angle formed by the intersection of a line drawn from the tuberculum sellae to the naison, with a line connecting the tuberculum with the anterior aspect of the foramen magnum. McGregor (18) has suggested that the basilar angle is normally 140° or less. The bimastoid line connects the tips of the mastoid processes. Decker et al. (23) have reported that the tip of the odontoid process normally lies

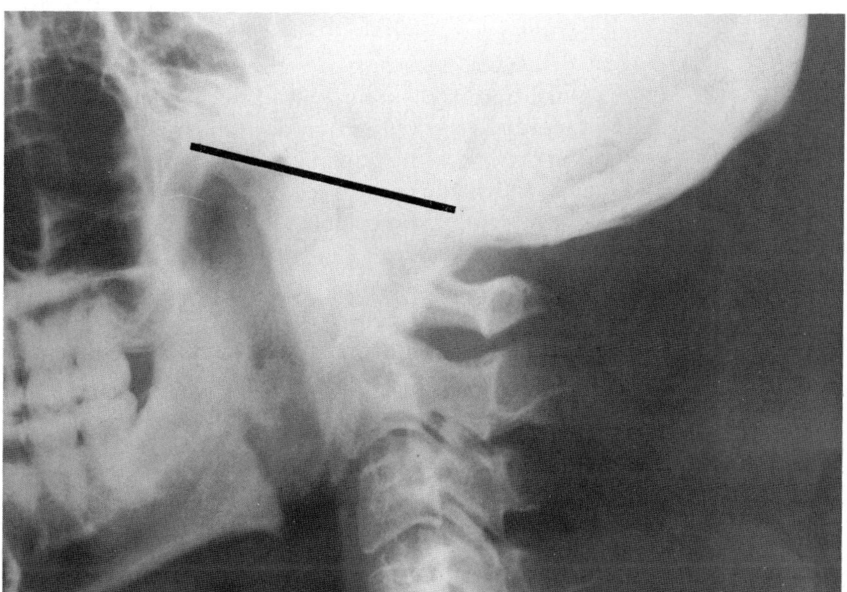

Figure 17.3. Lateral radiograph illustrating McRae's line which approximates the opening of the foramen magnum.

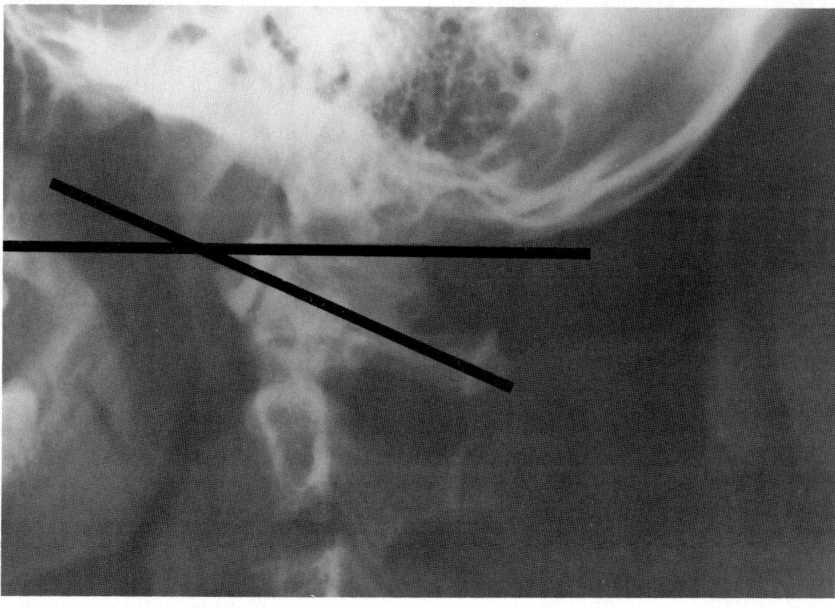

Figure 17.4. Lateral radiograph showing the construction of Bull's angle by the intersection of a line along the plane of the hard palate with a line along the plane of C1.

between 10 mm above and 3 mm below the bimastoid line. The temporomandibular line is used to measure the distance between the temporomandibular joint and the superior border of the anterior arch of C1 on either the anterior, posterior, or lateral radiograph. The distance in normal individuals is approximately 30 mm, but it becomes diminished with basilar impression (9, 24, 25). Finally, Klaus (26) described a height index, measuring the height of the line from the tip of the odontoid perpendicular to a line connecting the tuberculum sellae to the most superior aspect of the internal occipital protuberance. A Klaus height index of 30–36 mm is suggestive of basilar impression (26), although the normal range varies widely (9).

Treatment

The treatment of basilar impression depends on neurologic symptomatology and not radiographic findings. Anterior impingement from a hypermobile odontoid process is best treated with stabilization of the occipital cervical junction in extension (2). Anterior excision of the odontoid following initial stabilization in extension is indicated in cases with an irreducible odontoid. Impingement posteriorly is best treated with suboccipital craniectomy, and decompression with stabilization of the posterior arch of C1 (±C2). DeBarros et al. (10) have stressed the importance of opening the dura mater in order to lyse all constrictive posterior dural and arachnoid bands.

ATLANTO-OCCIPITAL FUSION

Atlanto-occipital fusion (occipitalization of the atlas) is a congenital condition of partial or complete fusion of the ring of C1 and the base of the skull (Fig. 17.5). Anterior fusion of the atlas and rim of the foramen magnum with an intact posterior arch is common. The position and/or size of the odontoid process is often abnormal, and the odontoid may be displaced posteriorly.

Additional anomalies of the proximal cervical spine are not uncommon. Fusion of the second and third cervical vertebrae was seen in 68% of McRae's patients with atlanto-occipital fusion (19). Fusion of the lower cervical vertebrae is less common but does occur in conjunction with occipitalization of the atlas.

The etiology of atlanto-occipital fusion has received much attention. Gladstone and Erichsen-Powell (27) suggested that occipitalization was a result of environmental factors. Gladstone and Wakey (28) attributed the anomaly to a genetic "weakness of germ cells." A number of authors (19, 29, 30) have suggested that failure of segmentation of somites may be the underlying factor.

Clinical Findings

Patients with atlanto-occipital fusion consistently display abnormal neck features which include short neck, low hairline, torticollis, and restricted range of motion (2, 5, 19, 31). Approximately one in four individuals with occipitalization displays associated congenital anomalies including jaw anomalies, cleft palate, cervical ribs, anomalies of the nasal cartilage, external ear deformities, hypospadias, and urinary tract anomalies (5, 19, 31).

Much like basilar impression, the signs and symptoms of atlanto-occipital fusion are related to bony impingement on neuronal tissue. A number of authors have commented that an odontoid of abnormal size, position, or mobility is the offending structure in symptomatic patients with occipitalization (19, 31–33). McRae and Barnum (19) have suggested that if the tip of the odontoid process is inferior to McRae's line, the patient will likely be asymptomatic. These authors believe that if the tip of the odontoid is in a position superior to McRae's line and angled posteriorly, crowding of anterior neurologic structures is likely. This idea is consistent with the clinical findings of pyramidal track signs (muscle wasting, weakness, spasticity, abnormal reflexes, and ataxia) which are commonly found in patients with occipitalization (19, 31). Dysphasia, diplopia, and tinnitis are less common complaints and are thought to result from compression of the cranial nerves.

Signs and symptoms of involvement of the posterior columns (loss of proprioception and vibration) are less common and result from posterior compression by the posterior margin of the foramen magnum or a dural band. Dull headache and scalp tenderness in the distribution of the greater occipital nerve are both common clinical findings. Vertical and/or horizontal gaze nystagmus is not uncommon and is suggestive of tonsillar herniation. The onset of symptoms in atlanto-occipital fusion is insidious and generally occurs between ages 20 and 40 years (34). Mild trauma has been associated with the gradual onset of symptoms in a significant portion of cases (19, 31, 33). Sudden onset of symptoms and sudden death associated with the anomaly have been reported (35).

As is the case with basilar impression, progressive ligament laxity with aging has been implicated as the etiology for the late onset of symptoms in occipitalization. Several authors have suggested that repeated neck flexion and extension leads to progressive ligament laxity about the odontoid (19, 31–33). Additionally, aging neurologic structures may become less tolerant of episodic compression by the odontoid process. Likewise, aging sclerotic vertebral vessels may become less compliant and more susceptible to extrinsic compression.

Radiographic Evaluation

Radiographic evaluation of the atlanto-occipital articulation is often difficult. Laminograms are useful in delineating bony fusion of the anterior arch of the atlas and the base of the skull. Computed tomographic (CT) scan, myelography, or magnetic resonance imaging (MRI) are useful

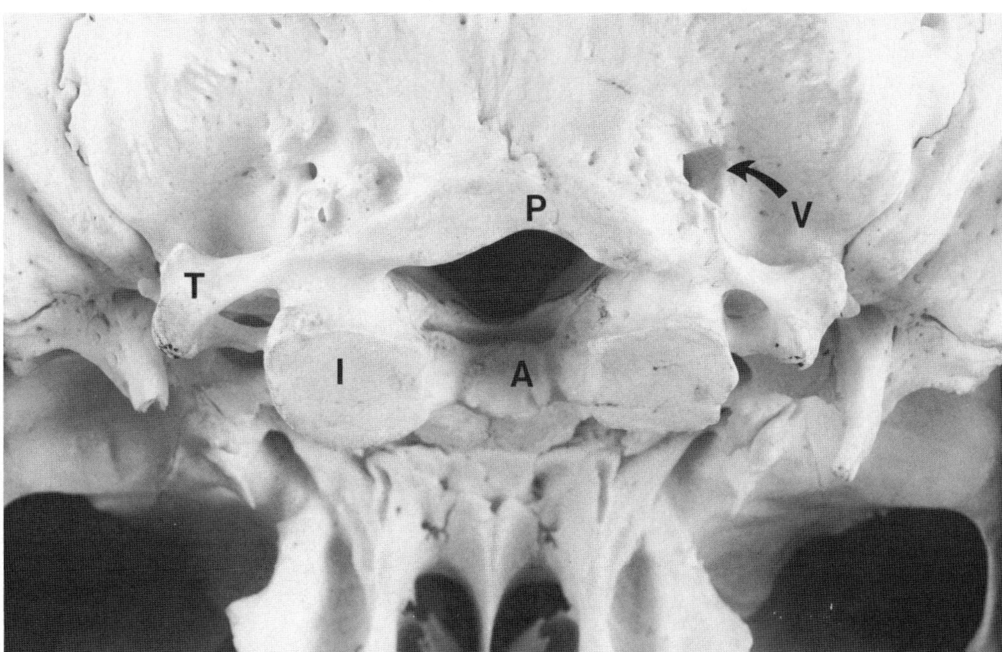

Figure 17.5. Photograph of the inferior aspect of a skull with occipitalization of the atlas. (*T*) is a transverse process; (*I*) is an inferior articular facet; (*P*) is the posterior arch of the atlas; (*A*) is the anterior arch of the atlas. Occipitalization of the atlas has caused the vertebral artery to enter the cranial cavity through the "vertebral foramen" (*V*).

in delineating impingement of the cord by the posterior ring of C1, the odontoid process, and narrowing of the spinal canal secondary to posterior positioning of the atlas.

In occipitalization, evaluation of the shape, length, and orientation of the odontoid process is of utmost importance. McRae and Barnum (19) have stated that approximately 60% of patients with the anomaly will have greater than 3 mm of displacement of the odontoid with respect to the anterior arch of the atlas. The authors have stated that a neurologic deficit is likely if the space available for the cord (SAC; the distance between the odontoid process and the posterior limb of the foramen magnum) is less than 19 mm on lateral radiograph (Fig. 17.6). Additionally, McRae and Barnum (19) have stated that patients typically develop neurologic complications when the odontoid projects superior to the opening of the foramen magnum.

Radiographic examination of atlanto-occipital fusion must include evaluation for associated pathology. Congenital fusion of C2–C3, and abnormalities in the inferior facets and transverse processes are common findings (34, 36). Myelography with post-contrast CT scanning is useful in delineating posterior dural bands. Blockage of myelographic material at the level of the foramen magnum is suggestive of cerebellar herniation (5). Vertebral angiography demonstrating a posterior inferior cerebellar artery in the cervical canal is also highly suggestive of herniation.

Radiographic evaluation of the atlanto-occipital region is difficult in the young child. At birth there are 5–9 mm of radiolucency in the posterior arch of the atlas (34). Ossification begins in the lateral masses and progresses posteriorly, ossifying by 4 years of age (37). Ossification of the anterior arch of the atlas typically is from the midline, gradually extending to the lateral masses by 3 years of age.

Treatment

Nonoperative treatment of symptomatic atlanto-occipital fusion consists of immobilization. Failure of conservative therapy necessitates surgical intervention. Posterior spinal fusion from the occiput to C2 is the treatment of choice in the case of a hypermobile odontoid process compressing anterior structures (2). Reduction of the odontoid should be obtained via skeletal traction prior to surgery. Operative reduction is associated with an unacceptably high mortality rate and is to be avoided (33, 38). Suboccipital craniectomy with excision of the posterior arch of C1 and dural bands are recommended in cases of atlanto-occipital fusion where posterior symptoms predominate.

CONGENITAL ANTLANTO-AXIAL INSTABILITY

Congenital atlanto-axial instability may arise from (1) laxity of the transverse ligament; (2) abnormalities of the odontoid process; and (3) atlanto-occipital fusion. Episodic neurological abnormalities may result from even minor trauma and may progress to become totally disabling. The clinical significance of the instability is the potential for reduction in size of the spinal canal with impingement of

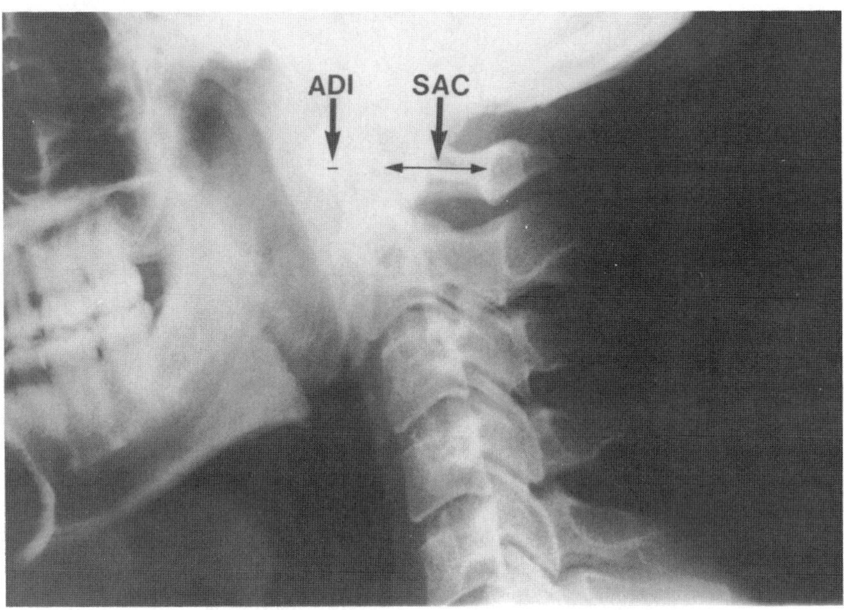

Figure 17.6. Lateral radiograph of the proximal cervical spine showing the *SAC* (space available for the cord) and the *ADI* (atlas dens interval).

neural structures. Atlanto-axial instability has been associated with a number of conditions including: Down's syndrome, congenital scoliosis, osteogenesis imperfecta, neurofibromatosis, Morquio's syndrome, Larsen's syndrome, short or webbed neck, Sprengel's deformity, and congenital heart defects. Associated spinal anomalies often result in scoliosis.

Approximately one-half of all rotational motion in the cervical spine occurs between C1 and C2. Extension between the atlas and axis is normally limited to approximately 10°; flexion is limited to 5°. In conjunction with rotational motion, the atlas and axis tend to shift laterally with respect to one another (2). The joint accounts for a great deal of motion and is consequently the least stable articulation of the cervical spine. The lack of stability of the atlanto-axial joint is accentuated by the fact that it is surrounded by two relatively immobile joints (atlanto-occipital and C2–C3).

Clinical Findings

Fielding et al. (39) have stated that "the patient with atlanto-axial instability leads a precarious existence." Indeed, the result of anterior or rotary displacement of C1 on C2 results in symptoms ranging from mild neurologic involvement to death. Symptoms typically manifest in adulthood and are rare before age 20 (2). Progression of symptoms with age is likely the result of increasing ligament laxity and less forgiving neural structures. Because of the changing relationship of C1 and C2, symptoms are inconsistent and transient and include paresthesia, tetraparesis, torticollis, blindness, and unconsciousness. With anterior impingement, signs and symptoms of muscle weakness and wasting, pyramidal tract irritation, hyporeflexia, ataxia, and spasticity are seen (40). With impingement of neural structures posterior to the odontoid process, posterior column symptoms become manifest. Nystagmus and coordination problems are observed with cerebellar herniation. Compromise of flow through the vertebral arteries results in dizziness, syncope, and seizures (41).

Nagashima (42) divided clinical manifestations of atlanto-axial dislocation in patients with congenital anomalies of the odontoid into acute (traumatic), delayed (traumatic), and chronic (nontraumatic). Immediate death may occur with the acute-type dislocation if bony displacement is great and there is severe damage to the cervical cord or vertebral arteries (42, 43). Survivors of acute atlanto-axial dislocation typically manifest symptoms of spinal shock. In the delayed type, onset of symptoms occurs months to years following the inciting trauma (42). Neurologic symptoms are of gradual onset and often progress to become totally disabling. In the chronic type there is no history of trauma, but symptoms progress to permanent cervical myelopathy (42).

Signs and symptoms in children with atlanto-axial instability are variable. Generalized weakness is seen in a great number of patients. Syncope, tetraplegia, torticollis, and dysesthesia have also been reported (42).

Radiographic Evaluation

The stability of the atlanto-axial joint may be assessed via lateral radiograph. The atlanto-dens interval (ADI) is the distance between the posterior edge of the anterior arch of the atlas, and the anterior portion of the odontoid process (Fig. 17.6). This interval is useful in assessing the space available for the cord (SAC). The internal span of the ring of the atlas on the lateral radiograph (anterior/posterior span) of an adult measures approximately 30 mm (44, 45). Steel (46) has suggested that the odontoid and spinal cord each occupy 10 mm of the 30 mm ring, and that there is a 10 mm area of "free space" available for displacement.

The normal ADI in adults is less than 3 mm (40). Even a small increase in the ADI in neutral is suggestive of disruption of the transverse ligament. Fielding et al. (39) have suggested that an ADI of 3–5 mm implicates disruption of the transverse ligament. An ADI of 5–10 mm suggests additional ligamentous damage, and an ADI of 10 mm or more represents disruption of all ligaments. Fielding et al. (39) have recommended flexion-extension radiographs in all suspected cases of atlanto-axial instability where there are no signs of cord involvement. Flexion and extension of the cervical spine should be performed by the patient alone. Changes in the ADI and SAC with flexion-extension are important in assessing degree and direction of displacement.

The ADI is of little value in evaluating patients with anomalies of the odontoid process. In this patient population, measurement of the SAC is of greater clinical value. The SAC represents the distance from the posterior ring of the atlas to the posterior aspect of the odontoid process or posterior aspect of C2 (whichever value is less). In the patient with atlanto-axial instability and a freely mobile odontoid process (as in os odontoideum), flexion and extension result in a reduction in the SAC with no change in the ADI.

McRae (36) studied the relationship between neurologic involvement and SAC and suggested that a measurement of less than 19 mm was always accompanied by symptomatology. Greenberg (32) suggested that in the adult cervical spine, cord compression always occurs if the anterior/posterior diameter behind the odontoid is 14 mm or less and never occurs if the diameter is 18 mm or more. More recently, Spierlings and Braakman (47) have reported that 13 mm or less of SAC is associated with neurologic sequelae. Fielding et al. (45) have suggested that anterior displacement of the atlas on the axis is less dangerous in the patient with an abnormal odontoid which may be carried forward with the atlas.

The normal ADI interval in children is believed to be less than 4 mm (39, 48). Locke et al. (48) studied lateral radiographs of 200 normal pediatric patients and reported no cases of ADI greater than 4 mm. The authors recommended radiographs be performed in the neutral position and caution that an ADI greater than 4 mm was suggestive of atlanto-axial subluxation. Normal values for the SAC in children vary with age (40, 49). The diameter of the SAC on the lateral radiograph is greatest at the atlas and progressively narrows to C5.

Myelography is of value in defining areas of impingement in atlanto-axial instability. Several authors have recommended the use of gas or water-soluble contrast rather than oil contrast (36, 50–52). CT scan in conjunction with myelography may be useful in evaluating the SAC (50, 52). If available, magnetic resonance imaging in flexion and extension is a useful diagnostic test.

Treatment

Treatment of atlanto-axial instability is dependent upon the etiology and extent of the instability as well as the patient's activity level (2, 39). Fielding et al. (39) have stated that "even when there is minimum instability, trivial trauma superimposed on an already weakened and compromised structure can be catastrophic."

Fielding et al. (39) suggest that the indication for spinal fusion in atlanto-axial instability is instability with persistent cervical symptoms, evidence of cord or brain involvement, or an ADI (or atlanto-axial distance in cases of odontoid pathology) greater than 5 mm. Intraoperative reduction is associated with an unacceptably high rate of mortality and morbidity (31, 33). Preoperative skeletal traction is useful for preoperative reduction or for intraoperative control of the atlanto-axial joint. Fielding et al. (39) do not employ preoperative traction in asymptomatic patients with less than 7 mm of displacement. Fielding et al. (39) have reported favorable results in their series of

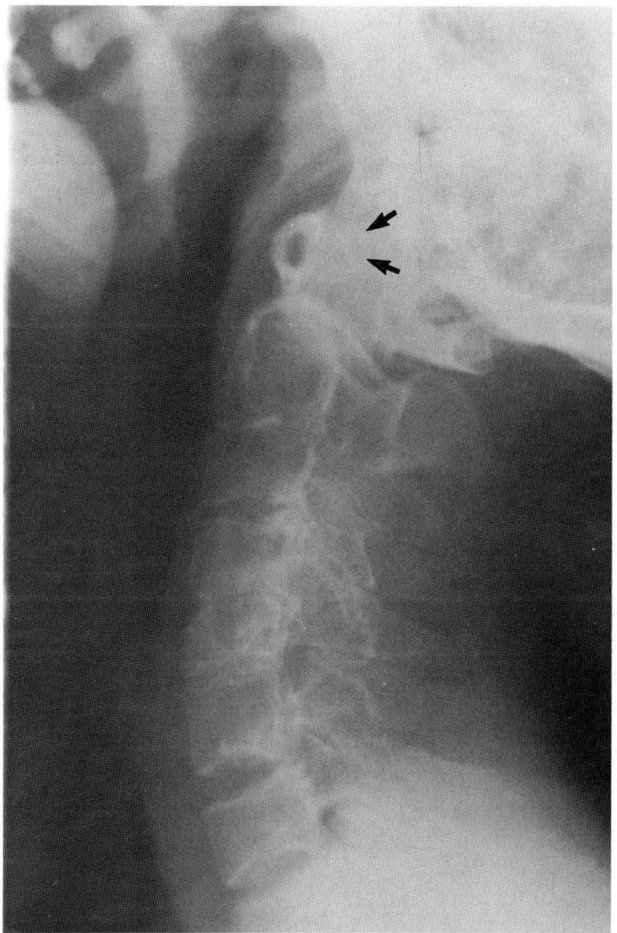

Figure 17.7. Lateral radiograph of a case of os odontoideum. Arrows indicate oval free ossicle in the orthotopic position.

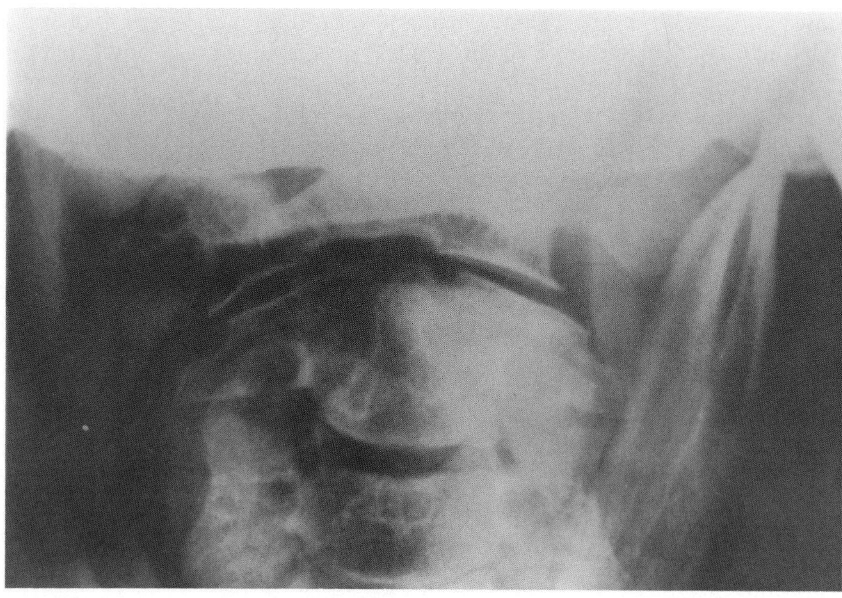

Figure 17.8. Anteroposterior radiograph of a 66-year-old white male who presented with a complaint of progressive parasthesia to the upper extremities over a 2-year period. Radiograph shows hypoplastic odontoid process.

46 patients receiving atlanto-axial fusion and suggest more extensive fusion in patients with: widespread bone destruction, deficient posterior arch of C1, widespread infection, odontoid herniation into the foramen magnum, additional congenital anomalies of the base of the skull and proximal cervical spine, or significant irreducible anterior displacement of C1 on C2.

CONGENITAL ANOMALIES OF THE ODONTOID PROCESS

Three types of congenital anomalies of the odontoid process have been described in the literature (41, 42, 53–70). Odontoid aplasia (or agenesis) is an uncommon anomaly characterized by complete absence of the odontoid process. Odontoid hypoplasia is characterized by partial absence of the odontoid process with a short, stubby odontoid whose superior border is typically at the level of C1–C2 articulation. Os odontoideum, the most common anomaly of the odontoid, is characterized by a smooth-bordered, round ossicle of bone separated from the axis. If the ossicle is located where the odontoid tip normally would be, it is said to be orthotopic; if the ossicle is located near the base of the occiput in the region of the foramen magnum, it is termed "dystopic." In practical terms, distinguishing aplasia, hypoplasia, and os odontoideum is of limited value. The three conditions typically manifest as an atlanto-axial instability with identical clinical signs, symptoms, and treatment. The distinction between the three anomalies is based on radiographic findings.

The frequency of anomalies of the odontoid process is uncertain. Fielding et al. (53) have suggested that the odontoid abnormality is often discovered on radiographic examination following head or neck trauma or following spontaneous onset of symptoms. Recognition of odontoid anomalies is essential as they result in atlanto-axial instability with neurologic involvement and even death. With an increasing index of suspicion, odontoid lesions are being recognized more commonly. In 1963, Wolin (57) reported an average age of diagnosis of 30 years in a series of patients with os odontoideum. By comparison, Fielding et al. (53) reported an average age at diagnosis of 18.9 years in their 1980 report. Odontoid anomalies are particularly more common in individuals with Down's syndrome, the Klippel-Feil syndrome, and certain skeletal and spondyloepiphyseal dysplasias (33, 47, 71–81).

The etiology of os odontoideum remains uncertain. Theories for a congential origin include failure of fusion of the apex of ossiculum terminale to the odontoid and failure of fusion of the odontoid process to C2. Arguments against these theories are that the ossiculum terminale is significantly smaller than the ossicle seen in os odontoideum and that failure of fusion of the odontoid to C2 would result in a significant defect in C2 (because a substantial portion of the axis comes from the odontoid) which is not seen in os odontoideum (2, 80).

Several authors have suggested that os odontoideum and odontoid hypoplasia may arise as a result of trauma or infection (36, 53, 57, 76, 82–86). Fielding et al. (53) reported a series of patients with os odontoideum who previously had normal cervical spine radiographs following a traumatic episode. The authors suggest that the etiology of os odontoideum is trauma rather than a congenital malformation and that an unrecognized odontoid fracture with a precarious blood supply results in a nonunion of the odontoid. The authors also suggest that following fracture of the odontoid, the alar ligaments contract, pulling the proximal odontoid fragments superiorly, and significantly separating the fragments.

Clinical Findings

Patients with anomalies of the odontoid may present with local neck pain, stiffness or spasm, upper or lower extremity weakness, episodes of paresis or paresthesias, headaches, torticollis, or gait disturbances (33, 53, 87). Neck pain, torticollis, and headaches may be due to local irritation of the atlanto-axial articulation (2). Neurologic symptoms arise as a result of displacement of C1 on C2 with spinal cord compression. Trauma is often associated with the onset of symptoms, and the anomaly is discovered upon radiographic examination.

When clinical symptoms are due to local joint irritation (neck pain, torticollis, headaches) the likelihood of a favorable outcome is excellent (53, 55, 69, 88). Patients exhibiting transient weakness of the extremities following trauma usually do not suffer any permanent loss of function (2). Fielding et al. (53) have stated that patients who experience an insidious onset of symptoms with progressive neurologic impairment are at a significant risk for permanent neurologic deficit. The neurologic insult may involve anterior and posterior structures, and weakness and ataxia are not uncommon findings (2). Sensory defects, spasticity, clonus, deep tendon reflex abnormalities, and loss of proprioception are less common findings. Rarely, patients present with signs and symptoms of cerebral and brainstem ischemia, mental deterioration, syncope, vertigo, visual disturbances, and seizures (39, 62, 69, 89).

Radiographic Evaluation

Os Odontoideum

Radiographic evaluation in os odontoideum reveals a radiolucent gap between the body of the axis and the odontoid process (Fig. 17.7). In children less than 5 years of age, the radiolucent gap of os odontoideum may be mistaken for the normal epiphyseal line. In young children, radiographic evidence of motion between the odontoid and the body of the axis confirms the diagnosis of os odontoideum (90).

A number of authors have noted that the radiographic appearance of a traumatic nonunion of the odontoid process is often quite similar to that of os odontoideum (36, 57). The radiolucent gap in os odontoideum typically appears to be wide with smooth margins and extends above the level of the superior facets of C2. In the case of a traumatic nonunion, the gap between the fragments is typically narrow with an irregular border. In os odontoideum, the free ossicle is typically oval in shape with a uniform rounded-off cortex (55, 90).

Radiographic evaluation should include lateral views in flexion and extension and an open mouth (odontoid) view. Tomograms may be of value when plain films are difficult to interpret. Stress views with the patient actively flexing and extending should be obtained, and the displacement of C1 on C2 should be noted. Displacement is obtained by measuring the anteroposterior distance between the posterior aspect of the body of C2 and the posterior aspect of the anterior arch of C1. Hensinger et al. (90) have suggested that a measurement greater than 3 mm indicates pathology. Additionally, the SAC should be measured and documented.

Aplasia and Hypoplasia of the Odontoid

Aplasia of the odontoid process may be diagnosed with a standard radiographic series. The odontoid is typically absent on the open mouth view, and a depression may be seen between the superior articular facets (2). In odontoid hypoplasia, a short osseous remnant of the odontoid process is observed (Fig. 17.8). Lateral laminographs may be of value in evaluating the odontoid process when surrounding bone obscures visualization.

Treatment

There is no consensus of opinion as to the preferred treatment of the asymptomatic or once symptomatic now

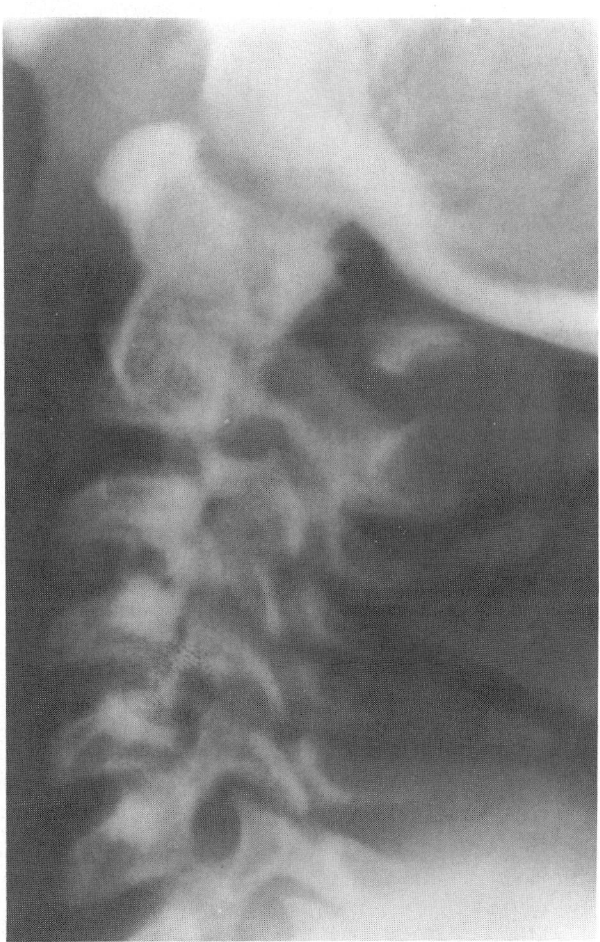

Figure 17.9. Lateral radiograph of an asymptomatic patient with failure of fusion of the neural arches of the atlas.

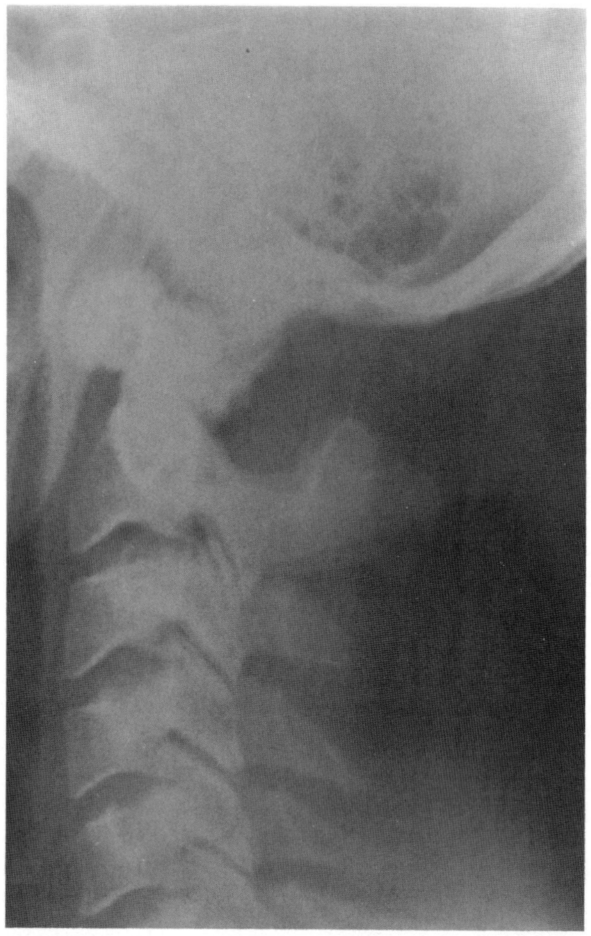

Figure 17.10. Lateral radiograph of a 34-year-old white male who presented with a complaint of diffuse back pain for 1 week. Radiograph reveals complete absence of the posterior arch of C1.

asymptomatic patient that has an anomaly of the odontoid. Shepard (91) believes that risk of neurologic catastrophe in patients with anomalies of the odontoid is significant enough that he recommends surgical stabilization in all cases. Other authors (55, 88, 92, 93) have suggested that surgery is associated with a significant risk of mortality and increasing neurologic deficit. These authors recommend surgical intervention only in those patients with progressive or recurrent neurological symptoms; all other patients should be instructed to avoid activities associated with head or neck trauma.

Most authors agree that surgical intervention is indicated with persistent neck complaints, or instability greater than 5 mm, or progressive instability (2, 53). Reduction of the atlanto-axial joint should be obtained via careful positioning of the patient or skeletal traction prior to surgery. Surgical reduction is associated with morbidity and mortality and is not recommended (92). Hensinger and MacEwen (2) have recommended that the patient remain in the reduced position for 1 to 2 weeks preoperatively in order to allow return of neurologic function.

Fielding et al. (94) have recommended surgical stabilization via posterior cervical fusion of C1–C2, with wire fixation and iliac bone graft. Arthrodesis of the occiput to C2 (with postoperative immobilization in extension) has been recommended in the patient with significant neurologic deficit (2, 55). An unreducible dislocation of C1 on C2 is a difficult problem and is beyond the scope of this discussion.

CONGENITAL ANOMALIES OF THE RING OF THE ATLAS AND AXIS

Ossification of C1 begins during the 7th week of intrauterine development (95). At birth, the anterior arch of the atlas is cartilaginous. Formation of the anterior arch occurs via extension from the lateral masses. The anterior arch of C1 normally fuses to the lateral masses by 6 to 8 years of age (96, 97). Ossification of the posterior arch of the atlas proceeds dorsally from the lateral masses. Cartilage separates the neural arches in the midline posteriorly at the time of birth. The ossification center for the posterior tubercle of C1 appears between the neural arches in the second year (95). Fusion of the posterior arches occurs during the 3rd or 4th year (96–98). Defects in the posterior arch of C1 range from midline cleft to partial or complete arch absence (unilateral or bilateral) (99). The arch and spinous process of the axis arise from a pair of cartilage centers (100).

Congenital defects of the ring of the atlas and axis are caused by failure of fusion of the synchondroses of the developing cervical vertebrae. Defects of the anterior arch of the atlas are extremely rare (95–97, 101). Geipel (101) reported a 0.1% incidence of clefts in the anterior arch of the atlas in 2749 postmortem specimens, and found no cases of anterior arch aplasia. While defects of the posterior arch of the atlas are extremely rare, they occur at least four times as often as those of the anterior arch (95, 96) (Figs. 17.9 and 17.10). Schulze and Buurman (99) have suggested that congenital defects of the posterior elements of the axis are far more rare than those of the atlas (100) (Fig. 17.11).

Congenital defects in the ring of the atlas and axis may be asymptomatic or may present with neurologic symptoms secondary to atlanto-axial instability. Radiographic evaluation of the cervical spine is often performed following minor trauma to the head and neck with or without symptoms. Malrotation and instability between C1 and C2 are not an uncommon finding in the case of an arch defect. Radiographs of the cervical spine which include oblique views are helpful in demonstrating arch defects. Lateral radiographs often show soft tissue swelling anterior to C1 with congenital absence of a portion of the anterior arch (95). CT scan is useful in delineating the location and extent of bony defects. Careful radiograph evaluation is

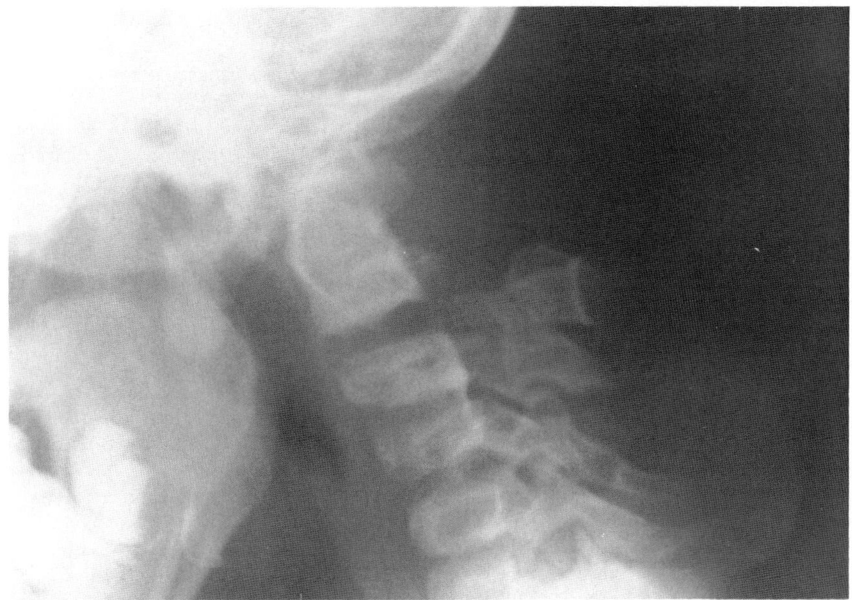

Figure 17.11. Lateral radiograph of the cervical spine (in extension) shows absence of the posterior arch of C1, failure of fusion of the posterior arch of C2, and fusion of the posterior elements of C2 and C3.

also useful in differentiating an arch fracture from a congenital defect.

Treatment in patients with arch defects of C1 and C2 is dependent upon instability and neurologic symptoms. When nonsurgical treatment is the chosen therapy, careful follow-up evaluation is mandatory.

ACKNOWLEDGMENT

The authors wish to acknowledge Charles M. Nice, M.D., and Edward H. Tan, M.D., of the Department of Radiology, Tulane University School of Medicine, for assistance in preparation of this chapter. The authors also wish to acknowledge Judi Clay for editorial assistance.

REFERENCES

1. Raynor RB. Congenital malformations of the base of the skull: the Arnold-Chiari malformation. The cervical spine. 2nd ed. Philadelphia: J.B. Lippincott, 1989:226–235.

2. Hensinger RN, MacEwen GD. Congenital anomalies of the spine. In: Rothman RH, Simeone FA, eds. The spine. 2nd ed. Philadelphia: W.B. Saunders Company, 1982:188–216.

3. Dolan KD. Cervicobasilar relationships. Radiol Clin North Am 1977;15:155–166.

4. Luyendij KW, Matricoli B, Thomeer RT. Basilar impression in an achondroplastic dwarf. Causative role in tetraparesis. Acta Neurochir 1978;41:243–253.

5. Spillane JD, Pallis C, Jones AM. Developmental abnormalities in the region of the foramen magnum. Brain 1957;80:11–48.

6. Dirheimer Y, Babin E. Basilar impression and hereditary fragility of the bones. Neuroradiology 1971;3:41–43.

7. Chakrabarti AK, Johnson SC, Samantray SK, Reddy ER. Osteomalacia, myopathy and basilar impression. J Neurol Sci 1974;23:227–235.

8. Epstein BS, Epstein JA. The association of cerebellar tonsillar herniation with basilar impression incident to Paget's disease. AJR Am J Roentgenol 1969;107:535–542.

9. Hinck VC, Hopkins CE, Savara BS. Diagnostic criteria of basilar impression. Radiology 1961;76:572–585.

10. DeBarros MC, Farias W, Ataide L, Lins S. Basilar impression and Arnold-Chiari malformation — a study of 66 cases. J Neurol Neurosurg Psychiatry 1968;31:596–605.

11. Hertel G, Nadjmi M, Kinze J. A statistical comparative study of the basilar impression in syringomyelia. Eur Neurol 1974;11:363–372.

12. Bernini F, Elefante R, Smaltino F, Tedeschi G. Angiographic study of vertebral artery in cases of deformities of the occipito-cervical joint. AJR Am J Roentgenol 1969;107:526–529.

13. Scoville WB, Sherman IJ. Playbasia, report of 10 cases. Ann Surg 1951;133:496–502.

14. DeBarros MC, Da Silva WF, Filho HCDA, Spinelli C. Disturbances of sexual potency in patients with basilar impression and Arnold-Chiari malformation. J Neurol Neurosurg Psychiatry 1975;38:598–600.

15. Taylor AR, Chakravorty BC. Clinical syndromes associated with basilar impression. Arch Neurol 1964;10:475–484.

16. Chamberlain WE. Basilar impression (platybasia) — a bizarre developmental anomaly of the occipital bone and upper cervical spine with striking and misleading neurologic manifestations. Yale J Biol Med 1939;11:487–496.

17. McRae DL. The significance of abnormalities of the cervical spine. AJR Am J Roentgenol 1960;84:3–25.

18. McGregor M. The significance of certain measurements of the skull in the diagnosis of basilar impression. Br J Radiol 1948;21:171–181.

19. McRae DL, Barnum AS. Occipitalization of the atlas. AJR Am J Roentgenol 1953;70:23–46.

20. Fischgold H, Metzger J. Etude radiotomographique de l'impression basilaire. Rev Rhum 1952;19:261–264.

21. Bull JWD, Nixon WLB, Pratt RTC. Radiological criteria and familial occurrence of primary basilar impression. Brain 1955;78:229–247.

22. Bergerhoff W. Uber die messtechnische beurteilung der basilaren impression im rontgenbild. Zentralbl Neurochir 1958;18:149–162.

23. Decker K, Fischgold H, Hacker H, Metzger J. Entwicklungsstorungen am atlanto-okzipitalen ubergang. Fortschr Geb Rontgenstr 1956;84:47–57.

24. Fischgold H, Lievre JA, Simon J. Indice radiographique de profil de l'impression basilaire. Rev Rhum 1959;26:72–75.

25. Fissore O. Arc anterieur de l'atlas et articulations temporo-maxillaires dans l'impression basilaire. Paris: These, 1958.

26. Klaus E. Roatgendiagnostik der platybasie und basilaren impression. Weitere Erfahrungen mit einer never untersuchungsmetnode. Fortschr Geb Rontgenstr 1957;86:460–469.

27. Gladstone RJ, Erichsen-Powell W. Manifestations of occipital vertebrae and fusion of the atlas with the occipital bone. J Anat Physiol 1914–1915;49:190–209.

28. Gladstone RJ, Wakely PG. Variations of the occipito-atlantal joint in relation to the metameric structure of the cranio-vertebral region. J Anat 1924–1925;59:195–216.

29. Hadley LA. Atlanto-occipital fusion, ossiculum terminale and occipital vertebra as related to basilar impression with neurological symptoms. AJR Am J Roentgenol 1948;59:511–524.

30. Moore KL, ed. The developing human. 3rd ed. Philadelphia: W.B. Saunders, 1982.

31. Bharucha EP, Dastur HM. Craniovertebral anomalies (a report of 40 cases). Brain 1964;87:469–480.

32. Greenberg AD. Atlanto-axial dislocations. Brain 1968;91:655–684.

33. Wadia NH. Myelopathy complicating congenital atlanto-axial dislocation. Brain 1967;90:449–472.

34. Hensinger RN. Anomalies of the atlas. The cervical spine. 2nd ed. Philadelphia: J.B. Lippincott, 1989:244–247.

35. Hadley LA, ed. The Spine. Springfield, IL: Charles C. Thomas, 1956.

36. McRae DL. Bony abnormalities in the region of the foramen magnum: correlation of the anatomic and neurologic findings. Acta Radiol 1953;40:335–354.

37. VonTorklus D, Gehle W, eds. The upper cervical spine. New York: Grune and Stratton, 1972.

38. Sinh G, Pandya SK. Treatment of congenital atlanto-axial dislocations. Proc Aust Assoc Neurol 1968;5:507–514.

39. Fielding JW, Hawkins RJ, Ratzan SA. Spine fusion for atlanto-axial instability. J Bone Joint Surg 1976;58-A:400–407.

40. Hinck VC, Hopkins CE, Savara BS. Sagital diameter of the cervical spinal canal in children. Radiology 1962;79:97–108.

41. Glannestras NJ, Mayfield FH, Provencio FP, Maurer J. Congenital absence of the odontoid process. A case report. J Bone Joint Surg 1964;46-A:839–843.

42. Nagashima C. Atlanto-axial dislocation due to agenesis of the os odontoideum or odontoid. J Neurosurg 1970;33:270–280.

43. Watson-Jones R. ed. Fractures and joint. 4th ed. Injuries. Baltimore: Williams and Wilkins, 1952.

44. Greenberg AD. Atlanto-axial dislocations. Brain 1968;91;655–684.

45. Fielding JW, Cochran GVB, Lawsing JF, Hohl M. Tears of the transverse ligament of the atlas. A clinical and biomechanical study. J Bone Joint Surg 1974;56-A:1683–1691.

46. Steel HH. Anatomical and mechanical considerations of the atlanto-axial articulations. J Bone Joint Surg 1968;50-A:1481–1482.

47. Spierlings ELH, Braakman R. Os osdontoideum: analysis of 37 cases. J Bone Joint Surg 1982;64-B:422–428.

48. Locke GR, Gardner JI, Van Epps EF. Atlas-dens interval (ADI) in children: a survey based on 200 normal cervical spines. AJR Am J Roentgenol 1966;97:135–140.

49. Naik DR. Cervical spinal canal in normal infants. Clin Radiol 1970;21:323–326.

50. Geehr RB, Rothman SLG, Kier EL. The role of computed tomography in the evaluation of upper cervical spine pathology. Comput Tomogr 1978;2:79–97.

51. Perovic NM, Koppits SE, Thompson RC. Radiologic evaluation of the spinal canal in congenital atlanto-axial dislocations. Radiology 1973;109:713–716.

52. Resjo M, Harwood-Nash DC, Fitz CR. Normal cord in infants and children examined with computed tomographic metrizamide myelography. Radiology 1979;130:691–696.

53. Fielding JW, Hensinger RN, Hawkins RJ. Os odontoideum. J Bone Joint Surg 1980;62-A:376–383.

54. Gwinn JL, Smith JL. Acquired and congenital absence of the odontoid process. Am J Roentgenol 1962;88:424–431.

55. Minderhoud JM, Braakman R, Penning L. Os odontoideum. Clinical, radiological, and therapeutic aspects. J Neurol Sci 1969;8:521–544.

56. Schiller F, Neida I. Malformation of the odontoid process. Report of a case and clinical survey. Calif Med 1957;86:394–398.

57. Wolin DG. The os odontoideum. Separate odontoid process. J Bone Joint Surg 1963;45-A:1459–1471.

58. Bachs A, Barraquer-Bordas L, Barraquer-Ferre L, Canadell JM. Modolell A. Delayed myelopathy following atlanto-axial dislocation by separated odontoid process. Brain 1955;78:537–553.

59. Dastur DK, Wadia NH, Desai AD, Sinh G. Medullospinal compression due to atlanto-axial dislocation and sudden hematomyelia during decompression. Pathology, pathogenesis and clinical correlations. Brain 1965;88:897–924.

60. Karlen A. Congenital hypoplasia of the odontoid process. J Bone Joint Surg 1962;44-A:567–570.

61. Kline DG. Atlanto-axial dislocation simulating a head injury: hypoplasia of the odontoid. J Neurosurg 1966;24:1013–1016.

62. Ford FR. Syncope, vertigo and disturbance of vision resulting from intermittent obstruction of the vertebral arteries due to defect in the odontoid process and excessive mobility of the second cervical vertebra. Bull Johns Hopkins Hosp 1952;91:168–173.

63. Fromm GH, Pitner SE. Late progressive quadriparesis due to odontoid agenesis. Arch Neurol 1963;9:291–296.

64. Greenberg AD, Scoville WB, Davey LM. Transoral decompression of atlantoaxial dislocation due to odontoid hypoplasia. Report of two cases. J Neurosurg 1968;28:266–269.

65. Ivie J McK. Congenital absence of the odontoid process. Report of a case. Radiology 1946;46:268–269.

66. Miyakawa G. Congenital absence of the odontoid process. Case report. J Bone Joint Surg 1952;34-A:676–677.

67. Nievergelt K. Luxatio atlanto-epistrophica bei aplasie des dens epistrophei. Schweiz Med Wochenschr 1948;78:653–657.

68. Roberts SM. Congenital absence of the odontoid process resulting in dislocation of the atlas on the axis. J Bone Joint Surg 1933;15:988–989.

69. Rowland LP, Shapiro JH, Jacobson HG. Neurological syndromes associated with congenital absence of the odontoid process. Arch Neurol Psychiatry 1958;80:286–291.

70. Weiler HG. Congenital absence of odontoid process of the axis with atlantoaxial dislocation. J Bone Joint Surg 1942;24:161–165.

71. Finerman GA, Sakai D, Weingarten S. Atlanto-axial dislocation with spinal cord compression in a mongoloid child. J Bone Joint Surg 1976;58-A:408–409.

72. Blaw ME, Langer LO. Spinal cord compression in Morquio-Brailsford disease. J Pediatr 1969;74:593–600.

73. Lipson SJ. Dysplasia of the odontoid process in Morquio's syndrome causing quadriparesis. J Bone Joint Surg 1977;59-A:340–344.

74. Melzak J. Spinal deformities with paraplegia in two sisters with Morquio-Brailsford syndrome. Paraplegia 1969;6:246–258.

75. Langer LO, Jr. Spondyloepiphyseal dysplasia tarda. Hereditary chondrodysplasia with characteristic vertebral configuration in the adult. Radiology 1964;82:833–839.

76. Curtis BH, Blank S, Fisher RL. Atlanto-axial dislocation in Down's syndrome. JAMA 1968;205:464–465.

77. Dzenitis AJ. Spontaneous atlanto-axial dislocation in mongoloid child with spinal cord compression. Case report. J Neurosurg 1966;25:458–460.

78. Hensinger RN, Lang JR, MacEwen GD. The Klippel-Feil syndrome: a constellation of associated anomalies. J Bone Joint Surg 1974;56-A:1246–1253.

79. Martell W, Tishler JM. Observations of the spine in mongoloidism. Am J Roentgenol 1966;97:630–638.

80. Schiff DCM, Parke WW. Arterial blood supply of the odontoid process (dens). Anat Rec 1972;172:399–400.

81. Tredwell SJ, O'Brien JP. Avascular necrosis of the proximal end of the dens. A complication of halo-pelvic distraction. J Bone Joint Surg 1975;57-A:332–336.

82. Fielding JW. Disappearance of the central portion of the odontoid process. J Bone Joint Surg 1965;47-A:1228–1230.

83. Fielding JW, Griffin PP. Os odontoideum: an acquired lesion. J Bone Joint Surg 1974;56-A:187–190.

84. Freiberger RH, Wilson PD, Jr, Nicholas JA. Acquired absence of the odontoid process. A case report. J Bone Joint Surg 1965;47-A:1231–1236.

85. Hawkins RJ, Fielding JW, Thompson WJ. Os odontoideum: congenital or acquired. J Bone Joint Surg 1976;58-A:413–414.

86. Ricciardi JE, Kaufer H, Louis DS. Acquired os odontoideum following acute ligament injury. J Bone Joint Surg 1976;58-A:410–412.

87. Stratford J. Myelopathy caused by atlanto-axial dislocation. J Neurosurg 1957;14:97–104.

88. McKeever FM. Atlanto-axial instability. Surg Clin North Am 1968;48:1375–1390.

89. Shapiro R, Youngberg AS, Rothman SLG. The differential diagnosis of traumatic lesions of the occipito-atlanto-axial segment. Radiol Clin North Am 1973;11:505–526.

90. Hensinger RN, Fielding JW, Hawkins RJ. Congenital anomalies of the odontoid process. Orthop Clin North Am 1978;9:901–912.

91. Shepard CN. Familial hypoplasia of the odontoid process. J Bone Joint Surg 1966;48-A:1224.

92. Garber JN. Abnormalities of the atlas and axis vertebrae: congenital and traumatic. J Bone Joint Surg 1964;47-A:1782–1791.

93. Gillman EL. Congenital absence of the odontoid process of the axis: report of a case. J Bone Joint Surg 1959;41-A:345–348.

94. Fielding JW, Hawkins RJ, Ratzan S. Spine fusion for atlanto-axial instability. J Bone Joint Surg 1976;58-A:400–407.

95. Mace SE, Holiday R. Congenital absence of the C1 vertebral arch. Am J Emerg Med 1986;4:326–329.

96. Gehweiler JA, Daffner RH, Roberts L. Malformations of the atlas vertebra simulating the Jefferson fracture. AJR Am J Roentgenol 1983;140:1083–1086.

97. Truex RC, Johnson CH. Congenital anomalies of the upper cervical spine. Orthop Clin North Am 1978;9:891–900.

98. Bailey DK. The normal cervical spine in infants and children. Radiol 1952;59:712–719.

99. Schulze PJ, Buurman R. Absence of the posterior arch of the atlas. Am J Roentgenol 1980;134:178–180.

100. Morizono Y, Sakou T, Maehara T. Congenital defect of posterior elements of the axis. Clin Orthop 1987;216:120–123.

101. Geipel P. Zur kenntnis der spaltbildungen das atlas und epistropheus. Teil IV. Zentralbl Allg Pathol 1955;94:19–84.

18

Cervical Angina, Dysphagia Due to Anterior Spondylotic Spurs, and Vertebral Artery Syndrome Due to Compression by Spondylotic Spurs

Alexander E. Brodsky and Momtaz A. Khalil

Cervical Angina

Pseudoangina pectoris, which represents chest pain that mimics the pain of coronary artery ischemia but is attributable to various visceral affections, has been described for many years implicating the gallbladder, esophagus, and stomach. It can also be caused by a number of skeletal conditions such as cervical discopathy, dorsal spine osteoarthrosis, and thoracic outlet syndrome.

History

In 1927, Phillips (1) called attention to cervical root compression causing anginal pain.

Gunther in 1928 and 1929 (2), and later with Kerr (3) and again with Sampson (4), analyzed first 30 and then 50 cases, distinguishing those cases of true coronary ischemia from those attributable to hypertrophic osteoarthritis of the spine.

In 1934, Nachlas (5) reported three cases of precordial pain arising from cervical spine conditions which responded to traction and physical therapy. One of his patients developed a Horner's syndrome, and Nachlas suggested ventral motor root compression as responsible for producing "protopathic pain" which arises in the same distribution as the affected ventral motor root.

Hanflig (6–7), in 1936, reported six cases of cervical arthritis associated with anginal and chest and shoulder pain.

In 1938, Reid (8) described four cases of brachial plexus pressure due to thoracic outlet syndrome, which caused chest wall pain similar to that of coronary pain.

Oille (9), in 1937, analyzed 617 cases of chest pain and found that 36.5% were of cardiac origin (92% due to coronary disease); while 392, or 63.5%, were noncardiac in origin. Of these, 51.3% were due to spondylosis, no cause was found in 52 cases, 14 had gallbladder disease, and 25 were due to miscellaneous illnesses such as pleurisy, aneurysms, breast carcinoma, or pneumonia.

In 1942, Smith and Kountz (10) reported 15 patients with pseudoangina, which they attributed to affections of the dorsal spine. They further described cadaver experiments to show that hyperflexion or hyperextension of the dorsal spine causes the spinal cord to move in a cephalad direction, which caused tension of the dorsal spinal roots.

Starting in 1947, David Davis (11–15), in a number of publications, did much to clarify the syndrome and delineate the causes and mechanisms of pain production. He considered most of his earlier cases as being due to dorsal spine radiculitis. He recognized the occurrence and possible mechanism of the autonomic symptoms, such as respiratory distress simulating cardiac asthma and the feeling of shortness of breath or inability to take a deep breath, sweating, diplopia, and pallor.

In 1953, Frykholm et al. (16) described experiments in human subjects to show that ventral or motor roots when manipulated can cause pain, either of the "neuralgic" or "myalgic" type, provided the dorsal root ganglia are intact. Response was more severe in patients in whom the roots were abnormal, such as in cases where the roots had been compressed for some period of time. Pain response was abolished by sectioning the dorsal root.

In 1964, Master (17) published an excellent study of 200 consecutive cases of chest pain due to coronary artery disease and another 200 consecutive patients with chest wall pain who were found free of coronary disease. His study showed that it was not possible to distinguish between the two groups using classic criteria, such as character of chest pain, presence of autonomic symptoms, duration of pain, response to nitrites, types of precipitation factors (exercise, cold, emotions) and the resting electrocardiogram (EKG). He emphasized the importance of doing

Table 18.1. Pseudoangina, 1960–1979

	# Cases
Nonoperated Cases	350+
Operated Cases	88
Cervical Spine Surgery	87
Posterior — with fusion	4
Posterior — not fused	3
Anterior	78
Combined Anterior-Posterior	2
First Rib Resections*	1

*(Two patients had unsuccessful first rib resections before neck surgery; one patient had chest pain relieved by first rib resection.)
With permission, Brodsky AE. Cervical angina: a correlative study with emphasis on the use of coronary angiography. Spine 1985;10:700.

Table 18.2. Patients According to Sex, Race, Age, and Average Follow-up

	# Patients
Sex:	
Male	47
Female	41
Race:	
Caucasian	83
Black	5
Average Age:	51.2 years
Average Follow-up: (3 months to 11.5 years)	22 months

With permission, Brodsky AE. Cervical angina: a correlative study with emphasis on the use of coronary angiography. Spine 1985;10:700.

Table 18.3. Differential Diagnosis of Chest Pain

Coronary Ischemia (Infarction or Insufficiency)
Other Cardiac Diseases
- Pericarditis
- Subaortic stenosis
- Aortitis
- Dissecting aneurysm

Gastrointestinal Conditions
- Esophagitis or cardiospasm
- Esophygeal reflux
- Hiatus hernia
- Gallbladder disease
- Peptic ulcer

Affections of the Ribs
- Bone lesions (metastasis, primary tumors, infection, osteomalacia)
- Tietze syndrome or costochondritis

Pulmonary
- Lung cancer including Pancoast syndrome
- Mediastinal tumors or cysts

Thoracic Outlet Syndrome
Muscular Fibrositis or Myofascitis
Psychosomatic Causes

With permission, Brodsky AE. Cervical angina: a correlative study with emphasis on the use of coronary angiography. Spine 1985;10:701.

exercise EKG's as an aid in ruling out coronary disease. This resulted in the treadmill stress test, but we will show that this alone is not sufficient and that coronary arteriography is necessary for a more accurate diagnosis in many patients.

Forrester et al. (18) in 1970 studied 253 patients who underwent coronary angiography to determine if coexistent noncardiac conditions, such as gallbladder disease, cervical arthritis, or hiatus hernia, contributed to or magnified the symptoms of coronary disease. They concluded that none of these conditions contributed to the development or magnification of the symptoms of angina pectoris. They further pointed out the overlap of autonomic pathways for transmission of pain stimuli from the gallbladder, esophagus, stomach, and heart.

In the last decade, the literature on this subject has been meager, until the publication of Booth and Rothman's (19) article in 1976 presenting seven cases, three of which were treated surgically by anterior cervical discectomy and fusion.

In 1980, Ockene et al. (20) reported a group of patients with chest pain and negative coronary arteriograms that they attributed to psychosomatic causes. However, they do not mention any workup to rule out visceral or musculoskeletal pathology that might have been responsible for this pain. However, it is unquestionable that psychosomatic factors can be paramount in the production of pseudoangina.

Our interest in pseudoangina, especially cervical angina, began over 25 years ago (21). In the 19 years, from 1960 to 1979, we documented 438 patients with pseudoangina pectoris due to a variety of causes (Tables 18.1–18.3). The majority of these were judged to be due to cervical spine pathology, with a small number attributable to thoracic outlet syndrome and moderate to upper gastrointestinal disorders. We have not included the nonsurgical cases in the study, since most of these cases are scattered in various parts of the United States and foreign countries and adequate follow-up has been impossible.

Eighty-eight of these patients were treated surgically by us and have been followed sufficiently to record the effects of surgery and other data. These 88 patients were divided into three categories:

Class A consists of 30 patients admitted for possible aortocoronary bypass surgery with a diagnosis of firmly established coronary artery ischemia. These patients were on cardiac regimens including medications and activity restrictions for long periods of time, some as long as 10 years. Subsequent studies at the Texas Heart Institute with coronary arteriography, ruled out coronary artery disease as the cause of their chest wall pain, although in many instances the pain was classical anginal pain with crushing substernal pain, autonomic symptoms, relief with nitroglycerine, etc.

Class B consisted of 25 patients admitted with angina pectoris and the diagnosis of coronary insufficiency but who were not on cardiac treatment regimens and were admitted primarily for diagnostic studies. Again, coronary arteriography ruled out coronary artery disease as the cause of their chest wall pain.

Class C consisted of 33 patients whose chest wall pain, while quite real, was incidental to a cervicobrachial pain syndrome. These were not admitted primarily for cardiac studies; most of them were younger, and only two required arteriography to rule out heart disease. In the other 31 patients, routine cardiac workup was enough to rule out coronary artery insufficiency as the cause of the chest pain.

Therefore, of the 88 patients, 55 were admitted to the cardiac service with the diagnosis of heart disease made by competent physicians and were referred for consideration of aortocoronary bypass surgery to alleviate anginal pain. We have separated Class B from Class A because the Class A patients have each had chest wall pain for a number of years, as many as 10 in some instances. This should answer any speculation that we are dealing with a self-limited disease, although in some cases I am sure that this might be correct. All of these Class A patients were treated by competent cardiologists and were referred to the Texas Heart Institute for open heart surgery. Only after negative coronary arteriography studies were carried out, was the cardiac diagnosis disproved.

The severity of the pseudoangina and its response to conservative treatment will depend upon the severity of the underlying pathology in the cervical spine and the pain threshold of the individual. The majority of our patients were adequately relieved by reassurance that the pain was not of cardiac origin and also by traction, physical therapy, soft neck collars, etc. These are the patients that we sent home on a conservative program. Others, however, did not respond adequately to such measures, and, in fact, some got worse with the passage of time and became candidates for surgical treatment of their neck problem.

Coronary Arteriography

Coronary angiogram proved to be the most reliable means of ruling out organic coronary artery disease, especially in questionable cases and even more so in instances where some heart disease was actually present, along with cervical spine pathology (22, 23) (Table 18.4). Coronary catheterization was carried out in a total of 55 patients and found to be negative in 44. There was insufficient pathology in an additional 11 patients to account for the anginal pain. In the Class A and B series of 55 patients, the coronary arteriogram was negative in 42 patients. Coronary catheterization was not done in two of the patients who were treated in the early 1960s before such studies were commonly done.

In the Class C group of 33 patients, arteriogram was needed only in two cases, both of which were clearly negative. In the other patients, heart disease was ruled out by more conventional criteria.

We recommend that coronary arteriogram must be performed to rule out significant coronary artery disease in cases of pseudoangina, if there is any question as to diagnosis (Figs. 18.1–18.5).

This is graphically delineated when one surveys the large number of patients who have been diagnosed and treated as having coronary insufficiency prior to their arrival at our hospital. Most of these were already on prescribed treatment programs of exercise, diet, and various medications including Isordil, Inderal, nitroglycerin, digitalis, and quinidine. Many were completely disabled from their usual occupation by the anginal pain and had retired or been retired by their employer. Symptoms and findings vary. They included arm pain, with or without numbness and tingling, and tender areas over the anterior chest wall. Neurologic findings in the upper extremities were more

Table 18.4. Coronary Arteriogram

	# Cases
Class A and B:	55
Positive	0
Negative	42
Positive (but not sufficiently to explain chest pain)	11
Not done (early 1960 cases ruled out by TMT and EKG)	2
Class C:	33
Positive	0
Negative	2
Positive (but not enough)	0
Not done	31

With permission, Brodsky AE. Cervical angina: a correlative study with emphasis on the use of coronary angiography. Spine 1985;10:702.

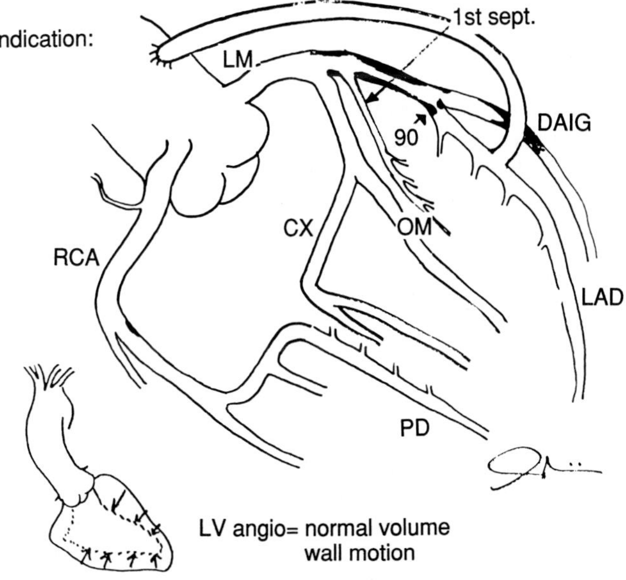

Figure 18.1. J.S. The patient had previous bypass surgery but continued to have chest pain. The arteriogram shows excellent patency of the LAD bypass. *RCA*, mild plaquing (dominant); LCA, severe proximal LAD obstruction. (With permission, Brodsky AE. Cervical angina: a correlative study with emphasis on the use of coronary angiography. Spine 1985;10:706.)

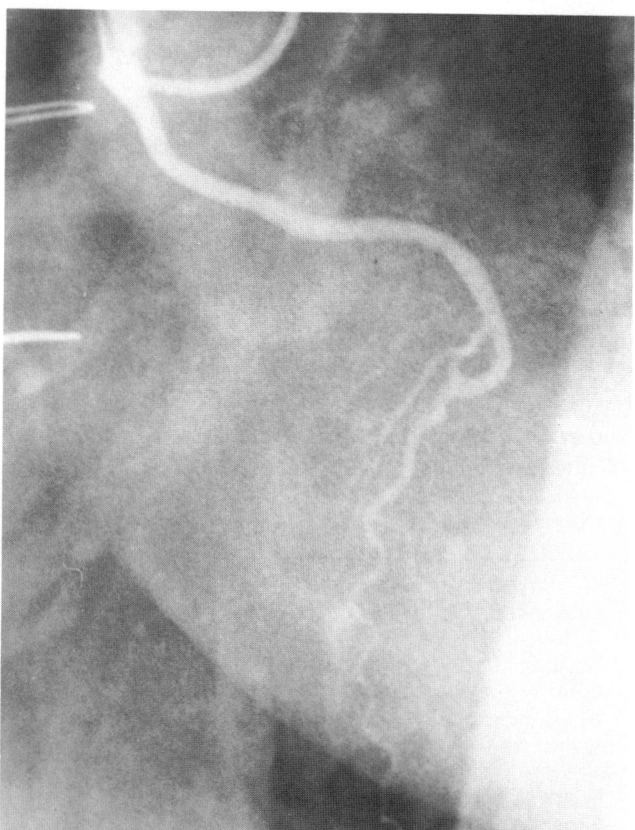

Figure 18.2. Same patient as Figure 18.1. The patient's pain cleared-up with anterior cervical discectomy and fusion at C5–C6 where both the myelogram and discogram were positive, with reproduction of chest pain on discogram. (With permission, Brodsky AE. Cervical angina: a correlative study with emphasis on the use of coronary angiography. Spine 1985;10:706.)

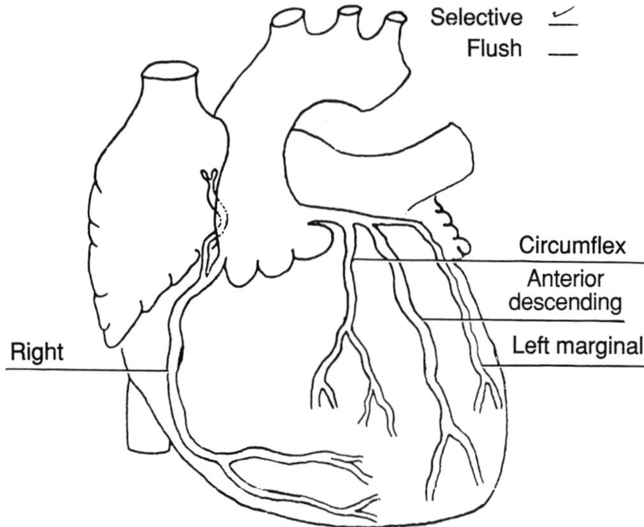

Figure 18.3. B.P., 67-year-old male with a longstanding history of angina and a history of having sustained a number of acute myocardial infarctions, has been on various medications including nitroglycerin and Isordil. (With permission, Brodsky AE. Cervical angina: a correlative study with emphasis on the use of coronary angiography. Spine 1985;10:707.)

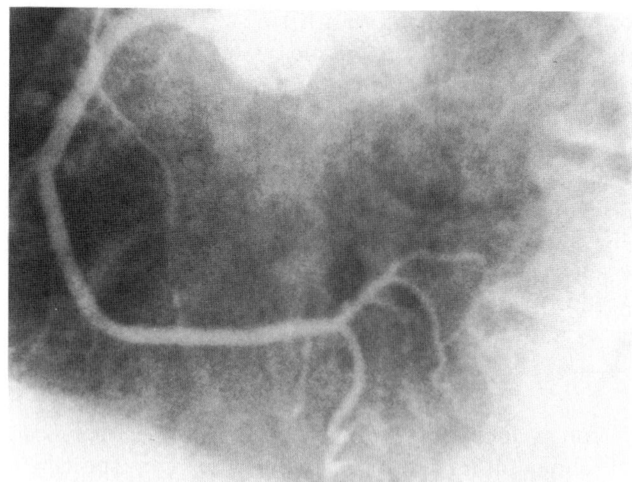

Figure 18.4. Same patient as Figure 18.3, retired from the U.S. Army service and civil service because of chronic heart condition. Coronary arteriogram shows a minor plaque in the right coronary and a normal left coronary. (With permission, Brodsky AE. Cervical angina: a correlative study with emphasis on the use of coronary angiography. Spine 1985;10:707.)

often absent than present. A few had some neck symptoms; usually these were occipital headaches and occasional vertigo and interscapular pain. Many had autonomic symptoms at the time of chest pain attacks, including nausea, dyspnea, diaphoresis, or pallor. Response to nitroglycerin has often been considered to be critical to the diagnosis of coronary ischemia. However, both in Master's (17) series and our own (21), there was a significant discrepancy as to the subjective test. Twenty-five of our 33 pseudo-angina patients who used nitroglycerin reported some degree of relief with that drug.

In our series of Class A and B "cardiacs," there was an excellent response to nitroglycerin in nine patients and an additional 16 who had a partial or delayed response. Eight had no response at all; in three cases the drug was not used, and in 19 we found no mention of its use in the records. This would tend to indicate that the nitroglycerin test is an unreliable diagnostic test.

In the Class C group of cervicobrachial pain syndrome patients, nitroglycerin was not used in 23 cases and was not mentioned in ten. These people were not seriously considered as cardiacs, and the purpose of their inclusion in this series was to document fully our experience with chest wall pain as a result of cervical root compression. Further statistical data show that resting EKG's were clearly abnormal in 18 patients and considered normal in 69, although the latter group included such minor abnormalities as bundle branch block and nonspecific S-ST wave changes (Table 18.5). Treadmill stress testing in Class A and B cervical angina patients was positive in three, indeterminate in 11, and negative in 19. It was not performed

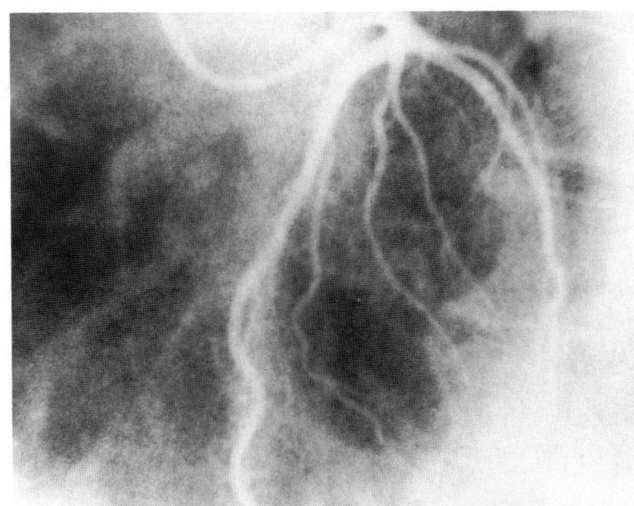

Figure 18.5. Same patient as Figures 18.3 and 18.4. The patient's chest wall pain completely relieved by successive posterior decompressive foraminotomies and anterior fusions, C4–C7. (With permission, Brodsky AE. Cervical angina: a correlative study with emphasis on the use of coronary angiography. Spine 1985;10:708.)

in 22 for a variety of reasons, often because the patients could not tolerate the test due to fatigue. In others, it was decided to proceed directly with coronary arteriography considered safer.

In the Class C group, the treadmill tests were done in 11 of the 33. The test was positive in one, indeterminate in three, negative in seven. It was deemed unnecessary in 22 patients (Table 18.6).

In this series of pseudoangina patients, coronary arteriography was necessary and decisive to the diagnosis. It is our opinion that this type of study should be performed more often, especially if precordial pain attacks persist after adequate coronary regimens and medications have been instituted, or in those cases in which there might be some doubt as to the diagnosis for a variety of reasons, usually in the absence of clear objective proof.

Table 18.5. Electrocardiogram (EKG)

Results:	# Cases
Abnormal	18
Normal (includes minor changes: nonspecific S-ST wave changes, sinus bradycardia)	69

With permission, Brodsky AE. Cervical angina: a correlative study with emphasis on the use of coronary angiography. Spine 1985;10:703.

Table 18.6. Treadmill Stress Testing (TMT)

	# Cases
Class A and B:	55
Positive	3
Indeterminant	11
Negative	19
Not done	22
Class C:	33
Positive	1
Indeterminant	3
Negative	7
Not done	22

With permission, Brodsky AE. Cervical angina: a correlative study with emphasis on the use of coronary angiography. Spine 1985;10:703.

Type of Chest Pain

The type of chest pain varied considerably from so-called classical pain of angina, which is a crushing type of severe substernal pain with or without arm or shoulder pain and which is also associated with nausea, diaphoresis, or dyspnea, up to a mild dull aching nagging discomfort which is suspected as being due to noncardiac causes. We, therefore, agree with Master (17) that in coronary artery disease physical findings may be entirely normal, and, on the other hand, the contrary is true: the presence of chest pain does not necessarily bespeak the presence of heart disease.

It is of further interest that 25 of our patients with cervical angina had documented organic heart disease. Twelve had had documented myocardial infarctions, three had had prior valve replacement or pacemaker insertions, and ten had had aortocoronary bypass procedures with relief of a portion of chest wall pain, which was attributable to the coronary insufficiency but with persistence of some degree of pain which proved to be due to cervical spine pathology. Seven other patients had achieved excellent relief of chest pain after neck surgery, and then subsequent persistent symptoms and follow-up studies showed that they had later developed symptomatic coronary artery disease that necessitated aortocoronary bypass surgery. Five others with similar scenarios were managed on a medical cardiac regime.

Pseudoangina Due to Visceral Causes

Twenty-nine patients in our series had gastrointestinal studies (upper gastrointestinal, gallbladder, and esophagram studies) preoperatively. In eight, there were some positive findings, most commonly, a hiatus hernia. However, in these cases, it was felt that the gastrointestinal condition was not responsible for chest wall pain. Unquestionably, in other cases such conditions can cause pseudoangina.

Thoracic Spine Radiculitis

We were unable to implicate, in any of our cases, the thoracic spine, although some of the patients had some varying degrees of thoracic osteoarthrosis. It is important to note that earlier investigators, including David Davis (11–15), attributed the pseudoangina in most of their cases to thoracic spine osteoarthrosis, but they based it chiefly upon tenderness present over the thoracic spinous processes (1–4, 10).

In this vein, many of our patients had interscapular or

scapular pain and tenderness attributable to cervical discopathy, which are usually considered to be due to involvement of the cervical nerve roots innervating the thoracic and scapular areas, much as they do the anterior chest wall and its musculature.

Psychosomatic

When coronary arteriograms fail to explain the patient's anginal syndrome one often thinks first of functional overlay and seeks a psychosomatic cause of the pain. This is understandable, since most of these patients manifest varying degrees of nervousness and anxiety about the condition. Several of our "poor" results and some of those classified as "fair," we think are at least in part attributable to functional factors. However, most such patients have chest wall pain due to organic causes. We consider it the clinician's responsibility to investigate the various organic systems capable of reproducing pseudoangina, such as the cervical spine and gastrointestinal tract, before settling upon a psychosomatic basis as the only diagnosis even if the patient has psychosomatic content in his or her past history.

Mechanisms of Pain Production

There has been considerable speculation as to the mechanism by which chest wall pain is mediated in the cases of cervical angina. We submit four postulates as to mechanisms which are capable of causing the symptoms of cervical angina:

1. Radicular pain secondary to root compression by a herniated disc, osteoarthritic spurs, or compression of nerves in a narrow intervertebral foramen — this may produce classical findings of root compression with motor reflex and sensory changes, along with chest pain. The cervical roots from C4 to C8 contribute to the sensory and motor innervation of the anterior chest wall.
2. Pressure on the ventral (motor) root area may cause ill-defined deep "protopathic" pain in the area of innervation of that root.
3. Referred pain, which we consider distinct from root compression — this would be secondary to painful foci in the neck, such as degenerated discs, facet arthrosis, degenerated disc without herniation, myofascial trigger points, pain arising from anterior and posterior longitudinal ligaments, etc.
4. Autonomic symptoms (dyspnea, nausea, diaphoresis, diplopia, pallor) — these are thought to be mediated through the sympathetic nervous system, and the exact pathway or mechanism is not fully understood in connection with cervical angina.

First Rib Resection

Two of our 88 surgical cases had undergone prior first rib resections for thoracic outlet syndrome, with partial or temporary benefit. However, it was necessary in both cases to do neck surgery later to relieve the chest wall pain more adequately. In one additional patient, a first rib resection adequately relieved the pain permanently.

Conservative Treatment

All patients were given initial treatment with neck traction, physical therapy, soft neck collar, small neck pillows, and postural exercises. Many of them were quite content to accept some discomfort once they were assured of the absence of coronary artery disease. Others were benefitted by conservative measures, and their pain remained under control with this type of treatment intermittently. Others may have come to neck surgery elsewhere.

Selection of Levels of Surgery

The most critical problem from a surgical standpoint, aside from diagnosis, is selection of the level or levels. This is often a vexing problem, as there are times when one cannot be certain that the choice is correct. Re-operation for additional levels proved to be necessary in five patients after either temporary or incomplete relief of chest wall pain was secured. Discography was frequently of considerable help in making this decision (21, 24–31). In general, three types of studies contributed to this decisionmaking: survey roentgenograms, myelograms, and discograms. Electromyographic studies were carried out in many of the patients but were of little help in selecting levels, although, occasionally they confirmed a positive myelogram revealing a single root lesion (Figs. 18.6–18.9). Table 18.7 shows that routine roentgenograms were positive in 70 cases, the myelogram in 66 patients, and the discogram in all 64 patients in which they were done (23 had no discogram, either because the cases were done before 1972 or because the myelogram and plain films were considered adequate for localization). It is noteworthy that in 20 patients (31.2%) the discogram reproduced the chest wall pain at one or more levels. Since the mechanism and pathways by which pain is reproduced on discography are unknown, failure to reproduce chest pain did not necessarily disqualify the discogram from being taken into consideration.

Rarely was a level selected from one study or modality alone. Usually all of the tests were positive, but the myelogram and discogram often added additional levels to those that were noted to be abnormal on plain films. More recently, magnetic resonance imaging (MRI) examination of the cervical spine has proven to be very helpful in this regard and has, in some cases, eliminated the need for myelograms. We tried to ignore the extra levels disclosed on discography on several occasions, but in five patients we had to go back and do a second operation for an additional level because of inadequate relief of symptoms. Our studies on determining appropriate levels for surgery continue and are being refined with increasing expertise

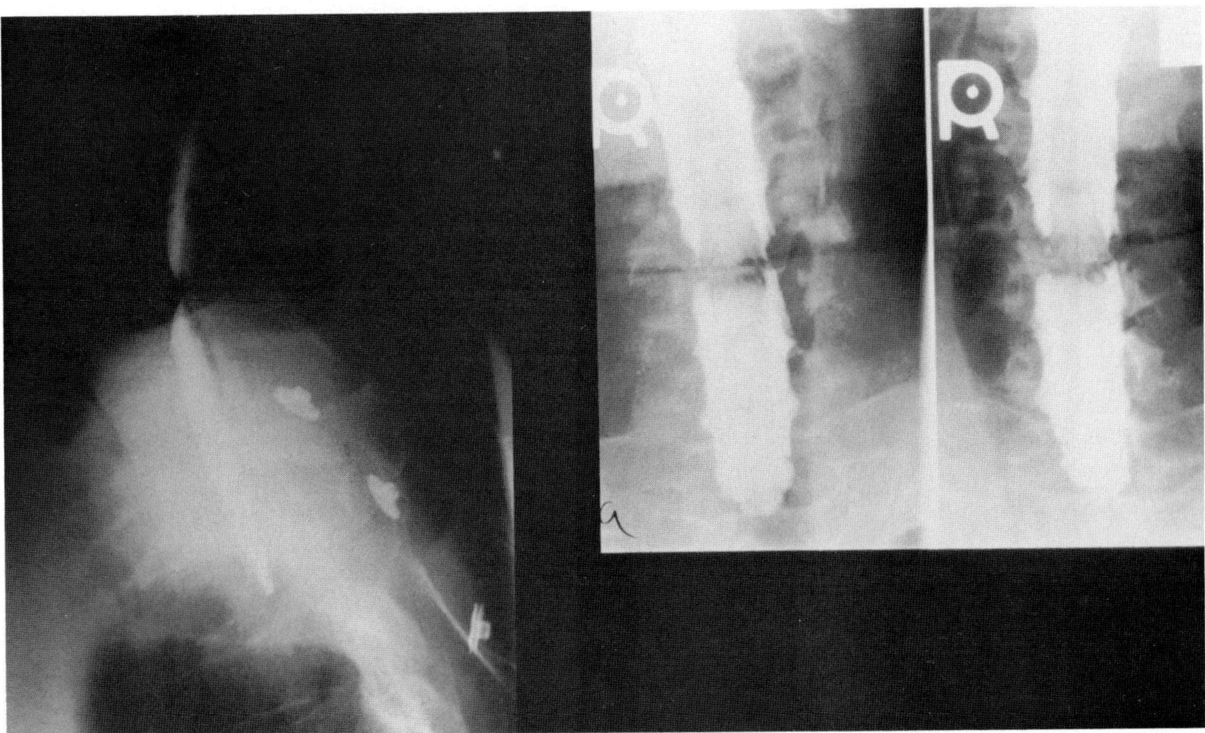

Figure 18.6. K.B., 48-year-old male. Preoperative myelograms. Frequent angina responding to nitroglycerin with small inferior wall myocardial infarct indicated on EKG. Coronary arteriogram showed minimal change but not enough to explain anginal pain. (With permission, Brodsky AE. Cervical angina: a correlative study with emphasis on the use of coronary angiography. Spine 1985;10:700.)

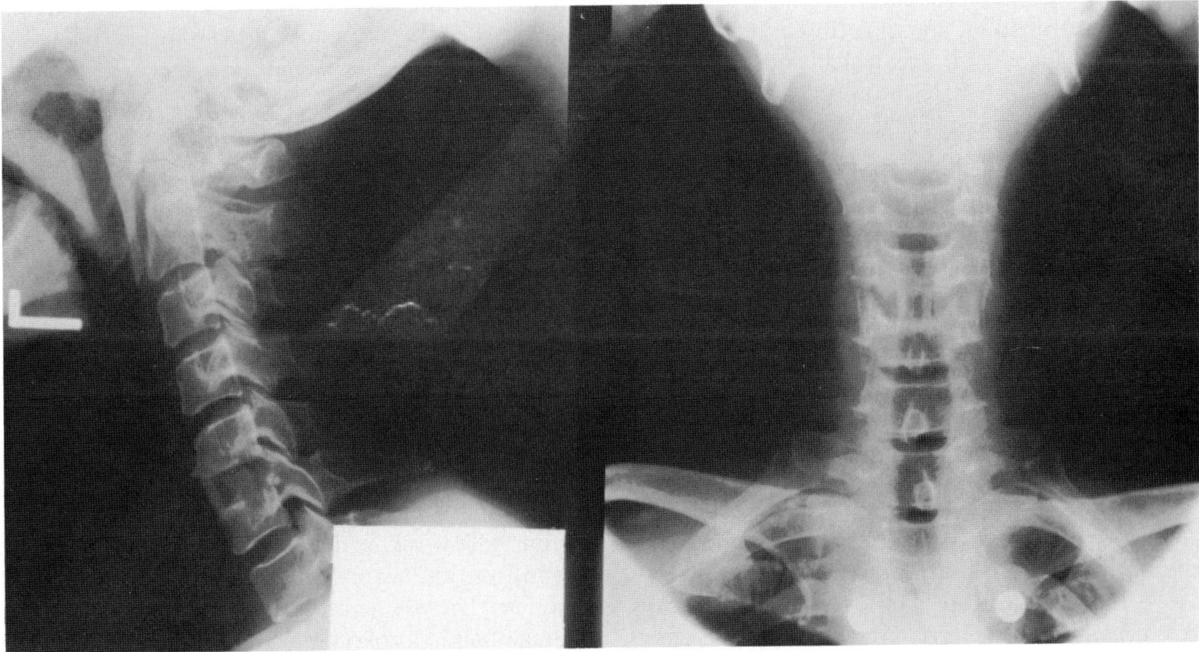

Figure 18.7. Same patient as Figure 18.6. Chest pain and numbness and tingling in both arms, worse in the right, relieved by anterior cervical discectomy and fusion at C5–C6. Chest pain and arm pain reproduced by head compression test. (With permission, Brodsky AE. Cervical angina: a correlative study with emphasis on the use of coronary angiography. Spine 1985;10:701.)

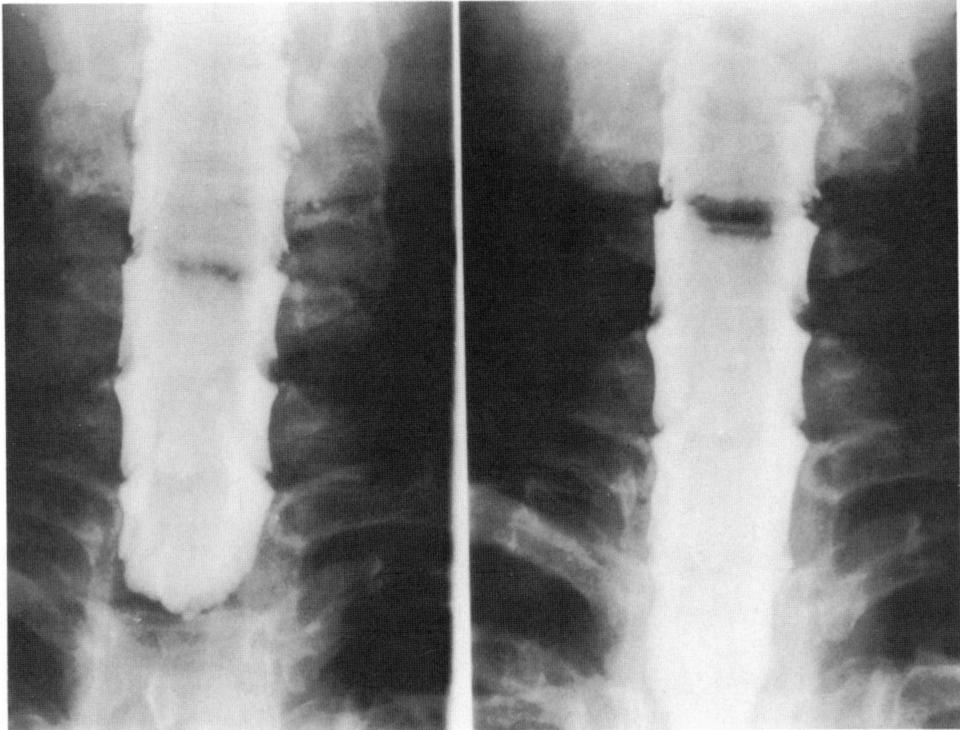

Figure 18.8. A.L., 49-year-old female. Six-year history of severe crushing substernal chest wall pain with multiple emergency room visits. Cardiac catheterization was negative. Three-month history of neck trouble without injury. Preoperative myelogram with severe changes at C5–C6 and root sleeve defects at C6–C7. (With permission, Brodsky AE. Cervical angina: a correlative study with emphasis on the use of coronary angiography. Spine 1985;10:704.)

in performing discography and the use of the MRI, although pain response in discography is not always completely accurate. This test is by no means as worthless as Holt (32–33) would have us believe. In many cases, the discogram has led us to an abnormal disc that was contributing to the anginal syndrome, which would have otherwise remained undetected. There are still some who will reject discography as being unreliable and misleading. Their numbers are dwindling with increasing experience with this test, refinement in technique, and a better understanding of its limitations (Figs. 18.10–18.12).

Surgery

Surgery was recommended and performed when adequate relief of pain was not obtained by conservative measures. In the early years of this series, the posterior approach was used exclusively in a small series. Posterior surgery was done in a total of nine cases with laminectomy and foraminotomies. In two of these there was a cervical spinal stenosis, and we combined the decompressive laminectomy with anterior interbody discectomy and fusion. The remaining 78 patients were operated upon by the anterior approach, namely, discectomy and the use of an interbody bone graft (34). There were a total of 95 operations. One patient had three operations (Table 18.8). Pseudoarthrosis repair was carried out in three, and removal of an additional disc, with anterior fusion, was done in five patients. A total of 205 levels were operated on in 95 operations, with a single level being done in 20, two levels in 44, three levels in 27, and four levels done in four patients in a single sitting. The most common level was C5–6, with C6–7 being the next most frequent and C4–5 a close third (Table 18.9).

Prior Neck Pain

Retrospectively, some history of prior neck pain was secured in 70 of our patients (80.5%), although in the vast majority it was minor in degree, often forgotten. Thirty-six of these people recalled a prior neck injury, usually a rear-end collision.

Results

The average follow-up on these patients, from the time of the study, was 22 months and is now stretched out in many cases for as long as 14 years.

For follow-up, patients were evaluated by clinical examination and history taking and by telephone and postal inquiry. The results of cervical spine surgery for cervical angina were as follows: "excellent" or "good" (relief of preoperative chest pain), 68 patients (78%); "fair" (occasional or mild atypical chest pain requiring no medicines), 12 patients (14%); "poor" (continued chest pain more or less severe requiring occasional medication), 4 patients (5%); follow-up inadequate or too brief in 3 patients (3%) (Tables 18.10 and 18.11).

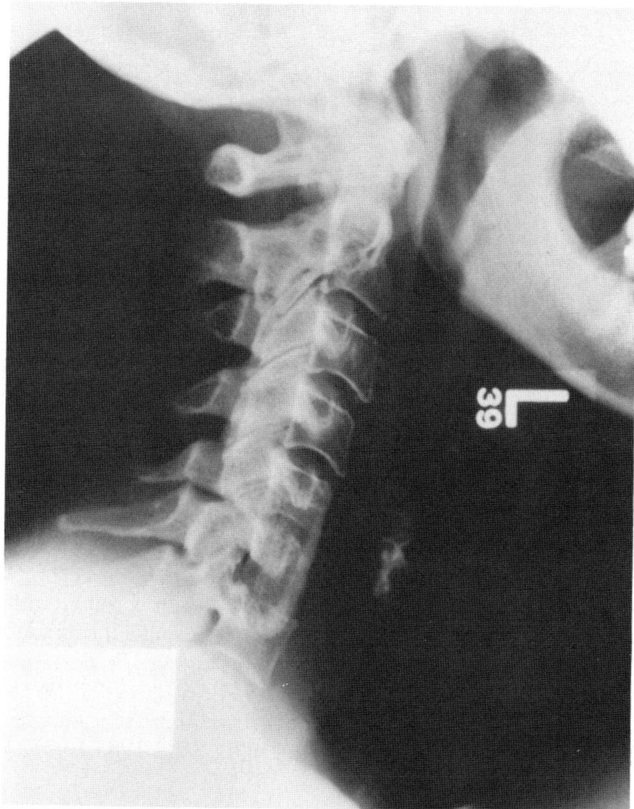

Figure 18.9. Same patient as Figure 18.8. Postoperative film showing single bone graft from C5 to C7 with resection of a portion of the body of C6. The patient achieved complete relief of chest pain. (With permission, Brodsky AE. Cervical angina: a correlative study with emphasis on the use of coronary angiography. Spine 1985;10:705.)

Table 18.7. Studies to Determine Level or Levels of Surgery

	# Studies
History and physical examination	
Cervical spine x-rays	
Positive	70
Negative	17
Cervical myelogram	
Positive	66
Negative	19
Not done	2
Cervical discogram	
Positive	64
Negative	23
Chest pain reproduced on discogram	20 (31.2%)
EMG — not useful	

With permission, Brodsky AE. Cervical angina: a correlative study with emphasis on the use of coronary angiography. Spine 1985;10:706.

Pseudoarthrosis

There were 17 patients who developed pseudoarthrosis of the bone grafting procedure in the 80 patients who were operated upon. Ten of the 17 presented some mild symptoms of neck and trapezius pain, and three had slight chest pain. Seven others were completely asymptomatic. In three patients, repair of pseudoarthrosis was carried out in conjunction with fusing another level. In the other 14 patients, we did not think that additional surgery was warranted, since no motion was detectable on bending films, and relationship of the roentgenographic changes to the symptoms was at best questionable. There is a significant group of surgeons who have been managing symptomatic cervical discopathy by simple disc excision anteriorly without fusion, and they have reported good results, comparable to those with fusion. We have continued to do a routine fusion.

Conclusions

Results of treatment of refractory cases of chest wall pain have been presented in over 400 cases, 87 of whom came to neck surgery. Cervical angina, based upon our studies, must be considered a major cause of pseudoangina and should be considered in differential diagnosis of chest wall pain (7, 21–22, 35–37). We have further emphasized and pointed out the value of coronary arteriography and the exclusionary process of diagnosis and assessment of the source of pain. Less invasive studies such as EKG, nitroglycerin response, and treadmill testing cannot be completely relied upon. Further conclusions would be that cervical angina is more prevalent than the old literature would indicate and that its recognition by primary physicians and cardiologists be increased when encountering cases of atypical chest wall pain or those in which routine cardiac treatment has been less than adequate in relieving symptoms.

Further studies on the mechanisms of pain production and pain transmission in this class of patients are necessary and also on methods with which to identify the level or levels in the cervical spine responsible for chest wall pain prior to surgery. This is often difficult to determine and can be a vexing problem. Invasive diagnostic studies, such as myelography and discography, are considered essential in the diagnostic process in most cases. MRI studies can frequently obviate the need for myelography. Discography, however, remains a very valuable tool, especially in cases with negative roentgenograms and myelograms. Flexion-extension films have been of little value, although in the past others have used them as criteria for surgery of the neck.

Eighty-eight cases of pseudoangina treated surgically were studied, and 87 of the 88 proved to be of cervical spine origin. One was relieved by first rib resection. Fifty-five of the 88 were admitted with a diagnosis of coronary insufficiency with angina pectoris, and 30 of these had been

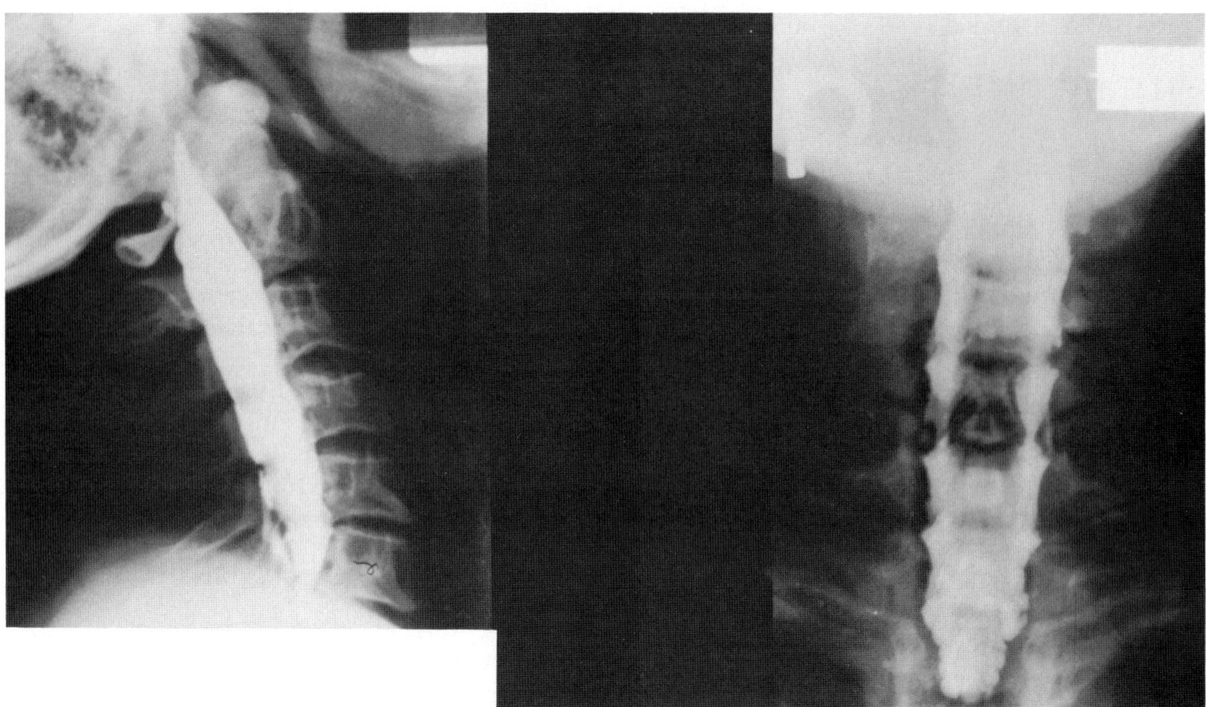

Figure 18.10. H.M., 57-year-old diabetic male with long history of severe anginal attacks chiefly at night. Initial diagnosis of acute myocardial infarction with 3-week hospitalization in 1975, with subsequent progressive increase in angina. Inconstant response to Nitroglycerin, attacks chiefly at night with severe chest and bilateral arm pain and autonomic symptoms. Coronary arteriograms showed a 100% occlusion of the right coronary with some mild changes in the LAD that did not explain the attacks. Complete relief of chest and arm pain by surgery. Preoperative myelogram with root sleeve defects at C5–C6 and C6–C7. (With permission, Brodsky AE. Cervical angina: a correlative study with emphasis on the use of coronary angiography. Spine 1985;10:702.)

treated for as long as 10 years as cardiac patients. The remainder were presenting varying degrees of cervicobrachial pain due to cervical radiculopathy with associated chest wall pain.

Historically, diagnosis of coronary insufficiency and angina was based upon clinical examination and routine EKG's. The accuracy has been improved with the advent of stress EKG's, coronary arteriography, thallium stress testing, and positron emission tomography.

DYSPHAGIA DUE TO ANTERIOR SPONDYLOTIC SPURS

Dysphagia due to anterior cervical osteophytes is not commonly encountered in spine practice, but when it is correctly recognized and treated the results are quite gratifying.

The etiology of dysphagia may be due to one or more of a variety of pathologic states, among them are: carcinoma of the esophagus; achalasia associated with failure of relaxation of the lower esophageal sphincter; spasm of the cricopharyngeal muscle at one of the two points of fixation of the esophagus at the level of C6; neurologic diseases affecting motor motility such as multiple sclerosis or amyotrophic lateral sclerosis; scleroderma; inflammatory moniliasis; strictures usually due to chemical ingestants (lye); and, lastly, psychiatric syndromes (globus hystericus).

Thus, a careful workup on patients presenting with dysphagia as a chief complaint is mandatory. It should include a very careful history and physical examination, x-rays of the cervical spine, an esophagram with barium swallow, and, often, a 2.5 cm barium tablet to simulate a solid food bolus. Esophagoscopy should be carried out in selected cases chiefly to rule out carcinoma.

History

Zahn (38–39) first reported dysphagia due to thoracic "ecchondritis" in 1905. In 1926 Mosher (40) reported two cases of dysphagia due to cervical osteophytes. In 1938 Iglauer (41) performed the first surgical removal of cervical osteophytes for dysphagia. A total of about 70 cases have been reported in the literature to date (42–48; B Jacobs, personal communication).

A small number of patients, usually elderly, present with dysphagia due to large anterior cervical osteophytes producing mechanical obstruction to the passage of food. Usually this involves solid food, but in later stages it may include the passage of liquids if the obstruction is great with a very narrow lumen.

The most frequent cause of the osteophyte formation is

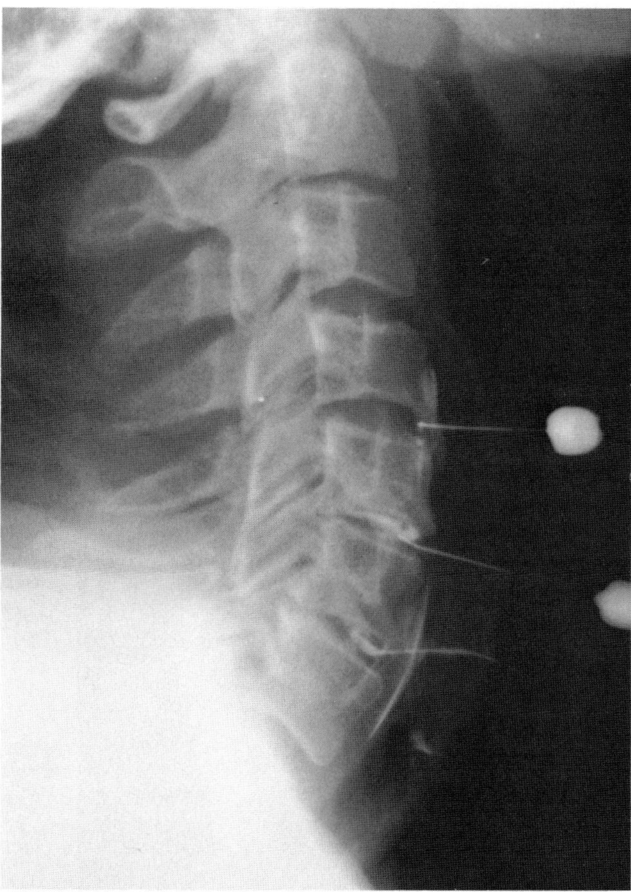

Figure 18.11. Same patient as Figure 18.10. Discogram with degeneration at C5–C6 and C6–C7 and reproduction of chest wall pain on injection of C6–C7.

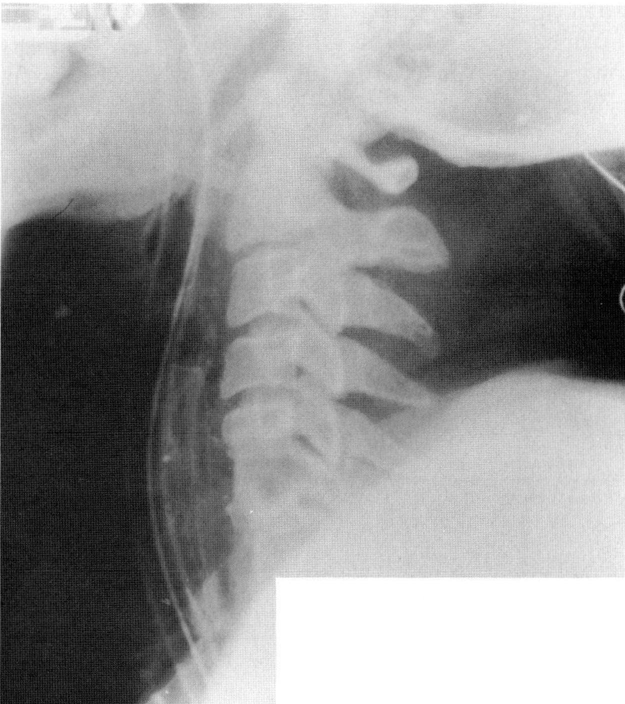

Figure 18.12. Same patient as Figures 18.10 and 18.11. Postoperative view with anterior bone grafts at C5–C6 and C6–C7. (With permission, Brodsky AE. Cervical angina: a correlative study with emphasis on the use of coronary angiography. Spine 1985;10:703.)

a condition called "DISH" (Diffuse Idiopathic Skeletal Hyperostoses) as described by Resnick et al. (49–52). It is also called "Forestier's disease" first described in 1950 (53–54). In this disorder, affecting the entire spinal column but most commonly the lower thoracic and lumbar areas, the discs are usually unaffected and the patients present a stiffness with little or no discogenic pain. The spurs usually involve multiple segments and are associated with ossification across the longitudinal ligaments but without ankylosis of the sacroiliac or facet joints (Figs. 18.13–18.15).

Some cases of degenerative spondylosis of the cervical spine may present with a single large spur, most often at C5–6, impinging upon the esophagus and usually associated with degeneration of that disc or discs and sometimes with discogenic symptoms of neck pain radiating to the scapula or arm as well as the presenting complaint of dysphagia (Fig. 18.16).

In the DISH syndrome one usually removes two or more spurs without any disc surgery. In the case of spondylotic spur or spurs, anterior cervical discectomy and fusion is often necessary along with the spur resection to alleviate discogenic pain as well as the dysphagia.

Chronic pressure on the esophagus may cause thinning

Table 18.8. Reoperations

95 cervical operations performed in 87 patients:
- 6 patients had 2 operations
- 1 patient had 3 operations

Repair of symptomatic pseudoarthrosis in 3 patients.
Removal of disc at an additional level in 5 patients.

With permission, Brodsky AE. Cervical angina: a correlative study with emphasis on the use of coronary angiography. Spine 1985;10:705.

Table 18.9. Levels of Discopathy

Most Common Level:	# Levels
First C5–6	75
Second C6–7	62
Third C4–5	55
Fourth C3–4	9
Fifth C7–D1	3
Sixth C2–3	1
Total	205

With permission, Brodsky AE. Cervical angina: a correlative study with emphasis on the use of coronary angiography. Spine 1985;10:705.

of the posterior wall and an inflammatory reaction to pressure. In some cases, there have been reports of favorable relief of symptoms with conservative treatment including nonsteroidal antiinflammatory drugs and antibiotics. The authors report that this enabled them to avoid surgical intervention. We have not been so fortunate in our experience, and surgery has remained the definitive treatment if esophageal pressure was sufficient to interfere with swallowing. Large spurs compressing the esophagus may occur in ankylosing spondylitis along with ankylosis of the sacroiliac joints and of the apophyseal joints.

Etiology of DISH is not known. Some have postulated

Table 18.10. Results of Neck Surgery in Relieving Chest Pain

Results:	# Cases	%
Excellent/Good	68	78
Fair	12	14
Poor	4	5
Unknown (Inadequate follow-up)	3	3
Total:	87	100

With permission, Brodsky AE. Cervical angina: a correlative study with emphasis on the use of coronary angiography. Spine 1985;10:708.

Table 18.11. Analysis of the Four Cases with Poor Results

Patient	Age	Level	Chest Pain at Night
C.C.	46	2	Yes; suspect additional level, but patient refused further studies
J.H.	56	2	Incomplete fusion C6–7; drug dependent
E.G.	57	3	Incomplete fusion C6–7; residual mild atypical pain
P.R.	56	3	Mild residual atypical chest and interscapular pain — functional overlay thought to be responsible

With permission, Brodsky AE. Cervical angina: a correlative study with emphasis on the use of coronary angiography. Spine 1985;10:708.

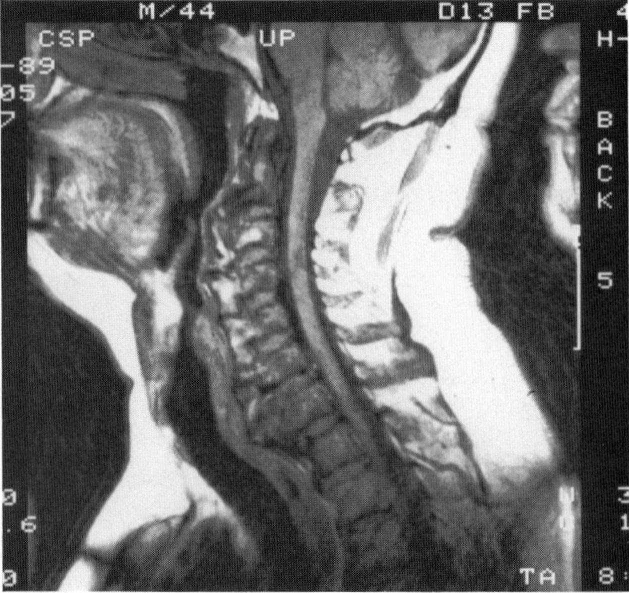

Figure 18.13. J.M., 44-year-old male with dysphagia of 2-year duration. Severe DISH. Large ossifications anterior to the cervical vertebra resected, C3 to C7. MRI, cervical spine. (Courtesy of John Berry, M.D., Houston, Texas.)

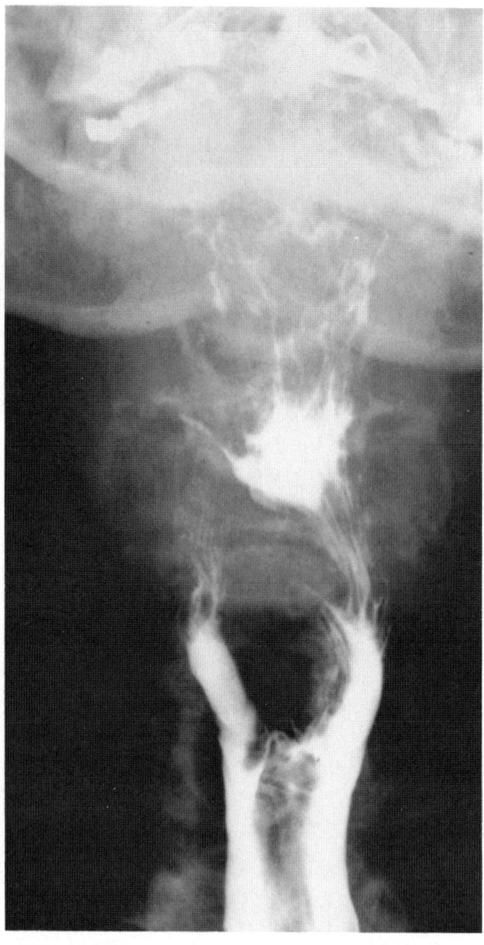

Figure 18.14. Same patient as Figure 18.13. AP film of esophagram with Solupate.

that this is an idiopathic ossification of the anterior longitudinal ligament associated, in some cases, with spurs of the calcaneous and olecranon and ossification of various ligamentous attachments to the bone (iliolumbar, patellar, and sacrotuberous ligaments). Resnick (50–52) found an 18% or more incidence of dysphagia in his cases of DISH.

The effect of the spur compression of the esophagus is magnified if it occurs at a site of esophageal fixation such as the cricopharyngeal muscle area at C6. The other point of immobility is at the diaphragm at the lower esophageal sphincter.

In the thinned-neck individual, one may palpate a mass anteriorly, but this is not usual. Esophagoscopy is optional and should be employed if one needs to rule out carcinoma. It should be performed with considerable care in these cases in order to avoid perforation.

Some of these patients may present with some degree of dysphonia (55). The mechanism is not clear but may involve pressure on the cricopharyngeal nerve or inflammatory changes around the spurs extending to the nerve or to the larynx.

The surgical approach is usually by the anterolateral route, either with a vertical or transverse incision. Some authors

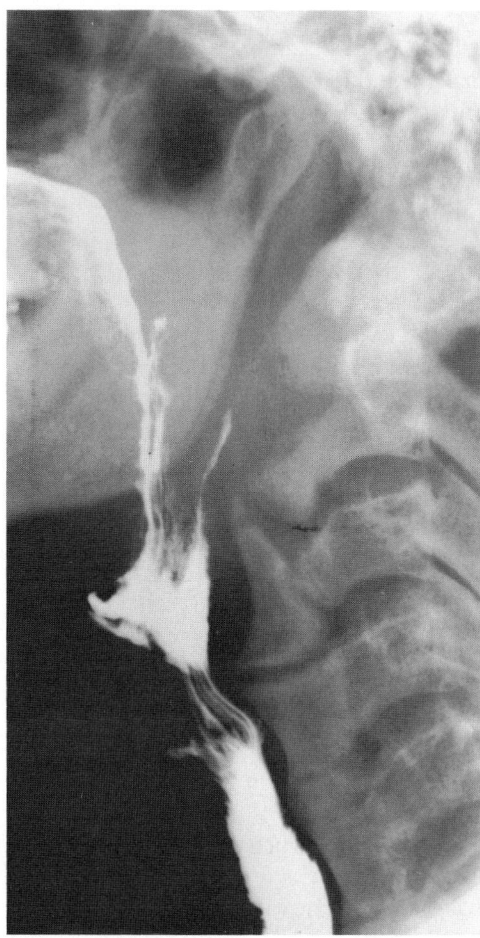

Figure 18.15. Same patient as Figures 18.13 and 18.14. Lateral film of esophagram with Solupate.

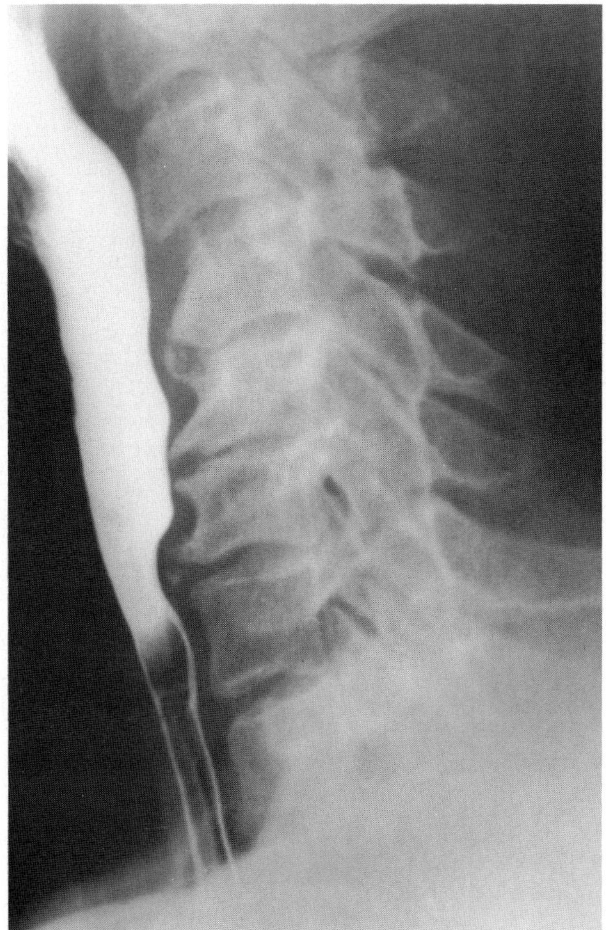

Figure 18.16. Another case of difficulty with deglutition due to large spondylotic anterior spurs at C6–C7. Patient was completely relieved by resection of the anterior spurs at C5–C6 and C6–C7. (Courtesy of Bernard Jacobs, M.D., Hospital for Special Surgery, New York.)

have advocated a trans-oral route to resect spurs at the upper three or four vertebra. We find this both unnecessary and possessed of a higher postoperative morbidity, particularly with regard to infection. There are reports in the literature of several postoperative deaths following this surgery, usually due to apnea. We have had no major complications in a small series and have experienced uniformly good results with anterior resection and meticulous postoperative care with special attention to the airway and to postoperative edema.

VERTEBRAL ARTERY SYNDROME DUE TO COMPRESSION BY SPONDYLOTIC SPURS

There has been an increased awareness and surgical interest in lesions compromising the arterial blood flow in the vertebral arteries from a variety of causes (56). These include: arteriosclerotic occlusion, thrombotic or embolic occlusion leading to vertebrobasilar insufficiency (Wallenberg syndrome) (57); arteriovenous fistulas and tears of the artery (often due to minor closed neck trauma); penetrating wounds; spontaneous dissection; congenital kinking or narrowing; fibromuscular dysplasia; and, last but not least, external compression by spurs from the uncovertebral or Luschka's joints plus fibrous bands compressing the artery (Fig. 18.17); rarely by massive disc extrusions and by tumors, especially dumbbell neurofibromata (58–59).

Surgery on the vertebral artery, especially the second and third portions, is technically demanding but reasonably safe in experienced hands (Spetzler — zero mortality in 40 cases) (60).

Our interest lies in those lesions produced by spondylotic spur compression usually in the second part of the artery, between C2 and C6. The first part lies from its origin at the subclavian artery to its entry into the foramen transversarium, usually at C6. The second portion is in the foramen transversarium up to C2. The third part is from C2 to the foramen magnum where it penetrates the basilar fascia and it becomes intracranial. The artery is surrounded by a number of thin-walled vertebral veins which one usu-

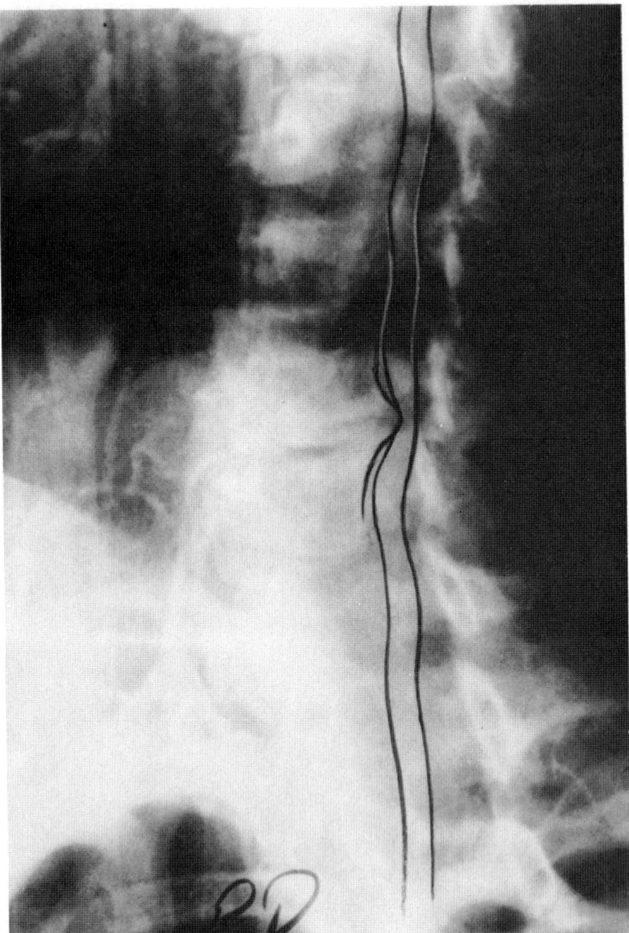

Figure 18.17. Vertebral arteriogram showing compression of the vertebral artery by a spondylotic spur, cervical spine. Patient was relieved by resection of this spur through an anterior approach. (Courtesy of Bernard Jacobs, M.D., Hospital for Special Surgery, New York.)

ally coagulates on exposure of the vessels. The fibrous bands which also compress the artery and run between transverse processes are carefully divided, and the spurs are then removed with a diamond burr and rongeurs, leaving the tip of the transverse process which protects the underlying spinal nerves.

Symptoms

Transient ischemic attacks (drop attacks or syncope); orthostatic vertebrobasilar ischemic strokes or combinations of the two; and dizziness, tinnitus, and nystagmus are the usual early symptoms of vertebral artery compression along with syncope or drop attacks.

The symptoms are usually aggravated or precipitated by movements of the head and neck. There have been cases reported of vertebrobasilar artery insufficiency or stroke following manipulation of the neck in patients with spondylosis of the cervical spine (61–62).

Wallenberg Syndrome Includes (63)

1. Dysphagia and palatal weakness (nucleus ambiguous);
2. Impaired sensation to pain and temperature on the ipsilateral face (descending root of 5th cranial nerve);
3. Horner's syndrome in the homolateral eye (sympathetic fibers);
4. Nystagmus (vestibular nuclei);
5. Cerebellar dysfunction in the ipsilateral arm and leg (restiform body and cerebellum);
6. Impaired sensation to pain and temperature on the opposite side of the body (spinothalamic tract).

Diagnostic Tests

1. Careful history and physical;
2. Plain x-rays of the cervical spine, plus bending films;
3. Vertebral angiography including films with flexion, extension, and rotation; As a rule, both vertebral arteries should be studied;
4. Ultrasound examination very carefully performed by an experienced technician may outline the caliber of the vertebral artery as well as its compromise;
5. Myelography should be done when indicated as when one suspects a coexistent spinal stenosis, disc herniation, or tumor;
6. MRI examination which is especially useful for identification of tumors;
7. CT scans are of some value in delineating osseous anatomy.

Surgical Approach

One can approach the lesion either anterolaterally along the anterior border of the sternocleidomastoid or along the posterior border of the sternocleidomastoid. The former is the more popular and less demanding approach and involves retraction of the carotid sheath and its contents laterally and the trachea, thyroid, and esophagus medially. The longus colli muscle is exposed and carefully transected, preserving the sympathetic chain which is retracted laterally, thus exposing the transverse process. A transverse skin incision is used for one or two segments, or a longitudinal incision for three or more. The transverse process is removed by diamond burr and rongeurs, leaving the tip; this protects the spinal nerves which lie just posterior to the tip. This exposes the vertebral vessels. The veins are then carefully coagulated with bipolar coagulation current. The artery is exposed and then retracted laterally. The vertebral spur or spurs are then resected using diamond burr with small, angled Kerrison punches and rongeurs (Fig. 18.18).

The posterolateral approach exposes the spinal nerves and the sympathetic chain and involves removal of the entire transverse process. It is somewhat more demanding.

Postoperative angiograms are done when indicated.

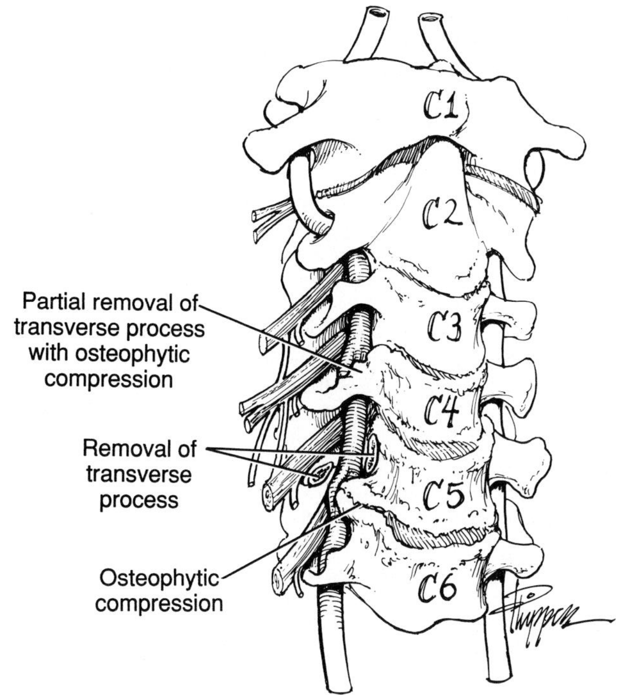

Figure 18.18. Artist's representation of the anatomy of the compromised vertebral artery showing not only the anatomy of the second part of the vertebral artery and the relationship of the exiting nerve roots to the artery into the spondylotic spurs, but at C4–C5 there has been partial resection of the transverse process prior to removing the offending spur beneath and adjacent to it. At C5–C6 the transverse process and spur have been completely removed, decompressing the artery. At the level below this, we see the large spondylotic spur projecting laterally and compressing the medial half of the vertebral artery. (From Spetzler R. Journal of Neurosurgery, Vol. 66, 1987.)

Postoperative anticoagulants are often used at the discretion of the team.

The results of appropriate cases are gratifying.

References

1. Phillips J. The importance of examination of the spine in the presence of intrathoracic or abdominal pain. Proc Int Postgrad M A North Am 1927;3:70.

2. Gunther L. Radicular syndrome and hypertrophic osteoarthritis of the spine. Calif West Med 1982;29:152–160.

3. Gunther L, Kerr WJ. Radicular syndrome and hypertrophic osteoarthritis of the spine, an analysis of 30 cases. Arch Intern Med 1929;43:212–248.

4. Gunther L, Sampson JJ. Radicular syndrome and hypertrophic osteoarthritis of the spine: root pain and its differentiation from heart pain. JAMA 1929;93:514–517.

5. Nachlas IW. Pseudoangina pectoris originating in the cervical spine. JAMA 1934;103:323–325.

6. Hanflig SS. Pain in the shoulder girdle, arm, and precordium due to cervical arthritis. JAMA 1936;106:523–526.

7. Hanflig SS. Pain in the shoulder girdle, arm, and precordium due to foraminal compression of nerve roots. Arch Surg 1943;46:652–663.

8. Reid WD. Pressure on the brachial plexus causing simulation of coronary disease. JAMA 1938;110:1724–1726.

9. Oille JA. Differential diagnosis of pain in the chest. Can Med Assoc J 1937;37:209–216.

10. Smith JR, Kountz WR. Deformities of thoracic spine as a cause of anginoid pain. Ann Intern Med 1942;17:604–617.

11. Davis D, Ritvo M. Osteoarthritis of the cervical dorsal spine (radiculitis) simulating coronary artery disease. N Engl J Med 1948;238:857–866.

12. Davis D. Radicular syndromes with emphasis on chest pain simulating coronary disease. Chicago: Year Book Publishers, 1957.

13. Davis D. Respiratory manifestations of dorsal spine radiculitis simulating cardiac asthma. Am Heart 1948;35:954–959.

14. Davis D. Spinal nerve root pain (radiculitis). Am Intern Med 1950;32:954–959.

15. Davis D. Spinal nerve root pain (radiculitis) simulating coronary occlusion, a common syndrome. Am Heart J 1948;35:70–80.

16. Frykholm HJ, Norlen G, Skoglund CR. On pain sensations produced by stimulation of ventral roots in man. Acta Physiol Scand 1953;29:[Suppl. 106]455.

17. Master AM. The spectrum of anginal and non-cardiac chest pain. JAMA 1964;187:894–899.

18. Forrester JS, Herman MV, Gorlin R. Noncoronary factors in the anginal syndrome. N Engl J Med 1970;282:786–789.

19. Booth RE Jr, Rothman RH. Cervical angina. Spine 1976;1:28–32.

20. Ockene IS, Shay MJ, Alpert JS, Weiner BH, Dalen JE. Unexplained chest wall pain in patients with normal coronary arteriograms. N Engl J Med 1980;303:1249–1252.

21. Brodsky AE. Cervical angina. A correlative study with emphasis on the use of coronary arteriography. Spine 1985;10:699–709.

22. Kemp HG, Elliott WC, Gorlin R. The anginal syndrome with normal arteriography. Trans Assoc Am Physicians 1967;80:59–70.

23. Sones FM Jr, Shirey EK. Sine coronary arteriography. Mod Conc Cardiovasc Dis 1962;31:735–738.

24. Cloward RB. Cervical discography. Am J Roent 1958;79:563–574.

25. Cloward RB. New method of diagnosis and treatment of cervical disc disease. [Proceeding of the Congress of Neurological Surgeons, Chicago, Ill. 1960]. Clin Neurosurg 1962;8:93–132.

26. Collis JS Jr. Lumbar discography. Springfield, IL: C.C. Thomas, 1963.

27. Hirsch C. An attempt to diagnose level of disc lesion clinically by disc puncture. Acta Orthop Scand 1948;18:132–140.

28. Klafta LA Jr, Collis JS Jr. The diagnostic inaccuracy of the pain response in cervical discography. Cleve Clin Q 1969;36:35–39.

29. Lindblom L. Diagnostic puncture of intervertebral discs in sciatica. Acta Orthop Scand 1948;17:231–239.

30. Meyer RR. Cervical discography, a help or hindrance in evaluating neck, shoulder and arm pain? AJR Am J Roentgenol 1963;90:1208–1215.

31. Roth DA. Cervical analgesic discography, a new test for definitive diagnosis for the painful disc syndrome. JAMA 1976;235:1713–1714.

32. Holt EP Jr. Fallacy of cervical discography. Report of 50 cases in normal subjects. JAMA 1964;188:799–801.

33. Holt EP Jr. Further reflection on cervical discography. JAMA 1975;231:613–614.

34. Smith GW, Robinson RA. The treatment of certain cervical spine disorders by anterior removal of the intervertebral disc and interbody fusion. J Bone Joint Surg 1958;40A:607–624.

35. Friedenberg ZB, Miller WT. Degenerative disc disease of the cervical spine. J Bone Joint Surg 1963;45:1171–1178.

36. Reeves TJ, Harrison TR. Problems in the evaluation of pain in the chest. Mod Conc Cardiovasc Dis 1958;27:461–466.

37. Semmes RE, Murphey F. The syndrome of unilateral rupture of the sixth cervical intervertebral disc with compression of seventh nerve root. Report of four cases with symptoms simulating coronary disease. JAMA 1943;121:1200–1214.

38. Zahn H. Ein fall von abknickung der speiserohre durch vertebrale ecchondrose. Munch Med Wochenschr 1905;52:1680.

39. Zahn H. Ein zweiter fall von abknickung der speiserohre durch vertebrale eccondrose. Munch Med Wochenschr 1906;53:906.

40. Mosher HP. Exostoses of the cervical vertebra as a cause for difficulty in swallowing. Laryngoscope 1926;36:181–182.

41. Iglauer S. A case of dysphagia due to an osteochondroma of the cervical spine — osteotomy recovery. Ann Otol Rhinol Laryngol 1938;47:799–801.

42. Bauer F. Dysphagia due to cervical spondylosis. J Laryngol Otol 1953;67:615–630.

43. Brain L. Some unsolved problems of cervical spondylosis. Br Med J March 23, 1963;771–777.

44. Bulos S. Dysphagia caused by cervical osteophytes. J Bone Joint Surg 1974;56B:148–152.

45. Coventry MB. Calcification in a cervical disc with anterior protrusion and dysphagia. J Bone Joint Surg (Am) 1970;52:1463–1466.

46. Gamache FW, Voorhies RM. Hypertrophic cervical osteophytes causing dysphagia. J Neurosurg 1980;53:338–344.

47. Lipson SJ, Muir H. Vertebral osteophyte formation in experimental disc degeneration. Arthritis Rheum 1980;23:319–324.

48. Nevill GE, Kirkaldy-Willis WH. Dysphagia due to osteoarthritis of the cervical spine. Can J Surg 1959;2:191–192.

49. Carlson MJ, Stauffer RN, Payne WS. Ankylosing vertebral hyperostosis causing dysphagia. Arch Surg 1974;109:567–570.

50. Resnick D, Niwayma G. Radiologic and pathologic features of spinal involvement in diffuse idiopathic skeletal hyperostosis (DISH) Radiology 1976;119:559–568.

51. Resnick D, Shapiro RF, Wiesner KB. Diffuse idiopathic skeletal hyperostosis (DISH). Semin Arthritis Rheum 1978;7:153–187.

52. Resnick D, Shaul S, Robins J. Diffuse idiopathic skeletal hyperostosis (DISH). Forestier's disease with extraspinal manifestations. Radiology 1975;115:513–524.

53. Forestier J, Lagier R. Ankylosing hyperostosis of the spine. Clin Orthop 1971;74:65–83.

54. Forestier J, Rotes-Querol J. Senile ankylosing hyperostosis of the spine. Ann Rheum Dis 1950;9:321–330.

55. Heck CV. Hoarseness and painful deglutition due to massive cervical exostoses. Surg Gynecol Obstet 1956;102:657–660.

56. George B, Laurian C. The vertebral artery. Pathology and surgery. New York: Springer-Verlag Wien, 1987.

57. Wallenberg A. Acute bulliar affection (embolic der art cerebellar post, inf sinister). Arch Psychiatr (Berlin) 1895;27:504.

58. Verbiest H. Intracranial and cervicoarterio-venous aneurysms of the carotid and vertebral arteries. Report of a series of 12 personal cases. Johns Hopkins Med 1968;122:350–357.

59. Verbiest H. A lateral approach to the cervical spine: technique and indications. J Neurosurg 1968;28:191–203.

60. Spetzler RF, Hadley MN, Martin NA, Hopkins LN, Carter LP, Budny J. Vertibrobasilar insufficiency. J Neurosurg 1987;66:648–661.

61. Hardin CA. Vertebral artery insufficiency produced by cervical osteoarthritic spurs. Arch Surg 1965;90:629–633.

62. Schmidek HH. Cervical spondylosis. Am Fam Phys 1986;33:89–99.

63. Macnab I. Cervical spondylosis. Clin Orthop 1975;109:69–77.

19

Syringomyelia

J. Lobo Antunes

Syringomyelia remains one of the most fascinating disorders of the spinal cord: its clinical presentation is often mystifying; its pathophysiology is still puzzling; and its treatment is always challenging.

The term syringomyelia, which literally means cavity within the spinal cord was coined by Charles P. Ollivier d'Angers in 1827 (1), but this phenomenon was first described by Estienne in 1546 (2). Gull (3) was among the first to note that in some cases the condition resulted from the pathological dilation of the central canal, and called this hydromyelia. Later, cases were described in whom the pathological cavities had no anatomical relationship with the central canal, and were associated with tumors or areas of gliosis. Simon (4) suggested that these were the true syringomyelias, whereas the term hydromyelia should be reserved for the cases with a dilated central canal.

Another important observation was made by Chiari in 1896 (5), who recognized the frequent association of syringomyelia with ectopia of the cerebellar tonsils, a condition now called Chiari malformation type I. We owe to Gardner (6) the first logical theory on the development of this disorder and rational therapeutic approach.

Classification

Syringomyelia is not a single entity but a pathological condition with multiple etiologies. These cause variable clinical pictures and often determine specific therapeutic approaches. Following the classification first proposed by Barnett (7), three main types may be considered.

I. Communicating Syringomyelia

In this type, also commonly referred to as *hydromyelia*—by analogy with hydrocephalus—the syrinx cavity results from the dilation of the central canal and communicates with the fourth ventricle. Within this variety there are two main groups of pathological entities.

I.1 *Secondary to congenital abnormalities*—Among these, the most common is the Chiari malformation type I (Fig. 19.1). The incidence of syringomyelia in patients with this disorder varies from series to series. In our group of 60 patients (8) with syringomyelia without demonstrable spinal neoplasm or previous trauma, the incidence of a Chiari I malformation was 26%. Three patients had basilar invagination, and another had a complex bony anomaly at the craniovertebral junction. Less frequently, a syrinx may develop in patients with Chiari II malformations and is a cause of late deterioration of patients with myelodysplasias (9, 10).

I.2 *Secondary to acquired lesions*—Syringomyelia may be seen in association with basal arachnoiditis (11), posterior fossa tumors such as cerebellar astrocytomas (12), midbrain gliomas (13), and meningiomas (14), posterior fossa cysts, hydrocephalus secondary to meningitis (15), or neurocutaneous melanosis (16) and acquired Chiari malformations. This disorder deserves further comment. Fischer et al. (17) first noted the development of syringomyelia in patients who had lumboureteral shunts for treatment of communicating hydrocephalus, but the position of the tonsils in these cases was not investigated. Later, Welch et al. (18) postulated that the syrinx could have resulted from impaction of the tonsils secondary to the drainage of the spinal subarachnoid space. More recently, Sullivan et al. (19) reported a case of syrinx and tonsillar herniation in a patient with a pseudotumor cerebri who had received a lumboperitoneal shunt. This was ligated and a ventriculoatrial shunt implanted, which resulted in improvement of the clinical picture. Resolution of the syrinx and tonsillar herniation was documented by magnetic resonance imaging (MRI).

II. Noncommunicating Syringomyelia

In this situation, the syrinx cavity has no relationship with the central canal and may be due to several pathological processes:

Posttraumatic (20, 21). Syringomyelia may develop as a late sequel of a severe spinal cord injury in 3.2% of the cases, and it is more common in tetraplegics (4.5%) than paraplegics (1.7%) (21). (Fig 19.2)

Spinal arachnoiditis.

Spondylotic cervical myelopathy. Syrinx cavities have now been demonstrated quite often with computerized tomography (CT) and MRI in patients with cervical spon-

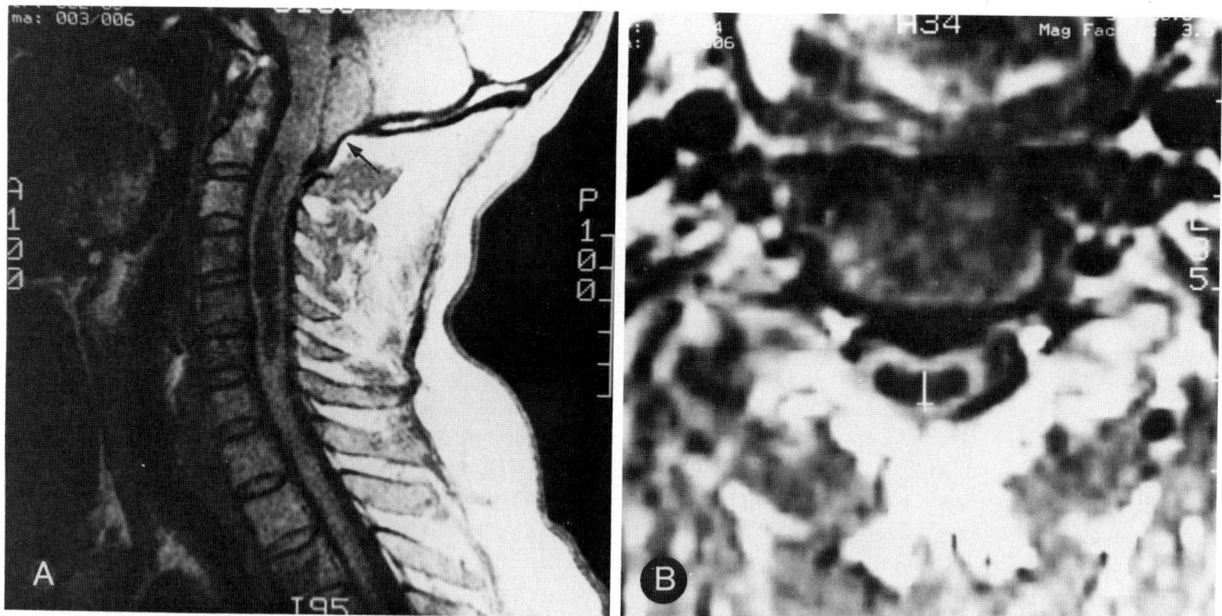

Figure 19.1 **A**, cervical syringomyelia associated with a Chiari type I malformation (*arrow*) (TR = 600 msec; TE = 20 msec). **B**, transverse cut (TR = 600 msec; TE = 20 msec).

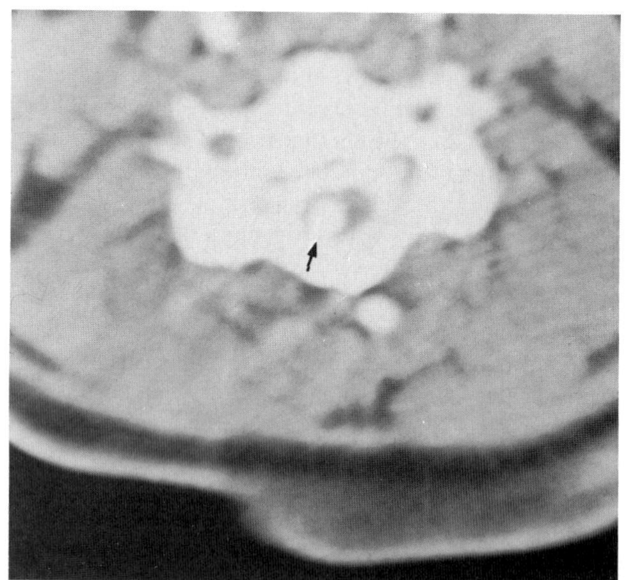

Figure 19.2. Posttraumatic cervical syringomyelia (*arrow*) demonstrated by CT scan with subarachnoid instillation of metrizamide.

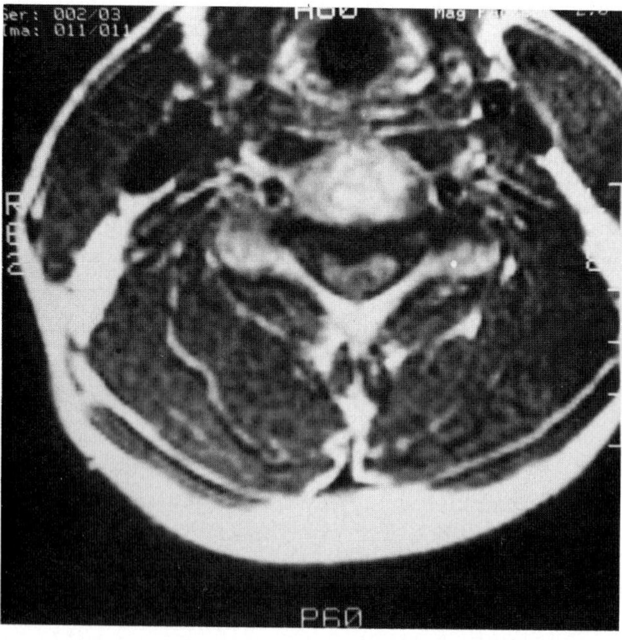

Figure 19.3. Syrinx associated myelopathy secondary to cervical spondylosis (TR = 600 msec; TE = 20 msec).

dylosis (Fig. 19.3). These lesions are probably responsible for some unusual clinical presentations, such as a "syringomyelic" type of neurological involvement or atrophy of the intrinsic muscles of the hand. This also may explain why some of these patients do not improve following decompressive laminectomy (22).

Spinal cord tumors. This association has been extensively analyzed by Poser (23). Its incidence has been estimated between 25 and 57.6% of the intrinsic spinal cord tumors (24). It is more often associated with glial neoplasms, or tumors secondary to familial disorders like the von Recklinghausen or von Hippel-Lindau diseases (Fig. 19.4). It has also been described in other conditions such as an intramedullary lymphoma (25), or a neurofibroma of the filum terminale (26). It is exceedingly rare to see this type of syndrome in cases of extramedullary tumors, or compressive spinal column pathology such as Paget's or Pott's diseases, or metastatic tumors.

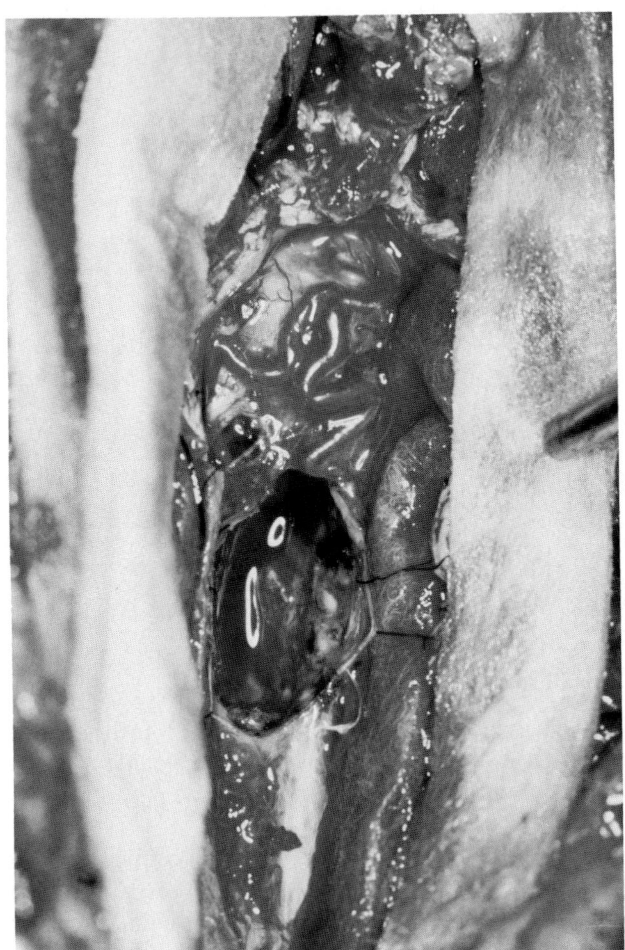

Figure 19.4. Syringomyelia associated with a hemangioblastoma, surgical view following removal of the tumor.

III. Idiopathic Syringomyelia

In a number of patients it is not possible to identify a causal entity. It is likely, however, that the use of MRI will substantially reduce the number of patients previously included in this category.

PATHOLOGY

Pathologically communicating syringomyelia is characterized by the presence of a cavity located in the central grey matter, usually just anterior to the posterior columns (27). Interestingly, it has been demonstrated in an experimental study by Rascher (28), that the ependyma and subependymal tissues of the ventral midline area are more able to resist the progressive dilation of the central canal than the dorsal midline zone, perhaps because the posterior median septum is the part of the canal where, during the embryological development, obliteration occurs the latest.

The cavity is usually not symmetrical and may be lined with ependymal cells. This layer may not be continuous, so that the wall may be covered in some places just by glial cells or connective tissue (Fig. 19.5). There may be other cystic areas, totally independent from the preserved central canal.

Surrounding the central cavity there may be a thick wall of proliferated glial cells and fibers. Quite often it also contains abnormal vessels with thickened hyalinized walls. Old or fresh foci of hemorrhage may occasionally be found. Extensive areas of gliosis are sometimes encountered rostrally or caudally to the areas of cavitation. These are more often located in the lower cervical region and usually spare the first cervical segments.

Areas of neuronal loss and edema are observed adjacent to the syrinx. The lesion also causes demyelination of the long ascending and descending tracts, in part due to impingement upon the decussating fibers (Fig. 19.6). Extension of the process to the medulla is rare.

In the posttraumatic type, the lesion is also located just anterior to the dorsal columns and appears as a single area of cystic degeneration, or multiple, coalescing small cysts.

When a tumor is present, tumor cells may be partially investing the syrinx, and a tumor nodule can actually protrude into it. The wall is usually quite thick, and an abundant network of Rosenthal fibers is a characteristic finding (24).

PATHOPHYSIOLOGY

A number of pathophysiological theories have been advanced to explain the development of communicating syringomyelia. It was Gardner (6, 29) who in a series of landmark papers first established a causal relationship between this entity and certain development anomalies of the posterior fossa, suggesting that the Chiari malformation, the Dandy-Walker malformation, "arachnoid cysts" of the cerebellum, and syringomyelia were just different pathological expressions of the same anomaly, namely "embryonal atresia of the IV ventricle." In 1965 he proposed his "hydrodynamic theory" of syringomyelia, pointing out that the impermeability of the rhombic roof present in these situations would not allow the pulsatile egress of spinal fluid, which normally occurs as a consequence of the rhythmical arterial pulsation of the choroid plexus. In cases of syringomyelia this "water-hammer" effect would originate a progressive enlargement of the central canal through its communication with the fourth ventricle.

Gardner's theory would account for the frequent association between hindbrain abnormalities and syringomyelia, and the similarity of composition of the spinal subarachnoid fluid and the fluid contained in the syrinx cavity. However, a number of criticisms have also been offered. Indeed, it is not always possible to demonstrate the communication between the fourth ventricle and the central canal, and, on the other hand, the foramina of Luschka are often patent in these patients. It is also intriguing why hydrocephalus is present only in a minority of

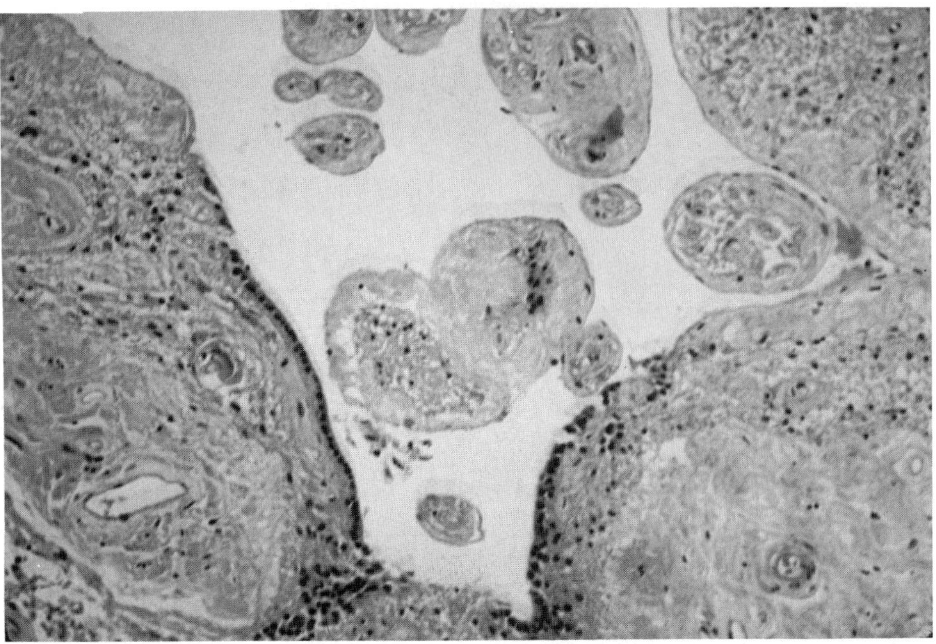

Figure 19.5. Microscopic view of an enlarged central canal in a case of communicating syringomyelia. Note that the cavity is partially lined with ependymal cells, and note the presence of vascular changes (H&E).

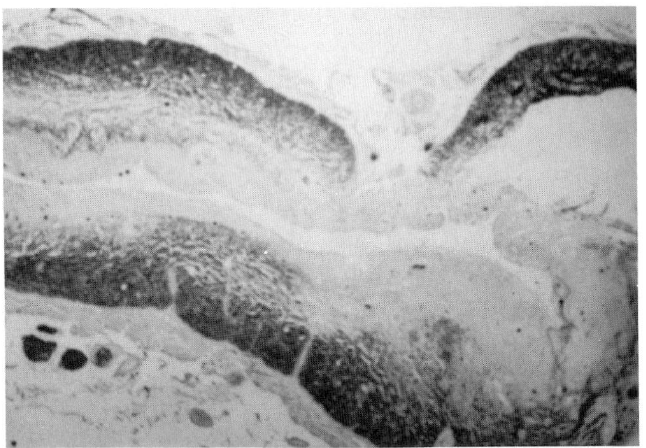

Figure 19.6. Cervical syringomyelia, microscopic view. Note the presence of a large canal, the destruction of the grey matter, and the associated demyelination (Myelin stain).

these patients. Williams (30) and others have cast some doubt on the role of the arterial pulsations, feeling that they are not strong enough to distend the central canal. In very elegant studies, Du Boulay et al. (31) demonstrated that with cough or Valsalva maneuvers, 4–8 ml of spinal fluid flowed rostrally across the foramen magnum, but only 0.6 ml were exchanged with each heartbeat.

Williams (32) also emphasized the role of the obstruction at the level of the foramen magnum, arguing that it caused a "craniospinal pressure dissociation." According to this author, intermittent raises of venous pressure, due to instance of cough impulses, could cause an increase in intraspinal fluid pressure, which would determine a secondary flow wave, thus temporarily dislocating the ectopic tonsils, allowing spinal fluid to enter the fourth ventricle through its exit foramina. The fluid wave would propagate down the central canal and determine the reimpaction of the tonsils.

Ball and Dayan (33) also accepted the obstruction at the foramen magnum but felt that the increase in intraspinal pressure would cause the penetration of the fluid through the Virchow-Robin spaces, and this would lead to the development of the cystic cavities. A transmedullary passage of fluid was also proposed by Aboulker (34). It is also conceivable that the glial cells that line the wall of the syrinx may also contribute to the formation of the cystic fluid.

The genesis of the posttraumatic syrinx or the varieties related to inflammatory spinal pathology is probably multifactorial. Very rarely has a communication been demonstrated between the subarachnoid space and the injured area. The syrinx thus probably results from degeneration of the damaged cord tissue, but there may be contributions from the glial cells and vascular structures. In these cases the protein content of the cystic fluid usually exceeds the subarachnoid values.

The origin of the fluid in the cases associated with intraspinal neoplasms may again be multiple: from tumor cells themselves, from damaged tissues (due, e.g., to ischemia secondary to pressure) or even from leakage from abnormal blood vessels.

CLINICAL PICTURE

The clinical manifestations of syringomyelia depend not only on its location and extension, but also from the underlying causal disorder. A syrinx secondary to a Chiari malformation is obviously different in its presentation and course from the posttraumatic type. We will take the first variety as paradigm.

It is important to emphasize that the great majority of cases will present initially with relatively few signs or symptoms, and one should not wait for the classical neurological syndrome to order the appropriate imaging studies to confirm the diagnosis. One should be aware that there are patients who run a fluctuating course quite similar to a demyelinating disorder.

The age of onset goes from the first to the sixth decade, but, as a rule, the disorder usually affects patients in the third or fourth decade. There is no sexual preference. Familial cases are exceedingly rare (35).

Most patients will suffer from combined motor and sensory symptoms affecting one upper extremity. Distal weakness, or loss of dexterity to perform fine movements associated with dysesthesias or disturbances of proprioception are common complaints.

Pain was the initial symptom in about ⅓ of the patients in the series of Anderson et al. (36). Later in the course of the disease, it afflicts almost ⅔ of the cases. Patients with Chiari malformations often suffer from headaches or neck pain, often precipitated by coughing or sneezing. The syrinx may be responsible for other types of pain, particularly in the interscapular region or with a radicular distribution. These may be at times quite severe or have a most unpleasant burning or itching quality. Pain or paresthesias in the trigeminal territory may also be present.

Other initial symptoms include ataxia, visual disturbances, paralysis of the lower cranial nerves, Horner's syndrome, or even syncope (37). Scoliosis is not uncommon in the younger individuals, and was present in about 40% of our cases.

We have previously reported the different patterns of motor weakness in this condition. It is present in about 85% of the patients, and more frequently affects only one upper limb, particularly the more distal segments. Hemiparesis, tetraparesis, or involvement of both upper extremities have also been observed. These changes are associated with alteration of the deep reflexes, which show diminution in the upper limbs, contrasting with marked enhancement in the lower. Muscle wasting and trophic changes occur in the long standing cases, but the classical "Charcot joints" are now seldomly encountered.

Sensory findings were present in 90% of our cases. In general, the thermal and pain modalities are more affected than tactile sensation or proprioception. The classical suspended level was detected in 40% of the patients; a radicular type of distribution was the next most common pattern. Sphincter disturbances are quite rare and appear usually only when the syrinx extends to the conus medullaris.

Involvement of the cranial nerves is often present. The most frequently affected is the sensory component of the trigeminal nerve, but palatal weakness, hoarseness, and atrophy of the tongue are not uncommon (38). Nystagmus is observed in 23% of the cases (39), but pure cerebellar syndromes are rare.

Autonomic disturbances are the result of the involvement of the sympathetic pathways due to compromise of the intermediolateral columns. Sweating abnormalities, Horner's syndrome, and trophic changes have all been described. Some patients will complain of postural hypotension, and impairment of the cardiovascular reflexes or of the ventilatory responses to CO_2 changes may be clinically relevant (40). We were able to demonstrate in some of these patients periods of hypoventilation and even apnea during sleep, and these may be the cause of unexpected death after an uneventful surgical decompression of the foramen magnum.

The evolution of the disease is extremely variable, but in almost half of our cases a stable clinical picture was established within 2 years of the onset, while in the other half, the disease progressed very slowly. It is our feeling that the course is a bit faster in the younger individuals. The fact that a good number of these patients remain with quite acceptable levels of functions over long periods of time was also emphasized by Boman et al. (41). In rare instances, sudden clinical deterioration follows episodes of transient increase of venous pressure, such as after sneezing or trauma, which may cause hemorrhage in the syrinx—the so-called "Gower's syringal hemorrhage" (42).

In the posttraumatic variety, the symptoms may appear as early as 3 months following the injury or as late as 32 years. The symptoms are, in order of increasing frequency, pain, an ascending level of sensory loss, or an increase in muscle weakness or spasticity (21). Deterioration of a previously fixed neurological deficit is also the hallmark of a syrinx in young patients with myelodysplasia (10).

Among the ancillary studies one should mention electromyography which may help by demonstrating involvement of the anterior horn cells in the brachial segments (43). Somatosensory evoked potentials show two types of changes: reduced amplitude or absent cervical potentials and an abnormal central conduction time (44).

Spinal fluid protein in our series of patients with communicating syringomyelia averaged 60 mg/dl and only rarely exceeded 100 mg/dl. The protein content of the fluid obtained from the syrinx cavity was invariably lower than the subarachnoid sample.

Diagnosis

The diagnosis of syringomyelia depends on the demonstration by imaging techniques of a cavity within the spinal cord. Let us emphasize from the start that this is an area in which MRI has made a decisive impact.

Until some years ago myelography with air or positive

contrast media was the only technique available (45). The diagnosis was based on the demonstration of a widened spinal cord—although there are cases of syringomyelia with a normal or even small cord—which would collapse when the patient's position was changed. This indicated that there was fluid within the cord which could exit, probably through the communication between the central canal and the fourth ventricle. Occasionally, when using positive contrast media, one could visualize the cavity within the cord; this could also be demonstrated by injecting the contrast directly within the syrinx, the so-called endomyelography. Quite often, the syrinx would have a beaded appearance, due to septations within the cyst, sometimes suggesting a metameric narrowing, an image also seen with MRI. This septation may be a sign of increased pressure within the syrinx and should not be interpreted as indicating loculations within the dilated canal (46). A major difficulty with these techniques was due to the fact that in a certain number of cases, 15% in our series (8), the syrinx cavity could not be demonstrated, and patients were operated on with the diagnosis of an intrinsic spinal cord tumor, only to find a flat, collapsed cord.

With the advent of CT the diagnosis was further refined, particularly with the help of instillation of water soluble contrast media in the subarachnoid space (47). With this technique one could demonstrate the enlarged spinal cord, and with delayed images (4–6 hours after the introduction of the contrast) the syrinx cavity was clearly visualized. In one series, the sensitivity of the technique was 91%, and its specificity 87% (48). Penetration of contrast within the cord may also be seen in areas of cystic myelomalacia secondary to spinal cord trauma or cervical spondylosis, or in cavities associated with spinal cord tumors, such as hemangioblastomas or astrocytomas (49). Some have advocated the combination of endomyelography and CT (50), which allows the demonstration of the extent of the cavity. Knowing whether or not the contrast flows through it may give some useful information when considering the various surgical alternatives.

The CT is also helpful in identifying the various etiologies of the syrinx—such as the Chiari malformation, hydrocephalus, posterior fossa pathology, etc.—which has obvious therapeutic implications.

The MRI has made all the above techniques obsolete, and has simplified dramatically the diagnosis of this entity (51–56). This method gives an excellent sagittal visualization of all the neuroaxis, including the craniovertebral junction. It demonstrates the presence of the cavity, the relationship between the width of the cavity, the cord, and the subarachnoid space, and any associated pathology.

MRI has confirmed data obtained from other techniques that there is no correlation between the clinical picture and the extension of cyst, its diameter, or the relationship between the width of the cord and cyst (55).

Using appropriate methods—long TR, long TE sequences—the pulsatility of the fluid within the cord or the subarachnoid space can be demonstrated as areas of signal loss. It has been suggested that, in general, the wider the cord, the more marked is the pulsation within the cyst; in this situation, the subarachnoid space is narrower and its signal is higher, indicating a decrease in its pulsation.

Occasionally on T2-weighted images areas of increased signal may be seen. These may be related to static fluid, or foci of malacia or gliosis (57, 58). In addition, the use of paramagnetic substances such as the Gd-DTPA may help to distinguish between areas of gliosis, or edemas, or even demonstrate an unsuspected tumor. One should be aware, however, of possible artifacts (59).

MRI is quite useful in the analysis of the changes in the cord following treatment. When the syrinx is effectively drained the cavity collapses and the subarachnoid space regains its normal appearance.

TREATMENT

The goal of treatment in syringomyelia is to improve the neurological symptoms or signs that are either the result of a dilated spinal cord, or of the associated pathology, such as the impairment of the lower cranial nerves when a Chiari malformation is present, or at least to try to arrest the progression of the disease. It is therefore essential to restore, as much as possible, normal spinal fluid dynamics. This can be obtained by eliminating the causal abnormality, or by draining the spinal cord cavity by making it communicate with the subarachnoid space, or with another body cavity, such as the peritoneum. Unfortunately, the matters are not always this simple, as the neurological abnormalities may not be due solely to the cystic cavity itself but may be related to other pathological changes secondary to vascular insults or gliosis, which do not respond to any operative maneuvers.

The number of procedures that have been proposed over the years to deal with this challenging disorder clearly indicate that none of them represents an absolute answer. The first therapeutic attempt to drain a cystic spinal cord through a myelotomy was reported by Abbe and Coley in 1892 (60), and over the years there have been numerous reports concerning this procedure. The problem has always been the difficulty in keeping an open communication between the syrinx and the subarachnoid space, and to this effect a number of materials such as silk, tantalum, or silastic sheaths have been tried, but they all have proven to be of a dubious value (61, 62). Alvisi et al. (63) have even proposed the marsupialization of the cystic cavity with apparent success.

Better results have been obtained with syringosubarachnoid (Fig. 19.7) or syringoperitoneal shunts (61, 64–69). The latter have the advantage of creating a larger differential pressure. In addition, a free flow of fluid may not be possible in cases in whom arachnoiditis is present, so

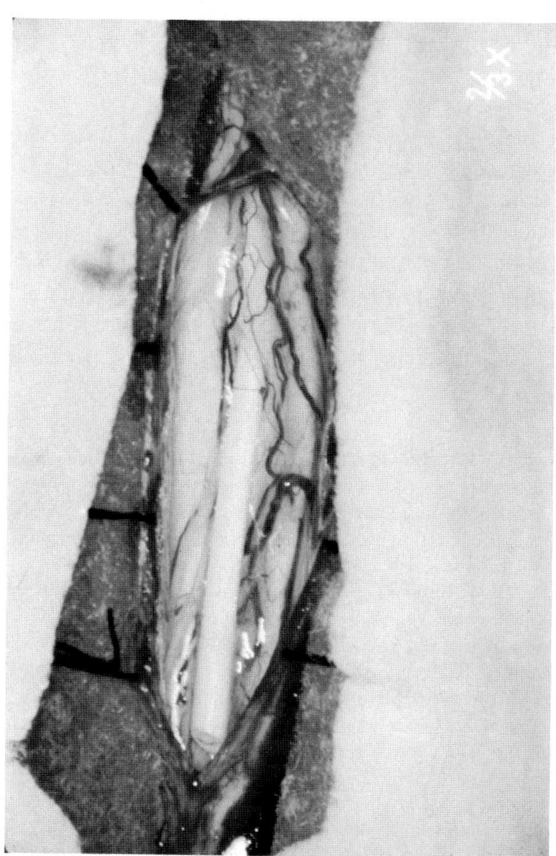

Figure 19.7. Posttraumatic syringomyelia treated with a syringo-subarachnoid shunt.

the effectiveness of syringosubarachnoid shunts may be limited.

One other question to be raised is where to perform the myelotomy. Rhoton (70) has suggested the zone of entry of the posterior roots as the safest location for the myelotomy, but we prefer the thinnest area of cord. In this regard, the information obtained by intraoperative ultrasonography may be of great help. In cases where there is already a total deficit, such as in posttraumatic syringomyelia, a cordectomy may be of value (71).

The terminal ventriculostomy proposed by Gardner (72) is another type of syringostomy and has been adopted in cases where the cavity extended all the way down to the filum terminale. This procedure which consists of the section of this structure is, however, of a rather limited usefulness and has been practically abandoned (32).

Of the techniques mentioned above, the syringoperitoneal shunts are the most valuable and are indicated in cases without pathology at the posterior fossa or craniovertebral junction, such as in the idiopathic variety or when associated with spinal pathology, either neoplastic or posttraumatic. They are also useful as a second alternative after a craniovertebral decompression has failed to achieve a satisfactory relief.

The decompression of the craniovertebral junction in cases of syringomyelia associated with a Chiari malformation was first suggested by Gardner (6) and was the natural corollary of his theory on the pathophysiology of this variety of the disorder. In general, we perform a limited occipital craniectomy and remove the posterior arches of C1 and C2, although in certain cases, particularly in the presence of Chiari type II malformation, one may have to go lower to decompress the tonsils adequately. In this regard the MRI is extremely useful in providing the relevant anatomic information. The dura is then opened and a plasty is performed using lyophilized dura to minimize the unpleasant aseptic meningitis that sometimes occurs. Like Logue (73), we have, in cases where the arachnoid membrane was kept intact, just covered the area with a large piece of Gelfoam. We have avoided extensive dissections of the arachnoid around the tonsils and the fourth ventricle, and have not attempted to plug the obex of the fourth ventricle to interrupt the communication between this structure and the dilated central canal.

This maneuver first proposed by Gardner (6) and adopted by others, seems not to add much to the effectiveness of the procedure and is a clear factor of morbidity. In most cases, we do not feel justified in performing a syringostomy at the same time.

The morbidity and mortality of this procedure have been estimated by some at around 5–10% (74), but this value is, in our view, unacceptably high. One should, however, emphasize that these are fragile patients and ventilatory and cardiovascular disturbances may occur both during and following surgery (75). For this reason we prefer to operate in the prone position. Careful postoperative monitoring is therefore mandatory. A cause of later deterioration is the development of hydrocephalus, which may be due to inflammatory changes, or to a shift of the intracranial structures.

A relatively small percentage of patients (less than 10%) will have hydrocephalus "ab initio," and this should be treated before any other procedure is tried (76, 77).

Another therapeutic modality first proposed by Vitek (78) and subsequently developed by others, in particular Schlesinger (8), is the percutaneous aspiration of the cystic cavity (Fig. 19.8). This is quite useful for the cervical syrinx, and can be safely performed under local anesthesia. Why it sometimes affords a long lasting benefit is unclear, but its simplicity and the possibility of repeating it makes it a helpful alternative in selected cases.

Radiotherapy was used in the past, and the benefits noted in some patients were probably due to the reduction of the bulk of an undiagnosed radiosensitive tumor. It has, nowadays, no role to play in the primary treatment of syringomyelia.

A question that has to be raised concerns the indications for surgery in syringomyelia. As it was mentioned before, the natural history of this disorder is quite unpredictable,

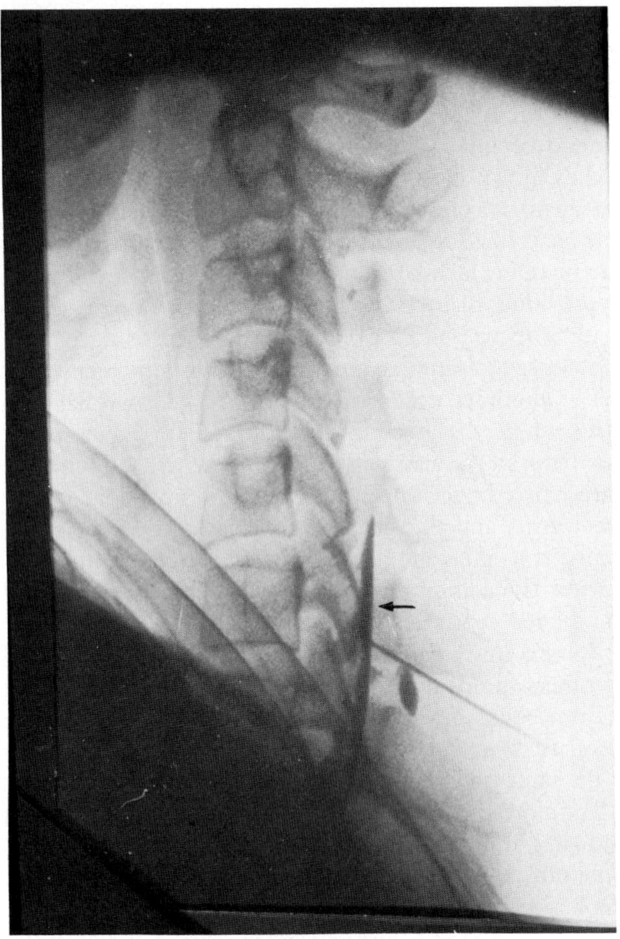

Figure 19.8. Percutaneous aspiration of a cervical syrinx. Note the presence of contrast medium within the central canal (*arrow*).

and many patients will present stable pictures for long periods, and these should only be followed closely. We, like Logue (73), do not believe in prophylactic surgery in this situation. Furthermore, sudden deterioration is very uncommon, so surgery should probably be left for patients who show progressive deterioration of their symptoms or who complain of unbearable pain. On the other hand, some authors suggest that early surgery is indicated because of the possibility of irreversible damage to the cord. We believe also that one should be particularly cautious with patients with severe, fixed neurological deficits, particularly the ones suffering from bulbar involvement.

Evaluation of results obtained with the different therapeutic modalities is, unfortunately, quite difficult because of the variability of the clinical syndromes, the capricious nature of natural history, and the different methods of appraising the possible benefits. Moreover, not all the symptoms and signs respond the same way. Quite often, the pain, the cranial nerve dysfunction, or the motor performance improve more than the sensory complaints or the trophic changes. When we analyze our own experience and the results reported in the published series, we come to the conclusion that there is an overall percentage of improvement or stabilization of the picture of 60–70% (8, 73, 79–83).

As time goes by, recurrences do occur, and these are difficult to deal with. In general, there is no benefit in reoperating in the posterior fossa in a patient who had previously undergone a foramen magnum decompression. In this situation a syringostomy and placement of syringoperitoneal shunt is probably the treatment of choice. In cases in whom a shunt was the first procedure, one has to check the patency of the system and revise it if necessary.

REFERENCES

1. Ollivier d'Angers CP. Traité de la Moelle Épinière et de ses maladies. Paris: Chez Crevot, 1827.
2. Estienne C, quoted by Foster JB, Hudgson P. Historical introduction. In: Barnett HJM, Foster JB, Hudgson P, ed. Syringomyelia. London: WB Saunders, 1973:3–10.
3. Gull WW. Case of progressive atrophy of the muscles of the hands: enlargement of the ventricle of the cord in the cervical region with atrophy. Guys Hosp Rep 3rd series. 1862;8:244.
4. Simon T. Uber Syringomyelie und Geschwultstbildung im Rückenmark. Arch Psychiatrie und Nervenkrankheiten 1875;5:120.
5. Chiari H. Uber Veränderungen des Kleinhirns infolge von Hydrocephalie des Grosshirns. Deutsche Medizinische Wochenschrift 1891;17:1172.
6. Gardner WJ. Hydrodynamic mechanism of syringomyelia: its relationship to myelocele. J Neurol Neurosurg Psychiatry 1965;28:247–259.
7. Barnett HJM. The epilogue. In: Barnett HJM, Foster JB, Hudgson P, ed. Syringomyelia. London: WB Saunders, 1973:303–313.
8. Schlesinger EB, Antunes JL, Michelsen WJ, Louis KM. Hydromyelia: clinical presentation and comparison of modalities of treatment. Neurosurgery 1981;9:356–365.
9. Hall PV, Campbell RL, Kalsbeck JE. Meningomyelocele and progressive and progressive hydromyelia. Progressive paresis in myelodysplasia. J Neurosurg 1975:43:457–463.
10. Hoffman HJ, Neill J, Crone KR, Hendrick EB, Humphreys RP. Hydrosyringomyelia and its management in childhood. Neurosurgery 1987;21:347–351.
11. Appleby A, Bradley WG, Foster JB, Hankinson J, Hudgson P. Syringomyelia due to chronic arachnoiditis at the foramen magnum. J Neurol Sci 1969;8:451–464.
12. Kumar C, Panagapoulos K, Kalbag RM, McAllister V. Cerebellar astrocytoma presenting as a syringomyelic syndrome. Surg Neurol 1987;27:187–190.
13. Williams B, Timperley WR. Three cases of communicating syringomyelia secondary to midbrain gliomas. J Neurol Neurosurg Psychiatry 1976;40:80–88.
14. Hirata Y, Matsukado Y, Kaku M. Syringomyelia associated with a foramen magnum meningioma. Surg Neurol 1985;23:291–294.
15. McClone DG, Siqueira EP. Post-meningitic hydrocephalus and syringomyelia treated with a ventriculoperitoneal shunt. Surg Neurol 1976;6:232–325.
16. Leaney BJ, Rowe PW, Klug GL. Neurocutaneous melanosis with hydrocephalus and syringomyelia. Case report. J Neurosurg 1985;62:148–152.
17. Fischer EG, Welch K, Shillito J. Syringomyelia following lumboureteral shunting for communicating hydrocephalus. J Neurosurg 1977;47:96–100.
18. Welch K, Shillito J, Strand R, Fischer EG, Winston KR. Chiari I "malformation"—an acquired disorder? J Neurosurg 1981;55:604–609.

19. Sullivan LP, Stears JC, Ringel SP. Resolution of syringomyelia and Chiari I malformation by ventriculoatrial shunting in a patient with Pseudotumor cerebri and a lumboperitoneal shunt. Neurosurgery 1988;22:744–747.

20. Shannon N, Symon L, Logue V, Cull V, Kang J, Kendall B. Clinical features, investigation and treatment of post-traumatic syringomyelia. J Neurol Neurosurg Psychiatry 1984;44:35–42.

21. Rossier AB, Foo D, Shillito J, Dyro FM. Posttraumatic cervical syringomyelia. Brain 1985;108:439–461.

22. Middleton TH, Al-Mefty O, Harkey LH, Parent AD, Fox JL. Syringomyelia after decompressive laminectomy for cervical spondylosis. Surg Neurol 1987;28:458–462.

23. Poser CM. The relationship between syringomyelia and neoplasm. Springfield: CC Thomas, 1956.

24. Barnett HJM, Newcastle NP. Syringomyelia and tumours of the nervous system. In: Barnett HJM, Foster JB, Hudgson P, ed. Syringomyelia. London: WB Saunders, 1973:261–301.

25. Landan I, Gilroy J, Wolfe DE. Syringomyelia affecting the entire spinal cord secondary to primary spinal intramedullary central nervous system lymphoma. J Neurol Neurosurg Psychiatry 1987;50:1533–1535.

26. Gooding MR. Syringomyelia in association with a neurofibroma of the filum terminale. J Neurol Neurosurg Psychiatry 1972;35:560–564.

27. Schliep G. Syringomyelia and syringobulbia. In: Vinken PJ, Bruyn GW, eds. Handbook of clinical neurology. Amsterdam: North-Holland Publishing Co, 1978;32:255–327.

28. Rascher K, Booz K-H, Donauer E, Nacimiento AC. Structural alterations in the spinal cord during progressive communicating syringomyelia: an experimental study in the cat. Acta Neuropathol 1987;72:248–255.

29. Gardner WJ, Abdullah AF, McCormack LJ. Varying expressions of embryonal atresia of fourth ventricle in adults. Arnold-Chiari malformation, Dandy-Walker syndrome, "arachnoid" cyst of the cerebellum and syringomyelia. J Neurosurg 1957;14:591–607.

30. Williams B. The distending force in the production of "communicating syringomyelia." Lancet 1969;2:189.

31. Du Boulay G, O'Connell J, Currie J, Bostik T, Venty P. Further investigations on pulsatile movements in the CSF pathways. Acta Radiol (Diagn) 1972;13:496–523.

32. Williams B, Fahy G. A critical appraisal of "terminal ventriculostomy" for the treatment of syringomyelia. J Neurosurg 1983;58:188–197.

33. Ball MJ, Dayan AD. Pathogenesis of syringomyelia. Lancet 1972;2:799.

34. Aboulker J. La syringomyélie et les liquides intra-rachidiens. Neurochirurgie 1979;25:1–144.

35. Busis NA, Hochberg FH. Familial syringomyelia. J Neurol Neurosurg Psychiatry 1985;48:936–938.

36. Anderson NE, Willoughby EW, Wrightson P. The natural history and influence of surgical treatment in syringomyelia. Acta Neurol Scand 1985;71:472–479.

37. Hampton F, Williams B, Loizon LA. Syncope as a presenting feature of hindbrain herniation with syringomyelia. J Neurol Neurosurg Psychiatry 1982;45:919–922.

38. Bleck TP, Shannon KM. Disordered swallowing due to a syrinx: correction by shunting. Neurology 1984;34:1497–1498.

39. Thrush DC, Foster JB. An analysis of nystagmus in 100 consecutive patients with communicating syringomyelia. J Neurol Sci 1973;20:381–386.

40. Nogués MA, Newman PK, Male VJ, Foster JB. Cardiovascular reflexes in syringomyelia. Brain 1982;105:835–849.

41. Boman K, Iivanainen M. Prognosis of syringomyelia. Acta Neurol Scand 1967;43:61–68.

42. Sedzimir CB, Roberts JR, Occleshaw JV, Buxton PH. Gowers' syringal hemorrhage. J Neurol Neurosurg Psychiatry 1974;37:312–315.

43. Schwartz MS, Stalberg E, Swash M. Pattern of segmental motor involvement in syringomyelia: a single fibre EMG study. J Neurol Neurosurg Psychiatry 1980;43:150–155.

44. Anderson NE, Frith RW, Synek VM. Somatosensory evoked potentials in syringomyelia. J Neurol Neurosurg Psychiatry 1986;49:1407–1410.

45. Heinz ER, Schlesinger EB, Potts DG. Radiologic signs of hydromyelia. Radiology 1966;86:311–318.

46. Lederhaus SC, Pritz MB, Pribram HFW. Septation in syringomyelia and its possible clinical significance. Neurosurgery 1988;22:1064–1067.

47. Aubin ML, Vignaud J, Jardin C, Bar D. Computed tomography in 75 clinical cases of syringomyelia. Am J Neuroradiol 1981;2:199–204.

48. Gates PC, Fox AJ, Barnett HJM. CT metrizamide myelography in syringomyelia: sensitivity and specificity. Neurology 1986;36:1245–1248.

49. Kan S, Fox AJ, Vinuela F, Barnett HJM, Peerless SJ. Delayed CT metrizamide enhancement of syringomyelia secondary to tumor. Am J Neuroradiol 1983;4:73–78.

50. Blumenkopf B. Percutaneous minidose metrizamide endomyelographic computed tomography in syringomyelia. Neurosurgery 1987;20:434–438.

51. Modic MT, Hardy Jr RW, Weinstein MA, Duchesneau PM, Paushter DM, Boumphrey F. Nuclear magnetic resonance of the spine: clinical potential and limitation. Neurosurgery 1984;15:583–592.

52. Kokmen E, Marsh WR, Baker Jr HC. Magnetic resonance imaging in syringomyelia. Neurosurgery 1985;17:267–270.

53. Wilberger Jr JE, Maroon JC, Prostko ER, Baghai P, Beckman I, Deeb Z. Magnetic resonance imaging and intraoperative neurosonography. Neurosurgery 1985;20:599–605.

54. Enzmann DR, O'Donohue J, Rubin JB, Shuer L, Cogen P, Silverberg G. CSF pulsations within nonneoplastic spinal cord cysts. Am J Radiol 1987;149:149–157.

55. Grant R, Hadley DM, MacPherson P, Condon B, Patterson J, Bone I, Teasdale GN. Syringomyelia: cyst measurement by magnetic resonance imaging and comparison with symptoms, signs and disability. J Neurol Neurosurg Psychiatry 1987;50:1008–1014.

56. Sherman JL, Barkovich AJ, Citrin CM. The MR appearance of syringomyelia: new observations. Am J Radiol 1987;148:381–391.

57. Al-Mefty O, Harkey LH, Middleton TH, Smith RR, Fox JL. Myelopathic cervical spondylotic lesions demonstrated by magnetic resonance imaging. J Neurosurg 1988;68:217–222.

58. MacDonald RL, Findlay JM, Tator CH. Microcystic spinal cord degeneration causing posttraumatic myelopathy. Report of two cases. J Neurosurg 1988;68:466–471.

59. Bronskill MJ, McVeigh ER, Kucharczyk W, Henkelman RM. Syrinx-like artifacts on MR images of the spinal cord. Radiology 1988;166:485–488.

60. Abbe R, Coley WB. Syringomyelia, operation-exploration of cord, withdrawal of fluid, exhibition of patient. J Nerv Ment Dis 1892;19:512.

61. Love JG, Olofson RA. Syringomyelia: A look at surgical therapy. J Neurosurg 1966;24:714–718.

62. Faulhauer K, Loew K. The surgical treatment of syringomyelia. Long-term results. Acta Neurochir 1978;44:215–222.

63. Alvisi C, Cerisoli M. Long-term results of the surgical treatment of syringohydromyelia. Acta Neurochir 1984;71:133–140.

64. Peerless SJ, Durward QJ. Management of syringomyelia: a pathophysiological approach. Clin Neurosurg 1982;30:531–576.

65. Tator CH, Meguro K, Rowed DW. Favorable results with syringosubarachnoid shunts for treatment of syringomyelia. J Neurosurg 1982;56:517–523.

66. Barbaro NM, Wilson CB, Gutin PH, Edwards MSB. Surgical treatment of syringomyelia. Favorable results with syringoperitoneal shunting. J Neurosurg 1984;61:531–538.

67. Suzuki M, Davis C, Symon L, Gentili F. Syringoperitoneal shunt

for treatment of cord cavitation. J Neurol Neurosurg Psychiatry 1985;48:620–627.

68. Lesoin F, Petit H, Thomas III CE, Viaud C, Baleriaux D, Jomin M. Use of the syringoperitoneal shunt in the treatment of syringomyelia. Surg Neurol 1986;25:131–136.

69. Vaquero J, Martinez R, Salazar J, Santos H. Syringosubarachnoid shunt for treatment of syringomyelia. Acta Neurochir 1987;84:105–109.

70. Rhoton Jr AL. Microsurgery of Arnold-Chiari malformation with and without hydromyelia. J Neurosurg 1976;45:473–483.

71. Durward QJ, Rice GP, Bell MJ, Gilbert J, Kaufmann JCE. Selective spinal cordectomy: clinicopathological correlation. J Neurosurg 1982;56:359–367.

72. Gardner WJ, Bell HS, Poolos PN, Dohn DF, Steinberg M. Terminal ventriculostomy for syringomyelia. J Neurosurg 1977;46:609–617.

73. Logue V, Edwards MR. Syringomyelia and its surgical treatment. J Neurol Neurosurg Psychiatry 1981;44:273–284.

74. Calliauw L, Dehaene I. The surgical risk in the treatment of Arnold Chiari malformation. Acta Neurochir 1977;39:173–179.

75. Williams B. A critical appraisal of posterior fossa surgery for communicating syringomyelia. Brain 1978;101:223–250.

76. Krayenbühl H, Benini A. A new surgical approach in the treatment of hydromyelia and syringomyelia: the embryological basis and the first results. JR Coll Surg Edinb 1971;16:147.

77. Ogilvy CS, Borges LF. Treatment of symptomatic syringomyelia with a ventriculoperitoneal shunt: a case report with magnetic resonance scan correlation. Neurosurgery 1988;22:748–750.

78. Vitek J. La ponction dorsal thérapeutique et diagnostique des cavités syringomyéliques. Brux Med 1929;9:311–312.

79. Garcia-Uria J, Leunda G, Carillo R, Bravo G. Syringomyelia: long term results after posterior fossa decompression. J Neurosurg 1981;54:380–383.

80. Cahan L, Bentson JR. Considerations in the diagnosis and treatment of syringomyelia and the Chiari malformation. J Neurosurg 1982;57:24–31.

81. Levy WJ, Mason LP, Mahn JF. Chiari malformations presenting in adults: A surgical experience in 127 cases. Neurosurgery 1983;12:377–390.

82. Paul KS, Lye R, Strang FA, Dutton J. Arnold Chiari malformation. Review of 71 cases. J Neurosurg 1983;58:183–187.

83. Filizzolo F, Vesari P, D'Aliberti G, Arena O, Scotti G, Mariani C. Foramen magnum decompression versus terminal ventriculostomy for the treatment of syringomyelia. Acta Neurochir 1988;93:96–99.

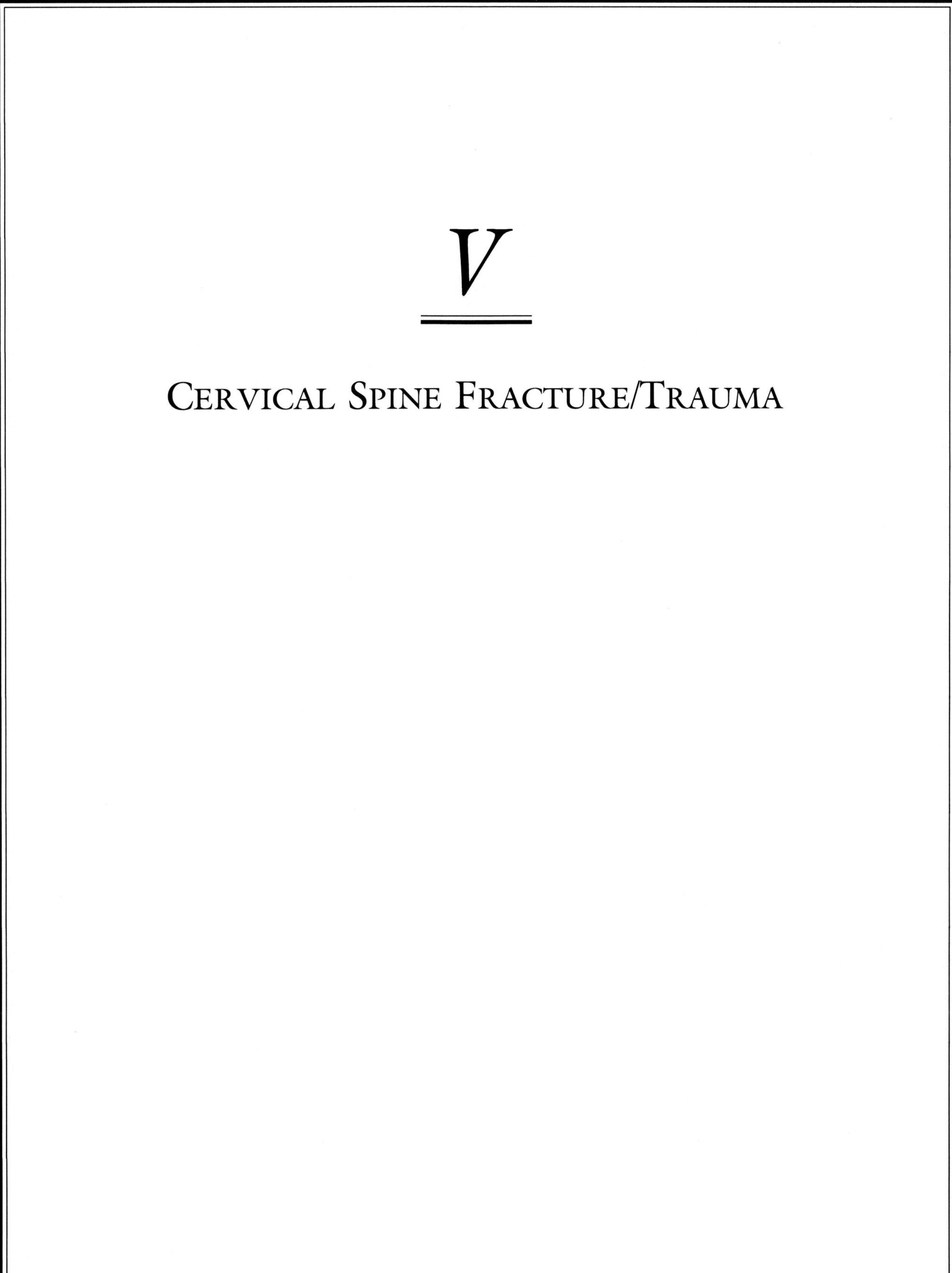

V

Cervical Spine Fracture/Trauma

20

Classification of Lower Cervical Spine Injuries

David R. Chandler, Michael A. Kropf, and Robert L. Waters

Classification systems of cervical spinal column injuries are clinically useful insofar as they contribute to understanding the mechanism and extent of injury, prognosis, and direct appropriate therapy. The classification system should also be simple so it can be easily taught, recalled, and applied. This discussion is confined to injuries of the lower cervical spinal column resulting from indirect trauma. These comprise the largest group of cervical spinal column injuries. Upper cervical spine injuries, injuries from direct trauma, and neurologic injuries have been addressed in other chapters.

The first recorded clinical description of a cervical spine injury is found on the Edwin Smith papyrus and is by an Egyptian medical author in 2500 BC (1). The Egyptian author listed six cases of spinal injury including a sprain, a dislocation, and a crushed vertebra. Spinal injuries were considered an ailment not to be treated.

Mortality from spinal injuries remained very high until the twentieth century. In addition to improved methods of manipulation and immobilization, Durbin attributed the decline to the discovery of x-rays by Roentgen in 1895 which enabled the diagnosis of a spinal column injury when the clinical findings were not marked (2). It is certain that x-rays allowed a much more detailed examination of the various vertebral elements and their alignment. Much of the discussion of cervical spinal column injuries was done within the classification framework of fractures, fracture-dislocations, and dislocations. This is essentially the system employed by the Egyptians 4500 years previously, and, as noted by Ellis in 1946, it is not of much use clinically (3).

Most cervical spine injuries were thought to result from a flexion compression mechanism, but formal classification systems based on differing mechanisms of injury were not popularized until the 1960s. These mechanistic systems are based primarily on the lateral x-ray, but anteroposterior, obliques, and odontoid views are also recommended for initial assessment of possible cervical spine injuries. The clinical situation may dictate the use of additional views and imaging modalities.

Roaf experimentally analyzed the mechanics of spinal injury in 1960 (4). Whitely and Forsyth reported a classification system based on the dynamics of injury, attempting to correlate the radiographic findings with pathologic anatomy (5). Both flexion and extension injuries with or without compression were recognized radiographically. Holdsworth in 1970 noted that the prognosis and treatment of spinal fractures were related to the type of injury based on its mechanism (6). Braakman and Penning, 1968 (7), recognized the importance of compressive and distractive forces in addition to the previously accepted flexion, extension, and axial rotation forces. Taylor and Blackwood, Forsyth, and Burke described and emphasized the importance and frequency of cervical injuries in which extension predominated (8, 9, 10).

Most recently, Allen et al. identified six lower cervical spine injury patterns which are divided into stages according to the extent of the spinal column damage (11). This classification system is useful because it indicates the extent of injury and distinguishes injuries with a stable prognosis that can be treated nonoperatively from those injuries with an unstable prognosis that may require operative intervention. The key features of this classification system are displayed in Figures 20.1–20.5 and summarized as follows:

Distractive Flexion (Fig. 20.1)

Stage 1 This lesion consists of failure of the posterior ligamentous complex, as evidenced by facet subluxation in flexion with abnormal divergence of the spinous process.

Stage 2 This lesion is a unilateral facet dislocation. Beatson (12) serially divided the posterior or interspinous ligaments, facet capsule, posterior or longitudinal ligament and found that unilateral facet dislocation may occur following rupture of the posterior interspinous ligaments and the facet capsule with only minimal damage to the posterior longitudinal ligament. Beatson's work was conducted in spines dissected free of all musculature. In cadaver work conducted on whole-body specimens with intact musculature (13), additional section of the ipsilateral posterior longitudinal ligament and annulus were found to be necessary for production of a unilateral facet dislocation. A component of rotation in addition to distraction and flexion was also necessary.

Stage 3 This is a bilateral facet dislocation. Beatson

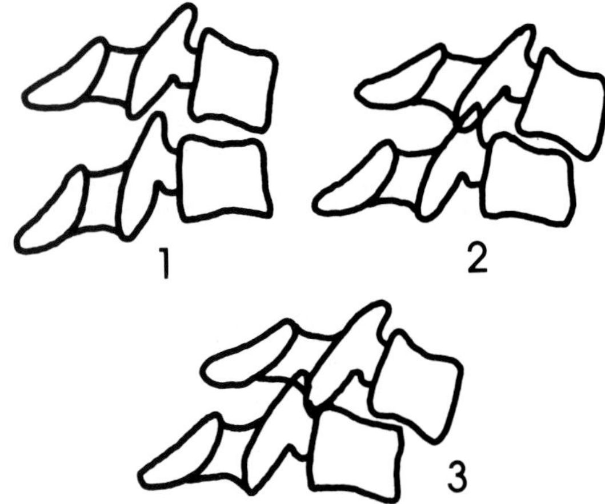

Figure 20.1. Distractive flexion injury: *Stage 1* — facet subluxation; *Stage 2* — unilateral facet dislocation, forward displacement less than 50% of vertebra; *Stage 3* — bilateral facet dislocation, forward displacement 50% or more of vertebra; *Stage 4* (not shown) — full vertebral body width anterior displacement or grossly unstable segment with appearance of a floating vertebra.

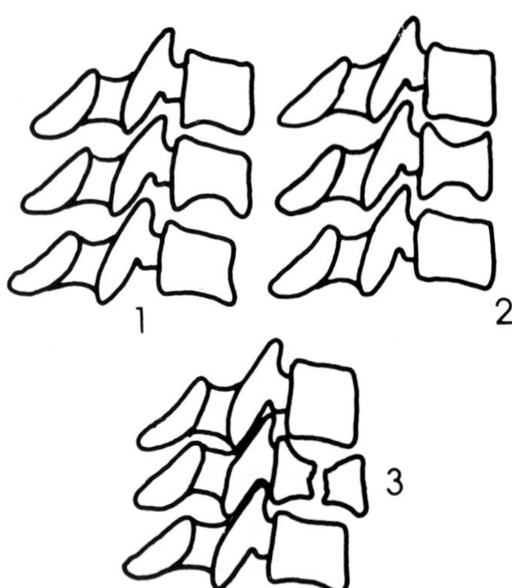

Figure 20.2. Vertical compression injury: *Stage 1* — superior or inferior endplate cupping; *Stage 2* — superior and inferior endplate cupping with possible centrum fracture but essentially no displacement of the posterior vertebral into the spinal canal; *Stage 3* — comminuted centrum with posterior displacement into the spinal canal.

demonstrated that rupture of the interspinous ligament, the capsules of both facet joints, the posterior longitudinal ligament, and the annulus fibrosus was necessary for production of this injury.

Stage 4 The stage 4 lesion is full vertebral body width displacement anteriorly or a grossly unstable segment giving the appearance of a floating vertebra.

VERTICAL COMPRESSION (FIG. 20.2)

Stage 1 This lesion consists of a fracture of either a superior or inferior end-plate with a cupping deformity.

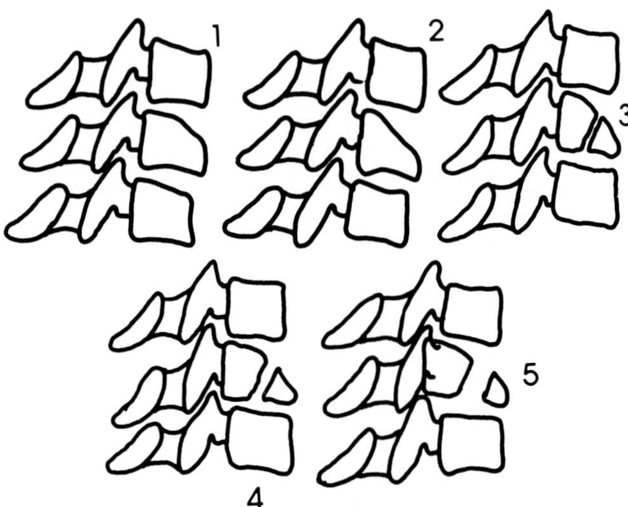

Figure 20.3. Compressive flexion injury: *Stage 1* — anterior blunting; *Stage 2* — wedge compression with "beak" appearance; *Stage 3 — centrum fracture through "beak"; Stage 4* — less than 3 mm posterior displacement into the spinal canal; *Stage 5* — more than 3 mm displacement into the spinal canal.

The initial end-plate failure is central rather than anterior, and there is no evidence of ligamentous failure.

Stage 2 This lesion consists of fracture of both vertebral end-plates with cupping deformities. There may be fracture lines through the centrum, but displacement of the posterior body wall into the spinal canal is minimal.

Stage 3 This lesion shows fragmentation of the centrum, and its residual pieces are displaced peripherally in multiple directions. The posterior portion of the vertebral body is fractured and may be displaced into the neural canal. In some cases, the vertebral arch is completely intact, and there is no evidence of ligamentous failure, while in others there is comminution of the vertebral arch with gross failure of the posterior ligamentous complex.

COMPRESSIVE FLEXION (FIG. 20.3)

Stage 1 This lesion consists of blunting of the anterosuperior vertebral margin to a more rounded contour. There is no evidence of failure of the posterior ligamentous complex.

Stage 2 This lesion shows obliquity of the anterior vertebral body and loss of some anterior height of the centrum. The result is a "beak" appearance of the anterior-inferior vertebral body. The concavity of the inferior endplate may be increased, and there may be a vertical fracture of the centrum.

Stage 3 This lesion has a fracture line passing obliquely from the anterior surface of the vertebral body through the centrum and extending through the inferior subchondral plate; a fracture of the beak is also present.

Stage 4 This lesion additionally demonstrates a 3 mm or less displacement of the inferior-posterior vertebral margin into the neural canal.

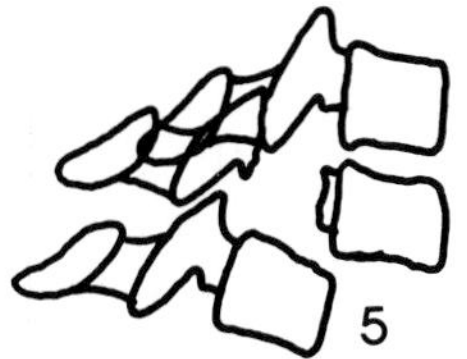

Figure 20.4. Compressive extension injury (stages 1–4 not shown): *Stage 1* — unilateral vertebral arch fracture; *Stage 2* — bilaminar fractures; *Stage 3* — bilateral pedicle, facet, or arch fractures; *Stage 4* — stage 3 with partial displacement; *Stage 5* (shown) — stage 4 with gross displacement.

Stage 5 This lesion demonstrates the features listed above and a more than 3 mm displacement of the inferior-posterior vertebral margin into the neural canal. The vertebral arch characteristically remains intact. The articular facets are separated, and there is increased distance between the spinous processes at the injury level, indicative of posterior ligamentous disruption under tension.

Compressive Extension (Fig. 20.4)

Stage 1 This lesion consists of a unilateral vertebral arch fracture with or without anterorotary vertebral body displacement. The fracture may be a linear fracture through the articular process, a compression of the articular process, or an ipsilateral pedicle and laminar fracture.
Stage 2 This lesion consists of bilaminar fractures without evidence of other tissue failure in the vertebral motion segments. Usually the posterior element fractures are seen at multiple contiguous levels.
Stage 3 This lesion consists of bilateral posterior element fractures including articular processes, pedicles, lamina, or some combination thereof without vertebral body displacement.
Stage 4 This lesion consists of bilateral vertebral arch fractures with partial vertebral body width displacement anteriorly.

Compressive-extension stages 3 and 4 were not observed in Allen's original series but were postulated as transitional forms between stage 2 and stage 5.
Stage 5 This lesion consists of bilateral arch fractures with full vertebral body width displacement anteriorly. The most posterior vertebral elements remain posteriorly, while the more anterior of the posterior elements are displaced anteriorly with the vertebral body. Ligamentous failure occurs posteriorly between the fractured vertebra and the level above and anteriorly between the fractured vertebra and the level below. The displaced vertebral body commonly shears off the anterosuperior portion of the vertebral body below.

Distractive Extension (Fig. 20.5)

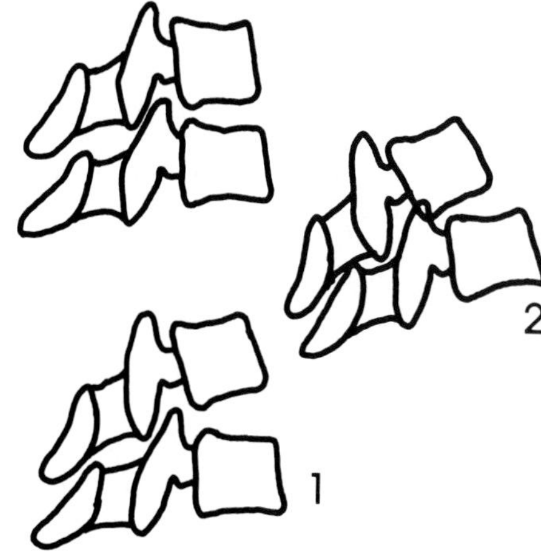

Figure 20.5. Distractive extension injury: *Stage 1* — rupture of the anterior ligamentous complex or transverse centrum fracture; *Stage 2* — rupture of the posterior ligamentous complex with posterior displacement.

Distractive extension injuries are the opposite of distractive flexion injuries with initial failure occurring in the anterior longitudinal ligament. The key radiographic feature is anterior widening of the disc space on extension.
Stage 1 A transverse nondeforming fracture of the vertebral body may be observed in addition to anterior longitudinal ligamentous failure. There is no posterior vertebral body displacement.
Stage 2 This lesion also displays posterior ligamentous failure with posterior displacement of the upper vertebral body. This displacement often reduces spontaneously with the head in the neutral or flexed position, and initial cross-table supine films usually show displacement of 3 mm or less.

Lateral Flexion

Lateral flexion injuries consist of asymmetric, unilateral compression fracture of the centrum plus the vertebral arch.
Stage 1 This lesion consists of asymmetric fracture of the centrum with vertebral arch fracture on the ipsilateral side as seen in the anteroposterior radiograph. The vertebral arch fracture may include compression of the articular process or comminution of the corner of the vertebral arch. The vertebral body fracture may include a uncovertebral fracture with superior end-plate compression, and there may be a vertical fracture of the centrum.
Stage 2 This lesion also consists of displacement of the vertebral arch fracture or contralateral ligamentous as seen on the anteroposterior radiograph.

Clinical Frequency and Observations

In addition to the original series by Allen et al., another large series of cervical spine injuries utilizing this mechanistic classification has been compiled at the Rancho Los Amigos Medical Center by Waters et al. (14). The series of Allen et al. consisted of 165 closed, indirect fractures and dislocations of the lower cervical spine, and that at

Rancho Los Amigos consisted of 151 fractures and dislocations.

Questions may arise about the correlation of the radiologic classification of the cervical injury with physical examination observations, e.g., how one resolves the radiographic appearance of a distractive flexion injury with physical observations of forehead abrasions which suggest extension. Resolution lies in consideration of complex clinical loading situations, materials failure criteria, and force vectors at the site of injury. Many cervical injuries result from motor vehicle accidents in which the craniocervical unit is subjected to a variety of complex loading situations occurring in rapid succession. Lack of pure loading situations which occur in the laboratory setting account for injuries which contain elements of different cervical injury classifications. In addition, paradoxical sagittal motion, i.e., snaking, has been observed during flexion extension maneuvers in radiographic studies of cervical orthoses (15, 16, 17, 18, 19). It must therefore be appreciated that forces producing extension on the craniocervical unit as a whole may result in flexion moments with compression or extension loading within the cervical spine itself. The location of the cervical injury will depend upon the location where the complex external loading situation results in internal stresses which exceed the local osseoligamentous failure criteria.

DISTRACTIVE FLEXION

Distractive flexion injuries comprised 37% of the Allen series and 32% of the Rancho Los Amigos series (11, 14). Within this injury classification in each of these series, stage 1 injuries accounted for 20% and 31%; stage 2 injuries accounted for 41% and 29%; stage 3 injuries accounted for 28% and 35%; and stage 4 accounted for 11% and 6%.

Allen et al. noted that some of these injuries had a minor compressive element in the anterosuperior portion of the centrum below which may suggest a primary axis of rotation placed in the anterior disc. This anterior compression was observed with decreasing frequency as the stage of injury increased, which suggests the primary axis of rotation lies more anteriorly in the more severe injuries.

Bauze and Ardran experimentally reproduced distractive flexion injuries and demonstrated that rotation was not necessary for ligamentous failure (20). However, a rotational element is necessary for lateralization of ligamentous injury. The cadaver injury model at Rancho Los Amigos by Chandler demonstrated that rotation was necessary for production of stage 2 injuries (13). Furthermore, the ligaments contralateral to the dislocated facet were observed to display varying degrees of attenuation. Also, after complete bilateral facet dislocation, subsequent reduction may occur to a unilateral facet dislocation position; therefore, stability of cervical injuries which present as unilateral facet dislocation must be questioned and extensive ligamentous damage should be assumed.

As noted by Ellis above, the injury to the ligamentous structures must be stressed. Failure of adequate ligamentous healing is not uncommon after knee and ankle injuries and results in difficulty with stability. In the series at Rancho Los Amigos, conservative management of cervical injuries in a halo-vest was followed by assessment of stability. Because bony injury was uncommon in this type of injury, residual instability was common, with failure of adequate healing observed in 71% of cases. Serious consideration should be given to surgical stabilization of these injuries.

VERTICAL COMPRESSION

Vertical compression injuries comprised 8% of the Allen series and 21% of the Rancho Los Amigos series (11, 13). Within this injury classification in each of these series, stage 1 injuries accounted for 36% and 6%; stage 2 injuries accounted for 29% and 48%; and stage 3 injuries accounted for 36% and 45%.

Allen et al. observed associated posterior arch fractures which increased in frequency from 16% in stage 1 injuries to 40% in stage 3 injuries. Ligamentous failure was not a prominent feature of vertical compression injuries, and in the Rancho Los Amigos series conservative halo management resulted in 71% bony ankylosis and only one case of residual instability.

COMPRESSIVE FLEXION

Compressive flexion injuries comprised 22% of the Allen series and 42% of the Rancho Los Amigos series. Within this injury classification in each of these series, stage 1 injuries accounted for 17% and 16%; stage 2 injuries accounted for 19% and 25%; stage 3 injuries accounted for 11% and 21%; stage 4 accounted for 22% and 21%; and stage 5 accounted for 31% and 17%.

Allen et al. observed that the ligamentous failure occurred between the fractured vertebra and the subjacent vertebra. However, Ellis pointed out that ligamentous damage does not always correspond to the level of dislocation, and the series at Rancho Los Amigos also observed ligamentous failure at the level above the fractured vertebra. Allen et al. emphasized ligamentous failure in stage 5 of compression flexion injuries, but at Rancho Los Amigos significant posterior ligamentous disruption was observed to occur beginning in stage 3 injuries. In fact, associated bony injury resulted in ankylosis in 92% of stage 4 injuries and 91% of stage 5 injuries, while residual instability was observed in 54% of the stage 3 injuries at Rancho Los Amigos. Mazur and Stauffer also warned about unrecognized spinal instability associated with seemingly "simple" cervical compression injuries (21). The exact mechanisms of the injuries were not well-detailed but were described to result from compression in flexion. Exclusion criteria were very strict and included not only flexion-extension radiographs but also exclusion of any patient with loss of cervical lordosis. Of 27 patients meeting their criteria, 7 patients, or 26%, demonstrated significant residual instability.

Compressive Extension

Compressive extension injuries comprised 24% of the Allen series but only 4% of the Rancho Los Amigos series. Within this injury classification in Allen series, stage 1 injuries accounted for 80%; stage 2 injuries accounted for 13%; and stage 5 injuries accounted for 8%. No stage 3 or 4 injuries were observed in either the Allen or Rancho Los Amigos series. Allen et al. postulated stages 3 and 4 as transitional stages between stages 2 and 5.

Ligamentous failure was observed by Allen et al. at two different levels in stage 5 injuries. Failure occurs posteriorly between the suprajacent and fractured vertebra, and anteriorly between the subjacent and fractured vertebra. Infrequency of this injury with the series at Rancho Los Amigos precludes any significant conclusion about residual instability.

Distractive Extension

Distractive extension injuries comprised only 5% of the Allen series and 1% of the Rancho Los Amigos series.

Lateral Flexion

Lateral flexion injuries comprised only 3% of the Allen series and 1% of the Rancho Los Amigos series.

Implications for Treatment

Once the particular injury classification is identified and the osseous and ligamentous damage assessed, attention must be focused on particular aspects of the injury to direct appropriate therapy. Issues of acute instability are important to emergency stabilization and initial treatment (22). Recognition of components contributing to chronic instability may allow definitive therapy to be instituted initially and obviate conservative failure.

Recognition of acute instability is crucial. It has been estimated by Cloward that up to 25% of spinal cord injuries are sustained during emergency extrication, transport, and evaluation of the patient subsequent to the precipitating accidental event (23). The work of White and Panjabi may be particularly helpful in alerting the physician to an acutely unstable spine requiring circumspect evaluation and treatment (24). In their assessment system, 1 point is assigned for abnormal disc narrowing, 1 point if large physiologic loading is anticipated in the patient's lifestyle, and 2 points are assigned for each of the following findings: *a*) anterior elements destroyed or unable to function, *b*) posterior elements destroyed or unable to function, *c*) relative sagittal plane rotation on any x-ray of more than 11°, *d*) relative sagittal plane translation of 3.5 mm, *e*) a positive stretch test, and *f*) spinal cord damage. A total of 5 points is considered an unstable spine.

The three column structural model as proposed by Denis for thoracolumbar injuries could be extrapolated to the cervical spine (25), but division into anterior and posterior columns or elements as discussed by Holdsworth is sufficient for conceptualizing cervical spine injuries (6). Quite simply, injury to both the anterior and posterior elements results in acute instability.

In the field, cervical spine injuries and instability often can only be suspected. Extreme caution should be exercised to avoid irreversible and devastating spinal cord injury, but the realities of extrication situations make this most difficult (22). Emergency cervical spine immobilization has been and continues to be an important area of research. In cadaver work by Chandler, a bilateral facet dislocation allows 82° of sagittal rotation and full body width translation. Placement in a cervical extrication collar only reduces this to 25° of sagittal rotation and 30% body width translation. Secure control of the head and shoulders can reduce motion to 4° sagittal rotation and 3% body width translation. These findings as well as photographic and radiographic studies in live subjects reinforce the recommendations for extrication and transport of accident victims as outlined by the American Academy of Orthopaedic Surgeons (22). Specifically, extrication collars themselves do not provide sufficient cervical spine immobilization, so that the addition of a short spine board with additional tape is a requisite.

Integrity of the posterior ligamentous complex has important implications for both acute and chronic instability. As noted by Ellis, the integrity of the soft tissues is crucial to maintenance of stability (12). As indicated above from the review of conservative treatment of cervical injuries at Rancho Los Amigos, data on conservative treatment failures supports early surgical stabilization of distraction flexion stage 1 and 3 injuries as well as compression flexion stage 3 injuries.

Halo management is successful for the majority of injuries with extensive anterior osseous damage, since this often leads to intervertebral ankylosis as noted in the series at Rancho Los Amigos. However, concomitant damage to posterior bony structures, specifically the facets, may so severely compromise the cervical spine structure that maintenance of stability is difficult even in a halo-vest. Whitehill et al. noted this failure of the halo-vest to maintain cervical spine fracture reduction (25, 26).

Conclusion

Disruption of the posterior ligamentous complex is the primary reason for late instability of cervical injuries treated conservatively. In general, injuries in which the posterior ligamentous complex is disrupted and in which there is minimal or no associated bony injury result in 31% bony ankylosis and 42% late instability. All other types of injury result in less than 5% late instability. The classification system of Allen et al., although somewhat complex, is clinically useful because it contributes to understanding the extent of injury and it identifies the probability of chronic instability for specific subclasses of injury for which the prognosis indicates conservative management and other subclasses for which the prognosis suggests surgical management.

REFERENCES

1. Power D. The Edwin Smith papyrus. Br J Surg 1934;21:385.
2. Durbin FC. Fracture dislocations of the cervical spine. J Bone Joint Surg 1957;39B:23–38.
3. Ellis VH. Injuries of the cervical vertebra. Proc R Soc Med 1946;40:19.
4. Roaf R. A study of the mechanics of spinal injuries. J Bone Joint Surg 1960;42B:810–823.
5. Whitely JE, Forsyth HF. The classification of cervical spine injuries. AJR 1960;83:633–644.
6. Holdsworth FW. Fractures, dislocations, and fracture-dislocations of the spine. J Bone Joint Surg 1970;52A:1534–1551.
7. Braakman R, Penning L. Injuries of the cervical spine. Amsterdam: Excerpta Medica, 1971:53–62.
8. Taylor AR, Blackwood W. Paraplegia in hyperextension cervical injuries with normal radiographic appearances. J Bone Joint Surg 1948;30B:245–248.
9. Forsyth HF. Extension injuries of the cervical spine. J Bone Joint Surg 1964;46A:1792–1797.
10. Burke DC. Hyperextension injuries of the spine. J Bone Joint Surg 1971;53B:3–12.
11. Allen BL, Ferguson RL, Lehman TR, O'Brien RP. A mechanistic classification of closed, indirect fractures and dislocations of the lower cervical spine. Spine 1982;7:1–27.
12. Beatson TR. Fractures and dislocations of the cervical spine. J Bone Joint Surg 1963;45B:21–35.
13. Chandler DR, Nemejc C, Adkins RH, Waters RL. Unpublished data from Rancho Los Amigos Medical Center, 1989.
14. Waters RL, Adkins RH, Nelson R, Garland D. Cervical spine cord trauma: evaluation and nonoperative treatment with halo-vest immobilization. Contemp Orthop 1987;14:35–45.
15. Fisher SV, Bowar JF, Awad EA, Gullickson G. Cervical orthoses effect on cervical motion: roentgenographic and goniometric method of study. Arch Phys Med Rehabil 1977;58:109–115.
16. Hartman JT, Palumbo F, Hill BJ. Cineradiography of the braced normal cervical spine. Clin Orthop 1975;109:97–102.
17. Johnson RM, Owen JR, Hart DL, Callahan RA. Cervical orthoses: a guide to their selection and use. Clin Orthop 1981;154:34–45.
18. Jones MD. Cineradiographic studies of the collar-immobilized cervical spine. J Neurosurg 1960;17:633–637.
19. Lind B, Sihlbom H, Nordwall A. Forces and motions across the neck in patients treated with halo-vest. Spine 1988;13:162–167.
20. Bauze RJ, Ardran GM. Experimental production of forward dislocation in the human cervical spine. J Bone Joint Surg 1978;60B:239–245.
21. Mazur JM, Stauffer ES. Unrecognized spinal instability associated with seemingly "simple" cervical compression fractures. Spine 1983;8:687–692.
22. American Academy of Orthopaedic Surgeons: Emergency care and transportation of the sick and injured. 3rd ed. Menasha, Washington: George Banta, 1981.
23. Cloward RB. Acute cervical spine injuries. Clin Symp 1980;32:15.
24. White AA, Johnson RM, Panjabi MM, Southwick WO. Biomechanical analysis of clinical stability in the cervical spine. Clin Orthop 1975;109:85–96.
25. Denis F. The three column spine and its significance in the classification of acute thoracolumbar spinal injuries. Spine 1983;8:817–831.
26. Whitehill R, Richman JA, Glaser JA. Failure of immobilization of the cervical spine by the halo vest. J Bone Joint Surg 1986;68A:326–332.

21

Basic Principles for Treatment of Cervical Spine Trauma/Experimental Trauma

Thomas G. Saul

Introduction

The primary objective of this chapter is to review the basic principles of treating cervical spine and spinal cord injury. The other chapters in this section will address specific types of injuries and their management. This chapter will present a more holistic approach to the initial management of cervical spine injury, concentrating on the nonsurgical management principles. While there is no single right way to deal with these problems, there are basic principles of management which if adhered to will increase the chance of optimal outcome for the patient. These principles are based on the pathophysiological events that follow cord injury. These pathophysiological processes have been documented over the past 2 decades through experimental cord injury models and recorded by a multitude of investigators. These investigations will be referenced when appropriate to support the pathophysiological principles. The pathophysiology of spinal cord injury can be divided into the following: (*a*) the mechanical insults, (*b*) hemodynamic changes, (*c*) biochemical derangements, and (*d*) ancillary medical problems.

Mechanical Insults

Three types of mechanical insults accompany spinal cord injury. (1) direct cord tissue disruption, (2) continued movement of an unstable spine after the injury, and (3) persistent compression of neural tissue secondary to bone or soft tissue material (intervertebral disc and/or ligament, hematoma).

Tissue Disruption

The spinal cord possesses no inherent regenerative capacity that results in *functional recovery* of anatomically disrupted tissue. The regenerative efforts of the cord produce only meager sprouts and no new distal growth. The irreversible damage begins in the central gray. Electron microscopic studies in the monkey have shown that the venules in the gray substance distend within 5 minutes of impact. Red cells can be seen in the perivascular space of the capillaries and venules within 15–30 minutes. Hemorrhages occur in the gray matter within 1 hour. Progressive vacuolation and swelling of the endothelium of the capillaries are marked within the first few hours (1). Within 48 hours posttrauma, central ischemic and hemorrhagic lesions are present on histological sections. There is progressive gray matter necrosis. White matter changes do not begin until 3 or 4 hours after injury. The cord periphery is initially spared except for the occasional flame-shaped hemorrhage that occurs with the original impact (2). In white matter there is initially edema. This causes abnormal perfusion, and the white matter undergoes destruction over the next few days. The total amount of destruction is generally related to the amount of trauma inflicted (3).

Man can withstand the initial gray matter injury. This alone represents a segmental, affordable loss of only a small portion of the total gray matter neuronal pool. If this were the limit of injury, neurological deficit would be minor. Man cannot tolerate segmental loss of the peripheral white matter. This disrupts ascending and descending fiber tracts and results in loss of distal functioning of those tracts. Neurons are rendered useless, and cord function is lost in varying degrees.

Regeneration of the spinal cord after traumatic disruption has been investigated extensively for many years (4, 5). Wolman demonstrated at autopsy well-developed axon regeneration in and around the damaged cord segments in 12 patients who died with traumatic paraplegia. These were small axon bundles found above and below the level of maximum cord damage. However, the origins of these nerve fibers were the posterior nerve roots and ganglia (6). Efforts have been made to induce a regenerative process in damaged spinal cords. Windle demonstrated that the brief phase of active regeneration that normally takes place after cord transsections may be extended by the administration of Piromen, a polysaccharide that reduces connective and glial scar formation. This work was done in cats

(7). Subsequently there were attempts to diminish scar tissue formation in spine injured dogs and rats by administering trypsin intrathecally (8). These works demonstrated no functional value in their findings.

In 1973, the Russian monograph by Matinian and Andreasian was published that reported enzyme therapy to be efficacious in the treatment of experimental paraplegia in rats. The substances employed were: trypsin, hyaluronidase, elastase, and Piromen. This study documented a 27–47% functional recovery in the treated group compared to controls who remained paraplegic. Moreover, these authors presented histological evidence of nerve fiber regeneration and electrophysiological evidence of conduction between sciatic nerve and cerebral cortex (9). Attempts were made to reproduce the Russian findings by a number of different investigators. These demonstrated (*a*) no recovery from paraplegia, (*b*) no impulse conduction across the injury site, (*c*) no histological evidence of nerve fiber regeneration (10–12).

In spite of the continued work in the area of cord regeneration, there is to date no effective intrinsic spinal cord regenerative process, nor is there any treatment available to induce such a process that could result in effectively reversing direct tissue disruption.

More recently, various neural transplantation techniques have been attempted to induce some type of regeneration process in injured spinal cord. This work has all been done in animal models and to date has not produced any promising results. David et al. used interposition grafts with peripheral nerve segments in order to promote axonal regrowth (13). Embryonic neural tissue has been attempted for intraspinal transplantation with the same hopes (14, 15). Some sprouting of selective fibers has been demonstrated by planting dorsal root ganglia into the dorsal column of embryonic implants (16). Certainly, in spite of the very slow progress of these experiments, this work will continue and hopefully lead to a viable treatment option for spinal cord injury.

Therefore, the only effective way to combat this aspect of cord insult is through primary prevention of these injuries. Approximately 10,000 new spinal cord injuries occur each year. The majority of these are caused by vehicular accidents and falls. They are also due to recreational and industrial accidents. Physicians in all medical disciplines as well as other medical personnel need to encourage and promote public and personal safety standards whenever possible. Recognizing this, the American Association of Neurological Surgeons and the Congress of Neurological Surgeons have undertaken the National Head and Spinal Cord Injury Prevention Program.

The other forms of mechanical insults (mobility and compression) can cause additional irreversible damage that can worsen a given neurological deficit or prevent the recovery of a marginal deficit. These phenomena, however, *can* be altered by therapeutic intervention.

Spinal Mobility Around an Injured Spinal Cord

Vertebral immobilization following injury to the spine has been a rule observed for many years. The obvious purpose of vertebral immobilization is that of preventing movement of an unstable vertebral column with consequent damage to the enclosed spinal cord. The fact is that physical movement at the site of a spinal cord injury can accentuate the pathology and have a detrimental affect on the clinical course. Ducker et al. demonstrated this experimentally by subjecting monkeys to variable degrees of spinal cord contusion at the T11/T12 level (17). The control group consisted of animals whose injury was inflicted with up to 500 g-cm but without vertebral immobilization. The experimental group received injuries from forces in the 500–800 g-cm range and rigid vertebral immobilization immediately following in every case. Clinical neurological evaluation of the animals was made at 6 hours and on each day for 7 days. The results of this experiment revealed that rigid immobilization of the vertebrae surrounding an injured spinal cord altered the clinical course of that lesion. A 500 g-cm injury consistently produced paraplegia in the non-immobilized animal. However, injuries of 750–800 g-cm are required to consistently produce paralysis when the animal is treated with vertebral immobilization. The mechanisms that account for this better outcome associated with immobilization are unknown. It is possible that further stretch injury is prevented, thus maintaining the integrity of surviving fiber tracts, glia, and neurons. In addition, the immobilization may optimize the vascular supply to the cord preserving marginally injured regions.

Therefore, the proper management of a cord-injured patient should include immediate immobilization of the spine.

In the early phase of management at the scene and in transit, this can be accomplished by utilizing rigid cervical collar, spine board, sand-bags, and tape. After the exact nature of the spine injury has been delineated by radiographic studies, more definitive immobilization should be done. Skeletal traction with one of the various types of cranial tongs can be used to immobilize the spine. After the tongs are inserted, weights are applied for traction force. Except for the rare cranio-cervical junction injury, the initial poundage is around 2–3 pounds per veretebra down to the level of the fracture. The weight is increased in 5- or 10-pound increments, depending on the age and weight of the patient as well as the fracture itself. As traction is being increased, the patient's head and neck can be appropriately positioned (mild hyperextension or flexion) in order to adequately align the bone. Frequent x-rays must be obtained during this time in order to assess the consequences of each maneuver.

In addition to immobilizing the fracture site, skeletal traction also reduces the fracture. That is to say, it realigns the spine and hopefully returns the spinal canal to its normal anatomic dimensions. This gives the injured cord optimal room. It "decompresses" the cord with respect to bony compression. As we will see later, cord compression has deleterious effects on function. This process of immobilizing and realigning the spine with skeletal traction is important especially if the injury has produced an incomplete cord lesion. An incomplete lesion has promise for recovery (18), and early attention to this aspect of the pathophysiology may benefit the patient.

If adequate realignment cannot be achieved by this method, open surgical reduction should certainly be considered in patients with incomplete lesions.

The timing of this procedure is a controversial issue. Some people maintain that operation within the first several days of injury is associated with significant morbidity (19). Others feel that the hope of improving a patient's incomplete cord lesion justifies the early operation. Still others justify early operation on the basis of a demonstrated lower incidence of systemic complications (20).

This author's approach would be to operate early if the lesion is incomplete and if the spine could not be realigned. It should be noted that under these circumstances, the surgical approach is dictated by where the compression and/or instability is located. If the injury is a unilateral facet fracture with posterior and lateral ligamentous injury and the vertebral bodies remain significantly subluxed after skeletal traction, I would recommend a posterior operation designed to: (*a*) "unlock" the facet and thus realign the spine, (*b*) assure adequate decompression of the exiting nerve root at the fracture site, and (*c*) definitively stabilize the spine.

The problem that is sometimes encountered is persistent bony compressions anteriorly associated with ligamentous disruption posteriorly. If early decompression of this type of fracture is indicated, maintaining postoperative stability is very difficult. A small percentage of patients therefore may require both anterior and posterior procedures. The point is this: any surgeon treating these types of spine injuries should be comfortable performing anterior as well as posterior procedures as described in the other chapters of this volume. The choice of procedure is dictated by the location of the compression and the instability. Most people would agree that any time a decompressive procedure is done in the presence of posttraumatic spinal instability, the stabilization procedure should ideally be performed simultaneously.

Persistent Compression of Neural Tissue

Extra-axial compression of spinal cord tissue can cause both anatomic and physiologic changes. This can result in partial or total loss of function. In spinal cord injuries, there is an initial acute compression of the cord due to the abnormal excursion of the spinal bony structures. The resultant cord contusion leads to the pathological changes described earlier in this chapter. However, it is also possible that bone and/or soft tissue (intervertebral disc, ligament, hematoma, etc.) may remain in the spinal canal and cause focal compression. During such compression, the blood vessels are often occluded. This observation has led to some debate as to whether the subsequent dysfunction is the result of the ischemic changes or mechanical distortion. This remains unanswered, which probably indicates that it is a combination of the two processes.

Experimental studies have documented the changes that accompany cord compression. Griffiths, using intradural balloon catheters in dogs, examined the effects that acute and chronic compression had on the electrical conductivity and vascular permeability of the cord (21). He found that evoked potentials through the dorsal column stopped abruptly with acute compression. If the compression was released, these potentials reappeared within 5–15 minutes. The same was true for chronically applied compression, except the cessation of the evoked potential was delayed. There was marked leakage of Evans blue albumin from the intermediate gray matter in the acute compression. Chronic compression did not increase vascular permeability until after the compression was released, at which time it resembled that of the acute compression. Histologically, all of the animals demonstrated perivascular hemorrhages in the gray matter. Disruption of the gray neuropil was also seen. Neuronal degeneration characterized by pallor of staining and loss of the Nissl substances was noted. The white matter changes consisted of separation of the myelinated fibers and disruption of normal architecture. Other investigators have noted similar neurophysiological and anatomical changes and showed that compression, in association with ischemia, produced an additive effect in cord pathology (22, 23). Kobrine et al. presented further descriptions of the pathophysiology of cord compression (24). They conducted experiments with acute balloon compression of varying duration on monkey spinal cords. The disappearance and return of spinal evoked responses, as well as the spinal cord blood flow (SCBF) were measured. They concluded that the major pathological cause for the neural dysfunction is physical injury to the neural membrane, irrespective of blood flow changes. They concluded further that the ability of that membrane to recover appears to be related to rapidity and length of time of compression and that focal blood flow changes may not be significant in this mechanism.

It would therefore seem logical that treatment of spinal cord injuries should include an early diagnostic search for any surgically amenable compression of the cord which, if treated, may result in a better recovery for that patient. This is especially true with incomplete cord lesions which have a better prognosis for return of neurological function (25). The judicious use of plain x-rays, tomography, CT scanning, or MRI are the tools used to identify bone or soft tissue causing cord compression. If such compression is present, the surgical decompression can be performed.

The timing of the diagnostic tests and any subsequent surgery has and will remain controversial. Certainly any associated injuries would affect this decision. In addition, there has never been any conclusive demonstration that immediate or early decompression results in better outcome (19, 20). There are certainly anectodal reports of enhancing recovery with urgent decompression, but nothing is conclusive. Saul and Ducker have reported 90 acute cervical cord injuries who underwent the now obsolete pantopaque mini myelogram (26). Twenty-three of the patients had abnormal myelograms (seven complete blocks and 16 anterior filling defects). Twelve of the 23 patients were operated upon. Only three of the patients showed greater neurological improvement (greater than two standard deviations) than that predicted by the recovery rates of Lucas and Ducker (25). This represented 3.3% of the total patients studied. It should be noted that patients were operated upon whether they had complete or incomplete spinal cord lesions. The yield of improving neurological outcome by immediate diagnostic and subsequent surgery is low. However, such an aggressive approach may be appropriate for certain patients.

At the present time, this author follows the following guidelines. If the patient sustains an apparently complete cord injury, the patient is immobilized and diagnostics are done on an elective basis to plan definitive treatment.

If a patient has an incomplete cervical cord lesion, the patient is immobilized in skeletal traction and realigned. A water soluble contrast CT scan is performed after the patient's spine is realigned i.e., the CT scan is performed with the patient in traction. When feasible and if MRI compatible tongs are employed an MRI scan can be performed in lieu of water soluble contrast CT scan. If either of these tests demonstrate persistent soft tissue compression, the patient is operated upon at that time.

It should be noted that this is one author's approach. It does not constitute the only right way to treat these problems. It is based upon *a*) pathophysiology of cord compression, *b*) the documented "recoverability" of incomplete cord lesions, *c*) the author's own philosophical approach to spinal cord injury.

HEMODYNAMIC CHANGES

When the spinal cord is injured, hemodynamic changes take place that profoundly affect cord function. These hemodynamic alterations involve the microscopic vasculature of the cord, as well as the microcirculation. Moreover, changes in the systemic hemodynamics can occur which can effect the intrinsic cord pathology (27).

Marked changes take place in spinal cord vasomotor responses, blood flow, oxygen tension, and autoregulation (28, 29). These hemodynamic abnormalities demand attention during the management of these patients.

The vasomotor reactivity of experimentally injured spinal cord is lost almost immediately after injury (30, 31). As in the brain, an increase in the partial pressure of carbon dioxide in arterial blood causes vasodilatation of the spinal cord vascularity and results in increased blood flow (32, 33). However, when the cord is injured, this response is impaired. In addition, other studies have demonstrated that circulation time is prolonged in the injured cord segment. The most marked increase is seen in the capillary and venous phases.

The xenon saturation techniques in animal spinal cords demonstrated a quantitative decrease in blood flow 2–3 hours after injury (34). Microangiographic studies of injured spinal cord blood vessels confirm that there may be an initial ischemic phase which involved both gray and white matter of the cord (35).

In summary, experimental cord injury studies seem to indicate that in general: *a*) following acute cord injury, there is a short delay before spinal cord blood flow diminishes to dangerously ischemic levels; *b*) the reduction of SCBF is more marked in the central gray matter than the peripheral white matter; *c*) the loss of vasomotor responsiveness and autoregulation has a profound effect on the development of the pathologic lesion; *d*) because of these losses, alterations of blood pressure can dramatically affect the evolution of the lesion; *e*) concomitant with these SCBF changes, there are parallel changes in the tissue oxygen tension which will ultimately affect cord metabolic function.

These pathophysiological changes—although they are not completely delineated or understood—have important implications in regard to the treatment of acute spinal cord injuries. Since all of these studies show a delay in the onset of the deleterious circulatory changes, strict attention should be paid to assuring adequate spinal cord perfusion and oxygenation. This begins at the scene of the injury with the paramedic personnel, as discussed earlier. These general principles of management should be imposed throughout the patient's acute and subacute phases of hospitalization. Assuring systemic normotension and optimal oxygenation should be the goal of the treatment team. By doing this, one is optimizing the physiological state for spinal cord recovery—at least based on the experimental evidence.

Intravenous lines should be inserted at the first convenient opportunity for vascular volume expansion in the event of hypotension. This may be necessary because of actual blood loss due to associated injuries or to vasomotor paralysis from the cord injury itself. Disruption of descending sympathetic pathways results in loss of vasomotor tone and subsequent hypotension. Concomitantly, the unopposed parasympathetic activity causes a bradycardia in face of hypotension (27). Fluid expansion should be managed cautiously because the cardiopulmonary response to fluid challenge may vary. A patient with a cervical cord injury may quickly develop pulmonary complications due to cardiovascular instability. One should be prepared to progress to pressor agents if the desired therapeutic effect is not realized with fluid administration.

Cervical cord injuries cause paralysis of intercostal respiration. Under these conditions, the patient is prone to respiratory distress and hypoxia on the basis of: *a*) inability to clear secretions, *b*) inability to cough or sigh, *c*) development of apnea, secondary to loss of diaphragmatic innervation if spinal cord edema involves the upper cervical segments (C3/C5). Therefore, in the treatment of these patients, the protocol should call for meticulous pulmonary therapy, including frequent suctioning, chest physiotherapy, and oxygen administration to maintain normal arterial blood gases. Careful nasotracheal intubation should be performed if these measures above do not effectively support the patient. A nasogastric tube should be inserted in order to prevent abdominal distension, secondary to a paralytic ileus. If untreated, this can result in vomiting and aspiration. Also, respiratory embarrassment can occur due to upward displacement of the diaphragm. It should be noted that all of these initial therapeutic interventions are aimed at optimizing spinal cord oxygenation and perfusion.

From a pharmacological point of view, there is at present no drug that is known to effectively alter these hemodynamic aspects of the pathophysiology of cord injury. The agents that have been utilized clinically and experimentally will be reviewed in a later section of this chapter following the discussion of biochemical abnormalities.

BIOCHEMICAL DERANGEMENTS

Over the past two decades many investigators have elucidated abnormalities in biochemical and cellular function that occur in the spinal cord following traumatic injury. Locke demonstrated increased lactate levels in injured spinal cord tissue (36). This was consistent with the known ischemic changes and increase in anaerobic metabolism.

The blood-brain barrier is the central nervous system's device for keeping itself clean and free of toxic substances. Normally, it allows only oxygen, sugar, and a few select amino acids to cross over into central nervous system tissue. Injury to the blood-brain barrier has been demonstrated in spinal cord trauma (37). The use of Evans blue as a fluorescent tracer demonstrated neuronal staining and extravasation of this tracer into the neuropile of injured canine spinal cords. When the blood-brain barrier is defected as they demonstrated, blood-borne substances and chemicals have access to the cord tissue.

Prompted by this attention to the biochemistry of spinal cord injury, some investigators began to examine the changes at the cellular and organelle level. Kao and Chang demonstrated massive accumulation of lysosomes and release of lysosomal hydrolases in canine spinal cords completely transected by a subpial microscopic technique (38). They demonstrated that the lysosomal activity peaks for 3–7 days and is associated with autolysis and subsequent cavitation of the cord stumps. Ito, Allen, and Yashon demonstrated mitochondrial alterations as an early manifestation of experimental spinal cord injury (39). They showed a drop in cytochrome oxidase activities in the center of the traumatic site. Cytochrome oxidase is the terminal and rate-limiting enzyme of the electron transport series and is located on the inner membrane of the mitochrondria. Furthermore, Clendendon et al. showed prompt and significant decrease at the center of the site of experimental cord injury of $Na^+ - K^+$ activated ATPase (40). This enzyme is thought to be localized to the plasma membrane of cells. These studies support the idea that irreversible spinal cord injury may be related to damage to the cell membranes and subsequent metabolic derangements (41). The etiology of the membrane damage remains an enigma. Some hypotheses include: altered platelet function via abnormal free radical productions (42); and disruption of long-chain fatty acid moieties of membrane phospholipids due to free radical reactions (43, 44). These investigations into the biochemical derangements accompanying spinal injury have not produced any well-accepted therapeutic regimen. What they have accomplished is to direct our thinking and research toward metabolic and biochemical manipulations as possible therapies.

PHARMACOLOGICAL TREATMENTS FOR SPINAL CORD INJURY

Over the years many pharmacological interventions have been suggested in an attempt to reverse and/or halt hemodynamic and biochemical processes that mediate spinal cord pathophysiology. Many of these measures show promise when applied to animal studies. Many have a logical application based on the documented pathophysiology. However, none are associated with documentable efficacy in human clinical trials.

Ducker et al. could demonstrate no significant beneficial effect on experimental cord injury by using Dextran, Phenobarbital, methyldopa, Phenoxybenzamine, or vasopressors (45). Others confirmed the inability of Dextran to be helpful in cord injury even though theoretically—by decreasing sludging and blood viscosity—there should be an increase in arterial bed perfusion (46). Antifibrinolytic agents such as epsilon aminocaproic acid (Amicar) have also been studied (47, 48). The rationale for use of these agents is that they interfere with the proteolytic enzymes that lead to spread of hemorrhagic necrosis. However, these studies do not demonstrate any significant efficacy.

The anti-edema and diuretic agents have been associated with a higher degree of efficacy than other drugs. Mannitol as an osmotic diuretic decreases spinal cord edema rapidly (49, 50).

Corticosteriods are probably the most widely accepted agents in use. Ducker and Hamit showed statistically significant improvement and recovery of neurological function associated with dexamethasone in experimental canine studies who had incomplete cord injury (51). The exact mechanisms by which steroids reduce cord edema or improve cord functions remain debated. Possible mechanisms include: *a*) edema reduction, *b*) protection from free radicals, and *c*) increase from spinal cord blood flow. Most of the studies demonstrating steroid efficacy in spinal cord injury are experimental. Moreover, whether steroids are beneficial in the real clinical setting is not settled. No human trial has documented significant beneficial effect. Nonetheless, many centers still employ steroids in the treatment of acute cord injury. The dose used varies from center to center. A recent multicenter double-blind randomized trial reported no difference in neurological recovery in patients treated with "megadose" versus standard dosing regimens of patients with spinal cord injury (52).

The present author utilizes the following scheme: Dexamethasone, 1 mg/kg/day or methylprednisolone, 5 mg/kg/day in divided doses. It is our opinion that if a cord injury is complete and remains so for 2–3 days, the steroids therapy should be stopped because the risks of continuous steroids treatment (i.e., gastrointestinal bleeding, hyperglycemia, interference with wound healing) may outweigh possible benefit. However, in patients with incomplete cord lesions or who are showing neurological improvement, steroid treatment is continued for 1 week and then the dose is tapered quickly.

Dimethyl sulfoxide (DMSO) is a solvent which has been studied and found to have some properties that may be beneficial in treating spinal cord injuries. DMSO appears to diminish adhesiveness and aggregation of platelets and thrombus formation in blood vessels; there is a diuretic effect, as well as an antiinflammatory effect associated with DMSO. It is also possible that one of the effects is to increase oxygen diffusion in injured tissue (53). Experimental paralysis in dogs injured by a 500 gm-cm force has been reversed with DMSO administration (54). At present the efficacy of this agent has not been established in either human or experimental studies.

In 1969, Hartzog, Fischer, and Snow reported recovery from experimentally induced paraplegia in baboons treated with hyperbaric oxygen therapy (55). Kelly et al. also reported that tissue PO_2 in traumatized spinal cords of dogs was significantly increased by hyperbaric oxygen treatments and that neurological recovery in the animals was greater than control groups (56). Hyperbaric oxygen therapy increases the tissue oxygen and decreases the tissue edema. Both of these effects would theoretically be advantageous during the early phase after spinal cord injury. Although some reports were initially promising, to date the efficacy of this modality is unproven. This, along with the unavailability of this modality in most centers makes this treatment impractical (57–59).

Albin et al. introduced early operative localized cooling (hypothermia) of the injured spinal cord (60, 61). The temperature reduction theoretically decreases metabolic activity, increases ischemic and hypoxic tolerance, and possibly reduces inflammation and edema. Ducker confirmed Albin's studies but pointed out that the good results with hypothermia did not differ significantly from those obtained using steroids (51). Theinprasit et al. demonstrated an impressive functional recovery rate in cats whose cords were traumatized resulting in paraplegia and loss of cortical evoked response for over 6 hours post injury (62). The animals treated with laminectomy and cooling recovered enough to be able to walk compared with inability to walk in both the control animals and those treated with laminectomy alone. The literature contains only small numbers of human trials of local hypothermia (63, 64). Many questions remain unanswered in regard to this form of treatment. In particular, are the cases of reported beneficial effects with truly complete spinal cord lesions; for if not, spontaneous and gradual improvement is possible regardless of treatment (65). The fact is that although local hypothermia has theoretical validity, experimental efficacy, and a number of strong advocates, it has not found wide acceptance and implementation among most neurosurgeons. The reasons are mainly that the technique requires a large expenditure of time, personnel, and equipment, and the results are not significantly better than other forms of therapy. Normothermic perfusion of experimentally injured animal cords has been shown to be as effective as hypothermic perfusion (66).

Endogenous opiates, endorphins, have been implicated as pathophysiologic agents in the production of secondary injuries following spinal cord injury (69). It is believed that this secondary injury is mediated by a decrease in spinal cord blood flow by acting on the microcirculation of the spinal cord (68). Therefore Faden et al. theorized that administering an opiate antagonist, naloxone, could possibly prevent these pathophysiological changes and improve outcome of spinal cord injury (69). Animal studies have been presented that suggest efficacy of naloxone in treatment of cord injury (70, 71). On the other hand, some studies suggest that the results may not be as promising (72, 73). Flamm et al. reported a Phase I trial of naloxone administration to spinal cord injury patients. They found no statistically significant differences in neurological outcome in varying doses of naloxone (74). There were no reported adverse reactions or complications, and further clinical trials are underway. At present, the efficacy of naloxone is unknown in the treatment of human spinal cord injury.

Thyrotropin-releasing hormone TRH has been found to partially block endogenous opiate. TRH is able to alter the adverse autonomic effect of the opiate but not the analgesic properties (75–77). Animal studies have confirmed its efficacy in experimental cord injuries (78) and its apparent superiority to naloxone and high-dose steroids (79, 80). At the present time there are no reports of efficacy in human studies available.

Calcium channel blockers have been shown to increase spinal cord blood flow in animals after experimental cord trauma. Guha et al. demonstrated this in rats (81, 82). Other investigators demonstrated similar results in a canine model (83). In these studies it was emphasized that because of the hypotensive effect of the calcium blockers, the subjects often needed the systemic blood pressure supported. Further studies are certainly required to make even preliminary statements regarding the role of these agents in the treatment of spinal cord injury.

The above-cited therapeutic modalities are directed primarily at the hemodynamic insults of spinal cord injury. The investigations into the biochemical derangements of spinal cord injury have not produced any well-accepted specific therapeutic interventions. Strict attention should be directed to maintaining the patient in good homeostatic balance. Avoiding high energy consumption states such as fever, infection, and extreme agitation may be appropriate. Endogenous or exogenous toxins should be minimized. This is important since the blood-brain barrier (BBB) is known to be defective. Therefore, infection with subsequent sepsis should be warded off. The use of pharmacological agents that may have an adverse effect on cord functions should be avoided. Attempts have been made to reduce the metabolic requirements and activity in the injured cord. This is one of the principles of local hypothermia as discussed previously.

ANCILLARY SYSTEMIC CHANGES

This chapter would not be complete if some mention were not made of the changes in other organ systems that are caused by cord injury and which in turn can affect the function of that injured cord. These will be discussed according to systems.

Pulmonary

As mentioned earlier, in cervical and high thoracic cord injuries, the patient's respiratory pattern is altered and at risk to such things as developing apnea, atelectasis, pneumonia, etc. Furthermore, pulmonary embolus is a very real danger to cord-injured patients during their hospitalization. Active physical therapy with frequent range of motion of all extremities begun early in a patient's course can be preventative. Also, pneumatic compression cuffs may decrease this possibility. The use of low dose anticoagulants is advocated by some. Whatever course is chosen, a high index of suspicion is required and aggressive diagnostic evaluation should be employed if the clinical situation is compatible with potentially fatal complications. In the patient's acute phase, pulmonary edema is not an uncommon finding. This can result from autonomic changes within the pulmonary system itself as a result of physiological cord transection. It can also be caused by large amounts of fluid replacement in treating hypotension that may on the basis of peripheral vasomotor paralysis, be due to the cord transection. It should be emphasized that all of these pulmonary changes can result in hypoxia, sepsis, fever, etc., which can have adverse effects on the already compromised cord function.

Genitourinary

After the acute phase of injury, the patient should be started on a program of intermittent bladder catheterization to prevent bladder dysfunction secondary to overdistention and also to prevention infection that could lead to sepsis and primary renal disease. Early urological consultation will provide a proper regimen and antibiotic coverage.

Gastrointestinal

The patients should be started on a bowel regimen of stool softeners and laxatives to maintain good bowel function. When steroids are used, antacids and/or ranitidine should also be used. Gastrointestinal hemorrhage can be a fatal complication of the cord-injured patient. However, it should also be remembered that the hypotension and debilitation resulting from this complication can aggravate the cord pathology. Intraabdominal events can account for up to 10% of fatalities in cord-injured patients. A perforated viscus with peritonitis is the most common. The sensory deficit makes the routine abdominal exam virtually useless. Certain clinical signs should draw attention to the possibility of this impending disaster. Persistent nausea and vomiting, tachycardia or bradycardia when the pulse has been normal, pain in the shoulder or clavicular regions referred from subdiaphragmatic irritation may all be signs of intraabdominal problems. If any of these occur, one should perform the appropriate diagnostic tests.

Integument

Special measures from meticulous skin care should be instituted when the patient arrives. Decubiti begin in the emergency room. As soon as possible, the patient should be removed from the full spine board used for transporting. The patient can be safely cared for during the initial emergency room phase on a firm stretcher being transferred "like a log" as needed. Infection and subsequent sepsis from decubitis may impede a patient's progress. Paralyzed anesthetic body parts should be moved and repositioned at least every 2 hours. Specialized foam or rubber mattresses or horizontally rotating frames can be employed. Skin should be washed, massaged, and powdered at least once a day. Bedding should always be dry and meticulous. Perineal and sacral skin care is obligatory.

SUMMARY

The treatment of acute spinal cord injury should be guided by the basic principles based on the pathophysiology creating the neurological deficit. This chapter has summarized those pathophysiological changes and their nonsurgical treatment interventions. At the present time, prevention of cord injury is the only treatment for the initial irreversible tissue disruption that occurs at the time of injury. The remainder of any current treatment protocol consists of minimizing secondary injuries to spinal cord tissue which occur as a result of inadequate immobilization, persistent spinal cord compression, and poor oxygenation and blood flow. The goal is to optimize the environment in order to allow the spinal cord to recover as much as possible depending on the severity of the initial injury.

The experimental work that is being conducted in the areas of biochemical and cellular manipulations, as well as regenerative studies, are to be encouraged in hopes that in the future a protocol may be adopted that is directed to reversing some of the neurological deficits.

Finally, physicians and researchers in all medical disciplines should encourage and promote public and personal safety standards whenever possible. For if we do not, we will continue to experience the high incidence of needless death and disability secondary to spinal injuries.

REFERENCES

1. Dohrmann GT, Wagner FC, Bucy PC. The microvasculature in transitory traumatic paraplegia. An electron microscopic study in the monkey. J Neurosurg 1981;35:263–271.
2. Assenmacher DR, Ducker TB. Experimental traumatic paraplegia: the vascular and pathologic changes seen in reversible and irreversible spinal cord lesions. J Bone Joint Surg 1971;53:671–680.
3. Ducker TB. Experimental injury of the spinal cord. In: Vinken PJ, Bruyn GW, eds. Handbook of clinical neurology. Chapter 2; Vol. 25. New York: American Elsevier Publishing Co., Inc., 1976.
4. Guth L, Bright D, Donati EJ. Functional deficits and anatomical alterations after high cervical spinal hemisection in the rat. Exp Neurol 1978;58:511–520.
5. Guttman L. Spinal cord injuries: comprehensive management and research. Chapter 2. London: Blackwell Scientific Publications, 1973.
6. Wolman L. Axon regeneration after spinal cord injury. Paraplegia 1966;4:175–188.
7. Windle WF. Regeneration of axons in the vertebrate CNS. Physiol Res 1956;36:427–440.
8. Freeman LW, MacDougall J, Turbes CC, Bowman DE. The treatment of experimental lesion of the spinal cord of dogs with trypsin. J Neurosurg 1960;17:259–265.
9. Matinian LA, Andreasian AS. Enzyme therapy in organic lesions of the spinal cord. Akademia Nauk American SSr, 1973:94. (English Translation: Los Angeles: Brain information service, Univ. of California, 1956:156.
10. Feringa ER, Kowalski TF, Vahlsing HL, et al. Enzyme treatment of spinal cord transected rats. Ann Neurol 1979;5:203–206.
11. Knowles JF, Berry MD. Effect of enzyme treatment of CNS lesions in rats. Exp Neurol 1978;59:450–454.
12. Pettegrew RK. Trypsin inhibition of scar formation in cordotomized rats. Anat Res 1976;184:501.
13. David S, Aguayo AJ. Axonal elongation into peripheral nervous system "bridges" after central nervous system injury in adult rats. Science 1981;214:931.
14. Reier PJ, Bregman BS, Wujeck JR. Intraspinal transplantation of embryonic spinal cord tissue in neonatal and adult rats. J Comp Neurol 1986;247:275.
15. Reir PJ, Perlow MJ, Guth L. Development of embryonic spinal cord transplants in the rat. Brain Res 1983;312:201.
16. Tessler A, Himes BT, Houle J, Reier PJ. Regeneration of adult dorsal root axons into transplants of embryonic spinal cord. J Comp Neurol 1988;270:537.
17. Ducker TB, Salcman M, Daniell HB. Experimental cord trauma, III: therapeutic effect of immobilization and pharmacologic agents. Surg Neurol 1978;10:71–76.
18. Ducker TB, Lucas JT, Walleck CA. Recovery from spinal cord injury. Clin Neurosurg 1983;30:495–513.
19. Marshall LF, Knowlton S, Garfin SR, et al. Deterioration following spinal cord injury. J Neurosurg 1987;66:400–404.
20. Wilberger JE, Layman S, Diamond DL, Maroon JC. Timing of surgical spinal stabilization after spinal cord injury. Adv Man Spinal Cord Inj 1991;2:13.
21. Griffiths IR. Varsogenic edema following acute and chronic spinal cord compression in the dog. J Neurosurg 1975;42:155–165.
22. Brodkey JS, Richards DE, Blasingame JP, et al. Reversible spinal cord trauma in cats. Additive effects of direct pressure and ischemia. J Neurosurg 1972;37:591–593.
23. Gooding MR, Wilson CB, Hoff JT. Experimental cervical myelopathy. Effects of ischemic and compression of the canine cervical spinal cord. J Neurosurg 1975;43:9–17.
24. Kobrine AE, Evans EE, Rizzoli HV. Experimental acute balloon compression of the spinal cord: factors affecting disappearance and return of the spinal evoked response. J Neurosurg 1979;51:841–845.
25. Lucas JT, Ducker TB. Motor classification of spinal cord injuries with mobility, morbidity and recovery indices. Am Surg 1979;45:151–158.
26. Saul TG, Ducker TB. Early myelography in acute cervical injury in early management of acute spinal cord injury. Tator CH, ed. NY: Raven Press, 1982.
27. Piepmeier JM, Lehmann KB, Lane JG. Cardiovascular instability following acute cervical spinal cord trauma. Cent Nerv Sys Trauma 1985;2:153–160.
28. Janssen L, Hansebout RR. Pathogenesis of spinal cord injury and newer treatments. A review. Spine 1989;14:23–32.
29. Young W. Blood flow, metabolic and neurophysiological mechanisms in spinal cord injury. Central Nervous System Status Report: 463–473.
30. Ducker TB, Kindt GW. The effect of trauma on the vasomotor control of spinal cord blood flow. Curr Top Surg Res 1971;3:163–171.
31. Smith AJ, McCreery DB, Bloedel JR, et al. Hyperemia, CO_2 responsiveness and autoregulation in the white matter following experimental spinal cord injury. J Neurosurg 1978;48:239–251.
32. Kindt GW, Ducker TB, Huddlestone J. Regulation of spinal cord blood flow. In: Russell RW, ed. Brain and blood flow. New York: Pitman Medical and Scientific Publishing Co., Ltd, 1971:401–405.
33. Smith AL, Pender JW, Alexander SC. Effects of PCO_2 on spinal cord blood flow. Am J Physiol 1969;216:1158–1163.
34. Ducker TB, Salcman M, Perot PL, et al. Experimental spinal cord trauma. I: Correlation of blood flow, tissue oxygen and neurologic status in the dog. Surg Neurol 1978;10:60–63.

35. Fairholm DJ, Turnbull IM. Microangiographic study and experimental spinal cord injuries. J Neurosurg 1971;35:277–286.

36. Locke GE, Yashon D, Feldman A, et al. Ischemia in primate spinal cord injury. J Neurosurg 1971;34:614–617.

37. Vise WM, Yashon D, Hunt WE. Mechanisms of norepinephrine accumulations within sites of spinal cord injuries. J Neurosurg 1974;40:76–82.

38. Kao CC, Chang LW. The mechanisms of spinal cord cavitation following spinal cord transection. Part I. A correlated histochemical study. J Neurosurg 1977;46:197–209.

39. Ito T, Allen M, Yashon D. A mitochondrial lesion in experimental spinal cord trauma. J Neurosurg 1978;48:434–442.

40. Clendenon NR, Allen N, Gordon WA, et al. Inhibition of $NA^+ - K^+$ activated ATPase activity following experimental spinal cord trauma. J Neurosurg 1978;49:563–568.

41. Hall ED, Braughler JM. Role of lipid peroxidation in post-traumatic spinal cord degeneration: A review. Cent Nerv Sys Trauma 1986;3:281–294.

42. Brody JS, Richard DE, Blasingame JP, et al. Interaction of Na – K ATPase with chlorpromazine for radical and related compounds. Ann N Y Acad Sci 1974;242:527–542.

43. Kimelberg HK, Papahadjopoulos D. Effects of phospholipedacyl chain fluidity phase transections, and cholesterol on $Na^+ - K^+$ – stimulated adenosine triphosphatase. J Biol Chem 1974;449:1071–1080.

44. Milvy P, Kakari S, Campbell JB, et al. Paramagnetic species and radical products in cat spinal cord. Ann N Y Acad Sci 1973;222:1102–1111.

45. Ducker TB, Salcman M, Daniell HB. Experimental cord trauma. III. Therapeutic effect of immobilization and pharmacologic agents. Surg Neurol 1978;10:71–76.

46. Killen DA, Edwards RH, Tinsley EA, et al. Effects of low molecular weight dextran, heparin CSF drainage, and hypothermia on ischemic injury of the spinal cord, secondary to mobilization of the thoracic aorta from the posterior parietec. J Thorac Cardiovasc Surg 1965;50:882–886.

47. Brodner RA, Vangilder JC, Collins WF. The effect of antifibrinolytic therapy in experimental spinal cord trauma. J Trauma 1977;17:48–54.

48. Campbell JB, DeCrescito V, Tomasula JJ, et al. Effects of antifibrinolytic and steroid therapy on the contused spinal cord of cats. J Neurosurg 1974;40:726–733.

49. Parker AJ, park RD, Stowater JL. Reduction of trauma-induced edema of spinal cord in dogs given mannitol. Am J Vet Res 1973;34:1355–1357.

50. Yashon D. Spinal injury. New York: Appleton-Century-Crofts, 1978.

51. Ducker TB, Hamit HF. Experimental treatments of acute spinal cord injury. J Neurosurg 1969;30:693–697.

52. Bracker MB, Collins WF, Freeman DF, et al. Efficacy of methylprednisolone in acute spinal cord injury. JAMA 1984;251:45–52.

53. Jacob SW, Herschler R. Biological actions of dimethyl sulfoxide. In: Conference on the Biological Action of Dimethyl Sulfoxide. New York: New York Academy of Science, 1974.

54. de la Torre JC, Kawanga HM, Rowed DW, et al. Dimethyl sulfoxide in central nervous system trauma. Ann N Y Acad Sci 1975;243:362–389.

55. Hartzog JT, Fischer RG, Snow C. Spinal cord trauma: effect of hyperbaric oxygen treatment. Proc Annu Clin, Spinal Cord Inj Conf 1969;17:70.

56. Kelly DL, Lassiter KZL, Vaon Svivut A, et al. Effects of hyperbaric oxygenation and tissue oxygen studies in experimental paraplegia. J Neurosurg 1972;36:425–429.

57. Gamache FW Jr, Myers RAM, Ducker TB, et al. The clinical application of hyperbaric oxygen therapy in spinal cord injury: A preliminary report. Surg Neurol 1981;15:85–87.

58. Holbach KH, Wassmann H, Linke D. The use of hyperbaric oxygen in the treatment of spinal cord lesions. Eur Neurol 1977;16:213–221.

59. Jones RF, Unsworth IP, Marosszeky JE. Hyperbaric oxygen and acute spinal cord injuries in humans. Med J Aust 1978;2:573–575.

60. Albin MS, White RJ, Acosta-Rua GJ, et al. Study of functional recovery produced by delayed localized cooling after spinal cord injury in primates. J Neurosurg 1968;24:113–130.

61. Albin MS, White RJ, Yashon D, et al. Effects of localized cooling on spinal cord trauma. J Trauma 1969;9:1000–1008.

62. Thienprasit P, Bantli H, Bloedel JR, et al. Effect of delayed local cooling on experimental spinal cord injury. J Neurosurg 1975;42:150–154.

63. Bricolo A, Alle Ore G, DaPian R, et al. Local cooling in spinal cord injury. Surg Neurol 1976;6:101–106.

64. Blume H. Management of acute spinal cord injuries with local hypothermia and decompression. Presented at the Fifth International Congress of Neurological Surgeons, Tokyo, 1973. Excerpta Med Int Congr Serv 1973;293:194.

65. Schneider R, Crosby E, Russo H, et al. Traumatic spinal cord syndromes and their management. Clin Neurosurg 1973;20:424–492.

66. Tator CH, Deeke L. Value of normothermic perfusion, hypothermic perfusion, and decotomy in the treatment of experimental acute spinal cord trauma. J Neurosurg 1973;39:52–64.

67. Faden AI. Neuropeptides and central nervous system injury. Clinical applications. Neurol Rev 1986;43:501–504.

68. Faden AI, Jacobs TP, Holaday JW. A possible pathophysiologic role for endorphins in spinal injury, abstracted. Fed Proc 1980;39:762.

69. Faden AI, Jacobs TP, Holaday JW. Opiate antagonist improves neurologic recovery after spinal injury. Science 1981;211:493–494.

70. Flamm ES, Young W, Demopoulos HB, et al. Experimental spinal cord injury: treatment with naloxone. Neurosurgery 1982;10:227–231.

71. Young W, Flamm ES, Demopoulos HB, et al. Naloxone ameliorates posttraumatic ischemia in experimental spinal contusion. J Neurosurg 1981;55:209–219.

72. Black P, Markowitz RS, Keller S, Wachs K, Gillespie J, Finkelstein SD. Naloxone and experimental spinal cord injury: Part 1. High dose administration in a static load compression model. Neurosurgery 1986;19:905–908.

73. Black P, Markowitz RS, Keller S, Wachs K, Gillespie J, Finkelstein SD. Naloxone and experimental spinal cord injury: Part 2. Megadose treatment in a dynamic load injury model. Neurosurgery 1986;19:909–913.

74. Flamm ES, Young W, Collins WF, Piepmeier J, Clifton GL, Fischer B. A phase I trail of naloxone treatment in acute spinal cord injury. J Neurosurg 1985;63:390–397.

75. Horita A, Carino MA, Chesnut RM. Influence of thyrotropin releasing hormone (TRH) on drug-induced-narcosis and hypothermia in rabbits. Psychopharmacology (Berlin) 1976;49:57–62.

76. Holaday JW, D'Amato RJ, Faden AI. Thyrotropin-releasing hormone improves cardiovascular function in experimental endotoxic and hemorrhagic shock. Science 1981;213:216–218.

77. Faden AI, Jacobs TP, Smith Mt. Thyrotropin-releasing hormone in expermental spinal injury: dose response and late treatment. Neurology 1984;34:1280–1284.

78. Faden AI, Jacobs TP, Holaday JM. Thyrotropin-releasing hormone improves neurologic recovery after spinal trauma in cats. N Engl J Med 1981;305:1063–1067.

79. Faden AI, Jacobs TP, Smith MT, Holaday JW. Comparison of thyrotropin releasing hormone (TRH), naloxone and dexamethasone treatments in experimental spinal injury. Neurology (Cleveland) 1983;33:673–678.

80. Arias MJ. Treatment of experimental spinal cord injury with TRH Naloxone, and Dexamethasone. Surg Neurol 1987;28:335–338.

81. Guha A, Tator CH, Piper I. Increase in rat spinal cord blood flow with the calcium channel blocker, nimodipine. J Neurosurg 1985;63:250–259.

82. Guha A, Tator CH, Piper I. Effect of a calcium channel blocker on posttraumatic spinal cord blood flow. J Neurosurg 1987;66:423–430.

83. Hall ED, Wolf DL. A pharmacological analysis of the pathophysiological mechanisms of posttraumatic spinal cord ischemia. J Neurosurg 1986;64:951–961.

22

The Use of Halo Vest in Management of Cervical Fractures

Michael L. Schwartz, Stanley D. Gertzbein, and Mahmood Fazl

As of 31 December, 1989, the Acute Spinal Cord Injury Unit at Sunnybrook Medical Centre had treated a total of 963 patients with cervical injuries, of whom 522 had spinal injuries only and 441 suffered spinal cord damage. The halo-vest apparatus has been in use for 15 years in the Acute Spinal Cord Injury Unit (1). The cumulative experience is shown in Figure 22.1, where the proportion of patients with and without spinal cord injury is indicated.

Principles of Treatment

When a spinal cord injury is present, the primary objective of treatment is to optimize recovery of spinal cord function. For partial spinal cord lesions with persisting compression, we attempt to realign the spinal column by in-line halo traction. Open surgical decompression is reserved for cases that fail to reduce with traction or when spinal cord compression and neurological deficit persist despite correct alignment. When there is no spinal cord injury or when there is no prospect of recovery, as in complete lesions of the cervical spinal cord, stability and prevention of further injury are the major considerations.

Risk Reduction

These general indications have lead to surgical procedures in approximately 25% of patients with cervical spinal injuries since 1974. The same principles of treatment, that is, the relief of spinal cord compression, spinal realignment, and stability have more often required operative reduction and internal fixation (ORIF) and have led to an operative rate of just over 50% in patients with thoracic and lumbar fractures as there is no reliable method of closed reduction and no easy method of external fixation that allows mobility while fracture union occurs. Appropriate use of halo traction and the halo-vest apparatus results, therefore, in a 50% reduction of the need for surgical intervention, reducing cost and risk to the patient.

This chapter will present the method of applying the halo ring and vest, provide an algorithm with examples of how treatment decisions are made, and indicate possible complications and advice for their avoidance.

Halo Program

The treatment of patients using the halo-vest apparatus is best accomplished as part of a coordinated program, as there are many details that must be attended to that might otherwise tend to be overlooked. At Sunnybrook Medical Centre we have two nurse practitioners who are skilled in the supervision of halo pin sites, checking pin tensions, and applying and removing the vest portion of the apparatus, that is, the technical aspects of the device. They also advise patients on aspects of personal hygiene in the halo-vest, how to modify clothing so it will fit over the apparatus, and so on. The Acute Spinal Cord Injury Unit provides a booklet that is useful to patients, nurse practitioners, and physicians and that is available on request.

Technique of Halo-Vest Application

Halo Application

Figure 22.2 shows a halo ring being applied. Unbroken rings in several sizes, adjustable rings, and a crownlike device, open at the back, are available from several manufacturers. Our preferred supplier is Bremer Orthopedics, Jacksonville, Florida. It is important to select the smallest ring that will permit access to the pin sites on the scalp. Minimizing the length of the pin projecting inward from the ring provides the greatest stability and results in the least likelihood of bony erosion of the skull at the tip of the pin. This reduces the risk of dislocation of the halo. The ring should be applied as low as possible on the skull. It may be possible to impale the eyebrow, taking care to draw it upward so as to avoid plunging into the orbit, as this obviates unsightly scars on the forehead when the ring is removed. The posterior pins should be placed so that the lower edge of the ring is at the level of the upper edge of the pinna. On application of the ring, the pins are tightened to a torque of 8 inch-pounds (0.9 nm). Twenty-four hours later they will require tightening, as the pressure will have diminished. A dressing of gauze soaked in Hibitane (chlorhexidine gluconate), 1/2000 solution is initially applied.

Halo Traction

If the spinal column is correctly aligned, the vest may be applied directly once the halo ring has been applied. If malalignment persists, then in-line traction, by means of a system of weights and pulleys attached to a bail affixed to the halo ring, is established (Fig. 22.3).

One begins with the appropriate amount of weight, lower weights being required for the reduction of dislocations nearer the top of the cervical spinal column and greater weights at the lower cervical levels, as indicated in Figure 22.4. A maximum of 1 kg per vertebral level is a good starting weight. The amount should be adjusted downward for smaller, older, or less muscular subjects. Once traction is begun, a lateral cervical spine radiograph is obtained to determine whether or not the dislocation has reduced. The traction weight and the time that the radiograph was made should be written on each x-ray. The patient should be under close observation for neurological deterioration, as distraction of the spinal column may impair spinal cord function. In our hospital, ordering, obtaining, and then viewing the lateral cervical spine radiographs takes at least an hour. If the malalignment persists, one may then increase the amount of weight. The weight applied to the pulley system is generally increased in 3- to 5-pound increments (approximately 1 and 3 kg, respectively). On occasion, we have applied as much as 30 kg of weight, without untoward effects. In general, fracture dislocations of the lower cervical spine, especially in muscular individuals, take more weight to reduce.

Vest Application

Once the fracture dislocation reduces, the vest is applied, as illustrated in Figure 22.5. Radiographs are obtained to be certain that spinal column alignment is maintained with the patient in the horizontal position after traction is removed. Adjustments of the rods connecting the halo to the vest may have to be made to correct minor malalignment. If satisfactory alignment is maintained in the horizontal position, the patient is allowed up and radiographs are repeated to be certain that correct alignment is maintained with the patient vertical. Open reduction with in-

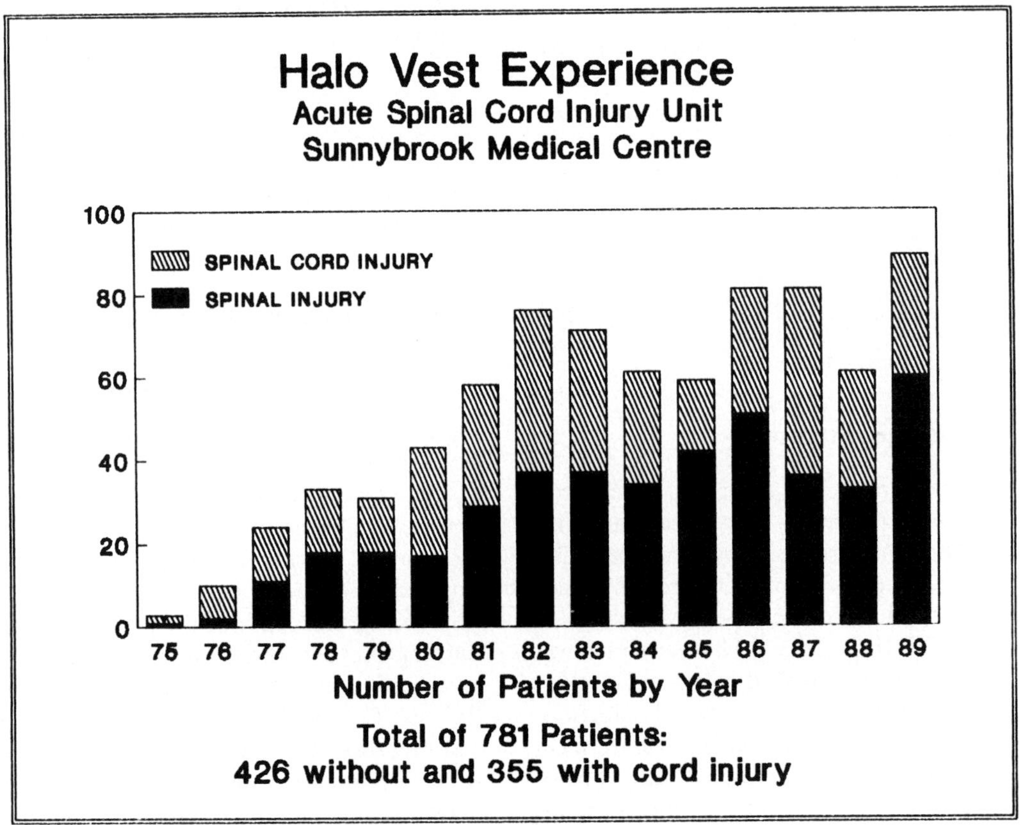

Figure 22.1. Out of a total of 963 patients with cervical spine injuries, 781 patients were treated with the halo-vest apparatus. The cumulative experience to the 31st of December, 1989, and the proportion of patients without and with spinal cord injury is indicated.

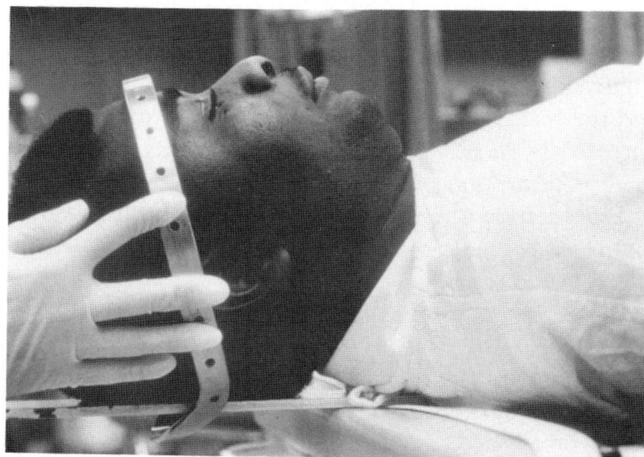

Figure 22.2. The halo ring is applied as low as possible on the skull so as to minimize the possibility of its dislodging.

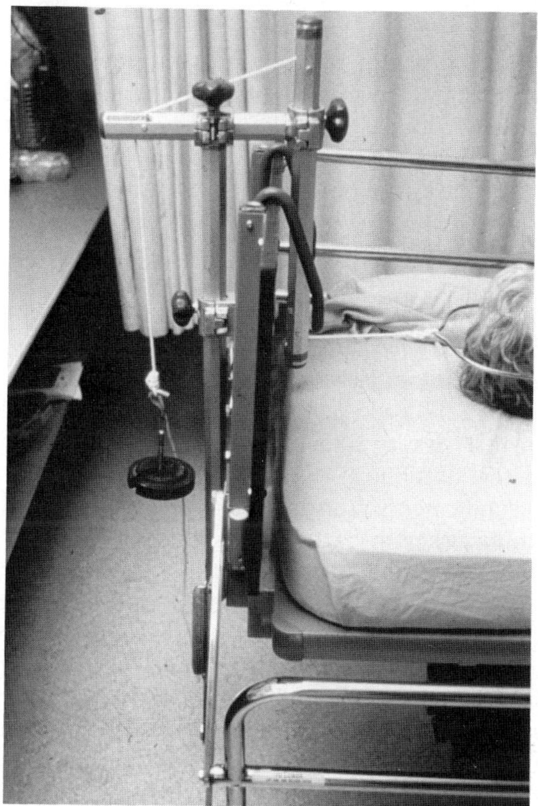

Figure 22.3. In-line traction, by means of a system of weights and pulleys, is attached to a bail affixed to the halo ring.

ternal fixation is reserved for the approximately 20% of our patients in whom reduction by means of in-line traction cannot be obtained or who reduce on traction but whose alignment cannot be maintained with the halo-vest apparatus.

If correct alignment is maintained by the halo-vest apparatus, patients without spinal cord injury may be discharged home, and those with a spinal cord injury may be transferred to a rehabilitation facility.

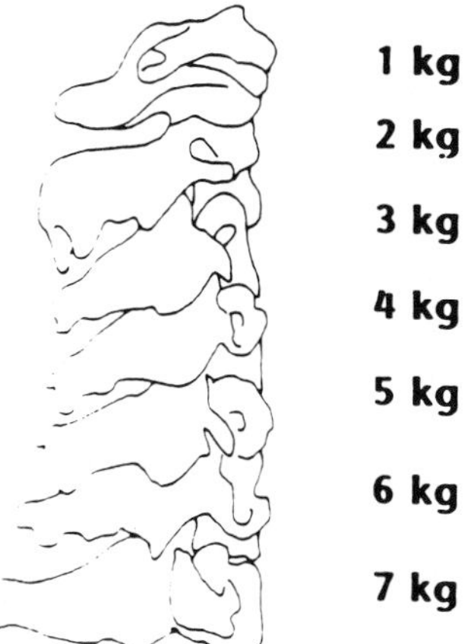

Figure 22.4. Maximum starting weight for in-line traction is 1 kg/vertebral level.

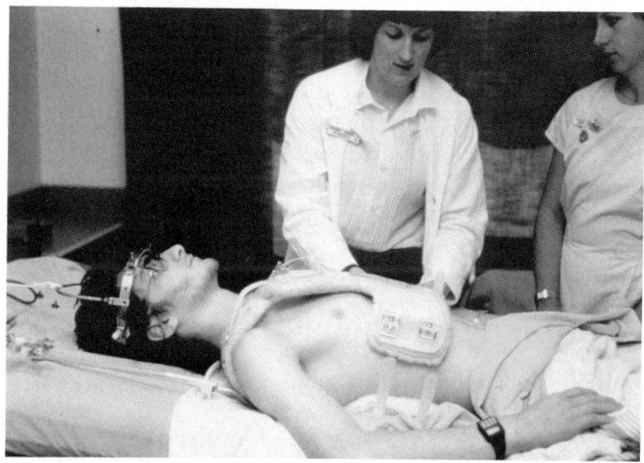

Figure 22.5. Application of the vest. Once the spinal column is correctly aligned, the vest may be applied. When the halo has been connected to the vest by means of stiff rods, the traction is disconnected and a radiographic check of the spine is obtained.

Follow-up

Monthly follow-up visits are arranged. At each visit, spinal radiographs are obtained to check alignment and to look for radiological evidence of bony union. The pin sites are checked by the nurse practitioner, who adjusts the pin torque to 8 inch-pounds. Reduction of pin pressure is normal, as the outer table tends to erode as a result of the continued pressure applied by the pin. If the pins loosen, the halo becomes uncomfortable, and discharge from the pin site may develop. If sufficient loosening occurs, the entire ring may dislodge. It is important not to tighten the pins too much or too frequently, as this will accelerate erosion of the underlying skull and may even result in penetration of the pin through the inner table of the skull. The physician or the nurse practitioner should be available to respond to problems arising between follow-up visits, as patients can correctly judge when their pins are loose or when something is amiss with the halo-vest device. At the 3-month follow-up visit, the halo and vest are disconnected. Lateral radiographs are obtained in flexion and extension, and the stability of fusion is assessed. All but approximately 3% of patients will have fused at 3 months.

If the fracture is solidly healed, the ring is removed and the patient is given a stiff collar to wear when traveling in a car or when in situations where he might fall, for example, walking on icy surfaces. The patient is instructed to wear a collar inside the house only when his neck becomes tired. In this way, the patient tends to wear the collar less and less as his endurance improves. In fact, many patients have virtually ceased wearing the device by the time of the 4-month follow-up visit. A radiograph is obtained once again at the 4-month follow-up visit to be certain that alignment has not changed. Further follow-up is maintained only as required.

Quadriplegic or severely quadriparetic patients will continue to require supervision and rehabilitation directed by the physiatrist. Patients with little or no neurological deficit very often require no physiotherapy, as the neck muscles generally recover strength and suppleness with normal use.

Needless to say, departures from the ideal situation just presented do occur. An algorithm for decision making with specific case examples is presented below.

ALGORITHM FOR DECISION MAKING IN MANAGEMENT

Early Operation

The algorithm (Fig. 22.6) is drawn in the style of Weinstein and Fineberg (2). Faced with an unstable fracture, the clinician has a choice of operating immediately to reduce the fracture if that is necessary to produce fixation or to apply traction. If the pattern of injury is such that even with immobilization in the halo-vest a stable union is unlikely, the halo-vest apparatus may be applied for support while the patient is positioned on the operating table and, if necessary, to provide some immobilization if wiring or instrumentation cannot immediately be relied upon for the maintenance of stability. For example, if diastasis of the lateral masses of the atlas is greater than 6 mm, one assumes that the transverse ligament is disrupted and stable union will not occur. The 18-year-old hockey player whose axial loading injury is illustrated in Figure 22.7 was operated upon in the halo-vest apparatus, and the device was removed immediately after the procedure. If, at node A in Figure 22.6, traction is applied and the fracture remains aligned or reduces, then one proceeds through node B, and the vest is applied. Hangman fractures, for example, virtually always heal in the halo-vest apparatus, even when there is disruption of the anterior longitudinal ligament and subluxation of C2 with respect to C3, as illustrated in Figure 22.8.

Increased Neurological Deficit

At node B there are three possible outcomes. As indicated by the path proceeding via node C, the patient's deficit may worsen, necessitating further investigation and operative treatment. Figure 22.9A shows the C5 burst fracture suffered by a 16-year-old girl who dove through an inner-tube in a swimming pool and struck her head on the bottom. She was initially motor complete but had well-preserved posterior column sensation. Her sensory function worsened slightly on the fourth day after her injury, and, accordingly, a myelogram was obtained. Figures 22.9B and C show computerized tomographic (CT) cuts at C5 and 6, indicating compromise of the spinal canal and swelling of the spinal cord resulting in obliteration of the subarachnoid space and a complete myelographic block. It was elected to decompress the spinal cord by an anterior approach. A bony graft was fashioned from the iliac crest. As no instrumentation was used, continuing immobilization in the halo-vest apparatus was relied on to maintain alignment. Early and late postoperative films are illustrated in Figures 22.9D and E. In this way, the halo-vest apparatus may serve as an adjunct to surgery obviating the need for internal fixation.

A second case also serves to illustrate the treatment of worsening deficit in traction as illustrated at nodes B and C of the treatment algorithm. In this case, a 28-year-old man attempted a back-flip off a coffee table and suffered a flexion injury producing a bilateral facet dislocation as illustrated in Figure 22.10A. Traction was begun. Figure 22.10A shows the effect of 27 pounds in-line traction. Figure 22.10B shows the effect of increasing the weight to 37 pounds. At this point, the patient, who had suffered only a minor partial injury, had a dramatic worsening in his spinal cord function. It is possible that an even greater distraction of the C6–7 level had occurred than is illustrated in the radiographs, because as soon as his spinal cord function worsened, the traction was immediately reduced without waiting for further x-rays. He was taken to the operating room and an open reduction and internal fixation by sublaminar wiring as illustrated in Figures 22.10C and D was carried out. In this case, as there was virtually no fracturing, and the wire held the relatively intact facet joints in place; the spine was considered immediately stable, and the halo-vest apparatus was removed without delay.

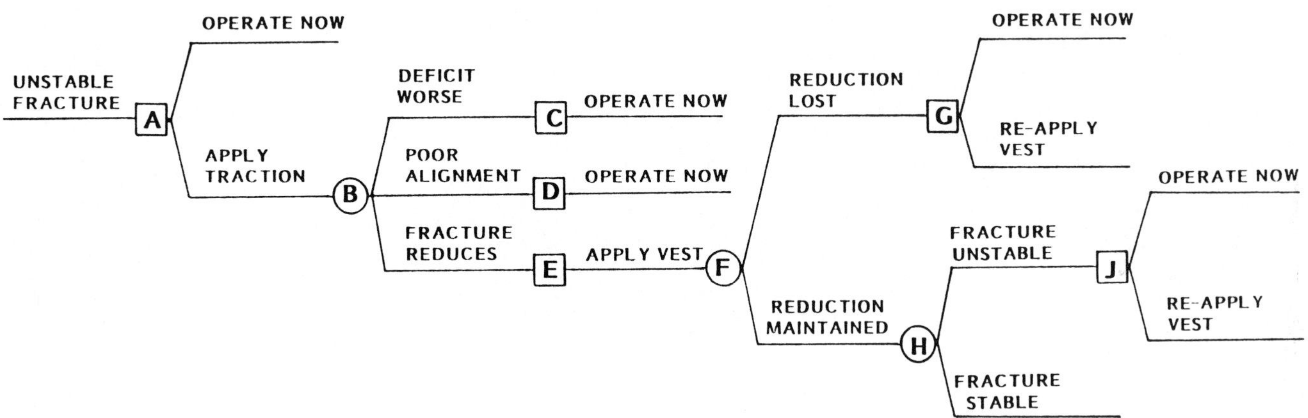

Figure 22.6. Treatment algorithm for patients with unstable cervical spine fractures. Decisions about the use of the halo-vest apparatus are made in a logical and consistent way.

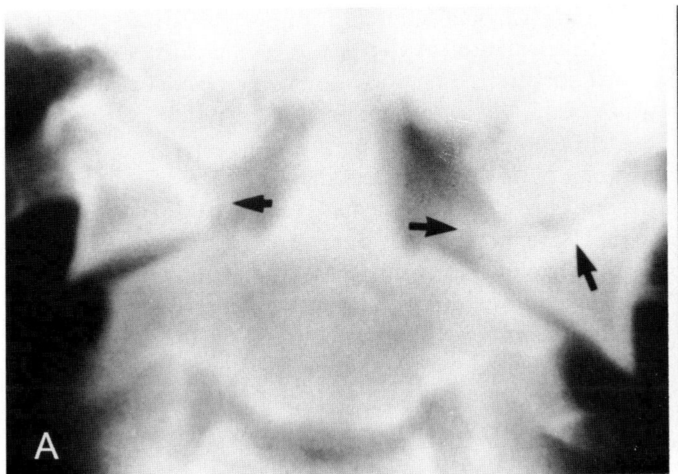

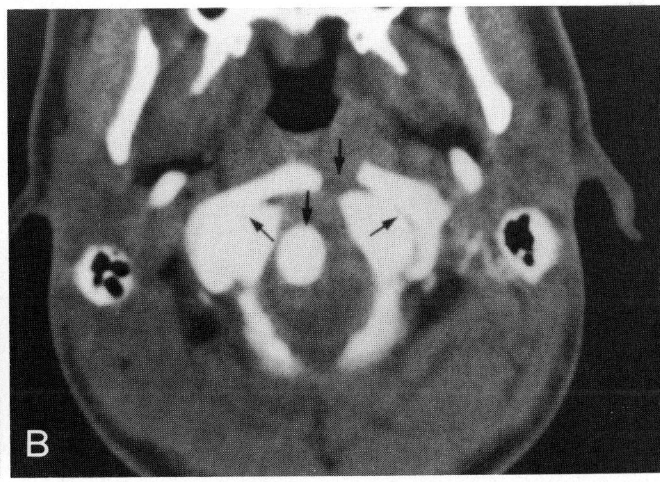

Figure 22.7. **A**, AP tomograms showing a Jefferson fracture with diastasis of the lateral masses of C1 greater than 6mm. **B**, CT scan showing fracture and diastasis of the anterior arch of C1 and lateral displacement of the lateral masses. The gap between the anterior arch of C1 and the odontoid process is increased, indicating rupture of the transverse ligament.

Failure to Reduce

As illustrated at nodes B and D in Figure 22.6, the fracture may fail to reduce despite traction. Figure 22.11 illustrates the case of a 41-year-old man who dove into shallow water and suffered a right C5–6 jumped facet with a right C6 radiculopathy. Despite maximal traction, he failed to reduce. Figures 22.11C and D show the postoperative radiographs. He was maintained in the halo-vest apparatus for 6 weeks to be certain of stability. The wiring illustrated was, of necessity, more complex than the previous case, as, in addition to the jumped facet, there was a laminar fracture.

We have recently reviewed a series of 173 consecutively treated patients in our unit in an effort to identify the features which predispose to successful realignment of the cervical spine and maintenance of reduction resulting in spinal stability and a good anatomical outcome (3). It was concluded that the entire patient population could be divided into two separate groups; those with and those without facet joint fracture dislocation. Only 44% of the patients with facet dislocations achieved stability using conservative management in the halo-vest without surgery and almost half of these failed to retain good anatomical alignment. In contrast, of patients without facet joint fracture dislocations, 70% achieved stability with the halo-vest alone, and 75% of them healed in good anatomical alignment.

Preservation of Mobility

Figure 22.12 illustrates a 33-year-old patient who suffered his injuries by the same mechanism, that is, diving into shallow water. As illustrated in Figure 22.12, there are

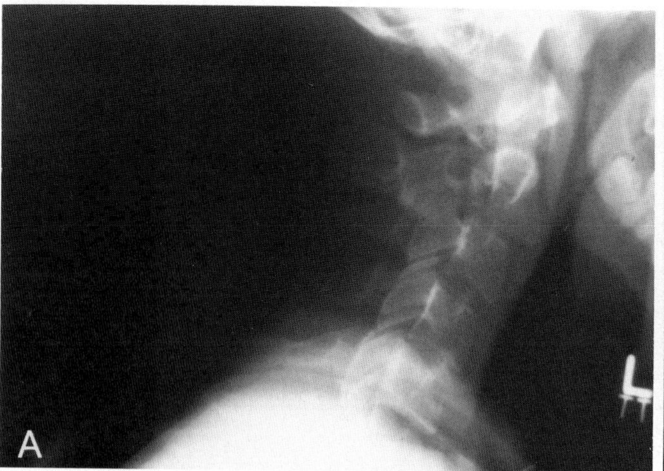

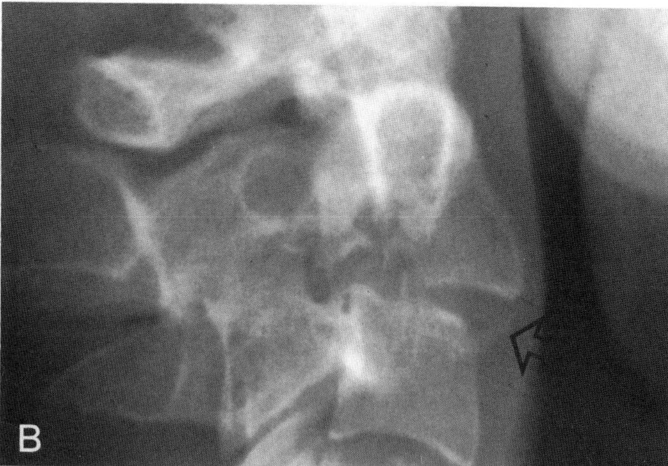

Figure 22.8. **A**, Hangman's fracture. There is a bipedicular fracture of C2 and displacement of the body of C2 forward upon C3. The alignment in the halo-vest apparatus is imperfect but adequate. **B**, After 3 months' immobilization in the halo-vest, the bipedicular fracture has healed. The *arrow* indicates a bony bridge between the anterior edge of C2 and C3, just visible on lateral plain x-rays. The fracture was stable on flexion-extension views.

fractures through both the laminae and vertebral bodies of C4 and C5. There was a partial spinal cord injury in this case. Were one to carry out an operative fusion, it would be necessary to fuse from the 3rd to the 6th cervical vertebra, resulting in greatly diminished cervical movement. Figure 22.12C shows the result after 3 months of immobilization in the halo-vest, that is, loss of movement at a single intervertebral joint and excellent cervical mobility.

Loss of Reduction

As illustrated in Figure 22.6 at node F, reduction may be maintained successfully or lost in the halo-vest. One has the option of readjusting the head position with respect to the vest as illustrated at node G. In fact, the nurse practitioners in our unit are very experienced at making minor adjustments to optimize bony alignment. We routinely keep patients for 2 or 3 days in hospital after the application of the vest to be certain that alignment is maintained as they resume their activities and move around the ward. If alignment cannot be maintained, then ORIF is carried out. Although one would suppose that the greater the in-line traction weight required for reduction, the less likely redislocation would be to occur, we have not actually been able to prove this (3). Although there was a tendency for patients who enjoyed a good anatomical result to require higher traction weights, 31 as opposed to 25 pounds, the standard deviations were too high (22 pounds) for statistical significance. As noted above, patients with facet dislocations were less likely to remain correctly aligned than were patients with other types of fractures.

Failure to Fuse

As previously reported from our unit (4), the halo-vest apparatus is our primary method of treating odontoid fractures. Although the Gallie fusion, that is, a posterior wiring of C1 to C2, as illustrated in Figure 22.13B, is safe and effective, rotation of the head is limited by about 50% when rotation about the odontoid peg is curtailed. For this reason, we favor nonoperative treatment. On review, we have found that patient age, fracture type, and the amount of dislocation affect the likelihood of solid union. In our review, older patients (greater than 55 years) with type II fractures, that is across the base of the dens and with greater displacement of the distal fragment, were least likely to fuse solidly. Nevertheless, as illustrated at node F in the treatment algorithm (Fig. 22.6), we usually treat patients with odontoid fractures for 3 months in the halo-vest apparatus. As illustrated at node H, halo and vest are disconnected and stability assessed. We have reapplied the vest and kept patients in the apparatus as long as 6 months (node J) before they healed solidly or conservative therapy was abandoned for a Gallie fusion. Figures 22.13A, B and C illustrate the case of an octogenarian who suffered a fractured odontoid in a motor vehicle accident. Figure 22.13A illustrates his type II odontoid fracture with some rarefaction of the fracture line after 6 months. Figure 22.13B shows the Gallie fusion. Figure 22.13C illustrates the radiograph taken yet another 6 months later. Although he never developed a bony union of either his odontoid or his graft, he had sufficient stability to avoid injury to his spinal cord.

Halo-Vest as an Adjunct to Surgery

The use of halo-vest immobilization may simplify operative treatment of complex fractures. The 21-year-old exotic dancer whose C4 burst fracture is illustrated in Figure 22.14A and B was still unstable after 3 months of immobilization in the halo-vest. Nevertheless, the fractured vertebral body had healed sufficiently to serve as a fulcrum. The factor creating her instability proved to be ruptured posterior

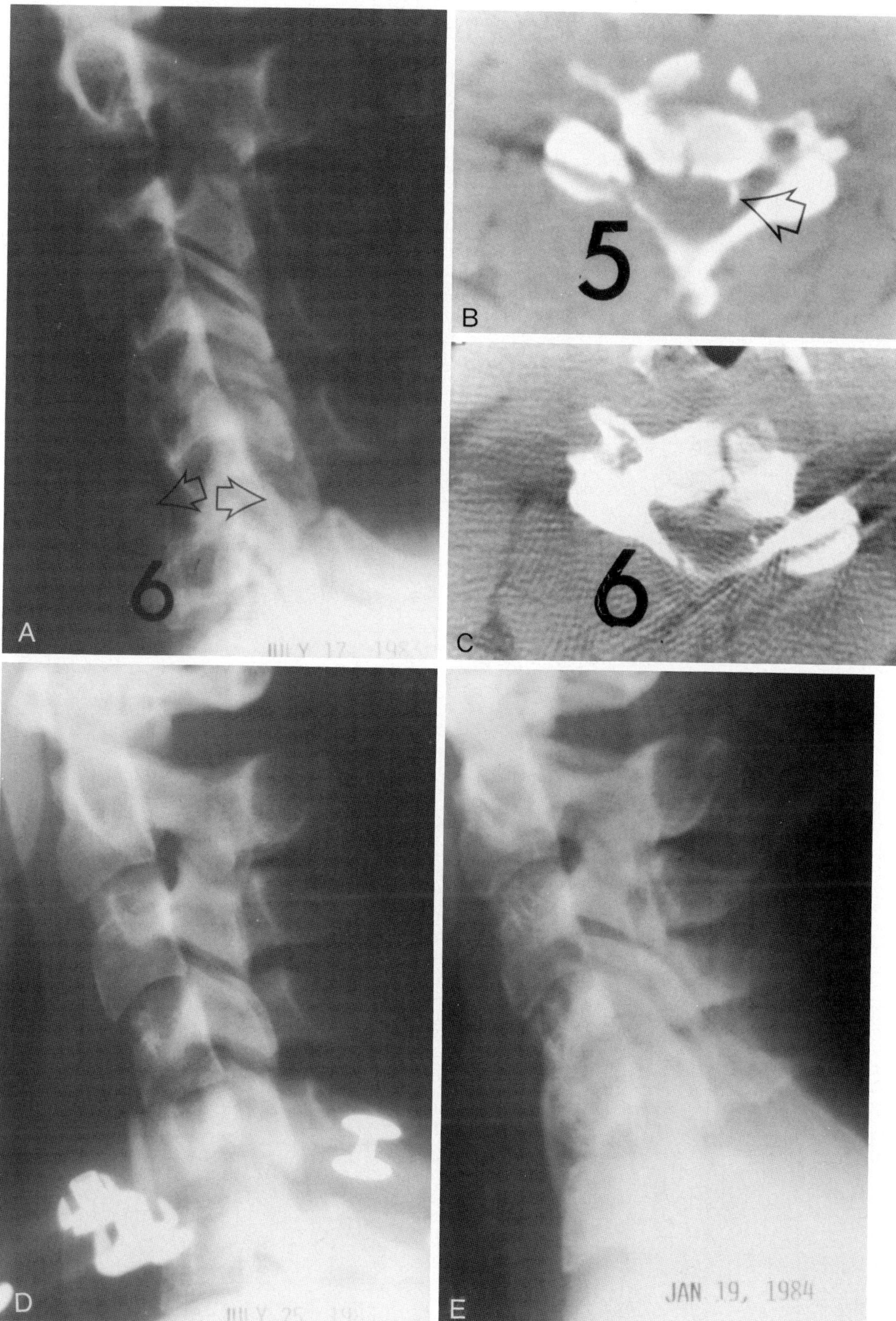

Figure 22.9. **A**, A lateral cervical spine x-ray illustrating a burst fracture of the body of C5 caused by axial loading. The *arrows* indicate bony fragments driven anteriorly and posteriorly. **B**, CT scanning through the body of C5 shows a sagittal fracture and two anterior fragments. The *arrow* indicates a fleck of soluble myelographic contrast material. **C**, The vertebral body of C6 is also split, and there is a complete block of myelographic contrast material at its superior edge. **D**, Immediate post-op film. The C5 vertebral body has been excised and replaced by an iliac crest graft. One cortical edge of the graft can be seen just anterior to the line of the vertebral bodies. **E**, A 6-month follow-up film shows solid fusion of C4, 5, and 6.

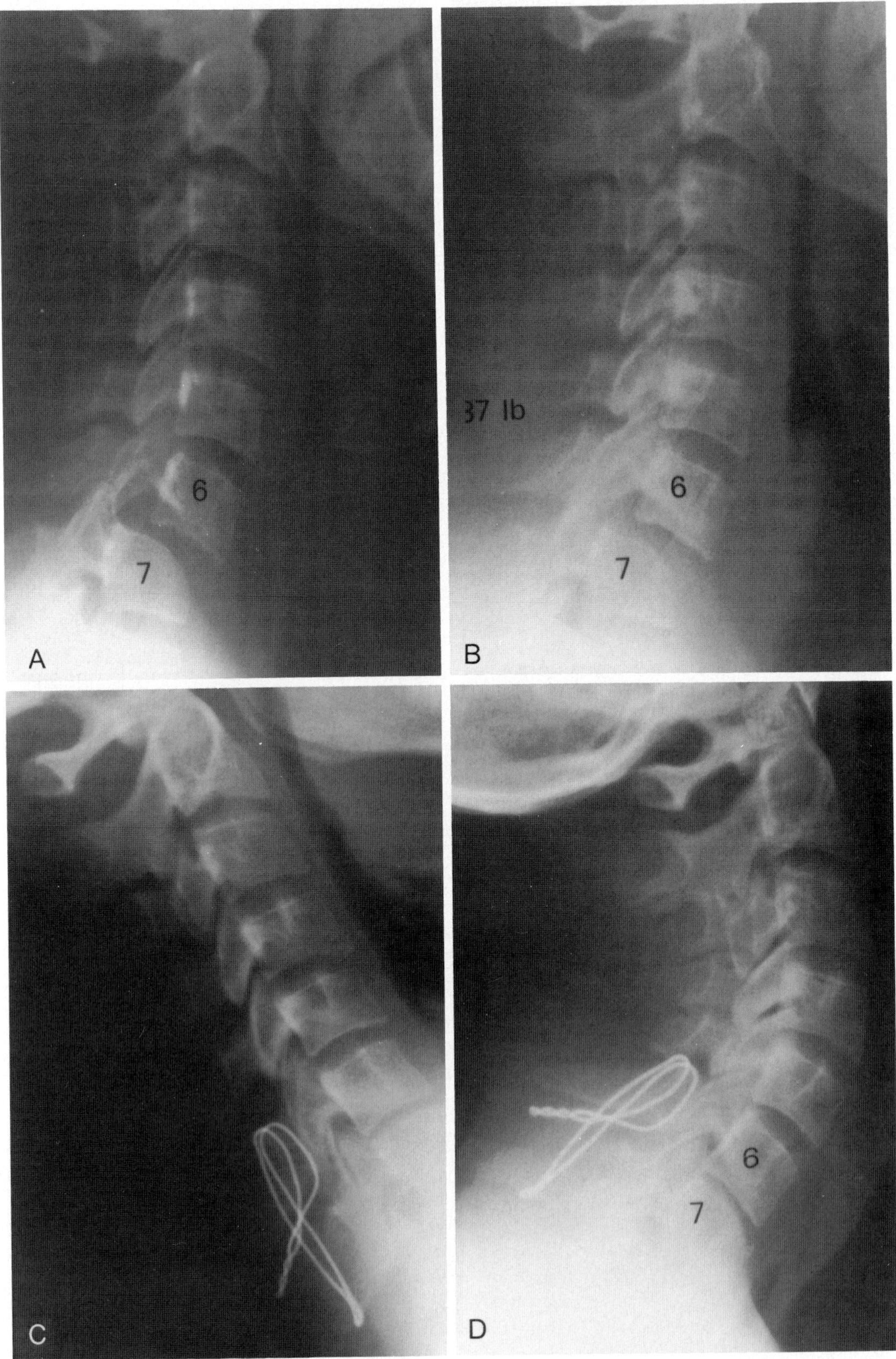

Figure 22.10. **A**, Lateral cervical spine films showing bilateral facet dislocation at C6–7. Twenty-seven pounds of traction have been applied. **B**, Thirty-seven pounds of traction have been applied, and there is slight distraction of C6 from C7. At this point, the patient's neurological deficit increased, and the traction was released. **C**, Sublaminar wiring of C6 and 7 shown in flexion. **D**, Sublaminar wiring of C6–7 shown in extension. The halo-vest apparatus was removed immediately after the surgery.

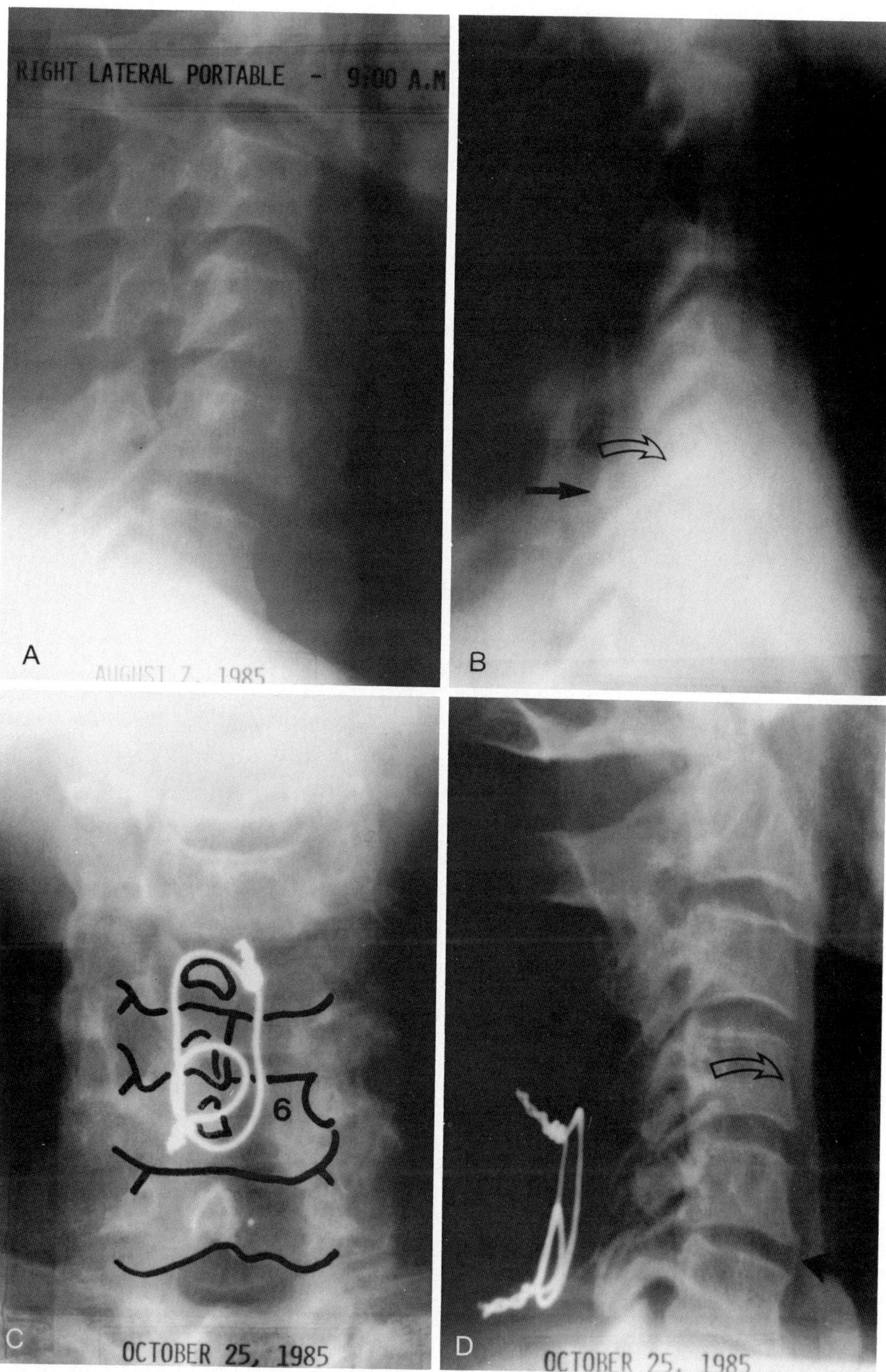

Figure 22.11. **A**, Lateral cervical spine film showing a right C5–6 fracture dislocation that failed to reduce with traction. **B**, Lateral tomograms showing the facet joints. The *open arrow* indicates the right C5 facet displaced anteriorly. The *solid arrow* indicates a facet fracture fragment. **C**, A more complex wiring was required to achieve stability as the right C5 lamina and facet were completely disconnected from the pedicle. The fragment could not be incorporated into the fusion. **D**, Lateral cervical spine film. The patient is flexing forward as indicated by the *open arrow*. The solid arrow shows an anterior bony bridge across the C5–6 interspace 3 months after ORIF and 6 weeks after removal of the halo-vest.

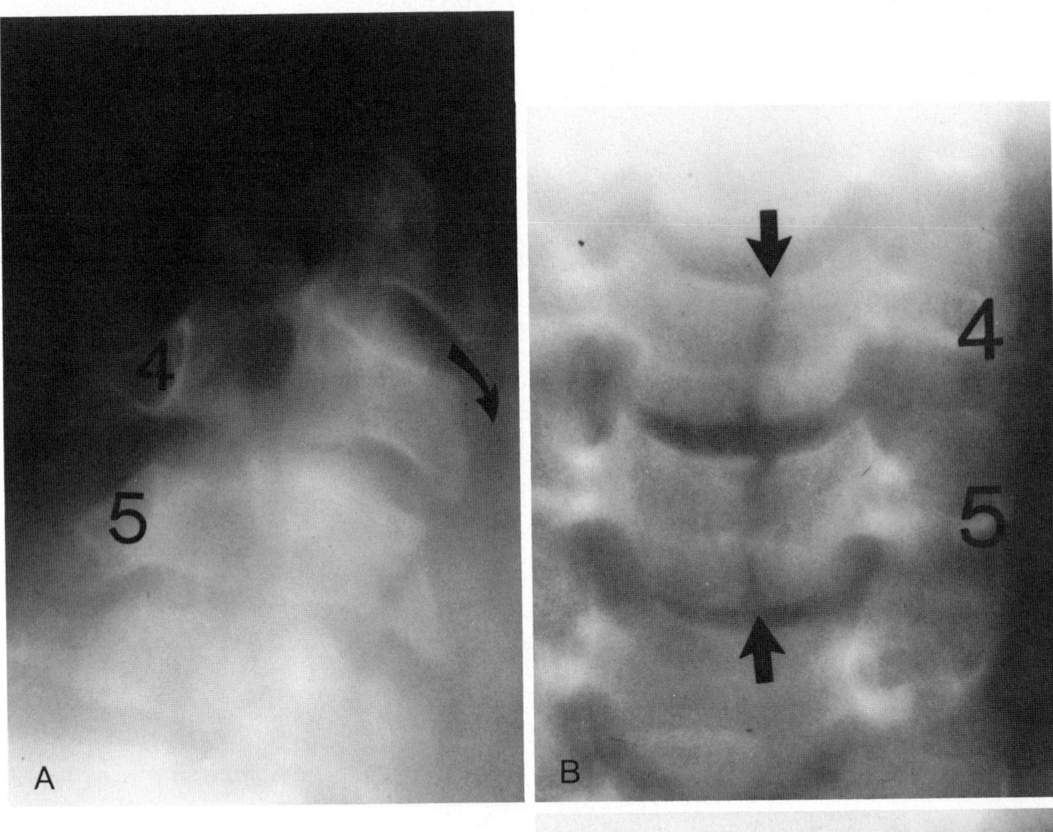

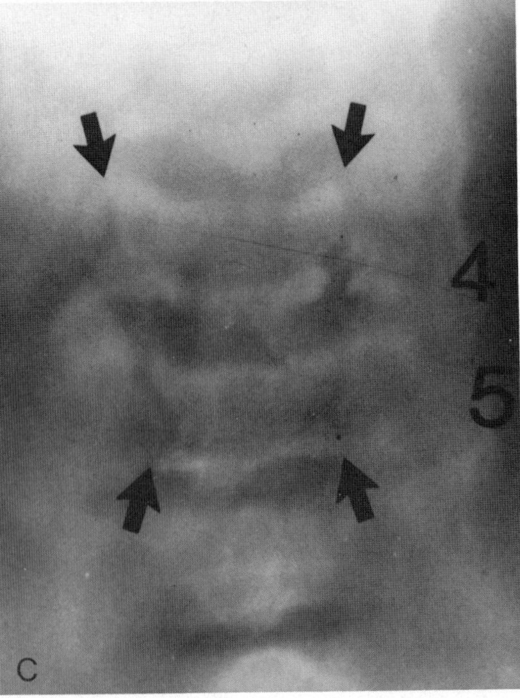

Figure 22.12. **A**, Lateral cervical spine film showing a C4–5 fracture dislocation caused by axial loading in flexion. A teardrop fragment anterior to the body of C5 is shown. The alignment in the halo-vest apparatus is good. **B**, AP tomography through the vertebral bodies shows sagittal splits of C4 and C5. **C**, AP tomography through the laminae shows bilateral fractures through the laminae of C4 and C5. **D**, With the halo-vest apparatus removed, a lateral cervical spine film obtained in flexion shows a solid bony fusion. The *arrow* indicates the bony bridge between C4 and C5. **E**, Lateral cervical spine film in extension indicates stability.

soft tissue elements, permitting too much flexion. Accordingly, Halifax interlaminar clamps (5) were applied posteriorly and stability obtained. Had ORIF been undertaken immediately, it is likely that a more complex surgical procedure would have been required.

In the treatment of patients with ankylosing spondylitis the halo-vest apparatus alone may be insufficient to maintain adequate stability so that bony union may occur (6). When coupled with ORIF a solid bony union can be obtained. Figure 22.15 illustrates the case of a 59-

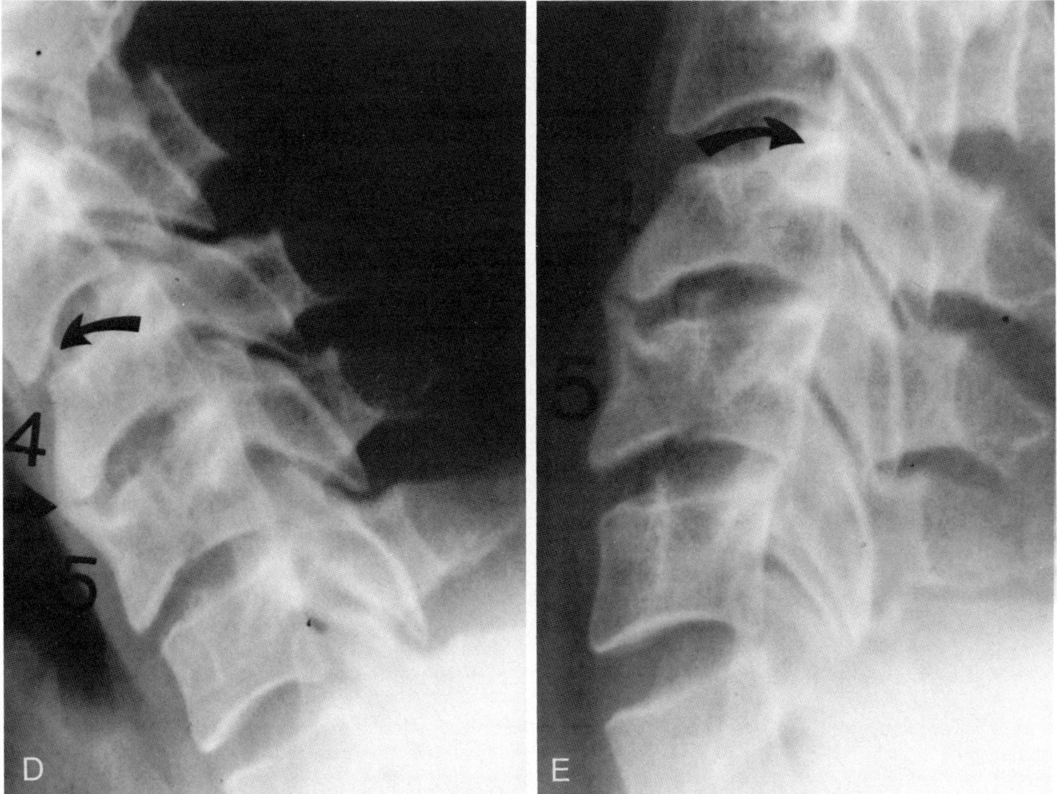

Figure 22.12. D–E.

year-old man with ankylosing spondylitis who slipped on the ice beside his car, striking the back of his head and forcing his neck into flexion. Following the fracture, he was unable to raise his head off his chest. He could not be realigned in the halo-vest. An open reduction and fixation was carried out, utilizing Halifax clips. The lamina of C7 was excised, and the clips were applied between C6 and T1. The patient was maintained for 3 months post-op in the halo-vest. An improved alignment and a solid bony fusion were achieved.

COMPLICATIONS

Halo Complications

The complications associated with the use of the halo-vest apparatus are most commonly related to the pins that affix the halo ring to the skull. Purulent discharge is common and can usually be managed by twice daily cleaning of the pin sites with Hibitane and dressing with gauze soaked in Hibitane solution. Osteomyelitis is rare. Occasionally, swelling of a particular pin site requires withdrawal of the pin. It is often possible to place a second pin through an adjacent threaded hole in the ring without removing the ring. As a rule, pins loosen as time progresses but usually do not require tightening more frequently than at the monthly visits. Occasionally, especially in active patients, the pins may loosen more frequently and require tightening. The ring may even dislodge completely. When fixation to the skull is lost, there is painful traction on the scalp. We have had no patients suffer a neurological deficit because of dislocation of the halo.

It has been necessary to reapply the ring during the course of treatment in about 12% of patients. In 1989, 89 patients had halos applied. One patient, who required two reapplications, was very restless and on one occasion fell out of bed, dislodging the pin fixation crown. A second patient, who also required two reapplications, had the crown pop off when his arms were pulled down for x-rays. This same patient removed his own crown at home. Four patients required a single reapplication because too large a ring was initially applied. Two patients required reapplication because all the pins migrated. One patient had the ring reapplied for frequent pin-loosening; one patient's crown "popped off" for no identifiable reason, and one diabetic patient developed cellulitis at pin sites, requiring reapplication of the ring.

It is important to avoid too frequent tightening of the skull fixation pins, as progressive erosion of the skull may lead to intracranial penetration. This occurred in one recent case. If a particular pin is torqued but there is diminished resistance, it should be withdrawn and a new pin placed in an adjacent hole or the ring entirely reapplied. At times, we have removed the halo-vest apparatus after less than 3 months when there were scalp complications and radiographic evidence of bony healing.

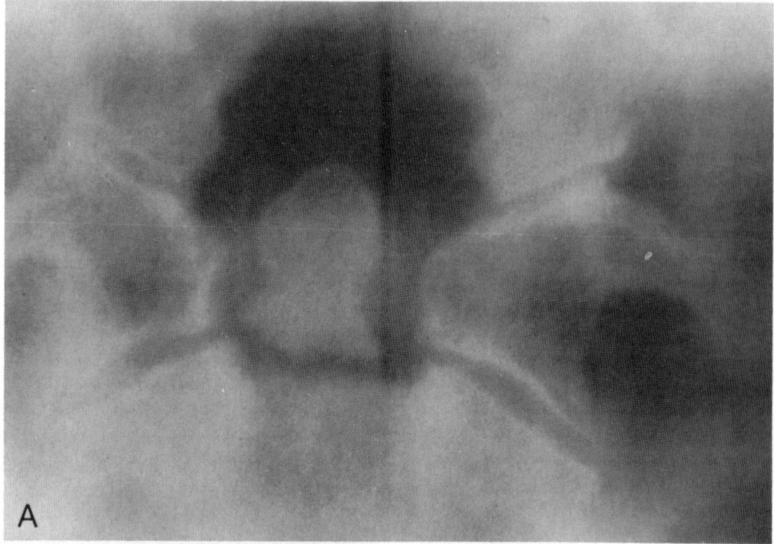

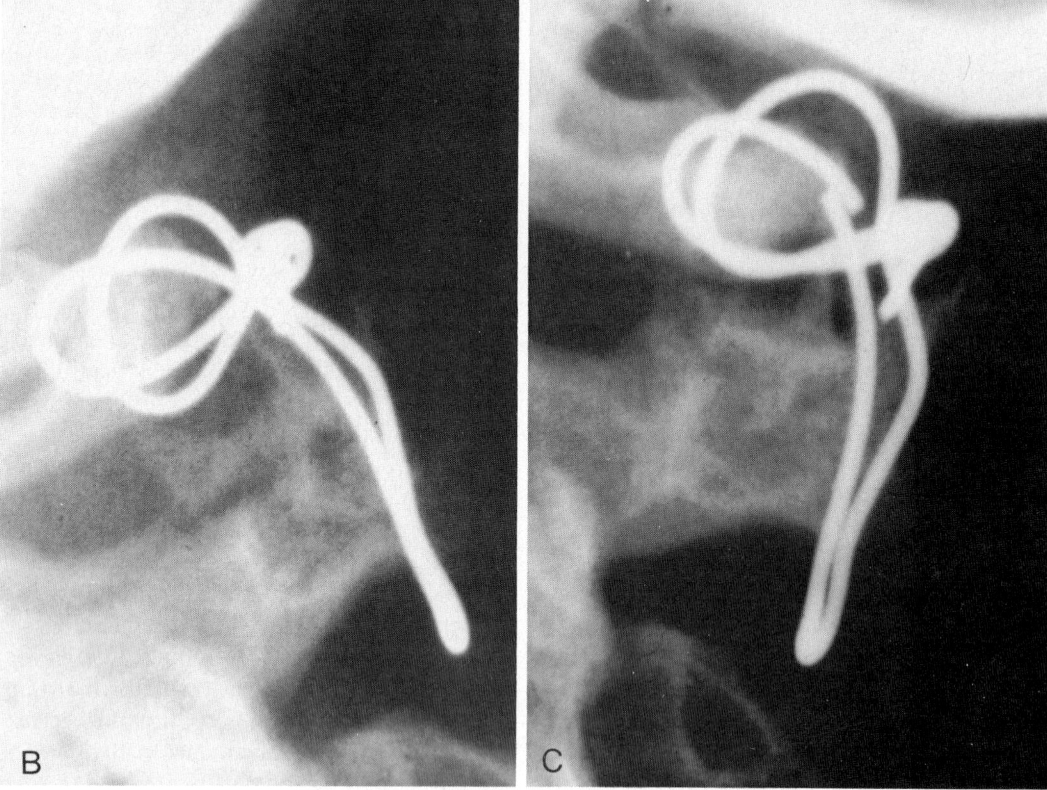

Figure 22.13. **A**, Anterior cervical spine film after 6 months in the halo-vest apparatus shows rarefaction at the site of a type II odontoid fracture. Flexion-extension views (not shown) showed angulation at the fracture site. **B**, A Gallie fusion has been carried out. There has been some settling of C1 upon C2. A solid fusion has not been obtained. **C**, At 6 months post-op there has been no solid bony union. Nevertheless, there is no abnormal movement. The wire has fractured, but the patient is asymptomatic.

Vest Complications

Pressure sores under the vest occur in fewer than one percent of our patients. Elderly or debilitated patients with multiple injuries who have little subcutaneous tissue are most susceptible to this complication. Pressure sores can usually be avoided by meticulous hygiene, resourceful trimming of the vest, and building up the padding to relieve pressure on bony prominences.

Conclusion

The halo-vest is an extremely useful apparatus in the management of patients with cervical spine injuries. Because

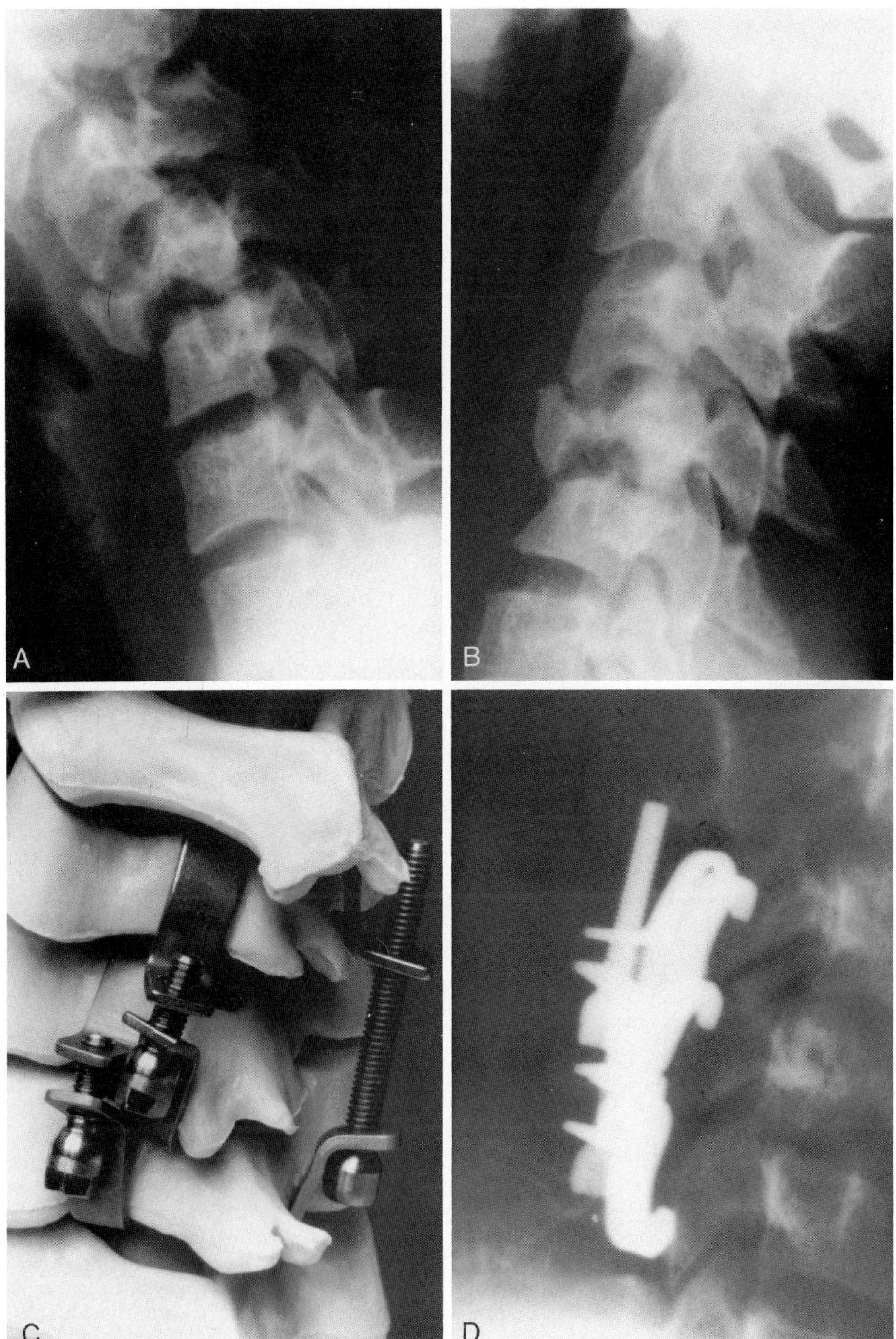

Figure 22.14. **A**, Lateral cervical spine film in flexion showing angulation. The larger fragment serves as a fulcrum. **B**, Lateral cervical spine film in extension. **C**, Halifax interlaminar clips have been applied to an anatomical model to illustrate their application in this patient. **D**, Lateral cervical spine film showing Halifax clips in situ. There was no movement on flexion and extension.

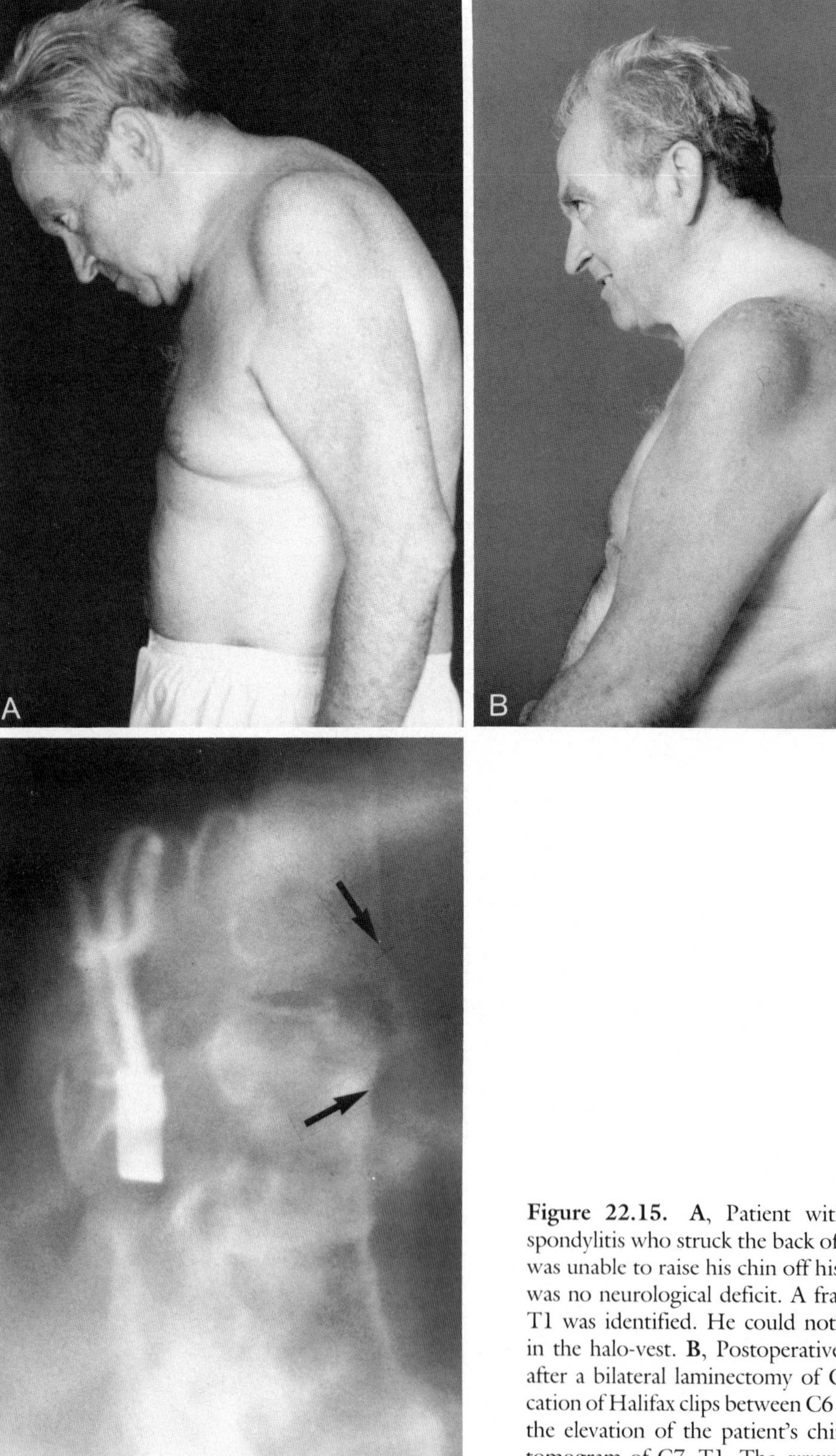

Figure 22.15. **A**, Patient with ankylosing spondylitis who struck the back of his head. He was unable to raise his chin off his chest. There was no neurological deficit. A fracture of C7–T1 was identified. He could not be realigned in the halo-vest. **B**, Postoperative photograph after a bilateral laminectomy of C7 and application of Halifax clips between C6 and T1. Note the elevation of the patient's chin. **C**, Lateral tomogram of C7–T1. The *arrows* indicate the edge of an anterior fusion mass.

in many cases operation is obviated by the use of the device, cost and risk are reduced. Where surgical operation is required, the halo-vest apparatus is a useful adjunct that enhances safety and may result in simplification of the procedure required.

ACKNOWLEDGMENT

The authors would like to acknowledge the major contributions of our "halo-nurses," Mrs. Kathi Colwell and Mrs. Maureen Starnes. They are essential to the formal management and operation of the Acute Spinal Cord Injury Unit, and their kindness to our patients is greatly appreciated.

REFERENCES

1. Tator CH, Ekong CEU, Rowed DW, Schwartz ML, Edmonds VE. Halo devices for the treatment of acute cervical cord injuries. In: Tator CH, ed. Early management of acute spinal cord injury. New York: Raven Press, 1982.
2. Weinstein MC, Fineberg HV. Clinical decision analysis. Toronto: W.B. Saunders Company, 1980.
3. Sears W, Fazl M. Prediction of stability of cervical spine fracture managed in halo-vest and indication for surgical intervention. J Neurosurg 1990;72:426–432.
4. Ekong CEU, Schwartz ML, Tator CH, Rowed DW, Edmonds VE. Odontoid fracture: management with early mobilization using the halo device. Neurosurgery 1981;9:631–637.
5. Holness RO, Huestis WS, Howes WJ, Langille RA. Posterior stabilization with an interlaminar clamp in cervical injuries: technical note and review of the long term experience with the method. Neurosurgery 1984;14:318–322.
6. Simmons EH. The surgical correction of flexion deformity of the cervical spine in ankylosing spondylitis. In: Sherk HH, ed. The cervical spine. Philadelphia: J.B. Lippincott Company, 1989:573–598.

23

Traumatic Injuries of the Occipital-Cervical Articulation

Paul A. Anderson and Pasquale X. Montesano

Atlanto-occipital fractures and dislocations are rare injuries which are difficult to diagnose and which present a major treatment challenge for physicians. Unfortunately, neurologic deficits associated with these injuries are usually not compatible with survival. In this chapter, the relevant anatomy and biomechanics of the occipital-cervical junction will be reviewed followed by discussion of occipital condyle fractures and atlanto-occipital dislocations.

Anatomy

The upper cervical spine is the transition between the rigid cranium and the remaining mobile spinal column (Fig. 23.1). It consists of the foramen magnum, the paired occipital condyles, the atlas, and the axis. These structures together should be thought of as the cranio-cervical articulation. Protected within this articulation is the lower portion of the medulla oblongata, the upper spinal cord, and the vertebral arteries. As a result of the large brain size in humans, large forces and moments are applied to the bony structure and restraining ligaments. Despite this biomechanical requirement, the cranio-cervical articulation has been designed for large ranges of motion.

Bony Anatomy

The foramen magnum is a large opening in the posterior aspect of the base of the skull in the occipital bone, through which passes the spinal cord. The basion is the anterior aspect of foramen magnum and is normally located within 5 mm and directly above the tip of the odontoid process (1). The opisthion is the posterior rim of foramen magnum. The occipital condyles are located on the inferior surfaces of the occipital bone and along the anteriolateral edges of foramen magnum. Viewed from the side, the condyles are convex, semilunar in shape, and describe an arc of approximately 180°. Viewed from the front, the occipital condyles are wedge-shaped, extending farther distally on their medial aspects. These condyles articulate with the corresponding concavities in the superior aspect of the lateral masses of the atlas (Fig. 23.1.**A**).

The atlas obtains its name because it supports the "globe of the head." It consists of two lateral masses which are connected by anterior and posterior bony arches. The atlas has no body or spinous process. In many ways the atlas functions as an ossified meniscus between the occiput and axis. The superior surface of the atlas has two concave facets for articulation with the condyles of the occiput. This allows for flexion and extension of the head. The inferior facets of the atlas are concave and oval, which allows for rotation of the atlas on the axis. Each transverse process of the atlas contains a bony transverse foramen through which the vertebral artery passes. Both the anterior and posterior arches have medially flared tubercles where ligaments are attached. The medial aspect of each lateral mass has a small tubercle for attachment of the transverse ligament. Occasionally, in the posterior arches of the atlas a deep groove or canal forms, which contains the vertebral artery. The canal, when present, is referred to as the ponticulus posticus (2).

The axis or C2 is distinguished by a large vertical process connected to its body. This odontoid process or dens represents the body of the atlas that has been embryologically separated from the atlas and later unites with the axis. The odontoid provides a pivot around which the axis rotates. The superior facets of the axis are anterior alongside the odontoid and are slightly convex to aid in atlanto-axial rotation. The inferior facets of the axis are located posteriorly and are in the same orientation as those in the remaining lower cervical spine.

Ligamentous Anatomy

The major restraining ligaments between the occiput and cervical spine bypass the atlas and span from the occiput to the axis. The atlas merely acts as a bushing or spacer. This arrangement allows the large ranges of motion present in the upper cervical spine but maintains stability.

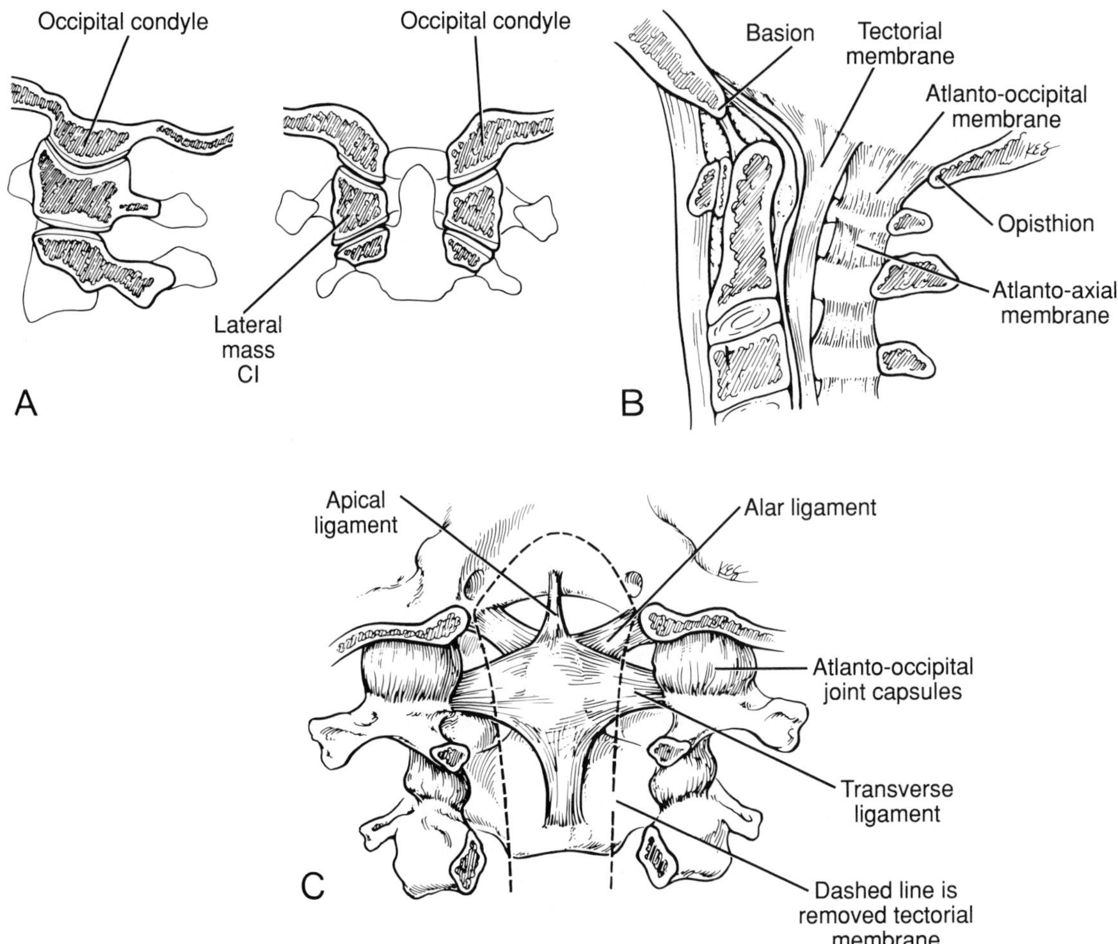

Figure 23.1. **A**, Osseous anatomy of occipital-cervical articulation. **B**, Sagittal view of occipital-cervical articulation. **C**, Posterior view of internal cranial cervical ligaments.

The important ligaments can be classified as external cranial cervical ligaments, which lie outside of the vertebral canal, and internal cranial cervical ligaments which lie within the vertebral canal (Fig. 23.1.**B** and **C**).

External Cervical Cranial Ligaments

The ligamentum nuchae extends from the external occipital protuberance to the posterior tubercle of the atlas and all other spinous processes of the cervical vertebra. In quadrupeds, this ligament is a very well-developed structure.

The yellow elastic fibers which connect the lamina of adjacent vertebrae are referred to as the ligamentum flavum. Such fibers are not found in the cranio-cervical articulation. There is also no intervertebral disc in the cranio-cervical articulation.

The anterior atlanto-occipital membrane is a fibro-elastic band located between the anterior margin of the foramen magnum and the upper border of the anterior arch of the atlas. Similarly, the posterior atlanto-occipital membrane is located between the posterior margin of the foramen magnum and the upper border of the posterior arch of the atlas. The atlanto-axial membrane is a thin structure between the posterior arch of the atlas and the lamina of the axis. In addition, there are capsular ligaments surrounding the atlanto-occipital and the atlanto-axial facet articulations.

Internal Cranial Cervical Ligaments

There are several ligaments on the posterior aspect of the vertebral bodies which are arranged to prevent excessive movement and provide strength to the articulations (3). The most important is the tectorial membrane which is the cranial prolongation of the posterior longitudinal ligament. It is a thin, flat ligament located on the posterior aspect of the body and odontoid process of the axis and attaches to the anterior aspect of foramen magnum. The transverse ligament is a thick cord-like structure which passes posterior to the odontoid processes and attaches to tubercles located on the inner aspect of each lateral mass of the atlas. The alar ligaments are two strong bands stretching obliquely outward from the superior lateral aspect of the odontoid processes to the inner aspect of the occipital condyles. The apical ligament is a rudimentary structure extending from the apex of the odontoid process to the anterior midpoint of the foramen magnum.

Biomechanics

Werne (3) has performed extensive anatomic, radiographic, and biomechanical analysis of ligaments of the upper cervical spine. He concluded that the tectorial membrane checks extension of the occiput on the atlas. Flexion was limited by impingement of the basion on the anterior arch of the atlas. The alar ligaments were found to check both atlanto-occipital and atlanto-axial lateral flexion and rotation. On lateral flexion to one side, the contralateral alar ligament was noted to tighten and limit further flexion (Fig. 23.2.**A**). On rotation, the ipsilateral alar ligament was noted to tighten first. On extreme rotation, the ipsilateral alar ligament shortened by winding around the dens (Fig. 23.2.**B**). The allows the contralateral alar ligament to tighten and limit further rotation. This work has recently been substantiated by the work of Dvorak and Panjabi (4). Distraction between occiput and C1 or C1 and C2 is limited by both the tectorial membrane and alar ligaments. The apical ligament, atlanto-occipital membranes, and joint capsules have little effect on stability of the cranio-cervical articulation.

The cranio-cervical articulation accounts for a significant portion of neck motion. Using cadaver specimens, Werne (3) determined the range of motion between the occiput and C1 and between C1 and C2. Occipital-C1 motion averaged 13° of flexion-extension, 8° of lateral bending and 0° of rotation. Atlanto-axial rotation was 10° of flexion-extension, 0° of lateral bending, and 47° of rotation.

Occipital Condyle Fractures

Fractures of the occipital condyle were first described in 1817 by Bell (5). Kissinger (6) then reported an additional case in 1900. Wachenheim (7), in 1974, described a series of six occipital condyle fractures, but no follow-up was reported. Four were avulsion injuries of the occipital condyle, while two cases were compression injuries. Since that time, other authors have reported additional cases of occipital condyle fractures (8–17). The most common clinical features were loss of consciousness or cranial nerve

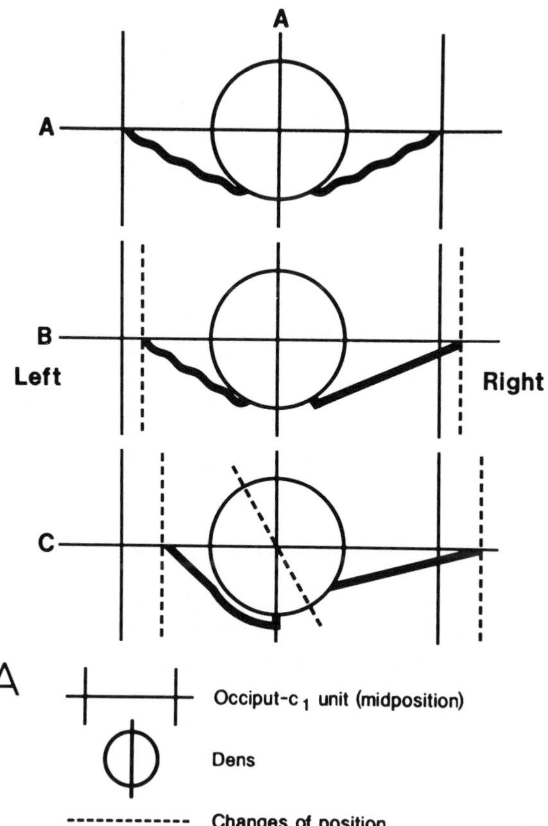

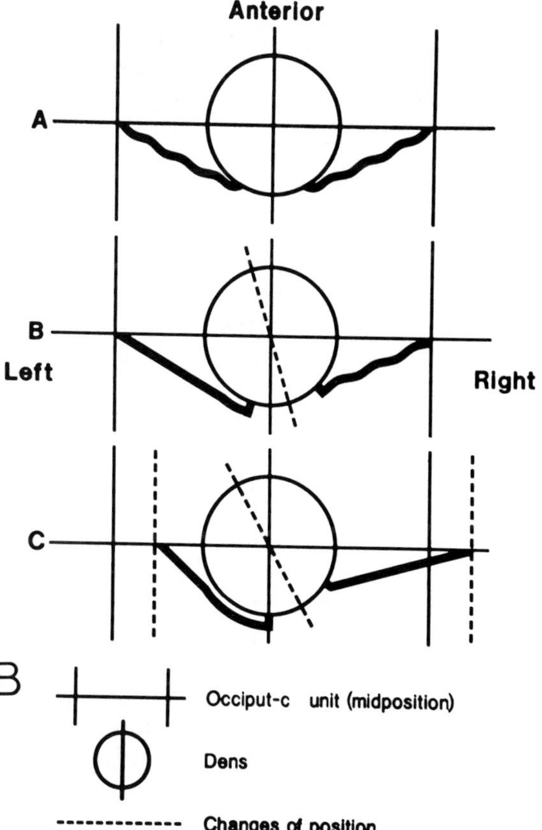

Figure 23.2. **A**, On lateral flexion to one side, the contralateral alar ligament becomes tight, limiting further flexion. **B**, On rotation, the ipsilateral alar ligament tightens first. On extreme rotation, the ipsilateral alar ligament shortens by winding around the dens. This allows the contralateral ligament to tighten, thereby limiting further rotation.

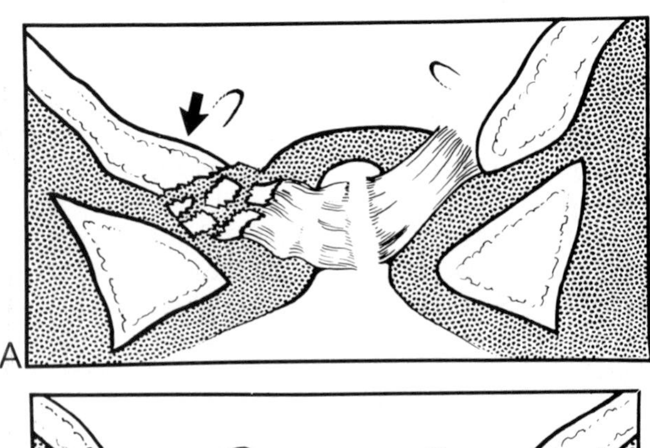

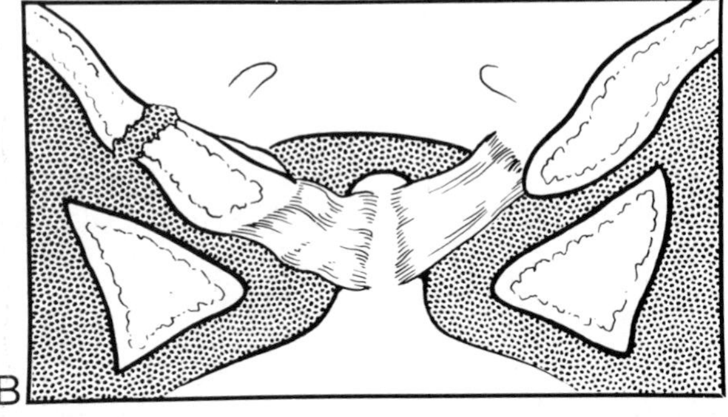

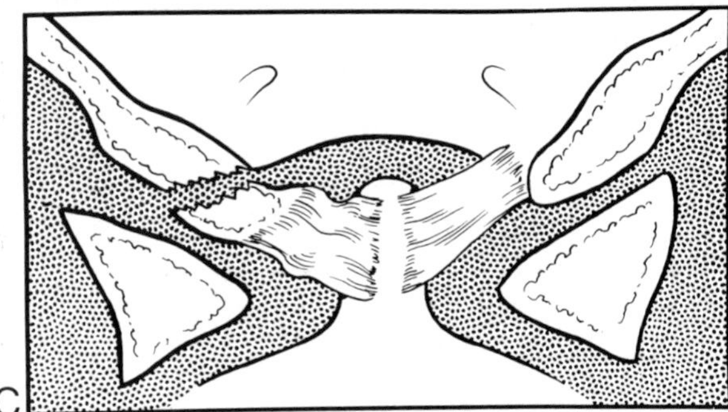

Figure 23.3. Classification of Occipital Condyle Fractures. **A**, Type I—Impacted type occipital condyle fracture. **B**, Type II—Basilar skull type occipital condyle fracture. **C**, Type III—Avulsion type occipital condyle fracture.

Table 23.1. Occipital Condyle Fractures

Type I	—	Impacted
Type II	—	Basilar skull fracture
Type III	—	Avulsion

damage. It appears that this injury is often overlooked and is not obvious on plain radiographs. The diagnosis requires a high index of suspicion and is easily confirmed by computerized axial tomography with reconstructions or conventional tomography. In July of 1988 the authors (18) reported a series of six occipital condyle fractures. A classification of occipital condyle fractures was devised, based on fracture morphology, pertinent anatomy, and biomechanics (Fig. 23.3 and Table 23.1).

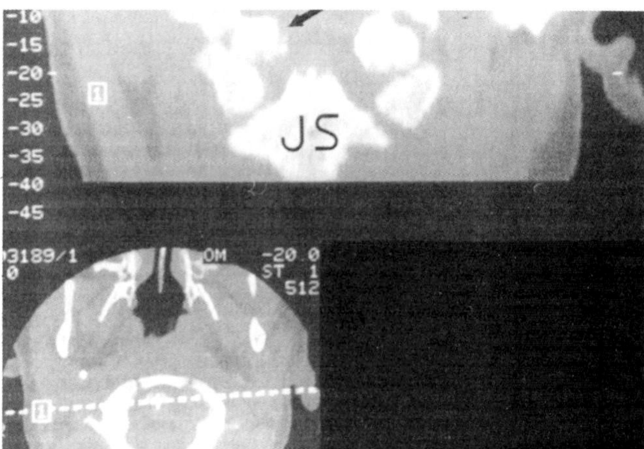

Figure 23.4. Case 1 Three-year-old boy involved in MVA sustaining closed head injury. CT scan reveals an impaction fracture of the right occipital condyle. Plain radiographs were negative. Treatment consisted of hard collar for 2 months. At follow-up 18 months later the patient has full range of motion and is pain free.

Type I Occipital Condyle Fracture

A Type I injury is an impacted occipital condyle fracture occurring as the result of axial loading of the skull onto the atlas, similar to the mechanism for a Jefferson fracture. Morphologically, there is comminution of the occipital condyle with minimal or no displacement of fragments into the foramen magnum (Fig. 23.4). Although the ipsilateral alar ligament may be functionally inadequate, spinal stability is assured by the intact tectorial membrane and contralateral alar ligament.

Case 1

A 3-year-old boy was involved in a motor vehicle accident, sustaining a closed head injury. His initial plain cervical radiographs were negative. CT scan of the brain (Fig. 23.4) revealed an unrecognized comminuted fracture of the right occipital condyle. The patient was noted to be neurologically intact including the cranial nerves and was placed in a hard collar. At follow-up 18 months later, the patient had full range of motion and was pain free.

Type II Occipital Condyle Fracture

A Type II occipital condyle fracture occurs as part of a basilar skull fracture. A fracture line can be seen on axial sections of the base of the skull that exits the occipital condyle and enters the foramen magnum. The mechanism of injury is a direct blow to the skull. Stability is maintained by intact alar ligaments and tectorial membrane. Morphologically, a fracture line can be seen on axial sections of CAT.

Type III Occipital Condyle Fracture

A Type III occipital condyle fracture is an avulsion fracture of the occipital condyle by the alar ligament. The alar ligaments are primary restraints of occipito-cervical rotation, lateral bending, and vertical translation. Therefore, we believe the mechanism of this injury is rotation, lateral bending, or rapid deceleration with the head thrown forward.

Following avulsion of the occipital condyle, the contralateral alar ligament and tectorial membrane are progressively loaded and may be injured. Therefore, the Type III occipital condyle fracture is a potentially unstable injury. Morphologically, a small fragment from the inferior and medial aspect of the occipital condyle is displaced toward the tip of the odontoid.

Case 2

A 23-year-old female was an unrestrained passenger in a motor vehicle accident. She was initially treated for a closed head injury. Her lateral cervical radiographs were normal. Forty-eight hours later, her head injury resolved, and she complained of upper cervical neck pain and occipital headache. CT scans of the upper spine revealed bilateral avulsion Type III occipital condyle fractures (Fig. 23.5.**A**, **B**). She was treated with a Minerva brace for 2 months. At follow-up after 9 months, she had returned to work without any neck complaints.

In our series there were 6 cases of occipital condyle fractures, one Type I fracture, one Type II, and four Type III fractures. The patients with the Type I and Type II healed with 8 weeks of immobilization in a rigid orthosis. At follow-up of 24 and 12 months respectively, the patients were pain free and had a full range of neck motion.

Of the four patients with Type III fractures, two were immobilized in a rigid orthosis, and one in a halo vest for 12 weeks. The other patient with a Type III fracture died as a result of brainstem injury from the displaced occipital condyle fragment. At follow-up of 12 to 36 months, the three surviving patients were pain free and had a full range of neck motion.

Type I and Type II injuries are considered stable injuries and are both thought to be secondary to axial loading. Type III injuries are avulsion fractures of the occipital condyle. Since occipital condyle avulsion fractures may result in a loss of integrity of the alar ligaments, they may be potentially unstable injuries. While healing may occur in a halo or rigid cervical orthosis, these injuries deserve close follow-up. Furthermore, flexion-extension radiographs should be obtained after a 12-week immobilization to determine healing. Should persistent instability be documented, then we recommend that an occipito-cervical fusion be performed.

TRAUMATIC ATLANTO-OCCIPITAL DISLOCATIONS

Traumatic occipito-cervical dislocations are usually fatal and therefore rarely present as a clinical problem. Improvement in the care of the trauma victim by on-site intubation, immediate resuscitation, and early transport to hospital facilities has led to survival of patients with these injuries. Despite increased awareness of this injury, the majority of surviving patients with occipito-cervical dislocations have had significant delays in diagnosis and treatment (19, 20). Overlying shadows from the base of the cranium and mastoid processes, and inadequate understanding of the bony anatomy make radiographic diagnosis difficult.

Forensic studies reveal an alarming incidence of atlanto-occipital (AO) injuries in deaths following vehicular accidents. Davis et al. (21) performed comprehensive autopsies on 50 victims who died of craniospinal injuries. Injuries between the occiput and C2 were found in 20% of cases. Ligamentous injuries were especially prominent in the upper cervical spine, whereas bony injuries were much more common below C2. Bucholz (22) roentgenographically studied the cervical spine in 112 fatalities of multiple trauma. Atlanto-occipital dislocation was the sin-

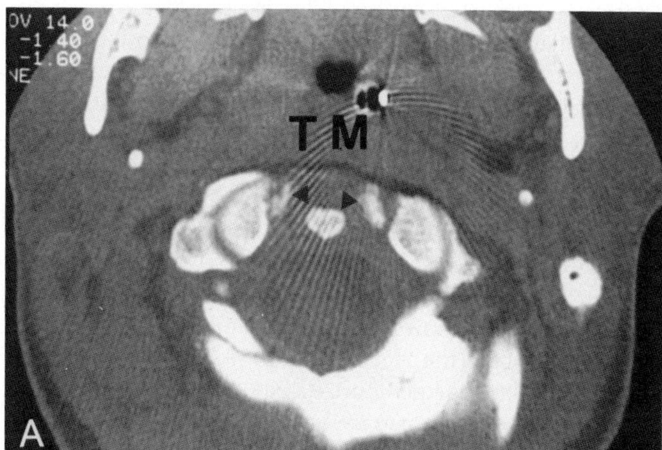

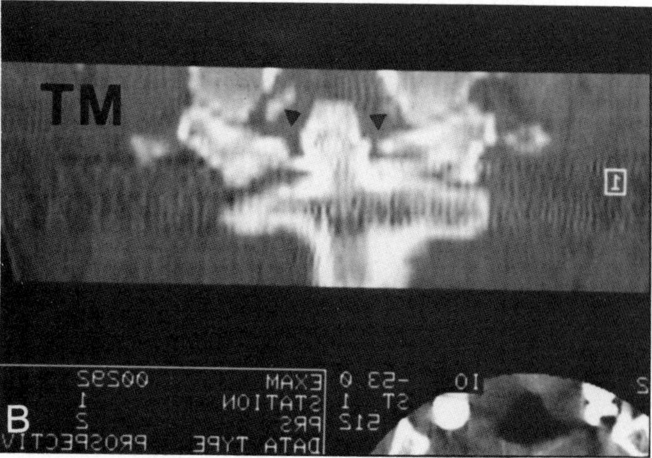

Figure 23.5. **Case 2** Twenty-three year-old female who was involved in a motor vehicle accident. **A**, Axial CT demonstrates bilateral avulsion Type II occipital condyle fractures. **B**, Coronal CT reconstruction demonstrating displacement of occipital condyle fractures medially.

Table 23.2. Classification of Atlanto-Occipital Instability

Type I	Anterior displacement occiput on atlas
Type II	Vertical displacement occiput and cervical spine **A.** Between occiput and atlas **B.** Between atlas and axis, associated with transverse ligament rupture
Type III	Posterior displacement occiput on atlas

gle most common spinal injury in these trauma victims. Nine cases of AO dislocations were discovered, and six were autopsied. Three of these cases had total disruption of all ligaments between the skull and cervical spine. In two cases only the alar ligaments were spared, and they were associated with avulsion fractures at their attachment to the occipital condyles. In one case the posterior atlanto-occipital membrane was the only structure left intact. Bucholz felt that the mechanism of injury was hyperextension and distraction. Consistent with other reports, there was a higher incidence of this injury among children (15%) than adults (6%). Werne (3) found total ligamentous disruption in five cases of AO instability. He emphasized that there were avulsion type fractures of the alar ligament attachments to the occipital condyles in each case.

Case Reports of Atlanto-Occipital Dislocations

There have been upwards of 20 case reports (3, 19, 23–27) of survivors of AO dislocation. The majority of patients have had deceleration motor vehicular injuries or were pedestrians struck by cars. Over 70% of patients have evidence of head injury. Noncontiguous spinal fractures are common. Delayed diagnosis or misdiagnosis was frequently seen with several patients deteriorating neurologically during hospitalization. Cranial nerve palsies, especially of the sixth, eleventh, and twelfth nerves, are seen in 50% of cases. Complete quadriplegia or brainstem injuries usually resulted in death. Incomplete quadriplegia was frequently of the Brown-Sequard or central cord type. Successful treatment consisted of reduction and subsequent posterior occipito-cervical fusion with postoperative immobilization in a halo brace or Minerva cast. However, at least two patients were treated nonoperatively with no apparent long-term sequelae (19).

Classification

Traynelis (20) in an excellent review has classified AO injuries according to the primary direction of displacement of the occipital and C1 articulation (Table 23.2 and Fig. 23.6).

Type I Atlanto-Occipital Instability

Type I injuries are the most common in reported survivors. This type is an anterior atlanto-occiput dislocation with both occipital condyles subluxated anterior on their corresponding atlantal facets (Fig. 23.6.**B**). Biomechanical studies have demonstrated rupture of all major ligaments is required to produce this injury.

Case 3

A 23-year-old female was admitted with multiple injuries secondary to a motor vehicle accident. She complained of upper cervical neck pain and occipital headaches. Neurologically the cranial nerves and extremities were intact. Lateral cervical radiographs revealed an anterior Type I atlanto-occipital dislocation (Fig. 23.7.**A**). CT reconstructions showed anterior subluxation of both occipital condyles (Fig. 23.7.**B**). The axial CT demonstrated absence of occipital condyle articulation with lateral masses of the atlas (Fig. 23.7.**C**). Closed reduction was performed using careful head positioning and tong traction. Ten days postinjury she underwent posterior occipital cervical fusion and postoperative halo vest immobilization. Six months later, the patient had a solid arthrodesis and had returned to previous employment (Fig. 23.7.**D**).

Type II Atlanto-Occipital Instability

Type II injuries are direct vertical displacement of the occiput on the cervical spine and represent rupture of all restraining AO ligaments (Fig. 23.6.**C**,**D**). Type II injuries are recognized by wide distraction between the occiput and C1. Radiographically an empty space is identified above the atlas where normally the occiput should lie (Fig. 23.8**A**). Biomechanically, Werne (3) has shown vertical displacement of the occiput on C1 is limited normally to less than 2 mm. Displacements greater than this amount represent failure of the tectorial membrane and probably alar ligaments. Similarly, vertical distraction between C1 and C2 is prevented by these same ligaments.

We have observed a variant of Type II injury where vertical displacement occurs between C1 and C2, rather than atlanto-occipitally (Fig. 23.6.**D**, 23.8.**B**). We classify this as atlanto-occipital instability because in both patterns the primary ligamentous restraints, the alar ligaments and tectorial membrane, are damaged. However, in this latter kind of Type II injury the secondary restraints such as the atlanto-axial joint capsules and membranes are damaged rather than those between the occiput and atlas.

Atlanto-occipital instability may be associated with injuries to the transverse ligament of the axis (28). Continued forward translation of C1 on C2 after rupture of the transverse ligament stresses the alar ligaments and tectorial membrane. When the atlanto dens interval exceeds 7–10 mm these secondary ligaments are damaged. We have observed this combined injury pattern in 75% of patients who have an initial diagnosis of traumatic transverse ligament rupture and in 50% of patients with initial diagnosis of atlanto-occipital instability. Treatment of the combined injury pattern requires posterior occipital-cervical fusion.

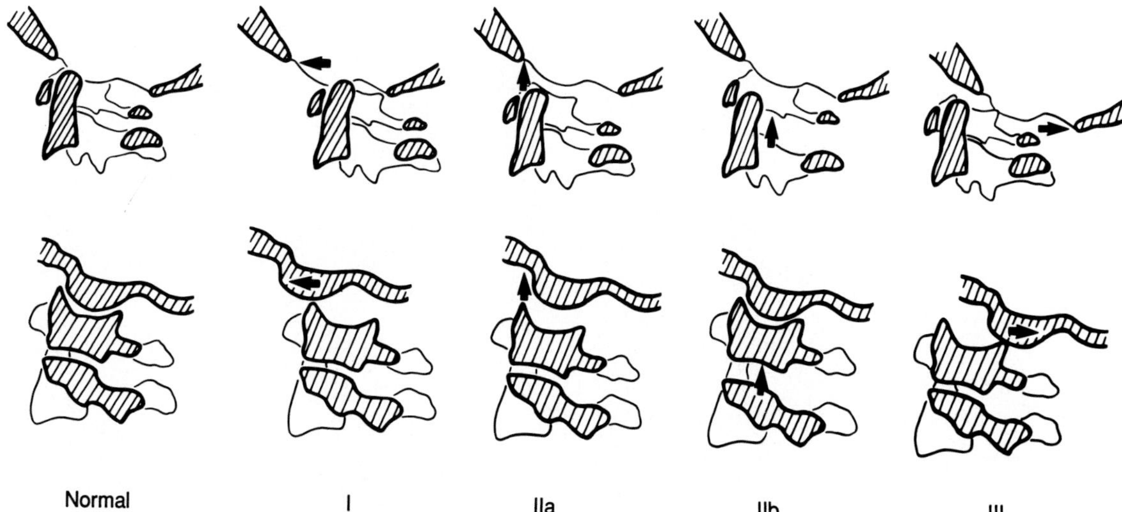

Figure 23.6. Classification of traumatic occipital-cervical dislocations as modified from Traynelis VC, Marano GD, Dunker RO, Kaufman HH. Traumatic atlanto-occipital dislocation: Case report. J Neurosurg 1988;65:863–870. **A, Normal; B, Type I** Anterior translation between occipital condyles and atlas; **C, Type IIa** Vertical displacement between occiput and atlas; **D, Type IIb** Vertical displacement between C1 and C2; **E, Type III** Posterior displacement of the occipital condyles and atlas.

Case 4

A 24-year-old female was involved in a high speed motor vehicle accident. She sustained a mild closed head injury and open left supracondylar fracture. She complained of occipital headaches and upper cervical pain and was neurologically intact. The initial lateral cervical radiograph in traction demonstrated distraction between C1 and C2, and fracture of the anterior arch of C1 (Fig. 23.9.**A**). A second radiograph demonstrates increased atlanto-dens interval, indicating rupture of the transverse ligament of the atlas (Fig. 23.9.**B**). Upper cervical CT following reduction revealed a displaced occipital condyle fracture and normal bony alignment (Fig. 23.9.**C**,**D**). Because of the vertical displacement noted on her traction film we felt she had Type IIb anterio-occipital instability. She underwent a posterior occipital cervical fusion with postoperative halo-vest immobilization.

Type III Atlanto-Occipital Instability

In Type III injuries the occiput is displaced posterior to the atlas. Only two survivors have been reported with this pattern. In one case (27) the Type III injury was associated with displaced laminar fractures of C1 accounting for the patient's survival. Although diagnosis was significantly delayed until transferred to the care of the authors, the patient had a successful closed reduction and posterio-occipital cervical fusion.

RADIOGRAPHIC DIAGNOSIS

Routine lateral cervical radiographs are required on all trauma patients and should include visualization of the occiput and cervical-thoracic junction. Type II injuries with vertical displacement are readily diagnosed by the obvious diastasis between occiput and atlas. Less obvious and frequently unrecognized are Type I and III injuries.

When examining cervical radiographs the status of the articulations between the occipital condyles and atlantal lateral masses should be considered. Unfortunately, because orientation of these joints lies oblique to the x-ray beam they are not easily seen on lateral views. Also overlying shadows from the cranium, mastoid processes and maxilla obscure these joints on both open mouth and lateral radiographs. However, indirect evidence of atlanto-occipital injury may be present (Table 23.3).

Wholey (1) reviewed 600 radiographs to determine the normal relationships at the cranio-spinal junction. He found that the retropharyngeal space anterior to the body of C2 averaged 3.7 mm and never exceeded 7 mm. Massive prevertebral soft tissue swelling has been noted in most survivors of AO dislocations. He also evaluated the relationship between the occiput and atlas by determining the distance between the basion (anterior lip of foramen magnum) and the tip of the dens. This averaged 5 mm and was more reliable than either Chamberlain's or McGregor's line. Unfortunately, the basion is difficult to visualize because of overlying shadows.

The clivus is a long bony plate starting at the sella turcica and ending at the basion. Normally the basion lies directly above the tip of the dens, but it is difficult to locate its exact position. However, a line drawn down the clivus should intersect with the tip of the dens. When this line is offset, atlanto-occipital subluxation should be strongly suspected. Less sensitive is the relationship between the mastoid process and the dens, as seen on lateral radiographs. Normally, the mastoid projects over the posterior one-half of the dens.

Powers (19) used the ratio of the distances from the basion to posterior arch of C1 and the opisthion (posterior edge of foramen magnum) to the anterior arch of C1 to determine presence of atlanto-occipital dislocation. A nor-

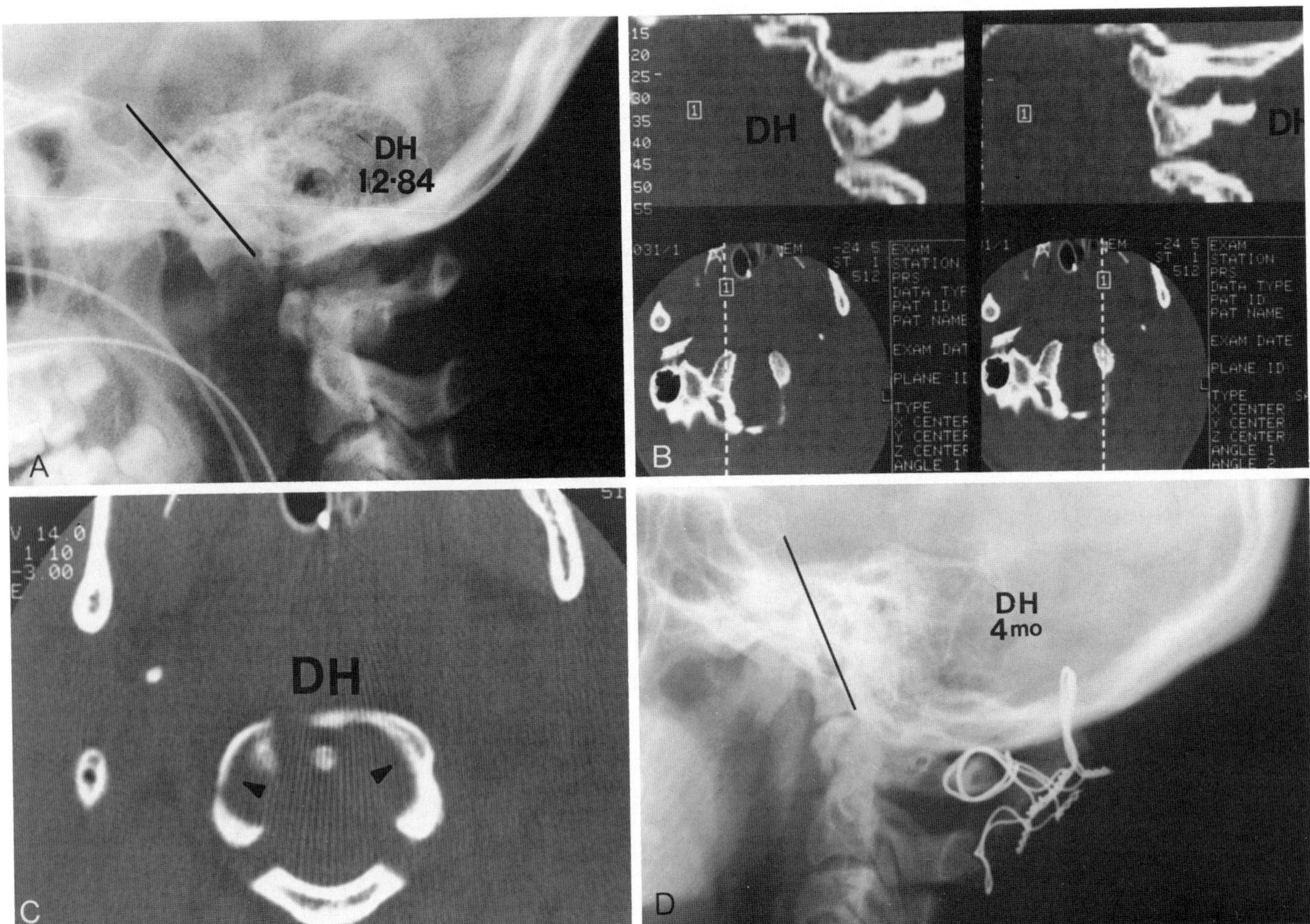

Figure 23.7. Case 3. A 23-year-old female with multiple injuries secondary to motor vehicle accident. **A**, Lateral view demonstrates anterior displacement of the occiput on atlas. Note the black line representing the clivus points well anterior to the tip of the dens. **B**, CT reconstruction in sagittal plane through articulations show anterior subluxation of occipital condyles and atlantal lateral masses. **C**, Axial CT scan. Black *arrows* represent missing occipital condyles. **D**, Lateral radiograph 4 months following closed reduction, posterior occipital–C2 fusion and halo immobilization. Clivus now points toward dens.

mal value is 0.77 and never exceeds 1.0. He states that values greater than 1.0 are seen in all cases of anterior atlanto-occipital dislocation. This ratio is not useful when the atlas is fractured or when C1–2 translation is present. Unfortunately, overlying shadows make the exact identification of the basion and opisthion difficult and limit the usefulness of this technique.

Computerized axial tomography (CT) is far more accurate in analyzing the relationships between the occiput and cervical spine. We recommend CT scanning using 3 mm slice thickness and routine multiplane sagittal and coronal reconstructions to evaluate all patients with suspicious upper cervical radiographs. Patients with signs of brainstem injury, unexplained quadriparesis, or cranial nerve palsies should undergo upper cervical spine CT scanning. Sagittal reconstructions performed through the level of the occipital condyles and C1–2 articulations will demonstrate definitively the presence or absence of atlanto-occipital subluxation or dislocation. Less clear may be those injuries with minor degrees of vertical translation manifested by increased joint space. Comparison of the joint diastasis between the level in question and adjacent ones will determine the presence or absence of injury.

TREATMENT

Successful treatment results only after early accurate diagnosis. In all injured patients, a lateral cervical spine radiograph is mandatory. This needs to be scrutinized for the subtle findings suggestive of AO dislocations. When indicated from this radiograph or from presence of pain, neurologic deficits, or cranial nerve palsies, CT from the occiput to C2 should be performed.

As in any spinal injury, the goals of treatment are to protect the neural tissue, reduce and stabilize the spinal column, and provide long-term spinal stability. Skeletal traction is effective in treating most cervical spine injuries.

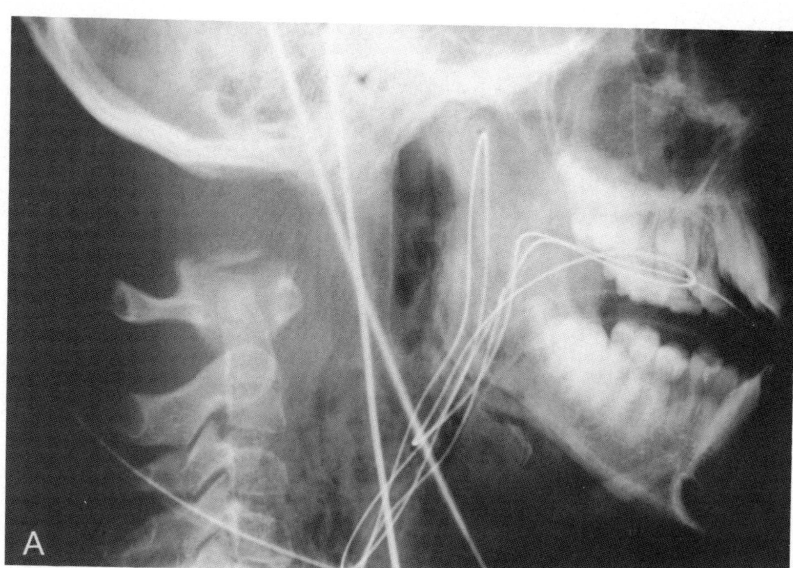

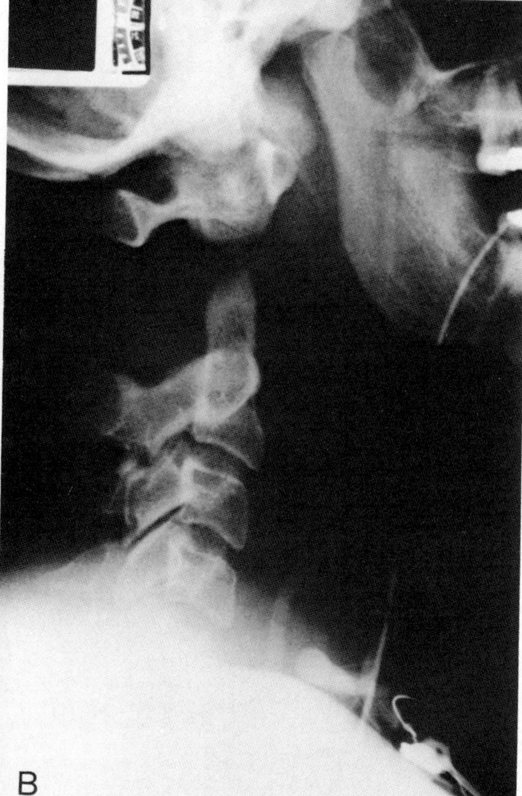

Figure 23.8. **A**, Lateral radiograph from fatal victim showing Type IIa AO injury. **B**, Lateral radiograph from fatal victim showing Type IIb AO injury. Note that displacement is between C1 and C2.

Biomechanically, skeletal traction applies tension to the ligaments, especially the posterior longitudinal ligament, and thereby realigns the spinal column. In patients with atlanto-occipital instability, traction should be used with extreme caution. All stabilizing ligaments are potentially damaged, and small amounts of weight can cause distraction and resultant brainstem injury. We recommend using skeletal tong traction limited to 2–5 pounds.

More important than traction, one needs to consider the relative position of the head and neck. As in the young child, where the head is larger than the thorax, the spine will be in a flexed position when lying on a flat board. If atlanto-occipital instability exists under these conditions, displacement will invariably be anterior. Consequently, to help align these dislocations, one needs to adjust the position of the head and thorax until reduction is achieved. Blanket rolls are placed under the thorax elevating the neck to help reduce anterior dislocations. In patients with vertical translations, elevation of the head of the bed will allow gravity to reduce the injury. Posterior dislocations can be reduced by placing blankets behind the occiput.

After reduction the patient is placed in a halo vest. Repeat radiographs in both supine and upright positions are required as these injuries may displace despite halo vest immobilization. For long-term stability we recommend posterior occipital cervical fusion. The neurologic consequences of loss of position and poor capacity for spinal ligamentous injuries to heal warrant this surgical approach despite the expected loss of range of motion.

Surgical Technique

Ideally the patient is brought to the surgical site in a reduced position in a halo vest. Awake nasotracheal intubation is performed aided by fiberoptic scope. The patient is then turned prone on a regular operating table with the head held by the horse-shoe cerebellar head rest. A lateral radiograph is taken to assure proper spinal alignment. After positioning, a neurologic check is performed and then the patient is placed under general anesthesia. Although some surgeons recommend removal of the posterior half of the halo vest for surgery, we have had no difficulty performing upper cervical posterior arthrodesis with both halves of the vest in position.

The technique for posterior cervical fusion has been recently reported by Bohlman (29). A midline incision is made exposing the occiput and upper two cervical lamina. At the external occipital protuberance where the bone is thick, two parallel holes for wire placement are made separated by a 3–4 mm bridge of bone. A tunnel is created with angled curettes connecting the holes creating a bony bridge. It is not necessary to enter the cranium, as one can

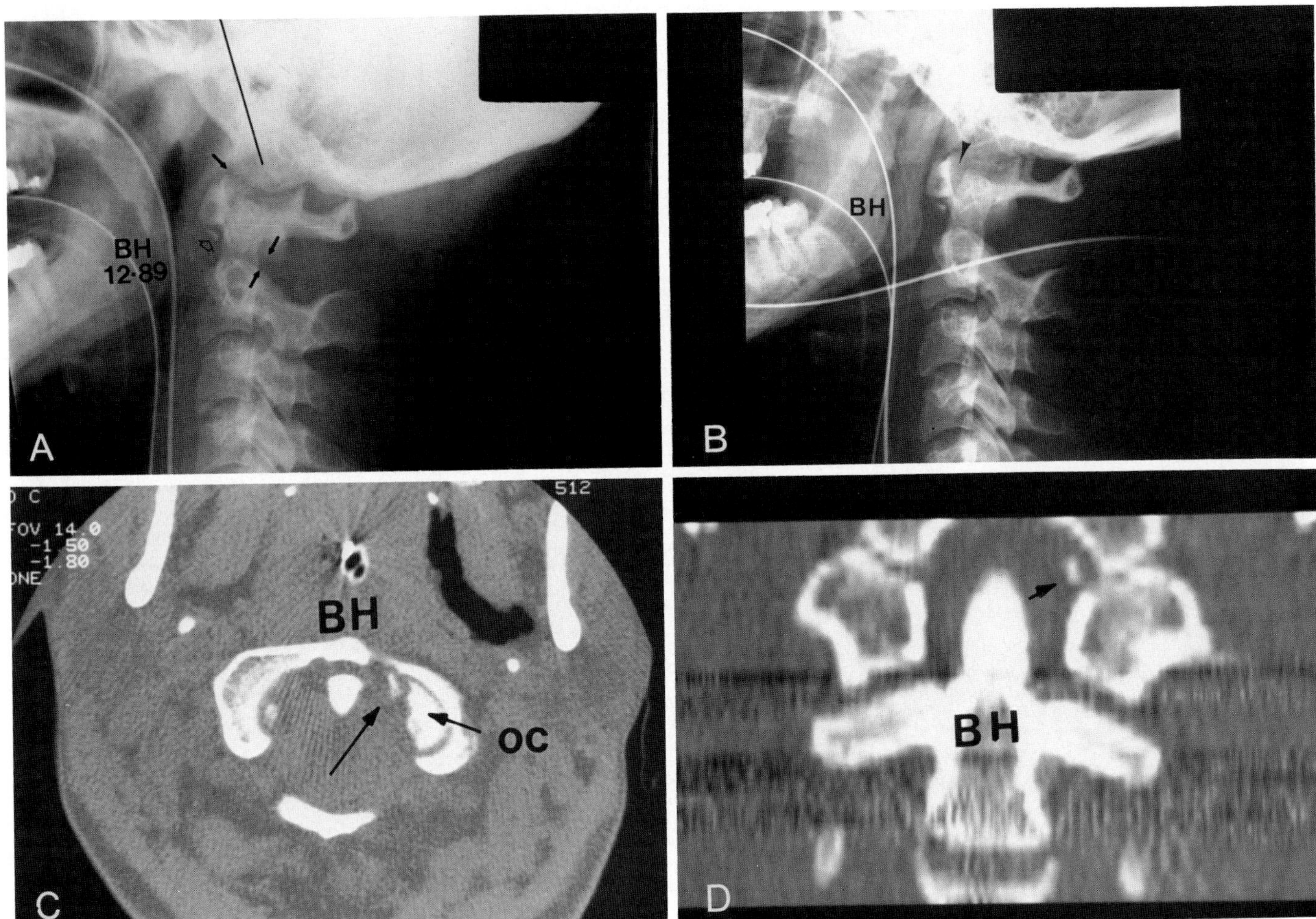

Figure 23.9. Case 4. A 37-year-old female involved in a motor vehicle accident sustaining multiple injuries. **A**, Initial lateral radiograph demonstrating Type IIb injury between occiput and cervical spine. There is increased joint space between C1 and C2. *Open arrow* shows avulsion fracture of anterior arch of C1. *Black line* representing clivus points posterior to dens. **B**, Lateral view in 3 pounds of skeletal traction. Black area shows an increase in atlantodens interval and increased vertical translation between C1 and C2. The anterior arch of C1 is cranial to dens. **C**, Axial CT showing avulsion type occipital condyle fracture. **D**, Coronal reconstruction showing avulsion fracture of left occipital condyle.

Table 23.3. Radiologic Signs of Atlanto-Occipital Injuries

Prevertebral soft tissue swelling
Basion to dens distance >5 mm
Clivus not pointing to dens tip
Mastoid not overlying dens
Powers ratio >1.0

generally stay above the inner table. A 20-gauge wire is double looped around this bony bridge. Another 20-gauge wire is placed sublaminarly around C1. A third wire is passed through a drill hole in the base of the spinous process of C2 and looped around the caudal edge of the spine.

Two cortico-cancellous strips of iliac bone graft, 4 cm long, 12 mm wide and approximately 7 mm thick are harvested. Three holes are placed in the grafts to accept the previously placed wires. The wires are passed through the grafts, and then the grafts are placed down onto the lamina. The wires are tightened holding the grafts in place. Dural tears should be anticipated in any patient with initial wide displacement or neurologic deficits. Postoperatively the halo vest is worn for a minimum of 3 months and until bony consolidation occurs.

CONCLUSION

Injuries to the cranio-cervical articulation are highly unstable and frequently cause significant neurologic injuries or death. These injuries usually involve only the major restraining ligaments and therefore are easily overlooked on plain radiographs. High resolution CT with reconstructions will demonstrate the cranio-cervical articulations and occipital condyles. Halo-vest immobilization and posterior occipital fusion are recommended for injuries involving the tectorial membrane and alar ligaments. Occipital condyle fractures can be treated successfully with halo-vest or cervicothoracic braces.

ACKNOWLEDGMENT

We would like to thank Ms. Kate Sweeney, our medical illustrator, and Mr. Edward Kohnstamm, photographer for the Department of Orthopaedics at Harborview Medical Center in Seattle, Washington, for their help with and dedication to this project.

REFERENCES

1. Wholey MH, Bruwer AJ, Hillier LB. The lateral roentgenogram of the neck (with comments on the atlanto-odontoid-basion relationship). Radiology 1958;71:350–356.

2. Erickson LC, Greer RO. Ponticulus posticus; an anomaly of the first cervical vertebra as seen on the cephalonetric head film. Oral Surg Oral Med Oral Pathol 1984;57:230.

3. Werne S. Studies in spontaneous atlas dislocation. Acta Scand Orthop 1957;(Suppl)23:1–150.

4. Dvorak J, Panjabi MM. Functional anatomy of the alar ligaments. Spine 1987;12:183–189.

5. Bell C. Surgical observations. Middlesex Hosp J 1987;4:469.

6. Kissinger P. Luxationsfraktur in atlantocipitalgelenke. Zentralbl Chir 1900;37:933–934.

7. Wackenheim A. Roentgen diagnosis of the craniovertebral region. 1974;Berlin, Springer-Verlag.

8. Bolander N, Cromwell LD, Wendling L. Fracture of the occipital condyle. AJR Am J Roentgenol 1978;131:729–731.

9. Comassa NW, Casavola C, Castelli M, Scapati C. Fraturra del condilo occipitale. Radiol Med (Torino) 1983;63:154–155.

10. Goldstein SJ, Woodring JH, Young AB. Occipital condyle fracture associated with cervical spine injury. Surg Neurol 1982;17:350–352.

11. Harding-Smith J, MacIntosh PK, Sherbon KJ. Fracture of the occipital condyle. J Bone Joint Surg 1981;63A:1170–1171.

12. Hollerhage HG, Renella RR, Becker H. Fracture of the occipital condyle. Case description review of the literature. Zentralbl Neurochir 1986;47:250–258.

13. Peeters F, Verbeeten B. Evaluation of occipital condyle fracture and atlantic fracture, two uncommon complications of cranial vertebral trauma. ROFO 1983;138:631–633.

14. Schliack H, Schaefer P. Hypoglossal and accessory nerve paralysis in a fracture of the occipital condyle. Nervenarzt 1965;36:362–364.

15. Spencer JA, Yeakley JW, Kaufman HH. Fracture of the occipital condyle. Neurosurgery 1989;15:101–103.

16. Spirig P. A case of the fracture of the occipital condyle. Unfallchir Versicherungsmed Berufskr 1985;78:119–122.

17. Von Ahlgren P, Dahlerup JV. Fractura condylus occipitalis. Fortschr Roentgenstr 1964;101:202–204.

18. Anderson PA, Montesano PX. Morphology and treatment of occipital condyle fractures. Spine 1988;13:731–736.

19. Powers B, Miller MD, Kramer RS, Martinez S, Gehweiler JA. Traumatic anterior atlanto-occipital dislocation. Neurosurgery 1979;4:12–17.

20. Traynelis VC, Marano GD, Dunker RO, Kaufman HH. Traumatic atlanto-occipital dislocation: case report. J Neurosurg 1988;65:863–870.

21. Davis D, Bohlman H, Walker E, Fisher R, Robinson R. The pathologic finding in fatal cranio-spinal injuries. J Neurosurg 1971;34:603–615.

22. Bucholz RW, Burkhead WZ. The pathologic anatomy of fatal atlanto-occipital dislocations. J Bone Joint Surg 1979;61-A, 248–250.

23. Gabrielsen TO, Maxwell JA. Traumatic atlanto-occipital dislocation. AJR Am J Roentgenol 1966;97:624–629.

24. Evarts CM. Traumatic occipito-atlantal dislocation: report of a case with survival. J Bone Joint Surg 1970;52A:1653–1660.

25. Page CP, Story JL, Wissinger JP, Branch CL. Traumatic atlanto-occipital dislocation. Case report. J Neurosurg 1973;39:394–397.

26. Woodring JH, Selke AC Jr, Duff DE. Traumatic atlanto-occipital dislocation with survival. AJR Am J Roentgenol 1981;37:21–24.

27. Eismont FJ, Bohlman HH. Posterior atlanto-occipital dislocation with fractures of the atlas and odontoid process: report of a case with survival. J Bone Joint Surg 1978;60A3:397–399.

28. Anderson PA. Occipital cervical instability associated with traumatic tears of the transverse ligament. Orthop Trans 1988;12:41.

29. Wertheim SB, Bohlman HH. Occipitocervical fusion: indications, technique, and long-term results in thirteen patients. J Bone Joint Surg 1987;69A:833–836.

24

Atlantoaxial Injuries

Thomas A.S. Wilson, Jr., and J. Michael McWhorter

The atlantoaxial complex is one of the most complicated joint structures in the body. Its peculiar articulations provide a significant portion of the mobility of the cervical spine. Injuries to this complex, particularly those sustained in high-speed motor vehicle accidents, are an important cause of long-term morbidity and occasional mortality. Common injuries include atlantoaxial rotatory dislocations, Jefferson's fractures, hangman's fractures, and odontoid fractures. We shall discuss each of these, placing particular emphasis on their anatomy, pathogenesis, classification, and management.

Atlantoaxial Rotatory Subluxations

Atlantoaxial rotatory subluxation is an uncommon disorder that was first described by Corner in 1907 (1). The term applies to a spectrum of rotatory abnormalities ranging from simple rotatory fixation in which the atlantoaxial joint is fixed in a position of normal rotation, to rotation accompanied by subluxation, implying ligamentous injury and instability.

The atlantoaxial complex comprises four synovial joints: Two are between the inferior articular masses of the atlas and the superior articular masses of the axis. The third is the anterior articulation of the odontoid process with the posterior surface of the anterior arch of the atlas. The fourth is the articulation between the posterior surface of the odontoid and the transverse ligament. The transverse ligament extends between the medial aspect of the lateral masses of the atlas and secures the odontoid against its anterior arch (Fig. 24.1). The paired alar ligaments pass from the posterolateral portion of the odontoid tip superiorly and laterally to the medial aspect of the occipital condyles. On examination of cadaveric specimens, Wortzman and Dewar found that sectioning of the transverse ligament resulted in forward subluxation of 4–7 mm, with further subluxation being prevented by the alar ligaments (2). They further noted that sectioning of the alar ligaments resulted in excessive atlantoaxial rotation.

The normal atlantoaxial joint rotates up to 40–50°, accounting for 50% of the rotation of the cervical spine. Coutts discovered that complete bilateral dislocations of the articular masses occurred at 65° when the transverse ligament was intact; when the transverse ligament was incompetent, complete unilateral dislocation occurred at 45° of rotation (3). The degree of dislocation and subluxation determines the extent of spinal canal compromise and thus the likelihood of cord injury.

In 1978, Fielding and colleagues proposed a classification system for rotatory dislocations based on a series of 17 cases, which has been helpful in determining prognosis and appropriate management of these lesions (4) (Fig. 24.2). Type I refers to rotatory fixation without anterior displacement of the atlas (predental space of 3 mm or less). In this condition, the transverse ligament is intact, but the joint is fixed in a normal state of rotation. This was the most common type of dislocation encountered in their series. The type II refers to rotatory fixation with anterior displacement of 3–5 mm and unilateral displacement of one lateral mass, implying deficiency of the transverse ligament. The opposite lateral mass remains nondisplaced, acting as a pivot. In type III lesions, there is rotatory fixation with a predental space greater than 5 mm, anterior displacement of both lateral masses, and associated deficiency of both the transverse and the secondary ligaments. Type IV injuries, rotatory fixation with posterior displacement, were the least common; they occurred with defi-

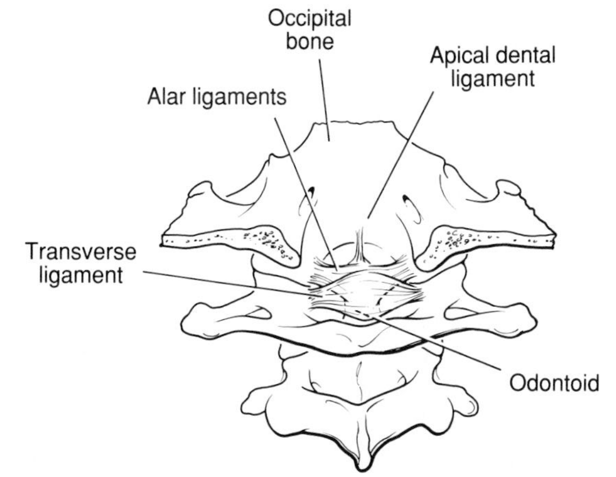

Figure 24.1. Diagram of occipito-atlanto-axial complex as viewed posteriorly, with important ligamentous structures.

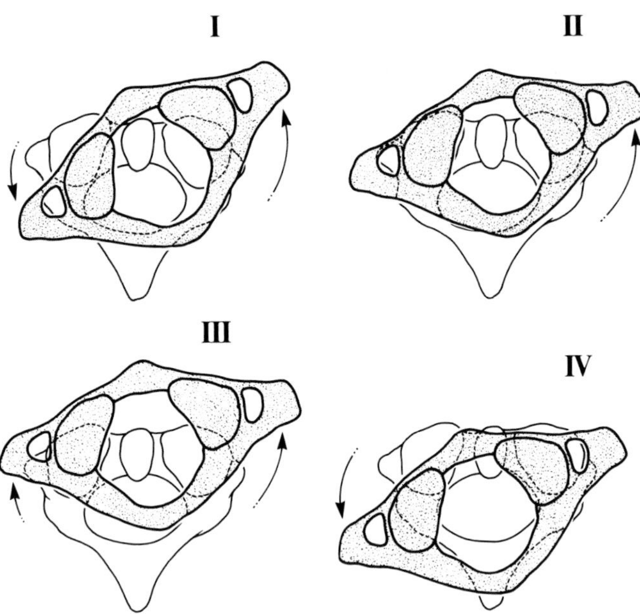

Figure 24.2. Fielding and colleagues' four types of atlantoaxial rotatory dislocations.

ciencies in the dens, allowing one or both lateral masses to sublux posteriorly.

Patients complain of neck pain; the chin is rotated toward one side and the head tilted in the opposite direction. This is the so-called "Cock-Robin" position described by Fielding and colleagues. The sternocleidomastoid muscle on the side to which the chin is rotated frequently is in spasm, suggesting an attempt at reduction (4, 5). Rotation is restricted in both directions and causes pain. Neurologic deficits are uncommon (4, 5), but when present should prompt close investigation of the remainder of the cervical spine.

The rotatory deformity can be demonstrated on a plain anteroposterior through-the-mouth odontoid view. Normal rotation of the atlas on the axis results in several typical changes. The lateral mass of the atlas on the side opposite the direction of the head rotation is closer to the odontoid process, is broader, and has a widened joint space. Conversely, the lateral mass on the side of rotation appears less broad, and its joint space is narrowed.

The diagnosis, however, is dependent on dynamic studies in which the relationships remain unchanged despite rotation to the normal position (2). Lateral films should be scrutinized closely to determine presence and extent of anterior atlantoaxial subluxation by measuring the predental space. More recently, computed tomography (CT) has also proved to be useful in diagnosis. Patients are scanned as they present, i.e., with their heads in the "Cock-Robin" position. Subsequent scans are obtained with the head turned maximally contralaterally. Again, persistence of the deformity is diagnostic of this abnormality (6). In contrast, dynamic studies with either plain films or CT of patients with benign torticollis will demonstrate partial or full resolution of the rotational deformity.

These subluxations may be present, particularly in children, after a mild upper respiratory tract infection, or after relatively minor trauma. Coutts suggested that there were synovial fringes that prevented the reduction of the deformity (3). Others have proposed joint effusions or incompetence of the alar ligaments as etiologic agents. However, studies have shown that simple incompetence of ligaments does not explain persistence of the deformity (2). Furthermore, no definitive pathologic studies have been undertaken to support these theories. Thus, the exact pathogenesis of atlantoaxial rotatory subluxation remains obscure.

For type I injuries, patients should undergo axial traction for a period of approximately 2 weeks. The likelihood of reduction seems to be related to the latency between onset and treatment (5). When significant facial trauma is not involved, halter traction will suffice; otherwise, tong traction is indicated. If these fail to reduce the subluxation, wire and bone fusion of C1–2 should be undertaken. When ligamentous instability is present, the subluxation should be stabilized initially by axial traction, followed by surgical fusion.

JEFFERSON'S FRACTURES

In 1920, Geoffrey Jefferson reviewed 42 fractures of the atlas, to which he added four from his experience (7). In this article, Jefferson described the pertinent anatomy, proposed mechanisms of injury, discussed associated injuries, and suggested treatment strategies for these fractures. Since that time, all atlas fractures have come to bear his name. This discussion will concentrate on the so-called "burst" fracture of the atlas.

Anatomically, several points are important in an understanding of atlas fractures. The atlas consists of an anterior and posterior arch and two lateral masses. The anterior arch is shorter, broader, and stronger than the posterior arch, which has grooves on either side through which the vertebral arteries pass. Structurally, these grooves are the weakest point in the ring. Each lateral mass has a superior and an inferior articular facet. The superior facets, facing superiorly and medially, articulate with the occipital condyles; the inferior facets, facing inferiorly and medially, articulate with the superior facets of the axis. The transverse ligament, as pointed out in the previous section, passes between the medial aspects of the lateral masses, articulating with the odontoid process anteriorly and securing it in place against the anterior arch.

Jefferson surmised that with axial loading injuries, the atlas is subjected to two forces; these pass through it in opposite directions and on divergent lines. The sum of the force vectors results in laterally directed forces (7). Thus, when a force is applied to the vertex of the skull, the atlas

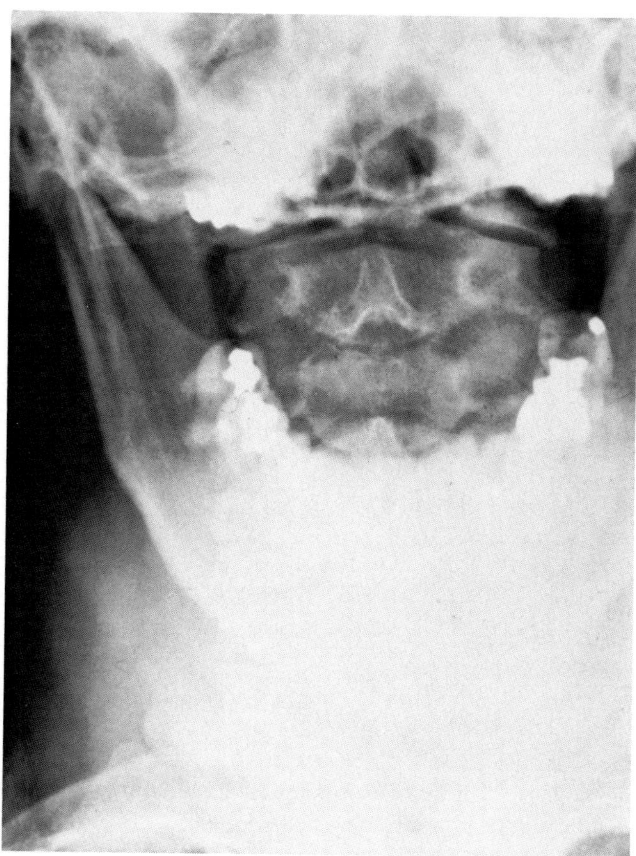

Figure 24.3. Through-the-mouth odontoid view demonstrating a Jefferson's fracture.

experiences horizontal forces which, if great enough, result in fracture of the arches at one or more points.

Atlantal fractures represent 2% to 13% of all cervical spine fractures. Falls and automobile accidents account for the vast majority of the atlantal fractures (8). Other associated injuries include closed head injury, scalp lacerations, and additional cervical spine fractures, most commonly, fractures of the axis. Conscious patients complain of neck pain and have limited range of motion in the cervical spine. Neurologic deficits are uncommon.

The diagnosis of a burst fracture usually is easily made on the basis of routine cervical spine films. The through-the-mouth odontoid view demonstrates lateral displacement of the lateral masses of the atlas with respect to the axis (Fig. 24.3). Lateral films frequently show no bony abnormality but may demonstrate prevertebral soft tissue swelling. No further diagnostic studies are needed to evaluate isolated fractures, although axial CT or tomograms may more clearly define the anatomy of the fractures.

Through the years, a variety of therapeutic regimens have been employed. Prolonged bedrest with or without cervical traction gave way to earlier mobilization with the fracture in an external fixation device, most notably the halo (7, 9, 10). More recently, more conservative management has been advocated (11). Hadley et al. recommend a Philadelphia collar for isolated Jefferson's fractures when the spread of the lateral mass is less than 6.9 mm and halo external immobilization when that spread exceeds 6.9 mm. The distinction is made on the basis of cadaveric studies which demonstrated that if spread of the lateral masses of the atlas with respect to the axis exceeded 6.9 mm, there was a significant incidence of transverse ligament rupture, thereby implying atlantoaxial instability (12).

A recent review of records at our institution revealed ten patients with isolated fractures of the atlas. All were treated with a Philadelphia collar for an average of 3 months, regardless of the degree of lateral mass displacement. Follow-up x-rays, including flexion and extension views, demonstrated good healing without evidence of instability in any case. No patients developed delayed neurologic complications, and the only complaints were intermittent neck pain and some limited range of motion. We therefore recommend conservative management of all isolated atlas fractures, using the Philadelphia collar with close clinical follow-up.

Hangman's Fractures

The term, hangman's fracture, refers to bilateral fracture through the posterior arch of the axis; the term, traumatic spondylolisthesis of the axis, has also been used. Wood-Jones, in 1913, published a classic article entitled "The Ideal Lesion Produced by Judicial Hanging," in which he discussed the results of subaural (angle of the mandible) and submental knots (13). Wood-Jones concluded that the submental knot produced a fracture dislocation of the neural arch of the axis with transection of the spinal cord. In 1965, Schneider noted the similarity of these fractures to eight that had resulted from motor vehicle accidents (14). It was he who termed these injuries hangman's fractures.

The anatomy of the axis is distinct from that of the other cervical vertebrae, and the axis serves as a transition between the more mobile occipito-atlantoaxial complex, or cervicocranium, and the relatively rigid remainder of the cervical spine. The superior facets of the axis are located in the same vertical plane as the body of the axis and the odontoid. The inferior facets are located posteriorly, in line with the facets of the remainder of the cervical spine (15). The narrow isthmus between superior and inferior facets, or pars interarticularis, represents a point of structural weakness in the neural arch, a point vulnerable to injury. This weakness may be accentuated by the juxtaposed foramen transversarium (15).

There are two basic mechanisms by which hangman's fractures occur, hyperextension/distraction and hyperextension/compression. Distraction is thought to be a more violent injury than compression and one that is more likely to result in a catastrophic neurologic event (16). Hyperextension distraction, which was originally described by Wood-Jones as causing the injury in association with punitive hangings, occasionally is seen today in the patient whose rapidly moving torso was restrained under the chin (17).

As for hyperextension/compression, because the superior and inferior facets do not lie in the same vertical plane, hyperextension coupled with axial loading results in a shearing force that acts on the axis and is maximal at the pars interarticularis, thereby causing it to fracture. Further hyperextension will result in rupture of the anterior longitudinal ligament, the first disc space, and, finally, the posterior longitudinal ligament (16). Following injury, the body of the axis is displaced anteriorly, thereby enlarging the spinal canal. This decompression, combined with a large spinal canal at this level of the vertebral column, is thought to account for the relatively low incidence of neurologic sequelae. It is hyperextension/compression that is responsible for the vast majority of today's hangman's fractures.

Several classification systems have been proposed; the one presented here is that of Effendi and colleagues (18). Type I refers to fractures of the ring of the axis with little or no displacement of the anterior fragment. Type II refers to fractures in which the anterior fragment is displaced. Type III fractures are those in which the anterior fragment is in a flexed position and the facets at C2–3 are locked. This type is believed to be the result of a primary flexion, which locks the facets, followed by extension, which causes the characteristic arch fracture. Type III fractures were by far the least common in the series of Effendi et al. Flexion and extension x-rays should be obtained in all patients to determine the degree of subluxation.

The incidence of these fractures ranges from 2% to 25% of all cervical spine fractures (19, 20). All age groups are affected, but the late teens and early twenties are the ages in which they most commonly occur. Automobile accidents account for the vast majority of hangman's fractures, and multiple trauma is common. Other cervical spine injuries are common, with Jefferson's fractures accounting for the greatest number of these.

Large series of hangman's fractures indicate a low incidence of neurologic deficits. Those that do occur are almost always transient. However, there is a sentiment shared by some that these fractures may result in a higher incidence of neurologic deficits. Bucholz found that 38 of 170 fatalities resulting from automobile accidents were associated with cervical spine injuries, of which eight were hangman's fractures, second only in incidence to atlanto-occipital dislocations (21). Autopsy performed in six of the eight patients with hangman's fractures showed three to have complete spinal cord transections. This finding implies that neurologic deficits are relatively common but are incompatible with survival.

The diagnosis of hangman's fractures routinely can be made on the basis of the lateral plain film (Fig. 24.4). The fractures are difficult to see on anteroposterior views. CT or tomography is seldom necessary and should be reserved for those instances in which the diagnosis is uncertain on the basis of the plain films.

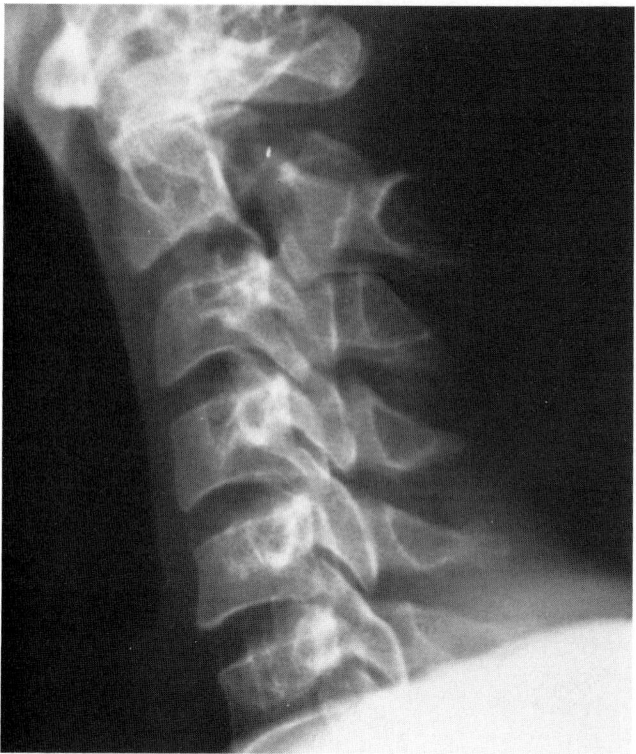

Figure 24.4. Lateral x-ray demonstrating a hangman's fracture.

As with Jefferson's fractures, the treatment of hangman's fractures has grown more conservative over the years. A recent study at our institution examined our experience with these fractures over a 10-year period (22). We found that satisfactory healing occurred regardless of the type of treatment used, which had included soft collar, Philadelphia collar, four-poster brace, and halo. Subluxation up to 6 mm did not affect healing, and none of these fractures were unstable on follow-up flexion and extension films. Of the 38 patients examined, 29 (76%) returned to their previous functional level, and none were disabled as a result of their hangman's fracture. It is our recommendation that all high cervical fractures with subluxation up to 6 mm should be treated with Philadelphia collar and early mobilization. Where C2–3 subluxation is greater than 6 mm, halo external immobilization should be used.

ODONTOID FRACTURES

Odontoid fractures were first described at the beginning of this century and today account for a major category of trauma to the cervical spine. These fractures can be difficult to diagnose, particularly when the index of suspicion is low, and treatment remains controversial.

The odontoid process projects superiorly from the body of the axis; its relationship to the transverse ligament and atlas is described in the section on atlantoaxial rotatory subluxations. The embryologic derivation of the odontoid process is complex. The base of odontoid is derived from the first cervical sclerotome together with the body of the atlas. The base migrates caudally to fuse with the body of the axis, which is derived from the second cervical sclerotome. However, the tip of the odontoid arises from the fourth occipital sclerotome with the rim of the foramen magnum, including the occipital condyles, and migrates caudally to fuse with the superior aspect of the base of the odontoid (23).

The blood supply of the odontoid is relatively constant. Paired anterior and posterior ascending arteries arise from the vertebral arteries of the foramina between the second and third vertebrae, course superiorly close to the odontoid, and form an apical arcade in the region of the alar ligaments. Cleft perforators arising from the internal carotid arteries anastomose with this network of vessels inferior to the apical arcade (24). The peculiar anatomy of this blood supply is thought to have an impact on the natural history of the different fracture types, as will be discussed shortly.

In 1974, Anderson and D'Alonzo proposed the classification system for odontoid fractures that is in use today (25) (Fig. 24.5). A type I fracture is an oblique fracture through the upper part of the odontoid, which Anderson and D'Alonzo considered to be an avulsion fracture at the point of attachment of the alar ligaments. Type II is a horizontal fracture of the junction of the odontoid process and the body of the axis. In type III, the fracture line extends into the body of the axis. Some have suggested that type III fractures occur at the embryologic fusion of the base of the odontoid process and the body of the axis (26).

In a laboratory investigation, Mouradian et al. were able to produce odontoid fractures by forward and lateral loading (27). The forward loading tended to produce type III fractures, and it was proposed that these resulted from forces exerted by the alar, apical, and posterior longitudinal ligaments acting in concert. These fractures were frequently associated with rupture of the transverse ligament. With lateral loading, type II fractures were typical. With these fractures, Mouradian et al. surmised that the lateral mass of the atlas acted as a "bony hammer," striking the odontoid process and shearing it at its base. On the basis of their clinical experience, they proposed rotational injuries as an alternate mechanism (27). Others have suggested that pure hyperextension may cause odontoid fractures. It seems, then, that the relatively liberal translation and rotation afforded by the atlantoaxial joint results in tremendous forces bearing on the odontoid process at the extremes of motion. In type II and type III fractures, the odontoid process may sublux in conjunction with the atlas and occiput, resulting in damage to the upper cervical cord.

Odontoid fractures may account for up to 14% of all cervical spine fractures (27). Patients frequently complain of severe neck pain, which may be referred to the occipital region, and they may hold their heads with their hands to prevent any motion that accentuates their pain. However, in some instances, particularly when there is no displacement of the fracture, clinical signs and symptoms are few. The most frequent neurologic complication is damage to the greater occipital nerve with consequent occipital pain (26). Most deficits, however, are mild and resolve completely in time (25). In Bucholz's autopsy series of automobile fatalities with cervical spine fractures, odontoid fractures represented the third most common lesion, following atlanto-occipital dislocations and hangman's fractures, thereby implying that severe neurologic complications may be more frequent than suspected (21).

The diagnosis of odontoid fractures can usually be made on the basis of lateral and anteroposterior through-the-mouth plain films. However, if there is no displacement, the fracture line may be difficult to demonstrate. We routinely obtain either tomograms or thin section CT scans with reconstruction on any patients in whom we suspect an odontoid fracture. These studies determine the presence and type of fracture involved, and this determination will impact significantly on both prognosis and treatment (Fig. 25.6).

In terms of treatment, we have no experience with type I fractures and question their existence. We treat type III fractures with a halo for a period of approximately 3 months after initial stabilization and reduction in tong traction.

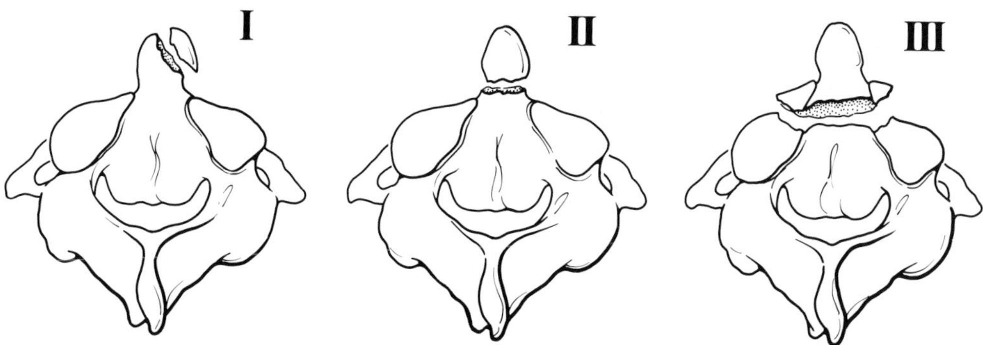

Figure 24.5. Anderson and D'Alonzo's three types of odontoid fractures.

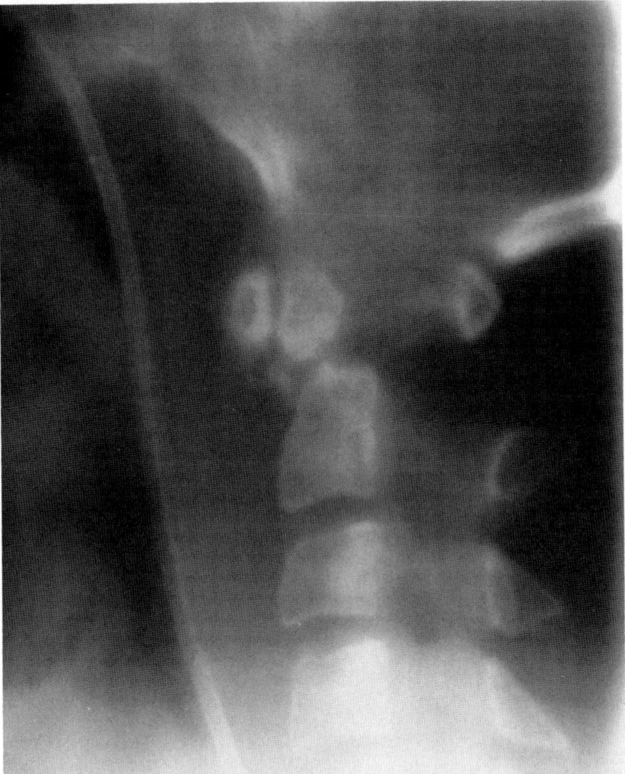

Figure 24.6. Lateral tomogram demonstrating type II odontoid fracture.

Several large series have demonstrated excellent fusion rates using the halo (19, 28–31), and this has been our experience as well. The controversy in treatment of odontoid fractures concerns the type II fractures. Various authors have reported the incidence of nonunion to be as low as 4.8% and as high as 100%. It has been suggested that a fracture at the base of the odontoid disrupts the arterial supply passing superiorly and contributes to its propensity toward nonunion (32). Several authors have attempted to identify which subpopulations tend not to heal, and age of the patient and/or degree of subluxation have been suggested as correlating with nonunion (30, 31, 33). Some groups favor early mobilization in a halo device, with surgery being reserved for those who fail to fuse (33). Others operate early on those considered at high risk for nonunion and treat the remainder with a halo (31). Surgery typically involves wire and bone fusion with halo application for a period of several months. We treat all type II fractures with C1–3 wire and acrylic internal cervical fixation after initial stabilization and reduction with tong traction. Our rates of fusion have been excellent, and this rigid internal construct allows early mobilization while avoiding the need for external fixation with the halo.

REFERENCES

1. Corner ES. Rotary dislocations of the atlas. Ann Surg 1907;45:9–26.

2. Wortzman G, Dewar FP. Rotary fixation of the atlantoaxial joint: rotational atlantoaxial subluxation. Radiology 1968;90:479–487.

3. Coutts MB. Atlanto-epistropheal subluxations. Arch Surg 1934;29:297–311.

4. Fielding JW, Hawkins RJ, Hensinger RN, Francis WR. Atlantoaxial rotary deformities. Orthop Clin North Am 1978;9:955–967.

5. Phillips WA, Hensinger RN. The management of rotatory atlantoaxial subluxation in children. J Bone Joint Surg 1989;71A:664–668.

6. Kowalski HM, Cohen WA, Cooper P, Wisoff JH. Pitfalls in the CT diagnosis of atlantoaxial rotary subluxation. Am J Roentgenol 1987;149:595–600.

7. Jefferson G. Fracture of the atlas vertebra: report of four cases, and a review of those previously reported. Br J Surg 1920;7:407–422.

8. Sherk HH, Nicholson JT. Fractures of the atlas. J Bone Joint Surg 1970;52A:1017–1024.

9. Zimmerman E, Grant J, Vise WM, Yashon D, Hunt WE. Treatment of Jefferson fracture with a halo apparatus. J Neurosurg 1976;44:372–375.

10. Schlicke LH, Callahan RA. A rational approach to burst fractures of the atlas. Clin Orthop 1981;154:18–21.

11. Hadley MN, Dickman CA, Browner CM, Sonntag VKH. Acute traumatic atlas fractures: management and long term outcome. Neurosurgery 1988;23:31–35.

12. Spence KF Jr, Decker S, Sell KW. Bursting atlantal fracture associated with rupture of the transverse ligament. J Bone Joint Surg 1970;52A:543–549.

13. Wood-Jones F. The ideal lesion produced by judicial hanging. Lancet 1913;1:53.

14. Schneider RC, Livingston KE, Cave AJE, Hamilton G. "Hangman's fracture" of the cervical spine. J Neurosurg 1965;22:141–154.

15. Brashear HR Jr, Venters GC, Preston ET. Fracture of the neural arch of the axis. A report of twenty-nine cases. J Bone Joint Surg 1975;57A:879–887.

16. Francis WR, Fielding JW, Hawkins RJ, Pepin J, Hensinger R. Traumatic spondylolisthesis of the axis. J Bone Joint Surg 1981; 63B:313–318.

17. Williams TG. Hangman's fracture. J Bone Joint Surg 1975;57B:82–88.

18. Effendi B, Roy D, Cornish B, Dussault RG, Laurin CA. Fractures of the ring of the axis. A classification based on the analyses of 131 cases. J Bone Joint Surg 1981;63B:319–327.

19. Hadley MN, Browner C, Sonntag VKH. Axis fractures: a comprehensive review of management and treatment in 107 cases. Neurosurgery 1985;17:281–290.

20. Chan RC, Schweigel JF, Thompson GB. Halo-thoracic brace immobilization in 188 patients with acute cervical spine injuries. J Neurosurg 1983;58:508–515.

21. Bucholz RW. Unstable hangman's fractures. Clin Orthop 1981;154:119–124.

22. Lee KS, Kelly DL Jr, Alexander E JR, Davis CH Jr, McWhorter JM. Satisfactory treatment of hangman's fractures without the halo apparatus [Abstract]. Neurosurgery 1987;21:120–121.

23. Greenberg AD. Atlanto-axial dislocations. Brain 1968;91:655–684.

24. Schiff DC, Parke WW. The arterial supply of the odontoid process. J Bone Joint Surg 1973;55A:1450–1456.

25. Anderson LD, D'Alonzo RT. Fractures of the odontoid process of the axis. J Bone Joint Surg 1974;56A:1663–1674.

26. Blockey NJ, Purser DW. Fractures of the odontoid process of the axis. J Bone Joint Surg 1956;38B:794–817.

27. Mouradian WH, Fietti VG Jr, Cochran GVB, Fielding JW, Young J. Fractures of the odontoid: a laboratory and clinical study of mechanisms. Orthop Clin North Am 1978;9(4):985–1001.

28. Maiman DJ, Larson SJ. Management of odontoid fractures. Neurosurgery 1982;11:471–476.

29. Dunn ME, Seljeskog EL. Experience in the management of odon-

toid process injuries: an analysis of 128 cases. Neurosurgery 1986;18:306–310.

30. Hadley MN, Sonntag V. Acute axis fractures. Contemp Neurosurg 1987;9:2.

31. Hensinger RN, Fielding JW, Hawkins RH. Congenital anomalies of the odontoid process. Orthop Clin North Am 1978;9(4):901–912.

32. Apuzzo ML, Heiden JS, Weiss MH, Ackerson TT, Harvey JP, Kurze T. Acute fractures of the odontoid process. An analysis of 45 cases. J Neurosurg 1978;48:85–91.

33. Ekong CEU, Schwartz ML, Tator CH, Rowed DW, Edmonds VE. Odontoid fracture: management with early mobilization using the halo device. Neurosurgery 1981;9:631–637.

25

Facet Injuries in the Cervical Spine

Alan M. Levine

Facet injuries involving the lower cervical spine form a diverse group of pathologic entities. As a result of their unique anatomic configuration, the nature of the injury and instability can cause a wide variation in patterns of both symptomatology and radiologic findings. In order to fully understand and appreciate this diverse and unique group of injuries and to rationally apply treatment modalities to them, it is important to fully understand the anatomic configuration of this area as well as the mechanisms of injury for the various fracture patterns.

These patterns of cervical facet injuries occur with varying frequency at six different levels from the junction of the upper cervical spine with the lower cervical spine at C2–3 to the junction of the lower cervical spine with the thoracic spine at C7–T1. In spite of the fact that the C2 vertebra has markedly different anatomic configuration from those caudal to it, the position and orientation of the inferior C2 facet joint is similar to the remainder of the lower cervical spine. The joints cephalad to C2–3 are anterior and have a completely different configuration than the joints of the lower cervical spine. The lower cervical facets are inclined at an angle of approximately 45° to the horizontal. In the upper segments at C2, C3, C4, and C5 they are canted slightly inward, whereas in the lower segments they are tipped slightly laterally. They are usually slightly elliptical in shape with the actual joint surface measuring slightly less than 1 cm in the vertical direction and slightly greater than 1 cm in the medial lateral direction. The facet joint forms the posterior border of the neural foramen with the anterior medial border of the foramen formed by the joint of Lushka. In close relationship to the facet is the vertebral artery, the location of which is critically important for certain types of posterior cervical fixation for facet joint injuries. Although the artery is anteromedial to the facet joints and not visualized from a posterior approach, the posterior boney landmarks give a good approximation of its location. At the junction of the medial edge of the facet and the lateral edge of the lamina is a slight vertical depression. Directly anterior to that depression lies the pedicle and then the vertebral foramen. The actual configuration of the posterior surface of the inferior facet is a dome shape. These are in fact diarthrodial joints with usual synovial membranes and fibrous capsules. The joint capsules are more lax than in other areas of the spine, thus permitting the wide range of motion which will be discussed. Both the multifidus and the short and long rotators of the neck muscles originate from the posterior tubercles of the transverse processes in the lower cervical spine. These muscles insert upon the spinous processes, and thus with surgical approaches to this area these muscles must be carefully dissected laterally in order to observe the entire width of the facet joint.

The lower cervical spine has a considerable range of motion in six different planes. These include flexion, extension, distraction, compression, lateral bending, and rotation. There are variations in the degrees of motion. The upper cervical facet joints have less flexion-extension than the middle range joints at C4–5 and C5–6 and roughly similar to the lower cervical facet joints. The upper spine (C2–3, C3–4) averages approximately 12°, whereas the most mobile segments (C4–5, C5–6) average 20° decreasing to 12–15° in the lower portion of the cervical spine (C6–7). Lateral bending averages approximately 6–7° throughout the entire cervical spine, and rotation ranges from 0–10°. There is noted to be, however, an inverse relationship between age of the individual and range of motion in the lower cervical spine, with motion decreasing as the age increases. It is measured by the stretch test of White and Panjabi (47); the maximum distraction is approximately 1.7 mm. Horizontal displacement similarly has an upper limit of approximately 3.5 mm. As described by Lysell (19) there is also coupled motion so that an amount of axial rotation is coupled with lateral bending at various levels in the spine. In the second cervical vertebra there are 2° of coupled rotation for every 3° of lateral bending; however, at C7 there is only 1° of rotation for every 7.5° of lateral bending. This gradual decrease in the amount of rotation associated with the lateral bending may be related to changes in the inclination of the facet joints as previously described. The increased compliance to rotation with lateral bending may account for the fact that in the upper portion of the cervical spine (C2–3, C3–4), unilateral facet fractures and dislocations are less common, whereas in the lower cervical spine they are somewhat more common.

The resistance to exceeding the extremes of motion is a combination of the bony architecture as well as the soft tissue restraints. These restraints consist of the compliance of the disc as well as the anterior and posterior longitudinal ligaments. In addition, the facet capsules as well as supraspinous and interspinous ligaments contribute to the posterior ligamentous complex. Any injury which results in exceeding the normal range of motion, by definition, is associated with significant disruption of either the bony architecture or the ligamentous restraints.

HISTORICAL PERSPECTIVE

Although the gravity of cervical injury was recognized by the Greeks, the recognition of the phenomenon of unilateral and bilateral locked facets has been attributed to Malgaigne as early as 1855 (21). The history of the treatment of facet injuries is punctuated by two major interrelated themes, the recognition of the various types of injuries and the evolution and application of treatment modalities. These two themes were not advanced dramatically by any single event or individual but, rather, slowly with the addition of bits and pieces. However, the real controversy began in the 1930s with Bohler (5) advocating the use of manual traction and manipulation to reduce fractured dislocations of the cervical spine. This was similarly advocated by Crooks and Birket (9) but with the use of a general anesthetic. However, others such as Crutchfield advocated the use of tongs for continuous skeletal traction (10). Definitive treatment was prolonged traction until healing of both bony and ligamentous injuries could take place. Little thought initially was given to operative stabilization or rapid mobilization. In fact, these early studies did not clearly differentiate the various types of injuries. Bilateral facet dislocations were differentiated from the remainder of the injuries which generally included fractures of the posterior elements as well as fractures of the body in a variety of different combinations. Rogers in 1942 (25) was the first to advocate the use of operative intervention in these patients. As a result of complications with Crutchfield tongs, and patients with dislocations irreducible in traction, he suggested that open reduction and internal fixation with wire provided a reliable method of treatment of these injuries. The use of manipulation for reduction of these injuries became a less evident theme in the United States in the 1950s and 1960s. However, these techniques continued to be actively used in Europe. The majority of North American surgeons used continuous skeletal traction as the means of reduction, and the controversy continued as to whether traction and reduction were satisfactory or whether open operative stabilization was also indicated (12, 14). The major indication for surgical intervention during this period was neurologic involvement. The implications of nonoperative treatment for those patients without neurologic injury were not fully appreciated.

Radiologically the differentiation between facet subluxations and facet dislocations was quite clear and easily differentiated in the majority of studies. The differentiation between unilateral facet injuries and bilateral facet injuries both in terms of pathomechanics and radiologic differentiation was further elucidated by both Roaf (23) and Beatson (4). However the differentiation both in terms of the pathomechanics of injury and subsequent stability was not clear between unilateral facet fractures and dislocations as well as between bilateral facet fractures and dislocations. These differences would not become clearly evident until somewhat later. Rogers, in fact, in 1957 (26) was the first to realize the difference between unilateral facet fractures and dislocations. He suggested that dislocations could be adequately fixed with a wire loop and fused without loss of position. However patients in whom the superior articular facet was fractured would not maintain the reduction and therefore were fused in the unreduced position. Bilateral fracture dislocations were evidently so unusual that Rogers did not comment upon them. His bilateral facet dislocations or "anterior dislocations" did not have either inferior or superior facet fractures.

The earliest delineation of the various types of facet injuries and treatment tailored to the nature of the instability appears to be work done by Robert Judet and Raymond Roy-Camille in Garche in approximately 1970 (22, 28, 29). The technique of posterior cervical plating allowed reduction of deformities and maintenance of the reduction irrespective of the type of injury. However the injuries were in fact treated differently, with facet injuries requiring the use of a tile plate which essentially restored the stability compromised by the fractured articular facet whether it was the superior facet or inferior facet. With intact facets (dislocations and subluxations) the tile plate was not used and standard cervical spine plates were used. This treatment was advocated irrespective of the presence or absence of neurologic deficit. However, in the presence of neurologic deficit it allowed laminectomy and decompression when necessary.

A drive towards various types of operative treatment of facet injuries was more prominent in Europe than in North America during the 1970s. In the United States the controversy continued to smolder over the relative advantages of nonoperative treatment, and, in contradistinction from Europe, there was a less frequent role for operative stabilization. In North America concern was expressed over the various classifications of cervical spine injuries, and in fact in the mechanistic theories the cervical facet fractures and dislocations were lumped with compression fractures and tear drop fractures (17). The concern over the ability to achieve a closed reduction of facet injuries was expressed in a number of articles, with varying degrees of success with unilateral "dislocations"; no differentiation was made between unilateral facet fractures and unilateral facet dislocations. Without that differentiation, the discrepancy in the results cannot be clearly explained. It became evident that some unilateral injuries could be reduced with traction, whereas others required manipulation. The skill with manipulation and the various techniques were subsequently analyzed by Cotler et al. (8). They were successful at reducing approximately 70% of the true bilateral and unilateral facet *dislocations*. These were clearly defined as not having *any* facet fractures associated with them. Patients were treated nonoperatively. At a similar time, other approaches were being contemplated to deal with facet injuries including anterior reduction and plating (11) as well as methods of posterior stabilization aimed at counteracting the rotational deformity and instability associated with facet fractures. These techniques included the oblique wire (13), the Magerl hook plate (20), and the triple wire technique (30). It is only extremely recently that there has been a direct comparison of the operative and nonoperative results, demonstrating that in fact in patients treated nonoperatively there was a higher degree of persistent pain. Those patients treated operatively had substantially improved longterm results (27); in addition, there was a realization again that external immobilization including the halo (32) cannot maintain alignment and reduction, especially in unilateral facet fractures. Even in bilateral facet dislocations there is a certain amount of "snaking" or "toggling" which results in less than anatomic maintenance of position with these injuries.

CLASSIFICATION AND MECHANISMS OF INJURY OF FACET FRACTURES AND DISLOCATIONS

Classification of injuries to the facets can be divided into two patterns. The first is the mechanistic pattern of classification, and the second is the anatomic pattern of classification. Classifications of these injuries should be relatively simple to use and should be helpful to the physician in terms of treatment and prognosis. Unfortunately, the mechanistic classifications are indirect classifications resulting from the assessment of either the hypothetical or proven patterns of force applied to the spine resulting in the injury. In fact they may be useful since knowing the mechanism of injury can allow extrapolation in order to arrive at an estimation of the extent and type of instability. One of the earliest classifications of cervical spine injuries was that of Whitley and Forsyth (33) based predominantly on a radiographic interpretation of the direct and indirect forces applied to the spine: flexion, extension, rotation, and occasionally lateral bending. Braakman and Penning in 1968 subclassified flexion injuries (6) into both distractive flexion and compressive flexion. In the distractive hyperflexion group they placed unilateral facet dislocations as well as bilateral facet dislocations. They suggested that unilateral facet dislocations had in addition an element of rotation (3). Roaf (24), on the other hand, suggested that lateral flexion was the predominant mechanism in unilateral facet dislocations. Allen and Ferguson further subdivided the classification of all spinal injuries into multiple categories (1). Distractive flexion consisted of four stages. Stage 1 was a facet subluxation and flexion; stage 2 was a unilateral facet dislocation; stage 3 was a bilateral facet dislocation with approximately 50% vertebral displacement; and stage 4 was a grossly unstable spine or floating vertebra. Compressive extension stages 3 and 4 were felt to be hypothetical but could consist of fractures of the articular processes. In addition, lateral flexion involved asymmetric compression of the vertebral body with the possibility of ipsilateral disruption of the articular processes. Such a mechanistic theory becomes somewhat confusing as it is in fact part hypothetical modeling divided into many artificial subsegments. In addition, the mechanistic classification theory does not describe the resultant instability nor clearly delineate the structures that are insufficient.

On the other hand, a descriptive classification system as suggested by Roy-Camille et al. (29) as well as Harris (15, 16) gives a limited number of types of injuries which have clearly defined instability patterns. Although the actual mechanisms of injuries may still remain suppositional, the critical factor for the determination of treatment and prognosis is the resultant instability. The effective instability determines the requirements for stabilization. The simplest and most direct classification is a progressive descriptive branching pattern which easily adapts to an algorithm for treatment. The injuries should be divided into bilateral and unilateral facet injuries (18). The initial injury in the bilateral group is a subluxation. Facet subluxation involves a flexion injury resulting in partial disruption of the interspinous and supraspinous ligaments as well as "sprains" of the facet capsules. There are no clearly defined parameters for the endpoints for bilateral cervical sprains, although a segmental kyphosis with overriding of the facet joints is about as precise a definition as has been available. The next more severe injury is bilateral "perched" facets. It is clear that all of these injuries of subluxations through dislocations are part of a spectrum of increasing disruption of the posterior ligamentous complex. However, classically, the bilateral "perched" facets involve significant disruption of the interspinous ligament, supraspinous ligament, and facet capsules as the tip of the inferior facet comes to rest upon the tip of the superior facet of the level below. The final stage of this continuum of flexion and distraction injuries is the bilateral facet dislocation. These involve a significant flexion and distraction force resulting in complete disruption of the interspinous ligament, supraspinous ligament, facet capsule, and ligamentum flavum, essentially the entire posterior ligamentous complex. It also requires disruption of the disc to allow the 50% translation which is evident in the roentgenographic studies. The inferior facet of the level above locks anterior to the superior facet of the level below.

Bilateral facet fractures, on the other hand, do not standardly have the same degree of flexion and distraction as the dislocation. They tend to have slight flexion but with a greater shear component, and instead of completely disrupting the posterior ligamentous complex the facets of the level above slide slightly cephalad and then translate anteriorly, shearing off the superior facet of the level below. There is far less ligamentous disruption and more significant bony disruption. The final bilateral facet injury is one facet dislocation and one facet fracture. This is the rarest of the facet injuries and most probably results from a combination of flexion rotation and shearing. The exact mechanism is difficult to discern; however, more importantly, it clinically exhibits a complex instability. It has rotational instability on one side and ligamentous disruption and flexion instability on the other.

The initial three injuries (bilateral facet subluxation, "perched" facets, and dislocations) are all a result of flexion and distraction with varying degrees of disruption of the posterior ligamentous complex. Once fully reduced, their instability is a flexion instability from the disruption of the posterior ligamentous complex, which is the restraint to flexion. Depending on the degree of disruption, a varying degree of flexion instability will result. Thus, both surgical and nonsurgical intervention in these injuries should be aimed at a primary complete anatomic reduction followed by a mode of treatment which will prevent further flexion with recurrence of deformity and which will restore or substitute for the posterior ligamentous complex. Bilateral facet fractures, on the other hand, have little flexion deformity but have a high degree of shear instability. They may also have a bilateral rotational instability because of the lack of the bony buttress as a result of the fracture of the superior facets. The facets in this type of injury are rarely dislocated but simply shear off. The superior facet remains in contact with the inferior facet of the level above as it translates forward. Intervention in this case should be aimed at preventing recurrent translational deformity. Obviously, the combination of a unilateral facet fracture and unilateral facet dislocation gives a deformity with rotational instability on one side and flexion instability on the other. Any interventional modalities should be able to prevent recurrence of deformity to both portions of the injury.

Unilateral facet injuries form a very diverse group. Unilateral facet dislocations are comparable in terms of their degree of instability and compromise of restraints to the spectrum of bilateral facet dislocations. Here, however, the predominant force is that of flexion, distraction, and rotation. Varying degrees of disruption of one side of the posterior ligamentous complex result. Although theoretically unilateral subluxations and "perched" facets may occur, they are exceedingly infrequent and do not enter into most treatment schema. On the other hand, a unilateral facet dislocation is a complex and often perplexing injury which has proven difficult to treat. To occur, disruption of the entire facet ligamentous complex with partial disruption of the interspinous ligament, partial disruption of the ligamentum flavum, and, in fact, partial disruption of the posterolateral corner of the disc including the uncinate process or the joint of Luschka are required. Once fully reduced, the resultant instability is a coupled flexion and rotation instability. Since the bony buttress remains intact, counteracting any additional deformity can simply be done by restricting any subsequent flexion.

Unilateral facet fractures form a diverse and interesting group and can be divided into three different types. The most common type of facet fracture is the fracture of the superior facet occurring at approximately 80% of all unilateral facet fractures. This most probably is a flexion rotation injury with shearing-off of the superior facet of the lower level. The fragment will generally remain to some degree attached to the inferior facet at the level above but rotates into the neural foramen. There is usually minimal to moderate disruption of the interspinous ligament, however, the contralateral capsule remains intact. The disc is also partially disrupted, which is probably proportional to the degree of instability. Classically, on lateral roentgenogram these fractures demonstrate only about 4 mm of translation. The second most common type of unilateral facet injury is the fracture of the inferior facet of the level above. Instead of the inferior facet shearing-off the superior facet, in this case, as the body rotates forward a fracture lines propagates through the inferior facet generally at the level of the tip of the superior facet. These are purely rotational injuries with a minimal flexion component. There is minimal to moderate disruption of the interspinous ligament and moderate disruption of the facet capsule. The subsequent instability is generally purely rotational. The final type of injury is a fracture separation of the articular mass. The mechanism of this type of injury is not clearly defined; it may be a combination of an extension/rotation injury with disruption of the pedicle and a vertical fracture through the lamina just medial to the articular mass. This isolates and separates the entire articular mass from both the level above the injury and the level below, thus creating two segments of instability. Generally one segment of instability is more dominant, and the translation will be apparent at that level. Although if the other is unrecognized and untreated, subsequent instability will occur at that level as well. Unlike the remainder of these injuries, this clearly has two levels of instability. The tilting ("horizontalization") of the lateral mass is a radiologic finding for which the mechanism is not clearly understood.

RADIOGRAPHIC EVALUATION

The complete evaluation of facet fractures and dislocations may require a number of radiographic modalities. Most of these injuries can be differentiated on the basis of plain roentgenograms, although the final definition of fracture lines generally requires adjunctive studies. The lateral cervical spine roentgenogram can help to differentiate and define facet injuries. The majority of facet injuries will affect a single spinal level by causing varing degrees of kyphosis and translation. The kyphotic component is more prominent with the flexion type injuries than with the rotational injuries. The degree of either real or apparent translation which is visible on the roentgenograms is directly proportional to the amount of soft tissue disruption. The rotation can be visualized most effectively on the plain roentgenogram. Specifically, the lateral roentgenogram of a patient with either bilateral "perched" facets or bilateral facet dislocations will show significant kyphosis and 50% or greater translation of the vertebral body above over the level below. In addition little or no rotation will be evident on either the plain lateral roentgenogram nor on the AP roentgenogram. On the AP roentgenogram, however, there will be widening of the distance between the spinous processes at the affected level. Bilateral facet fractures will tend to have the same degree of translation as bilateral facet dislocations but less kyphosis. The interlocking of the facets often seen on bilateral facet dislocations will not be present, although the facets may well be obscured and not clearly visualized on either lateral or AP roentgenograms.

Unilateral facet dislocations and fractures are difficult to differentiate among themselves, although they are usually relatively easily differentiated from bilateral facet problems. The hallmark of the unilateral facet fracture dislocation or fracture separation of the articular mass is the rotational component. In these injuries a lateral roentgenogram will demonstrate both edges of the biconcave surface of the posterior aspect of the vertebral body either above or below the level of the injury and a pure lateral view on the opposite side of the injury. In addition, an AP roentgenogram will frequently visualize an offset in the spinous processes, thus again demonstrating the rotational component of the injury. For some injuries, a pillar view may help to clarify the facet pathology. The pillar view is also helpful in differentiating superior facet fractures from inferior facet fractures and occasionally for definitively making the diagnosis of a fracture separation of the articular mass. In that particular injury the entire lateral mass is horizontalized, a feature not present in other types of injuries.

Final delineation of the nature of the injury can be done with one of two modalities. Since most facet fractures are in the coronal plane which parallels the cuts of a CT scan, the resolution of the fracture is dependent on a reformatted reconstruction. If there is any registration offset in various cuts, the diagnosis can be difficult. A set of lateral tomograms, although requiring the patient to be placed in the lateral position, is the most reproducible way to differentiate the various types of facet fractures and dislocations. Interestingly, an additional subtle diagnostic test is the use of skeletal traction. In unilateral facet injuries, if the translational/rotational deformity easily reduces with a small amount of traction (less than 20 pounds) the fracture is most frequently a unilateral facet fracture. Unilateral facet dislocations will not reduce with traction alone and require manipulation; thus, irrespective of the weight added, they remain rotationally displaced. We strongly recommend the use of tomography to make the differentiation of the site of fracture. The only pattern more easily seen on CAT scan is the fracture separation of the articular mass, since in that pattern the fracture lines are perpendicular to the coronal cuts of the CT scan and are thus well seen. The final imaging modality for which MRI scanning is most helpful is not the definition of the boney injury but, rather, in cases of neurologic injury. The degree of disc disruption varies with these types of injuries. The use of an MRI in cases of neurologic deficit or increasing neurologic deficit may define a large herniated disc requiring separate operative intervention. The use of MRI for routine imaging of facet injuries, however, is clearly not indicated at this time, as it does not give a high resolution of the bone detail. The goal of imaging facet injuries is to determine the exact anatomic type of injury and thus secondarily, once the type of injury is defined, to find the resultant instability. Treatment of these injuries is dependent on counteracting the resultant instability.

NEUROLOGIC INJURY

The occurrence and severity of neurologic injury with unilateral and bilateral facet injuries is in part the result of the initial size of the neural canal and the degree of translation experienced at the time of injury. The early studies of facet injuries and their treatment concentrated predominantly on those patients with neurologic injury, and therefore a representation of the total number of patients and the degree of neurologic injuries associated with each type of injury were really unclear (9, 10, 12). More recent studies have given a clearer indication of the spectrum and the occurrence of neurologic injury. In one of the larger series of facet fractures and dislocations reported, Roy-Camille found that 24% of the patients with unilateral facet dislocations had cord symptomatology and 68% had radicular symptomatology, for a total of 92% having some neurologic injury (29). Of the patients with bilateral facet dislocation there was a higher rate of cord symptomatology (41%) and a lower rate of radicular symptomatology (32%). In the patients with unilateral facet fractures 66% had radicular symptomatology and none had central neurologic symptoms. In fracture separations of the articular mass approximately 48% of patients had radicular symptomatology and 16% had cord symptoms in varying degrees. Cotler demonstrated that 9 of 13 patients with bilateral dislocations had complete injuries, whereas with the unilateral facet injuries 7 of 11 patients had some neurologic deficit (8). In Roraback's series, of 26 patients, all with unilateral injuries, 11 had root injuries and 3 had central injuries (27). Finally, Braakman and Vinken, in a series of unilateral injuries, had 8 of 37 with root injuries and 12 of 37 with some type of cord injury (7). Of the bilateral facet dislocations there were only 4 of 35 with root lesions and 28 of 35 with cord lesions (18 being complete cord lesions).

Thus the degree and type of neurologic deficit is very strongly related to the type of injury. Approximately 50% of patients with bilateral facet dislocations and bilateral facet fractures with a high degree of translation (greater than 50%) will have either complete neurologic deficits or a partial cord syndrome (some of which may be recoverable). Unilateral facet injuries, on the other hand, are in part related to the degree and type of instability. Although the unilateral facet dislocation and fracture appear to have the same degree of rotational/translational malalignment (approximately 4 mm), the unilateral facet dislocation requires more disruption of the ligamentous structure and a greater degree of deformity of the spine than the fracture. The amount of kyphosis necessary to achieve a dislocation and the disruption of the posterior corner of the disc results in a higher degree of cord symptoms than in patients with unilateral facet fractures. Facet fractures, on the other hand, will frequently have radicular symptoms as a result of the closure of the neural foramen on the affected side. The patients with unilateral facet fractures will predominantly have radicular compression and rarely have cord syndromes. The majority of the radicular symptoms are incomplete and vary anywhere from dysesthesias to motor and sensory loss.

TREATMENT

Although there have been a variety of opinions about the optimal treatment for injuries of the facets, establishment of a consistent treatment pattern is now possible. The goals of treatment should be a primary consideration in deciding on the treatment modality. Those specific goals are to reduce the deformity, restore a stable spine and, finally, achieve neural decompression when necessary. In order to achieve those goals, a clear understanding of the mechanism of injury, the extent of disruption of soft tissue and boney structures, and the resultant deformity is critical for achieving the goals with the least morbidity.

Therefore, for subluxations of the lower cervical facets, the force which has caused the injury is generally flexion and distraction with partial disruption of the interspinous ligament, supraspinous ligament, and facet capsules. Occasionally there will be some stretching of the ligamentum of flavum and posterior aspect of the disc. Achieving a reduction is generally reasonably straightforward and can be done with hyperextension of the cervical spine. In some patients with very minimal disruption of the posterior ligamentous complex holding the patient in hyperextension for approximately 6–12 weeks will allow sufficient healing to reestablish a stable cervical spine. However, in other patients with more severe disruption or in whom nonoperative treatment has failed, operative treatment is necessary. Since those patients have disruption of the posterior ligamentous complex, the construct to reestablish that intergerity requires a single level arthrodesis performed with any of a variety of techniques including Rogers' wiring or posterior cervical plating, etc. The goal should be to restore spinal stability and maintain alignment, but care must be taken to confine both the dissection and the fusion to only the single involved level.

The next entity in this progression is the bilateral "perched" facets. Again in this case, a flexion and distraction injury has occurred which has resulted in an impingement of the tip of the inferior facet and the tip of the superior facet with complete disruption of the facet capsules, interspinous ligament, and ligamentum flavum. However both these patients and those with subluxation rarely have significant neurologic deficit. However, the patients with "perched" facets will frequently require skeletal traction with Gardner Wells tongs to sufficiently unlock facets before achieving hyperextension for total reduction. The patients should be placed supine with a direct longitudinal pull of approximately 10–15 pounds to begin the reduction followed by carefully monitored increasing weight until the facets are visibly unlocked. Then, with slight extension of the neck and decrease in the amount of weight, the reduction should be easily completed. Although there is controversy concerning the rate of spontaneous arthrodesis after facet injuries, it is probably reasonable to consider primary single level fusion in these cases. The morbidity of a acute single level fusion followed by immobilization in an external orthoses is generally acceptable. It allows restoration of both anatomic alignment, thus preventing resubluxation and will reestablish a stable spinal segment, as generally healing of the posterior ligamentous complex is incomplete in injuries where a significant amount of soft tissue disruption has occurred.

The remainder of the facet injuries are generally somewhat more severe and require two phases to their treatment. The first is the acute phase, and the second is the definitive treatment. It is of note that more bilateral facet injuries will present acutely, in part, because a significant level of neurologic involvement occurs with those than with unilateral facet injuries. Unilateral facet injuries in a number of series have been documented to present secondarily (7, 28) after the patient has had persistent neck pain or development of late radiculopathy. Since the majority of symptoms with unilateral facet injuries are radicular, these may be missed early on, thus accounting for the late pickup. In addition, the accidents resulting in bilateral facet injuries are often more dramatic than those resulting in unilateral injuries, thus evoking a heightened sense of suspicion. Therefore the immediate treatment upon discovery of these bilateral facet injuries varies depending on whether the injury is seen acutely, the degree of initial displacement, and the presence or absence of neurologic deficit. All patients who present acutely with neurologic deficit or with significant displacement on the lateral roentgenogram (5 mm or greater) should have immediate skeletal traction applied as soon as the patient is taken off the emergency immobilization on which he arrived. The lateral roentgenogram should always be taken prior to this treatment decision, and thus the basic type of injury (burst versus facet injury) is evident. A more specific initial impression allows "fine tuning" of the initial phase of treatment. For the majority of the facet injuries, postoperative immobilization in a halo-vest will be unnecessary. Therefore in the acute trauma phase the use of Gardner Wells tongs for traction in the majority of these injuries will be optimal. This device allows immediate external immobilization as well as application of traction. It is easy to apply, and since the desired period of immobilization will be short (less than 10 days), it is applicable to these injuries. After immediate immobilization and prior to the definitive studies for these patients, approximately 10 pounds of weight should be added to the spine. A second lateral roentgenogram is taken immediately to ascertain that a pure distraction injury has not occurred and to rule-out that a small amount of weight has caused pathologic distraction of the spine. If the spine appears to be reducing with a small amount of weight, a slightly greater amount (in 5-pound increments) can be added. In those patients with neurologic deficit rapid achievement of reduction is a reasonable goal. For bilateral facet dislocations, weight should be added in 5-pound increments until the tips of the facets are unlocked. In a light patient (<120 lbs.) this may require placing the Stryker frame or bed in reverse Trendelenburg so that the patient is not drawn up the bed with further application of weight. Generally no more than 50 pounds of weight are required for any reduction, if the weight is appropriately applied and the patient adequately positioned in bed. Once the tips of the facets are unlocked, slight extension of the neck is applied by placing a towel roll underneath the neck. The weight is decreased, thus maintaining the reduction.

For unilateral facet injuries the application of initial traction is important to help resolve the dilemma of whether it is a facet fracture or dislocation. Generally unilateral *fractures* with application of small amounts of weight (less than 20 pounds) will generally achieve essentially complete reduction of the deformity without any manipulation. Care should be taken that the weight is not applied in flexion but is applied in slight extension by positioning of the weights with reference to the head. There are some exceptions. However, acute unilateral facet *dislocations* will generally not reduce with any amount of weight. If no reduction has occurred by the time that 40–50 pounds of weight have been applied, no further weight should be applied. At this point all injuries should be sent for secondary evaluation to determine the exact nature of the injury by use of tomography and or CT and or MRI.

The immediate immobilization of facet injuries discovered late (greater than 1 week) from the time of injury generally does not require acute immobilization unless just prior to admission the patient developed new onset of neurologic symptoms. Those patients with new onset of neurologic symptoms should be immobilized immediately, whereas those who are stable and have simply been discovered because of the persistent neck pain can be continued to be immobilized in the collar until institution of definitive treatment.

The definitive treatment of bilateral facet dislocations should be based on the goals of reducing the deformity and maintaining a stable reduction. In these patients the posterior ligamentous complex has been totally disrupted as has the disc. There is little evidence that restoration of the ligamentous complex can occur spontaneously. A spontaneous arthrodesis may occur in the reduced position. However, there is great difficulty, even in a halo-vest, preventing the spine from falling back into kyphosis as halo-vests do not prevent "toggling." Therefore it is reasonable that in a patient who has a reduced bilateral facet dislocation a Rogers wiring or posterior cervical plating be done across one interspace to reestablish spine stability. These patients can then be immobilized postoperatively in a cervical orthosis and do not require halo immobilization. Should the workup after reduction demonstrate that in fact either a bilateral facet fracture or a combination of a facet fracture and dislocation have occurred, appropriate constructs should be directed at those injuries.

The surgical stabilization should counteract the deformities which can potentially recur. In a patient with a bilateral facet fracture a Roger's wiring or interspinous wiring cannot prevent the recurrence of bilateral rotational deformities. With the absence of the facet buttress, the patient may experience both shear and rotation even in the face of a midline interspinous wiring. Therefore a posterior cervical plating, bilateral Magerl hook plates, or, in the presence of intact spinous processes, a triple wire or oblique wire technique will allow maintenance of the reduction even in the face of gross structural instability. This is similarly true in the case of a combined unilateral fracture and unilateral dislocation. Each side can be treated appropriately, thus reducing the deformity and maintaining the reduction. Postoperative immobilization can be a single external orthosis until fusion occurs.

The complex of unilateral facet dislocations and fractures should again be treated as is appropriate for the instability. Unilateral facet dislocations present the most difficult case for reduction. In this instance, the injury has occurred with flexion distraction and rotation applied in the appropriate amounts and sequence. This predominantly results in one-sided disruption, with attenuation of the interspinous ligament and ligamentum flavum, and complete disruption of the facet capsule on the side of the injury. Partial disruption of the disc on that side may also occur, depending on the extent of deformity. Generally the contralateral side is intact both radiographically and clinically. Reduction of these injuries will not occur with traction alone, irrespective of the weight applied. The reduction maneuver requires sequencing the various forces to take the injury in reverse. Therefore initially the patient needs to have traction and flexion applied to the neck to attempt to unlock the facet followed by increasing the rotation so that the intact inferior facet will tip and be able to be reduced above the superior facet without fracturing it. Once the flexion, rotation, and traction have been applied minimizing the direction of the injury, the neck is then derotated and extended and the traction is reduced, thus reducing the deformity. If insufficient reproduction has occurred, then the tip of the inferior facet will not clear the tip of the superior facet and reduction cannot occur. The degree of success of the reduction maneuver is in fact in part related to the degree of disruption of the ligamentous complex. The relative laxity of the complex will make the reduction easier. Therefore most series have found that reductions are only successful in approximately 50% of these patients. An appropriate approach to treatment of these patients is to allow the patient the choice of treatment. Clearly, in the case of radicular injury reduction it is necessary. The patient therefore has the choice of an attempted close reduction and if successful (50% of the time) then he can be maintained in external immobilization for 8–12 weeks to see whether either spontaneous arthrodesis or sufficient healing in the ligamentous complex occurs to reestabilize the neck. Should reduction not be successful or should the patient elect operative treatment, an open reduction should be achieved without sacrificing either portion of the facet. This will then fully decompress the neural foramen and allow restoration of stability. Since the facets remain intact, a simple plating or interspinous wiring will restore stability at the level. There is essentially no rotational deformity present here; therefore, a more complex technique such as an oblique wiring is not necessary in this instance.

Unilateral facet fractures, either inferior or superior, are grossly unstable injuries. Halo immobilization is not an adequate treatment alternative unless it is reasonable to allow the injury to heal in unreduced position. The only techniques which have been shown to adequately reduce the deformity and reestablish the stability predictably are those involving surgical stabilization techniques which counteract the rotation deformity. For fractures of the superior facet which are by far the more common injuries there are two schools of thought. In patients with neurologic injury, some surgeons suggest removal of the broken facet to decompress the root. Others feel that adequate reduction of the deformity will achieve reduction of the offending facet fragment. Generally the fragment remains attached to the inferior facet of the level above, as the facet joint itself is not significantly disrupted. The primary deforming force in this case is rotation, and therefore the technique to achieve reduction and stabilization should be able to counteract that rotational instability. The techniques capable of that at this point, then, are oblique wiring, Magerl hook plate, and posterior cervical plating with or without a tile plate. Again, these techniques only require immobilization of the two segments adjacent to the injured interspace. The fractured facet does not interfere with purchase on either of the injured levels. Postoperative immobilization is with a collar.

Fractures of the inferior facet present a different and less common problem. The deformity is again rotational. The facet fragment is easily visible and may be loose in the field. It therefore is easily removed; however, it does not need to be removed in order to decompress the neural foramen. It is generally removed simply because its removal doesn't compromise stability and it can be used for grafting. The major problem is that fracture of the inferior facet of the upper level of the dislocation compromises the purchase site for both an oblique wire and a posterior cervical plating. This particular injury which is reasonably rare will require immobilization of not only the injured level but also the level above in order to gain adequate control over the rotational deformity. This is one of the rare indications of a one-level instability, necessitating a two-level arthrodesis.

The final type of injury, the fracture separation of the articular mass, involves the facets at two levels and is a two-level instability. At the affected level, the pedicle and lamina are both fractured, thus allowing the articular mass on one side to be unstable in the articulations with both the adjacent vertebra above and below. Generally, however, this manifests as rotational instability on the roentgenogram at only one level. More commonly, this is the level below the fracture. However, immobilization of only that level will result in subsequent kyphosis at the level above; thus, this is in fact a two-level instability. Recognition is important and a two-level construct should be done. This can be accomplished with a triple wire technique, an oblique wire technique, or a posterior cervical plating plus or minus the tile plate.

The final occurrence is the rare instance of documented disc herniation in the presence of a facet injury (2). In those patients with either progressive neurologic deficit or those with high grade deficit initially, from bilateral facet dislocations or unilateral facet fractures with extreme instability, sufficient disruption of the disc may have occurred to have caused impingement on the dural sac. This is generally documented either by myelogram and CAT scan or by MRI. In that instance reduction without evacuation of the herniated disc can cause increased neural injury. This is especially true of techniques such as Rogers' wiring where tightening the wire requires compression of the interspace. This compression of the interspace at the time of reduction may in fact cause additional pressure on the already injured disc with extrusion of disc material against the dural sac. With the exception of this instance all facet injuries should logically be approached posteriorly. Since the posterior ligamentous complex is disrupted, the only structure maintaining some structural integrity at the level is the anterior spinal ligamentous complex. Surgical intervention should preferably not disrupt the remaining structures, as this increases instability and stress on the fixation. However, the presence of a documented herniated disc in the presence of a facet injury is one of the few indications for anterior approach to this problem. In that case, an anterior discectomy should be done prior to posterior fixation. Anterior discectomy and Smith-Robinson graft will give a satisfactory result both in terms of neural decompression and in terms of restoration of stability. There are a few series suggesting that anterior discectomy plus plating may give a satisfactory result as well. The experience with this technique is somewhat more limited.

RESULTS OF TREATMENT

There are two major concerns when evaluating the treatment of facet injuries. The first is the relative experience with the nonoperative reduction and treatment with restoration of alignment stability and normal function. The second is the success with reduction and operative stabilization in reference to the same parameters.

Closed reduction of facet injuries has been evaluated in a number of different papers. These studies have raised two basic questions. The first is an accurate assessment of the percentage of patients with the various types of facet injuries who are able to achieve an anatomic closed reduction. The second is the rate of spontaneous arthrodesis and thus a stable secondary result. In fact, the only patients for whom to even consider closed reduction appropriate are those patients who may end-up with a stable result post reduction and fixation. Clearly, this is not a satisfactory modality in the case of patients with facet fractures, as it is not possible to maintain an anatomic result with nonoperative treatment. Similarly, with bilateral facet dislocations prolonged immobilization in a halo-vest probably carries more morbidity than a simple interspinous wiring. The most appropriate injury for nonoperative treatment is probably the unilateral facet dislocation. It has been shown in a number of different studies that even with manipulation of success of reduction of unilateral facet dislocations ranges between 40 and 70%. If the reduction can be maintained, the majority of patients will have a satisfactory long-term result. For unilateral facet fractures, recently Roraback et al. (26) showed that patients who were treated nonoperatively had a higher incidence of pain and deformity than those patients treated operatively. The results with operative stabilization irrespective of the type of surgery demonstrate a high level of union, with excellent restoration of anatomic alignment if the proper construct is used to counteract the deforming forces.

Neurologic recovery from these injuries falls into two separate categories. Those patients with radicular signs and symptoms from unilateral facet injuries generally show a very high rate of recovery. Unfortunately those patients with bilateral facet injuries generally have a central neurologic syndrome. Those with incomplete injuries show excellent recovery, whereas those with complete injuries at the time of presentation rarely show any recovery with the exception of distal roots. This is the predominant result of the severe translation that occurs with intact neural arches translating one upon the other and essentially physiologically transecting the spinal cord.

COMPLICATIONS

The complications of treatment of facet injuries fall into several major categories. The first and probably most common is the failure to diagnosis. Unilateral facet injury is one of the more commonly missed injuries at initial examination. Often patients who would sustain this injury are involved in motor vehicle accidents and have multiple contusions or lacerations and other complaints about the head and neck. Uniltateral facet injuries, either fractures or dislocations, may have minimal translation and rotation and therefore may not be apparent on a first glance on a lateral cervical spine roentgenogram. They frequently present several weeks later because of persistent neck pain, and especially with unilateral facet fractures they may on secondary evaluation show increased deformity.

The second complication is related to the use of traction in the reduction of these injuries. It is reasonably common to use high weights which can cause secondary stretching and neurologic problems. Most of this is related to inappropriate application of weight and failure to recognize that certain of the facet injuries require manipulation and cannot possibly be reduced with straight traction alone. In addition, the direction of application of traction is critically important in attempting to reduce a facet dislocation. Slight extension will in fact lock the dislocation and make it more difficult to reduce. Judicious application of weight (generally less than 50 pounds) applied in a well-determined manner is most appropriate.

The next complication is loss of reduction; this has been especially well-documented with the use of a halo-vest. It, however, is not so much the fault of the device as of the individual applying the device. It has been well known that controlling the cervical spine with point of fixations only on the skull and very loose fixation about the thorax allows persistent toggling and rotational deformities to reoccur. It is therefore not logical to use such a device to attempt to control rotational deformities. The degree of loss of correction is to be expected. The final major complication is increase in neurologic injury during the course of reduction and/or stabilization. This has been reported by Arenas and Eismont (2). There is an under-estimation of the severity of disc involvement with these injuries. They demonstrated five cases where after reduction of several displaced unilateral and bilateral facet injuries, patients had increasing neurologic deficit because of extrusion of the disc. Care must be taken that all reductions be done with the patient awake (but sedated if possible) so that careful monitoring of the patients' neurologic function can occur at all times. Secondly, fixation should be done with techniques that minimize compression of the interspace. Finally, any case where the amount of initial neurologic symptomatology is out of proportion to the apparent degree of translation should be evaluated by MRI. In cases of disc extravasion, this should occur prior to posterior stabilization.

REFERENCES

1. Allen BL, Ferguson RL, Lehmann TR, O'Brien RP. A mechanistic classification of closed, indirect fractures and dislocations of the lower cervical spine. Spine 1982;7:1–27.

2. Arena MJ, Eismont FJ and Green BA. Intravertebral disc extrusion associated with cervical facet subluxation and dislocation. J Bone Joint Surg 1988;72A:43.

3. Babcock JL. Cervical spine injuries. Arch Surg 1976;111:646–651.

4. Beatson TR. Fractures and dislocations of the cervical spine. J Bone Joint Surg 1963;45B:21.

5. Bohler L. Die technick der knachenbruchbehandlung. 12e und 13e Auflage, Band 1. Wien: Wilhelm Maudrich Verlag, 1953.

6. Braakman R, Penning L. The hyperflexion sprain of the cervical spine. Radiol Clin Biol 1968;37:309–320.

7. Braakman R, Vinken PJ. Old luxations of the lower cervical spine. J Bone Joint Surg 1968;50B:52–60.

8. Cotler HB, Miller LS, DeLucia FA, et al. Closed reduction of cervical spine dislocations. Clin Orthop 1987;214:185–199.

9. Crooks F, Birkett AN. Fractures and dislocations of the cervical spine. Brit J Surg 1944;31:252.

10. Crutchfield WG. Treatment of injuries of the cervical spine. J Bone Joint Surg 1935;20:696.

11. De Oliveira JC. Anterior reduction of interlocking facets in the lower cervical spine. Spine 1979;4:195–202.

12. Durbin FC. Fracture-dislocations of the cervical spine. J Bone Joint Surg 1957;39B:23–38.

13. Edwards CC, Matz SO, Levine AM. The oblique wiring technique for rotational injuries of the cervical spine. Orthop Trans 1985;9(1):142.

14. Ellis VH. Injuries of the cervical vertebrae. Proc R Soc Med 1946;54:367.

15. Harris JH, Edeiken-Monroe B. The radiology of acute cervical spine trauma. Baltimore: Williams & Wilkins, 1987.

16. Harris JH Jr, Edeiken-Monroe B, Kopaniky DR. A practical classification of acute cervical spine injuries. Orthop Clin N Amer 1986;17:15–30.

17. Jacobs B. Cervical fractures and dislocations (C3–7). Clin Orthop 1975;109:20–32.

18. Levine AM, White JB, Edwards CC. Facet injuries in the cervical spine. Orthop Trans 1987;11:1.

19. Lysell E. Motion in the cervical spine. An experimental study on autopsy specimens. Acta Orthop Scand 1969;Supp 123.

20. Magerl F, Grob D, Seemann P. Stable dorsal fusion of the cervical spine C2–T1 using hook plates. In: Kehr P, Weidner A, eds, Cervical spine I. Vienna-New York: Springer Verlag, 1987:217.

21. Malgaigne JF. Traite des fractures et des luxations, Tome 2: Des luxations. Paris: JB Bailliere, 1855.

22. Marie-Anne S. Les fractures-separation des massifs articulaires du rachis cervical inferieur. In: Roy-Camille R, ed, Les journees d'orthopedie de la pitie. Masson, 1979.

23. Roaf R. A study of the mechanics of spinal injury. J Bone Joint Surg 1960;42B:810.

24. Roaf R. Lateral flexion injuries of the cervical spine. J Bone Joint Surg 1963;45B:36–38.

25. Rogers WA. Treatment of fracture-dislocation of the cervical spine. J Bone Joint Surg 1942;24:245–258.

26. Rogers WA. Fractures and dislocations of the cervical spine, an end result study. J Bone Joint Surg 1957;39:341–376.

27. Rorabeck CH, Rock MG, Hawkins RJ, Bourne RB. Unilateral facet dislocation of the cervical spine, an analysis of the results of treatment in 26 patients. Spine 1987;12:23–27.

28. Roy-Camille R, Mazel G, Mariambourg G, Saillant G. Les fractures-separation du massif articulaire. In: Rachis cervical inferieur, R Roy-Camille, ed, Sixiemes journees d'orthopedie de la pitie. Masson, 1988:104–107.

29. Roy-Camille R, Mazel G, Edourard B. Luxations et luxations-fractures. In: Rachis cervical inferieur, R Roy-Camille, ed, Sixiemes journees d'orthopedie de la pitie. Masson, 1988:94–103.

30. Stauffer S. Management of spine fractures C3–C7. Orthop Clin N Amer 1986;17:45.

31. White AA, Johnson RM, Panjabi MM, Southwick WO. Biomechanical analysis of clinical stability in the cervical spine. Clin Orthop 1075;109:85–96.

32. Whitehill R, Richmann JA, Glaser JA. Failure of immobilization of the cervical spine by halo vest. J Bone Joint Surg 1986;68A:326.

33. Whitley JE, Forsyth HF. The classification of cervical spine injuries. AJR 1960;83:633–644.

26

Athletic Cervical Spine Injuries

Jack Wilberger and Joseph C. Maroon

Introduction

The incidence of serious spine and spinal cord injuries associated with athletics has significantly decreased in the past 10 years. The development of sports-related spine injury registries, the elucidation of the pathophysiology involved, and the implementation of appropriate preventive measures have all contributed to this decrease. Nevertheless, virtually any athletic endeavor may be associated with spine injury, and spine surgeons must maintain proper vigilance for their occurrence and remain well versed in their management. Generally, few questions arise in regard to the management of the seriously spine- or spinal cord-injured athlete. Rarely, is it appropriate to consider allowing such individuals to return to any type of competitive athletic activity. However, considerable controversy exists over the management of the athlete with a "minor" or stably-healed spine fracture, athletes who suffer transient reversible neurologic symptoms, and athletes discovered to have asymptomatic cervical spinal stenosis. This chapter will review the incidence, pathophysiology, and common features of athletic spine injuries and attempt to devise an overall approach to their management.

Pathophysiology

The pathophysiology of spine injuries in athletics appears to be similar regardless of the sport involved. Previously, it has been held that hyperflexion of the cervical spine was the source of the most severe injuries. However, careful epidemiologic, cinematographic, and laboratory analyses have clearly shown that axial loading is the most important factor in athletic injuries. Cervical musculature normally absorbs energy transmitted to the cervical spine. This energy-absorbing capacity is greatest with the neck in the anatomic position—slight extension due to the normal cervical lordosis. However, the bones, discs, and ligaments may be subjected to tremendous energy inputs when the head, neck, and trunk are positioned in such a way that the forces are transmitted along the longitudinal axis of the cervical spine. During axial loading, the neck is slightly flexed to approximately 30°. The normal cervical lordosis is eliminated, and the cervical spine is converted into a straight segmented column. When the athlete's head comes in contact with another player, the ground, or the bottom of a pool, the cervical spine is compressed between the decelerated head and the force of the oncoming trunk (Figure 26.1). When this pathophysiology is taken into account, it appears that rather than accidents or freak occurrences, occasionally techniques and maneuvers are used by athletes that deliberately place the cervical spine at risk of injury.

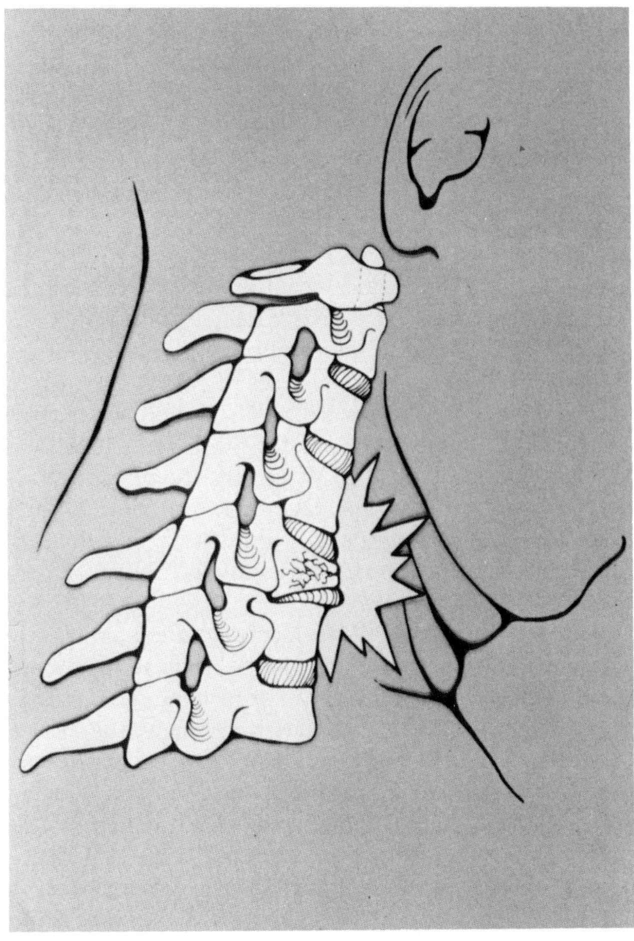

Figure 26.1. Axial loading with the neck in slight flexion is the predominant mechanism of athletic spinal injury.

EPIDEMIOLOGY

While the pathophysiology may be similar, the specifics of various spine injuries vary from sport to sport. Cervical spine injuries resulting from participation in gymnastics have become synonymous with the trampoline and mini-trampoline. From 1955 through 1978, 114 cases of quadriplegia from trampoline use were reported. This led to a rather strong reaction from groups such as the American Academy of Pediatrics, which in 1977 called for a ban on the trampoline. In 1978 the National Collegiate Athletic Association (NCAA) issued a series of guidelines for the trampoline, and the National Gymnastic Catastrophic Injury Registry was established (10). Since 1978, only 20 catastrophic spinal injuries have been reported, with 14 occurring on the trampoline.

In ice hockey, in the mid-1970s, a perceived significant increase in spine injuries led to the Canadian-organized Committee on Prevention of Spine Injuries Due to Hockey (4). The committee documented 42 spine injuries with 28 spinal cord injuries from 1976 through 1983. The most common causes were spearing and checking. As a result of its activities, in 1983 the committee issued a series of guidelines aimed at decreasing the incidence of spine injuries: better enforcement of rules against boarding and cross-checking, institution of rules against pushing or checking from behind, development of muscle conditioning programs, better player education in regard to neck injuries, better helmet design with regard to shape and shock absorbency. Since these changes were instituted, only 5 injuries have been reported in the Canadian hockey leagues.

The National Football Head and Neck Registry was established in 1975 to document the incidence of head and neck injury in organized football. From 1971 through 1975, there were 259 cervical spine injuries for a rate of 4.1 per 100,000 participants and 99 cases of permanent quadriplegia—a rate of 1.58 per 100,000 (6). This information provided the primary impetus for the 1976 NCAA rules changes which intended to abolish the use of the head as an offensive weapon—"spearing." The institution of these rules has resulted in a dramatic decrease in both the incidence of spine and spinal cord injury in football (Figure 26.2).

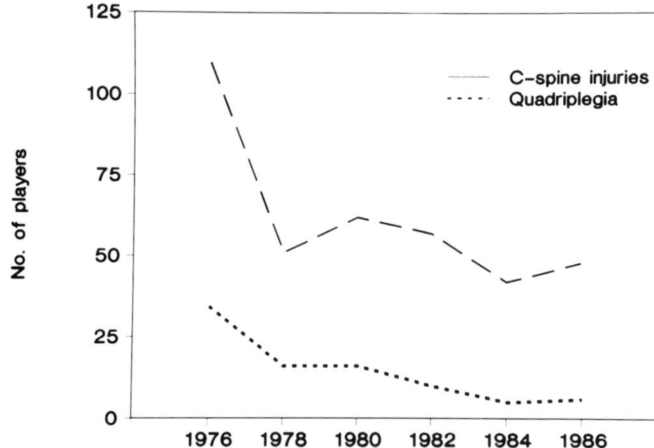

Figure 26.2. Spine and spinal cord injuries reported from the National Football Head and Neck Registry 1976–1986.

The careful study of the incidence, location, and mechanism of sports-related spine injuries brings to light many common features. The incidence of such injuries increased concomitantly with the increasingly violent and aggressive nature of the sport involved. Nonprofessional athletes appear to be at greater risk because of less conditioning, less protective equipment, and in general less regard for the rules of the sport. Improperly conditioned neck muscles put the athlete at significant risk when sustaining inadvertent or intentional blows to the head. Similar risk results from improper or inadequate training in the manner in which to sustain an impact or in the other techniques of the sport involved. Improper helmet fit coupled with the use of the helmet as an offensive weapon is another common feature of sports-related spine injury.

MANAGEMENT

From what is known of the incidence and pathophysiology of athletic cervical spine injury, it is possible to devise a scheme of management that is reasonable in regard to the spine and spinal cord integrity and the athlete's often overwhelming desire to return to his sport. Four situations are not infrequently encountered in sports medicine:

1. Should an athlete be allowed to return to his sport/any sport after a serious spine injury without associated neurological deficit?
2. When, if ever, should an athlete be allowed to return to his sport/any sport after a "minor" spine injury—ligamentous laxity, chip fractures, posterior element fractures?
3. When, if ever, should an athlete be allowed to return to his sport/any sport after sustaining a transient neurological deficit in connection with sports activity?
4. Should an athlete with known but asymptomatic spinal stenosis be allowed to compete?

Serious Spine Injury without Neurologic Deficit

Case Report: A 14-year-old sustained a C3–4 fracture/dislocation during competitive diving. No neurologic injury occurred. A posterior cervical wiring and fusion was performed and recovery was uneventful. The patient was not allowed to return to diving but was allowed to participate in other competitive sports. He developed a particular interest in gymnastics and went on to become a state high school champion by age 18. During one competition, while performing on uneven horizontal bars, he fell. Immediate quadriplegia secondary to an odontoid fracture resulted (Figure 26.3). He remains ventilator-dependent.

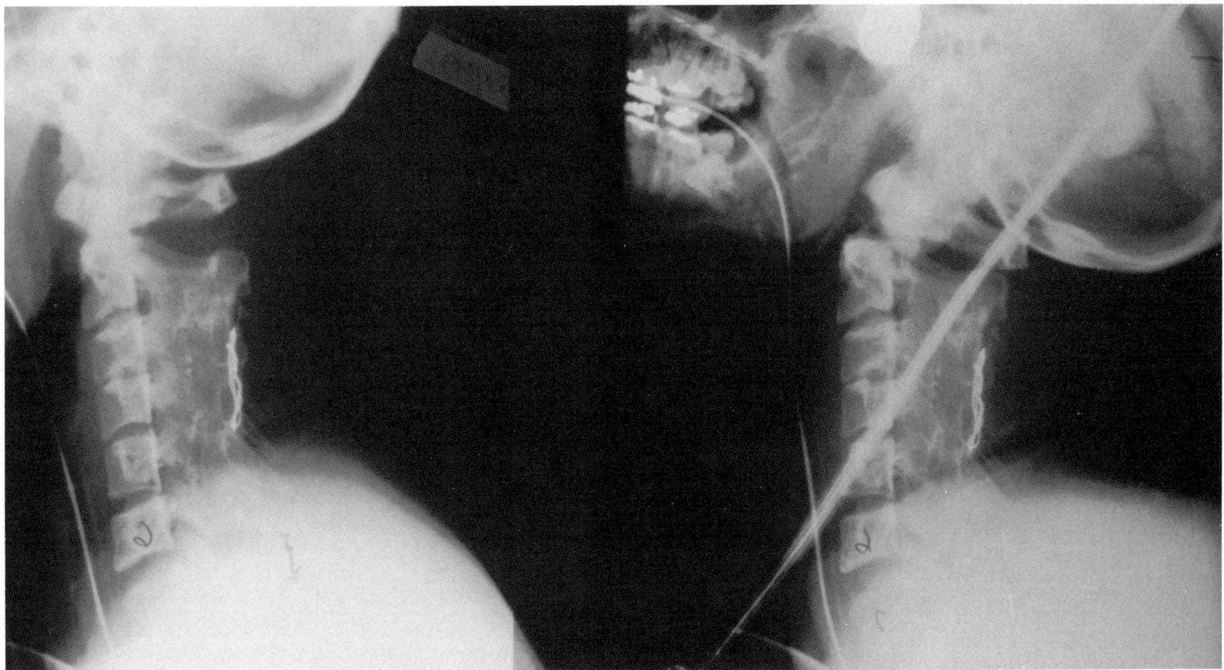

Figure 26.3. Type II odontoid fracture in an 18-year-old gymnast who 4 years previously underwent fusion for C3–4 fracture-dislocation.

In those athletes who have suffered a significant fracture or fracture/dislocation of the cervical spine and have undergone spinal fusion, a return to contact sports or any sport involving risk of further spine injury is not recommended. Even in the presence of a stable spine on flexion and extension radiographs, continued participation is not advised, as it is currently impossible to predict stability under the variety of stresses created by athletic involvement. There are no good experimental or clinical data to guide us in assessing the degree of stability following a healed fusion of the cervical spine when it is placed under extreme degrees of stress. Torg has estimated that the forces involved in football tackling can be in the range of 18 G (8). The response of the spine to movement has been studied in regard to what is known as the "functional spinal unit" or spinal motion segment (7). The spinal column has been considered as both a 2- and 3-column system for the determination of stability. The posterior elements—pedicles, facets, and laminae have been estimated to bear up to one-third of a compressive load to the spine. The disc combined with the anterior and posterior longitudinal ligaments are estimated to provide close to 50% of the stability with torsional forces. There is no definite data concerning individual vertebral body contributions to stability, especially when one includes the possibility of either partial or complete ligamentous injury, the healing process after fracture has occurred, the insertion of a bony graft, and the additional stress forces to which the athlete may be subjected. In addition, after a spinal fusion has occurred, the concept of the spinal motion segment is no longer valid. In the absence of any objective ability to measure the degree of dynamic stress stability, any healed fracture of the cervical spine (with the exception of chip fractures, isolated laminae or spinous process fractures) and any injury which has required internal stabilization may be considered to be unsuitable to safely withstand further challenges from contact sports.

Minor Spine Injury

Case Report: A 19-year-old linebacker developed neck pain during a college game after a hard tackle. Cervical x-rays were obtained several days later because of persistent neck pain; neurologic exam was normal. A C5 anterior wedge fracture was present. The athlete was treated with a cervical orthosis for 3 months and was kept out of football for the season. He returned to play the next season and subsequently went on to play for several National Football League and United States Football League teams over the next 6 to 7 years without incident. He presented at 27 years of age with neck pain and right arm tingling after a tackle on a kickoff play. Neurologic exam was normal. Cervical spine films with flexion and extension as well as a MRI in flexion and extension continued to demonstrate the old C5 wedge fracture, but no new traumatic abnormalities and no evidence of instability (Figure 26.4). He was allowed to return to football after his symptoms resolved.

As noted previously, there are no definite objective data to fully assess dynamic spinal stability and stress tolerance

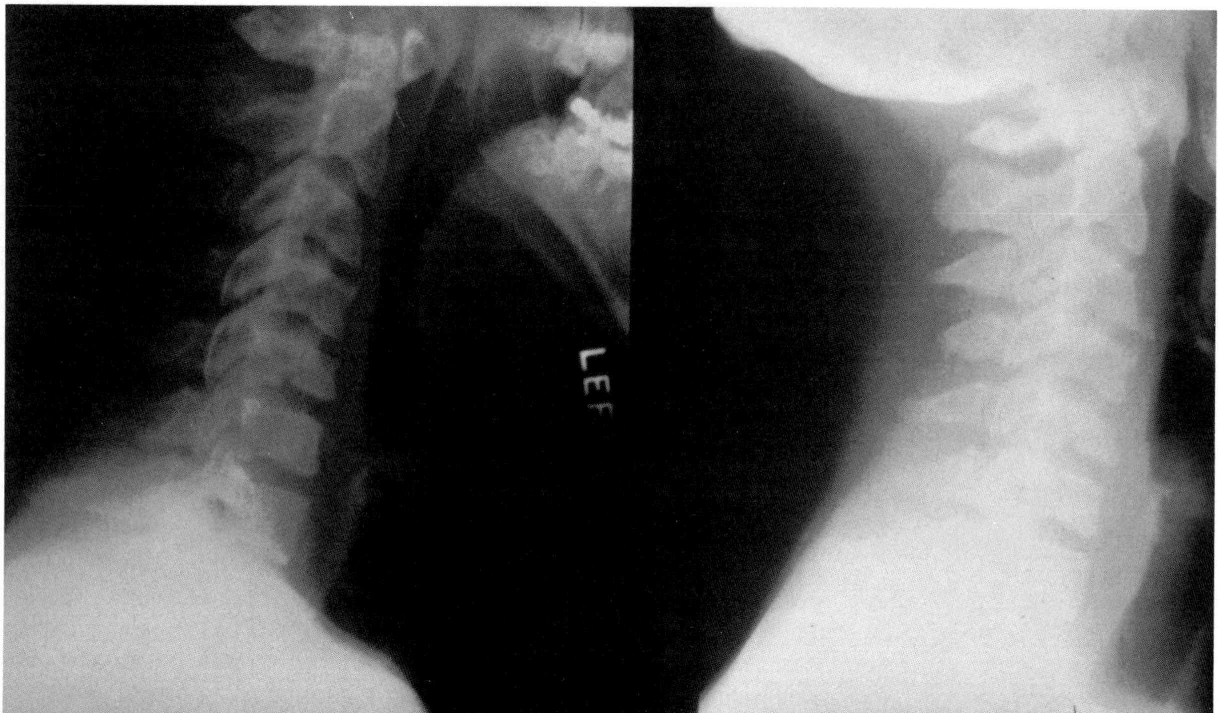

Figure 26.4. Old C5 anterior wedge fracture which had caused no symptoms during 7 years of NFL and USFL competition.

after bony injury. The wedge fracture in this particular incident was able to withstand repeat stresses without evidence of long-term instability. It does appear reasonable to conclude that isolated wedge and chip fractures of the vertebral body, laminar fractures, and spinous process fractures should pose no long-term problem once adequate healing has occurred. When such injuries do occur in an athlete, it is recommended that they be removed from all contact and competitive sports for at least 4 months. If the athlete is asymptomatic, has normal MRI of his disc, and dynamic films show fracture healing without evidence of instability, then return to competition is most likely safe and is unlikely to be associated with significant risks of further injury (9).

Case Report: A 22-year-old ice hockey forward complained of severe localized neck pain after being cross-checked into the boards during a game. Neurologic exam was normal. Cervical spine films in flexion and extension showed 5 mm of active movement at the C2–3 level. He was maintained in a hard cervical collar for 4 weeks at which time he was asymptomatic. Repeat cervical spine flexion/extension films showed no evidence of ongoing abnormalities. He was allowed to return to hockey after another 4 weeks and further repeated films continued to show no abnormality (Figure 26.5).

It is well-known that ligamentous damage may accompany a cervical spine injury and can occur in the absence of bone injury. Generally, this is a minor, self-limiting problem but on occasion may result in progressive instability, cervical spine deformity and potential spinal cord injury. Presently, there are guidelines to assist in determining ligamentous stability. Under normal conditions, the ligaments permit very little motion between the cervical vertebrae. In cadaver studies, with all ligaments intact, the horizontal motion of one vertebral body on the next does not exceed 3.5 mm, and the angular displacement of one vertebral body on the next is always 11° or less (7). Only when a majority of the restraining ligaments are injured or destroyed are motions in excess of this seen. In the clinical setting measurements of horizontal or angular displacement can be made on neutral or flexion/extension radiographs.

When any subluxation is seen following athletic-related injury it is recommended that the individual be maintained in a hard cervical collar. An MRI and dynamic flexion/extension films should be repeated 2–4 weeks after injury. If there is no evidence of progression or if there is a return to normal of the cervical spine films, it is unlikely that any significant injury has occurred, and generally the athlete can be allowed to safely return to his/her competitive sport.

Transient Neurologic Deficit

The development of transient neurological deficit—sensory changes, motor weakness, or paralysis—may occur frequently in association with athletic activity. In 1984, a survey of over 500 NCAA football programs with a total of over 39,000 players found a 1.3 per 10,000 participants incidence of transitory paresis and paresthesias. A 6.0 per 10,000 participants incidence of numbness and tingling was also found.

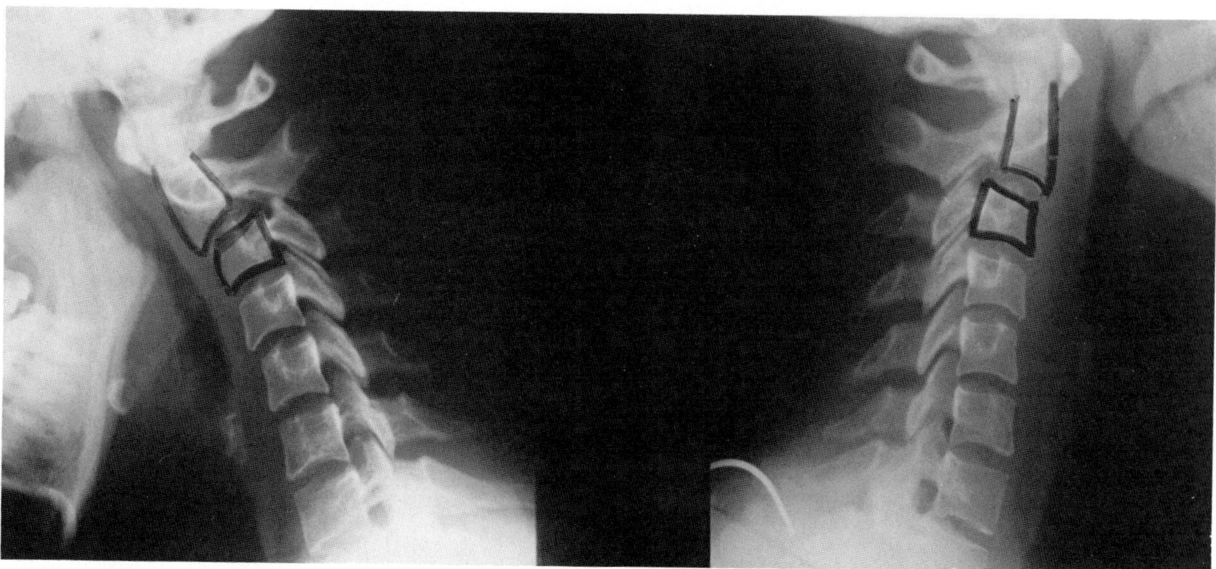

Figure 26.5. Flexion radiographs taken at the time of injury (5mm C2–3 subluxation) and 4 weeks after injury (2mm subluxation) in a 22-year-old hockey player demonstrating resolution of a minor ligamentous injury.

The burning hands syndrome is the most well-known of these entities. First described by Maroon in 1977, the syndrome has come to be recognized as a variant of the central cord syndrome (2). The characteristic complaint is that of burning paresthesias and dysesthesias in the arms or hands and occasionally the legs. This syndrome is to be distinguished from the "pinched nerve" or "stingers" due to brachial plexus traction commonly seen in football players (11). Burning hands syndrome was originally described to be associated with a bony or ligamentous spine abnormality in approximately 50% of the individuals so affected. Thus, the importance of recognizing the syndrome is that the athlete should be treated as having had a significant spinal cord/spine injury until proven otherwise. If a spine injury has been ruled out, somatosensory evoked potentials may be useful in documenting physiologic cord dysfunction. In some instances, MRI may document an anatomic cord abnormality such as swelling or a hyperintense lesion (Figure 26.6).

Torg et al. in 1986 reported on 32 athletes with what he termed neurapraxia of the cervical cord with associated transient quadriplegia (5). In all instances, abnormalities were found on cervical spine films. Seventeen of the 32 had developmental cervical cord stenosis. A ratio method of determining spinal canal dimensions was used, with a ratio of spinal canal to vertebral body of less than 0.8 indicating significant stenosis. Four of the 32 showed evidence of ligamentous instability, six of the 32 had acute or chronic intervertebral disc disease and five of the 32 had congenital cervical anomalies. The quadriplegia lasted from 1 minute to 48 hours and in all cases resolved completely. MRI was obtained in only one patient and no intrinsic cord abnormalities were demonstrated.

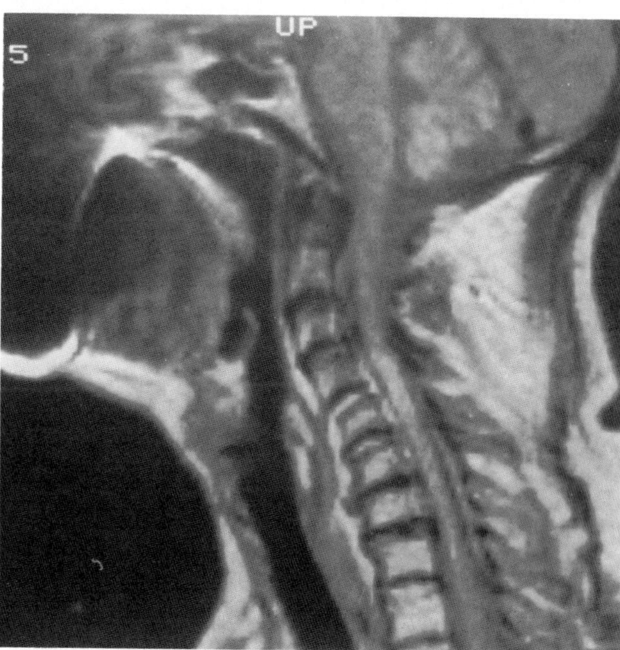

Figure 26.6. Cervical MRI in a 23-year-old football player with severe burning dysesthesias in both hands. A hyperintense intramedullary lesion extends from C4–C5. This is consistent with a cervical cord contusion.

In order to attempt to determine the relative risk of future neurologic consequences to these athletes, a retrospective analysis was accomplished on 117 quadriplegic athletes in the National Football Head and Neck Registry (6). None of these athletes reported any episodes of transient motor weakness prior to their permanent cord injury. Only one of this group reported prior transient sensory symptoms.

In Torg's series of the athletes with developmental stenosis, nine stopped all athletic activity after the first episode of transient quadraplegia. Three individuals returned to football but stopped playing after the second episode occurred and one continued on in spite of a second episode without subsequent problems. Three returned fully to their normal athletic activities without subsequent problems. A boxer who underwent a laminectomy after experiencing transient quadraplegia returned to boxing and had no further symptoms. The follow-up ranged from 3 to 5 years in this group. Of the five patients with congenital anomalies, four stopped athletic activity, and one continued without subsequent problems. Three of the six individuals with the degenerative disc disease left athletics. One returned without subsequent problems and two underwent anterior cervical discectomies without a return to their sport. Of the four with ligamentous instability, two stopped athletic activity, one patient had three further episodes before stopping, and one continued on without subsequent problems. The follow-up in this group of patients ranged between 1 and 5 years.

Based on these findings, Torg concluded "the young patient who has had an episode of neurapraxia of the cervical spinal cord with or without transient quadriplegia is not predisposed to permanent neurologic injury because of it" (5).

When faced with an athlete who has suffered a transient neurologic deficit a thorough workup must be undertaken to rule out a bony or ligamentous injury to the spine. Plain cervical spine radiographs with flexion and extension views are most helpful in this regard. CT scan and/or polytomography may be necessary to evaluate for subtle injuries. If no bony or ligamentous abnormalities are identified in the setting of a transient neurologic deficit, an effort may be made to rule out ongoing extrinsic cord or nerve root compression or intrinsic cord abnormality. This is most readily accomplished by MRI (Figure 26.6). Somatosensory evoked potentials (SSEPs) may also prove useful in documenting physiologic cord dysfunction. Special concerns should be raised if any intrinsic cord abnormalities are seen on MRI or documented SSEPs, as this provides direct evidence of an overt, although minor, spinal cord injury, and this should preclude return to athletics. If there is no evidence of spinal cord injury and no bony or ligamentous problem, then return to competition is probably safe. A second episode of transient neurologic deficit, however, should preclude further athletic participation.

Cervical Stenosis

Cervical spinal canal stenosis may be present in the athlete as a developmental or congenital condition or may occur due to acquired degenerative changes in the spine (Figure 26.7). It is well-known that long-term athletic participation predisposes to degenerative changes. However, most attention has been focused on the developmental variety of spinal stenosis as a result of dramatic cases of spinal cord injury occurring in association with a congenitally small canal in several athletes. In spite of this, however, there is little information concerning the risk of an asymptomatic narrow spinal canal in the athlete. Schneider has been quoted as collecting a "large series of cases of athletes who sustained an injury to the neck and were later discovered to have stenosis of the cervical spine. Permanent neurologic deficit, quadraplegia or death occurred in a high percentage of these athletes" (3). However, no published details are available from this series. Similarly, while the National Football Head and Neck Registry maintains excellent statistics, there is no specific information available on the rate of cervical stenosis in association with such injuries (6).

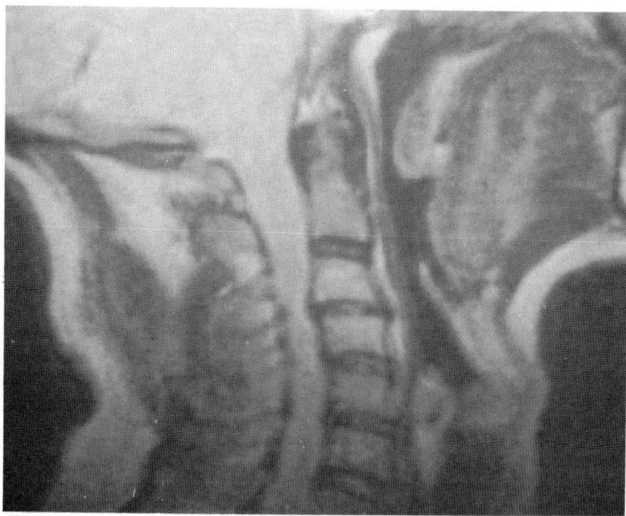

Figure 26.7. Mild degenerative stenosis at C3–4 level demonstrated on MRI in an asymptomatic 21-year-old football player.

It is well-known that, pathophysiologically, individuals with developmental or spondylitic narrowing of the spinal canal are especially at risk for neurologic injury during hyperextension. During hyperextension the sagittal diameter of the spinal canal is further compromised by as much as 30% by infolding of the ligamentum flavum and the interlaminar ligaments. However, as has been noted previously it appears that axial loading rather than hyperextension or hyperflexion is the most important factor in athletic-related spinal cord injury. In Torg's series, seven of 32 patients (53%) with transient quadriplegia associated with athletic activity had cervical stenosis (5). Spinal canal diameter in these individuals ranged from 10–17 mm at the C3–C6 levels with a mean of 14.17 mm. Torg developed a ratio method for determining the significance of any degree of spinal canal narrowing. This ratio compared the canal width with the anterior/posterior width of the mid-point of the corresponding vertebral body. His group felt that a ratio of the spinal canal to the vertebral body of less than 0.80 was indicative of significant stenosis. The ratio in his 17 patients ranged from 0.36 to 0.85.

None of Torg's 17 patients went on to develop any permanent neurologic problems. Nine of the 17 did not return to any athletic activity. Three of the 17 returned to football without subsequent problems. Three of the 17 returned but suffered a second episode and subsequently stopped playing, and one of the 17 continued playing after a second episode without subsequent problems. One of the individuals who was a boxer underwent a cervical laminectomy and returned to boxing without future problems. Based on such data, Torg felt that transient quadriplegia occurring in association with developmental stenosis does not predispose to permanent neurologic injury. At the same time, citing other factors, his group recommended precluding any individual with transient quadriplegia in association with a narrow cervical canal from further athletic competition.

Therefore, the question has yet to be resolved as to whether asymptomatic cervical stenosis in the athlete increases the risk of spinal cord injury. Increased attention may be further focused on this area in the near future as a number of National Football League teams are now requiring detailed investigations of the cervical and lumbar spine (some including MRI scan) as a prerequisite to their draft process.

CONCLUSIONS

Returning to the questions posed earlier on the management of specific cervical spine injury in athletes, the following guidelines are recommended:

1. Spinal cord injury or serious spinal bony injury without neurologic deficit—no return to any competitive sports activity involving contact or risk of subsequent spine injury;
2. Minor cervical spine bony injury—ligamentous, vertebral wedge, or chip fractures, posterior element fracture—without neurologic deficit—may return to competitive sports activity if asymptomatic and dynamic radiographs show no evidence of instability;
3. Transient neurologic deficits—may return to competitive sports activity if asymptomatic and no bony, ligamentous, or spinal cord abnormalities demonstrated on appropriate studies. A second episode should preclude further participation.
4. Asymptomatic cervical stenosis—individualized management is appropriate.

REFERENCES

1. Ladd AL, Scranton PE. Congenital cervical stenosis presenting as transient quadriplegia in athletics. J Bone Joint Surg 1986;68A:1371–1374.

2. Maroon JC. Burning hands and football spinal cord injury. JAMA 1977;238:2049–2051.

3. Schneider RC. Serious and fatal neurosurgical football injury. Clin Neurosurg 1966;12:226–236.

4. Tator CH, Edmonds VE. National survey of spinal injuries in hockey players. Can Med Assoc J 1984;130:875–880.

5. Torg JS, Pavlov H, Genuario SE, et al. Neurapraxia of the cervical spinal cord with transient quadriplegia. J Bone Joint Surg 1986;68A:1354–1370.

6. Torg JS, Vegso JJ, Sennett B, Das M. The national football head and neck registry: fourteen year report on cervical quadriplegia, 1971–1984. JAMA 1985;254:3439–3443.

7. White AA, Johnson RM, Panjabi MM, Southwick WO. Biomechanical analysis of clinical stability in the cervical spine. Clin Orthop 1975;109:85–96.

8. Torg JS. Epidemiology, pathomechanics and prevention of athletic injuries to the cervical spine. Med Sci Sports Exerc 1985;17:295–303.

9. Funk FJ Jr, Wells RE. Injuries of the cervical spine in football. Clin Orthop 1975;109:50–58.

10. Torg JS, Das M. Trampoline-related quadriplegia: a review of the literature and reflections of the American Academy of Pediatrics position statement. Pediatrics 1984;74:804–812.

11. Wilberger JE, Maroon JC. Burning hands syndrome revisited. Neurosurgery 1987;20:599–605.

27

Pediatric Spine Injuries

Mark N. Hadley[a]

Overview

Spinal column trauma is uncommon in the pediatric patient population (11, 19, 20, 24, 29, 33, 37). Only 5% of all spinal cord and vertebral column injuries involve patients between birth and 16 years of age. Hadley et al. reported 122 pediatric spine injured patients treated over a 14-year period (19, 20). This pediatric spine injury population represented only 4.7% of 1250 vertebral column injuries they managed. Ruge and associates documented an incidence of pediatric spine injury of 2.7% over a similar time period (33); however, their review included only those individuals between birth and 14 years of age. Other investigators have reported incidence estimates ranging between 1% and 11% (11, 20, 22, 24, 26, 30, 38), the variability presumably dependent upon the volume of spinal trauma at a given institution and regional referral patterns.

When the entire pediatric age range is examined, males more frequently sustain pediatric spinal trauma than do females (19, 20, 29, 33). These statistics, however, are inordinately influenced by an increased likelihood of vertebral column injury by the "more active" adolescent males in the 11 to 16-year-old age groups. Interestingly, females appear to sustain spinal cord and vertebral column injuries more frequently than males in the youngest age group patients, particularly those between birth and 5 years of age (20, 33).

The etiology of pediatric spine injuries differs according to the age of the patient. The youngest age group patients (0–9 years) have a high incidence of falls and pedestrian-automobile accidents, while their older counterparts have a higher incidence of motor vehicle accidents, motorcycle accidents, and sports-related injuries (19, 20, 33) (Table 27.1).

There are important differences between pediatric spinal cord and vertebral column injuries and those which occur in adult patients. The types of spinal injury, the levels of injury, and the frequency of injuries are distinctly different among pediatric patients. In addition, the incidence and degree of neurological compromise from the injury and the ultimate outcome from injury are age-related and are influenced by the maturity, elasticity, and strength of the vertebral segments and supporting muscular and ligamentous structures.

Anatomy

The immature spine has several anatomical and physiological features that, on the one hand, account for the relative resistance of the pediatric vertebral column to spinal trauma and that, on the other, help explain the many important differences between pediatric and adult spine-injured patients. The infant spine has increased physiological mobility and elasticity due to marked ligamentous laxity, underdevelopment of neck and paraspinous musculature, incompletely ossified, wedge-shaped vertebrae, shallow horizontally oriented facet joints, and absent uncinate processes (11, 19, 20, 24, 30, 33, 38). These features, in combination with the relatively large size of the head with respect to the torso in the younger pediatric patients increases the likelihood of cervical spine injuries, specifically between the occiput and the axis, compared to older more mature, physically developed individuals (11, 19, 20, 33). The relative fulcrum of the head on the vertebral column appears to be located at the C1–C2 level in infants. With development and maturation of the spine and supporting structures, force vectors are altered, lowering the relative

Table 27.1. Etiology

Injury Type	Total	Age Group (Years)		
		0–9	10–14	15–16
	%	%	%	%
MVA	39	17	26	52
Fall	15	39	13	9
Sports	11	11	11	12
Pedestrian/automobile	11	33	16	3
Motorcycle	9		13	11
Diving	8		13	7
Miscellaneous	7		8	6

Reprinted with permission, Hadley MN, Zabramski JM, Browner CM, et al. Pediatric spinal trauma: a review of 122 cases of spinal cord and vertebral column injuries. J Neurosurg 1988;68:18–24.

[a]The views of the author are his own and are not to be construed as official or reflecting the position of the United States Air Force or the Department of Defense.

fulcrum to the C5–C6 level in older pediatric patients and adults.

The strength of the ligaments and musculature increases with age, and the geometry and degree of ossification of the vertebral bodies and facets change with maturation (11, 19, 20, 21, 28, 33, 38). The uncinate processes are absent early and develop gradually by age 10 years. It appears that age-related maturation occurs earlier in the upper cervical spine and is usually completed by age 9 years (11, 19–21, 28, 33, 38). Maturation and development of the lower cervical spine occur more gradually and are usually complete by age 14 years (11, 19–21, 28, 33, 38).

The laxity, elasticity, and mobility of the young spine probably afford some protection against spinal trauma that might cause fracture or fracture-subluxation in the more mature, rigid spine (19, 20). In support of this concept, the youngest age group pediatric patients have been found to have a statistically significant lower incidence of injury compared to their older counterparts (19, 20). This same elasticity and mobility of the infant spine help to explain the relative resistance of the youngest age group patients to spinal cord and vertebral column trauma, yet also explain why, when an accident occurs with sufficient force, the youngest patients have a higher incidence of neurological injury than older children and adolescents (19–21, 28, 33) (Table 27.2).

Several congenital pathological states exist which predispose pediatric patients to spinal column instability or make them more susceptible to vertebral column and spinal cord injury (27). These include os odontoideum, occipitalization of the atlas, Down's syndrome, Warfarin syndrome, and Conradi's syndrome. These conditions must be kept in mind during the management of pediatric patients with suspected vertebral column trauma who have neurological deficits out of proportion to their apparent bony injuries.

INJURY PATTERNS

The relative maturity of the spine which distinguishes pediatric patients from adult vertebral column injury patients can be utilized to further subdivide the pediatric patient population into three age categories: 0 to 9 years of age, 10 to 14 years of age, and 15 to 16 years of age. This categorization scheme is based on known maturation milestones of the vertebral column and supporting structures and allows a comparison among pediatric patients between patient age, level and type of injury, the incidence of neurological compromise, and outcome after therapy (19, 20). Standard chi-square statistical methods have been employed by Hadley et al. to analyze potential differences in the above-mentioned factors between the various age groups as outlined (20).

In comparison with adult spine injured patients, individuals 0 to 16 years of age have a high incidence of cervical spinal cord and vertebral column injuries and have significantly fewer thoracolumbar junction vertebral injuries (2, 3, 11, 14–17, 19, 20, 23, 35, 38). Not only are cervical injuries more frequent among pediatric patients, but the level of injury is higher on the cervical vertebral column than that which occurs in adults (2, 3, 7, 16, 17, 19, 20, 33, 35). This has to do with the relative fulcrum of the head on the developing spinal column. When the three age categories within the pediatric patient population are compared, patients in the youngest age group appear uniquely susceptible to superior cervical spinal column trauma and have a statistically significant higher incidence of occiput through C2 level injuries than their older counterparts ($p<0.001$; $\times 2 = 11.107$) (Table 27.3) (19, 20). The oldest pediatric patients have injury levels similar to those observed in the adult population (11, 19, 20, 33). Patients in the 11 to 14 years age category have maturing, adolescent spines and represent an intermediate injury level group.

The type of vertebral column or spinal cord injury a pediatric patient will sustain is also age-maturation related. Four distinct injury patterns common to pediatric spine-injured patients have been identified (19–21, 28, 29, 33). Using radiographic criteria, injury types may be divided into:

1. Fracture of the vertebral body or posterior arch;
2. Fracture with subluxation;
3. Subluxation only; and
4. Spinal cord injury without radiographic abnormality (SCIWORA).

Younger patients have a relatively high incidence of SCIWORA and subluxation only and a lower incidence of fracture only than their older, more mature counterparts (19, 20, 33, 37). As expected, individuals in the 15 to 16-

Table 27.2. Age (Years) Versus Injury Type*

Age	Number	Fracture only	Fracture/subluxation	Subluxation only	No fracture/subluxation
(years)		%	%	%	%
0–9	18	5 (28)	3 (17)	4 (22)	6 (33)
10–14	38	18 (47)	11 (29)	3 (8)	6 (16)
15–16	66	27 (41)	26 (39)	5 (8)	8 (12)

Reprinted with permission, Hadley MN, Zabramski JM, Browner CM, et al. Pediatric spinal trauma: a review of 122 cases of spinal cord and vertebral column injuries. J Neurosurg 1988;68:18–24.

*NOTE: Difference in injury pattern among age groups not statistically significant ($p = 0.07$).

Table 27.3. Age Versus Level of Injury*[#]

Level	Age Group (Years) 0–9	10–14	15–16
	%	%	%
All cervical[+]	13 (72)	23 (60)	36 (55)
Occiput–C2[#]	9 (50)	7 (18)	9 (14)
All thoracic	3 (17)	12 (32)	17 (26)
All lumbar	2 (11)	3 (8)	11 (17)
Thoraco-lumbar	2 (11)	6 (16)	14 (21)
All sacral	0	0	1 (2)

Reprinted with permission, Hadley MN, Zabramski JM, Browner CM, et al. Pediatric spinal trauma: a review of 122 cases of spinal cord and vertebral column injuries.

*No significant difference in incidence of cervical spine injury among age groups ($p = 0.17$).

[#]Statistically significant difference in incidence of occiput–C2 injuries among age groups [($p \leq 0.001$, X × 2 = 11.107, df = 1(Yates)].

year-old age category have a higher incidence of fracture only and fracture with subluxation (Table 27.2). The latter distribution of injuries is consistent with that observed among adult spine-injured patients (2, 3, 14–17, 35).

Pediatric spine-injured patients have a lower incidence of neurological injury compared to adults who have sustained vertebral column trauma (3, 15, 19, 20, 33, 35). This appears particularly true for complete neurological injuries (19, 20, 33). Combined data from contemporary reviews by Hadley et al. and Ruge et al. reveal that nearly 50% of pediatric spine-injured patients will be neurologically intact and that only 18% will have complete neurological injuries (20, 33). These studies refute the reports by earlier investigators which indicate that the child with a spinal column injury has a higher incidence of complete neurological injury than the adult who has suffered vertebral column trauma (7, 25). Of adult spine-injured patients, 25% to 30% present neurologically intact, and approximately 35% have complete neurological injuries (2, 3, 15, 35).

SCIWORA

The incidence of spinal cord injury without radiographic abnormality among large populations of pediatric spine-injured patients is approximately 20% (19–21, 33). It has been documented as low as 16% by Hadley et al. (20) and 21% by Ruge et al. (33) and as high as 67% by Pang and Wilberger (28, 29). The lower incidence rates are probably most accurate and reflect contemporary radiologic diagnostic accuracy and eliminate potential referral bias which may have been present in earlier reviews.

SCIWORA appears to be a syndrome unique to the pediatric population (19–21, 28, 29, 31, 33, 37, 38). While spinal cord injury without radiographic evidence of fracture or subluxation does occur in adults, usually these patients will have spondylitic degenerative changes of the cervical vertebrae which result in spinal stenosis and may predispose these patients to neural injury after trauma without demonstrable fracture or subluxation.

Children of all ages are susceptible to SCIWORA. The youngest age group patients appear to have a higher incidence of SCIWORA but no statistically significant difference in incidence between the three pediatric age groups has been identified (20, 29, 31, 33). It appears that younger patients (0 to 9 years) suffer greater neurological trauma and have a worse prognosis than their older counterparts with SCIWORA (19, 20, 29, 31, 33). In the review by Hadley et al. older children with SCIWORA experienced incomplete neurological injuries which improved dramatically during their hospitalization (20). Among the youngest age group patients (0 to 9 years) neurological compromise was complete (or nearly so) and showed little evidence of recovery over time (20).

The onset of SCIWORA may be delayed by hours, even days, after vertebral column trauma (8, 28, 29, 31, 33, 37). Pang has described 15 children who had a delayed onset of SCIWORA (28). Nine of 15 patients had transient initial symptoms that were either missed or dismissed by their initial evaluators. In addition, delayed neurological deterioration has been reported in neurologically incomplete SCIWORA patients (8, 28, 29, 31, 33, 37). These occurrences are uncommon and raise suspicions about a vascular-ischemic etiology for the exacerbation of neurological compromise in affected patients (8, 29, 31).

Recurrent SCIWORA is a real and potentially lethal phenomenon which occurs in a small subset of SCIWORA patients (28, 29, 31). Pollack et al. documented eight children of 55 SCIWORA patients (14%) who developed recurrent neurological compromise 3 days to 11 weeks after the initial injury (31). It appears that patients with the most mild initial SCIWORA injuries are most likely to sustain recurrent SCIWORA. More seriously impaired patients will be unable to resume physical activity and are less likely to be reinjured. Those patients with transient symptoms, irrespective of how severe, often forget their temporary neurological deficits and their need for cervical immobilization and are more likely to resume potentially injurious physical exercise (28, 31). Four of the eight patients Pollack described were left with significant and severe neurological deficits following recurrent SCIWORA. A more stringent treatment plan including a 3-month period of immobilization is recommended for mildly injured SCIWORA patients to prevent recurrent injury (28, 31).

Evaluation

Pediatric spine-injured patients merit a complete radiological diagnostic assessment no different from that performed in adult spine-injured patients. Any patient with a potential spine injury should be immobilized until vertebral column and/or spinal cord injury can be excluded (12, 19, 20, 31, 32, 35, 36). Radiographic evaluation begins with routine lateral radiographs of the area(s) of suspected injury. That 11% to 20% of pediatric patients will have more than one level of vertebral column injury suggests the need for a full spinal column assessment in selected patients (4, 5, 19, 20, 32, 33). Thin section computerized tomography (CT) of the specific region of presumed fracture or dislocation is next obtained (4, 5, 19, 32, 35). In SCIWORA patients, the area of the spine to be examined with CT is determined by the patients' neurological injury level. Patients with significant cervical spine subluxation-dislocation as determined by the initial standard lateral and swimmer's x-rays are placed in Gardner-Wells tongs for rapid reduction and realignment prior to proceeding with CT or other diagnostic studies (19, 35).

Dynamic flexion and extension x-rays are obtained after the CT scan in patients without evidence of fracture or obvious subluxation (19, 20, 35, 38). Magnetic resonance imaging (MRI) and/or water soluble myelography in conjunction with CT have value for selected patients with neurological injuries that are unexplained by the radiographic studies already obtained (1, 9, 19, 20, 35). These studies are also of value for preoperative evaluation of patients with bone fragments, disc material, or persistent subluxation compromising the spinal cord or nerve root structures. For patients with congenital anomalies of the spine who have neurological deficits, three-dimensional CT studies with myelography are often helpful in deciphering the complexities of the vertebral column and neural impingement after traumatic injury (18). This is particularly true for patients with skull base-proximal cervical spine congenital deformities. MRI has been used in SCIWORA patients, but the results have been disappointing in all but patients with complete neurological injuries (19, 20, 28, 31). Patients with incomplete neurological injuries have had normal cervical MRI studies without evidence of white matter signal changes or edema. Patients with complete deficits have had MRI studies which reveal increased water signals from the spinal cord at the level of injury.

TREATMENT

The treatment of pediatric spinal cord and vertebral column injuries must be individualized and depends on several important injury factors. These include: the age of the patient, the severity and the level of vertebral column or spinal cord injury, the type of injury, the degree of neurological compromise, and the presence of associated, nonvertebral injuries. In general, early surgical intervention is not indicated (19, 20, 33). Hadley et al. operated upon 16% of 122 pediatric spine injured patients (20) (Table 27.4). Similarly, 27% of 71 patients reviewed by Ruge et al. required operative reduction or stabilization (33). Few of these patients were operated upon within the first 4 days after injury. Most pediatric spine-injured patients can be managed by nonoperative means. The type and the duration of external immobilization are dependent upon the type, level, and severity of the injury. Age is less of a consideration with respect to nonoperative immobilization of pediatric patients with cervical spine injuries due to the increased utilization of pediatric halo-vest immobilization devices (6, 19–21, 33).

Table 27.4. Treatment

	Age Group (Years)		
Level	0–9	10–14	15–16
Bed rest	5	12	12
Collar			
Foam	2	3	
Philly	6	7	7
Halo vest		7	22
Cervico-thoracic brace	1		
SOMI brace	1	1	1
4-Poster brace		2	
Hyperextension brace		1	6
Bivalve body jacket			7
Early surgery	3	5	11
Totals	18	38	66

Reprinted with permission, Hadley MN, Zabramski JM, Browner CM, et al. Pediatric spinal trauma: a review of 122 cases of spinal cord and vertebral column injuries. J Neurosurg 1988;68:18–24.

A small percentage of patients will be excluded from nonoperative treatment (the very young, 0 to 3 years). Few patients will fail nonoperative external immobilization; therefore, compulsive follow-up is essential. Persistant dislocation, nonunion of fractures, and/or progressive kyphosis are indications for late surgical stabilization. The indications for early surgical therapy in the pediatric patient population are not well-defined but include nonreducible fracture-dislocations, patients with markedly unstable injuries, significant subluxation injuries without fracture, and patients with incomplete neurological injuries with x-ray documentation of spinal cord or nerve root compression (3, 11, 19, 20, 33, 34). Neurologically intact patients with radiographic evidence of neural compression and patients with complete neurological injuries less than 24 hours after injury with documented spinal cord compression may also be considered for surgical decompression (15, 19, 35).

When early surgery is indicated, most authors advocate proceeding between 2 and 10 days after injury (3, 11, 15, 19, 20, 33, 34). When a thoracic or lumbar decompression is performed a direct decompression of the offending compressive pathology is advocated followed by stabilization in a single operative procedure (3, 15, 19). Frequently, a team approach is employed, utilizing both orthopaedic and neurological surgeons.

The treatment of SCIWORA patients has undergone evolution as investigators have learned more about the injury syndrome (19–21, 28, 29, 31, 33, 37, 38). An algorithm which depicts the evaluation and treatment of pediatric spine-injured patients is listed in Figure 27.1. SCIWORA patients, patients with neurological injuries

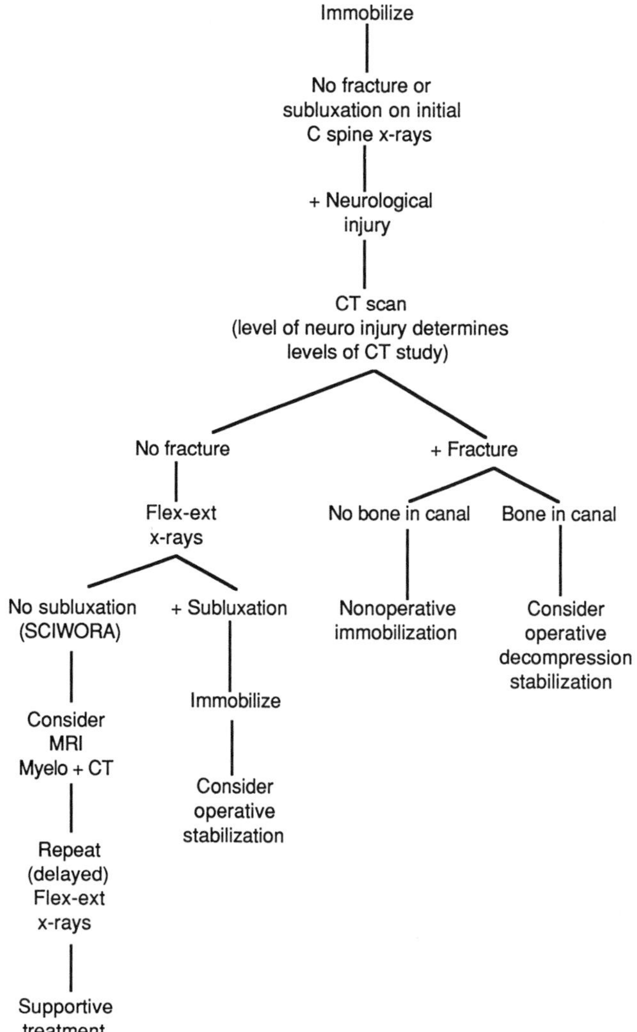

Figure 27.1. Treatment algorithm for suspected SCIWORA patients.

but without demonstrable radiographic abnormality, (by definition) require immobilization and aggressive supportive treatment. Close attention to patients with early, transient symptoms who appear neurologically intact must be maintained to assist with the identification of patients who will develop delayed SCIWORA. Delayed dynamic studies must be performed in all SCIWORA patients to rule-out subluxation and instability not appreciated at the initial assessment due to muscular guarding or rigidity (19, 28, 29, 31). Patients with mild to moderate SCIWORA who show signs of neurological recovery must be immobilized, restricted from activities and followed compulsively in the outpatient setting to prevent the occurrence of recurrent SCIWORA. Pollack, Pang, and Sclabassi have published a revised treatment protocol for these patients which includes the aforementioned measures and stresses the need for detailed follow-up with somatosensory evoked potential recording, parent-family education, and social worker participation to facilitate patient compliance (28, 31).

Outcome

In general, pediatric patients have a good prognosis after spinal cord and vertebral column injury (2, 19–21, 23, 33). Hadley et al. reported that 55 intact patients treated for fractures and/or subluxations remained intact at long-term follow-up (44 months, median) (20). Thirty-four of 38 patients (89%) with incomplete neurological injuries improved. Twenty-three of these patients were neurologically intact at last examination. Four of 20 patients with complete neurological injuries (20%) were improved at the time of the last examination; three regained significant motor and sensory function (20). Twenty patients, four incomplete and 16 with complete neurological injuries had no improvement in neurological function. These findings are similar to those reported by Hahn in which 90% of patients with incomplete injuries improved and 22% of patients with complete neurological injuries showed evidence of significant functional recovery with time (21, 33).

The relatively good outcome experienced by pediatric spine-injured patients when compared to adults probably relates to the rapid healing properties of the bony and ligamentous injuries in children (23), the plasticity of the nervous system in the young (10), the absence of underlying medical problems which are typical in adult patients, and the length of follow-up obtained (19, 20). Several of the patients who made neurological recoveries, particularly the patients with complete injuries, realized the improvements late after injury (improvements that may have been missed with a shorter follow-up) (19, 20, 33).

Summary

Children of all ages are susceptible to spinal cord and vertebral column injury. Approximately 5% of all spinal trauma will involve patients in the pediatric age population (0 to 16 years). The youngest patients (0 to 9 years of age) appear to be relatively resistant to vertebral column trauma due to several anatomical and physiological features of the immature spine. However, when they are injured they have a higher incidence of subluxation without fracture and SCIWORA, a higher incidence of occiput through C2 level injuries, and an increased incidence of neurological compromise compared to older children.

The frequency of SCIWORA is probably not as high as previously reported. Dangers with SCIWORA patients include delayed onset or delayed deterioration of neurological symptoms and recurrent episodes. Proper, compulsive evaluation and effective long-term immobilization can optimize the potential for recovery among SCIWORA patients. The treatment of pediatric spinal cord and vertebral column injuries must be individualized on the basis of the patient's age, neurological condition, and type and level of injury. Surgical therapy is infrequently required, and, in general, the prognosis for recovery after pediatric spinal trauma is good.

REFERENCES

1. Allen RI, Perot PL Jr, Gudeman SK. Evaluation of acute nonpenetrating cervical spinal cord injuries with CT metrizamide myelography. J Neurosurg 1985;63:510–520.

2. Beatson RT. Fractures and dislocations of the cervical spine. J Bone Joint Surg (Br) 1963;45:21–35.

3. Bohlman HH. Acute fractures and dislocations of the cervical spine. An analysis of three hundred hospitalized patients and review of the literature. J Bone Joint Surg (Am) 1979;61:1119–1142.

4. Brant-Zawadzki M, Miller EM, Federle MP. CT in the evaluation of spine trauma. AJR 1981;136:369–375.

5. Brown BM, Brant-Zawadzki M, Cann CE. Dynamic CT scanning of spinal column trauma. AJR 1982;139:1177–1181.

6. Browner CM, Hadley MN, Sonntag VKH, Mattingly LG. Halo immobilization brace care: an innovative approach. J Neurosci Nurs 1987;19:24–29.

7. Burke DC. Traumatic spinal paralysis in children. Paraplegia 1974;11:268–276.

8. Choi JU, Hoffman HJ, Hendrick EB, et al. Traumatic infarction of the spinal cord in children. J Neurosurg 1986;65:608–610.

9. Cooper PR, Cohen W. Evaluation of cervical spinal cord injuries with metrizamide myelography-CT scanning. J Neurosurg 1984;61:281–289.

10. Davis L. Treatment of spinal cord injuries. Arch Surg 1954;69:488–495.

11. Fielding JW. Injuries of the cervical spine in children. In: Rockwood CA Jr, Wilkins KE, King RE, eds, Fractures in children. Philadelphia: JB Lippincott, 1984.

12. Fischer RP. Cervical radiographic evaluation of alert patients following blunt trauma. Ann Emerg Med 1984;13:905–907.

13. Frankel HL, Hancock DO, Hyslop G, et al. The value of postural reduction in the initial management of closed injuries of the spine with paraplegia and tetraplegia. Paraplegia 1969;7:179–192.

14. Hadley MN, Browner CM, Sonntag VKH. Axis fractures: a comprehensive review of management and treatment in 107 cases. Neurosurgery 1985;17:281–290.

15. Hadley MN, Browner CM, Dickman CA, Sonntag VKH. Compression fractures of the thoracolumbar junction: a treatment algorithm based on 110 cases. BNI Quart 1989;5:10–19.

16. Hadley MN, Dickman CA, Browner CM, Sonntag VKH. Acute axis fractures; a review of 229 cases. J Neurosurg 1989;71:642.

17. Hadley MN, Dickman CA, Browner CM, Sonntag VKH. Acute traumatic atlas fractures: management and long term outcome. Neurosurgery 1988;23:31–35.

18. Hadley MN, Sonntag VKH, Amos MR, Hodak RTJ, Lopez LJ. Three-dimensional computed tomography in the diagnosis of vertebral column pathological conditions. Neurosurgery 1987;21:186–192.

19. Hadley MN, Sonntag VKH, Rekate HL. Pediatric vertebral column and spinal cord injuries. Contemp Neurosurg 1988;10:1–4.

20. Hadley MN, Zabramski JM, Browner CM, et al. Pediatric spinal trauma: a review of 122 cases of spinal cord and vertebral column injuries. J Neurosurg 1988;68:18–24.

21. Hahn Y. Pediatric cervical spinal cord injuries. Presentation at the Joint Section on Disorders of the Spine and Peripheral Nerves, AANS/CNS Meeting, Feb 13, 1989, Cancun, Mexico.

22. Henrys P, Lyne ED, Lifton C, et al. Clinical review of cervical spine injuries in children. Clin Orthop 1977;129:172–176.

23. Hubbard DD. Injuries of the spine in children and adolescents. Clin Orthop 1974;10:56–65.

24. Kewalramani LS, Kraus JF, Sterling HM. Acute spinal cord lesions in a pediatric population: epidemiological and clinical features. Paraplegia 1980;18:206–219.

25. Kewalramani LS, Tori JA. Spinal cord trauma in children: neurologic patterns, radiographic features and pathomechanics of injury. Spine 1980;5:11–18.

26. LeBlanc HJ, Nadell J. Spinal cord injuries in children. Surg Neurol 1974;2:411–414.

27. Menezes AH, Osenbach R. Spinal cord injuries in the young child (below age three years). Presentation at the Congress of Neurological Surgeons Annual Meeting, Sep 26, 1988, Seattle, WA.

28. Pang D. Spinal cord injury without radiographic abnormality. Presentation at the Joint Section on Disorders of the Spine and Peripheral Nerves, AANS/CNS Meeting, Feb 13, 1989, Cancun, Mexico.

29. Pang D, Wilberger JE Jr. Spinal cord injury without radiographic abnormalities in children. J Neurosurg 1982;57:114–129.

30. Papavasiliou V. Traumatic subluxation of the cervical spine during childhood. Orthop Clin North Am 1978;9:945–954.

31. Pollack IF, Pang D, Sclabassi R. Recurrent spinal cord injury without radiographic abnormalities in children. J Neurosurg 1988;69:177–182.

32. Roub LW, Drayer BP. Spinal computed tomography: limitations and applications. AJR 1979;133:267–273.

33. Ruge JR, Sinson GP, McLone DG, Cerulo LJ. Pediatric spinal injury: the very young. J Neurosurg 1988;68:25–30.

34. Sherk HH, Schut L, Lane JM. Fractures and dislocations of the cervical spine in children. Orthop Clin North Am 1976;7:593–604.

35. Sonntag VKH, Hadley MN. Nonoperative management of cervical spine injuries. Clin Neurosurg 1987;34:630–649.

36. Wales LR, Knopp RK, Morishima MS. Recommendations for evaluation of the acutely injured cervical spine: a clinical radiologic algorithm. Ann Emerg Med 1980;9:422–428.

37. Walsh JW, Stevens DB, Young AB. Traumatic paraplegia in children without contiguous spinal fracture or dislocation. Neurosurgery 1983;12:439–445.

38. Wilberger JE Jr. Spinal cord injuries in children. Mt Kisco, NY: Futura, 1986.

28

Penetrating Injuries of the Cervical Spine

Frank P. Cammisa, Jr., Frank J. Eismont, and Thomas Tolli

Although the incidence of penetrating injuries to the cervical spine continues to increase, controversy regarding the indications for surgical management persists. Gunshot wounds are the third most common cause of spinal cord injury (SCI), following only automobile accidents and falls (52). Treatment has largely been based on the military experience with war-time injuries secondary to high velocity missiles. However, in our society, the vast majority of penetrating injuries of the cervical spine are due to low velocity missiles and sharp instruments. This chapter will discuss the mechanism of injury and treatment of penetrating injuries of the cervical spine in the civilian population.

Mechanism of Injury

The extent of injury caused by a missile is dependent on several factors. Since kinetic energy is one-half the product of the mass and velocity squared, it becomes obvious that high velocity missiles have the ability to impart more energy and thereby cause more serious injury than low velocity missiles (9). However, one must also consider the interaction of the projectile and the type of tissue it has entered (12). Neurological injury due to high velocity missiles is not dependent on a direct penetration of neural tissues. Indirect injury occurs as shock waves transmit energy from adjacent tissues to the spinal cord. In contrast, many penetrating spinal cord injuries in the civilian population are caused by handguns which propel low velocity missiles. Therefore, the kinetic energy transmitted in such injuries is much lower, and direct injury to the spinal cord and adjacent structures is often required to produce neurological deficit. Usually, the bullet or a fragment does enter the spinal canal and may remain. Therefore, low velocity missiles are often associated with retained fragments and may be a major consideration in choosing surgical treatment.

In other penetrating trauma such as knife wounds, direct injury to neural tissues is the most likely mechanism of injury, and retained foreign bodies are not a major consideration.

Emergency Treatment

Treatment must address not only the vertebral column and neural elements but also the associated vital structures situated in the neck region. Therefore, treatment in the emergency setting must include a thorough examination. The tenets of emergency medical care ("ABC's"—airway, breathing, circulation) must be strictly adhered to. Serial physical examinations should be performed at regular intervals and changes of neurologic status should be documented. Knowledge of the anatomy and physiology of the nervous system is important for accurate interpretation of neurologic findings.

Radiographic Evaluation

Complete radiographic evaluation of the patient with a penetrating wound to the neck is essential. Initially, plain radiographs of the neck and chest should be obtained in all patients. Penetrating injuries may violate the pharynx; esophagus; trachea; vascular structures such as the carotid, vertebral arteries, and jugular veins; peripheral nerves; vertebral column; and the spinal cord. Therefore, plain radiographs may reveal such abnormalities as air in the soft tissues, widening mediastinum, or fracture of the vertebrae. Angiography may be beneficial in detecting occult vascular injuries. Overall, if arteriography is combined with surgical exploration, the mortality and morbidity related to vascular and visceral injuries in the neck may be decreased.

In terms of spinal injuries, plain radiography and tomography have been the primary methods employed in the evaluation of patients with penetrating wounds. These studies may indicate the extent of bony involvement, and may help assess the stability of the spine. Computed tomography (CT) is an efficient technique for localization of bony fragments as it allows imaging in the axial plane (33). As well as allowing identification of metallic or bony fragments in the canal, it may also determine the extent of soft tissue lesions. Magnetic resonance imaging (MRI) may prove to be helpful in the evaluation of penetrating injuries to the spine. However, one must realize that MRI may cause complications in patients who have fragments made of ferrous materials. MRI may cause fragment motion or migration as a result of the electromagnetic field generated. Furthermore, ferrous materials may cause distortion of the images obtained. Fragments containing lead may produce image signal loss in the fragment itself but may allow for clear imaging of the surrounding tissues (11).

Myelography in general is not recommended as part of the routine radiographic work-up. Bloody cerebrospinal fluid with contrast medium may increase the incidence of arachnoiditis.

SURGICAL EXPLORATION

Debate continues regarding surgical exploration of patients with penetrating injuries without obvious vascular or visceral damage. Penetrating injuries are defined as those deep to the platysma muscle. Roon et al. (37) recommended surgical exploration of the neck in all stable patients with wounds that penetrate the platysma. In contrast, Flax et al. (14) proposed specific indications for surgical exploration of the neck wounds that penetrate the platysma. Surgical exploration was performed for continued hemorrhage, subcutaneous emphysema, or progression of neurological deficits. Additional complications were sudden voice change; difficulty swallowing or breathing; large or expanding hematoma; and coughing, spitting, or vomiting blood.

If vascular damage is present in patients with penetrating injuries, then the appropriate vascular management is indicated. Repair of the carotid artery is generally recommended, while ligation is generally recommended for vertebral artery injuries. Roon et al. (37) did not recommend the use of prosthetic grafts in penetrating wounds, as they are all potentially contaminated. In the specific case of an extensively damaged carotid artery with ipsilateral severe focal neurological deficits, Roon et al. suggested ligation rather than repair.

After assessment and treatment of the neck wound, the treatment of the spinal injury ensues. The indications for surgical treatment of spinal injuries is controversial. In general, the goals of surgical treatment are prevention of infection and optimization of neurologic recovery. Surgery includes debridement with or without removal of retained fragments within the canal. Numerous reports have addressed these issues. Many reports, especially those based on the military experience, favor debridement and removal of bullet fragment from the canal. Others favor debridement of soft tissue but canal exploration only if neurologic deficits are progressive.

Debridement is generally indicated for prevention of infection, especially if the bullet has passed through a contaminated viscus. Removal of intracanal fragments is favored by many, as it potentially prevents complications such as cerebrospinal fluid leak, meningitis, lead toxicity, pain, and progressive neurologic deficit secondary to fragment migration or chronic fibrosis. Furthermore, many feel it enhances neurologic recovery.

Those who are against fragment removal feel that there is no evidence of neurologic recovery after bullet removal and that the risk of surgery outweighs the risk of a retained intracanal fragment.

The issue of debridement for prevention of infection will be addressed first. In the past, surgical exploration and debridement has generally been indicated in penetrating injuries of the cervical spine that initially traverse the pharynx, esophagus, larynx, or trachea prior to traumatizing the spinal column. Schaefer et al. (39, 40) reported osteomyelitis as a potential complication of a transesophageal cervical spine gunshot wound. In order to minimize the risk of cervical osteomyelitis, a strict treatment protocol was proposed. They perform endoscopy initially to confirm the transesophageal course of the missile and to assess the mucosal injury. Surgery includes primary repair of damaged viscera. Debridement includes removal of devitalized tissues such as ligaments, disc, and bone. Cultures for aerobic and anaerobic organisms are taken. Appropriate prophylactic antibiotics are instituted and maintained for a period of 7 to 10 days. A penrose drain is used for 2 to 3 days. Patients with spinal instability are placed in a halo-vest for approximately 6 weeks.

Craig et al. (7) reported two cases of osteomyelitis after gunshot wounds to the neck. The patients were initially treated nonoperatively, and both were later found to have esophageal injuries. Failure to diagnose esophageal injury was felt to have contributed to subsequent infections.

This situation is analogous to injuries in the thoracic and lumbar spine. It is felt that penetration of the colon prior to spinal injury is best treated by early surgical intervention. Romanick et al. (36) have reviewed 20 patients with thoracic and lumbar spine injuries secondary to low velocity gunshot wounds to the abdomen. All patients were treated conservatively with intravenous antibiotics for at least 48 hours. Maximum duration of antibiotics was 5 days. Infection was not present in any of the eight patients without associated gastrointestinal injury or in four patients in whom the small intestine or stomach was violated. In contrast, seven of eight patients with an associated colon injury prior to vertebral column trauma developed infection. It was felt that a nonoperative approach was satisfactory for gunshot wounds of the abdomen that did not involve the colon. However, perforation of the colon prior to injuring the vertebra was associated with a high incidence of infection. Therefore, it was felt that in such situations, early operative intervention was indicated. This experience further supports the view that penetrating cervical injuries involving the pharynx, the esophagus, larynx, and trachea should be surgically debrided.

Controversy now exists concerning these recommendations, however. Roffi et al. (35) reviewed 42 patients with low velocity gunshot wounds to the spine with an associated perforated viscus in order to assess the roles of initial antibiotic therapy and early bullet removal. Only three patients developed documented spinal or paraspinal infections. One patient developed acute meningitis after isolated stomach perforation, while two other patients developed psoas abscesses after colon injuries. In 21 of their 42 patients, adequate records were available to determine the type and duration of the initial antibiotic therapy. Three of the 21 patients developed infections as noted. In the 18 patients without infection, the average duration of initial intravenous antibiotics was 11 days. Eight cases with colon perforations had an average of 13 days of initial antibiotic therapy, and only the two paraspinal infections occurred as noted above. The initial antibiotics were always broad spectrum in coverage.

Concerning early bullet fragment removal, Roffi et al. (35) found that it did not appear to be a significant factor in prevention of infection. Thirty-five of the 42 patients had bullet fragments lodged within the spinal canal, disc space, or vertebral body. No bullet fragments in the disc space or vertebral body were removed. Seventeen patients had debridement and bullet removal from the spinal canal via a posterior approach. The rationale for removal was to enhance recovery in cases of incomplete neurologic injuries, except for one patient with meningitis and another with multiple abscesses, where removal was felt necessary for control of the infection. In one patient who developed a psoas abscess, both fragments were lodged in the spinal canal and never removed. Eighteen patients had bullet fragments left in and around the vertebral column without subsequent evidence of infection. Nine of these 18 cases had associated colon perforations, while six had isolated stomach injuries.

Based on this experience, it may not be necessary to debride every spinal injury caused by a bullet traversing a contaminated viscus. In comparison to the study of Romanick et al. (36), it appears that the longer course of antibiotic therapy accounted for the low incidence of infection and obviated the need for routine bullet removal in order to prevent infection. It is important that a prophylactic antibiotic regimen provide broad spectrum coverage of aerobic and anaerobic organisms, including gram negatives. It appears from this study of Roffi et al. (35) that early bullet removal and debridement does not significantly affect the infection rate.

The results of this study are further supported by the prospective study of Waters and Adkins (49). Of 90 cases of penetrating gunshot wounds to the spine, 19 had the bullet pass through the alimentary canal prior to entering the spinal canal. In 10 of these cases, the bullets were left within the canal, and in the remaining nine, the bullets were removed. No cases of meningitis or spinal infection were reported in either group, supporting the contention that with adequate antibiotic therapy, debridement for prevention of infection may not be necessary. Although it appears that debridement is not necessary in the civilian population, it may not be true for military gunshot wounds. Military injuries are often suffered in the field under conditions which are favorable for contamination. This, combined with the greater tissue destruction caused by high velocity missiles, increases the probability of contamination. Therefore, the data present above may not be applicable to military injuries.

The second issue of surgical treatment of penetrating cervical injuries for optimization of neurologic recovery is also controversial. Simpson et al. (42, 43), retrospectively reviewed a total of 160 cases of penetrating spine injuries affecting the cervical, thoracic, and lumbar spine. Associated injuries of the esophagus, trachea, bronchi, or bowel were present in 107 (67%) of the cases. Gunshot wounds accounted for 142 of the injuries, while only 18 cases were the result of knife wounds. The cervical spine was injured in 27% of the cases, while the thoracic spine and lumbosacral spine were involved in 54% and 19% of the cases, respectively. Surgical treatment was undertaken in 31 (20%) of the patients suffering from gunshot wounds and in 6 (33%) of patients with stab wounds, for a total of 37 patients. Laminectomy was performed in 34 patients, and 20 of these had intradural explorations. The remaining patients had wound exploration and debridement only. Of the surgically-treated patients with complete paraplegia or quadriplegia, only 2 (13%) improved, 13 (81%) were unchanged, and 1 (6%) worsened. Similar results were obtained with nonsurgical treatment was employed as 12 (15%) improved, 64 (82%) remained unchanged, and 2 (3%) worsened. Of the cases involving incomplete neurologic deficits, surgical treatment resulted in 6 patients (40%) improving, 6 (40%) remaining unchanged, and 3 (20%) worsening. Nonoperative management resulted in 19 (58%) patients improving, 8 (24%) with no change, and 6 (18%) deteriorating. Of 4 cases with complete neurologic deficits secondary to stab wounds, 2 were surgically treated, 1 had neurologic improvement, while the other showed no change. With conservative management, the remaining 2 patients showed no change. In the 4 stab wound patients with incomplete neurologic lesions treated surgically, 2 improved, 1 did not change, and 1 worsened postoperatively. Conservative management resulted in improvement in 7 patients and no change in 3. In this study, surgical treatment did not improve neurologic recovery.

Heiden et al. (17) studied 38 civilian cervical gunshot injuries. Of the 25 patients with complete neurologic deficits, 16 (64%) were treated with laminectomy and debridement. The remaining 9 (36%) patients were treated conservatively. The type of treatment provided did not affect recovery as none of the patients with complete lesions showed any significant improvement. The group of 9 patients with incomplete neurologic deficits included 8 with the Brown-Sequard syndrome and 1 with a progressive deficit. Laminectomy performed on 5 (62%) of the patients with the Brown-Sequard syndrome resulted in clinical improvement. Similar improvement was noted in the 3 patients treated conservatively. The single patient with the progressive deficit failed to improve despite the laminectomy. No neurologic deficit was reported in the final group of 4 patients who suffered from cervical spine fractures. They were treated in Minerva jackets, and neurologic deterioration did not occur. From these data, Heiden et al. concluded that surgical therapy did not affect neurologic recovery.

Yashon (51) analyzed the efficacy of surgical treatment in 42 patients with gunshot wounds injuring the spinal cord and 23 with similar injuries to the conus medullaris and cauda equina. The patients were separated into four groups depending on their neurologic deficit. Thirty-five patients suffered immediate complete loss of function above the level of the conus medullaris. In this group, the cervical cord was involved in 6 (17%) patients and the thoracic cord in 29 (82%). Laminectomy was performed in 24 (68%) of the cases, while the others were treated nonoperatively. Significant functional recovery was not reported regardless of treatment undertaken. The three other groups of patients studied (incomplete deficits, progressive deficits, conus/cauda injuries) did not include cervical injuries. However, in no group was surgery found to improve neurologic recovery.

Six et al. (44) evaluated 59 cases with gunshot wounds affecting the neural elements. The cervical spine was injured in 17 cases, while the thoracic, lumbar, and sacral areas were involved in 30, 11, and 1 cases, respectively. Operative treatment was employed in 43 (72.8%) of the patients. This consisted of debridement and laminectomy, with or without dural repair, as well as excision of fragments. Of the 23 patients with complete sensory and motor loss who underwent surgery, 2 (8.6%) improved, 15 (65%) had no change, and 1 (4.3%) worsened. Nonoperative treatment resulted in 1 (4.3%) patient improving. Evaluation of cases with incomplete neurologic deficits revealed partial recovery of function in all patients, regardless of whether surgery was performed. All patients with cauda equina lesions underwent surgery, and 8 (66%) improved, while 4 (33%) remained unchanged. Thus, neurologic recovery was again unrelated to the type of therapy provided.

Of the 185 patients with low velocity gunshot wounds studied by Stauffer et al. (45), 106 (57%) had complete deficits. Fifty-six (52%) underwent laminectomy. One patient in this group had return of some function. The remaining 50 patients with complete lesions were treated nonoperatively and had no functional improvement. Incomplete lesions were present in 45 patients undergoing laminectomy, of whom 32 (71%) improved. In contrast, nonoperative therapy was employed in 34 patients with incomplete lesions, and spontaneous recovery was evident in 26 (76.5%). Therefore, Stauffer et al. were unable to show any significant improvement in neurologic function in patients treated with laminectomy.

In an effort to determine the effects of removal of bullet fragments retained in the spinal canal, a collaborative study by the National Spinal Cord Injury Model Systems was conducted by Waters and Adkins (49). Serial neurologic examinations were conducted on 90 patients with bullet fragments lodged in the spinal canal. Annual follow-up examinations were completed on 66 patients. Detailed statistical analyses revealed that the removal of bullet fragments made no significant difference with regard to reducing pain and improving the recovery of sensation. However, bullet removal did have an effect on motor recovery, depending on the level at which the lesion occurred. The number of cervical cases was only 14. Specifically, the small proportion of cervical cases from whom the bullet was removed did not allow for adequate testing of the effect of bullet removal. Therefore, no specific recommendations could be made regarding cervical injuries with a retained bullet fragment, whether the lesion is complete or incomplete. However, it should be noted that among those patients with lesions between the vertebral levels T12 and L4, there was a significantly greater motor recovery in those patients from whom the bullet was removed compared to that in patients not have bullet removal. Bullet removal from the canal between T1 and T11 had no significant effect on motor recovery. Therefore, the indications for bullet removal in the cervical spine are unclear. In incomplete quadriplegia with plateau of function, it may be reasonable to remove a space-occupying bullet fragment to enhance root recovery. However, further clinical study will be needed to substantiate such an approach.

Only one review specifically addresses stab wounds of the spine. Peacock et al. (32) reviewed 450 stab wounds of the spinal cord with 20 patients (4.4%) having laminectomy for cerebral spinal fluid leakage and/or foreign body removal. No comparison was made between surgical and nonsurgical treatment. Overall, good results were noted in 65.6% of patients, as walking with minimal support was possible. Fair recovery was noted in 17.1% of patients, and 17.3% had no significant functional recovery. Their treatment included prophylactic antibiotics along with early mobilization and intense rehabilitation in an effort to obtain maximal independence.

It should be noted that spinal cord pathology at the time of laminectomy rarely provides useful information that will allow the surgeon to predict the ultimate neurologic recovery (45). The microvascular blood supply to the central gray matter is sensitive to trauma. Injury of the cord parenchyma results in decreased perfusion, hypoxia, and microhemorrhage in the gray matter of the cord. The external cord surface may appear anatomically intact, but within hours, irreversible hemorrhagic necrosis occurs in the central cord.

Postoperative complications may result after surgical

treatment of penetrating injuries to the spine. Stauffer et al. (45) reported deep wound infections in four patients and spinal fluid fistulae in six patients. This represents 10% of all surgically-treated cases. The nonoperative group did not encounter such problems. Although conservatively treated patients did not suffer from spinal instability, six (6%) of those who underwent laminectomy developed instability requiring fusion. Simpson (42, 43) reported meningitis, spinal fluid leakage, and wound infections in 22% of patients treated surgically, and only 7% of those treated nonoperatively. Waters and Adkins, however, found that secondary complications (within one year of injury) including cerebral spinal fluid leak, pain, meningitis, and lead toxicity were not influenced by surgery for bullet removal. In a previous study by Waters (48), no significant differences were found with regard to early complications (within 1 month of injury) such as cerebral fluid leak, meningitis, or pain between patients nonoperatively or operatively treated.

It is important that patients with irreversible neurologic dysfunction start an intense rehabilitation program as soon as possible (44).

SEQUELAE OF PENETRATING INJURIES

There are several uncommon sequelae of penetrating spinal injuries which have been reported in the literature. Although rare, traumatic aneurysms of the carotid or vertebral arteries are often due to direct penetration of the vessels. Diagnosing an arteriovenous fistula is usually simple, as a pulsatile mass and bruit may be present. However, distinguishing carotid from vertebral artery lesions is often difficult and requires angiography (34, 38, 41). Treatment includes excision of the aneurysms with possible grafting of the carotid or ligations of the vertebral artery.

Retained foreign bodies in the spinal canal may cause myelopathy. A rare cause of delayed cervical myelopathy was reported 17 years after an injury from a bombshell (1). The patient was asymptomatic for 17 years until left-sided weakness of the shoulder girdle and upper extremity developed. The fragment entered the right side of the neck and migrated to the left side of the subarachnoid space without causing spinal cord damage. The fragment was found intradurally with an envelope of fibrous tissue. The neurologic condition improved after removal of the fragment.

An interesting historical fact involves the assassination of President John F. Kennedy. Thornburn (47) reported that trauma to the spinal cord at the sixth cervical level results in abduction of the arms and flexion of the elbows. Lattimer et al. (21) concluded that the first bullet striking Kennedy injured the spine at the C6 level, causing the sudden upward jerk of his arms with elbows flexed, as seen on the Zapruder films. The cord injury was felt to be due to concussive force rather than a direct injury.

A rare case of acute lead intoxication from a bullet in the intervertebral disc space (16) has been described. Lumbar disc herniation secondary to a gunshot wound (25) has occurred. Spontaneous migration of bullets has also been known to occur (2, 20). Bullet fragments have been reported to migrate from the brain to the spinal cord (2), throughout the spinal canal (20, 46), and to other body cavities (22, 29).

SUMMARY

Penetrating injuries to the neck region must be treated aggressively by a multidisciplinary trauma team. Vascular and visceral injuries must be handled expeditiously by the appropriate surgical specialist. Although controversy exists concerning spinal injuries, it would appear from the most recent studies that wounds caused by bullets penetrating the esophagus, pharynx, larynx, or trachea do not need immediate spine debridement but do need appropriate prophylactic antibiotic care. Injuries to the bony vertebral column must be assessed for stability and treated accordingly. The indications for operative intervention for neurologic recovery are also controversial. In cases of progressive deficit, a cause of progressive compression of the cord must be identified which can be relieved by surgery. Otherwise, the cause of progressive neurologic loss is probably secondary to continued hypoxemia and necrosis. The removal of retained fragments within the canal has been shown to be efficacious only in the area of the cauda equina, not in the cervical cord. The only exceptions may be for relief of root compression or the rare case of late myelopathy secondary to migration of a fragment with resultant cord compression. The importance of early intense rehabilitation cannot be overemphasized.

REFERENCES

1. Amitani K, Tsuyuguchi Y, Hukuda S. Delayed cervical myelopathy caused by bombshell fragment: a case report. J Neurosurg 1976;44:626–627.

2. Arasil E, Tascioglu AO. Spontaneous migration of an internal intracranial bullet to the cervicospinal canal causing Lhermitte's sign. J Neurosurg 1982;56:158–159.

3. Arishita GI, Bayer JS, Bellamy RF. Cervical spine immobilization of penetrating neck wounds in a hostile environment. J Trauma 1989;29:332–337.

4. Benzel EC, Hadden TA, Coleman JE. Civilian gunshot wounds to the spinal cord and cauda equina. J Neurosurg 1987;20:281–285.

5. Christy JP. Complications of combat casualties with combined injuries of bone and bowel: personal experience with 19 patients. Surgery 1972;71:270–274.

6. Coleman JE, Benzel EC, Hadden TA. Gunshot wounds to the spinal cord and cauda equina in civilians. Surg Forum 1986;37:496–498.

7. Craig JB. Cervical spine osteomyelitis with delayed onset tetraparesis after penetrating wounds of neck. S Afr Med J 1986;69:197–199.

8. Das PB. Simultaneous penetrating injury of the trachea and esoph-

agus by knife jammed into the vertebral body. Int Surg 1976;61:160–161.

9. DeMuth WE. Bullet velocity and design as determinants of wounding capability: an experimental study. J Trauma 1966;6:222–232.

10. Ducker TB, Bellegarrigue R, Salcman M, Walleck C. Timing of operative care in cervical spinal cord injury. Spine 1984;9:525–531.

11. Ebraheim NA, Savolaine ER, Jackson WT, Andreshak TT, Rayport M. Magnetic resonance imaging in the evaluation of a gunshot wound to the cervical spine. J Orthop Trauma 1989;3:19–22.

12. Fackler ML. Wound ballistics: a review of common misconceptions. JAMA 1988;259:2730–2736.

13. Fife D, Kraus J. Anatomic location of spinal cord injury: relationship to the cause of injury. Spine 1986;11:2–5.

14. Flax RL, Fletcher HS, Joseph WL. Management of penetrating injuries of the neck. Am J Surg 1973;39:148–150.

15. Gordon DS. Surgery of violence: missile wounds of the head and spine. Br Med J 1975;1:614–616.

16. Grogan VP, Bucholz RQ. Acute lead intoxication from a bullet and intervertebral disk space. J Bone Joint Surg 1981;63A:1180–1182.

17. Heiden JS, Weiss MH, Rosenberg AW, Curze T, Apuzzo MLJ. Penetrating gunshot wounds of the cervical spine in civilians: review of 38 cases. J Neurosurg 1975;42:575–579.

18. Jacobson SA, Bor SE. Spinal cord injury in Vietnamese combat. Paraplegia 1970;7:263–281.

19. Jones RE, Bucholz RW, Schaefer ST, Carter HM. Cervical osteomyelitis complicating transpharyngeal gunshot wounds. J Trauma 1979;19:630–634.

20. Karim MO, Nabors NW, Golocobsky MN, Cooney FD. Spontaneous migration of a bullet in the spinal subarachnoid space causing delayed radicular symptoms. Neurosurgery 1986;18:97–100.

21. Lattimer JK, Schlesinger EV, Merritt HH. President Kennedy's spine hit by first bullet. Bull NY Acad Med 1977;53:280–291.

22. Ledgerwood AM. The wandering bullet. Surg Clin North Am 1977;57:97–109.

23. Linden MA, Manton WI, Stewart RM, Thal ER, Feit H. Lead poisoning from retained bullets: pathogenesis, diagnosis, and management. Ann Surg 1982;195:305–313.

24. Maier RV, Carrico CJ, Heimbach DM. Pyogenic osteomyelitis of axial bones following civilian gunshot wounds. Am J Surg 1979;137:378–380.

25. Mariottini A, Delfini R, Ciappetta P, Paolella G. Lumbar disk hernia secondary to gunshot injury. Neurosurg 1984;15:73–75.

26. McInnis WD, Cruz AB, Aust JB. Penetrating injuries to the neck: pitfalls in management. Am J Surg 1975;130:416–420.

27. Mektubjian SR. Low velocity gunshot maxillofacial injury combined with a "blind" wound of the neck: a case report. J Max-Fac Surg 1981;9:85–88.

28. Miller R, Davis B. Fracture of the odontoid from a gunshot wound: a case report. Contemp Orthop 1989;454–456.

29. Morrow JS, Haycock CE, Lazaro E. The "swallowed bullet" syndrome. J Trauma 1978;18:464–466.

30. Ohry A, Rozin R. Acute spinal cord injuries in the Lebanon War, 1982. Isr J Med Sci 1984;20:345–349.

31. Pattisapu JV, Al-Mefty O. Gunshot wound to the odontoid process: a case report. Spine 1987;12:1052–1054.

32. Peacock WJ, Shrosbreedtkey AG. A review of 450 stab wounds of the spinal cord. S Afr Med J 1977;51:961–964.

33. Plumley TF, Kilcoyne RF, Mack LA. Computed tomography in evaluation of gunshot wounds of the spine. J Comput Assist Tomogr 1983;7:310–312.

34. Robinson NA, Slotte CT. Traumatic aneurysms of the carotid artery. Ann Surg 1974;40:121–124.

35. Roffi RP, Waters RL, Adkins RH. Gunshot wounds to the spine associated with a perforated viscus. Spine 1989;14:808–811.

36. Romanick PC, Smith TK, Kopaniky DR, Altfield D. Infection about the spine associated with low velocity missile injury to the abdomen. J Bone Joint Surg 1985;67A:1195–1201.

37. Roon AJ, Christensen N. Evaluation and treatment of penetrating cervical injuries. J Trauma 1979;19:391–397.

38. Rothman SLG, Pratt AG, Kier EL, Allen WE. Traumatic vertebral-carotid-jugular arteriovenous aneurysm: a case report. J Neurosurg 1974;41:92–96.

39. Schaefer SD, Bucholz RW, Jones RE, Anderson RG, Carder HM. "How I do it"—head and neck. A targeted problem and its solution. Treatment of transpharyngeal missile wounds to the cervical spine. Laryngoscope 1981;91:146–148.

40. Schaefer SD, Bucholz RW, Jones RE, Carder HM. The management of transpharyngeal gunshot wound to the cervical spine. Surg Gynecol Obstet 1981;152:27–29.

40. Sherk HH, Giri N, Nicholson JT. Gunshot wound with fracture of the atlas and arteriovenous fistula of the vertebral artery. J Bone Joint Surg 1974;56A:1738–1740.

42. Simpson RK, Venger VH, Narayan RK. Penetrating spinal cord injury in a civilian population: a retrospective analysis (1980–1985). Surg Forum 1986;37:494–496.

43. Simpson RK, Venger VH, Narayan RK. Treatment of acute penetrating injuries of the spine: a retrospective analysis. J Trauma 1989;29:42–46.

44. Six E, Alexander E, Kelly DL, Davis CH, McWhorter JM. Gunshot wounds to the spinal cord. South Med J 1978;72:699–702.

45. Stauffer ES, Wood RW, Kelly EG. Gunshot wound of the spine: the effects of laminectomy. J Bone Joint Surg 1979;61A:389–392.

46. Tanguy BA, Chabannes J, Deubelle A, Vanneueville G, Dalens B. The intraspinal migration of a bullet with subsequent meningitis. J Bone Joint Surg 1982;64A:1244–1245.

47. Thornburn W. Cases of injury to the cervical region of the spinal cord: position of the elbows after injury to C6 (level confirmed at autopsy). Brain 1886–1887;9:510–543.

48. Waters RL. Spinal cord injuries due to gunshot wounds. J Am Paraplegia Soc 1984;7:30–33.

49. Waters RL, Adkins RH. The effects of removal of bullet fragments retained in the spinal canal: a collaborative study by The National Spinal Cord Injury Model Systems. Spine 1991;16:934–939.

50. Wu WQ. Delayed effects from retained foreign bodies in the spine and spinal cord. Surg Neurol 1986;25:214–218.

51. Yashon D, Jane JA, White RJ. Prognosis and management of spinal cord and cauda equina bullet injuries in 65 civilians. J Neurosurg 1970;32:163–170.

52. Young JS, Burns PE, Bowen AM, McCotchen R. Spinal cord injury statistics, experience of the Regional Spinal Cord Injury Systems. Phoenix, Arizona: Good Samaritan Medical Center, 1982:152 pp.

29

Brachial Plexus and Root Avulsion Injuries

Hanno Millesi

Etiology

The most frequent cause of traumatic brachial plexus lesions are motorcycle accidents. The high energy involved in these injuries produce the most severe damage to the brachial plexus. Usually, they are closed injuries, but they may or may not be accompanied by rupture of the subclavian or axillary artery or vein. Less severe damage results when the patient is involved in a motor vehicle-pedestrian or automobile accident. Infrequent causes are sports injuries (skiing, horseback riding), seat belts during car accidents, or job-related accidents. Open injuries with sharp transection such as gunshot wounds or by knife or glass lacerations are rare. In cases of transection by a sharp instrument such as knife or glass, usually the upper trunk is involved. Gunshot injuries produce a complete loss of continuity of those elements of the brachial plexus which are directly hit by the projectile. A shock wave caused by a high velocity projectile damages other parts of the brachial plexus, but this damage is to a lesser degree and has a better chance for spontaneous recovery. Stretch lesions develop after carrying heavy weights (1) especially in soldiers (paralysie du paguetage) (2–4).

Iatrogenic lesions may accidentally occur during surgery with transection of brachial plexus structures or after planned resection of segments during tumor surgery. A brachial plexus lesion may occur after plexus anesthesia or may be the result of compression intraoperatively due to positioning. Obstetric brachial plexus lesions may occur during normal delivery in cases of a narrow pelvis (5). Usually, though, they are the consequence of manipulations associated with complicated deliveries. Brachial plexus lesions caused by irradiation, tumors, chronic compressions, or inflammation will not be discussed in this chapter.

Pathogenetic Mechanisms

Most frequently the elements of the brachial plexus are damaged by traction. The whole length of the brachial plexus is involved if the skeletal protection against traction is lost as a result of a fracture of the humerus or a dislocation of the shoulder joint as the arm is displaced away from the body. If this movement has a purely lateral direction, C7 is more involved and sustains injury first. If the movement is in a downward direction, C5 and C6 are more exposed to traction, and if the movement is upward in direction C8 and T1 are affected first (6). The intradural course of the roots may contribute to a different sensitivity against traction. Increased growth of the cervical spinal cord is the reason why the root C5 crosses horizontally to the intervertebral foramen in contrast to the upper roots which descend to the foramen and the roots C6 through T1, which ascend to their intervertebral foramen (7).

Compression is another mechanism in brachial plexus injuries occurring between the clavicle and the first rib if the shoulder is hit directly by a heavy object or if the patient strikes an obstacle directly.

Compression and traction can be combined if according to the above mechanisms the brachial plexus is compressed between the clavicle and the first rib and the head of the patient moves in a contralateral direction. In this case the plexus segments proximal to the clavicle are exposed to traction. The brachial plexus can be damaged directly by bony fragments as a result of a fracture of the clavicle or by a transverse process of the spine. Additional damage might be caused by compression due to swelling or a hematoma with consequent fibrosis. Narakas (8) states that this may occur with associated vascular lesions which occur in 27% of all cases.

Clinical Diagnosis and Indications for Surgery

A brachial plexus lesion usually results from severe trauma. Frequently this patient has suffered multiple injuries, and therefore life-saving procedures have priority with the treatment of a brachial plexus lesion delayed for an early secondary repair. An open injury is an indication for immediate surgery. A clean transection can be assumed if there is a wound in the supraclavicular fossa with a corresponding functional loss. Usually, the upper trunk and rarely the middle trunk are involved. After a clean transection, nerve repair is performed as a primary neurorrhaphy. An open injury with vascular damage requires immediate vascular repair. At the same time the brachial plexus should be explored only if an expert in brachial plexus anatomy and surgery is available. Otherwise, additional damage may be caused. Frequently, patients are referred after primary vascular repair with the information that the concomitant brachial plexus has been explored and the transected stumps marked by silver clips. This is not helpful since the additional scar tissue caused by the primary exploration makes the secondary procedure more challenging.

Immediate exploration is indicated with signs of hematoma formation in the supra- and infraclavicular area and associated vascular insufficiency of the upper extremity. Evacuation of the hematoma and vascular repair should be performed expeditiously. Exploration of the brachial plexus with primary repair is indicated only if an expert in brachial plexus surgery is available and the condition of the patient allows a prolonged procedure.

Fractures of the clavicle and the transverse process with associated neurologic symptoms are indications for primary surgery to remove compression or irritation of the brachial plexus by bony fragments.

When there is a closed injury associated with a brachial plexus lesion, a decision must be made whether a primary exploration should be performed or the patient referred for a secondary repair. If the overall condition of the patient permits and an expert in brachial plexus surgery is available, a primary exploration may be considered, otherwise the procedure should be deferred. The arguments for primary exploration at a special center are (9):

1. No loss of time;
2. The exploration is easier because no fibrosis has developed yet.

The arguments against primary exploration at a center with an expert available are:

1. The amount of damage cannot initially be evaluated precisely.
2. The damaged nerves may be repaired but will develop secondary fibrosis.
3. The medical status of a patient may not be favorable for a long procedure.
4. In cases of 1st or 2nd degree lesions, although immediate exploration is not indicated, it may be difficult for the surgeon to exclude these cases from primary surgery.

In general, in a closed injury it is best to schedule the patient for early secondary surgery. In the interval the patient should receive adequate physiotherapy, have his neurologic parameters observed, and the exact clinical diagnosis confirmed. After several days to 1 week, Wallerian degeneration develops in all motor fibers having suffered damage of second degree or more, and conductivity is lost. Nerves suffering a 1st degree injury will have preserved conductivity, and this can be confirmed by an EMG study. Therefore, 1st degree lesions can be excluded at this time whereas they may not have been apparent immediately after injury.

In the case of a 2nd degree lesion, a Tinel Hoffmann sign will develop and proceed in a distal direction. After 2 to 3 months signs of early recovery may be noticed in proximal muscle groups. As long as there are signs of progressive recovery conservative treatment should be continued. When no further progress is noted and the Tinel Hoffmann sign stops at a certain point surgical exploration is considered. The reason for such a course in a 2nd degree lesion may be the development of fibrosis, and in those cases where neurolysis is performed an excellent prognosis can be expected.

In cases of a 3rd degree lesion, a Tinel Hoffmann sign will develop. It may progress beyond the site of the lesion, but the punctum maximum does not change, and no sign of recovery is noted in proximal muscles. If there is no improvement within 3 or 4 months, surgical exploration should be performed before 6 months have elapsed.

In a 4th degree lesion a strong Tinel Hoffmann sign will develop, but there will not be any progression in a distal direction. As with a 3rd degree lesion, surgery is indicated when there is no further improvement.

In a 5th degree lesion (loss of continuity), there may be an avulsion of the spinal root or interruption more distally.

Today, surgical exploration is indicated in all cases of brachial plexus lesions with or without root avulsion, and this exploration should be performed within 6 months from the time of the accident, but preferably earlier. When root avulsions are proven, it does not make sense to wait until cases with chances of spontaneous recovery can be excluded. On clinical examination there is flaccid paralysis of all muscles of the involved extremity. The arm is flail and the shoulder joint subluxated. In 5th degree lesions, especially in cases of root avulsion, severe muscle atrophy develops rapidly. If the function of the pectoralis major muscle is preserved, the lesion has a very peripheral location. If the sternal portion of the pectoralis major muscle is paralyzed, the inferior trunk or medial cord is damaged. If the clavicular portion is paralyzed, the lesion is located in the superior trunk or the lateral cord. If the supra and infraspinatus muscles remain innervated the lesion is located at the level of the divisions or cords. If the serratus anterior muscle is intact, the lesion is at the level of the trunks. If the serratus anterior muscle is denervated, the lesion is located at a very proximal level (spinal root, spinal nerve, C5, C6, C7). Paralysis of the rhomboideus muscle suggests involvement of the cervical plexus. The function of the subclavius muscle and the scalenius muscles can not be evaluated since they are usually directly involved by the trauma and may develop fibrosis.

In a complete brachial plexus lesion the whole arm, except the inner surface of the upper arm, is anesthetic. In an upper brachial plexus lesion there is a loss of sensitivity in the deltoid area on the lateral surface of the upper arm and on the lateral-radial surface of the forearm, especially if C7 is involved. If C8 and T1 are involved, the ulnar side of the hand, including the middle finger, loses sensitivity, and a Tinel Hoffmann sign develops only if the lesion is distal to the dorsal root ganglion. Spinal root avulsions do not develop a Tinel Hoffmann sign. In rare cases there may be an isolated lesion of the dorsal root with loss of sensitivity, but with intact motor function, or an isolated lesion of the ventral root with loss of the motor function but with intact sensitivity. A lesion of the rami communicans albus interrupts the preganglionic myelinated fibers to the ganglia of the sympathetic trunk (stellate ganglion), and this may result in a Horner's syndrome. A Horner's syndrome is usually associated with a lesion of C8 and T1, but it may result from direct trauma to the inferior cervical ganglion (stellate ganglion).

Somatosensory evoked potentials are useful to prove avulsed rootlets with an intraforaminal location of the roots (10–14). Lesions proximal to the rami dorsalis of the spinal nerve cause denervation of the deep muscles of the neck which can be proven by electromyography (15). Ultrasound studies of the trunks, especially the upper and middle trunks should also be obtained. Myelographic irregularities at the site of the root pockets, empty root pockets, or pseudomeningoceles are suggestive of root avulsion as well (15, 16). False positive and false negative results do occur. Postmyelographic CT scans provide an image of rootlets and root pockets. MRI scanning with and without contrast provides images of rootlets, spinal roots, and spinal nerves. Utilizing these techniques it should be possible to diagnose root avulsions and formulate the indications for surgical exploration.

Surgical Procedures at the Brachial Plexus

Exposure

There are two basic ways to expose the spinal roots:—The anterior and the posterior approach.

In the posterior approach the patient is placed in a semiprone position (17). The surgeon exposes the trunks by a parascapular incision, detaching the inferior trapezius and the rhomboid muscles, reflecting the scapula, and resecting the first rib. This approach was designed for patients with root or trunk lesions with irradiation damage or scarring to the anterior chest wall and to the supraclavicular fossa.

The anterior approach is performed with the patient lying in the supine position having support underneath the scapula of the involved side. The head is turned to the contralateral side so that the neck and shoulder can be spread apart. The ipsilateral thorax is included in the operative field, as well as the shoulder, the axilla, and the upper and the lower arm. The extremity is prepped and draped so that it can be moved as desired. The whole brachial plexus can be explored in this position. Spinal nerves can be followed into the intervertebral foramina, but the surgeon cannot visualize the spinal roots within or medial to the foramen. Reimplantation of avulsed roots into the spinal cord remains impossible, but this is not regarded as a major disadvantage. Frequently the avulsed roots are outside the foramen and there is no need for further dissection in this area. Only in cases in which the roots are avulsed but not extracted from the foramen is there a difficulty in differentiating this situation from non-avulsion.

The standard anterior skin incision follows the posterior border of the sternocleidomastoid muscle toward its insertion at the medial end of the clavicle then turns lateral to follow the clavicle. At the distal third of the clavicle it turns again to traverse the clavicular origin of the deltoid and pectoralis major muscle and then follows a lateral direction along the free lower border of the pectoralis major muscle to reach the upper arm. Finally it turns medially to reach the midline of the upper arm. This incision transects the skin, the subcutaneous tissue, and the platysma. After elevating the skin five different skin flaps can be created:

1) A triangular flap over the supraclavicular fossa with a dorsal base,
2) A triangular flap over the infraclavicular fossa with a medial base,
3) A flap over the distal portion of the major pectoralis muscle and the deltopectoral groove with a lateral base,
4) A flap at the level of the anterior axillary crease, and
5) A small laterally based flap on the upper arm.

This incision can be modified depending upon the area the surgeon wishes to expose. For exploration of the supraclavicular fossa, the incision posterior to the sternocleidomastoid and over the clavicle is sufficient. The infraclavicular fossa is exposed by an incision along the clavicle and across the pectoralis major muscle to elevate the medially based flap. One should always be prepared to lengthen the incision along the appropriate lines if additional exposure is required. This skin incision has one disadvantage which involves the angle between the sternocleidomastoid and the incision over the clavicle. If this angle becomes too acute, then the dorsally based flap may be very long, resulting in an insufficient blood supply to the distal end. To prevent this problem the incision behind the sternocleidomastoid muscle should be curved to traverse the medial aspect of the supraclavicular fossa. To avoid a hypertrophic scar this segment of the incision is performed in a "Z" fashion.

Alternatively, an incision which follows the skin tension lines in a sagittal direction over the supraclavicular fossa results in a better cosmetic appearance. This incision can be extended at its dorsal end to cross the lateral third of the clavicle and reach the deltopectoral groove to follow the distal portion of the incision, as outlined above. If exposure of C5, C6, and the cervical plexus is required, a transverse incision of the neck, paralleling the sagittal incision, may be utilized, lifting the skin between the incisions as a bipedicled flap.

SUPRACLAVICULAR FOSSA

With elevation of the skin and the platysma, the external jugular vein is identified and then transected to improve exposure. The supraclavicular fossa is entered in its medial part to define the scalenus anterior muscle and the phrenic nerve. Between the scalenus anterior and the scalenus medius muscle is the superior trunk. If this area is fibrotic, one follows the phrenic nerve to reach C4. From here it is not too difficult to define the spinal nerve C5. The superior trunk and the spinal nerve, C6, are next identified. The superficial cervical artery, the superficial branch of the transverse cervical artery, near the omohyoideus muscle is isolated but not transected. Caudal to the superior trunk, the middle trunk is identified, and then the lower trunk can be approached. In this exposure the inferior trunk may be difficult to visualize. At this point the surgeon has two options: He can perform an osteotomy of the clavicle or just isolate the clavicle and move it in the desired direction in order to facilitate further dissection. Personally I prefer the isolation of the clavicle. The next step, therefore, is dissection of the infraclavicular fossa.

INFRACLAVICULAR FOSSA

After elevation of the medially based flap, the deltopectoral groove is identified. The dissection is localized between the deltoid and the pectoralis major muscle. The cephalic vein is preserved. After transection of the fascia beneath the pectoralis major muscle and the sheath of its neurovascular bundle is performed the lateral cord can be visualized. Superiorly and dorsally the posterior cord is identified and inferiorly and dorsally the axillary veins are seen. The inferior cord is exposed by dissecting between the axillary artery and the lateral cord. The axillary veins are located inferiorly and medially. Usually this area is not involved and is therefore free of scar tissue, making the dissection easier.

Cranially between the deltoid muscle, clavicle, and pectoralis major muscle one enters the space superficially to the clavipectoral fascia with the branches of the thoracoacromial artery and branches of the lateral pectoral nerve. The fascia is transected, and the cephalic vein is isolated. In the depth of the fossa, again the lateral pectoral nerve is the first structure to be identified. The posterior cord is located cranially and posteriorly, and the axillary artery caudally and deeper to the lateral cord. Isolation of the medial cord, located under the artery may be difficult if this area is already scarred. It is therefore easier to isolate and lift the pectoralis minor muscle and to follow the structures previously identified laterally to the pectoralis minor muscle in a medial direction. The clavicular origin of the pectoralis major muscle is detached. Now it is possible to approach the fossa below the clavicle and reach the operative field previously exposed by the supraclavicular dissection. The clavicle is then isolated by separation of its connections to the cervical fascia, isolating the omohyoideus muscle, and detaching the subclavius muscle. The supraclavicular artery and vein are identified below the clavicle. With this technique the following structures are isolated:

1. —Cervical fascia with omohyoideus muscle,
2. —Supraclavicular vessels,
3. —Clavicle, and
4. —Subclavius muscle.

Several options are now available to explore the brachial plexus:

1. Within the supraclavicular fossa,
2. Between the remainders of the cervical fascia including the omohyoideus muscle and clavicle,
3. Between the clavicle and subclavius muscle,
4. Between the subclavius muscle and the detached pectoralis major muscle medial to the pectoralis minor muscle, and
5. Between the deltoid and the pectoralis major muscle lateral to the pectoralis minor muscle.

The brachial plexus, when imbedded in scar tissue, may be fixed down to the first rib. Angulation of the course of the brachial plexus may be caused by this fibrous tissue. Exploration should follow a medial direction along the inferior cord by lifting the clavicle maximally. The area where T1 passes the inner border of the first rib and the edge of the suprapleural membrane is then reached. The inferior trunk must be separated from the artery with care taken at this level to avoid damage to the profunda cervicalis artery (deep branch of the transverse colli artery) which runs between the middle and lower trunk, the intercostalis supreme artery, and the dorsal scapular artery (variation). As the exploration proceeds a diagnosis differentiating between a lesion in continuity or a severed nerve can be made at the level of the cords, division, or trunk. External compression by fibrous tissue or bony fragments should be relieved and the structures liberated from adhesions. A root avulsion may be suspected if the trunks or the cord show a relaxed state or if the trunks and spinal nerves deviate from their expected courses. By following such deviations it is possible to identify an avulsed spinal nerve showing thickening of the dorsal root ganglion followed by the small rootlets. The exit at the intervertebral foramen of such an avulsed spinal nerve is observed to be empty. Otherwise, one follows along the spinal nerve until the anterior and posterior spine of the transverse process is identified. The posterior intertransversarius muscle is resected (18) and the dorsal side of C5, C6, and C7 with the dorsal roots is exposed. The dissection of the ventral side is dangerous, as there is a possibility of an injury to the vertebral artery. With no cord, root, or spinal nerve lesion having been detected yet, a decision must be made whether the spinal nerve and the spinal root proximal to the level of dissection are intact or if there has been a root avulsion. A normal appearance and the lack of adhesions are arguments for an intact root. Fibrosis and adhesions may cause a suspension of a more proximal injury, and the conductivity of the rootlets can be studied intraoperatively by utilizing evoked potentials or central stimulation of the gyrus precentralis.

As dissection proceeds along the spinal nerves a cystic structure may be encountered representing a pseudomeningocele. The attachment to the dural cavity is then identified. The pseudomeningocele is resected and the communication closed in a watertight fashion.

Lesions with Preserved Continuity

As an exploration proceeds external neurolysis should be performed simultaneously. The degree of injury is assessed. If the nerve has no fibrosis on the surface, external neurolysis is sufficient, and no further manipulation is needed. If the surface is fibrotic and the nerve indurated, a microsurgical longitudinal incision of the superficial layers of the para and epifascicular epineurium is performed (epifascicular epineurotomy). If the nerve has suffered a first or second degree lesion and if the fibrosis is only superficially surrounding the nerve, decompression is achieved by this maneuver and the nerve tissue should expand to protrude between the margins of the incision. The epineurotomy has to be extended until normal tissue is reached proximally and distally. It is sometimes necessary to perform a second and third epineurotomy along the surface of a nerve. After the epineurotomy, the fascicular structures are visible. A diagnosis of a first degree or II/A lesion can be established. The differentiation between IA and II/A can be made only in retrospect. After a IA lesion, regeneration occurs quickly; after a IIA lesion it will require further time.

If the epineurotomy is not sufficient for decompression because of fibrous tissue entering the depths of the nerve, the epifascicular epineurium is resected completely in the involved segment (epifascicular epineurectomy). If this is sufficient to achieve decompression no further steps are undertaken. If there is additional fibrosis between the fascicles, that part of the fibrotic interfascicular epineurium is removed (partial interfascicular epineurectomy). No attempt is made to isolate all the fascicles, and dissection is limited merely to the space between the fascicle groups and is strictly limited to the fibrotic elements within the interfascicular space. If the fascicular structure is well-preserved and the fascicles still have turgor (meaning they expand after the removal of the fibrous tissue) a I or IIB type lesion is present. If the fascicular structure is still preserved but the fascicular structures do not show any turgor, a third degree lesion is present. An internal neurolysis is performed in the same way. In some cases the fascicular structure is still visible, but the fascicles are shrunken and indurated. In this instance, even preserved fascicular patterns and continuity will not result in regeneration. These fascicles are resected and continuity is restored (lesion of type IIIC). If, after epineurotomy and epineurectomy, no fascicular structure can be seen, we have a fourth degree lesion. Then resection is the best solution. There are some 3rd and 4th degree lesions where some fascicles are better preserved than others. In these cases intraoperative electrical stimulation is helpful to assist in determining whether neurolysis or resection with restoration of continuity should be considered.

Clean Transection

If there was a clean transection by knife or glass without any defect, an end-to-end neurorrhaphy is performed. This is a very rare condition, most likely involving either C5 or C6, the upper trunk, or middle trunk.

Loss of Continuity with a Defect

When the nerve has been severed, usually there is a major defect. This void increases further due to the necessity of resecting the two stumps until normal tissue is reached. Usually it is impossible to achieve an end-to-end repair of the prepared stumps. In our series all attempts at end-to-end anastomosis did not result in improvement; therefore, these defects are best treated by a bridging nerve graft. It was not until the development of microsurgical grafting techniques (19–23) that nerve grafting started to achieve reasonable success. The basic technique depends upon the restoration of continuity by free nerve grafts utilizing segments of cutaneous nerves. Sural nerve grafts provide a graft of 30–40 cm in length that can be divided into several segments or cables. An alternative to the sural nerve is the medial antebrachial cutaneous nerve which provides a 20–25 cm-long segment. A third choice for nerve grafting is the lateral femoral cutaneous nerve, which is 20 cm long. In addition, the superficial radial nerve of the ipsilateral extremity has been utilized.

In preparation for a surgical procedure a priority scheme needs to be formulated to determine which functions are more important and which functions have a better chance to regenerate. The most important function is *elbow flexion* and, therefore, the regeneration of muscles which perform elbow flexion or have the capacity to perform this, have the highest priority. These include the biceps muscle, the brachialis muscle, and secondarily the triceps brachii muscle. In spite of being an elbow extensor, it is easy to transfer the triceps and convert it into an elbow flexor. It may reinforce a weak biceps, especially in the case of cocontracture, or it may replace it. It is especially important because the triceps muscle innervation has the best chance for regeneration. Consequently, it is of greatest importance to graft the anterior division of the upper trunk (especially that portion which contains the musculocutaneous fibers), the lateral cord (especially the part containing the fibers of the musculocutaneous nerve), and the musculocutaneous nerve itself according to the level of injury. The caudal and the caudolateral segments of the radial nerve contain the fibers for the motor branches of the triceps. The motor branches of the triceps branch off the radial nerve early and can be isolated and grafted separately. The next most important function in an extremity is stabilization of the shoulder joint. If subluxation of the shoulder joint is avoided and the patient achieves control of the shoulder joint, a major function is preserved. This means partial regeneration of the suprascapular and/or the deltoid muscle by grafting of the suprascapular and the axillary nerve, respectively. The third most important function is adduction, which is provided by the pectoralis major and latissimus dorsi muscles.

In the case of a complete brachial plexus lesion the reconstruction of a primitive grip should be attempted. It is also desirable that some of the forearm muscles (brachioradialis, radial wrist extensors, radial wrist flexor, superficial finger flexors) function be restored by grafting of the median and radial nerve. It is also important to have some type of primitive sensitivity, especially in the median nerve distribution. The return of function of the deep finger flexors and the intrinsic muscles of the hand would be of greatest importance, but in adults the intrinsic muscles of the hand never recover when there is complete loss of continuity with a defect.

A sufficient length of nerve grafting material can be harvested if the ipsilateral ulnar nerve is used as a nerve graft. Due to the poor chances of the ulnar nerve innervated muscles recovering in case of complete loss of continuity at a proximal level, the ulnar nerve will be harvested only as a nerve graft if C8 and T1 are avulsed. The ulnar nerve can be applied as a free nerve graft but its thickness may result in central fibrosis secondary to poor revascularization. Two alternative methods are available to overcome this. The ulnar nerve is split into minor units by longitudinal dissection, separating fascicle groups. Since the ulnar nerve consists of several well-defined fascicle groups, this facilitates this maneuver. When doing this, some of the interconnecting fibers between the fascicle groups must be sacrificed. A changing fascicular pattern in a nerve does not allow separation of fascicles for the total length of the nerve. Usually, one is able to split nerve grafts for a sufficient length to cover the existing defects. The split nerve grafts with the reduced diameter then become revascularized to survive the free grafting procedure. Another method is to transpose the ulnar nerve with preservation or immediate restoration of its blood supply by microvascular anatostomosis. This vascularized nerve graft can then be transplanted along with the ulnar artery and the concomitant veins. Breidenbach and Terzis (24–26) report that the superior collateral ulnar artery, a branch of the brachial artery, which reaches the ulnar nerve in the proximal third of the upper arm is sufficient to maintain the circulation along the total length of the ulnar nerve. The ulnar nerve can be utilized as a vascularized nerve graft by microvascular anastomosis of the superior ulnar artery and the concomitant veins. Usually the superior collateral artery provides a pedicle of approximately 5 cm which descends along the upper arm to reach the ulnar nerve. By exploiting the length of this pedicle, it is possible to transpose the ulnar nerve as an "island flap" with the superior collateral artery and veins as a vascular pedicle. If this pedicle is long enough, the ulnar nerve can be transposed to the supraclavicular triangle and introduced into a defect between spinal nerves and distal structures as a double graft.

The technique for free nerve grafting is relatively simple. If the grafts are transplanted individually, a selected point of the cross-section of the proximal stump can be connected with a selected point of a distal stump. The proximal coaptation is maintained by one single 10–0 nylon stitch per graft. Grafts placed in the cavity at the external end of the intervertebral foramen require no sutures. These grafts adhere to each other and the surrounding soft tissue in a very short period of time by natural fibrin formation. Longitudinal traction must be avoided, and this is best achieved by selection of a proper length of graft that is longer than the real distance between the two stumps. With the introduction of fibrin glues (27–32) it is now easier to achieve coaptation. Narakas (33) suggested glueing the proximal ends of the grafts together and treating them as if they were an artificial nerve trunk. This allows for placement of more nerve grafts on the same surface.

Free nerve grafts survive by forming adhesions with the surrounding tissue and being revascularized from the recipient site. This occurs within a very short period of time if the recipient site is well vascularized. Due to the fact that free grafts form adhesions with the surrounding tissue, they are extremely sensitive to longitudinal traction. Any tension at the sites of coaptation can be avoided by selecting the proper length of graft.

Vascularized nerve grafts survive in a scarred bed, since they have a preserved perineurium and do not need to form adhesions. They too are less sensitive to longitudinal traction. The coaptation has to be performed as an end-to-end coaptation of two nerve trunks by epineural stitches which do not allow for a more precise coaptation of fascicles. The risk is that the vascularized graft may become necrotic if the microvascular anastomosis fails or if the circulation in the pedicle, an island flap transfer, becomes occluded. If the results of published data are analyzed, the majority of authors (34–40) are not convinced that the final results after vascularized nerve grafting is better than free nerve grafting. Only Breidenbach and Terzis (2, 26) claim to have achieved significantly better results.

Another alternative to increase the quantity of nerve tissue is using allografts. Allografts can provoke an immunologic reaction. This reaction can be diminished with the use of immunosuppressive therapy such as cyclosporine A (41, 42). Even with optimal survival of allografts, there may only be partial neurotization. It remains questionable whether this technique has developed to a level where it can be utilized in human patients. Alternatives to the application of nerve grafts are connecting the two stumps by conduits, especially if they are biodegradable (43), veins (44), or degenerated muscle after freezing (45). There is evidence that for short distances the growth of nerve fibers from the proximal stump takes place, but it seems that a neurotization is inferior to the application of an autograft nerve. In root avulsions no proximal stump is available, so neurotization can be achieved only by using nerves as axon donors. The proximal stump of the donor nerve and the distal stump of the recipient nerve are transposed to achieve direct coaptation. When this is not possible or not desired, the gap between proximal stump and distal stump of the recipient nerve is bridged by a nerve graft. Using this procedure, axons are transferred into the donor nerve directly or via a nerve graft to the recipient nerve in order to neurotize the nerve.

The first successful nerve transfers were performed by Seddon (46) utilizing the intercostal nerves to neurotize the musculocutaneous nerve for reinnervation of the biceps muscle. Tsuyama et al. (47) exposed the total length of the intercostal nerve and transposed this nerve to achieve direct end-to-end coaptation with the distal stump. These authors applied this technique without exploration of the brachial plexus itself after having proven root avulsion by one of the previously mentioned diagnostic tests. I disagree with these authors and feel that avulsion of the involved root must be proven by direct exploration. The distal end of the intercostal nerve of the upper segments (intercostal nerve II to V) contains mostly sensory fibers because the motor branches have already exited the nerve. I prefer to transect the intercostal nerves in the midaxillary line after the lateral cutaneous branches have left the nerve and then perform a nerve graft with the proximal stump which is then united with the recipient nerve at its distal end. I achieve better results with this technique than with utilizing the whole length of the intercostal nerve and avoid the application of a large graft. Celli et al. (48) transected the intercostal nerves dorsally to use the proximal stumps which contain more motor fibers. Nerve grafts connected with the stumps in this transfer are technically difficult and the results are not encouraging (49). Celli et al. also suggested the use of the lower intercostal nerves (8–12), connecting them to the proximal stumps of vascularized nerve grafts (50).

The accessory nerve was used by Kotani et al. (51, 52) as an axon donor. If this nerve is transected distal to the first branch of the trapezius muscle there is no significant loss of trapezius muscle function (37, 53).

Motor and sensory branches of the cervical plexus have been utilized by Brunelli (54) and Brunelli and Monini (55). By careful dissection of the cervical plexus, motor branches can be identified, transected, and used as motor axon donors. The proximal stumps of the supraclavicular nerves may be used as donors for sensory axons. Attempts have been made to transfer contralateral motor fibers of the brachial plexus to the paralyzed brachial plexus (56, 57). Sensory fibers derived from the intercostobrachial nerves of T2 are usually not involved in brachial plexus lesions, so transfer of long nerve grafts to the fascicles serving the thumb and the index finger can bring sensory fibers to this area (23).

Selection of Technique

In individual cases after a proper diagnosis is made by exploration, a plan should be formulated to achieve the greatest benefit for that particular patient. All available donor nerves should be utilized. Some authors have utilized intercostal nerves to restore as many functions as possible, but I feel that the intercostal nerve should be used for one or two synchronous functions and other donor nerves should be utilized for antagonistic functions.

Avulsion of all Five Roots

This is the worst possible scenario. The intercostal nerves III, IV, V, and usually VI must be anastomosed with the ulnar nerve which is utilized as an island flap and then connected with the distal stump of the musculocutaneous nerve. Alternatively, the intercostal VI, VII, VIII, or only VII and VIII are connected with the radial nerve which is transected at a very proximal level and then transposed to the thoracic wall. A severed intercostal nerve II is directly connected with the long thoracic nerve, and the accessory nerve is connected by a cutaneous nerve graft with the suprascapular nerve. The dorsal scapular nerve is connected by cutaneous nerve graft with the median nerve. C4 is sometimes utilized to neurotize the shoulder muscles or the biceps.

If there is avulsion of C6, C7, C8, and T1, the stump of C5 is connected with the ulnar nerve as a vascularized nerve graft or as a split trunk graft. If used as a vascularized graft, the ulnar nerve is transferred on the superior collateral ulnar artery and shaped into two trunk grafts, being sure to preserve their connective tissue connection with the blood supply. One of them is coapted distally to the musculocutaneous and the other to the median nerve. The intercostal nerve II is coapted to the long thoracic nerve if the serratus anterior muscle is paralyzed. The intercostal nerves III, IV, and V are coapted to the radial nerve which is transected at a very proximal level and then transferred to the thoracic wall. The accessory nerve is connected by one cutaneous nerve graft to the suprascapular nerve. The dorsal scapular nerve is connected by one graft to the axillary nerve.

If there is avulsion of C7, C8, and T1 with the root stumps of C5 and C6 available, again a vascularized nerve graft is formed using the ulnar nerve with the superior collateral ulnar artery forming two trunk grafts. The stump-C6 is connected with the two proximal ends; one distal end is grafted into the musculocutaneous and the other into the median nerve. The stump-C5 is connected by free cutaneous nerve graft with the axillary and the suprascapular nerve. The intercostal nerve II is coapted to the long thoracic nerve if the serratus anterior muscle is completely paralyzed. And the intercostal nerves III, IV, and V are connected to the radial nerve which is transected at a very proximal level and then transferred to the thoracic wall.

If there is avulsion of C8 and T1 with C5, C6, and C7 available, no transfer is performed. The stump-C5 is connected by cutaneous nerve grafts with the suprascapular, axillary, and the thoracodorsal nerve. The serratus anterior muscle should be intact in this case. The ulnar nerve is used as a vascularized nerve graft or as a split trunk graft and connected along with free cutaneous nerves with the lateral cord or used for neurotization of the musculocutaneous, median nerve, and radial nerve. If the root C8 or the root T1 are not avulsed, the ulnar nerve can not be used as a graft. Frequently, in those cases the inferior trunk with the roots C8 and T1 is in continuity. A neurolysis is performed, and the continuity between C5, C6, and C7 with the corresponding distal stumps is achieved by free cutaneous nerve grafts. In all other cases the proper technique is selected according to the site of the lesion, the extent of the lesion, and the degree of damage.

POSTOPERATIVE TREATMENT AND COMPLICATIONS

At closure, drains are utilized. When nerve grafts have been used suction drainage is contraindicated. The head and upper extremity are immobilized in a plaster cast to include the head, thorax, and upper extremity for 10 days. If the nerve repair has been performed without any tension, immobilization is no longer necessary after 10 days, and cautious mobilization may be started. After 21 days physiotherapy may begin; it consists of passive motion of all available joints and active exercises with the nonparalyzed muscles. Splints and other orthodeses are used to avoid hyperextension. Some authors recommend an abduction splint to avoid progressive stiffness of the shoulder joint. It is important to reintegrate the patient as soon as possible back to a normal lifestyle, since all these patients have considerable psychological problems to deal with. As motor recovery becomes apparent, active exercises focus on these muscle groups. Patients who undergo physiotherapy including electric stimulation with exponential current do better than those without. In cases with a nerve transfer, the patient must learn to activate the muscle which is innervated by a nerve with an original function that was completely different. In the case of intercostal nerve transfers to the biceps, early contractions of the biceps muscle occur if the patient breathes forcefully, coughs, or innervates the abdominal muscles. Utilizing this, the patient will learn to activate elbow flexion. This learning process can be enhanced by electrodes within the biceps muscle giving the patient an optical or acoustical signal when he has successfully innervated this muscle. In time the patient will be able to activate elbow flexion without conscious thought. This is easier in young patients.

COMPLICATIONS

Significant complications include a hematoma which requires immediate evacuation, superficial skin necrosis, and infections in spite of prophylactic antibiotics. In rare cases, osteotomy of the clavicle has resulted in nonunion or infection.

PAIN

Patients with brachial plexus lesions frequently suffer severe pain syndromes. They are more frequent in nonoperative cases and in patients with root avulsions, according to Bonard and Narakas (58). Surgery improved 25% of patients with root avulsions and cases of peripheral brachial plexus lesions (59). In most patients the pain syndrome progressively disappears with pain moving distally to finally concentrate in the hand and then eventually disappear. Persistent pain does occur and can be a significant problem. Sympathectomy helps only if the pain has a causalgic character. Chordotomy or coagulation within the dorsal root entry zone may also be helpful in pain syndromes.

FURTHER IMPROVEMENT BY RECONSTRUCTIVE SURGERY

If the reinnervated muscles during the second postoperative year have reached a certain strength, then further reconstructive procedures can be considered to optimize function. In addition, function or regenerated muscles may be improved by arthrodesis.

ELBOW FLEXION

Elbow flexion is the most important function in a paralyzed arm. If the biceps function is regenerated it must regain sufficient force to become functional. If the regenerated biceps is too weak, the efficiency of its force can be increased by transposing the insertion of the tendon in a distal direction to increase the lever arm. Efficiency can also be improved by transferring the tendon such that it becomes a pure elbow flexor without supination.

Elbow flexion unfortunately may be prevented by simultaneous cocontraction of the triceps muscle. If the triceps muscle is transferred and united with its biceps tendon both muscles may act as elbow flexors, and the available force is significantly increased. The transfer is performed by detaching the triceps tendon from the olecranon, isolating the distal half of the triceps, and transferring this muscle without impairing its blood supply and its innervation around the lateral side of the humerus by lifting the brachioradialis muscle and radial nerve. If the biceps does not regenerate but the triceps muscles have recoverd, then active elbow flexion can be achieved by the same transfer. In my experience the triceps recovers better than the biceps. Intercostal nerve transfer frequently leads to insufficient strength of the reinnervated biceps, and based on this experience we have a series of cases where the intercostal nerve transfer is performed to innervate the biceps and the triceps muscle in spite of the fact that they are antagonists. This sets the stage for the triceps muscle transfer to use the triceps as a flexor.

In lower brachial plexus lesions the elbow joint can not actively pronate, and the strong supinative effect of the biceps keeps the forearm and the hand in supination. This can be treated by a longitudinal splitting of the biceps tendon, transecting one-half proximally and one-half distally. The one-half which is attached distally is transposed around the radius to pull so that it now leads to pronation rather than supination. The other half is reattached to the proximal half of the biceps tendon with proper tension (60).

In upper brachial plexus lesions with an intact pectoralis major muscle, elbow flexion can be restored by transferring the lateral segment of the pectoralis major innervated by the branches of the medial pectoral nerve to the lateral side of the pectoralis minor (61, 62). This transfer, though, is very often too weak. Hovnanian (63) and Schottstaed et al. (64) suggested the use of the latissimus dorsi to replace elbow flexion. A detailed technique was elaborated by Zancolli and Mitre (65), and if the latissimus muscle is strong enough this transfer gives very good results. In an upper brachial plexus lesion with intact forearm flexors, a transfer of the complete origin of the forearm flexors, by transferring them from the medial epicondyle to the anterior surface of the shaft of the humerus, approximately 5 cm proximally, (66) usually gives excellent results.

SHOULDER JOINT

In order to achieve good elevation of the shoulder, one requires a strong deltoid and supraspinatus muscle. The force of these muscle after regeneration usually is not sufficient to provide good elevation of the shoulder in cases of complete brachial plexus lesions. However, it is sufficient to prevent subluxation which results secondary to denervation of the aforementioned muscles. If muscle function does not return, a trapezius muscle transfer (67) can help. The trapezius muscle is detached from its insertion at the scapular spine, acromion and clavicle and is transferred with the arm held in the maximum elevation to the surgical neck of the humerus and fixed there by a screw.

If the serratus anterior is functioning well, one can obtain good motion of the arm by moving the scapula if arthrodesis of the shoulder joint is performed. This is performed with 60° abduction, 30° of forward flexion, and 40° of external rotation (68). Many patients remain dissatisfied with this procedure in spite of satisfactory motion because of the uncomfortable position of the extremity in the position of rest.

Internal rotation usually returns due to the function of the pectoralis major muscle which at the same time adducts the arm. In contrast, external rotation is lacking in the majority of cases of brachial plexus injury. These patients, after good regeneration of the biceps, are able to flex the elbow joint in front of the body, but cannot use this limb in space. To achieve sufficient external rotation, a rotatory osteotomy of the humerus is performed, rotating the distal segment about 90° in external rotation before plating the osteotomy site. Active external rotation can be added by detaching the pectoral minor muscle from its insertion and origin. The muscle is rotated by 90°, and the origin is reinserted at the level of the second rib, and its insertion on the coracoid is transferred dorsally to the neck of the humerus.

GRIP RECONSTRUCTION

In partial brachial plexus lesions the classical techniques of tendon transfer for peripheral nerve lesions may be applied in a modified way. The major problem is to reconstruct a primitive grip if only one, two, and three muscles regenerate. If there is a good regeneration on the extensor side and dorsiflexion of the wrist is powerful, the grip can be reconstructed by tenodesis of the flexor tendons on the ventral aspect of the radius. If the patient now attempts dorsiflexion, the fingers can close to make a fist. A second available extensor tendon may be transferred to the thumb to achieve adduction.

If there is no dorsiflexion a wrist arthrodesis is performed in neutral position. The IP-joint of the thumb is arthrodesed. The flexor pollicis longus tendon is detached and transferred to the radial dorsal aspect of the basal phalanx of the thumb. The one functioning tendon is then connected to the distal stump of the flexor pollicis longus tendon, in order to achieve a key-grip function.

If there are two muscles available, one is used in the way described above, and the second is used to bring the fingers into a flexed position. If there are three muscles available, besides the arthrodesis of the wrist joint and tendon transfer in the above mentioned case, one tendon is transferred to the finger extensors to provide some finger extension.

If there are four muscles available, a similar procedure is performed and, in addition, one of the tendons is connected to the flexor digitorum superficialis tendons.

Govilar (69) and Berger et al. (70) transferred the latissimus dorsi muscle in a way that finger flexion can be achieved. The ipsilateral muscle may be used as an island flap or the contralateral muscle as a free tissue transfer. In cases in which the local muscles are already too degenerated, free muscle grafts innervated by intercostal nerves have been utilized to restore finger flexion (47).

RESULTS

If the patient has strong elbow flexion and some control of the shoulder joint in complete brachial plexus lesions with root avulsion, it can be regarded as a satisfactory result. These results can be achieved in more than 60% of the cases. If some forearm muscles become functional, allowing reconstruction of a primitive grip, the result is regarded as very good. In cases of a more peripheral injury to the brachial plexus and in cases of lesions with preserved continuity, the results are far better.

BRACHIAL PLEXUS LESIONS OTHER THAN POSTTRAUMATIC

During delivery, the brachial plexus may suffer similar injuries as in adult trauma. There may be an avulsion by longitudinal traction along the axis of the extremity or compression of the arm with or without traction of the clavicle during delivery. In the majority of cases, the lesions are not complete. If regeneration starts late, then the final results are usually less than satisfactory. Therefore, surgical exploration is indicated at the end of 3 months if the biceps muscle does not show any regeneration.

Damage to the brachial plexus may have four different etiologies:

1. Compression by fibrosis: In this case neurolysis has a satisfactory prognosis. The loss of function will not return but the progression of the process will be halted.
2. Direct damage to the nerves of the brachial plexus occurs with irradiation. After irradiation for cancer treatment, the brachial plexus may be damaged. This leads to a progressive loss of function and in many cases to the development of severe pain syndromes.
3. Deterioration of function may occur as a consequence of the surgical manipulation.
4. The loss of the brachial plexus function may be caused by metastatic cancer to the plexus or by primary nerve tumors such as neurofibromas or malignant schwannomas.

REFERENCES

1. Rieder H. Die "Steinträger-Lähmung". Eine Form der kombinierten Armnerven-oder Brachialplexus-Lähmung. Münch Med Wschr 1893;40:121–123.

2. Daube JR. Rucksack paralysis. JAMA 1969;208:2447–2452.

3. Jéquier M. Une forme rare de lésion du plexus brachial. "La paralysie du paquetage". Schweiz Med Wochenschr 1949;79:397–402.

4. Schüpbach D, Oettli M, Meier C. Katamnestische Untersuchungen mit Rucksacklähmungen. Wehrmed Mschr 1987.

5. Mürset G. Lähmungen des Neugeborenen in Folge intrauteriner Druckwirkung (Dissertation). Zürich:1957.

6. Taylor PE. Traumatic intradural avulsion of the nerve roots of the brachial plexus. Brain 1962;85:579–602.

7. Kubik S, Müntener M. Zur Topographie der spinalen Nervenwurzeln. II. Der Einfluß des Wachstums des Duralsackes, sowie der Krümmagen und der Bewegungen der spinalen Nervenwurzeln. Acta Anat 1969;74:149–168.

8. Narakas A. In: Mumenthaler M, Schliack H, eds. Läsionen peripherer Nerven. 5th ed. Stuttgart-New York: Georg Thieme Verlag, 1987:181.

9. Bonney G, Birch R, Jamieson AM, Eames RA. Experience with vascularized nerve grafts. Clin Plast Surg 1984;11:137–142.

10. Jones SJ. Investigation of brachial plexus traction lesions by peripheral and spinal somatosensory evoked potentials. J Neurol Neurosurg Psychiatry 1979;42:107–116.

11. Jones SJ, Wynn-Parry CB, Landi A. Diagnosis of brachial plexus traction lesions by sensory nerve action potentials and somatosensory evoked potentials. Injury 1981;12:376–382.

12. Siivola J, Myllylä VV, Sulg I, Hokkanen E. Brachial plexus and radicular neuropathy in relation to cortical evoked responses. J Neurol Neurosurg Psychiatry 1979;42:1151–1158.

13. Stöhr M, Riffel B, Buettner UW. Somatosensible evozierte Potentiale in der Diagnostik von Armplexuslähmungen. EEG-EMG 1981;12,195–197.

14. Synek VM, Cowan JC. Somatonsensory evoked potentials in patients with supraclavicular brachial plexus injuries. Neurology 1982;32:1347–1352.

15. Buffalini C, Pescatori G. Posterior cervical electromyography in the diagnosis and prognosis of brachial plexus injuries. J Bone Joint Surg 1969;51-B:627–631.

16. Rohr H. Untersuchungen über die Segmentinnervation des Hals-Schulter-Arm-Gebietes bei cervikalen Wurzelläsionen. Langenbecks Arch Chir 1962;103:873–879.

17. Kline DG, Kott J, Barner G, Bryant L. Exploration of selected brachial plexus lesions by the posterior subscapular approach. J Neurosurg 1978;49:872–880.

18. Herzberg G, Narakas A, Comtet JJ, Bouchet A, Carret TP, Goushe J. Microsurgical relationship of brachial plexus roots. Paper held at the Joint Meeting of the Groupe pour L'Avancement de la Microchirurgie (GAM) and the Deutschsprachige Arbeitsgemeinschaft für Mikrochirurgie der peripheren Nerven and Gefäße (DAM), Strasbourg, May 2–4, 1984.

19. Millesi H, Ganglberger J, Berger A. Erfahrungen mit der Mikrochirurgie peripherer Nerven. Chir Plastica 1967;3:34–55.

20. Millesi H. Zum Problem der überbrückung von Defekten peripherer Nerven. Wr Med Wochenschr 1968;118,9/10:182–187.

21. Millesi H. Die Eingriffe an den Hand- und Fingernerven. In: Wachsmuth W, Wilhelm A, eds. Allgemeine und spezielle chirurgische Operationslehre, Vol. 10, Part 3: Operationen an der Hand. Berlin-Heidelberg-New York: Springer Verlag, 1972:226–250.

22. Millesi H. Surgical management of brachial plexus injuries. J Hand Surg 1977;8:367–379.

23. Millesi H, Meissl G, Katzer H. Zur Behandlung der Verletzungen des Plexus brachialis. Vorschlag einer integrierten Therapie. Brun's Beitr Klin Chir 1973;220:429–446.

24. Breidenbach WB, Terzis JK. Vascularized nerve grafts. ASPRS Essay Contest 1983.

25. Breidenbach WB, Terzis JK. The anatomy of revascularized nerve grafts. Clin Plast Surg 1984;11:65–71.

26. Terzis JK, Breidenbach WC. The anatomy of free vascularized

nerve grafts. In: Terzis JK, ed. Microreconstruction of nerve injuries, part 1. Philadelphia: WB Saunders Co, 1987:101.

27. Matras H, Dinges HP, Lassmann H, Mamoli B. Zur nahtlosen interfaszikulären Nerventransplantation im Tierexperiment. Wien Med Wochenschr 1972;122:517.

28. Matras H, Kuderna HP. The principle of nervous anastomoses with clotting agents. Proceedings VIth Int Congress of Plastic and Reconstructive Surgery. Paris, Aug 24–29, 1975: Paris: Masson 1976:134.

29. Kuderna H. Discussional remark at the symposium: Indication, Technique and Results of Nerve grafting, Vienna, May 21–23, 1977. Handchir Suppl 2, 1977.

30. Kuderna H. Ergebnisse und Erfahrung in der klinischen Anwendung des Fibrinklebers bei der Wiederherstellung durchtrennter peripherer Nerven. Paper held at 17th Annual Meeting of the Deutsche Ges f Plastische u Wiederherstellungschir. Heidelberg, Nov 1–3, 1979.

31. Kuderna H. Erfahrungen mit der Fibrinklebung peripherer Nerven. Paper held at the Gesellschaft der Ärzte in Wien, Vienna, April 13, 1984.

32. Kuderna H. Die Fibrinklebung peripherer Nerven in: H. Nigst, ed. Nervenwiederherstellung nach traumatischen Läsionen. Stuttgart: Hippokrates Verlag, 1985:78.

33. Narakas A. Les greffes nerveuses—expérience clinique. Ann Chir Main 1989;8,4:302–311.

34. Birch R. Traction lesions of the brachial plexus. Br J Hosp Med 1984;Sept:140–143.

35. Alnot JY, Oberlin Ch, Bellaicke H. Vascularized ulnar nerve transfer in total palsy of the brachial plexus. Paper held at the Joint Meeting of the Groupe pour l'Avancement de la Microchirurgie (GAM) and the Deutschsprachige Arbeitsgemeinschaft für Mikrochirurgie der peripheren Nerven und Gefäße (DAM), Strasbourg, May 2–4, 1984.

36. Merle M, Lebreton E, Bour Ch, Mancaud M, Marin-Braun F. Free vascularized nerve transfer in brachial plexus injuries. Paper held at the Joint Meeting of the Groupe pour L'Avancement de la Microchirurgie (GAM) and the Deutschsprachige Arbeitsgemeinschaft für Mikrochirurgie der peripheren Nerven und Gefäße (DAM), Strasbourg, May 2–4, 1984.

37. Merle M. Neurotization of brachial plexus lesions with the spinal accessory nerve—functional results. Paper held at the Annual Meeting of the Am Soc for Surgery of the Hand, Las Vegas, February 1986.

38. Allieu Y. Personal communication at the Joint Meeting of the Groupe pour L'Avancement de la Microchirurgie (GAM) and the Deutschsprachige Arbeitsgemeinschaft für periphere Nerven und Gefäße (DAM), Strasbourg, May 2–4, 1984.

39. Millesi H. Eingriffe an peripheren Nerven. In: Gschnitzer F, Kern E. Chirurgische Operationslehre. Munich-Vienna: Urban & Schwarzenberg 1986;1–68.

40. Anderl H, Hussl H. Erfahrungen mit vaskularisierten Nerventransplantaten. Paper held at Annual Meeting of the Deutsch-sprachige Arbeitsgemeinschaft für Mikrochirurgie der peripheren Nerven und Gefäße, Berne, Dec 5–6, 1986.

41. Mackinnon SE, Hudson AR, Falk RE, Hunter DA. The allograft response, an experimental model in the rat. Ann Plast Surg 1985;14:334.

42. Berger A, Schaller E, Mailänder P, Walter A, Wonigeit K, Becker M. The effect of Cyclosporine A on free autologue and allogen grafts of the sciatic nerve in the rat. Paper held at the 3rd Congr. of Int Fed of Societies for Surgery of the Hand, Tokyo, Nov 3–8, 1986.

43. Mackinnon SE, Hudson AR, Bain JR. The nerve allograft response in the primate immunosuppressed with cyclosporin A. Presented at the Sunderland Society Meeting, Durham NC, June, 1988.

44. Chiu DTW, Janecka I, Krizek TJ, Wolff M, Lovelac RE. Autogenous vein graft as a conduit for nerve regeneration. Surgery 1982;91:226.

45. Glasby MA, Gschmeissner SE, Hitchcock RJI, Huang CLH, De Souza BA. A comparison of nerve regeneration through nerve and muscle grafts in rat. Neuroorthop 1986;2:21.

46. Seddon HJ. Nerve grafting. J Bone Jt Surg 1963;45-B:447.

47. Tsuyama NR, Sagakuchi T, Har T, Kondo S, Kaminuma M, Ijichi M, Ryn D. Reconstructive surgery in brachial plexus injuries. Proc 11th Ann Meeting Japanese Soc of the Hand, Hiroshima 1968;39.

48. Celli L, Mingione A, Landi A. Nuovo acquisizioni di tecnica chirurgica nelle lesioni del plesso brachiale: indicazioni alla neurolisi. Autoinnesti e trapianti nervosi. Atii del LIX Congresso della Società Italiana Ortopedia e Traumatologia, Cagliari, Sept 29–Oct 3, 1974.

49. Celli L. Paper held at the Giornate Internazionale di Chirurgia, Taranto, June 8–10, 1978.

50. Celli L, Balli A, de Luise G, Rovesta C. La neurotizzazione degli ultimi nervi intercostali, mediante trapiano nervoso peduncolato, nelle avulsioni radiculari del plesso brachiale (Nota preliminare di tecnica chirurgica). La Chirurgia degli Organi di Movemento, Vol LXIV, Fac.V. 1978;461.

51. Kotani PT, Toyoshima Y, Matsuda H, et al. The postoperative results of nerve transfer for the brachial plexus injury in root avulsion. Proceedings of the 14th Ann Meeting of the Society for Surgery of the Hand, Osaka, 1979;34.

52. Kotani PT, Matsuda H, Suzuki C. Trial of surgical procedures of nerve transfer to avulsion injuries of plexus brachialis. Abstracts SICOT XII, Israel, Oct 9–13, 1972;520.

53. Allieu Y, Privat JM, Bonnel F. Paralysis in root avulsion of the brachial plexus: neurotization by the spinal accessory nerve. Clin Plast Surg 1984;11:133.

54. Brunelli G. Neurotization of avulsed roots of the brachial plexus by means of anterior nerves of the cervical plexus. Int J Microsurg 1980;1:55.

55. Brunelli G, Monini L. Neurotization of avulsed roots of brachial plexus by means of anterior nerves of the cervical plexus. Clin Plast Surg 1984;1:149.

56. Millesi H. Unpublished observation 1983.

57. Gilbert A. Personal communication 1984.

58. Bonnard C, Narakas AO. Syndrome douloureux et lésions posttraumatiques du plexus brachial. Etude de l'influence de l'acte réparateur chirurgical sur le syndrome douloureux chez 211 patients opérés de lésion posttraumatique par arrangement ou rupture du plexus brachial. Helv Chir Acta 1985;52:621.

59. Narakas AO. The effects on pain of reconstructive neurosurgery in 160 patients with traction and/or crush to the brachial plexus. In: Siegfried J, ed. Phantom and stump pain. Berlin: Springer, 1981.

60. Zancolli EA. Paralytic supination contracture of the forearm. J Bone Joint Surg 1967;49-A:1275–1284.

61. Clark JPM. Reconstruction of biceps brachii by pectoral muscle transplantation. Br J Surg 1946;34:180.

62. Atkins RM, Bell MJ, Sharrard W. Pectoralis major transfer for paralysis of elbow flexion in children. J Bone Joint Surg 1985;67-B:640.

63. Hovnanian AP. Latissimus dorsi-transplantation for loss of flexion or extension at the elbow. Ann Surg 1956;143:493–497.

64. Schottstaed ER, Larsen LJ, Bost FC. Complete muscle transposition. J Bone Joint Surg 1955;37-A:897–919.

65. Zancolli E, Mitre H. Latissimus dorsi transfer to restore elbow flexion. An appraisal of eight cases. J Bone Joint Surg 1973;55-A:1265.

66. Steindler A. Transplantations of muscle and tendons at elbow. Am Acad Orthop Surg Lect 1944;276.

67. Saha AK. Surgery of the paralyzed and flail shoulder. Acta Orthop Scand 1967;Suppl. 97.

68. May VR. Shoulder fusion. A review of 14 cases. J Bone Joint Surg 1962;44-A:65–76.

69. Govilar A. The use of the latissimus dorsi muscle as an active motor unit for digital flexion. J Hand Surg (Br) 1989;14-B:70–71.

70. Berger A, Flory PJ, Schaller E. Muscle transfer in brachial plexus lesions. J Rec Microsurg 1990;6(2):113–116.

VI

Rehabilitation of Cervical Spine Injuries

30

Rehabilitation of Patients with Cervical Spine Disorders

Kristjan T. Ragnarsson

Introduction

Virtually every clinical condition which receives significant attention in this book will require an intervention by one or more members of the rehabilitation team. The disorders of the cervical spine which benefit from such intervention may range in severity from neck pain without any objective findings to serious traumatic or degenerative conditions with extensive neurological and skeletal deficits. The rehabilitation treatment may thus vary widely from simple exercise instructions to comprehensive inpatient rehabilitation involving all members of the rehabilitation team (Table 30.1).

Physical medicine constitutes one of the three main therapeutic approaches of traditional clinical medicine along with surgery and drug treatment. Physical medicine may be defined as that aspect of medicine which deals with the management of disease by means of physical agents, i.e., light, heat, cold, water, electricity, and various mechanical agents, i.e., massage, exercise, traction, manipulation, and a variety of mechanical apparatuses (1). Radiation grew in importance early this century, which led to the establishment of a new medical specialty, radiology. Rehabilitation medicine is a treatment concept which first became widely accepted during World War II when it was shown that individuals with physical disabilities would best benefit from a multidisciplinary intervention. Dr. Howard A. Rusk, an early pioneer of rehabilitation medicine defined it as the maximum restoration of physical, psychological, vocational, recreational, and economic function within the limits imposed by a physical disability. The American Board of Physical Medicine and Rehabilitation has been recognized by the American Board of Medical Specialties since 1949. The medical specialists practicing this field are now called physiatrists (phys-i-a'-trists), derived from the Greek word "phys" referring to physical agents and "iatros," meaning physician. More recently, the specialty has even been referred to unofficially as physiatry.

Evaluation

The patient with symptoms relating to the neck, head, shoulders, and upper limbs demands that the examining physician be knowledgable in anatomy and biomechanics, able to localize the pathology, and form an accurate diagnosis in order to determine and prescribe the most effective and safe treatment.

Medical History

It has been estimated that the majority of acute cervical spine disorders are related to trauma that was sustained in motor vehicle or sports accidents, falls, and violent acts. It is therefore important to obtain specific and detailed information about the type of accident, the power of impact, the patient's use of protective equipment, body position on impact, and all associated injuries. Whether acute or chronic, symptoms should be carefully documented with respect to onset, distribution, character, and course, as well as how these are affected by activity and interventions. When the symptoms do not appear to be related to trauma, the history should include information about previous injuries, major accidents, and neck symptoms as well as information about the patient's general health and presence of systemic disease which may affect the cervical spine. Since the field of Physical Medicine and Rehabilitation (PM&R) is not limited to a single organ system but is dedicated to the concept of the "whole person" and maximum restoration of func-

Table 30.1. Rehabilitation Medicine Multidisciplinary Team

Physician (physiatrist, consultants)
Rehabilitation nurse
Physical therapist
Occupational therapist
Speech pathologist
Psychologist
Social worker
Recreation therapist
Vocational counselor
Orthotist/prosthetist
Home economist (architect)
Driving instructor
Equipment coordinator/vendor
Educator

tion in the various aspects as stated above, the medical history has to include information on previous and current functional performance and lifestyle.

Physical Examination

A careful physical examination is most important and should be directed in particular to the musculoskeletal and nervous systems. Posture is affected by various factors, i.e., habit, genetic features, mood, physical condition, and disease but is biomechanically largely determined by the alignment of the pelvis with the spine. Segments higher in the spine make a compensatory adjustment which may be altered by any deviation, thus increasing or decreasing the normal lumbar lordosis, thoracic kyphosis, and cervical lordosis. Therefore, it is important to examine the entire spine although the symptoms may be confined to the cervical spine and upper limbs. The range of motion of the neck should be assessed in six different directions: flexion, extension, left and right lateral tilting, and left and right rotation. Although the upper cervical spine accounts for 30% of flexion/extension (occipital-atlantal-axial joints) and 50% of rotation (atlantal-axial joint), the most mobile segments are C4–5, C5–6, and C–7. In full flexion the chin should approximate or touch the sternum (45°), in extension the patient should be able to look straight up (45°), in rotation the chin should align with the shoulder (80–90°), and in lateral tilting the ear should move half-way towards the shoulder (45°). The physician should document all complaints during motor testing as well as the resistance given by the patient during passive and active motion. Palpation should include both bone structures and soft tissues, i.e., the various neck organs and musculature, and tenderness and muscle spasm should be documented (2). Various diagnostic maneuvers of the head, neck, and shoulder may be helpful when assessing cervical radicular symptoms (2). A gradually increasing axial compression of the head on the neck in the sitting position may lead to local or radiating pain or paresthesias. The Spurling test is done in a similar manner but with the head rotated to one side and a vertical blow delivered to the top of the head. A head distraction test may relieve compression and alter symptoms. Shoulder depression test is done by pushing the shoulder down while tilting the head to the opposite side. The Valsalva maneuver may also produce radicular symptoms which can be helpful in making a diagnosis. Swallowing should be observed, as various neuromusculoskeletal abnormalities may cause dysphagia. The presence of Horner's syndrome may indicate neck pathology. Several specific tests also exist for the assessment of thoracic outlet syndrome. A complete neurologic examination usually should be undertaken. The physiatric evaluation requires careful review of various radiological and imaging studies as indicated by clinical symptoms. These are discussed elsewhere in the book. Other diagnostic tests frequently employed by physiatrists include electromyography (EMG) and nerve conduction studies (NCS), xerography, and thermography. EMG and NCS are helpful to verify the presence or absence of radicular or peripheral nerve dysfunction, especially when clinical examination is inconclusive. Altered electrical potentials and conduction usually cannot be distinguished earlier than 3 weeks after onset of symptoms. Baseline electrodiagnostic studies however are often done earlier by some clinicians for all suspected radiculopathies in order to compare these with subsequent studies. This practice indeed may be helpful in order to allow dating of lesions, to assess acuity, and to detect changes caused by combinations of entrapment neuropathy and radiculopathy prior to treatment (3). Electrodiagnostic studies are generally considered noncontributory in the presence of muscle spasm, although it has been reported that patients with low back pain and palpable muscle spasm have EMG activity in paraspinal muscles during sleep, whereas controls have none (4).

Thermography is sometimes used to document objectively the presence of muscle spasm, trigger points, and even radiculopathy in disc disease (5). Although controversial as an accurate diagnostic technique, it is well-documented that thermography detects infra-red heat emission from the body and provides a thermal color image where 1°C heat difference accounts for a difference in color. Numerous extrinsic and intrinsic factors may influence the thermography image, including environmental temperature and local circulation, but, if taken into consideration, a definitely asymmetrical image may be clinically useful.

Functional Evaluation

An important part of the physiatrist evaluation is the accurate assessment of the functional consequences of an illness or injury. The World Health Organization defined three terms which are frequently used when functional deficits are discussed, i.e., impairment, disability, and handicap. *Impairment* is "any loss or abnormality of psychological, physical, or anatomical structure of function," e.g., paralysis. *Disability* is "any restriction or lack (resulting from an impairment) of an ability to perform an activity in the manner within the range considered normal for a human being," e.g., paralysis resulting in inability to walk. *Handicap* is "a disadvantage for a given individual, resulting from an impairment or disability that limits or prevents the fulfillment of a role that is normal (depending on age, sex, and social and cultural factors) for that individual," e.g., paralysed, unable to walk and therefore can't meet the requirements of the job and return to work (6).

The functional evaluation addresses a number of communication, self-care, and mobility activities, each rated according to the individual's level of independence, i.e., completely independent, independent with devices, requires assistance (supervision, "spotting," reminding, physical help) or completely dependent. The functional evaluation has become the guide against which the effec-

Table 30.2. Functional Independence Measure

LEVELS		
	7 Complete Independence (Timely, Safely) 6 Modified Independence (Device)	NO HELPER
	Modified Dependence 5 Supervision 4 Minimal Assist (Subject = 75%+) 3 Moderate Assist (Subject = 50%+) Complete Dependence 2 Maximal Assist (Subject = 25%+) 1 Total Assist (Subject = 0%+)	HELPER

	ADMIT	DISCHG	FOL-UP
Self Care			
A. Eating			
B. Grooming			
C. Bathing			
D. Dressing-Upper Body			
E. Dressing-Lower Body			
F. Toileting			
Sphincter Control			
G. Bladder Management			
H. Bowel Management			
Mobility			
Transfer:			
I. Bed, Chair, Wheelchair			
J. Toilet			
K. Tub, Shower			
Locomotion			
L. Walk/wheel Chair	w c	w c	w c
M. Stairs			
Communication			
N. Comprehension	a v	a v	a v
O. Expression	v n	v n	v n
Social Cognition			
P. Social Interaction			
Q. Problem Solving			
R. Memory			
Total FIM			

NOTE: Leave no blanks; enter 1 if patient not testable due to risk.

tiveness of rehabilitation services are gauged. Accurate comprehensive evaluation requires collection of numerous diverse data. Several evaluation scales have been developed for measurement; some are simple and easy to use but provide incomplete information, while others are detailed, extensive, complicated, and time-consuming, as they address not only performance and self-care, but also the quality of life with respect to such factors as employment, income, education, family activities, living arrangement, transportation, etc. Computer technology has made collection analysis and plotting of data much easier and thus has made it possible to document progress during both inpatient and outpatient rehabilitation. Currently, the functional evaluation scale which appears to be gaining wide acceptance is the Functional Independence Measure (FIM) (Table 30.2)(7).

Psychological Evaluation

It is important to keep in mind that many of the conditions which affect the cervical spine are associated with various psychological changes. Severe neck injury is often accompanied by cerebral concussion and residual cognitive deficits. Chronic pain may influence behavior and mood. Conversion reaction and emotional tension may play a role in the etiology of neck pain. The prospect of a permanent disability will cause some degree of reactive depression. A psychological assessment is thus most important, and when psychological abnormalities are suggested a more detailed evaluation and intervention by a clinical psychologist may be requested.

Table 30.3. General Indications for Heat Therapy

1. Analgesia
2. Relaxation of muscles
3. Sedation
4. Increased extensibility of collagen
5. Increased cutaneous blood flow
6. Increased phagocytosis

PHYSICAL AGENTS

Physical agents have been used therapeutically for thousands of years in the management of musculoskeletal and neurological disorders, although interest and belief in their therapeutic efficacy has fluctuated. The medical profession's view of many of these agents has been mixed with suspicion for the greater part of this century, partly due to the incomplete scientific foundation for the clinical use of many of these and partly because treatments with physical agents often can be provided by nonphysicians. The clinical use of physical agents is constantly being refined, and many that were frequently used previously are now rarely employed while new approaches are being evaluated or are already in use (laser beams, electronic devices, etc.).

This section will review the therapeutic application of various physical agents and approaches, their usefulness, indications, and contraindications, especially as they relate to disorders of the cervical spine.

Heat: The local application of heat is a time-honored and useful intervention, especially in the management of pain, whereas systemic hyperthermia (fever therapy) is no longer used. Local application of heat results in increased local temperature, metabolism, circulation, and membrane permeability, as well as in supply of oxygen, nutrients, antibodies, and leukocytes in the heated tissue, a reaction similar to an acute inflammatory response. This may be helpful in clearing metabolites and debris from a tissue with chronic low-grade inflammation. Additionally, heat results in mild analgesia, sedation, as well as decrease in gamma nerve fiber activity and in viscoelasticity of collagen, all of which combine to make physical activity and exercises easier to perform following heat application. The general indications for local applications of heat are listed in Table 30.3 and its contraindications in Table 30.4.

Heat may be applied superficially or deep in the tissues by various means. When heat therapy is prescribed, it is

Table 30.4. General Contraindications for Heat Therapy

1. Impaired circulation
2. Impaired sensation
3. Inability to communicate (infants, confused patients)
4. Metal implants
5. Edema
6. Acute inflammation, trauma, or bleeding
7. Poor cardiac reserve
8. Malignancy in treated area
9. Bleeding disorders
10. Heat intolerance (MS, SLE, adrenal insuff.)
11. Scarred and atrophic skin

necessary for the physician to state the source of the heat, the body part to be treated, frequency of treatment, and precautions, if any. The safe intensity of the heat source and duration of the heat application as well as the most appropriate position of the patient, should be well-known to the physical therapist and thus may not always need to be stated.

Superficial heating of tissues is more often used than deep heating and is administered by three different mechanisms, i.e., conduction, conversion, and convection. The penetration of superficial heat is small or less than 1 cm due to the skin's limited heat tolerance, poor tissue conductivity, and the body's physiological response to reduce local temperature elevation. Maximum heating is usually obtained in 15–20 minutes. Conductive heat is commonly applied as hot packs, hot water bottle, electric heating pads, or paraffin. The infra-red radiant energy from a heat lamp converted to superficial heat is a convenient and inexpensive way of providing local heat, but this method tends to dry the skin and is less preferred than moist heat. Convective heating modalities, i.e., whirlpools and Hubbard tanks, provide gentle massage and debridement of wounds by the action of warm, agitated water in addition to superficial heating. Safe water temperature depends on the patient's general health and the body parts to be treated, i.e., less than 39°–40°C for the whole body and lower limbs and 40°–43°C for the upper limbs.

Deep heating modalities, i.e., ultrasound and diathermy with short-waves or microwaves, are required to heat tissues at more than 1 cm of depth. Here different forms of energy are converted to heat deep in the tissues, but the actual depth of penetration depends on the exact modality, frequency of energy waves, techniques, and tissue composition.

Ultrasound (US), perhaps the most commonly used deep heating agent, consists of high frequency sound waves (standard 0.8—1MHz). Besides heating, some nonthermal biophysical effects, i.e., cavitation, media motion, and standing waves, may occur with use of US with potential beneficial or harmful effect (8). US is usually delivered by direct contact, stroking the skin over the affected body part with the head of the US device using intensity of 0.5 to 2 W/cm^2 and continuous or interrupted wave form for 5–10 minutes. A coupling medium, i.e., water, gel, or oil, is applied to the skin to increase effectiveness. Recently, a technique called phonophoresis has become popular. Here, pharmaceutical substances, i.e., cortisone, lidocaine, etc., are mixed with the coupling medium and presumably forced by the US into the tissues. US may be used for numerous subacute or chronic clinical conditions, i.e., tendonitis, bursitis, arthritis, etc. but should be avoided over a fluid-filled body cavity and the central nervous system.

Short-wave diathermy (SWD) another popular method of conversive deep heating employs radio waves of 27.12 MHz for tissue heating. Higher temperatures are usually reached in tissues rich with water (i.e., muscle) rather than in fat. Special care is required to reduce sweating of the skin and subsequent overheating by application of towels. Metals such as jewelry or surgical implants, should not be present in or on the patient's body, as these may distort the electromagnetic field and absorb excessive heat.

Microwave diathermy is not used very often in health care facilities but is effective to heat water-rich tissues, i.e., muscles and joints. Rather complicated dosimetry and guidelines for safe use along with numerous precautions have reduced its popularity, although focusing the heat waves is relatively easy.

Cold: Cryotherapy employs various simple cooling modalities, i.e., ice, cold water, vaporizing liquids, chemical packs, refrigerated units, etc., which are applied to the skin to produce superficial local effects and secondary distant changes. The effect of local cold application are essentially opposite to those of heat, which are described above, although with continuous cooling to 15°C of tissue temperature, vasodilatation occurs. In addition, cooling reduces spasticity, muscle tone, and pain perception. Effects can usually be obtained after 10 minutes of application, but 20–30 minute treatment periods are customary. The major indications for cold application is acute musculoskeletal trauma, where cold is applied intermittently during the first 24–48 hours after the injury in order to reduce pain, swelling, pressure, reflex muscle spasm, and the detrimental effects of hypoxia. Cold may also be used to reduce chronic musculoskeletal pain in conjunction with an exercise program, to reduce spasticity, and to preserve tissue viability. Prolonged cooling should be avoided as it may cause tissue damage. Acutely injured athletes should be examined carefully before being allowed to re-enter the game after application of cold, which by pain reduction may mask the symptoms of a serious injury.

Electrical Stimulation: Electricity has been used therapeutically for centuries for a variety of clinical conditions. Its current clinical use in physical medicine is mostly limited to neuromuscular stimulation, although iontophoresis and electrolysis are techniques that are occasionally employed. Iontophoresis is a process of transferring polarized ions into tissues by an electrical force. Since this is a slow and cumbersome process most physicians prefer to inject the chemically active substances into the tissues for treatment of various musculoskeletal conditions where iontophoresis might otherwise be helpful. Electrolysis refers to destruction of tissue lesions with the use of electricity.

Neuromuscular electrical stimulation has been used extensively to prevent atrophy and fibrosis of weak muscles, to reduce pain, spasticity, and muscle spasms, and in recent years, to provide function lost by upper motor neuron paralysis (functional electrical stimulation, FES). FES was first attempted 30 years ago (9), but its use has been enhanced during the last decade by technological development. Clinical application has included electrical stimulation of various organs, i.e., bowel, bladder, male sexual organs (for erection and ejaculation), inner ear, as well as pacing of the diaphragm and the heart for respiration and correction of cardiac dysrhythmia. Extensive research and clinical trials on the usefulness of FES in providing function for upper and lower extremities paralyzed by upper motor neuron lesions have been conducted for many years. This technique will be discussed further in this chapter in the section on cervical spinal cord injury.

Transcutaneous electrical nerve stimulation (TENS) has become a popular and often an effective way of treating various painful conditions of the musculoskeletal and peripheral nervous systems. Its use is based on the "Gate Theory" of Melzack and Wall (10) where nociceptive signals may be blocked in the substantia gelatinosa in the spinal cord ("The Gate") by certain afferent sensory signals generated by TENS. The TENS unit is small and easily portable and provides adjustable current (0–100mA), pulse rate (1–200Hz), and pulse width (10–300 microseconds). The electrodes are placed in a rather arbitrary fashion over the painful area, nerves, trigger points, etc. The clinician and the patient work together to find subjectively by trial and error the most effective parameters with respect to the stimulus strength, frequency, pulse width, and electrode placement. It is customary, however, to start with the device set at low amplitudes and high frequency. TENS use should be avoided in individuals with cardiac pacemakers or dysrythmias, as well as in close proximity to sensitive body organs, i.e., heart, carotid sinus, epiglottis, etc.

Biofeedback is a treatment method which uses nonphysiological information obtained by monitoring (feedback) various physiological functions in order to obtain better control of these. Biofeedback in its most basic form may be listening to and responding to the instructions and comments of a trainer, coach, or therapist, but in recent decades various sophisticated electronic equipment has allowed continuous monitoring and feedback of different intricate body functions, i.e., by EMG, EKG, thermometry, sphygmomanometry, etc. With respect to neck disorders, EMG biofeedback with both visible and auditory signals has been used with success for muscle relaxation in tension myalgia as well as for reeducation of paretic muscles. There are no specific contraindications or adverse effects for this kind of biofeedback.

Massage: Therapeutic manipulation of the soft tissues of the body in a systematic manner is an old remedy used to reduce pain, relax muscles, increase mobilization, diminish swelling, improve circulation, or simply to increase physical and emotional wellbeing. Numerous mechanical and electrical devices are available for this purpose, but the human hand, however, is still considered the most effective means of application. Manual massage is time-consuming and fatiguing for the therapist and should therefore not be prescribed rigidly by the physician but rather used in a limited fashion at the therapist's discretion. Massage also tends to become habit-forming or addictive for some patients, further emphasizing utmost care on the part of the prescribing physician. Several different massage techniques exist within the major categories of eastern and western massage. Eastern massage aims for reflex effect on various organs through the nervous system by stimulation of skin points along the meridians, i.e., acupressure, reflexology, etc., whereas western massage aims directly at the musculoskeletal and vascular systems by various approaches, i.e., stroking (effleurage), kneading (pétrissage), percussion (tapotement), and friction. Massage is optimally given after heat application with the patient completely relaxed and comfortable. It should never cause pain and is contraindicated at the site of thrombophlebitis, tissue infection, open wounds, hematomas, and malignant neoplasms.

Therapeutic exercise: Physical exercise is currently the most important therapeutic agent in physical medicine, an indispensable part of any longterm treatment of neck and back disorders. The exercise program may be designed for muscle strengthening, muscle re-education, and for improving general endurance, range of motion, or coordination. Muscle strengthening exercises may be isometric, isotonic, or isokinetic. Isometric exercise does not involve joint motion and therefore is indicated for painful or unstable body parts, whereas isotonic exercise involves motion with variable resistance given. Isokinetic exercise involves use of special equipment (Cybex) to provide constant resistance. Passive exercises to maintain or increase joint range of motion are performed by an assistant for stretching of muscles and joints. Other exercises include those that are task oriented, e.g., (ADL [activities of daily life] and ambulation) which by repetition may insure safety and enhanced function.

Traction: Cervical traction when properly applied is generally considered helpful in the management of certain painful conditions in the neck regardless of nerve root involvement, although scientific evidence supporting its efficacy is scant. It may relieve muscle spasm and widen the intervertebral foramina thus ameliorating new root compression. Traction should only be applied after careful medical history, physical examination, and diagnostic work-up has been completed. It is contraindicated in acute soft tissue injuries, spinal instability, myelopathy, and malignant or infectious disease of the spine. The physician needs to ensure that the traction is properly applied, whether it is given at a health care facility or at home. Various techniques of traction exist, each of which may be given in the sitting or supine positions, and may be continuous or intermittent, manual or mechanical. Cervical traction has been found to be most effective when the angle of the pull is 15–25°C of flexion. Whether sitting or supine, the force of traction should be applied to the occiput and not the jaw. Intermittent traction is generally better tolerated than continuous traction when similar loads are used. Usually 15–20 lbs are initially applied when traction is intermittent, and this is increased to 35–50 lbs as tolerated with each treatment session lasting 20–30 minutes. Horizontal continuous traction, commonly used in hospital settings for patients in acute pain, employs much lower weights (5–10 lbs) for progressively longer periods of time as tolerated, up to 24 hours per day.

Manipulation: Spinal manipulation, the principal treatment approach of chiropraxis, and to some extent, osteopathy, involves application of forces on the various components of the spine (muscles, tendons, ligaments, joints, bones, discs, etc.) in order to restore normal alignment and motion as well as to eliminate pain. Scientific proof of the benefits of spinal manipulations is lacking, but there is ample subjective evidence that it is helpful in treating acute and even chronic musculoskeletal back and neck pain (11); some even believe that it may result in relief of visceral symptoms. Few physicians have obtained the necessary skills of spinal manipulative therapy, which appears to be gaining some interest among physical therapists. Complications of this treatment are reportedly rare, but are most likely to occur with manipulation of the cervical portion of the spine. This may occasionally cause symptoms of vertebral artery insufficiency for shorter or longer periods of time especially when neck extension is employed. Nonetheless, the contraindications for spinal manipulation include all of those for cervical traction, as well as several others (11).

Cervical Orthoses: Spinal orthoses (12) can be classified according to the spinal segments involved, e.g., cervical orthoses (CO), cervical thoracic orthoses (CTO), head cervical orthoses (HCO), head cervical thoracic orthoses (HCTO), cervical thoracic lumbosacral orthoses (CTLSO), etc., or they can be described according to the restriction they provide, as flexible, semi-rigid, or rigid. COs (Fig. 30.1) are provided to restrict motion of the cervical spine either by mechanical means or by serving as a reminder to limit motion (sensory biofeedback). They are clinically useful in numerous cervical disorders i.e., acute soft tissue injury, muscle spasm, radiculopathy, bony instability, and neck pain for a variety of other reasons. Three basic designs

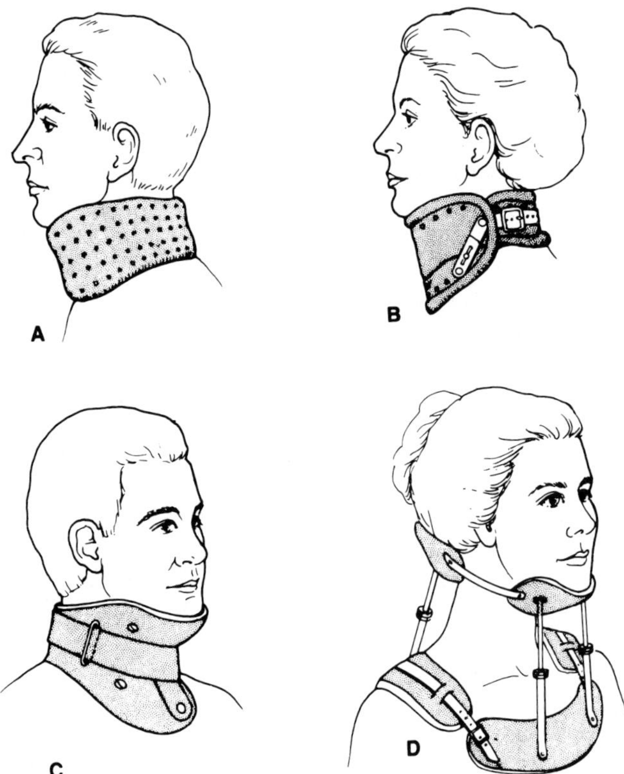

Figure 30.1. Cervical orthoses: **A,** cervical collar **B,** semi-rigid adjustable cervical collar **C,** semi-rigid thermoplastic two-piece cervical collar (Philadelphia collar) and **D,** cervical multiple poster appliance. (Reproduced with permission from Ragnarsson KT. Orthotics and shoes. In: DeLisa JA, ed. Rehabilitation medicine: principles and practice. Philadelphia: J.B. Lippincott, 1988).

are available: collars, poster appliances, and custom molded devices. The design of most COs is such that neck flexion and extension is restricted more than rotation and lateral flexion.

Soft collars made of cloth or foam rubber are usually comfortable to wear and limit motion mostly through sensory feedback, but provide little mechanical restriction. More *rigid collars* made of various plastic materials are available in different designs to provide greater support and restriction, i.e., the Philadelphia collar. *Poster appliances* usually have between two and four adjustable metal uprights which connect the chin and occipital pieces to the sternal and back plates. These devices restrict neck motion more effectively than collars. The sternal occipital mandibular immobilizer (SOMI) (Fig. 30.2) is lightweight, easily applied and fitted, comfortable, provides excellent neck support, and is the CTO which is generally preferred.

Custom molded total contact body appliances are usually made of plastic materials which are molded over a positive body cast. Best known of these is the Minerva type orthosis which encloses the trunk, neck, and the back of the head and may have a band around the fo-

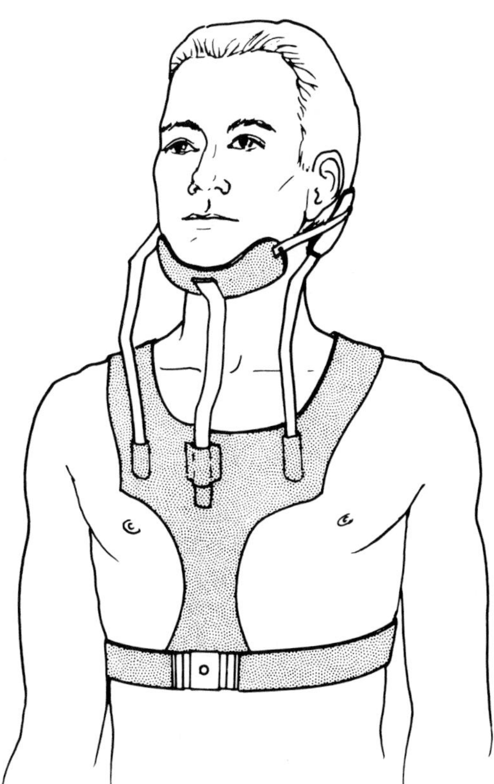

Figure 30.2. Sternal-occipital-mandibular immobilizer (SOMI orthosis). (Reproduced with permission from Ragnarsson KT. Orthotics and shoes. In: DeLisa JA, ed. Rehabilitation medicine: principles and practices. Philadelphia: J.B. Lippincott, 1988).

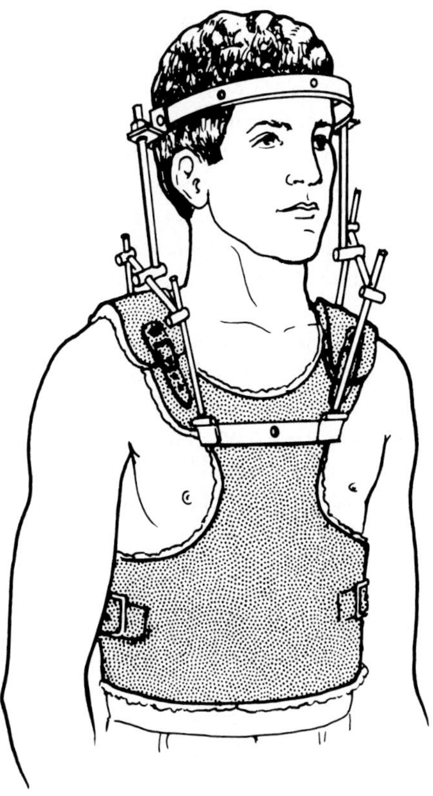

Figure 30.3. Halo-orthosis. (Reproduced with permission from Ragnarsson KT. Orthotics and shoes. In: DeLisa JA, ed. Rehabilitation medicine: principles and practice. Philadelphia: J.B. Lippincott, 1988).

rehead, thus providing excellent restriction of lateral and rotational neck motions in addition to the limitation of flexion and extension. The halo orthosis provides the maximum restriction of motion of the potentially unstable cervical spine (Fig. 30.3). Here a carefully placed metal halo ring is fixed to the outer table of the skull bones with four metal pins. The pins are optimally placed under local anesthesia, approximately one centimeter above the lateral third of each eyebrow and one centimeter above the top of each ear. Upright metal bars connect the halo ring to a rigid plastic thoracic jacket which is lined with sheepskin. In recent designs the metal used in halo orthoses is inert to minimize interference with diagnostic imaging techniques. Halo orthoses are generally well-tolerated, although skin problems may arise both from pin site infection and from excessive pressure over the bony prominences under the jacket. Frequent inspection and readjustment is required after application of the halo orthosis. A significant advantage of this orthosis is that the patient with unstable cervical spine may be mobilized out of bed and allowed to participate in physical activities whether ambulatory or confined to a wheelchair.

Different upper and lower limb orthoses and assistive devices may be indicated for the patient with disorders of the cervical spine and a host of associated different neurological deficits, but discussion of these is outside the scope of this chapter.

CLINICAL DISORDERS OF THE CERVICAL SPINE

The final section of this chapter will address the most significant clinical disorders that affect the cervical spine and will most benefit from nonsurgical intervention, including treatment with physical agents and rehabilitation intervention.

Acceleration Hyperextension Injury

In rear end car collisions, the vehicle hit and the occupant's body are both suddenly thrust forward, but in the absence of adequate headrest the head of the occupant will fall backward into a forceful extension ("whiplash"). Whereas sudden forceful neck flexion which often follows, is stopped by the chin hitting the sternum, there is no mechanical stop to forceful neck extension until the occiput strikes the upper thoracic spine far beyond the physiological extension excursion. Such hyperextension may result in minor or major tears of the various tissues anteriorly in the neck, e.g., muscles, anterior longitudinal ligament, esophagus, larynx, intervertebral discs, vertebral artery, sympathetic nerves, bones, and joints (13) and in compression of the spinal cord if the spinal canal is abnormally narrow. Not surprisingly, cerebral concussion and injury to the temporomandibular joint may occur as well. The severity of the injury depends on numerous factors, but especially the rate of acceleration of the struck vehicle after the impact, which in turn depends on the force applied and the inertia (13).

Symptoms are somewhat variable depending on the severity of the injury. Pain and stiffness are the primary complaints and may start immediately after the injury or be delayed as long as 1–2 days. The pain is usually diffuse, but mostly localized in the neck, shoulders, and suboccipital regions, or radiate, or referred to one or both arms. Headaches are common, and many patients later complain of back pain as well. Other common complaints include sensory deficits in the C7–8 root distribution, dizziness, tinnitus, dysphagia, hoarseness, and visual blurring. Duration of symptoms is extremely variable, or from a few days to several months or years, by which time they may have taken considerable emotional toll. Clinical examination may initially be entirely normal, but within a few hours (0–48) tenderness of the anterior and posterior cervical muscles is noted with muscle spasm and restriction of motion. Neurological examination is usually within normal limits. Radiological findings are insignificant, except for occasional subtle changes which should be interpreted with care i.e., loss or reversal of the normal cervical lordosis, widened disc space, prevertebral soft tissue swelling, and, rarely, anterior avulsion fracture or posterior facet joints fracture. When symptoms are severe or continue for weeks, new x-rays and additional imaging studies should be done.

Treatment: Appropriate and adequate early treatment is of great importance to ensure optimal results. The treatment should be based on good understanding of the pathomechanism and severity of the injury, both of which should be carefully and reassuringly explained to the patient. Early rest is most important. This may be accomplished by applying a cervical collar which may suffice exclusively for the milder cases, but for more significant injuries bedrest for 1–7 days is required. The cervical collar should not be used for more than 2 weeks (3), as prolonged use may cause neck muscle atrophy and weakness, reduction of the neck motions, dependency, and functional overlay. After no more than 2 weeks of collar use patients should be started on an exercise program and gradually weaned off the collar. Cervical isometric exercises for neck flexors, extensors and lateral flexors should be performed several times each day by having the patient alone, or with a therapist, contract the muscles against a firm resistance for 10 seconds and repeat each contraction up to 10 times as tolerated (Fig. 30.4). Range of motion or mobilization exercises should not be started until after the acute symptoms have subsided. Application of cold initially after the injury and of heat after at least 72 hours have passed, may help to relieve the pain and the muscle spasm. Analgesics and sedatives with muscle relaxing action may be given for a brief period of time especially during the acute period while bedrest is also recommended. Cervical traction may sometimes relieve pain but is rarely indicated in the acute period and, indeed, may be contraindicated. While the symptomatic patient should be given advice on "Neck Sparing Routine" (13) i.e., sleeping on the back in reclining or semi-sitting position for 10 hours per night and avoid symptom producing activities, i.e., sitting with the head tilted backwards ("tuck the chin in"), emotional tension, prolonged driving, reaching or looking up, lifting heavy objects, and participation in sports while symptomatic. Since various physical activities may cause or aggravate pain for a lengthy period of time, in order to reduce fear and emotional tension and to encourage full participation in beneficial activities the patient needs to be reassured that this does not signify further damage to neck structures.

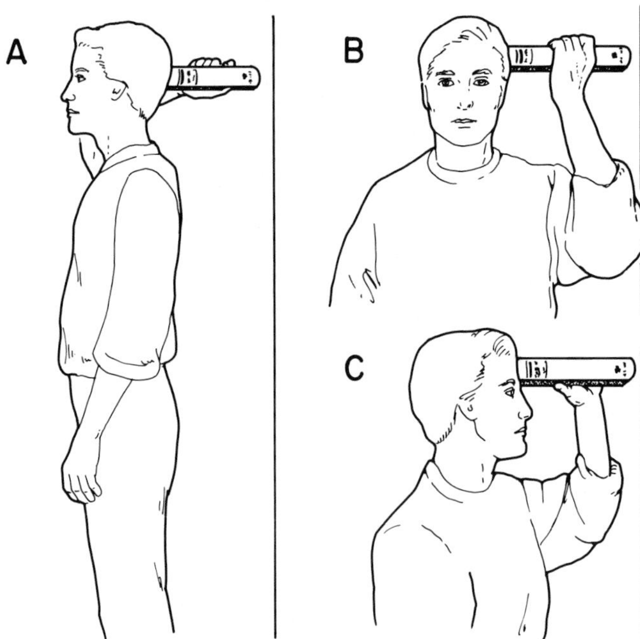

Figure 30.4. Cervical isometric exercises. A book is used to maintain neutral neck position while firm pressure is applied to isometrically strengthen neck extensor **(A)** lateral flexor **(B)** and flexor muscles **(C)**.

Duration of symptoms is highly variable and does not appear to be related to the assessed severity of the injury but, rather, to a host of other factors (14) i.e., arm numbness and pain, persistent pain, prolonged need for cervical collar and various other treatment, preexisting degenerative disease of the cervical spine, etc.

The role of emotional factors and pending litigation in

the chronicity of symptoms has been much discussed, especially because objective findings are usually scant. Various studies have provided conflicting views on this issue. In defense of the symptoms, MacNab (13) points out first, that patients with chronic symptoms have often sustained other even more serious injuries which do not result in lasting complaints, second, that flexion or lateral impact injuries of the neck rarely result in prolonged complaints, and third, that 45% of patients in his series of 266 patients had persistent symptoms 2 years after court settlement. Optimal outcome can best be assured by optimal treatment, both during the acute period and after symptoms have become chronic. When symptoms become chronic the physician needs to establish a close and trusting relationship with the patient, and to be cognizant and respectful of the original injury and of the symptoms, honest about the treatment provided, realistically optimistic about the prognosis, as well as concerned about the patient obtaining maximum function in every aspect within the limits of the disability, i.e., physical, psychological, social, vocational, recreational, and economic, the physician must be careful not to aggravate anger or litiginous behavior.

Cervical Myofascial Pain

Pain arising from the soft tissues in the neck and back, i.e., muscles, fascia, ligaments, and tendons, without neurological deficits or significant skeletal findings, has often been attributed to a condition which is variously called fibromyalgia (15), fibrositis (16), interstitial myofibrositis (17), tension myositis (18), and myofascial pain syndrome (19) as well as by several other terms. This condition typically affects women 20–50 years of age who complain of diffuse aches and pains in the neck, shoulders, back, and limbs. The symptoms have usually been present for several months or years, either continuously or recurrently. The pain is usually aggravated by numerous factors including cold, humid weather, different physical activities or, paradoxically, inactivity, poor work habits, anxiety, emotional stress, and poor sleep. The majority of patients also complain of fatigue, stiffness, chronic sleep disorder, a subjective feeling of numbness, headaches, anxiety, depression, and altered bowel habits similar to irritable bowel symptoms.

On physical examination, multiple tender spots, usually referred to as trigger points, are found on palpation in certain typical locations, i.e., in the trapezius, suboccipital, and sternocleidomastoid muscles, in the neck, thoracic and lumbar paraspinal muscles, iliosacral region, at the costochondral junction, and in the limbs at the medial fat pads of the knees and over the lateral and medial aspects of the elbows. The location of these trigger points usually correlates with the subjective complaints of pain and limitation of movement, and, in general, the more numerous these points are, the more common are the other subjective complaints. The examination may further reveal structural changes which affect posture and body mechanics and place increased stress on musculoskeletal structures, i.e., scoliosis, poor posture, large breasts, leg length discrepancy, etc. Frequency, the complaints of pain at the trigger points are limited to the neck and shoulders or, conversely, to the low back. It has been recommended that the term fibromyalgia be used for widespread presence of trigger points and the term myofascial pain when there is a regional localization (20).

There are no diagnostic, radiological, or laboratory findings, but thermography has been used to identify trigger points, and dolorimeter is often used to quantify local tenderness by measuring pressure threshold (5). The histopathological changes that have been described (17)(21) are relatively insignificant. Endocrine dysfunction, in particular hypothyroidism and menopause, have been described (22, 23) as a risk factor if not the direct cause of muscle pain (24). The etiology and pathophysiology of this condition remains unknown, although many contributing factors are well-known, both mechanical and psychological. Poor posture with increased cervical lordosis, round, sloping shoulders, increased thoracic kyphosis, flat or caved-in chest, lumbar lordosis, and protuberant abdomen are common findings, and a history of emotional tension, stressful events, low stress tolerance, perfectionistic personality traits, depression, etc. may often be elicited. Nonetheless, psychological abnormalities have been found to be absent in approximately 60% of patients (20). It has been postulated that muscle tension caused by mechanical strain or secondary to the autonomic effects of anxiety may generate ischemia within the muscle, altered muscle fiber contractility, and spasm resulting in pain and tender spots (25)(26).

Treatment: Myofascial pain tends to be chronic or recurrent. A successful management requires that a firm diagnosis be made, a diagnosis which the patient trusts and can rely on. This may require that any number of appropriate diagnostic tests be undertaken to eliminate any doubt that a destructive or crippling condition may be the underlying cause of the symptoms. Following a thorough physical examination and evaluation of all tests, the physician should carefully explain the symptoms to the patient, addressing both mechanical and psychological factors, and give the patient assurance that the condition is benign and not physically deforming or disabling. Most patients respond best to a treatment approach which includes reduction and recognition of stressful factors, both physical and psychological, judicious use of medications (tricyclic antidepressants, cyclobenzaprine (Flexoril) anti-inflammatory agents), use of various physical agents (heat, cold, exercise, TENS, massage, etc.) and trigger point injections. Although excessive physical activity should be avoided, a carefully designed graded exercise program which emphasizes muscle stretching as well as strengthening and endurance exercises for the neck, shoulders, trunk, and all limbs has been very successful. Ultimately, trunk strength, flexibility, and increased aerobic fitness maintained by regular exercise appears to correlate best with improvement of symptoms. It may be speculated that such exercise program may simultaneously both reduce emotional stress as well as improve strength and physical fitness. Injection of trigger points with 2–10 cc of lidocaine 1–2% solution is used extensively by some clinicians, often with excellent results (27). Caution should be taken not to inject the lidocaine into the blood vessel; also, the patient should rest for several minutes afterwards, as complaints of dizziness are frequent. Sometimes the lidocaine is mixed with depot corticosteroid solution for a longer lasting effect, although this is not generally recommended. When one treatment method proves to be unsuccessful, the clinician should modify or dramatically change the approach by use of different treatment techniques, since proper treatment of myofascial pain is more art than science and requires understanding, patience, trust, firmness, and a good doctor-patient relationship over a lengthy period of time.

Acute Cervical Disc Herniation

Although all intervertebral discs will eventually develop degenerative changes as substance is lost from the nucleus pulposus with resulting narrowing of the disc space, acute herniation of a cervical disc with development of distinct neurological signs is relatively rare. When neurological signs do develop due to root compression, nonsurgical treatment is successful for the majority of patients (28), whereas immediate surgical intervention is required for signs of acute cord compression. Persistent or progressive neurological signs, especially motor deficits, also warrant early surgical treatment. Surgical management for severe, persistent, or recurrent pain after other therapy has been attempted unsuccessfully, is often indicated, especially when diagnostic studies show conclusively the presence of a sizeable herniated disc.

The nonsurgical treatment frequently is protracted and time-consuming and thus requires good doctor-patient relationship. The physician must explain clearly to the patient the nature of the pathology, symptoms, and treatment to ensure complete understanding and confidence in this approach. Initially, rest and immobilization of the cervical spine is crucial to allow healing of the ruptured disc and reduction of swelling. While bedrest may be indicated for a few days, a well-fitting cervical orthosis which places the head and neck in slight flexion should be worn continuously for 2 to 3 weeks after which weaning off the orthosis may start. Cervical traction is controversial in the management of acute disc herniation but is probably of little additional value except in the most skillful hands. Manipulation of the neck is risky and should be avoided. Application of heat or cold may help to relieve pain and muscle spasm, but deep heating modalities are of little use. In the past absolute rest has customarily been advocated during acute care, but this concept is changing as it has been pointed out that rapid deconditioning of the body will occur which will impede subsequent rehabilitation efforts and the path to full recovery. If complete segmental rest of the cervical spine can be maintained, a carefully designed exercise program may help to maintain strength and endurance of trunk and extremity muscles. Isometric exercises of the neck muscles as previously described are started after the pain has mostly subsided, frequently 2–3 weeks after onset of the symptoms. Medications should be prescribed judiciously to reduce pain, muscle spasm, and inflammation. A short course of oral corticosteroids has been advocated, but the efficacy of this is not proven.

The treating clinician needs to monitor the patient carefully for any progression of neurological signs and to provide the patient with emotional support and reassurance during the course of management which may last for as long as 6–12 weeks before the patient recovers.

Cervical Spondylosis

Continued degenerative changes of the intervertebral discs result in classical pathological findings which are of varying degree. Some of these changes are easily noted radiologically, i.e., narrowing of disc space, instability with slight subluxation between spinal segments, osteophytes (spurs, ridges) which may encroach upon intervertebral foramina and spinal canal, and fusion between vertebrae as the osteophytes bridge across the discs. It is well-known that as age advances these changes become more visible radiologically and are thus seen in 75% of all people over 50 years of age and in almost 100% 70 years old or older (29)(30). Only a very small percentage of these, however, will have significant clinical symptoms. Correlation of radiological findings with the most common symptoms, i.e., pain, stiffness, crepitus, tenderness, and sensory disturbance in the absence of neurological signs may therefore be difficult and inaccurate. As the degenerative changes progress and the osteophytes in the cervical spine grow larger, encroachment may occur upon the nerve roots or, less commonly, the spinal cord, arteries, or esophagus, depending on the osteophyte's exact location and size. As a result, a variety of symptoms and signs may be produced.

Nonsurgical treatment is effective for most patients. The treatment should be directed in a fashion closely similar to that for acute cervical disc herniation when neurological signs are present or for that of myofascial pain when neurological signs are absent. The surgical treatment should be reserved for those with neurological signs, especially when these are rapidly progressive or, electively, if patients do not respond to nonsurgical therapy. Results of surgery tend to be better in acute cases when the location of a single large osteophyte correlates with the clinical findings.

When neurological signs are absent application of a cervical orthosis or traction for a brief period of time and use of superficial and deep heating modalities as well as a TENS unit may help to relieve pain. An exercise program should be prescribed with incremental efforts as the acute symptoms subside in order to improve mobility, posture, strength and endurance. Judicious use of nonnarcotic analgetics and anti-inflammatory medications may further be of value. As with most of the other chronic conditions affecting the cervical spine, understanding, patience, compliance, and confidence are of utmost importance for a successful management, since cure can usually not be found.

Thoracic Outlet Syndrome

The thoracic outlet syndrome is a collective term used to describe various clinical syndromes which cause neurovascular compression between the scalenus anterior and medius muscles above and the first rib below in the lower part of the neck. The exact pathology and the diverse symptomatology is described elsewhere in this book. Suffice it to say that symptoms and signs will include, in order of decreasing frequency, pain in the neck, shoulder, and/or arm, paresthesias in the C8–T1 root distribution, numbness, coldness, muscle fatigue, weakness, and, rarely, atrophy.

Nonsurgical treatment is indicated for all patients except for those who fail to respond to a thorough therapeutic attempt and for those cases that develop signs of acute circulatory impairment. The basis of the nonsurgical management rests on the hypothesis that elevation with slight abduction of the shoulder girdle decreases the compressive forces on the neurovascular bundle at the thoracic outlet (31). While mild symptoms may respond adequately to careful explanation, assurance, and avoidance of aggravating positions and activities, more severe symptoms usually require a therapy program which emphasizes graded strengthening exercises for the shoulder girdle elevators and postural training in order to obtain slight, but persistant, protraction and elevation of the shoulders in order to enlarge the outlet. Stretching of muscles in the neck and shoulders, especially the scalenus and pectoralis muscles, is also important. Adjunctive treatment with general fitness exercises, analgetic medications, application of heat, TENS, cervical traction, breast support, weight loss, etc. should also be considered to further ensure successful outcome.

Cervical Myelopathy

Cervical myelopathy presents a clinical challenge with respect to both diagnosis and management. The rehabilitation of individuals affected by this condition is equally challenging and is as varied as the extent of the neurological deficits. While some patients may have few neurological deficits and may not be in need of rehabilitation treatment, severe cases with quadriplegia will require comprehensive inpatient rehabilitation and subsequent lifelong follow-up.

There are multiple causes for cervical myelopathy, but these may be divided grossly into traumatic and nontraumatic causes. Cervical myelopathy of nontraumatic origin is caused by diverse pathology, i.e., tumors, vascular disturbances, spondylosis, degenerative nervous conditions, etc. These tend to have a relatively gradual progression and result in incomplete neurological deficits. Traumatic cervical spinal cord injury (SCI) with fracture or dislocation, on the other hand, results frequently in quadriplegia with complete loss of motor and sensory function below the injured cord level. Traumatic cervical SCI without fracture or dislocation may occur in individuals with the spinal canal abnormally narrowed by congenital or such acquired conditions as spondylosis and calcified ligaments. These may initially present with incomplete neurological deficits. The various syndromes of cervical myelopathy and the classification of cervical spine injuries are described elsewhere in this book. While it is impossible to actively estimate the incidence of nontraumatic myelopathy given the frequency of mild neurological symptoms due to spondylosis, the incidence of traumatic SCI is estimated to be approximately 30 per million each year, and more than half of these are due to cervical SCI. Almost 50% of these injuries are caused by motor vehicle accidents and 10–20% each by falls, sports activities including diving, and gunshot wounds. Most of the trauma victims are young, between the ages of 15 and 30, whereas patients with nontraumatic myelopathy tend to be significantly older (32).

Rehabilitation: For the sake of simplicity and space, this section will describe briefly the rehabilitation of individuals with traumatic quadriplegia, recognizing that in essence the rehabilitation of individuals with nontraumatic cervical myelopathy is similar.

As soon as the SCI has been identified, secondary prevention and rehabilitation interventions should be initiated. The neurological level and the extent of the injury should be accurately determined (see chapter written by Chandler, Kropf, and Waters). The early care of the patient with SCI is geared towards preventing further cord damage, whether related to spinal instability or to cord ischemia enhanced by various complications, i.e., hypotension, aspiration, and ventilatory failure. An unstable spine needs to be stabilized by external means (spinal traction or orthoses) or by surgical internal fixation. Respiratory dysfunction during the acute period in quadriplegics usually occurs due to paralyzed chest wall muscles and associated injuries, i.e., fractured ribs, bruised lungs, hemothorax, etc. Aspiration of blood or gastric contents may also occur. Atlectasis, pneumonia, and even respiratory arrest may easily occur, especially in quadriplegics and high level paraplegics demanding early aggressive intervention. Cardiovascular disturbances, i.e., bradycardia and hypotension, are frequently noted in quadriplegics and other high level SCI patients who have lost supraspinal sympathetic control, but treatment with medications is usually not necessary. Deep venous thrombosis occurs frequently and may result in pulmonary embolism and death and therefore needs to be aggressively prevented. Heparin, 5000 units subcutaneously every 12 hours, is customarily administered for up to 3 months after the injury, and elastic stockings are applied to the lower extremities. Acute gastrointestinal problems include paralytic ileus of a few days duration, peptic ulcer, and malnutrition, all of which require specific management. Management of the neurogenic bowel should be started as soon as practically possible with the establishment of a bowel routine with evacuation planned for a specific time of the day. Evacuation is facilitated by use of stool softeners, laxatives, and suppositories. The neurogenic bladder is usually of the flaccid type during the first several weeks after the injury and requires insertion of a foley catheter until an intermittent catheterization program can safely be started. Pressure sores, especially on the sacrum and heels, and joint contractures frequently develop during the acute phase when more attention is given to diagnosis and life saving measures than preventive skin and joint care. A good mattress, proper positioning, regular turning, and inspection will help to prevent the development of these complications. The patient should be seen as soon as possible after admission by the physiatrist and by a rehabilitation nurse, and under the direction of the physiatrist various members of the multidisciplinary team should become involved as judged appropriate by the patient's condition. The patient and the family are given psychological support and education in the medical aspects of SCI, and insurance issues are clarified.

When proper stabilization of the spine has been obtained and the patient is free of major medical complications, he is transferred to the inpatient rehabilitation service. This transition is made easier if the patient is well-informed and familiar with the physiatrist and the team of rehabilitation professionals. On the inpatient rehabilitation service, the SCI patient is again evaluated thoroughly by the physiatrist. A detailed medical and social history is obtained. The general medical and the precise neurological status is determined to establish the level and completeness of the spinal cord lesion as well as functional ability. Rehabilitation goals are established for the patient, and the physiatrist prescribes a specific and detailed evaluation and intervention program for the various members of the multidisciplinary rehabilitation team to follow. A number of conditions and complications associated with SCI may be noted which will require intervention (Table 30.5).

When the neurological deficit has been established it is possible to predict with reasonable certainty which functional goals the patient may realistically reach and which assistive devices will be required. Obviously, the lower the level of injury the greater will be the functional potential. A quadriplegic with C3 level or higher only survives if provided with continuous respiratory support by mechanical ventilation or diaphragmatic pacing. A C4 quadriplegic will be able to breathe independently and shrug his shoulders but lacks voluntary movements in his upper extremities. His function would be enhanced by teaching him to operate an environmental control system by mouth or voice which gives him control of the various commercial devices, i.e., television, radio, electrical bed, lights, automatic dialing telephone, door opener, computer, etc. A C5 quadriplegic will remain dependent in ADL although capable of operating an electric wheelchair with a joystick and of doing some limited writing, typing, and grooming using appropriate wrist/hand orthoses. A C6 quadriplegic can become independent for many upper extremity functions by the use of appropriate orthoses (grooming, feeding, writing, etc.) but in general will require assistance with dressing, transfers, bathing, and bowel and bladder management. A C7 quadriplegic who is otherwise healthy and well-motivated should obtain complete independence in an ADL although confined to a wheelchair. Persons with lower level of spinal cord injury should as a rule become totally self-sufficient at a wheelchair level unless impaired by a secondary disability or complication (weight, age, major organ system failure, severe spasticity, etc.). Ambulation, with or without crutches and orthoses is possible, but practically limited to those with grossly incomplete lesions. For severe myelopathy the metabolic cost of ambulation is too great and speed too slow to allow functional ambulation, but nonetheless orthoses for the lower limbs may be prescribed for cultural reasons, for exercise, and for psychological as well as potential physiological benefits.

Table 30.5. Conditions and Complications Associated with Spinal Cord Dysfunction

1. Loss of motor power
2. Loss of sensation
3. Pressure sores
4. Urinary dysfunction
5. Bowel dysfunction
6. Sexual dysfunction
7. Autonomic hyperreflexia
8. Pain
9. Spasticity
10. Joint contractures
11. Heterotrophic ossifications
12. Metabolic disturbances
    a) Negative calcium balance
    b) Negative nitrogen balance
    c) Hormonal imbalance
13. Circulatory disturbances
    a) Orthostatic hypotension
    b) Edema
    c) Deep vein thrombophlebitis
14. Respiratory disturbances
15. Psychological problems
16. Social problems
17. Vocational problems

In recent years, great interest has been generated by the investigative use of computer-controlled functional electrical stimulation (FES) on muscle groups in both the upper and lower extremities to improve hand function and ambulation potential. Bicycle ergometry has also been used clinically in order to improve bulk of the paralyzed muscles, strength, cardiovascular endurance, circulation, mental outlook, etc. (33).

Successful rehabilitation is not limited to the management of the various conditions and complications associated with SCI and obtaining maximum physical function as allowed by the neurological deficit and other limitations. The additional major goals of inpatient rehabilitation include thorough health maintenance education, psychological adjustment, obtaining appropriate adaptive equipment, accessible community housing, and transportation, formulation of vocational plans, referrals to community resources, i.e., physicians, nursing services, peer groups, Office of Vocational Rehabilitation, equipment vendors, and information networks, as well as solution of difficult financial issues.

At discharge each patient is provided with a plan for longterm care and follow-up. Since the major physical rehabilitation goals have generally been met at discharge, the patient may not always require intensive outpatient physical and occupational therapy. However, to ensure good health and successful community reintegration, the services of a physician, SCI nurse, social worker, and vocational counselor are needed. Evaluation of the neurogenic bladder and the kidneys are required annually for the first several years, but less often thereafter if the patient has been complication-free.

The life expectancy after SCI has increased significantly during the last half of the century but still depends to some extent upon the level and completeness of the cord lesion, as well as on age, general health, and social factors. Cardiovascular and respiratory disorders have replaced renal complications as the most common cause of death. It is difficult to assess psychological adjustment and social success, as many SCI individuals find disincentives in returning to work.

CONCLUSION

Most disorders of the cervical spine, whether affecting the soft tissue, the skeleton, or the nervous system, will benefit from treatment with physical agents and the services of the rehabilitation team. As soon as diagnosis has been made and appropriate surgical and medical interventions have been initiated, the physiatrist should be consulted with respect to further management. Hopefully, the main principles of the physical medicine and rehabilitation presented in this chapter will improve understanding and provide guidelines for clinicians in other medical specialties to follow.

REFERENCES

1. Krusen FA. Physical medicine. Philadelphia: W.B. Saunders Co., 1941.

2. Hoppenfeld S. Physical examination of the spine and extremities. New York: Appleton-Century-Crofts, 1976.

3. Lieberman JS. Cervical soft tissue injuries and cervical disc disease. In: Leek JC, Gershwin ME, Fowler WM, eds. Principles of physical medicine and rehabilitation in the musculoskeletal diseases. Orlando, FL: Grune and Stratton, 1986:263–286.

4. Fischer AA, Chang CH. Electromyographic evidence of paraspinal muscle spasm during sleep in patients with low back pain. Clin J Pain 1985;1:147–154.

5. Fischer AA. Documentation of muscle pain and soft tissue pathology. In: Kraus H, ed. Diagnosis and treatment of muscle pain. Chicago, IL: Quintessence Books, 1988;55–65.

6. World Health Organization. International classification of impairment, disabilities and handicaps: a manual of classification relating to the consequences of disease. Geneva: World Health Organization, 1980.

7. Research Foundation. State University of New York. Guide for use of the uniform data set for medical rehabilitation. Buffalo, NY: SUNY, 1987.

8. Coakley WT. Biophysical effects of ultrasound at therapeutic intensities. Physiotherapy 1978;64:166–169.

9. Liberson WT, Holmquest HJ, Scot D, Dow MJ. Functional electrotherapy: stimulation of the peroneal nerve synchronized with the swing phase of the gait of hemiplegic patients. Arch Phys Med Rehabil 1961;42:101–105.

10. Melzack R, Wall PD. Pain mechanism: a new theory. Science 1965;150:971–979.

11. Geiringer SR, Kincaid CB, Rechtien JJ. Traction, manipulation and massage. In: DeLisa JA, ed. Rehabilitation medicine, principles and practice. Philadelphia: JB Lippincott, 1988:276–294.

12. Ragnarsson KT. Orthotics and shoes. In: DeLisa JA, ed. Rehabilitation medicine principles and practice. Philadelphia: JB Lippincott, 1988:307–329.

13. MacNab I. Acceleration extension injuries of the cervical spine. In: Rothman RH, Simeone FA, ed. The spine. Philadelphia: W.B. Saunders Co., 1982:647–660.

14. Hohl M. Soft tissue injuries of the neck in automobile accidents: factors influencing prognosis. J Bone Joint Surg 1974;56A:1675–1682.

15. Goldenberg DL. Fibromyalgia syndrome. JAMA 1987;257:2782–2787.

16. Kraft GH, Johnson EW, LaBan MM. The fibrositis syndrome. Arch Phys Med Rehabil 1968;49:155–162.

17. Awad EA. Interstitial myofibrositis. Arch Phys Med Rehabil 1973;54:449–453.

18. Sarno JE. Chronic back pain and psychic conflict. Scand J Rehabil Med 1976;8:143–153.

19. Travell J, Rinzler SH. Myofascial genesis of pain. Postgrad Med 1952;11:425–434.

20. Bennet RM. Fibromyalgia. Editorial: JAMA 1987;257:2802–2803.

21. Kalyan-Raman UP, Kalyan-Raman K, Yunus MB, et al. Muscle pathology in primary fibromyalgia syndrome: a light microscopic histochemical and ultrastructural study. J Rheumatol 1984;11:808–813.

22. Golding DN. Hypothyroidism representing with musculoskeletal symptoms. Ann Rheum Dis 1970;29:10–14.

23. Wilke WS, Sheeler LR, Makarowski WS. Hypothyroidism with presenting symptoms of fibrositis. J Rheumatol 1981;8:626–631.

24. Sonkin LS. Myofascial pain in metabolic disorders. In: Kraus H, ed. Diagnosis and treatment of muscle pain. Chicago, IL: Quintessence Books, 1988:91–95.

25. Cailliet R. Neck pain originating in the soft tissues. In: Neck and arm pain. Philadelphia: F.A. Davis Co., 1972:40–43.

26. Sarno JE. Etiology of neck and back pain. An autonomic myoneuralgia? J Nerv Ment Dis 1981;169:55–59.

27. Kraus H. Trigger points. In: Kraus H, ed. Diagnosis and treatment of muscle pain. Chicago, IL: Quintessence Books, 1988:39–50.

28. Simeone FA, Rothman RH. Cervical disc disease. In: Rothman RH, Simeone FA, eds. The spine. Philadelphia: W.B. Saunders Co., 1982:440–499.

29. Elias F. Roentgen findings in the asymptomatic cervical spine. NY State J Med 1958;58:3300.

30. Pallis C, Jones AM, Spillane JD. Cervical spondylosis: incidence and implications. Brain 1954;77:274.

31. Phull PS. Management of cervical pain. In: DeLisa JA, ed. Rehabilitation medicine principles and practice. Philadelphia: J.B. Lippincott, 1988:749–764.

32. Stover SL, Fine PR, eds. Spinal cord injury. The facts and figures. Alabama: The University of Alabama at Birmingham, Alabama, 1986.

33. Ragnarsson KT. Physiologic effect of functional electrical stimulation—induced exercises in spinal cord injured individuals. Clinical Orthop 1988;233:53–63.

31

Management of Cervical Cord Lesions Including Advances in Rehabilitative Engineering

Barth A. Green, Frank J. Eismont, and K. John Klose

Introduction

The reader should understand that the management of cervical spinal cord injuries is based more on the art of the medicine than on science. Protocols for the systems approach to acute cervical spinal cord injury (SCI) presented in this chapter represent the present treatment program utilized by the University of Miami/Jackson Memorial Medical Center and the Miami Veterans Administration Medical Center. These protocols may differ in varying degree from care plans followed at other centers. Many types of specialists including neurological surgeons, orthopaedic surgeons, trauma surgeons, emergency room physicians, and even physiatrists manage cervical injuries at those different centers. It is the hope of these authors that the government will at some point fund a good prospective study to determine the relationship of the different care plans followed to their final outcome. The first step would include the establishment of a comprehensive data bank documenting the natural course of spinal cord injury lesions and providing normative data.

Spinal cord injury in the 1990s remains a disease of young people, with the majority being males in their second or third decade. The most common time for an injury to occur is between midnight and 4:00 AM. The most common causes of cervical spinal injury are vehicle accidents, including automobiles, motorcycles, and, more recently, a whole new group of accident injuries involving all-terrain vehicles, snowmobiles, etc. Industrial, agricultural, and sporting accidents account for most of the other victims except for the alarming increase in injuries as a result of handgun wounds. Gunshot wounds are most notable in large metropolitan areas where they can constitute a causal factor equal to vehicular accidents. The majority of cervical spinal cord injury patients have associated multisystem trauma which presents a significant challenge to the healthcare system. The most common injury site is in the mid to low cervical area which coincides with the most mobile segments of the cervical spinal column (1–4). Nationally, acute mortality has been estimated to be about 10%, although at major centers, it is about half of that. The most accurate information regarding the epidemiology of spinal cord injury in a geographical region has been collected by the Department of Labor, Division of Vocational Rehabilitation of the State of Florida. Florida has had a mandatory registration of spinal cord injuries for the last 15 years. Their data documents approximately 450 new injuries occurring each year in Florida. It has been estimated that 10–12 thousand new injuries occur annually in the United States with a prevalence of somewhere between 300–500,000 spinal cord injury patients presently living in this country. The prevalence numbers have increased rapidly in the last two decades as more sophisticated medical and surgical care has evolved.

Systems Approach

It is our contention that optimal treatment continuum for acute spinal cord injuries lies in a "systems approach" which features a multidisciplinary team of physicians, nurses, and allied health professionals who are committed to providing comprehensive care to a relatively rare subpopulation of trauma victims. The volume experience gained by this team translates into a lower morbidity and mortality as well as lower patient care costs. It also provides the patient with an identifiable health care team from the immediate through the lifelong follow-up phases (5).

A "systems approach" includes: *a*) prevention programs; *b*) prehospital management; *c*) acute inhospital care; *d*) rehabilitation; *e*) and lifelong medical follow-up. The major causes of death and morbidity in the prehospital and acute inhospital phases include aspiration, shock, and cardiopulmonary complications. In the rehabilitation and lifelong follow-up phases, morbidity and mortality were classically associated with renal complications and decubitus ulcers. More recently, as we enter the 1990s, the average spinal cord injured person that survives the acute phase has a relatively normal life expectancy and will probably die from the same causes as the able-bodied, i.e., heart disease, cancer, and stroke.

PREVENTION

In the absence of a serum containing common sense, which we could use to inoculate the American public, a concentrated effort is required to identify causal factors which might be minimized with better laws, engineering advances, or safety education. Safety equipment and laws requiring airbags, seat belts, helmets, and lowered speed limits have, in all probability, resulted in a reduction in incidence. However, in recent years these gains have been offset by an increase in the use of all-terrain vehicles, snowmobiles, ultralight aircrafts, hand-gliders, and recreational parachuting. One of the more effective prevention programs was created in the State of Florida and is entitled "Feet First, First Time." The theme of the program is to encourage the public to enter unknown waters feet first prior to engaging in head first diving. The program was started in Pensacola and has been utilized throughout the State of Florida. It has now been adopted by the various neurosurgical societies as part of a national prevention program, "Think First," and has been expanded to include head injury as well as spinal cord injury prevention. We have found it quite effective to take a team of SCI individuals along with allied health professional into the high schools to promote an awareness of risk situations and consequences to the highest at-risk target population, i.e., the teenagers. These programs have already made a significant impact within the state of Florida.

Although something as simple as the wearing of a seat belt would prevent many spinal cord injuries each year, in spite of mandatory seat belt laws, many Americans fail to use these very important safety restraint systems. An equally important causal factor unique to the United States involves the use and abuse of handguns. A visitor to Washington, D.C. will notice that the National Rifle Association (NRA) facilities are as large or larger than the White House and Pentagon. The NRA has created an uphill battle regarding effective handgun legislation. It is evident that any effective CNS trauma prevention program should emphasize the two most critical targets, handguns and vehicle accidents.

PREHOSPITAL MANAGEMENT

In the 1970s the majority of acute spinal cord injuries arrived at hospitals with complete deficits, having little or no chance of spontaneous recovery. Since the early 1980s, the majority of SCI patients arrived at hospitals with incomplete deficits and a good chance of at least some degree of neurological recovery. This change in presenting status has been attributed to the significant evolution of the emergency medical services (EMS) nationwide. Today, the first responder is no longer a good Samaritan, or a well-meaning highway patrolman, or a hearse driver from the local funeral home, but, instead, a highly skilled and trained paramedic. The EMS responders have played a tremendous role in the improved outcome for multisystem trauma victims, which includes the majority of spinal cord injuries. While it is obvious that the paramedics cannot change the primary amount of injury which is determined by the velocity and nature of the initial accident or insult, they can have a significant effect on preventing secondary damage. A secondary injury can result from a biochemical or mechanical insult that follows the initial trauma. The most common contributors to secondary injury include untreated hypotension or hypoxia and patient mishandling with regard to spinal immobilization. These possibilities have been minimized with the advent of the EMS accident scene specialist and the sophistication of new extrication devices and transportation equipment as well as the widespread implementation of telemetry monitoring and voice-to-voice consultation with the trauma physician in real time (6).

The paramedic at the scene follows the ABC's to establish adequate airway and ventilation and perfusion of the patient. They are taught to carefully handle the injured patients by moving them into a neutral supine position and immobilizing them on an appropriate spine board with sandbags on either side of their head and neck and tape across the forehead, leaving the mouth and airway free for access. We advocate transporting the patient in at least 15° of Trendelenburg position in order to minimize the chances of the two major causes of prehospital death, i.e., aspiration and shock. Usually this setup includes a loose strap across the chest and a firm one across the pelvis and knees and ankles for an adequate transport system. An important consideration for cervical injuries is that the neck, like other organs of the body, most often swells when injured. It is dangerous to place a restrictive collar around the neck unless it has an opening in the front to observe for expanding hematomas and subcutaneous edema. We recommend that the necklock or the Miami collar be used in the prehospital phase as an adjunct and not as a replacement for the sandbags and tape. The acute cervical spinal cord injury syndrome (neurogenic shock) is unique to cervical injuries. This is characterized by hypotension, bradycardia, and hypothermia. Patients often present with a systolic blood pressure of 70 or lower and a pulse in the range of 40 or lower and tend to exhibit extremely low body temperature. The accident scene goal should be to keep these patients as normal physiologically as feasible. This can be accomplished by using the Trendelenburg position for transport along with the administration of intravenous atropine for pulses below 60, and it should include the use of oxygen to optimize the arterial oxygen content. In the case of multisystem trauma patients, MAST or shock trousers can also be a valuable adjunct. Ideally, the patient should be transported with a Foley catheter inserted and a nasogastric sump tube inserted to drain and empty the stomach, and at least two major IV access sites started. A stethoscope is necessary for monitoring blood pressure and pulse, especially in noisy vibrating vehicles.

We have modified the University of Miami Neuro-Spinal Index (UMNI) (Fig. 31.1), as a neurological test which allows the paramedics to perform a good motor and sensory assessment which can provide an accurate baseline for comparison of deficit after admission (7). The prehospital initiation of a drug protocol has not been implemented in any of the major SCI trauma systems. However, we predict that in the near future we will implement the administration of high dose steroids at the accident scene to get a "headstart" on minimizing the secondary self-destructing chemical and biochemical changes occurring within the cord tissue. A final controversial area relates to prehospital care and involves the initiation of cervical traction prior to a baseline radiological assessment. It is our contention that spinal cord injured patients should never be placed in traction before x-rays are taken because of the significant risk of increasing the cervical cord injury. Even a small amount of traction can over-distract certain patients and exacerbate the neurological deficit. One example of a high risk cervical patient, who could very likely deteriorate due to traction, is a patient with ankylosing spondylitis. When placed in traction, a "bamboo" spine will often further dislocate and be associated with a worsening neurological deficit. For these reasons we strongly advise against a paramedic's application of traction at the accident scene, and in geriatric patients often the head and neck are best managed not in a true neutral position but in one that is most comfortable for the patient even if slightly flexed. The same advice applies to smaller hospitals not staffed by neurological or orthopedic surgeons who have been trained in the intri-

Patient Name:__________ Test Performed By:__________

Patient #__________ Date of Test:__________

Date of Admission:__________ Level of Injury:__________

	LEFT SCORE	RIGHT SCORE	TOTAL SCORE
SHOULDER ELEVATION			
ARM ELEVATION			
ARM HORIZONTAL ADDUCTION			
ELBOW FLEXORS			
ELBOW EXTENSORS			
WRIST FLEXORS			
WRIST EXTENSORS			
EXTRINSIC FLEXORS			
EXTRINSIC EXTENSORS			
THUMB OPPOSITION			
FINGER ABDUCTION			
UPPER ABDOMINALS			
LOWER ABDOMINALS			
HIP FLEXORS			
HIP EXTENSORS			
HIP ABDUCTION			
KNEE FLEXOR			
KNEE EXTENSORS			
FOOT DORSI-FLEXION			
FOOT EVERTER			
FOOT FLEXOR			
TOE EXTENSOR			
		Grand Total	

CODE:

0 = No function

1 = A visible or palpable flicker of contraction, but no resultant movement of limb or joint.

2 = The muscle can only move normally when the limb is so positioned that gravity is eliminated.

3 = The muscle is able to move normally against gravity, but not against additional resistance.

4 = The muscle, though able to move normally, is overcome by resistance.

5 = Normal muscle power.

Figure 31.1. University of Miami Neuro-Spinal Index (UMNI) Sensory Evaluation Form.

cacies of cervical biomechanics and the application of traction.

EMERGENCY ROOM MANAGEMENT

When an SCI arrives in the emergency room, a well-organized multidisciplinary team triage should include representatives from neurosurgery and orthopaedic surgery as well as the ER physician, who in some cases may be a trauma surgeon. It is essential that a good line of communication be established between the prehospital team i.e., the paramedic, and the emergency room staff, to insure that critical data pertaining to neurological status and vital signs as well as treatment procedures initiated at the scene or in transport are accurately documented. A description of the mechanism of injury and an estimate of the velocity of the insult can be quite helpful in developing a diagnosis, prognosis, and therapeutic plan. Emergency department baseline data, including the general physical examination as well as a detailed neurological assessment, must be accurately documented. A major legal issue in spinal injury cases often is based on a discrepancy between the initial examination at the accident scene or in the emergency department and some later point in time. Good documentation obviates unnecessary confusion and anguish for all involved. Once baseline assessments have been completed, a central venous line can be inserted, as well as a Foley catheter and a nasogastric sump tube (if not already done). Chest and abdominal x-rays as well as AP and lateral surveys of the entire spinal column are taken. It is estimated that 15–20% of all spinal injuries occur at multiple distant spinal levels, and the diagnosis of a single level of injury should raise a warning flag and mandate a careful assessment of other levels. During x-ray procedures the patient should be kept in a neutral supine position, and cervical spinal films should always include visualization of the C7–T1 junction, even if it means obtaining special "swimmer's" views, or in rare cases lateral tomograms may be necessary. Baseline arterial blood gases should be obtained and corrected to normal range. Adequate oxygenation can sometimes be achieved simply with a nasal cannula or face mask, but in certain cases intubation and ventilatory support is required. In multiple trauma cases, if abdominal visceral injury is suspected, the abdomen should be assessed with either peritoneal lavage or abdominal CT.

Once the x-rays, baseline examinations, and laboratory tests are analyzed and the results reviewed attention should shift to the cervical spine injury and to reestablishing the alignment of the head and neck with cervical traction. We recommend that all emergency rooms be stocked with CT- and MRI-compatible tongs and halo rings. In cases where a neurological deficit referable to a cervical level is noted and no obvious bony or soft tissue injury is seen on the initial x-rays, 10 pounds of cervical traction is applied. However, in cases where there is an obvious dislocation or fracture, traction is initiated following a formula of 5 pounds per interspace so that a C3–4 injury would have between 15–20 pounds of traction applied and a C5–6 between 25–30 pounds. This weight formula is modified in cases of young children with more flexible soft tissue support of the spinal column and is not applicable to certain cases such as ankylosing spondylitis or severe disruptive injuries. The reduction is accomplished under real time fluoroscopy or with serial plain film lateral x-rays. If adequate realignment cannot be accomplished within 30 minutes, utilizing when necessary intravenous and/or IM Valium, then our protocol requires that the anesthesia team be consulted. They nasotracheally intubate the awake patient, and we then administer a short-acting systemic paralyzing drug while assisting the patient with ventilation. The cervical spine is then manipulated under fluoroscopy until acceptable alignment is achieved without the resistance of cervical muscle tone. The vast majority of cervical spine injuries can be realigned with cervical traction, obviating the need for early surgery, which is associated with a higher morbidity and mortality. A small number of patients with a cervical burst fracture, epidural hematoma, or with a large herniated disc (which often will not retract from the canal with traction) require early surgical intervention which is outlined later in this chapter. However, we have been successful even with reducing bilaterally locked facets using this traction protocol. This aggressive realignment is implemented in all cervical spine injuries with significant neurological deficit. The exceptions to this rule are the intact or minimal deficit patients with a dislocation who are spontaneously recovering after low velocity spinal cord injury. These patients are treated less aggressively with traction while protected on a roto-rest treatment table. Generally, traction for reduction of a dislocation is best applied in a plane parallel to the table or bed that the patient is on. Linear traction is preferable to using flexion, extension, or rotation during reduction in order to accomplish the optimal distraction necessary to unlock the facets. The patient should be immobilized on a rigid structure, whether it is a padded spine board or a roto-rest treatment table, until the realignment is accomplished. Once the facets are unlocked, then a slight degree of flexion, extension, or rotation may be utilized. We never use weights totaling more than two times the initial starting level, i.e., 10 pounds per interspace. If this is not sufficient we go directly to the intubation and muscle relaxation protocol.

Once reduced, we place the patient in a Miami J-collar (Fig. 31.2) which allows us to visualize the front of the neck for any progressive swelling or hematoma or subcutaneous emphysema. This device acts as an adjunct to the traction for insuring maintenance of adequate spinal alignment and prevention of inadvertent flexation, rotation, or angulation. Also, once reduction is accomplished, the weights can be decreased to the minimal level necessary to adequately maintain alignment. Patients presenting with

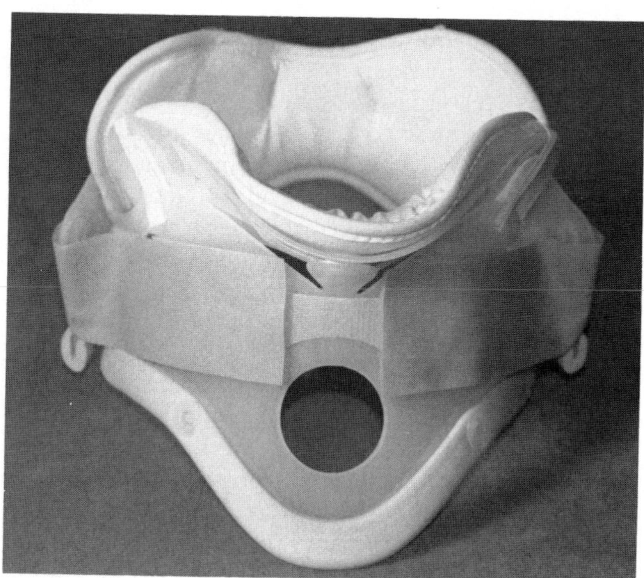

Figure 31.2. Miami J-collar.

an initially unstable injury, i.e., severely disruptive, bony or soft tissue injury, sometimes cannot tolerate any traction and need to be immobilized immediately either in a rigid Miami collar or cervical halo orthosis. Even the cervical halo orthosis is not always an effective immobilization device with ankylosing spondylitis, which remains one of the most treacherous injuries in the early acute phase.

NEUROLOGICAL ASSESSMENT FOR SCI PATIENTS

Our triage protocol does not differ for incomplete or complete injury patients with both types of injury treated equally aggressively. It is our experience that 3–5% of our "complete" injuries show significant improvement and may even end-up walking. The same experience has been reported by other large centers around the world. Since we are unable to discriminate which of the complete lesions will get better, we treat all of these patients aggressively. It is our working hypothesis that the patients with complete injuries who are not supposed to walk but do, are those individuals whose injury was caused by relatively low velocity trauma such as a diving accident or sports accident, rather than a high velocity vehicular accident or penetrating wound.

A detailed neurological assessment of the cervical spine injury begins with a standard motor and sensory evaluation. Motor function is scored on a 0–5 scale for each muscle tested, and the sensory exam should be multimodality and include assessment of the lateral and dorsal columns. The lateral columns carry pain and temperature sense and can be tested with a pinprick or an ice cube, and the dorsal columns carry touch, vibration, and position sense. We define a complete injury as one where no motor or sensory function exists below the zone of injury. The zone of injury includes up to three neurological segments below the point of damage. An important part of the initial neurological screening is the rectal exam, because of the importance of sacral sparing. Complete injuries can have rectal tone, so it is very important that it be a volitional contraction of the anal sphincter that determines incompleteness. Testicular sensation is also an important measure of sacral sparing. The most important senses prognostically are the ones carried in the lateral columns rather than the dorsal columns. Pain or temperature sparring in the perianal area is more significant than touch or vibration perception. It has been our experience that patients with sacral sparing, who are otherwise totally without motor and sensory function below the injury, may significantly improve even to the point of walking.

Reflex testing is the least reliable part of a neurological exam with regard to diagnosis and prognosis, since patients with high velocity injuries may never experience spinal shock and may be reflexive immediately and even have rectal tone. There is much confusion regarding the state of spinal shock and the designation of injury completeness. Spinal shock should be defined as a physiological transection of the cord associated with a lower motor neuron examination, i.e., flaccid and areflexive and without sensation below the level and zone of the injury. Therefore, all patients in spinal shock are by definition classified as complete injuries. The fact that 6 to 16 weeks after the traumatic event they spontaneously evolve into upper motor neurons lesions, (i.e., a reflexive state), does not change their prognosis. When they show upper motor neuron signs or spasticity, the bladder and bowel which initially are flaccid like their skeletal muscle, also become spastic and this changes their characteristic management needs. It is incorrect for a physician to tell a patient he cannot predict the outcome or give a prognosis because they are in spinal shock. In fact they should be told initially that since they are in spinal shock and have complete lesions, they have only a 3–5% chance of significant spontaneous recovery.

A thorough neurological examination often reveals a variety of incomplete injury types. The majority of incomplete injury patients have what we call mixed motor and sensory pictures. However, a significant number fit into classical categories or syndromes which relate to the diagnosis and prognosis. The most common syndrome seen in our center in South Florida which has a greater proportion of older people, is the Central Cord Syndrome (8). This syndrome is more common in patients of middle and older age groups that have a preexisting cervical spondylosis and stenosis. They classically present with a hyperextension injury and often have a bruise on their forehead as confirmation of the mechanism. Very often their x-rays show little or no bony abnormality other than spondylosis, i.e., most often not associated with a fracture or dislocation. These patients present with a clinical picture of upper extremity deficit greater than lower extremity. The most significant deficit is in their distal upper extremity where they not only have motor and sensory loss but also have a hyperesthetic picture with very significant hypersensitivity to touch especially in their hands and fingers. Initially they also present with a neurogenic bowel and bladder and with impotence but seem to recover naturally toward a greater state of incompleteness until at some point they plateau neurologically with an unacceptable level of deficit or pain. In the past, the dictum was to never operate on these patients, but today, once they plateau they are reclassified by most spinal cord injury centers as myeloradiculopathies rather than acute injuries. They are then reimaged and undergo a delayed decompression, which in our experience and that of other centers results in further neurological improvement and further relief of the pain problem. This syndrome, first described by Dr. Richard Schneider, was thought to be due to a hemorrhage of the central gray matter and swelling and hemorrhage of the surrounding adjacent white matter, which would explain why patients present with a classic pattern of disproportionate loss in the upper extremities, especially distally. Recent studies at the University of Miami and The Miami Project using actual human autopsy material from central cord syndrome patients have shown that this is indeed not the absolute case, since there seems to be more of a diffuse white matter injury noted in our central cord pathological specimens. This work is ongoing, but it has definitely changed our perception and understanding of this relatively more common clinical presentation syndrome.

The second most common classical syndrome seen in our center is the anterior cord syndrome (9, 10). These patients usually result from a flexion mechanism of injury which most often is associated with a fracture and/or dislocation. These individuals present with total loss of motor and lateral column sensory function below the level of injury, although they may have a local zone of one or two levels of incompleteness. However, they do have at least a patchy preservation of the dorsal columns below the lesion (i.e., proprioception, touch, and position sense). Unfortunately, most patients with an anterior cord syndrome do not have the same good prognosis as do central cord or other patients who are incomplete with pain or temperature, i.e., lateral column sensory sparing. Hypothetically the difference is because there is a different blood supply to the dorsal columns from that of the anterior and lateral columns with their motor and pain and temperature pathways. Some patients with incomplete pain and temperature function distally show recovery in motor function, whereas pure anterior cord syndromes rarely do.

The Brown-Sequard syndrome is usually associated with an anatomical hemisection of the cord. These patients present with an ipsilateral loss of dorsal columns, i.e., proprioception, touch, and vibration function and motor function and a contralateral pain and temperature loss which usually starts at least a couple of levels below the injury site. In our experience these patients usually improve dramatically over time and ultimately end up with the major residual deficit in their ipsilateral upper extremity. There is often a combination of spinal cord and nerve root or brachial plexus dysfunction, since they are laterally inflicted injuries. These injuries are usually caused by penetrating wounds or rotational closed injuries. A small percentage of Brown-Sequard syndrome patients demonstrate a progressive neurological deterioration that can evolve and ascend to a higher level of deficit or completeness. Patients who develop further deterioration are discussed later in this section.

The final cervical syndrome is a very rare type of injury termed the Posterior Spinal Cord Injury Syndrome. We have only admitted two such cases in this center over the last 15 years. These patients present with only dorsal column sensory loss but have preserved pain, temperature, and motor function. Although this type of injury might seem to be less compromising than other injuries, it can be devastating clinically because of the absence of position sense. These patients have great difficulty using their muscles and often require assistive devices for mobilization. The cases we have treated were both penetrating wounds that transversely crossed the posterior elements from side to side. Reports of closed injuries with these symptoms have also been documented and have been attributed to laminar fractures.

As we alluded to earlier (e.g., some Brown-Sequard patients), approximately 1% of the spinal injury population develops what is called an ascending cord necrosis syndrome. Although the at-risk population for this syndrome has not been clearly identified, our experience indicates that it occurs more commonly in young patients of the pediatric/adolescent age group. In contrast to the progressive deficit often noted in ankylosing spondylitis cervical injuries with fracture dislocation or epidural hematoma, these patients most often have no extrinsic cord compression at the time of their deterioration, which is usually in the first couple of weeks following injury. They usually are associated with a swollen cord noted on MRI or myelographic CT imaging studies. It is not certain whether this represents a problem of ischemia or progressive infarction, but it is thought by most clinicians that this is a vascular phenomenon. In our experience, this type of injury has been refractory to any type of treatment with pharmaceuticals, decompression, etc. In cases of cervical spinal cord injury this deficit may even ascend into the brainstem and become a fatal lesion, but there is no way to predict how many levels these patients will ascend. This syndrome can evolve from either complete or incomplete cervical spinal injuries.

IMAGING THE SPINAL CORD INJURY PATIENT

As stated earlier, an AP and lateral plain x-ray survey of the entire spinal column is obtained immediately after admission. The rationale for this approach can be demonstrated by examples from the last 6 month period. Two of our diving accidents had separate cervical and thoracic fractures, although according to witnesses, the patients hit only their heads on the bottom of the pool. In our center we are presently involved in a prospective study of acute SCI injuries comparing the relative benefits of high resolution CT scanning to MRI scanning. For the last 10 years, we have not performed myelograms or minimyelograms with CTs in the cervical area because we discovered that only rarely were the canals blocked once they were realigned, and there was no reason to do a myeloCT before they were realigned. We believed that the exceptionally large herniated disc or hematoma could be discriminated adequately with high resolution CT through the areas of suspicion. However, our initial review of our first 100+ MRIs on acute injuries has changed our minds. We have seen that a significant number of people with cervical spine injuries have herniated discs which were not well seen on high resolution CT or even identified in certain cases on myeloCT combinations. An example of this would be a patient with locked facets with a dislocation who has a disc concealed in front of the thecal sac and not visualized because of complete block of the myelogram. The MRI scan has been most advantageous in visualizing these soft tissue lesions, and we have recently developed a scale (Fig. 31.3) to grade MRI changes with regard to severity and are using this scale in a prospective clinical study. We expect that in the future most CNS trauma centers will have low magnetic field MRI machines capable of spinal cord imaging even in face of metal equipment such as a respirator. CT, however, is superior to MRI for bony anatomy or pathology. In the older age groups the CT scan is especially invaluable, but even in the younger patients CT can reveal fractures not seen on plain films and definitely not visible on MRIs. At this point we are still using a combination of high resolution unenhanced CT followed by MRI. In patients who present with a deficit or questionable canal compromise and have either a cardiac pacemaker or are intubated and supported on a respirator, an emergency myeloCT is performed with Iohexol via C1–2 puncture while maintaining the patient in a supine position. This limited myelogram is followed by a high resolution CT through the area of suspicion, but usually in cervical cases we survey the entire cervical spine with 5 mm cuts and then 2 to 3 mm overcuts through the area of injury. The majority of cervical cases do not show a block on the myeloCT or significant extrinsic pressure once they are reduced, but there are exceptions to this rule including the cervical burst fracture and the herniated disc which are seen much more commonly since the advent of high resolution MRI. Also, the rare case of traumatically induced epidural hematoma can be visualized in patients who have a cervical spinal cord injury with no significant evidence of bony disruption or disc herniation. They are maintained in traction and usually reimaged at a later date in 1 to 2 weeks. If there is no gross evidence of instability, carefully controlled flexion-extension movements are performed with real time fluoroscopy monitoring to ensure there is no instability. If there is none, then the patient's traction is removed. Reviewing our cases over the last several years, 98% of the patients who come in with closed cervical injuries do not require initial surgery and are placed on a roto-rest treatment table in traction for a 7–10 day period, while only those with instability are brought back for definitive stabilization. Only the severe case requires emergency surgery including a herniated disc, burst fracture, or epidural hematoma. There is no evidence in the literature that a myelotomy or a laminectomy for decompression of a swollen spinal cord alone or in combination have ever been effective in treating acute cervical spinal cord injuries.

Neurophysiological Assessment

A relative newcomer to the acute inhospital phase of care for spinal cord injury is the availability and sophistication of neurophysiological testing. Somatosensory evoked responses have been used in the emergency department by some but most commonly in the ICU or operating room for the diagnosis, monitoring, and, to some degree, for establishing prognosis in victims of paralysis. Very simply, by stimulating the legs and/or arms, one can make a recording off of the scalp. Using repetitive stimulation and an averaging computer, a waveform is created and analyzed. Much more predictable than the amplitude and frequency has been the latency from the time of stimulus to onset of waveform. The literature describes the classical W-waveform for somatosensory evoked responses, and of course the latency varies significantly between lower and upper extremities stimulation in relation to the distance from the stimulus to the scalp recording sites. Animal and human studies have indicated that the somatosensory evoked potentials most likely reflect the integrity of the dorsal columns of the spinal cord, which is important information but which is not as critical in the practical sense as the motor evoked responses. Motor evoked responses obtained by stimulating the scalp and recording off of the trunk or extremities musculature is still an investigational technique in most centers. Because of the discomfort associated with stimulation in the unanesthetized patient, inpatients and outpatients with spinal cord injury undergoing MEP evaluation are best stimulated with a magnetic coil rather than the transcortical (scalp) or electrical stimulation. Unfortunately, the magnetic coil has still not been well developed as a reliable clinical apparatus. Therefore, in the operating room for monitoring purposes, our group still utilizes electrical cortical (i.e., scalp) stimulation which has not been a problem in an anesthetized individual and has been much more reproducible and reliable. It is anticipated that motor responses will continue to rapidly develop as a very important part of the physiological monitoring protocol for spinal cord injury in the next several years. A more tra-

Patient name: ______________________

Patient #: ______________________

Date of admission: ______________________

Level of injury: ______________________

Code:

2 = present/normal

1 = present/abnormal

0 = absent

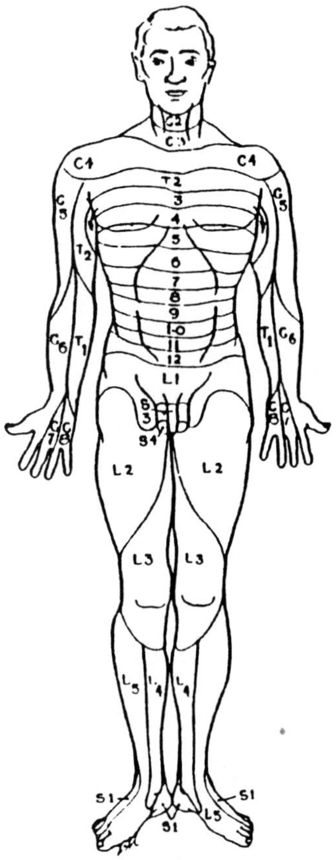

DORSAL COLUMN FUNCTIONS (DCF): vibration

LATERAL SPINOTHALAMIC TRACT FUNCTIONS (LSTF): Pain

LEFT	DCF	LSTF	CERVICAL	DCF	LSTF	RIGHT
			2			
			3			
			4			
			5			
			6			
			7			
			8			
			THORACIC			
			1			
			2			
			3			
			4			
			5			
			6			
			7			
			8			
			9			
			10			
			11			
			12			
			LUMBAR			
			1			
			2			
			3			
			4			
			5			
			SACRAL			
			1			
			2			
			3			
			4			
			5			
			COCCYGEAL			
			1			

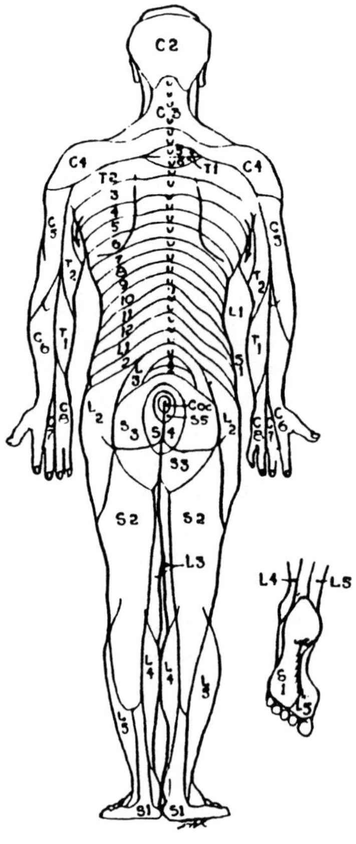

TOTAL ______________________

GRAND TOTAL: __________

Test performed by: __________

Date of test: __________

Figure 31.3. Motor evaluation form—muscle testing.

ditional tool used in outpatients and more recently in the operating room has been real time EMG monitoring. In the operating room real time EMG monitoring with visual and audio feedback has proved to be especially valuable to the surgeons working on a cervical and lumbar spinal level in and around the nerve roots. In a nonanesthetized in- or out-patient the use of needle or surface electrode EMGs has been sophisticated for diagnostic and therapeutic purposes when combined with a computerized multichannel EMG biofeedback system. Diagnostically this technology allows identification of motor units not seen clinically and potentially allows their enhancement or recruitment therapeutically. This will be discussed in further detail towards the end of this chapter in the research section. Finally, local reflexes such as the H-reflex have been used in spinal cord injury patients for diagnostic and prognostic purposes. It is our prediction that the use of multimodality evoked responses will play an increasingly important role as the technology develops as a viable tool for diagnosis, monitoring, and prognosis in acute spinal cord injury victims.

Surgical Management of Cervical Spinal Cord Injuries

In our protocol, the indications for surgical treatment in acute cervical spinal cord injuries include spinal column instability and refractory spinal cord and/or nerve root compression. Details of indications will be discussed under each major category of cervical spine injury in the following paragraphs and based on the combination of the neurological examination and imaging batteries described in the preceding paragraphs. The second major issue after indications involves timing, with two standard time slots being delegated to the acute cervical spinal cord injury patient. The first is early surgery which is performed within the first hours following injury in the relatively rare cases of burst fractures, herniated discs, and epidural hematomas compromising the canal and neural elements, and ankylosing spondylitis cases with dislocation. Also included in this group is the rare case of a cervical cord injury with locked facets unable to be reduced with the intubation/paralysis intravenous muscle relaxer protocol. What used to be considered a straight-forward issue and decision making process has now become more complex with the advent of MRI imaging. We now realize that just as important as the extent of a dislocation of the cervical spine are the preinjury spinal canal dimensions, the actual size of the spinal cord itself, and other canal contents including the ligamentum flavum. Even epidural fat has been suggested to play a pathological role. Our previous studies have shown that individuals with congenitally narrow canals who have a significant dislocation are most often quadriplegic, whereas those with "large bore" spinal canals preinjury rarely suffer a significant deficit with a similar degree of subluxation. Individuals with a normal size canal may go either way so to speak (11). In the early management of cervical spinal cord injury someone with a large, (e.g., 20 or 22 mm) canal who has a 2 or 3 mm offset even after attempts at reduction is most likely not compressing the spinal cord, and this fact can be confirmed with MRI imaging. However, a person with a 12 or 14 mm canal who has a 2 or 3 mm offset is very likely significantly compressing the spinal cord and may require more aggressive early intervention. The second time slot regarding timing of the surgery for cervical spinal cord injury would be what we call the delayed acute surgery. In these patients most often we are able to realign the spinal canal to an adequate degree to decompress the neural element and elect to delay surgery for 7–10 days and sometimes 2 weeks in cases of acute quadriplegia. The purpose of delay is to allow the patient to physiologically stabilize. Very frequently cervical injuries present in neurogenic shock, and for unknown reasons in many cases this seems to spontaneously resolve within the first week following injury. There is no doubt that a higher morbidity and mortality is associated with operating immediately in victims of major trauma including acute traumatic quadriplegia. Therefore, only the rare cases of intractable cord compression described above or cases of high risk for further deterioration are taken to the operating room immediately. The vast majority of cases are managed on the roto-rest treatment table in traction for a 7–10 day period. When presenting the early surgical protocol one must realize that the immediate versus 7–10 days timing decision is directed toward only ideal cases, and obviously accommodation has to be made for patients with multisystem injuries which are life-threatening and obviate surgical intervention at either time period. The protocols presented in the following paragraphs are specifically for injuries occurring with cervical level spinal cord neurological deficits which are less than 3 weeks following onset. This time period is critical because at approximately 3 weeks following an injury early spontaneous healing of the soft tissue occurs. This soft tissue bonding does not allow the same degree of intraoperative flexibility noted in the first days or week or two following injury with regard to manipulation and realignment. A very important surgical principle in all cervical spinal cord injury cases is that a decompression is never performed in isolation but always in tandem with a stabilization procedure. Although instability may not be the primary issue, i.e., neurological element compression is present without instability, decompression by itself often creates an unstable state requiring a fusion. The converse of this is that the patient may present with instability without compression. After traction is applied, the cord is decompressed via realignment of its spinal canal. These patients are stabilized (fused) surgically after 7–10 days, i.e., delayed until physiologically optimal. Delayed cases include the majority of the acute cervical injury patient population. These patients most often require a stabilization procedure without the decompression which has most often been accomplished with traction preoperatively. An important concept concerns the term "spinal fusion" which is often used synonymously with the term "stabilization," although in the true sense they are not the same. A stabilization procedure may have as its purpose a fusion of spine, which often may take several months to mature. Usually with an autograft, the earliest evidence of fusion is seen at 6–8 weeks, and with a heterograft it is even longer, although cadaver bone fusions may be supplemented with autograft to induce a more rapid healing process. Another important principle of cervical fusion is that metal instrumentation or cement does not create long-term stability by itself, and wires, plates, screws, clamps, or cement should never be used in isolation but always with autograft and/or heterograft. Metal and cement tend to fatigue with age and stress forces. For purposes of this discussion the surgical management of cervical injuries will be divided into two major categories: the occipital C1–2 level injuries and C3–7 injuries.

The majority of acute cervical injuries are approached surgically from the front or back. Lateral approaches to the cervical spine have been described and utilized, although technically they are tedious and complex and, in general, they are not necessary in the management of the acute cervical spinal cord injury patient. Occipital cervical dislocations and C1, 2 dislocations are rarely acutely treated through the anterior approach. Although the transoral approach gives a nice exposure to this area, it is not optimal with regard to stabilization. The transoral approach is accomplished by splitting the soft palate and posterior pharyngeal wall under fluoroscopic control. Acutely it is used only in rare cases of a bone or bullet fragment embedded in the anterior canal requiring a transoral decompression. When this procedure is utilized it is always followed in tandem or proceeded by a posterior cervical fusion of C1–2 or an occipital C1–2 fusion, depending on which members of the ligamentous and bony complex are disrupted. These procedures are always performed in cervical halo orthosis fixation (12). Occipital cervical instability is best determined on plain lateral x-rays. Essential in this assessment is the relationship of the top of the odontoid process to the tip of the basion. There should be approximately a 5 mm distance between them, with one being right above or below the other. Dislocation or distraction of this relationship is the most significant sign of occipital cervical ligamentous instability. These patients most often present intact or with incomplete deficits, since those with complete lesions most often are DOA (dead on arrival to the hospital). The appropriate surgical approach for these injuries is a halo cervical orthosis placement preoperatively and a posterior occipital cervical fusion from the occiput to C1 and C2 and, if necessary, C2 and C3 (i.e., if the dorsal arch of C1 is disrupted, which is not unusual in these injuries). Autografts and/or heterograft struts are used to bridge the decorticated suboccipital bone to the dorsal arches of C1 and C2 or C2 and C3 as described above. They are secured by number 22 braided wires or Luque wires attached from the skull to the graft and from the graft to the arches of C1–3. It is important to know technically that direct wiring of the occiput to the spine runs the significant risk of kinking the brainstem from hyperextension of the head and neck which is why preoperative halo placement is optimal for a safe surgical procedure. Technically the suboccipital bone and the dorsal arches of the upper cervical elements should be decorticated with a high speed drill which could also be used to create the appropriate holes for wire passage in the skull and the cervical spinous processes or lamina or even facet joints. The struts are best supplemented with small cortical cancellous bone fragments to help induce a more rapid fusion. Because of the dense cortical bone in the suboccipital bone as well as in the arch of C1, less rapid fusion takes place, and the patient is left in the halo a minimum of 3 to 4 months, in contrast to the 2 to 3 months used in lower cervical fusions. Halo fixation is followed by 4 weeks in a rigid Miami collar and then 4 weeks in a soft collar for a total immobilization period of 4–6 months; this is followed by serial radiographs.

Odontoid fractures may not always require surgical intervention, for example, a type 2 odontoid fracture through the base of the odontoid and type 3 through the body are quite adequately treated in a cervical halo orthosis in most individuals under 40 years but in fewer patients in the over-40 population. The alternative is a posterior cervical fusion from C1 to C2 with double number 22 wires or Luque wires and autograft and/or heterograft. We prefer the modified Brooks fusion with two wires placed on either side of the midline sublaminarly and a triangular bone wedge placed between the corticate arches of C1 and C2 so that the fusion wire will tie around the two dorsal arches and interposed bone grafts maintaining a relatively normal relationship between the C1 and C2 elements (13). Wiring C1 directly to C2 can often close down the foramen and create an intractable occipital neuralgia. In cases of Jefferson fractures with disruption of the arch of C1 with or without odontoid fractures, a halo orthosis is adequate treatment for both in most cases. Occasionally in severe disrupted unstable injuries, occipital cervical fusion may be required in addition to a halo orthosis, but in general, most Jefferson fractures are stable. In these cases stability is best confirmed by open mouth odontoid view x-rays. If the total overhang of both lateral masses is more than 7 mm, then instability is present. In simple Jefferson fractures without significant displacement, a Miami collar is often adequate. Hangmans fractures (C2–3 injuries) gap between the upper cervical and C3–7 lesions. These C2–3 injuries are, in the vast majority of cases, successfully treated in a cervical halo orthosis and only rarely require surgery. In cases of significant disruption and dislocation, an anterior cervical discectomy and fusion is performed and then protected by a halo orthosis. An adequate exposure can be made with a submandibular horizontal incision. Although C2–3 can be reached through a transoral approach, the bone graft is at risk because of the potential contamination of the surgical procedure through the oral cavity.

There are many schemes which have been proposed to evaluate cervical spine stability. One of the simplest and more useful is that a horizontal subluxation of greater than 3.5 mm or an angulation between adjacent vertebral bodies of greater than 11° are considered unstable in the C3–7 levels. In addition, severe disruption of the anterior and/or posterior elements are also important indicators of spinal column instability (White, 1975). Most injuries from C3–T1 which do not fulfill the criteria of instability can be simply treated in a cervical halo orthosis or even in certain cases with a rigid neck lock or Miami collar. In most cases of unstable subluxation or angulation without body disruption, anterior interbody fusion by means of the iliac bone graft techniques of Robinson and Smith or of Cloward are acceptable only if the patient is placed in a cervical halo orthosis as an adjunct (15–17). These fusions by themselves do not provide adequate immediate stability but do offer the optimal approach for decompression of the spinal canal from a ruptured disc and/or bone fragments. In cases with severe vertebral body disruption, anterior corpectomy is optimal with removal of the involved vertebral body and adjacent discs performed simultaneously with bilateral foramenotomies of each at the involved nerve root levels. This technique can be used to remove one or more bodies with the adjacent remaining vertebral bodies being bridged with an iliac autograft or fibula heterograft supplemented by vertebral body autograft. By hollowing out gutters in the inferior aspect of the body above and the superior aspect of the body below and applying extra distraction from the anesthesia end of the table the graft can be inserted and countersunk into place. These procedures are performed supine on either the roto-rest treatment table or a regular operating table with the head turned to the right with optimal exposure from the left side because of the decreased morbidity described in the literature. Like discectomy, the corpectomy does not provide any significant immediate stability, and the patient should be usually immobilized in a cervical halo orthosis or in certain cases a rigid neck lock or Miami collar can be used. The external orthoses are maintained for at least an 8–12-week period with 8 weeks usually being adequate with autografts and 12–16 weeks being required for heterografts. In cases of subluxation or angulation with instability due to posterior ligamentous disruption or posterior bony injury the posterior operative approach is optimal. These prone procedures or posterior approaches to the cervical spine are performed in our center using a Relton four bolster frame and a Mayfield head holder with cervical traction. It is imperative to make sure that the proper positioning is insured and that the position is checked serially throughout the case by anesthesia. The eyes must be well-protected, since there is no guarantee that the head position will not change during the case, especially with the surgical pulling and manipulations that often accompany these procedures. Either indirect mirrors or direct visualization should be used by anesthesia to closely monitor the patient's head and neck position and vital structures since the surgeon is not privy to this information with the patient under the drapes. We recommend the minimal amount of traction, i.e., 5–10 pounds, be used to maintain the head and neck during these procedures because more traction often places undue pressure on the forehead and can cause skin problems later. Muscle relaxation accompanying anesthesia most often reduces preoperative traction requirements, and one must be careful not to overdistract the patient. Serial x-rays are optimal in these cases intraoperatively, especially after positioning and anesthetic induction. Incomplete or unstable patients are most often nasotrachially intubated and positioned awake to prevent secondary injury. In cases without dorsal arch disruption, but with ligamentous injuries, a modified Roger's wiring technique is recommended which involves interspinous process wiring using braided number 22 wire passed through the base of the spinous processes. These wires are passed around an autograft of cortical cancellous bone. This edge is interposed between the decorticated spinous processes to maintain a normal relationship between the vertebral elements and to prevent the compromise of the foramen and intractable pain of radiculopathy, often due to tightly squeezing the dorsal spines together with wire but without a wedged graft. The decorticated dorsal arches of the involved levels are also covered with cortical cancellous graft before closure. In cases where a refractory facet subluxation is present and if there is any suspicion of a hidden anterior disc fragment, while the intraoperative realignment of the unilateral or bilaterally locked facets are performed, a small hemilaminotomy is used before final wiring and real time ultrasound are used to evaluate the anterior canal status. This technique can obviate a catastrophe from intraoperative disc herniation and displacement or additional spinal cord compression at the time of wire tightening. To some degree this catastrophe can be obviated with good preoperative MRI imaging. The ultrasound provides a safe means of confirmation of canal integrity intraoperatively without further violating spinal instability by using only a small 1½ cm window by means of a unilateral hemilaminotomy at the involved level. These cases are postoperatively managed in a neck lock or Miami collar for a 8–12-week period with serial x-rays being repeated every 4 weeks to determine maturity of the fusion. When the collar or a halo is removed after the surgical procedure, flexion and extension (dynamic) x-rays are obtained to insure that the fusion not only has the appearance of stability but actually is mechanically stable. This can be accomplished with a cervical halo orthosis without removing the ring but, rather, by simply disconnecting it from the jacket at a time thought to be appropriate for the dynamic radiological assessment.

In cases of lamina fractures facet wiring can be used as an adjunct to spinous process wiring. Another useful technique in cases with multilaminar fractures or hematomas is bilateral facet wiring using rib as a substitute for heterograft or iliac autograft struts with wires through each of the facets bilaterally to a level above and below the area of disruption. Facet wirings are always supplemented with autograft and/or heterograft, and the patient is placed in a halo or rigid neck lock or Miami collar for an 8–12-week period. Some cases of severe anterior and posterior interruption (i.e., a gross body comminution with laminar fracture or facet fractures) may require both anterior and posterior approaches in tandem, and in rare cases the lamina may actually be impacted into the spinal canal and neural elements and require laminectomy with and without repair of dural lacerations. In these cases various combinations of anterior and posterior decompression stabilization should be performed, and most often in our center the posterior decompression and stabilization is performed prior to logrolling the patient supine for the anterior decompression and fusion to obviate displacement of the anterior graft. Casper plates and screws provide an excellent instrumentation set-up for the C3–T1 level injury patients. However, since they are not yet available in MRI-compatible or CT-compatible metal alloys, it is this surgical team's practice not to use them in cervical spinal cord injury cases with deficits because they obviate postoperative non-invasive outpatient imaging to rule out spinal cord cysts, tethering, or other problems in the rarely encountered cases of delayed progressive neurological dysfunction or intractable pain. We believe it is optimal to serially image a quadraplegic's spinal cord following initial hospitalization and treatment, as it has become increasingly apparent that spinal cord injury is a dynamic process, not stabilizing within the first hours and days, as previously thought and reported in the literature. At this point it is important again to reiterate the fact that there is little real science but more an art with regard to the surgical management of these patients, and there is *more than one way to skin a cat* in the true sense when dealing with these complex injuries. What we presented in the preceding paragraphs were the surgical protocols utilized by these authors at the UM/JMH Medical Center. It does not mean that there are not other effective techniques to accomplish the same goals. However, regardless of the design of the surgical protocol, an acute cervical spinal cord injury treatment plan should include an adequately decompressed cord and stabilized spine. Early stabilization provides the opportunity for early mobilization which definitely decreases the morbidity and mortality in these acutely traumatized and paralyzed patients. Adequate decompression allows whatever neural functional recovery that is possible to occur.

INTENSIVE CARE MANAGEMENT

Following the emergency room triage and stabilization, physical and neurological exams and imaging studies, and, in certain selective cases, following surgery as well, patients are taken to the intensive care unit. Once in the ICU they should be carefully transferred from the spine board to a kinetic roto-rest treatment table using a logrolling maneuver. Each patient is optimally rotated continuously for at least 20 hours of each 24 hour period with recesses only for feeding, hygiene, physiotherapy, respiratory therapy, diagnostic testing, and x-rays (18). We contend that the kinetic roto-rest treatment table is the best equipment available to mobilize patients with unstable spinal columns during all phases of acute care. This also applied to postoperative, stabilized patients who are at high risk for cardiopulmonary, skin, and other systemic complications following their paralysis and early surgical intervention. Continuous motion decreases the complications associated with the state of immobility experienced by acutely paralyzed patients. A system of hatches and flaps permits access to all areas of the body without compromising spinal stability. Alternative devices sometimes used are the Striker frame and Circle electric bed as well as various types of airbeds or waterbeds which are inadequate, and, in most cases unsafe for acute spinal cord injured patients (19–21). Most of our patients remain in the roto-rest throughout their intensive care stay. Once they are ready to be removed from the roto-rest they are usually stabilized surgically or with an external orthosis and are able to be sat up in a wheelchair and actively participate in their rehabilitation program. Occasionally a surgically stabilized patient will be occasionally placed on a Biodyne, which is an oscillating airbed capable of continuously turning the patient. It does not offer the spinal stability of the roto-rest, but it does offer the systematic benefits of alternating movements and kinetic therapy. These special beds and treatment tables do not diminish the amount of time the ICU nurses spend caring for each patient but instead allow the nurses to concentrate on assessments and treatments rather than patient lifting, turning, and caring for preventable complications, including secondary cord injury from inadvertent spinal column motion.

Although cardiopulmonary complications are the major cause of death in acute in-hospital phase of care, every system in the human body is affected by immobility (22). This is especially true in SCI victims who most often have multisystem trauma associated with their paralysis. Atelectasis and stasis of respiratory secretions often lead to pneumonia as well as to other respiratory complications (23). Stasis in the cardiovascular system is demonstrated best in the universal presence of deep vein thrombus (24). Deep vein thrombosis translates into phlebitis and/or fatal pulmonary emboli in between 3 and 13% of the cases reported in the literature. Pressure on the insensitive skin can lead to decubitus ulcers. Extreme immobilization contributes to muscle atrophy and potentially severe contractures of the soft tissues around the joints (18). Stasis in the urinary tract system is associated with frequent infections and calculus formation (25). Immobility of the skeletal system is associated with massive mobilization of calcium and urinary tract stones, heterotopic bone formations, severe osteoporosis, and, ultimately a high risk of pathological fractures (26). Gastrointestinal tract paralysis can result in ulcerations, hemorrhage, and chronic constipation or obstruction. The single most striking evidence of the success of our kinetic therapy ICU protocol has been the fact that over the last 15 years we have treated over 1000 acute spinal cord injury patients, most of whom had associated multisystem trauma as well without a single occurrence of a pulmonary embolus in an acute patient nursed on a roto-rest treatment table. None of these patients received prophylactic heparin or variable compression extremity devices. Other multisystem benefits of kinetic therapy have been documented by other authors as well (27). We have well-established protocols for all the body systems which compliment the kinetic therapy protocol. In acute SCI patients over 40 years of age or in those who have cardiac arrhythmias or are in neurogenic shock or who have a past history of cardiac disease or direct injury to the heart, etc. Swan-Ganz catheter is inserted and they have their cardiac index monitored. In a younger, generally healthier patient multiport central venous pressure catheters are inserted in addition to peripheral IVs. Constant EKG monitoring is maintained for all acute spinal cord injured patients as well, because of the high incidence of arrhythmias and other cardiopulmonary complications seen in the ICU. The effectiveness of these protocols has minimized, but not eliminated, cardiovascular complications, and the most common complication with the SCI patient in the ICU is still related to the respiratory system. Pulmonary function is compromised because their intercostal muscles cannot assist in the respiratory efforts as well as because of the fact that the ribs and underlying lungs are often directly traumatized in these multitrauma patients. Prophylactic intubation is used frequently in high level quadriplegic patients as indicated by inadequate arterial blood oxygenation or respiratory distress in the form of a labored respiratory effort. Patients are routinely treated every 4 hours with chest physiotherapy. If needed, a 40% oxygen mask is used to maintain blood gas levels within normal ranges and, as in the emergency room, if intubation is necessary the nasotracheal route is most often used, with tracheostomy being avoided for as long as possible. The exception is the C1–4 quadriplegic without spontaneous respiration. In these cases, often early tracheostomy is ideal. Specific protocols for high quadriplegic patients without spontaneous respirations have been implemented and include chronic ventilatory support and periodic ultrasound and electrophysiological examinations of their diaphragm and phrenic nerve functions. In addition, vital capacity, tidal volume, and other respiratory parameters are closely monitored. If economically feasible, i.e., with good insurance coverage, high quadriplegics are sent home on a roto-rest treatment table with private duty around-the-clock nursing care and periodic visits from the rehabilitation teams as well as respiratory therapy, rehabilitation psychology, etc. We find that bonding the most severely disabled patients, such as the high quadriplegics to their families is really important for the long-term potential for family cohesiveness and support. These patients who are discharged early, i.e., at about 30 days postinjury, on a ventilator, are brought back every 3 months for a 1-day admission during which they are reevaluated with ultrasonography and electrophysiological and respiratory parameter assessment. At any point that they begin to show significant potential, they are readmitted for a ventilator weaning program. Our gastrointestinal system protocols no longer use intravenous hydrogen blockers or other IV agents because of the proven effectiveness of our acute GI protocol, which includes placement of a sump tube and constant drainage of nasogastric secretions. Every 4 hours we measure the pH and titrate it above 4.5. This protocol involves neutralizing the gastric acid and keeping it out of the stomach to minimize the possibility of GI bleeding as a major morbidity in the acute spinal cord injury patient. Because cervical level SCI patients often present in neurogenic shock, they have a sympathectomy-like syndrome with the opposite of a vagotomy, i.e., an increase of acid secretion. Also, their gut is ischemic because of the stress and is often flaccid because of the paralytic ileus associated with their spinal cord injury. Adding all these factors together, we have a set-up for stress ulceration, but again this problem has been, for the most part, eliminated with the above-described protocol. Another major GI complication seen in these patients is pancreatitis. It is questionable whether or not this is a true pancreatitis or a chemical hyperamylasemia. The elevated serum amylase is often associated with an ileus, abdominal distension, and spiking temperatures and requires intravenous hyperalimentation for maintaining an anabolic state. This protocol also includes close monitoring of serum and urine amylase levels and the constant acid suction and antacid neutralization techniques. The occurrence of pancreatitis decreases following the abandonment of the long-term high dose steroid or even lower dose steroid protocols. Once the GI system is functioning, i.e., good bowel sounds, etc., the sump tube is removed, the patient is started on an oral diet and routinely given suppositories every other day and stool softener/laxative combinations. A morbidity that has become increasingly evident more recently as a major cause of morbidity in intensive care SCI patients is urinary sepsis associated with urinary tract infection. The GU protocol starts by ER placement of an indwelling Foley catheter in all acute spinal cord injured patients for monitoring urine output and for evaluation of gross and/or microscopic blood.

Cultures are taken routinely from the Foley catheter every 4 days while the patient is in the ICU because of the high incidence of urosepsis. Almost all spinal cord injured patients will have a significant colonization of bacteria in their paralyzed bladders for the rest of their lives and seem to live in symbiosis with these organisms. However, in the ICU with all the invasive lines including catheters in the vascular system and sometimes A-lines and tongs, etc., they are at an especially high risk for sepsis. Therefore, the urine is kept sterile as much as possible by using a Q 4 hour sterile intermittent catheterization program as soon as the patient is felt to be physiologically stabilized, i.e., usually within a few days of admission. This intermittent catheterization program can be successfully implemented with a minimal infection rate but can only work in conjunction with a careful I and O management program because of the tendency to "flood" ICU patients with fluids, which in turn makes even the every 4 hour program impractical. The urinary output should not be more than 500 cc every 4 hours and optimally should be less. Another major systemic consideration in intensive care patients is their metabolic status. Patients with multisystem trauma classically enter into a major catabolic state as do patients with acute paralysis or spinal cord injury. Therefore we have sort of a "double whammy" with the combination of the multisystem trauma and paralysis creating a most significant insult to the metabolic system. The worst thing to do to an ICU patient, especially to one with a spinal cord injury, is to "starve" him. We recommend that within 24 hours of admission, all acute spinal cord injury patients be started on central intravenous hyperalimentation. This IV feeding program should be maintained with high caloric input until the bowel sounds return following the initial ileus which almost universally occurs in cervical injuries. Once bowel sounds return, we usually start them on oral Gatorade and clear liquids and then advance them to full liquids and then a regular diet within a few days. Then we start them on their stool softeners and suppositories every other day, as described above. Skin integrity represents another major ICU issue in these patients, with the average pressure sore (decubitus ulcer) costing upwards of $75,000.00 not to mention the significant delaying of rehabilitation. The use of a roto-rest kinetic treatment table by skilled nurses has virtually eliminated this problem as a major issue in the intensive care unit, although unfortunately some patients arrive with an impending breakdown from the prolonged pressure of a wooden spine board in transport and in the emergency room, X-ray, CT, and MRI suites. This is especially evident in patients who have been left for more than a few hours supine on a hard plywood board without being padded or rotated. Education of prehospital personnel and emergency room and X-ray personnel can minimize this morbidity so that what may start as a small lump or bruise may not always end up being a 6–8 week treatment program for a lesion which often requires major surgical intervention.

EARLY REHABILITATION IN THE ICU

Within the first 24 hours of admission, the multidisciplinary team from the rehabilitation center evaluates and creates a short-term treatment plan for the cervical spinal cord injured patient in the ICU. This team includes a physical therapist, occupational therapist, rehabilitation psychologist, social service specialist, and a primary rehabilitation physician. All intensive care spinal cord injured patients seem to experience a series of psychological sequela starting with a denial phase. This is followed by an anger phase and then a depression phase and then eventually by the final one termed coping phase. In this final phase, the patients make the decision not to resign themselves to a permanent seat in a wheelchair, but to make the best of their situation by coping with it on a day to day basis. At this point effective rehabilitation can be initiated. The family and significant others related to the patient experience the same psychological sequela to the injury, but often in a delayed fashion. It is imperative that the physicians, nurses, and allied health professionals dealing with these seriously injured patients fully understand the basis for their behavioral patterns and not react inappropriately. They should freely communicate with the rehabilitation psychology staff to smooth out the rough edges as much as possible during this difficult period of transition. These individuals have been transformed in seconds from healthy walking persons into critically-ill and quite probably chronically paralyzed individuals.

REHABILITATION OVERVIEW

Interposed between the intensive care stay and transfer to the rehabilitation center, the cervical spine injured patient will usually spend a period of time in the acute hospital ward in either the neurosurgical or orthopaedic ward. This period is necessary to ensure that the patient is adequately stabilized both skeletally and physiologically. Generally, the time from the day of injury to transfer to the rehabilitation center is usually about 2–3 weeks in most simple, i.e., uncomplicated, cervical injuries. The patient should at this time be able to sit up in a wheelchair, stabilized and braced in most cases with a external orthosis such as a Miami collar or a halo, and begin a full rehabilitation program. Realistically for a quadriplegic with multisystem injuries or those with higher injury levels requiring ventilatory support, the stay in the acute hospital may be significantly extended. Our acute care hospital protocol is based on rapid triage and definitive treatment with the idea of early stabilization for early mobilization to minimize the morbidity/mortality and cost of care. The rehabilitation inpatient phase of care is provided by a multispecialty team of physicians, nurses, and allied health personnel. Allied health professionals include the staff rehabilitation nurses as well as nurse clinicians, physical therapists, occupational therapists, recreational therapists, educational therapies, rehabilitation technicians, psychologists, social service specialists, vocational rehabilitation counselors, sexuality counselors, dieticians, education program instructors, aerodynamic technicians, and various administrative personnel. It must be emphasized that while physical restoration is part of the rehabilitation process, the total process also involves the psychological, social, sexual, educational, recreational, and vocational aspects of rehabilitation which are all necessary to achieve maximal independence. The overall goal of the rehabilitative phase is to return each patient to society with an optimal degree of independence and mobility. The average stay for a quadriplegic in such a facility has been 4–6 months, but recently this period has been drastically reduced by increasing the opportunity for more extensive but less expensive outpatient programs. Therefore, most patients at the time of discharge do not permanently separate from the rehabilitation team but, rather, participate in continuous outpatient therapy for months and sometimes years following their discharge. It is our experience that the majority of neurological recovery occurs in the first year following injury, and by 2 years after injury about 95% of what is to be expected is seen on a careful neurological evaluation of cervical spinal cord injured patients. The exception to this rule are the evolving incomplete deficit patients who can improve significantly for many years following their injury. Special facilities such as transitional living facilities have been designed to help smooth the transition from rehabilitation to a more independent and normal living environment with the family or significant others. In the case of the communal living facilities, they are designed to allow severely disabled and sometimes respiratory dependent quadriplegics to share expenses and resources and remain out of a nursing home environment, i.e., experience a better quality of life. Upon discharge from the rehabilitation center a lifelong follow-up care program is instituted for the cervical spinal cord injury victim. They are seen at least twice annually in a multidisciplinary clinic where all body systems as well as the spine and spinal cord function are reevaluated. It has been shown that such frequent follow-up visits dramatically decrease the number of days of readmissions due to systemic complications. Today, the average cervical spinal cord injured person who survives the acute period has a relatively normal life expectancy with a good lifelong follow-up care program.

Rehabilitative Engineering Advances in Cervical Spinal Cord Injuries

Over the last 2 decades, and more specifically over the last 3 years, there has been a tremendous proliferation of interest in individuals with severe disabilities both by the federal government and the private sector. This focus of attention has resulted in a significant evolution of technology available to improve the quality of life of quadriplegics and in certain cases to increase their functional capacities. At our center we routinely evaluate quadriplegic patients, whether they are classified as complete or incomplete, with a computerized multichannel EMG biofeedback apparatus. The purpose of the initial testing is to establish a baseline measure which can be compared to serially monitored measures over time to assess outcome success following different interventions. Muscles that are nonfunctional or weak in the zone of injury, i.e., adjacent to or near the injury level, are sampled for any evidence of motor unit electrical activity. Application of surface electrodes provides visual and auditory feedback of the electrical activity within a particular muscle group and often motor unit activity can be found in muscles which appear to be grossly nonfunctional under visual and tactile evaluation. This method is capable of identifying muscle motor activity that is beyond the ability of traditional motor testing methods to identify. Our experience indicates that computerized multichanneled EMG biofeedback training has been effective as an adjunct to other interventions such as functional electrical stimulation and conventional physiotherapy or even following surgical decompression.

Patients who have motor recruitment potential below their functional level of paralysis, clinical evidence of a local asymmetry of function, or local incompleteness in their zone of injury are reevaluated with MRI imaging. If metal instrumentation or wires are present and too much artifact exists, then a myelogram/CT is utilized. If evidence of significant canal compromise and neural element compression is documented, then the patients are counseled regarding their potential for a delayed surgical decompression. Results on the first 100 patients evaluated showed that the majority of them had some significant motor and/or sensory recovery when surgery was performed for that purpose. These results were most evident in quadriplegic level injuries because of the fact that even recovery of one nerve root level and even unilateral recovery can significantly alter their functional capacity and quality of life. For example, a C5 quadriplegic can rub his nose when it itches and even feed himself with certain splinting, whereas a C6 quadriplegic with a one level difference, can drive a car, help dress himself and do much more with regard to the activities of daily living. The addition of C7 function allows them to transfer and be much more independent, and some C7 quadriplegics even live independently. Another indication for delayed decompression has been intractable cervical radiculopathy in quadriplegics. When bone or soft tissue compresses the neural elements and compromises the canal, and is associated with an intractable local and/or radiating pain syndrome, we have been very successful in relieving this pain more than burning deafferented pain, although both have improved somewhat in these cases. The one patient problem that has not benefited from a delayed decompression except in some instances is intractable spasticity. In our experience this has been the least favorable to respond to delayed decompression. Besides being used as a tool to evaluate patients and to screen them for delayed decompression, the EMG biofeedback apparatus is also used therapeutically in our center as applied by a physical therapist in conjunction with conventional resistive exercises and FES (functional electrical stimulation).

A combination of more than one rehabilitative engineering modality into a system is termed a hybrid rehabilitation system. An example of hybrid systems now available include apparatuses which integrate biofeedback and functional electrical stimulation. A new device being developed in our center combines three modalities: biofeedback, functional electrical stimulation, and resistive exercise with an upper extremity ergometer. Functional electrical stimulation has been around since the days of the Pharaohs when their physicians used electrical eels to shock people with Bell's palsy and stroke. Today, thanks to bioengineers, sophisticated functional electrical stimulation systems are now being used by thousands of paralyzed individuals. Open loop FES with just a muscle stimulation component are available as small, portable or more sophisticated larger units. These are able to initiate movement against gravity and sometimes against resistance of paralyzed upper and lower extremities, especially when the muscles are spastic or upper motor neuron. Combined with resistive exercise this movement can result in increased muscle bulk and strength. At Wright State University this technology was advanced by adding a closed loop component to functional electrical stimulation and by combining a hybrid system of ergometry bicycle and FES. These closed loop functional electrical stimulation bicycle ergometers are now commercially available and are being used in hundreds of centers across the nation and around the world. They are especially beneficial to quadriplegics who are not able to achieve cardiopulmonary conditioning like able-bodied individuals with running, rowing, etc. and are not even able to condition as well as the paraplegics whose upper bodies can be used for such training. Further, physiological benefits of these bicycle ergometry systems are still being evaluated with regard to other complex systemic issues. There is no doubt, however, that in two areas they are extremely effective: *a*) with regard to reversing lower extremity atrophy and giving the patient an adequate mass of muscle over the bony prominence which minimizes the chance of a decubitus ulcer or a pressure sore. In addition, these hypertrophied muscles replacing atrophic ones provide the quadriplegic individual with a tremendous psychological advantage and a feeling of well-being. Body image is very important, especially when one considers that most of the victims of quadriplegia are young males; and *b*) closed loop FES bicycle ergometry reverses the cardiac atrophy that occurs in quadraplegics, although it is unclear whether it is secondary to denervation or disuse. Clearly, with the use of closed loop FES ergometry we will begin to answer some of the questions such as at which time exercise should begin following acute injury and whether it is able to limit or reverse osteoporosis and other negative changes which are much more devastating to the quadriplegic than to the paraplegic spinal cord injured individual. At the same time that the lower extremity walking systems and bicycle systems were evolving, upper extremity bioengineering advanced with equal strides. Today, several implantable and nonimplantable units are being evaluated in centers and probably in this decade will become commercially available. These combinations of hybrid systems with FES and in some cases combined with an orthosis enable higher level quadriplegics to have increased functioning of their distal upper extremities, which translates again into a significant improvement in the quality of life. A major thrust and focus of rehabilitative engineering has been to evaluate and develop safer and better implantable electrode systems which hopefully will not have long-term negative effects on the nerves on which the electrodes are placed. Simultaneously, development is ongoing for better and longer life battery systems and microprocessors and miniaturized systems. Other hybrid systems include the combination of functional electrical stimulation of the lower extremities with a new generation of reciprocating braces or other types of orthoses which may even allow ambulation in certain of the lower quadriplegics who are often called "superquads" because their functional capacity is much more than it should be in a classical sense, considering their level of disability. This level of engineering has advanced to include both noninvasive and invasive and implantable systems and surface systems. The best example of an invasive system which has evolved over the last decade is the implantable bladder stimulation apparatus which is being used widely in Great Britain by paraplegics and quadriplegics. There is a subcutaneous button which activates an implanted stimulator system with electrodes hooked to the appropriate sacral nerves or directly to the bladder wall, which in turn empties the bladder on command. The system is now being evaluated in this country. It has great potential to help alleviate the morbidity and the tremendous logistical problems associated with a neurogenic bladder. Another important urological engineering advance is in the sophistication of equipment for reproduction, including the combination of electrical ejaculation with artificial insemination which will allow many quadriplegic men to have their own children. Another important advance in the basic functions category by bioengineers has been the development of the Avatar system which is a bowel evacuation system which can turn a several-hour unpleasant bowel program into a 5-minute, no touch, reasonable experience for the quadriplegic patient with the neurogenic bowel. It has been compared to a sort of combination of bidet and vacuum cleaner but in reality may become a very important contribution to the disabled consumers' quality of life.

From the more creature comfort and labor intensive viewpoint, the bioengineers have also delivered a new generation of environmental control systems that function with the use of sip and puff straws or laser beams, etc. and which allow even the highest level of quadriplegics to control their lights and television and radios and room temperature. This can be done without any movement of the extremities. New communication systems have also evolved which allow the use of computers and word processors by these severely disabled quadriplegics. An older technology, phrenic nerve pacemakers for respirator-dependent quadriplegics, has really not advanced in the last 20 years, and due to the limited guarantee and life of this apparatus, we have been hesitant at this center to implant any more of these devices in our patients. A further step toward greater independence for severely disabled quadriplegics involves a new generation of driving assistive devices. These are now extremely light-touched and sensitive and easily controlled and are now adapted for high quadriplegics to the point where even C5 quadriplegics can drive their own vans. Even the vans themselves have undergone tremendous improvements with a new generation of vehicles for the disabled which have suspension systems which drop the vehicle to street level, obviating the previous requirement of hydraulic or electrical mechanical lifts and ramps.

Rehabilitative engineers have more recently extended their technology beyond the basic needs of paralyzed patients to include recreational requirements as well. Sailboats have now been developed that are especially equipped to be sailed by quadriplegics with special spring-loaded swiveling but secure seats which allow the quadriplegic to sail the boat with light touch and line control and even to tack to alternate sides of the boat with only partial use of their upper extremities. A new generation of light weight wheelchairs have also become available for competitive sports as well as for use in activities of daily living which allow the quadriplegic with a significant deficit to propel himself, whereas in the past they required motorized chairs because of bulk and sheer weight of their vehicles. Electric chairs have also been developed which allow patients to mobilize in a sitting or standing position, whichever they choose. The standing chairs allow the quadriplegic the advantage of eye-to-eye contact when reentering a very competitive able-bodied society. All in all, quadriplegics can continue to look to the rehabilitative engineer as an ever-enlarging source of evolving technology which can impact their lives most positively on a daily basis.

The diagnosis, treatment, and prognosis of cervical spinal cord injuries have undergone many significant changes in the last several years, with more technology and resources being focused upon this severely disabled group of patients and consumers. There is no reason to suspect that this rapid progress will not continue. Any reasonable basic science strategy involving central nervous system regeneration will also incorporate rehabilitative engineering technology, present and future, in developing a balanced approach toward long-term reversal of deficit.

REFERENCES

1. Ducker TB, Perot PL. National Spinal Cord Injury Registry. Div. of Neurosurgery, Medical Univ. of South Carolina, 80 Barre St., Charleston, SC 21401.
2. Mesard L, Carmody A, Mannarino E, and Ruge D. Survival after spinal cord trauma. Arch Neurol 1978;35:78–83.
3. Stover SL, Fine PR, ed. Spinal cord injury: the facts and figures. Birmingham: University of Alabama at Birmingham, 1986.
4. Young JS, Northrup NE. Statistical information pertaining to some of the most commonly asked questions about spinal cord injury. SCI Dig 1979;1:11.
5. Young JS. Initial hospitalization and rehabilitation costs of spinal cord injury. Orthop Clin North Am 1978;9:263–270.
6. Hall WJ, Green BA, Colodonato JP. Spinal cord injury: emergency management. Emerg Med Serv 1976;5:28–36.
7. Klose KJ, Green BA, Smith RS, Adkins RH, MacDonald AM. University of Miami Neuro-Spinal Index (UMNI): a quantitative method for determining spinal cord function. Paraplegia 1980;18:331–336.
8. Schneider RC, Thompson JM, Bebin J. The syndrome of acute central cervical spinal cord injury. J Neurol Neurosurg Psychiatry, 1958;21:216–227.
9. Schneider RC. The syndrome of acute anterior spinal cord injury. J Neurosurg 1955;12:95–122.
10. Schneider RC. Chronic neurological sequelae of acute trauma to the spine and spinal cord. Part II. The syndrome of chronic anterior spinal cord injury or compressed herniated intervertebral discs. J Bone Joint Surg 1959;41A:449–456.
11. Eismont FJ, Clifford S, Goldberg ML, Green BA. Cervical sagittal spinal canal size in spine injury. Spine 1984;9:663–666.
12. Cooper PR, Maravilla KR, Sklar FH, Moody SF, Clark WK. Halo immobilization of cervical spine fractures. J Neurosurg 1979;50:603–610.
13. Griswold DM, Albright JA, Schiffman E, Johnson RM, Southwick WO. Atlanto-axial fusion for instability. J Bone Joint Surg 1978;60A:285–292.
14. White AA, Johnson RM, Panjabi MD, Southwick WO. Biomechanical analysis of clinical stability in the spine. Clin Orthop 1975;109:85–96.
15. Robinson RA, Smith GW. Anteriolateral cervical disc removal and interbody fusion for cervical disc syndrome. [Abstract] Bull Johns Hopkins Hosp 1955;96:223–224.
16. Cloward RB. Treatment of ruptured intervertebral discs by vertebral body fusion: indications, operative technique and aftercare. J Neurosurg 1953;10:154–168.
17. Cloward RB. The anterior approach for removal of ruptured cervical discs. J Neurosurg 1958;15:602–617.
18. Green BA, Green KL, Kose KJ. Kinetic nursing for acute spinal cord injury patients. Paraplegia 1980;18:181–186.
19. Coppola AR. Stryker-frame death. Va Med 1977;104:475–476.
20. Slabaugh PB, Nickel VL. Complications with use of the Stryker frame. J Bone Joint Surg 1978;60A:1111.
21. Smith TK, Whitaker J, Stauffer ES. Misuse of the circular electric turning frame. J Bone Joint Surg [Abstract]. 1974;56A:205.
22. Dietrick JE, Whedon GD, Shorr E. Effects of immobilization upon various metabolic and physiologic functions of normal men. Am J Med 1948;4:3–32.
23. Bellamy R, Pitts FW, Stauffer ES. Respiratory complications in traumatic quadriplegia. J Neurosurg 1973;39:596–600.
24. Wolman L. The disturbance of circulation in traumatic paraplegia in acute and late stages. Paraplegia 1965;2:213–226.
25. Walsh JJ. Urinary calcium and kidney stones in paraplegia. Paraplegia 1974;12:31–32.
26. Bergman P, Heilporn A, Schoutens A, Paternot J, Tricot A. Longitudinal study of calcium and bone metabolism in paraplegic patients. Paraplegia 1977;15:147–150.
27. Whedon GD, Dietrick JE, Shorr E. Modification of the effects of immobilization upon various metabolic and physiologic functions of normal men. Am J Med 1949;6:684–710.

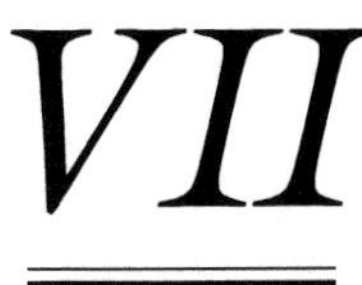

Surgical Management—Approaches and Techniques

32

Surgical Approaches to the Cervical Spine

Robert G. Watkins and William H. Dillin

Introduction

In this chapter we will attempt to describe in detail the surgical techniques used in alternative exposures of the cervical spine. Since many lesions may be approached by several routes we will only summarize the anatomy and techniques used to expose anterior, lateral, and posterior pathologic lesions of the cervical spine. The specific approach to be chosen will be left up to the familiarity and expertise of the individual surgeon.

Posterior Approach to the Cervical Spine

For the posterior cervical exposure at any level, the patient's head is positioned in the Gardner/Mayfield three-pin device that is then attached to the operating table. An alternate positioning method for the posterior approach is to use the Mayfield horseshoe frame. Positioning consists of rolling the patient from supine to prone onto chest rolls that are fixed firmly to the operating table by strapping velcro strap around a post on the table so that caudal sliding of the chest pad is prevented. The surgeon turns the patient using spine precautions. He holds the head and the trapezius area of the shoulders, cradling the head between his forearms. An assistant will hold the forearms to the head. Therefore, the side pressure of the forearms is reinforced by the assistant. This keeps the head immobile in position with the shoulders. In turning the patient over, this contact is maintained until the patient is on the chest rolls, then the surgeon's hands can be shifted to hold the head. Additional assistants bring the horseshoe to the patient's head. Great care is taken to have the horseshoe wide enough so there is no direct pressure on the eyes, and a general horseshoe shape from the lateral cheek around the forehead to the opposite cheek is maintained; the airway open, the eyes totally clear (5).

The neck generally is positioned with enough flexion to allow an adequate exposure, usually there will be no wrinkles in the skin on the back of the neck. Depending on the patient's condition, the amount of flexion has to be adjusted to the pathology. The legs are flexed at the knees, and the upright table attachment is used to provide support for the shins, with the knee flexed to 90°. The table is then put into reversed Trendelenberg position with the head up. Pressure is borne on the patient's knees and shins on the prepared foot rest. This positions the posterior cervical spine up to the surgeon. Additional readjustments of the horseshoe should be made, as the body might have slid slightly back. To visualize the lower cervical spine on the x-ray, Boger straps are secured on the wrists but not connected around the foot of the table until needed. Adhesive drapes are then positioned on the patient's neck.

A lateral radiograph with a needle inserted into a spinous process may be used for localization. Then, the skin and subcutaneous tissues are incised in the midline down to the fascia. The deep cervical fascia is exposed as it inserts into the ligamentum nuchae and supraspinous ligament. The incision is deepened with the electrocautery, staying within the thin, white median raphe. Cutting muscle is to be avoided so that the incision should follow the wandering, wavey median raphe. The median raphe is opened down to the spinous processes. Exposure is limited to the necessary levels to avoid spontaneous fusion at adjacent levels, especially in children and at the occiput.

The bulbous tips of the spinous processes are exposed with the electrocautery or with a #15 blade. The prominent spinous process at C2, C7, and T1 are easily identified. Their ligamentous attachments are important and should be reattached at closure. Spina bifida of the cervical spine should be identified on the preoperative x-ray as well as at surgery. The paraspinous muscles are stripped laterally to the facets and, if indicated, from the transverse processes.

When the occiput is to be fused, it is exposed subperiosteally as well. The self-retaining retractors are inserted to increase the exposure and aid in dissection of the base of the skull and the dorsal spine of C2. The area between the occiput and C2 will contain the ring of C1. This may be very deep when compared with C2. Feel for the posterior tubercle of C1. Identify and dissect soft

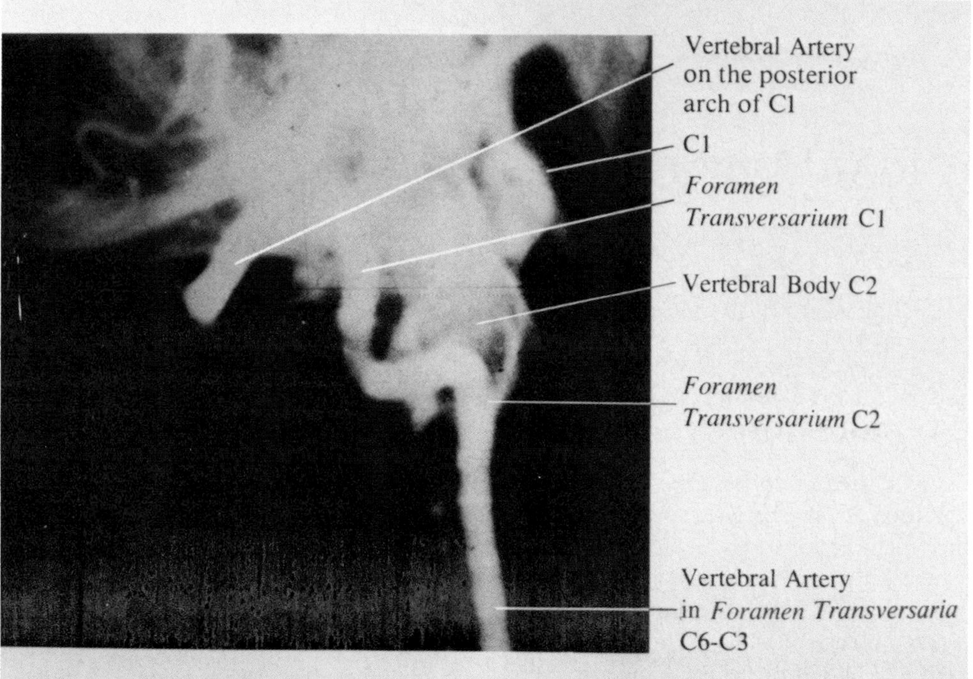

Figure 32.1. The course of the vertebral artery is from the foramen transversarium of C1 posteriorly in the region of the C1–2 articulation through the transversarium of C1, then posterior-medially to the posterior rim of C1.

tissue from it transversely from the midline with a sharp periosteal elevator.

The posterior arch of C1 is often very thin, and direct pressure can fracture it or cause the surgeon to slip off the ring penetrating the atlanto-occipital membrane. The underlying dura may be vulnerable to injury at both the superior and inferior edge of the ring of C1. Lateral dissection on the posterior arch should be limited to 1.5 cm.

The second cervical ganglion is an important lateral landmark on the ring of C1. It can be identified approximately 1.5 cm from the midline on the lamina of C1 or between the laminae of C1 and C2 prior to reaching the vertebral artery between C1 and C2.

The vertebral artery enters the foramen transversarium at the sixth vertebra and progresses cephalad through each successive foramen transversarium until it exits through the foramen transversarium of C1 and passes posteriorly and medially in a groove on the superior border of C1 toward the midline. It then turns cephalad along the spinal cord to enter the foramen magnum (Fig. 32.1). The vertebral artery can be damaged by deep penetration of the atlanto-occipital membrane above the ring of C1 more medial than the usually safe 1.5 cm from the midline. The most medial aspect of the groove for the vertebral artery and vein should be carefully identified on the superior border of the C1 ring (4). The bluish color of the vein is visualized first. By identifying the initial ridge of the groove, damage to the artery can be avoided. There is seldom any indication for dissection lateral to the groove of the vertebral artery on C1. The vertebral artery and vein are not only vulnerable in the groove (Fig. 32.2), but as the artery passes from the foramen transversarium of C2 to that of C1, it is in close lateral and posterior proximity to the C1–C2 facet joint (17).

The operative procedure may require exposure of the dura of the posterior fossa (8, 15, 16). After exposure of the ring of C1 and the bone of the posterior occiput, no attempt should be made to decompress the posterior fossa by removing bone from caudad to cephalad under the edge of the foramen magnum. Removal of the posterior rim of the foramen magnum and the suboccipital bone is best accomplished by placement of two burr holes, one to the left and another to the right of the midline. A suboccipital craniotomy can then be performed using multiple sized rongeurs. There is a venous sinus in the midline and the fascial attachment of the periosteum of the skull to the dura may at times contain an emissary sinus as well (Fig. 32.3).

For a more lateral approach to the C1–2 facet joint, the vertebral artery between C1 and C2 must be identified. In rotatory dislocations of C1–2, the artery is stretched tightly across the joint on the side where C1 is anterior to C2 and could easily be damaged (17).

For lower cervical exposure of a cervical nerve in an intervertebral foramina, identify the junction of the lamina and the inferior facet. Then identify the junction of the interlaminar area and the facet joint. Expanding these areas with a burr and a microkerrison allows entry into the intervertebral foramen and exposure of the nerve root.

Anterior Approaches to the Cervical Spine

The significant anatomic landmarks in differentiating approaches to the cervical spine are the sternocleidomastoid muscle, the carotid sheath, and the longus coli muscle. Categorization of the approach is based on the direction of approach relative to these specific structures. For example, approach Number 1 is medial to the sternocleidomastoid muscle and medial to the carotid sheath. Approach Number 2 is lateral to the sternocleidomastoid muscle and lateral to the carotid sheath. The significant differentiating feature of these approaches is whether to approach the carotid sheath medially or laterally. We prefer the anterior medial Smith-Robinson, Cloward approach for pathology from C2 to T1 (3, 7, 14). For T2 pathology a third rib under the arm approach is usually used.

The skin incision should be cosmetically acceptable (Fig. 32.4). Superficial landmarks used to help place the incision over the appropriate spinal level are: C3–4, which is above the thyroid cartilage; C5–6, which is at the cricoid cartilage (12). Alternately, 2 fingerbreadths above the clavicle can be used for C5–6 and 1 fingerbreadth for C6–7. For best cosmesis, make a 3 cm transverse incision in a skin crease from midline to the anterior border of the sternocleidomastoid muscle. A longer transverse incision allows adequate exposure for three vertebral bodies and two disc levels (2). It is best to open the platysma muscle along the line of its fibers. The platysma muscle should be opened carefully to avoid damage to underlying veins and the sternocleidomastoid muscle (12). The sternocleidomastoid must then be identified; for anterior medial approaches, the medial border of the sternocleidomastoid, and for the lateral approaches, the lateral border of the sternocleidomastoid. The carotid sheath is first identified by finger palpation of the carotid pulse. From there to the next landmark structure is the longus coli muscle, which must be identified under the prevertebral fascia over the vertebral body. Often the anterior tubercle of the transverse process is mistaken for the vertebral body. Inadvertent dissection in this more lateral area can damage the sympathetic plexus and cause bleeding from the longus coli. The more avascular area of the spine is the midline. Opening the prevertebral fascia in the midline allows lateral dissection and retraction of the longus coli and causes less bleeding.

In any approach to the anterior cervical spine the esoph-

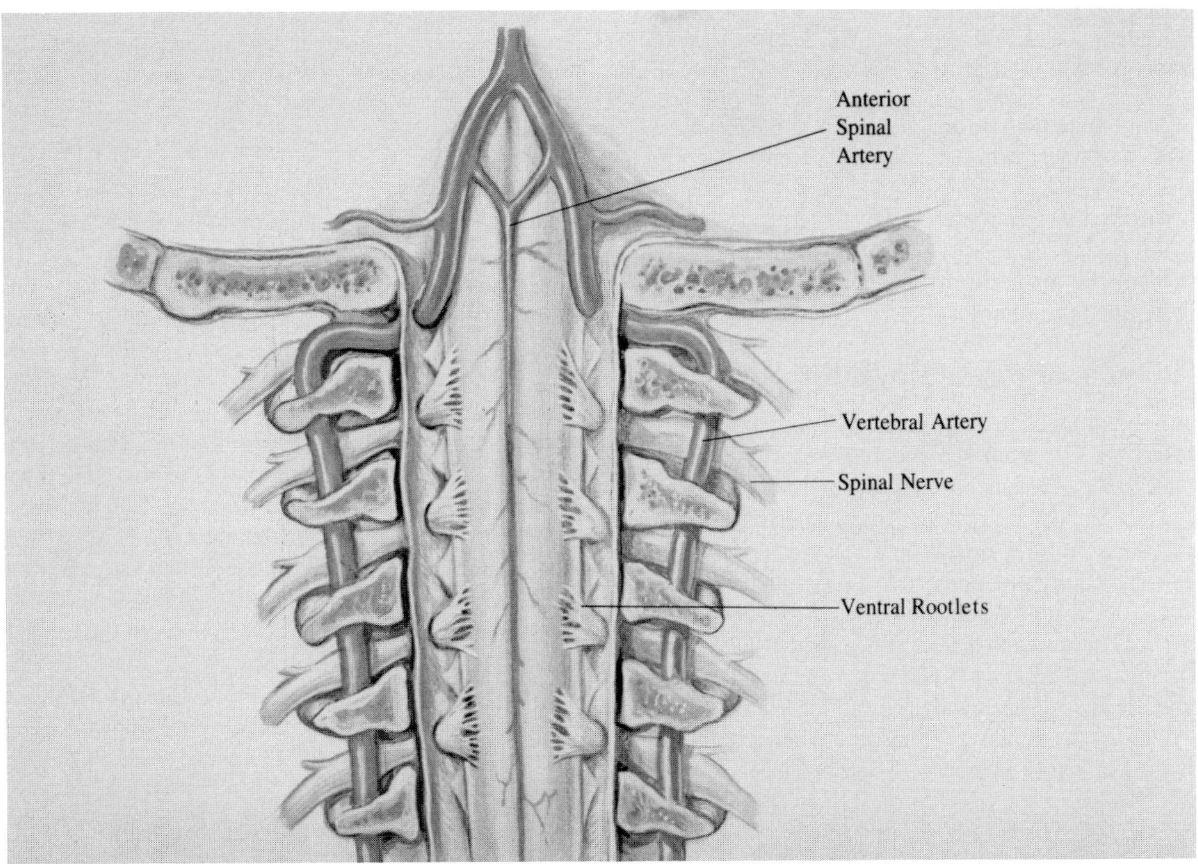

Figure 32.2. The anterior view without vertebral bodies emphasizes the formation of the anterior spinal artery. There are numerous variations in this formation, ranging from a unilateral vertebral artery contribution to no contribution.

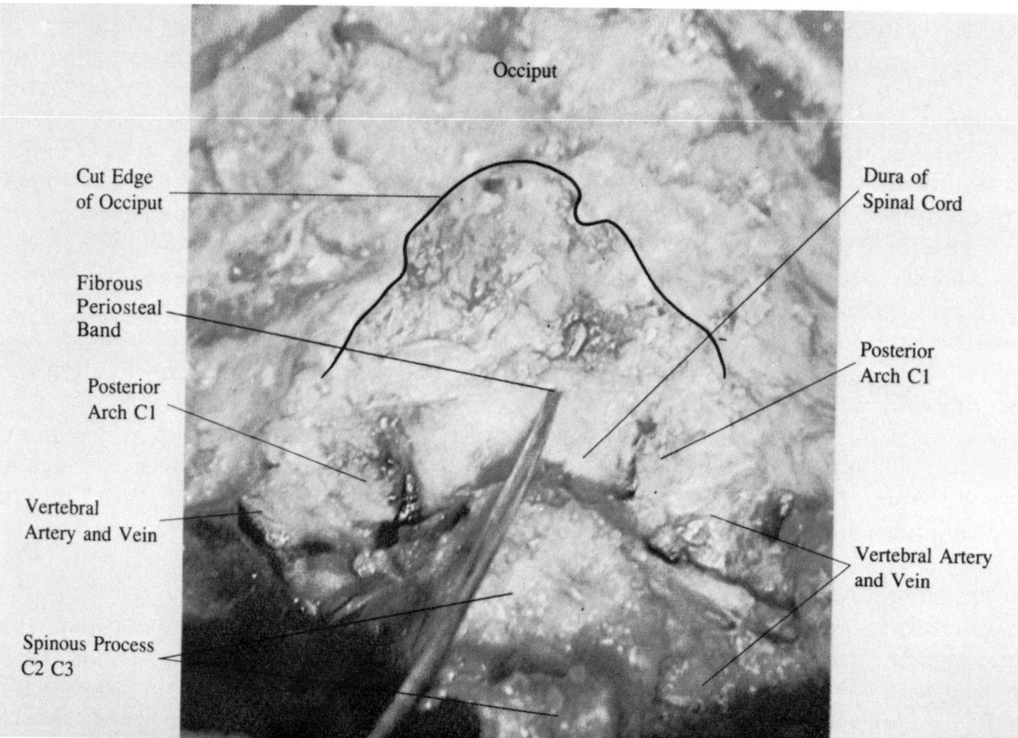

Figure 32.3. In the posterior approach to the foramen magnum, one must first place burr holes in the occiput above the foramen magnum. Two parasagittal holes allow removal of bone from the dura with a Harrison-type rongeur. Careful dissection medially from the burr holes protects one from the often significant fragile sinus, and dissection caudally approaches the foramen magnum. After removal of the occiput, including the boney rim of the foramen magnum, which is a sharp-lipped structure projecting directly anterior in the transverse plane, one encounters the fibrous attachment of the inner periosteum of the skull to the dura at the rim of the foramen magnum. There is sometimes a transverse venous sinus in this area that produces bleeding which can be significant when torn. Attachment to the dura in this area may produce a dural leak unless the area is carefully dissected.

agus is identified as a flat ribbon-like structure overlying the anterior prevertebral fascia. Use finger dissection to progress from the medial border of the sternocleidomastoid muscle to the midline of the spine.

Retraction of Neurovascular Structures

Vessels may be either ligated or retracted, depending on their size and location. The retraction of nerves and arteries varies, but general guidelines can be used. In more cephalad exposures, retract the hypoglossal nerve, glossopharyngeal nerve, and the digastric muscle cephalad. The superior laryngeal nerve and superior thyroid artery and vein are often retracted caudad for C1–C3 approaches and cephalad for C4–C7 approaches (7). The middle thyroid vein is ligated when necessary. The inferior thyroid artery and vein are retracted caudally for C7 and above exposures and cephalad for levels distal to T1. In addition, the omohyoid muscle crosses around C6 and is divided or retracted for C6–7 and below.

Right or Left Approach?

To determine whether to approach the spine from the right or the left, consider the following. When approaching from the left in the supraclavicular area one must beware of the point of entry of the thoracic duct into the jugular vein-subclavian vein junction (Fig. 32.5). A large fatty meal the day prior to surgery in this area is an aid to identify the duct, but the majority of approaches will be well medial to this area and will not require definitive identification. Approaches on the right from C4 and below may traumatize the right recurrent laryngeal nerve. This nerve passes from the area of the carotid sheath to the medial musculovisceral column in the C5–7 area. The left recurrent laryngeal nerve is in the tracheoesophageal groove throughout the neck. It can be injured by using a sharp angled retractor in the tracheoesophageal groove. For this reason we use blunt finger dissection from the medial border of the sternocleidomastoid muscle to the midline of the spine. Then place the nonlipped, hand-held Cloward retractor directly on the spine and avoid rigorous retraction into the soft tissue.

Traction During Surgery

Head halter traction or Gardner-Wells tongs are standard during all interbody grafting operations to allow for dis-

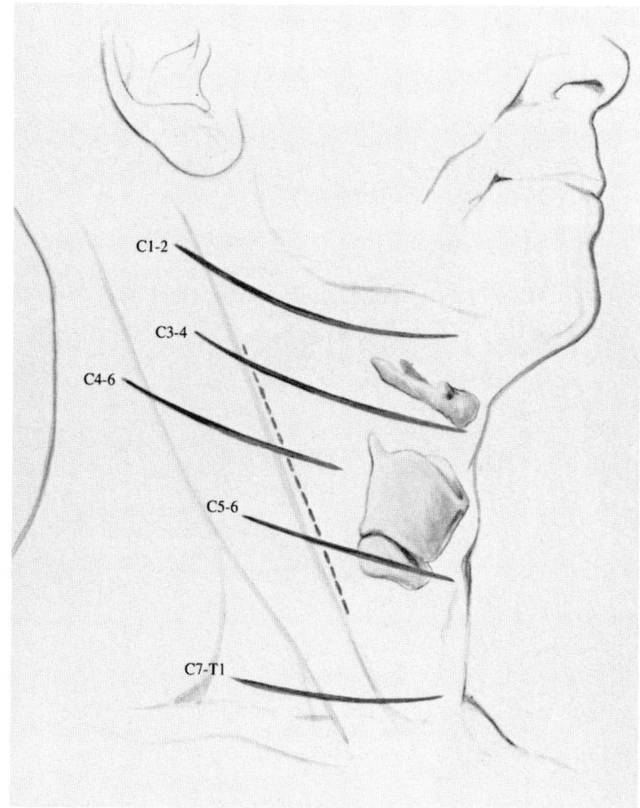

Figure 32.4. The approximate skin areas for approaches. Specific spinal levels are usually indicated by palpable subcutaneous structures.

traction of the interspace and resulting compression after the bone graft has been placed.

Positioning for Anterior Approaches

The head must be extended enough to allow exposure of the cervical spine. Patients will vary from a fixed kyphotic deformity to a short built neck to no neck. The amount of extension is altered according to the stiffness of the neck and the pathology (care should be taken in hyperextending a myelopathy patient, as this further closes the spinal canal). Holding the head with spinal cord precautions, place a rolled towel under the shoulders. Allow the head to extend gently to find its limit of extension. Then flex to less than this limit and observe the amount of anterior clearance. Assess the distance of the cricoid and thyroid cartilages from the sternal notch. Rotation of the head away from the side of the approach may be needed to provide adequate exposure. Remember, extension and rotation closes the intervertebral foramina opposite the approach. The Boger straps are positioned loosely around the patient's wrists in order to provide traction on the arms when needed during the case to visualize C-7 on an intra-operative radiograph. The straps are released after the x-ray.

TRANSORAL APPROACH TO C1–2

This approach will be discussed in great detail in the following chapters by Crockard-Menezes (1).

ANTEROMEDIAL APPROACH TO C1, C2, AND C3 (EXTENSION OF THE SMITH ROBINSON)

The skin incision is made under the angle of the jaw. It may be "T"ed along the medial border of the sternocleidomastoid muscle to allow a longer exposure of the spine (Fig. 32.6). The superior thyroid artery and vein and superior laryngeal nerve are identified. The superior thyroid artery arises from the external carotid artery at approximately the level of the hyoid bone. The hypoglossal nerve is identified and retracted. The hypoglossal nerve is found passing from lateral to medial superficial to the external carotid, lingual, and facial arteries. Positive identification of the hypoglossal nerve must be carried out prior to ligation of any structure. It is a superficial structure, first coursing vertically and parallel to the carotid sheath, then horizontally, crossing medially over the carotid. Both the lingual and facial arteries are identified and ligated. The digastric muscle is identified. This is usually retracted cephalad but may be transected. When necessary, divide the stylofacial band running from the stylohyoid process to the posterior pharynx. Difficulties may be encountered with the superior laryngeal nerve, both external and internal branches, and the pharyngeal branches of the vagus nerve. These should be identified and retracted but frequently suffer from retraction. The carotid sheath and the ligated stumps of the lingual and facial arteries are retracted laterally and the musculovisceral column retracted medially with deep right angle, hand-held blunt retractors.

A Kitner or peanut is used to dissect bluntly, to assist in identifying the prevertebral fascia and the midline of the vertebrae. The fibers of the longus colli muscle and fascia are elevated off the vertebral body from the midline laterally. Then use curved Cloward elevators to dissect a flap of the longus colli muscle from the vertebral body. The blades of the Cloward retractor are inserted under the longus colli muscle. Deep hand-held Cloward retractors are preferred by other surgeons (Fig. 32.7).

ANTERIOR MEDIAL APPROACH TO THE MIDCERVICAL SPINE

After a transverse skin incision at the appropriate level, dissect through the subcutaneous tissue to the platysma muscle (Fig. 32.8). The platysma muscle is opened carefully in line with the fibers. Under the platysma is the external jugular vein which is divided and ligated only when its presence interferes with the procedure. With

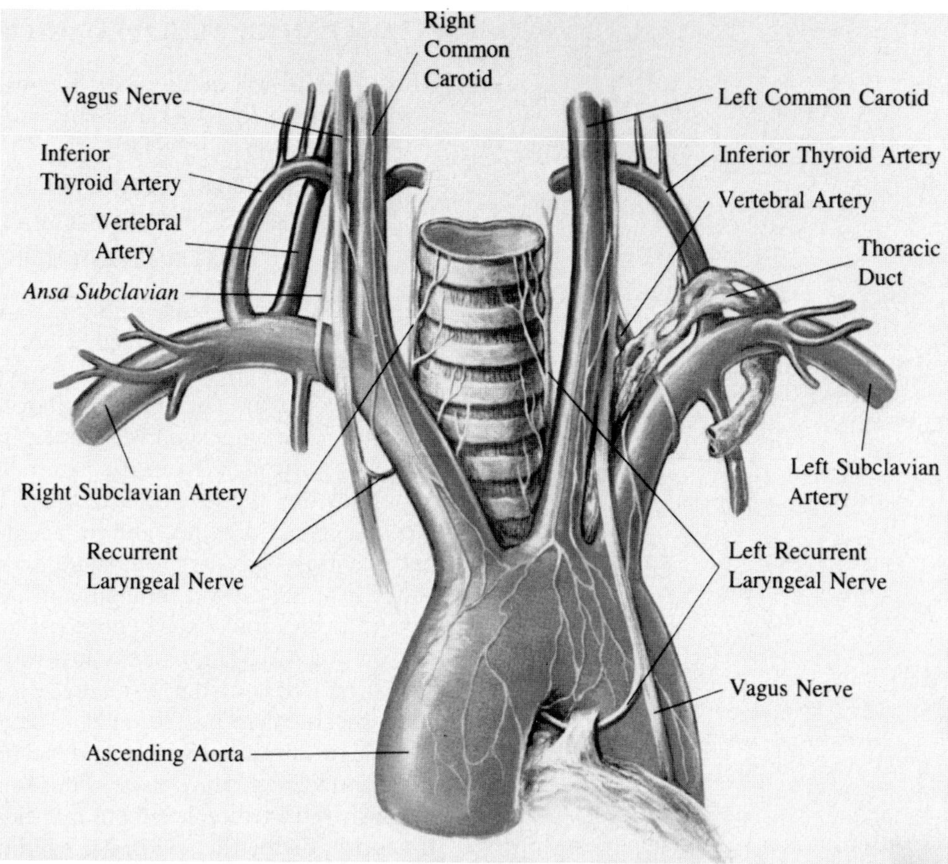

Figure 32.5. Neuroclavicular structures of the base of the neck. In approaching the spine from the right side of the neck, the prominent recurrent laryngeal nerve must be identified in the area between the musculovisceral column medially and the carotid sheath laterally. When one is approaching the spine from the left side, the thoracic duct may be damaged at the base of the neck as it enters the subclavian vein. Both vagus nerves seen here are in the carotid sheath.

identification of this medial border of the sternocleidomastoid then bluntly develop the interval between the sternocleidomastoid muscle and the musculovisceral column (13). The middle cervical fascia invests the sternocleidomastoid medially. This may be opened with scissors and spread vertically or the wound developed with blunt dissection only. The sternocleidomastoid is retracted laterally and the strap musculature medially (Fig. 32.9). The omohyoid muscle crosses from proximal medial to lateral distal through the middle cervical fascia at around C6–7. Retract the omohyoid, or if necessary, divide it laterally, tag it and repair it later. Vertical finger dissection spreads the middle cervical fascia just medial to the carotid sheath (12). The inconstant middle thyroid vein crossing at approximately C5 is identified, ligated, and divided when needed. The anterior surface of the vertebral body is identified with a finger. The blunt, nonlipped Cloward hand-held retractor is then inserted into the wound directed down to the spine. The retractor is held on the right longus colli. Beware of entering the tracheoesophageal groove with the retractor tip and thereby damaging the left recurrent laryngeal nerve (10). Retract distally the inferior thyroid artery and vein at the C6–7 level and retract proximally the superior thyroid artery and vein and the superior laryngeal nerve at C3–4 (Fig. 32.10). Do not mistake the transverse process for the midline of the vertebral body, as an incision deep in this area will damage the longus colli muscle, the sympathetic chain, and possibly the vertebral artery. An incision into the longus colli muscle produces bleeding. The key to avoiding this is to stay in the midline.

A disc is palpated in the midline of the spine and the prevertebral fascia opened with a small dissector longitudinally until the disc can be identified. The elevator exposes the disc horizontally. The retractor is inserted, and the esophagus should never be seen. The esophagus, trachea, and anterior strap muscles are retracted medially, and the carotid sheath and sternocleidomastoid muscle laterally. With the prevertebral fascia opened in the midline and the disc identified, a needle is inserted into a disc for lateral x-ray confirmation of the level.

Then the very important phase of developing a flap of longus colli muscle begins, as described earlier. The clawed blades of the Cloward self-retaining retractor are then inserted under the flap of the longus colli on both sides of the spine. If vertical exposure is needed to expose the de-

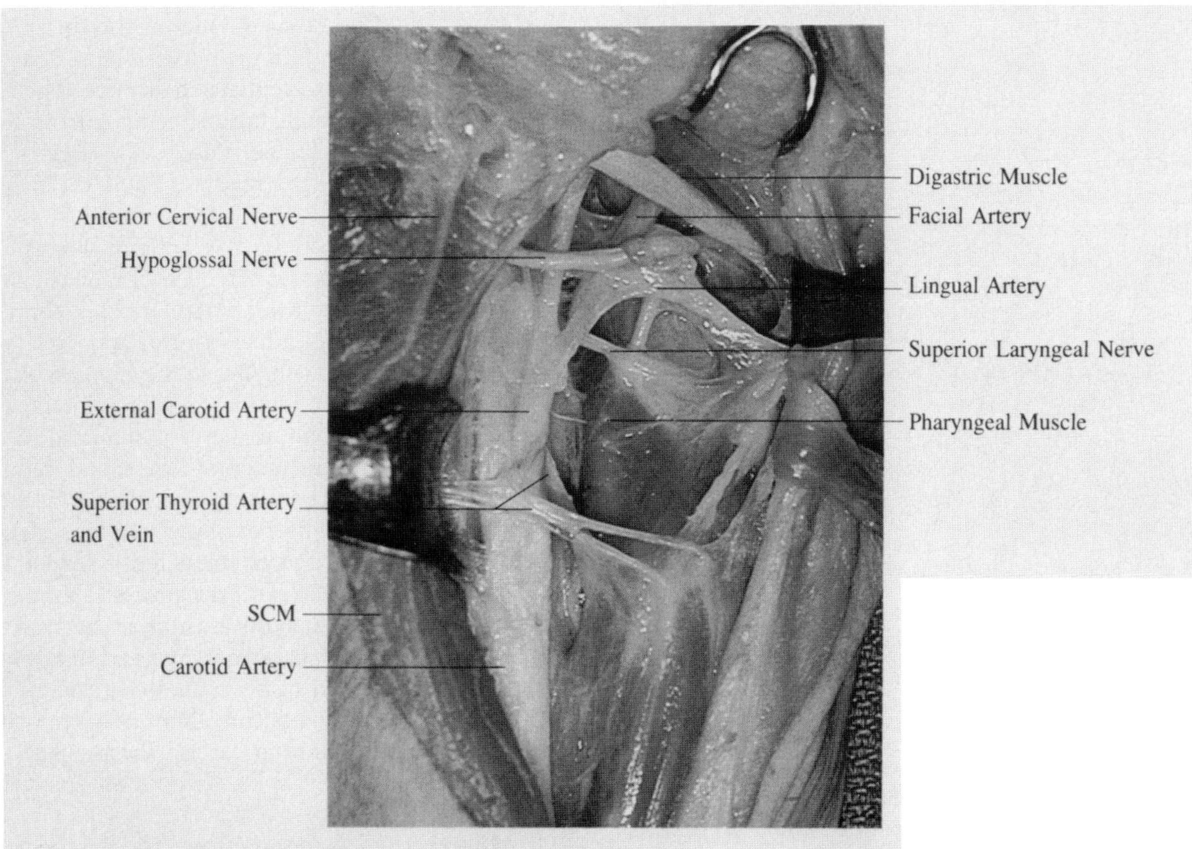

Figure 32.6. Dissected anatomy of the carotid triangle and area just below emphasizes the importance of identification of the hypoglossal nerve prior to ligation of the arterial structures in this area. The most common approach is cephalad to the superior thyroid artery and caudad to the digastric muscle.

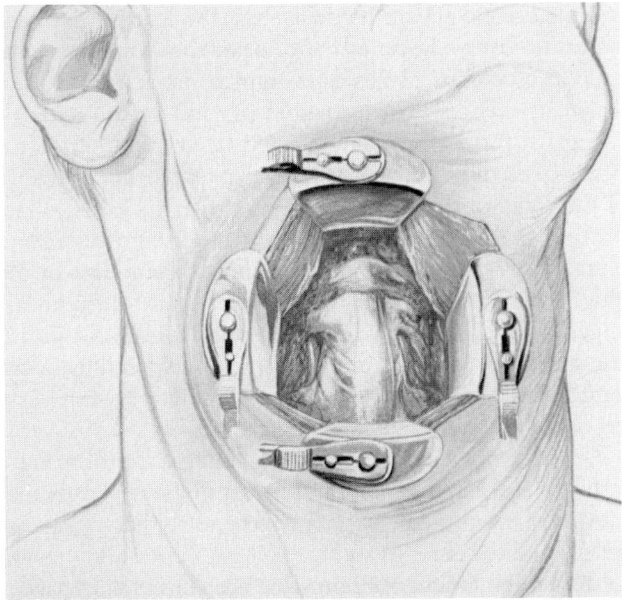

Figure 32.7. The spine exposed with deep retractor blades.

sired disc, use the blunt tipped Cloward self-retaining retractor longitudinally. The hand-held lipped Cloward retractor can also be used to retract as needed within the wound. Once the desired exposure is obtained the formal procedure may begin.

After completion of the procedure and hemostasis has been achieved, the deep wound closes with removal of the retractors. Close the subcutaneous tissue and use a subcuticular skin closure. We prefer to use a hemovac adjacent to the spine.

SUPRACLAVICULAR APPROACH

The patient is positioned supine. The neck is slightly hyperextended, rotated away from the side of the approach. A roll under the shoulder helps to extend the neck and a sand bag or the inflatable cervical pillow is used for additional support. Location of the thoracic duct and recurrent laryngeal nerve becomes even more important at this level. Approaches from the left for C6–T2 exposure are directly in the vicinity of the thoracic duct. Identify the thoracic duct when possible and protect it. If it is inadvertently divided, double ligate both ends well. With ap-

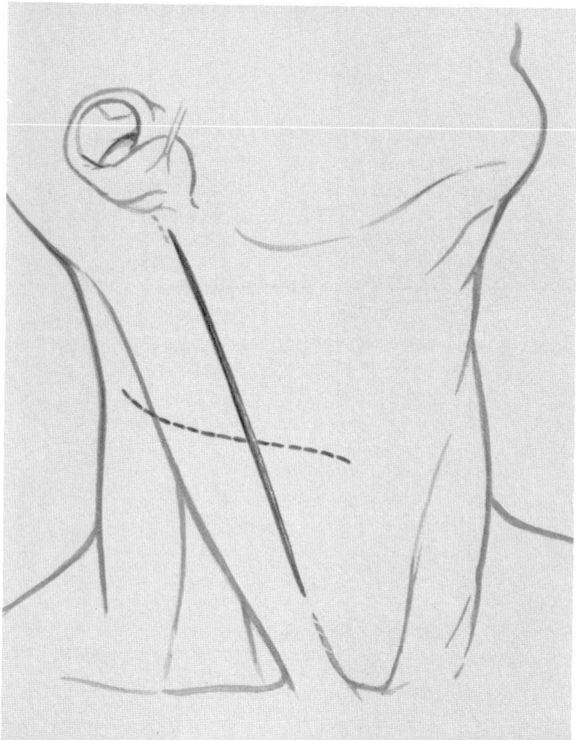

Figure 32.8. The more cosmetically suitable transverse incision is made at the appropriate level and should allow exposure of up to two discs and three vertebrae. A vertical incision can be used for an even greater exposure.

proaches from the right one should identify the recurrent laryngeal nerve and protect it. We recommend the left supraclavicular approach to avoid injury to the right recurrent laryngeal nerve.

A transverse incision is made approximately one finger-breadth above the clavicle from the midline to the posterior border of the sternocleidomastoid muscle. The platysma muscle is then incised in the line of the incision. Identification of the borders of the sternocleidomastoid is imperative. The external investing fascia is incised. A finger is passed laterally from the medial border of the sternocleidomastoid clearing off the venous structures underneath the clavicular head of the sternocleidomastoid. The sternocleidomastoid is divided laterally to medially, watching for the internal jugular vein (6). If required for visualization, the sternal head of the sternocleidomastoid muscle is reflected. Eventually reattachment depends on suturing the fascial covering of the muscle. The divided sternocleidomastoid is retracted in a cephalad-caudad direction with self-retaining blunt retractors. The floor of the incision, at this point, consists of the middle cervical fascia, which contains the omohyoid and the sternohyoid muscles. The middle cervical fascia is entered lateral to the carotid sheath. Bluntly dissect to the surface of the anterior scalene muscle. The superficial surfaces of the anterior scalene are composed of the outer layer of prevertebral fascia. Lying on the surface of the anterior scalene is the phrenic nerve. The phrenic nerve crosses lateral to medial, cephalad to caudad. The phrenic nerve is retracted medially after freeing it from the surface of the anterior scalene muscle. The large internal jugular vein is identified medially, and the carotid is palpated.

In the previous section, the anterior medial Smith Robinson approach can be extended distally to allow for exposure of the upper thoracic spine. This approach is medial to the carotid sheath. With this approach, you retract the carotid sheath laterally. In the supraclavicular approach, you retract the internal jugular vein and carotid sheath medially. The phrenic nerve is retracted to obtain good visualization of the anterior scalene and middle scalene. The brachial plexus and suprascapular nerves are more superficial at the lateral border of the anterior scalene. The medial and lateral borders of the anterior scalene muscle are delineated. The fascia on the deep surface of the anterior scalene is Sibson's fascia, a continuation of the prevertebral fascia. The apex of the parietal pleura and lung form the undersurface of Sibson's fascia. Dissect medially on the surface of the anterior scalene. Blunt dissection is now medially under the retracted carotid sheath. Stay on the prevertebral fascia to the spine. Expose the spine seeking the midline.

If more exposure is needed, carefully approach under the anterior scalene without violating the major portions of Sibson's fascia and divide the anterior muscle. The scalene can be retracted cephalad-caudad with self-retaining blunt retractors. The wound now consists of Sibson's fascia in the floor of the wound, the large internal jugular vein and the carotid sheath medially, and the apex of the lung beneath Sibson's fascia in the floor of the wound and laterally the brachial plexus as it courses superficially to the scaleneus medius. The proximal portion of the anterior scaleneus muscle may be dissected from the anterior tubercle of the transverse processes to allow greater exposure of the spine or brachial plexus (11).

Sibson's fascia is incised at the transverse processes and bluntly retracted inferiorly. This retracts the pleura of the lung, which is usually at the T1 level. The recurrent laryngeal nerve is mobilized medially with the carotid sheath and medial visceral column. The spine is exposed by opening the fascia in the midline over the body. The transverse processes and rib heads can be exposed (9).

Dissect to the second and third rib heads, producing a rather lateral exposure of the spine from the rib heads that must be carried medially to enter the retropharyngeal fascial cleft on the anterior surface of the spine without having to dissect the longus colli muscle. The vertebral artery entering the spine at C6 is identified. The subclavian vein courses on the floor of the wound.

If the approach is done from the left, the junction of the internal jugular veins and the subclavian veins will

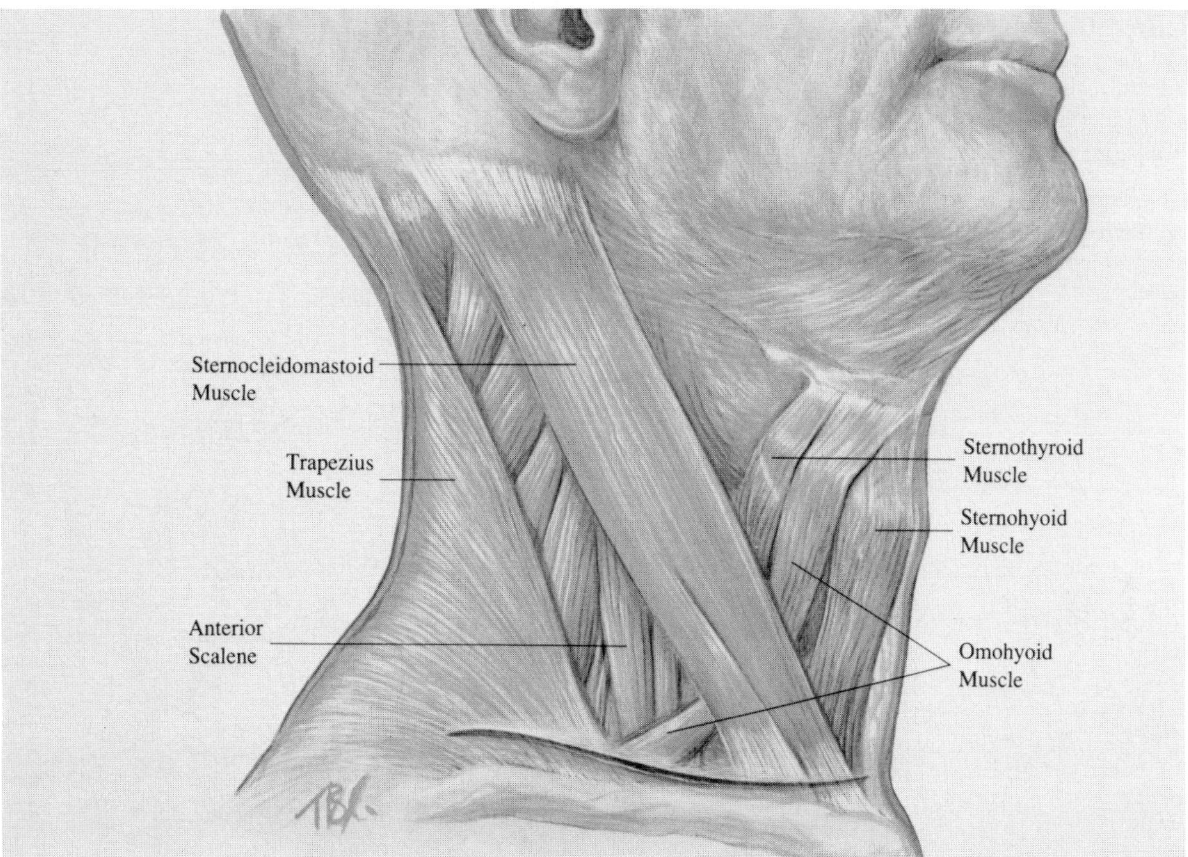

Figure 32.9. The key to the dissection at this point is to identify the medial border of the sternocleidomastoid muscle. With lateral retraction of the sternocleidomastoid, the interval between this muscle and the medial strap is delineated.

contain the thoracic duct. Identify the thoracic duct. In cases of damage, double-tie proximally and distally. Chylothorax may be prevented with proper ligation. Often a more judicious approach involves blunt dissection, progressing cephalad to caudad, as has been described for the transverse processes of C5, C6, and C7 to the rib head of the first rib down on the spine. This will sweep most of these structures cephalad to caudad. The danger, of course, lies in cutting restraining structures that cross the field. The sympathetic chain (stellate ganglion at C7) lies on the rib heads in a lateral position. Avoid damage by dissecting more medially.

Anatomy of External, Middle, and Prevertebral Fascia

The external investing fascia forms the anterior and posterior sheaths of the sternocleidomastoid muscle and the fascial covering of the visceral structures of the neck. This investing layer of cervical fascia is attached inferiorly to the acromion, clavicle, and manubrium of the sternum in an outer and inner layer superiorly to the hyoid bone, posteriorly to the mandible and mastoid processes, and superior to the nuchal line. The interval between the two laminae of the external investing fascia is called the suprasternal space or the space of Burns. This space contains the anterior jugular veins and sternal head of the sternocleidomastoid and is referred to as the cul-de-sac of Bruger. Communication between the anterior and external jugular veins is channeled through this inner laminar area.

The middle cervical fascia attaches to the carotid sheath and joins the external investing fascia at the posterior border of the sternocleidomastoid muscle. Inferiorly, the middle cervical fascia attaches to the posterior surface of the sternum, as do the muscles that they cover. It is the middle cervical fascia that attaches to the clavical and forms the loop for the inferior belly of the omohyoid muscle.

The prevertebral fascia is continuous with the endothoracic fascia caudally and laterally covers the levator scapuli and splenius muscles. It extends posteriorly to attach to the spinous processes of the vertebrae. In the neck and throughout the spinal column it covers the longus colli and capitus muscles and is secured to the tips of the transverse processes.

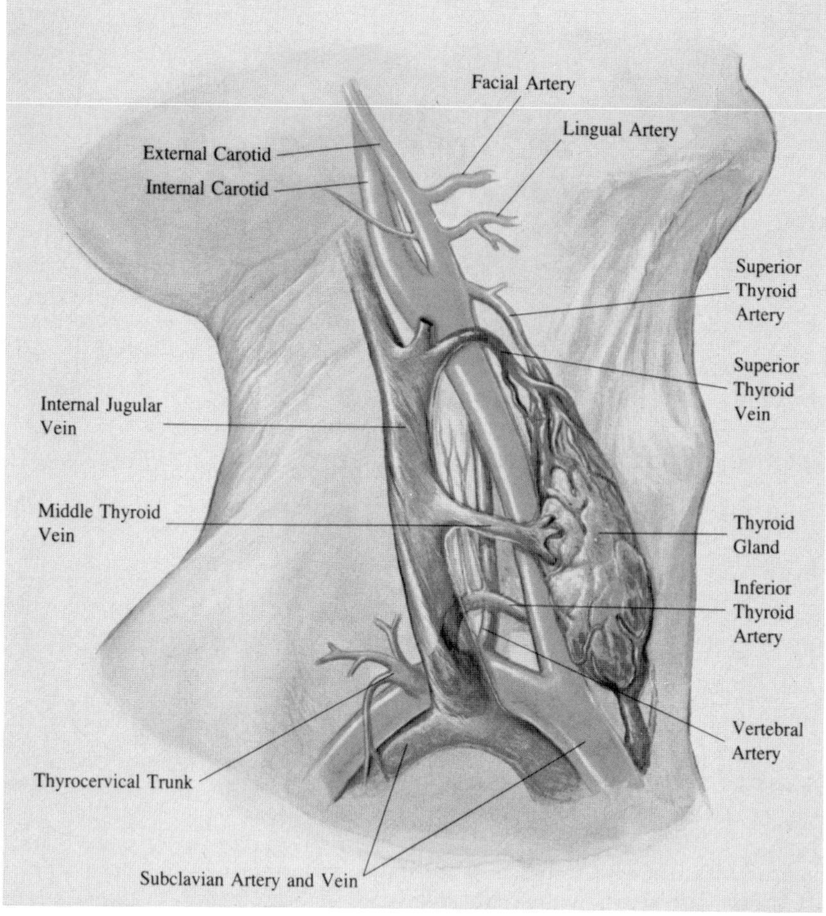

Figure 32.10. After retracting the sternocleidomastoid muscle laterally and the strap musculature medially, the arteriovenous structures of the middle cervical fascial layer must be identified. Palpate the carotid pulse. Open the midline cervical fascia medial to the carotid artery. Ligate and tie the medial thyroid vein. Retract the superior thyroid artery cephalad and the inferior thyroid artery caudad to expose the midcervical spine.

REFERENCES

1. Apuzzo MJ, Weiss MH, Hyden JS. Transoral exposure of the atlanto-axial joint. J Neurosurg 1978;3:201.

2. Bailey RW, Bagley CD. Stabilization of the cervical spine by anterior fusion. J Bone Joint Surg 1960;42:565.

3. Cloward R. Ruptured cervical intervertebral discs. Codman Signature Series 4. Randolph, MA: Codman and Shurtleff, 1974.

4. Fang HSY, Ong BG. Direct anterior approach to the upper cervical spine. J Bone Joint Surg 1962;44-A:1588.

5. Fielding JW. Personal communication.

6. Henry AK. Extensive exposure. Baltimore: Williams & Wilkins, 1959.

7. Hodgson AR, Rau ACM. Anterior approach to the spinal column. Recent Adv Orthop 1969;9:289.

8. Logue V. Compressive lesions at the foramen magnum. In: Ruge D, Wiltse L, eds. Spinal disorders: diagnosis and treatment. Philadelphia: Lea and Febiger, 1977.

9. Nanson EM. The anterior approach to the upper dorsal sympathectomy. Surg Gynecol Obstet 1957;104:118.

10. Perry J. Surgical approaches to the spine. In: Pierce D, Nichols V, eds. The total care of spinal cord injuries. Boston: Little, Brown & Co., 1977.

11. Riley L. Surgical approaches to the cervical spine. Clin Orthop 1973;91:16.

12. Riley L. Surgical approaches to the anterior structures of the cervical spine. Clin Orthop 1973;91:10.

13. Robinson RA. The craft of surgery. 2nd ed. Boston: Little, Brown & Co., 1971.

14. Robinson RA. Approaches to the cervical spine C1–T1. In: Schmidek HH, Sweet WH, eds. Current techniques in operative neurosurgery. New York: Grune & Stratton, 1978.

15. Robinson RA, Southwick WO. Surgical approaches to the cervical spine. A.A.O.S. Instruct. Course Lectures 1960;17:299.

16. Rothman R. The Spine, Vol. I. Philadelphia, W.B. Saunders, 1975.

17. Watkins RG, O'Brien JP. Anatomy of the cervical spine (sound/slide program). Atlanta: American Association of Orthopaedic Surgery, 1980.

33

Anterior Approaches to the Craniocervical Junction

H. Alan Crockard

Introduction

Modern imaging techniques have allowed unparalleled views of the base of the skull and spine, and nowhere has it been more valuable than at the craniocervical junction (Fig. 33.1). All but gone are the hazy views of polytomography, and with the availability of three-dimensional imaging packages, which may interrogate the original scanning data in any plane, one may have information comparable to that seen at autopsy. Dynamic scanning techniques and careful clinical assessment have revealed that some patients have been made worse by conventional posterior or posterolateral surgical approaches (Fig. 33.2). The increasing understanding of craniocervical junction throughout the medical fraternity places demands on the surgeon to correct that which hitherto was considered uncorrectable. At the same time as the improvements in imaging, the widespread use of the operating microscope and a generation widely skilled in microsurgical techniques have provided the surgical opportunity for more and more extensive surgery. Another factor is the availability of instruments designed specifically for transoral microsurgical procedures. Improved preoperative assessment and postoperative intensive care associated with good surgical technique have meant that infection is not a major problem and have allowed more and more surgeons to try and then to use, on a regular basis, a transoral approach (4, 7, 8).

Taking all this together, it is the author's contention that anterior approaches to the skull base and craniocervical junction have an important place in the armamentarium of the surgeon who would treat such pathology. In this chapter the basic anatomy, the investigations, and general comments on the various anterior approaches will be given. It will concentrate, however, on transoral surgical techniques for lesions placed below the foramen magnum.

Surgical Anatomy

The craniocervical junction is bounded by the anterior rim of the foramen magnum, the occipital condyles, the arch of C1, the odontoid peg, and the base of the second cervical vertebra. (Fig. 33.3). The minimum distance between the vertebral arteries at C1 is about 30 mm (range 26–31 mm). The distance from the foramen magnum to the base of C2 is about 40 mm, and that between the lateral masses of C1 is 27 mm (range 24–29 mm).

The key to the surgical exposure of the craniocervical junction is the detection of the anterior tubercle on the arch of C1. To this are attached the longus coli muscles and the anterior longitudinal ligament, and so a midline raphe can be seen extending up to this point. Above are attached the longus capitis and the rectus capitis anterior muscles; behind is the pharyngobasilar fascia. The vertebral arteries run about 14 mm on each side lateral to the tubercle. The surgical boundaries, therefore, of the anatomical exposure for the region are shown in Figure 33.4.

Deep to the bones will be the tectorial membrane and the posterior longitudinal ligament and the dura which is often attached to the anterior rim of the foramen magnum in the same sort of fashion as one experiences during occipital craniectomy. In a significant number of people, the marginal sinus, again a source of bleeding during a posterior fossa exploration, may provide the same problem during the anterior exposure.

Within the exposure described, and provided there is no rotation of C1, there are no major neural or vascular structures which cross the operative field.

Anterior Approaches in General

Figure 33.5 illustrates some of the approaches that have been described to the area. The **TRANSBASAL**, described by Derome (6), affords an excellent view of the whole of the midline base of skull including the ethmoids, sphenoid, and clivus; it is too extensive for the craniocervical junction. The **TRANSMAXILLARY** approach (1), in which a Le Fort osteotomy "brings down" the hard palate, allows an excellent view of the upper and middle third of the clivus but severely limits the exposure of the craniocervical junction below the rim of the foramen magnum. We have recently described an **EXTENDED MAX-**

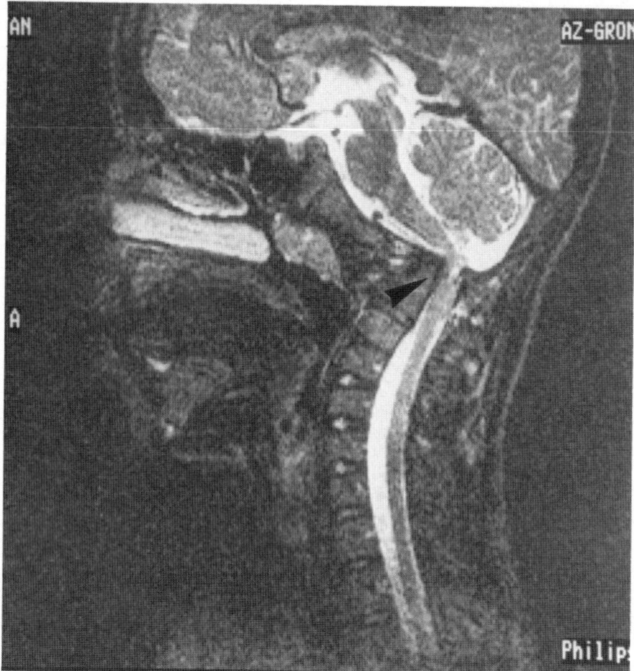

Figure 33.1. Magnetic resonance image (MRI) of congenital basilar invagination with craniocervical developmental anomaly showing the marked compression of the brainstem by the malformation.

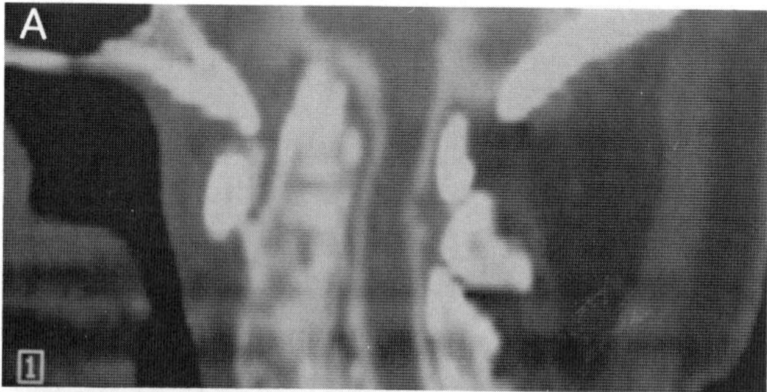

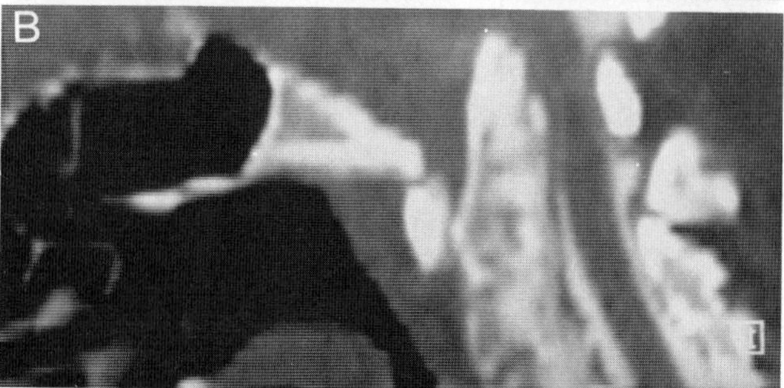

Figure 33.2. Dynamic scanning techniques are essential to understand craniocervical junction pathology. Computed myelotomography in **A,** extension and **B,** flexion illustrates the increased translocation and brainstem compression in a rheumatoid patient with intact odontoid peg. The studies illustrate the occipito-atlantal instability so often noted in this disease.

ILLOTOMY which combines the transmaxillary and transpalatal approaches. The **TRANSCERVICAL** route allows a completely extra-oral and "clean" approach to the craniocervical junction but requires a great deal of retraction of cranial nerves; the carotid artery and vertebral arteries are also in direct line during this procedure. It is, however, perhaps one of the most widely-utilized approaches to the region and has stood the test of time. The **SUPRAHYOID TRANSGLOTTIC** approach, in theory, is the shortest route from skin to the craniocervical junction, but the incision through the tongue has little to commend it in view of the amount of bleeding that ensues.

The **TRANSORAL** route is the author's choice for most midline pathology in this region. Provided there is no rotation of the atlas and the anatomy is relatively normal, there are no major neurovascular structures at risk from a direct midline approach. Without good visualization, adequate retraction, and proper instrumentation, however, the procedure is fraught with difficulties.

Radiological Investigations

PLAIN LATERAL RADIOGRAPHS of the craniocervical junction in flexion and extension and an anteroposterior view will allow the surgeon to define the bony limitations of the surgical field. Follow-up radiographs can be compared to these preoperative ones for rapid "office" assessment. Our unit uses conventional polytomography only occasionally.

In our experience, **COMPUTED TOMOGRAPHY (CT)** and more especially, **COMPUTED MYELOTOMOGRAPHY,** is the most accurate method for identifying bony abnormalities and for providing absolute measurements of the structures involved, as well as providing easy assessment of the craniocervical angles and the angle of the neuraxis (Fig. 33.2). **MAGNETIC RESONANCE IMAGING (MRI)** provides exquisite details of intradural pathology, as well as extradural and bony abnormalities but, with present software packages, cannot provide the absolute measurements which may be necessary for the surgeon during a procedure (Fig. 33.1). **VERTEBRAL ANGIOGRAPHY** is required only occasionally; the path of the vertebral arteries can usually be well-defined on the CT myelogram or the MRI, but in congenital malformations, and particularly where there is an element of C1 rotation, a vertebral angiogram may be extremely helpful to alert the surgeon as to the vascular hazards that he may encounter during the procedure. Obviously, if there are tumors in the area, angiography will define the vascularity.

PREOPERATIVE ASSESSMENT FOR TRANSORAL SURGERY

The Mouth

Paramount to a transoral operation is a careful preoperative evaluation of the mouth, its dentation, the size of the tongue,

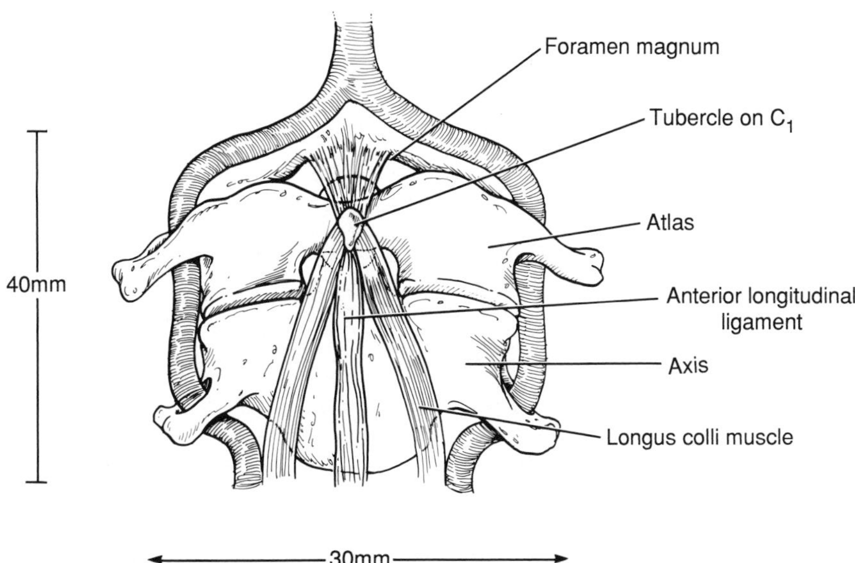

Figure 33.3. The surgical anatomy of the craniocervical junction. Provided there is no rotation or significant lateral mass destruction, a direct midline approach will not encounter any major hazards.

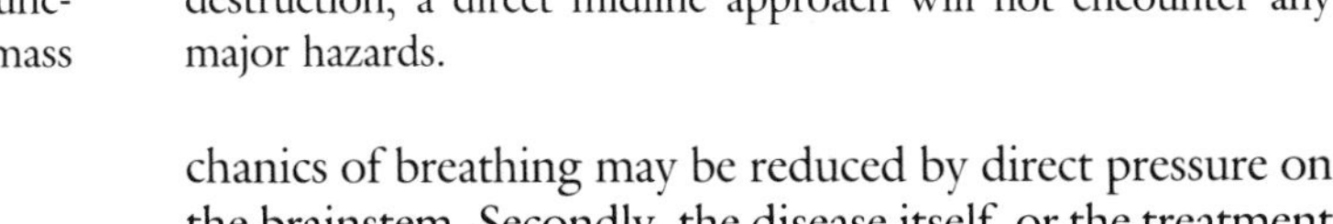

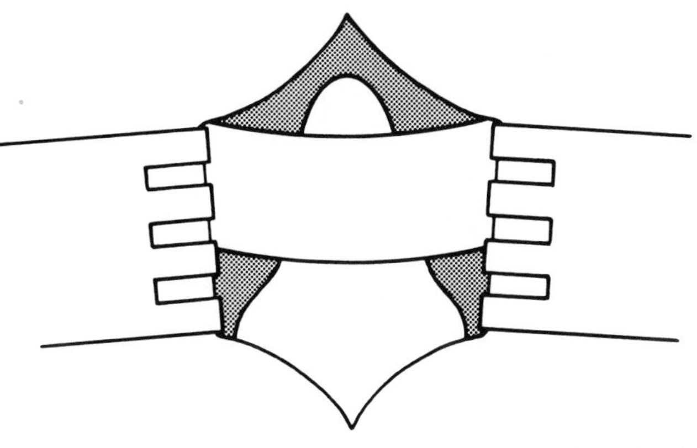

Figure 33.4. A midline pharyngeal incision over the tubercle on C1 will allow adequate access. A pharyngeal retractor will convert the vertical incision to a hexagon, expose C1 and C2, and protect the carotid arteries.

and the length of the mandible. Most important, however, is the amount of mouth opening. If the interdental distance is less than 25 mm, with the patient opening his mouth as widely as possible, it is unlikely that a conventional transoral procedure will be possible. The transoral route may still be used, however, by splitting the symphysis of the mandible in the midline and laterally retracting the two parts of the mandible; the author has found that the tongue can be retracted down out of the way to effect a reasonable exposure of the area.

General Physical Examination

Many of the patients with degenerative disease, particularly "endstage" rheumatoid arthritis, are not physically fit people and, therefore, full systemic evaluation is necessary if they are to withstand the rigors of major surgery. Pulmonary function assessment is important. Firstly, the mechanics of breathing may be reduced by direct pressure on the brainstem. Secondly, the disease itself, or the treatment of the disease, may have compromised pulmonary function. The vital capacity, arterial blood gases, oxygen saturation, and sleep studies are performed routinely on these patients. In general terms, those with a vital capacity of less than 1.2 liters may not be able to breath on their own after the operation. Cardiac status is obviously important, as many of the patients requiring the procedure are elderly. Renal function is also important in that many of the patients have had long-term therapy with steroids or immunotherapy.

Bacteriological swabs of the nose and throat and sputum and skin flora are also taken preoperatively and the appropriate antibiotic given with the anesthetic and into the first 4 or 5 days post-operatively.

Electrical Studies

Somatosensory evoked potentials (SSEP) and motor evoked potentials (MEP) have been performed on some patients pre- and postoperatively. In general terms, even though the radiological compression is dramatic and the neurological recovery striking, we have not seen huge changes in central conduction time. Perioperative assessment has been difficult.

ANESTHESIA

Airway

Critical decisions are required about whether or not to do a tracheostomy, whether to insert an orotracheal tube or a nasotracheal tube for anesthesia, and at what stage to remove the anesthetic airway. There are advantages and disadvantages to each route, and the important point is

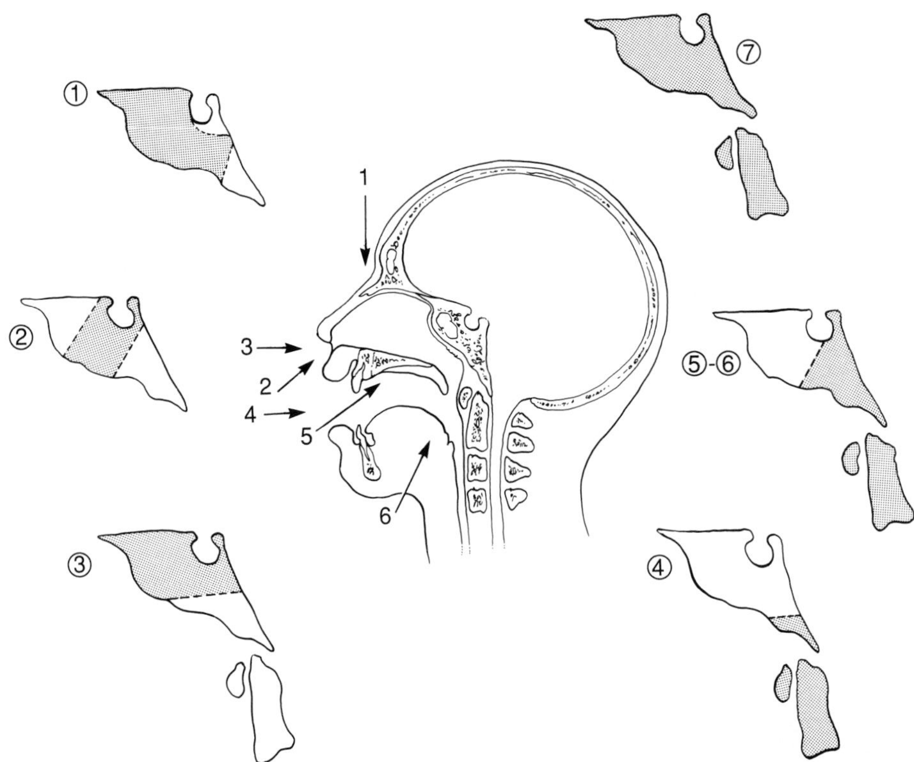

Figure 33.5. Various approaches to the craniocervical junction and clivus are illustrated: 1. Transbasal; 2. Transsphenoidal; 3. and 7. Transmaxillary; 4. Transoral; 5. Transpalatal; 6. Transglottic.

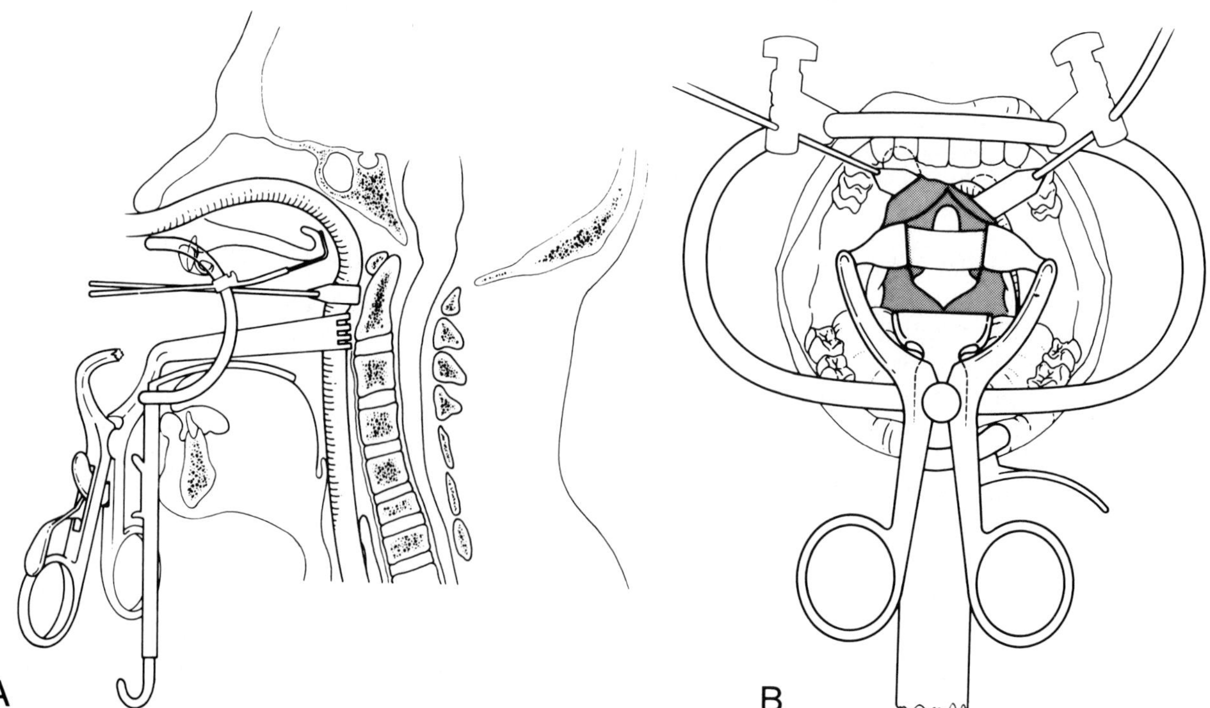

Figure 33.6. The transoral instruments in position to allow palatal retraction and protection of the nasotracheal airway. The palatal, pharyngeal, and the tongue retractors expose the operative area but also provide a "ring of steel" to protect underlying structures.

that it is a team decision and one that suits the local experience best. In our own experience, we have moved from routine tracheostomy in all our early cases to less than 15% tracheostomy in all our patients. In some of our patients with neck deformities, tracheostomy would be impossible technically due to an associated midcervical kyphus reducing the distance between the mandible and the manubrium to less than 3 cm. In others, for instance when a transoral transdural procedure is performed for intradural tumour, a tracheostomy is almost routine; firstly, to remove the airway from the direct area of surgery and, secondly, to divert all possible contaminants and minimize the risk of postoperative meningitis. An orotracheal tube is routinely used by the Phoenix group (7), and with a suitable tongue plate it can be shielded and retracted from the operative site. In our own experience, while not interfering with the surgery, the postoperative maintenance of an orotracheal tube is much less comfortable for the patient than a nasotracheal, and we are unhappy about changing from one form of airway to another at the end of the operative procedure. A nasotracheal airway is preferred by our group (3); it provides a more comfortable postoperative airway for the patient but requires a great deal of skill in its passage. (Fig. 33.6). The smaller tubes, 5.5 mm and less, add significantly to the work of breathing, and then a tracheostomy or orotracheal tube may be used.

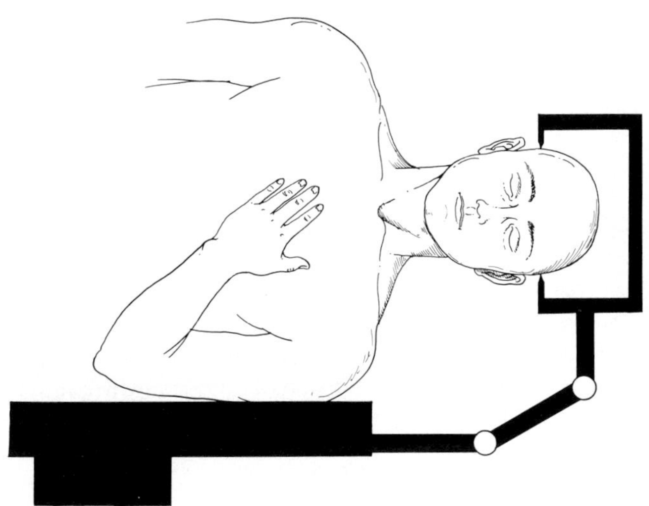

Figure 33.7. The lateral operative position provides a seated position for the surgeon and gravity drainage of blood and drill washings from the operative site.

The decision to extubate postoperatively again varies with experience and the pathology. For lesions of the clivus, where the incision is above the soft and hard palate, there is a strong argument for early post-operative extubation. In those patients with an incision down to C3, there may be a great deal of post-operative swelling, and our practice is to leave the airway in at least for 24 hours and to perform a lateral cervical radiograph to evaluate the amount of swelling prior to the decision to remove the airway.

Ventilation

Sleep is induced by inhalation agents using an oropharyngeal airway. Then the fiberoptic laryngoscope is used routinely to prevent any excessive movement in the unstable cervical spine. Tidal volume, respiratory rate, oxygen, and oxygen saturation have, for us, been the most immediate indices of brainstem compression. Controlled ventilation may not be maintained for the whole of the operative procedure. Thus, for many patients with severe craniocervical junction compression, muscle relaxation is reversed and the patient breathes spontaneously during the critical anterior and posterior surgical maneuvers.

Postoperative ventilation is employed in all those with

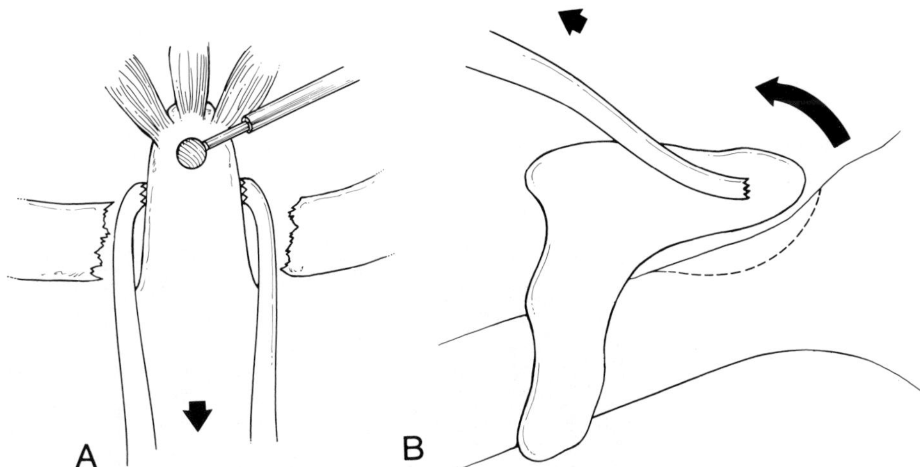

Figure 33.8. The odontoid peg may be "steadied" during drilling to prevent further neuraxial compression. **A,** transoral view. **B,** lateral view.

a compromised preoperative vital capacity, in patients who showed marked variation in respiratory pattern during the surgery, in the patients who have become cold on the operating table, or in those in whom the surgery has taken an inordinate time. The period of ventilation is usually 12 hours or less. The nasotracheal tube is left in position for a minimum of 24, and some up to 7, postoperative days, not only to prevent compromise of the airway and to allow ready access for tracheal toilet, but also to divert secretions away from the operative site.

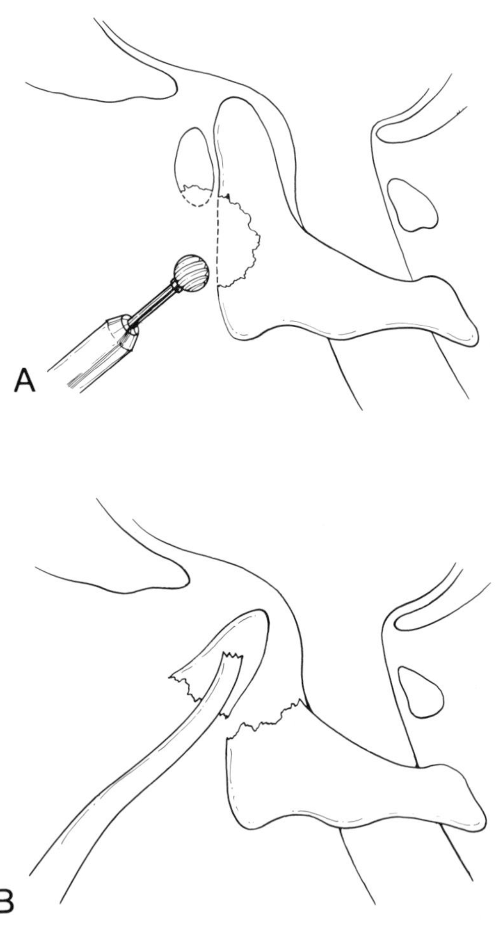

Figure 33.9. Removal of translocated odontoid. **A,** the base of the peg and anterior rim of C1 is removed. **B,** the distal fragment is then "delivered" out of the foramen magnum by traction and without removal of the anterior rim.

Nasogastric Tube

A nasogastric tube is inserted preoperatively, firstly, because it is easier to do so before the pharyngeal surgery and, secondly, to allow emptying of the stomach in the immediate recovery period to prevent regurgitation or vomiting soiling the wound. Repeated aspiration is carried out until bowel sounds have returned, and then the tube is used for fluid replacement and alimentation. This tube is removed at 5–7 days and is another means whereby potential mechanical or bacteriological soiling of the wound is avoided.

Perioperative Monitoring

Blood pressure, heart rate, the respiratory cycle and oxygen saturation, and end-tidal CO_2 provide good second to second indices of brainstem function. SSEPs are of more value during posterior upper cervical surgery, and MEPs are extremely difficult to obtain and have not given the immediacy that the cardiorespiratory changes have provided.

Drugs

Antibiotics, usually Cefuroxime and Metronidazole are given with induction of anesthesia and maintained for 5 days postoperatively. An antiemetic (Metoclopramide) and H2 blocking agents are used in the postoperative period to reduce regurgitation, vomiting, and stress ulceration. Pain is controlled with a pump infusion of a morphine derivative with careful attention to respiratory rate and function. Details of all are given elsewhere (3).

SURGERY

Positioning the Patient

It has been conventional surgical practice to lay the patient flat on his back and work around the "natural" position adopted by the sleeping patient. With modern tables and fixation techniques, it is possible to rotate the patient into a position suitable for the surgeon as well as the patient. In the author's experience, the **LATERAL POSITION** has been adopted with the head held in the Mayfield retractor (Fig. 33.7) (5). The advantage is that blood and

Figure 33.10. An intradural schwannoma at the craniocervical junction.

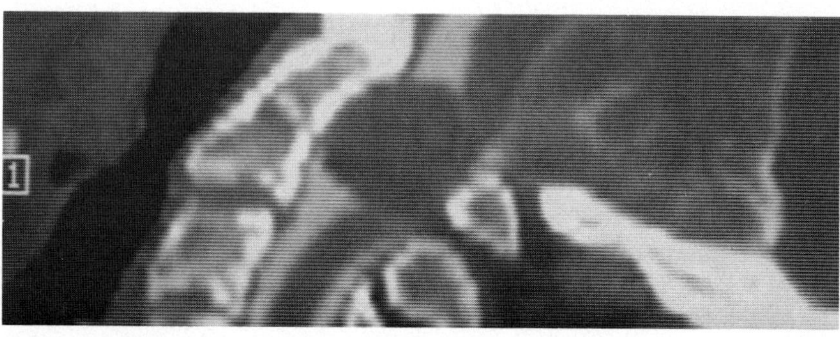

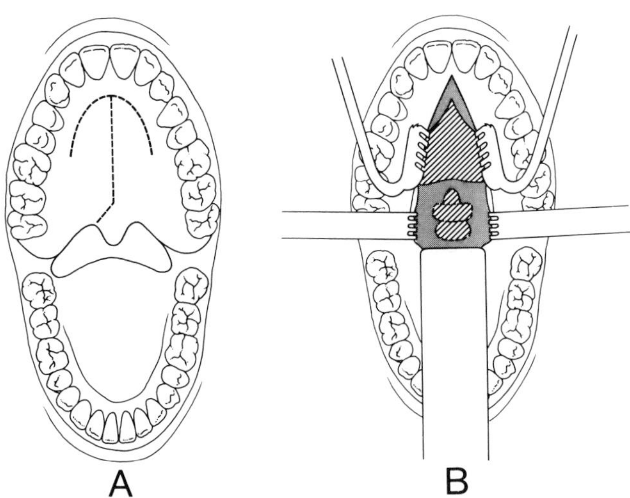

Figure 33.11. Incision of the soft and hard palate (**A**) will allow exposure of the lower one-third of the clivus as well as C1 and C2 (**B**).

washings drain away from the operative site, improving exposure. In addition, the operator may be seated and comfortable for an exacting procedure. Using this technique it is possible to perform an anterior craniocervical decompression and a posterior occipitocervical fusion with the patient fixed in the same position and using the lateral tilt facility to expose both areas sequentially. The disadvantage of the approach is that it makes perioperative x-rays difficult to obtain and interpret, and, in our own practice, any doubtful position or anatomy is evaluated with the patient asleep prior to the incision, supine with needle markers outlining the anatomical structure which is the subject of the surgeon's concern.

Preparation

The mouth is cleansed with an aqueous chlorhexidine solution, and after that, the transoral retractor is inserted with a tongue blade of suitable length. If there is deficient dentition in the upper jaw or loose teeth, a "gum guard" made from flexible dental cement (Optosil) can be prepared to fit over the teeth and into the upper denture guard. (Fig. 33.6). Great care is taken to ensure that the tongue is not caught between the lower dentures and the tongue retractor, and the mouth is opened as far as possible. The soft palate is "hooked up" using the curved soft palatal retractor, and this is held firmly in position with the locking nut. The other palatal retractor is employed to retract the nasogastric and nasotracheal tubes out of the operative field in the tonsillar fauces. The combination of both palatal retractors provides exposure up to the foramen magnum and well laterally.

Hydrocortisone cream is applied liberally to the lips and tongue before and immediately after surgery to minimize the postoperative swelling. If there is a degree of basilar invagination, the soft and the hard palate may have to be incised. The hard palate retractor is inserted in position to provide exposure.

Incision

The tubercle on the arch of C1 is identified, and local anesthetic with adrenaline 1 in 200,000 is injected at this area to create a plane of cleavage between the pharynx and the prevertebral tissues. A midline incision from above the tubercle down to the base of C2, in the midline, will not encounter any major bleeding or hazard, and after separating the pharyngeal mucosa the tissue can be retracted laterally using the pharyngeal retractor. (Fig. 33.4). The combination of the palatal retractors, the pharyngeal retractor, and the tongue retractor provides a "ring of steel" around the operative site and protects the soft tissues behind them from inadvertent slippage of the airdrill during bony removal.

The insertion of the longus coli and the anterior longitudinal ligament into the tubercle is divided with the cutting diathermy, and the outlines of C1 and that part of C2 requiring removal are identified with sharp dissection and the cutting monopolar diathermy.

Bone Removal

If at all possible the arch of C1 should at least be partly preserved. This will prevent the lateral masses being "squeezed" laterally between the weight of the skull and the vertebral body of C2. Obviously, in some situations the arch of C1 must be removed to effect a good decompression of the area, and then a very powerful posterior stabilization will be required to prevent late onset problems between C1 and C2. The arch of C1 and the odontoid peg are removed using a 3–4 mm cutting burr on an angled high-speed airdrill. If there is a great deal of instability of the odontoid peg, the arch of C1 will have to be removed, and, having removed soft tissues laterally, a specially designed grasping instrument has been developed which will hold the unstable peg in position during the drilling procedure and may actually pull it out of the foramen magnum (Fig. 33.8). The odontoid peg is "hollowed out" using the cutting burr, and when the color changes, indicating that cortical bone is exposed, a similar sized diamond drill is used. In this technique, the tip of the odontoid peg is not defined at this stage, and there is usually no reason to remove the anterior rim of the foramen magnum. Having "hollowed out" the odontoid peg and as much of C2 as is necessary, the 1 mm and 2 mm-long Kerrison "upcuts" will remove bone and fracture the remaining peg across. The distal tip can then be manipulated down into the wound and into the exposed field without removing the anterior rim of the foramen magnum (Fig. 33.9). The alar and apical ligaments can be visualized and divided using the cutting diathermy applied directly to the ligament on its insertion on the odontoid peg. Great care is made during this dissection that the dura is protected to prevent unnecessary CSF leaks. No attempt is made to remove all of the apical and altar ligaments; the decompression is usually adequate to allow soft tissue on the dura to bulge forward. Having removed the odontoid peg, the remainder of the basal part of the peg and the base of C2 is removed following drilling, curettes, and rongeurs. The posterior longitudinal ligament and the tectorial membrane may be removed if they are involved in the inflammatory mass and the tissues are thick and nonpulsatile. Very often, however, in the noninflammatory condition, the removal of the bone itself will allow good pulsation of the dura without the risk of a dural tear. The lateral bony removal is over the "equator" on both sides. Only when there are good free pulsations of the dura, is the area known to be satisfactorily decompressed. If the transverse ligament is intact and if it is not itself causing a significant compressive force, again the structure is left intact in an effort to preserve the position of the lateral masses of C1. If there is bleeding from the bone, bone wax on a pattie may be rubbed into the bone, and the diamond burr may further impact it into the structure of the bone. For more major arterial bleeding, such as inadvertent damage to the vertebral artery, a plug of Surgical and bone wax firmly impacted into the bony defect will usually control the bleeding. Venous bleeding in the area at times can be troublesome; there may be major epidural veins, and these may give great trouble during the removal of the posterior longitudinal ligament. Here, the laser may have a part to play.

If the C2/C3 disc is exposed, it must be removed and the end-plate of the upper surface of C3 also removed.

For a straightforward decompression of the area, the work is now complete, and the wound is closed in two layers. The muscle and fascial layer is closed with at least 2 sutures of 3/0 Vicryl; the mucosa is closed with 4 sutures of interrupted 3/0 Vicryl sutures.

CSF Leak

If there has been a CSF leak, then the wound is closed with layers of fascia and fat obtained from the thigh or abdomen and Surgicel; thrombin, fibrin glue will waterproof the area. A lumbar drain is inserted before the patient leaves the operating room using a Tuohy needle with a size 16 epidural catheter allowed to drain cerebrospinal fluid for a minimum of 48 hours to reduce the pressure and encourage healing at the site.

If there is a deliberate dural incision for a transdural procedure, the procedure is carried out as mentioned above. In addition, the lumbar drain will have been inserted prior to surgery, occluded until the surgery is over, and left draining for a period of 5 days to remove blood products and debris. After this, in addition to the waterproof repair already described, the lumbar drain is converted to a lumboperitoneal shunt, effectively reducing CSF pressure for a month or 6 weeks to allow a good dural closure.

Bone Grafts

In our early experience, bone grafting was not carried out anteriorly because we were afraid of infection, but, with increased experience, bone grafting has been carried in a variety of conditions with surprising success (2).

In patients in whom there is subaxial subluxation or osteophytes at C2/C3, the author has employed the transoral approach to allow a decompression at the C2/C3 joint, and a bone graft obtained from the right iliac crest is fashioned into a "Cloward" type dowel and with skull retraction is hammered firmly into position. In our experience this is a safe technique with good bony union (2, 5).

Some impacted bone struts from the clivus to the base of C2 have been used in our experience, but our experience of this or transoral screw fixation in the area is minute in comparison to Abe and Rene Louis.

Intradural Surgery

For intradural lesions in the midline at the craniocervical junction, the transoral route has been shown to be a satisfactory experience for schwannomas (Fig. 33.10). With meningiomas the exposure is somewhat limited, and it has been difficult to effect a total removal by this route. It must be added, however, that lesions anterior to the neuraxis in the midline at the craniocervical junction are difficult by any route, and it may well be that the transoral procedure is one of several used to effect an excision of the lesion in that area. The importance of dural closure following the surgery has already been stressed in the previous section.

Division of the Soft Palate

Occasionally, because of the local conditions, basilar invagination or other problems, the soft palate should be divided to give good exposure up to the anterior rim of the foramen magnum (Fig. 33.11). This is particularly so in patients with Klippel-Feil deformities which are often associated with some basilar assimilation. For them, the incision is along the midline raphe and then continued to one side of the uvula. Occasionally, the incision is carried up onto the hard palate which can be "infractured" into the nasopharynx following the removal of the vomer and lateral incisions in the hard palate on the anterior aspect of the hard palate.

For closure, the bone flaps are returned to their position using a Howarth dissector through the nose. Ribbon gauze packs are placed in the nose to hold them in position and the mucosa sutured with interrupted Vicryl sutures. The soft palate must be closed very carefully with 2 layers of sutures; a breakdown of the palate or poor suture technique will result in poor phonation and difficulty in swallowing. In our experience there is no need to remove part of the hard palate.

POSTOPERATIVE CARE

With careful attention to the pharyngeal tissues and a careful suture technique, wound infection has not been a major problem. The diversion of food and pulmonary secretions is also a significant part of the care of the area. Mouth care is instituted on a 4 hourly basis for 5 days. Swelling in the area is controlled by topical application of hydrocortisone cream on a 4 hourly basis.

Pain control is by a pump infusion of morphine with careful observation of the respiratory rate, the pump being discontinued if the respiratory rate falls below 10/min. Antibiotics, as mentioned earlier, are continued for a period of 5 days. It is our aim to mobilize patients as soon as possible; they are usually sitting out of bed on the second postoperative day. The care of the airway has already been mentioned.

CONCLUSIONS

The anterior approach to the craniocervical junction is now a well-defined technique which has significant possibilities in the management of craniocervical junction compression. It is not the only means whereby surgery is carried out to the area and should be considered as an important adjunct to the armamentarium of the surgeon interested in the base of skull and craniocervical junction.

ACKNOWLEDGMENT

The author is grateful to Michelle Green for all preparation of this manuscript.

REFERENCES

1. Archer DJ, Young S, Uttley D. Basilar aneurysms: a new transclival approach via maxillotomy. J Neurosurg 1987;67:54–58.
2. Ashraf J, Crockard HA. Transoral transpharyngeal fusion in high cervical fractures. J Bone Joint Surg (Br) 1990;72B:76–79.
3. Calder I. Anaesthesia for transoral surgery and craniocervical surgery. In: Jewkes D, ed Balliere's Clinical anaesthesiology. London: W B Saunders, 1987:441–457.
4. Crockard HA. Anterior approaches to lesions of the upper cervical spine. Clin Neurosurg 1988; 34:389–416.
5. Crockard HA, Clader I, Ransford AO. One stage transoral decompression and posterior fixation in rheumatoid atlantoaxial subluxation: a technical note. J Bone Joint Surg (Br) 1990;72B:682–685.
6. Derome PJ. The transbasal approach to tumours invading the base of the skull. In: Schmidek HH, Sweet WH, ed. Operative neurosurgical techniques, Vol 1. Florida: Grune and Stratton, 1988:619–633.
7. Hadley MN, Spetzler RF, Sonntag VK. The transoral approach to the superior cervical spine: a review of 53 cases of extradural cervicomedullary compression. J Neurosurg 1989;71:16–23.
8. Menezes AH, VanGilder JC. Transoral-transpharyngeal approach to the anterior craniocervical junction: ten-year experience with 72 patients. J Neurosurg 1988;69:895–903.

34

Anterior Cervical Discectomy and Fusion for the Treatment of Cervical Radiculopathy

David H. Clements and Patrick F. O'Leary

Historical Review

The posterior approach to the cervical spine was initially the only option available to a surgeon whose patients with cervical radiculopathy had failed conservative treatment. Dr. Ralph Cloward, in 1957 (4), described the anterior approach for cervical discography that had first been proposed by Dr. Exum Walker of Atlanta Georgia. Dr. Cloward came to the conclusion that the pathology, a ruptured cervical disc and/or a marginal osteophyte, could be approached directly and safely via the anterior approach. Removal of the osteophytes and disc fragments was easily accomplished using straight and angled curettes. He pioneered an approach which is similar to that currently used, and since he believed that fusion of the degenerative segment was important to the patient's final result, he designed a drill with a guard and depth gauge to create a hole in the intervertebral space into which a premeasured cylindrical bone dowel could be inserted. Drs. Bailey and Bedgley (1) also described indications for anterior cervical fusion when lesions rendered the spine unstable, such as fracture dislocations, traumatic disc herniations, post-laminectomy instability, or tumors. They recommended that an iliac crest strut graft combined with cancellous strips be packed in the disc space. Drs. Smith and Robinson (22) were also proponents of the anterior approach after developing and refining the technique in dogs. They first utilized their technique in a patient in February of 1954. Their technique differed by employing curettes and pituitary rongeurs instead of a Cloward drill, and they did not attempt to remove the posterior osteophytes. They favored placing a tricortical horse-shoe-shaped iliac crest graft into the intervertebral space. Modification of this approach to ventral cervical spine pathology continues to be one of the common surgical procedures for cervical spondylosis, tumors, and degenerative disc disease.

Epidemiology

Kelsy et al. (13) investigated the epidemiology of prolapsed cervical discs in an attempt to provide descriptive statistics on the characteristics of patients diagnosed with this disorder and to identify possible risk factors. They found the largest percentage of these patients to be in the fourth and fifth decades of life. Their male to female ratio of 1.4 to 1 was similar to that noted in other studies. The majority of patients, 75%, had involvement at either the C5–C6, or the C6–C7 disc spaces. A high degree of correlations was observed between current cigarette smoking or lifting heavy objects and an increased risk of developing a prolapsed cervical disc. The association between cigarette smoking and disc prolapse was theorized to relate to the increased frequency of coughing in these patients.

Signs and Symptoms

The differentiation between soft cervical disc degeneration as opposed to cervical nerve root impingement from cervical spondylosis and osteophyte formation can be overlapping and difficult to distinguish. Disc degeneration without prolapse or osteophyte formation can in itself be responsible for mechanical neck pain that radiates to the occipital region causing headaches, or to the shoulder, scapula, or arm. Not until a piece of disc actually herniates or an osteophyte appears in the foramen to impinge on a root, do these symptoms consistently localize to an anatomic distribution in the upper extremities. The longterm gradual progression of disc degeneration and osteophyte formation is of such ubiquity, up to 76% of the population by age 56 (10), that it can be considered to be a normal process of aging. Why certain patients are affected and others not has yet to be determined. The noxious stimulation of the sinovertebral nerve which innervates the anulus and posterior longitudinal ligaments may be a source of the discogenic pain, similar to that seen in the lumbar region. When a cervical root is impinged upon by a herniated disc or an osteophyte, the pain and/or numbness which occurs is found in the dermatome of that cervical root. The duration of symptoms and the consistency of localization are indications that cervical root irritation is the etiology of the patient's symptoms.

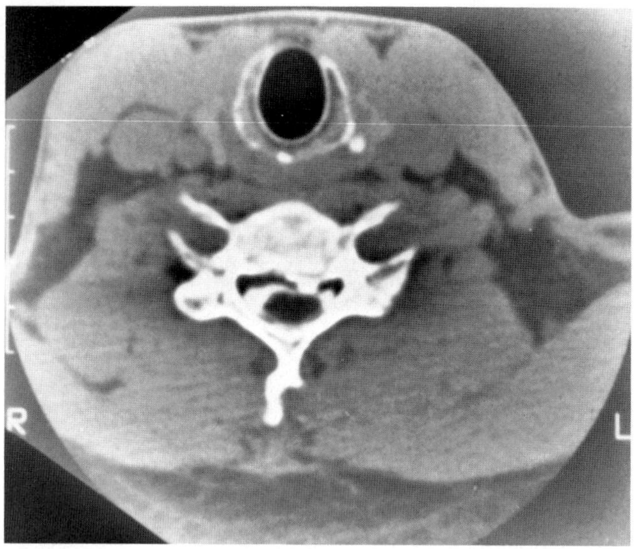

Figure 34.1. Postmyelogram CT scan of cervical spine demonstrates a posterolateral osteophytic spur adjacent to the foramen.

Intermittent shooting pain may more often be due to a discogenic nonradicular etiology, while a constant throbbing pain that is easily localized and identifiable by the patient may be more consistent with root irritation. Biceps tendonitis should be considered in the differential diagnosis in the patient complaining of shoulder and arm pain. Pain in the shoulder from this entity may radiate from the shoulder to the neck and also radiates down the arm to the elbow along the course of the biceps muscle. Usually the patient will complain of exacerbations of pain related to use of the shoulder, and a physical exam will confirm the suspicion. Other entities in the differential diagnosis of cervical radiculopathy are peripheral nerve entrapment syndromes. Median and ulnar nerve entrapment may have unilateral upper extremity pain and numbness that is confirmed by a careful physical examination and EMG findings. Osteophyte formation occurs in the foramen due to degeneration of the zygapophyseal joints, the joints of Luschka, or both (Fig. 34.1). Characteristically, symptoms develop over a period of time, in an insidious fashion, usually with no definable initiating event. These patients tend to be older, while disc herniations characteristically occurs in a more acute fashion usually in a younger patient with an initiating event being present, such as lifting a heavy object. Disc herniations protrude postolaterally into the foramen trapping the nerve, or in the midline compressing the thecal sac. Midline herniations may cause a myelopathic picture. Root irritation provokes pain which can be described as burning, tingling, or even aching. It follows the dermatomal distribution of the involved root, is usually worse in the morning, and, when severe, causes the patient to hold the arm at the side or over the head. Reflex changes and weakness relate to the root involved. Sensory changes generally follow the dermatomal pattern of the involved root (11). Acute radicular pain can be increased or decreased by head and neck positioning. One test which has a high degree of reproducibility is neck extension with subsequent tilting or rotating to the affected side. This will frequently reproduce or aggravate the patient's radicular symptoms. Moderate flexion of the neck in some patients can relieve the symptoms, as can manual traction on the head in a vertical fashion. Abducting the affected arm and placing the hand on top of the head will also frequently relieve the patient's radicular symptoms. This maneuver decreases traction on the inflamed root as it exits the neural foramen. Compression on the top of the head may reproduce a discogenic-type symptom of neck, shoulder, and scapula pain. The more closely the patient's sensory, motor, and reflex changes approximate the appropriate root distribution, the more certain is the diagnosis of cervical radiculopathy.

RADIOLOGY

It is almost axiomatic that the degree of degenerative changes on cervical spine roentgenograms can have little or no correlation with the patient's signs and symptoms. A completely normal-appearing film can be seen in a patient with acute disc herniation, and prominent osteophytosis can be seen in older asymptomatic patients. The findings of cervical disc degeneration on roentgenograms include sclerosis of the bone end-plates, anterior vertebral body osteophytes, and disc space narrowing. Posterolateral foraminal osteophytes may not be as obvious on AP and lateral radiographs but may be more apparent on oblique views of the cervical spine. The zygapophyseal joints may show narrowing and sclerosis with subluxation backward and downward as the disc is unable to preserve intervertebral height. CT scans demonstrate the bony detail of the osteophytosis but are not as sensitive to the disc and neurostructures. MRI is best for visualizing the anatomy of the disc and demonstrating a suspected disc herniation (Fig. 34.2). Unfortunately multiple herniations or degenerated disc levels can be visualized on MRI, and these must be correlated with the patient's history and physical exam. For this, cervical discograms have been successful to localize the correct level (5). Discectomy plus fusion of the symptomatic disc has, in this situation, a success rate of 70% (28).

If surgery is planned, myelography utilizing a water-soluble contrast agent and a postmyelogram CT scan remains the gold standard in confirming the diagnosis (Fig. 34.3). These studies show in multiple planes the relationship of the neural elements to the disc and the surrounding bone. The future need for myelography may be obviated with newer generation MRI scans. Choosing the appropriate levels to decompress anteriorly and fuse is straightforward in the patient whose signs and symptoms agree anatomically with their radiologic studies. However, prob-

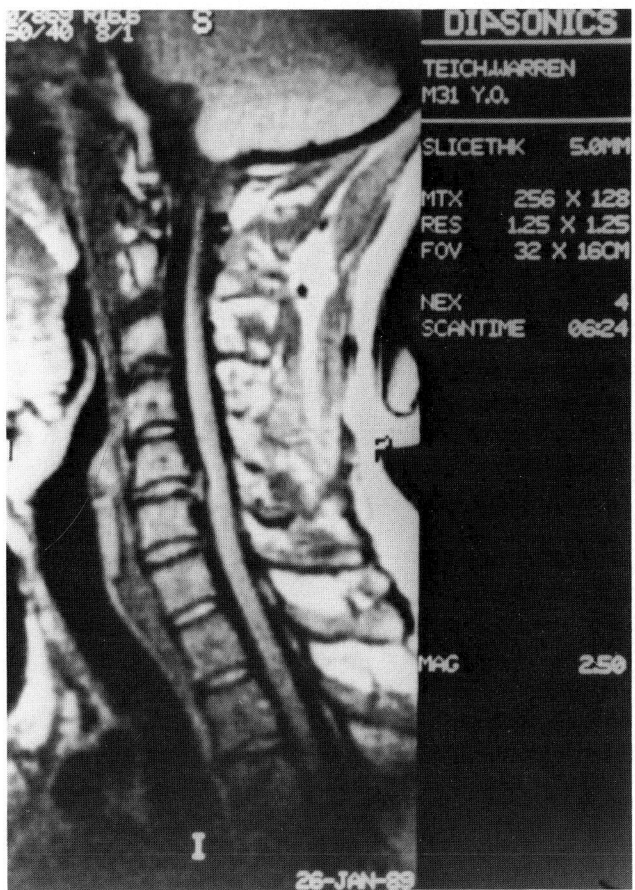

Figure 34.2. MRI of cervical spine showing herniated nucleus pulposis at C5–6.

lems arise in the patient who has symptoms referable to a specific level but has multiple levels of involvement, either from disc herniation or osteophyte spurring, as seen on the myelogram. In these patients, when only the symptomatic level is addressed, the outcome (60% good or excellent results) may not be as good as when no additional levels of involvement are present (88% good or excellent results) (3).

Electromyography

The value of electromyography lies in its ability to assist in localizing the level of cervical root compression. It does this by demonstrating a lower motor neuron lesion confined to the muscles supplied by a few adjoining spinal segments. It also aids in separating radiculopathy from neuropathy, and peripheral versus central nerve entrapment.

Surgical Technique

The anterior surgical approach, which is elegant in its simplicity, has not changed in any great degree since devised by Smith, by Cloward (4), or by Smith and Robinson (22). After induction, the patient is positioned supine on the operating table with the head either in halter traction or Gardner-Wells tongs placed with approximately 10 pounds of weight. The head rests on a horse-shoe-shaped Mayfield head support with the neck in a neutral or slightly hyperextended position. The arms are usually at the side. A roll is placed under the neck to act as a counter-force when tapping in the bone graft. Somatosensory-evoked potentials are used routinely in some centers as a means of monitoring the spinal cord during the procedure.

The surgical approach can be either from the right or the left side. The possibility of injury to the recurrent laryngeal nerve is more common with the right-sided approach; however, this approach is usually more comfortable for the right-handed surgeon. A skin incision is made transversely along the skin crease. The appropriate level of the incision can usually be identified by laying one's left hand on the right side of the neck with the index finger resting on the clavicle. Each finger then corresponds to a vertebral body with the index corresponding to C7. After the incision is made, the platysma may be divided, usually in line with the incision. Blunt dissection separates the sternocleidomastoid muscle and carotid sheath laterally from the strap muscles, trachea, esophagus, and thyroid medially. The prevertebral fascia is then exposed, and the anterior longitudinal ligament is found over the cervical discs and vertebral bodies in the midline. A needle is then placed in the appropriate disc space (Fig. 34.4), and a lateral cervical spin x-ray is taken to confirm the correct level. Discs from C2–C3 to C7–T1 can be easily exposed in this approach, with the fascia being divided in a vertical fashion when the exposure to a higher vertebral level is desired. Retractors are then placed. The anterior longitudinal ligament and anterior annulus fibrosus are incised in a rectangular fashion and the disc removed with a pituitary ronguer. Pituitary rongeurs and curettes are used to remove the disc material back to the posterior longitudinal ligament. Then a high speed burr can be used to remove the end-plates above and below back to the posterior cortices. A small angled curette is then used to remove the posterior longitudinal ligament. Defects in the posterior longitudinal ligament usually alert one to the possible pathway of a sequestered or extruded disc fragment which can be removed with a pituitary ronguer or currets. At this point a sizing instrument or ruler is used to measure the height of the disc space to be filled with the graft. A tricortical iliac crest graft should be taken of the appropriate size usually 10–15 mm high. The tricortical graft should be slightly oversized by 1 to 2 mm, depending on the height of the vertebral body at that level. After decorticating the vertebral body end-plates, the graft is gently tapped into place while a cooperative anesthesiologist augments the 10 pounds of traction on the tongs or head halter. Once seated flush with the anterior cortex of the vertebral bodies above and below, the manual traction is released, and an x-ray is taken

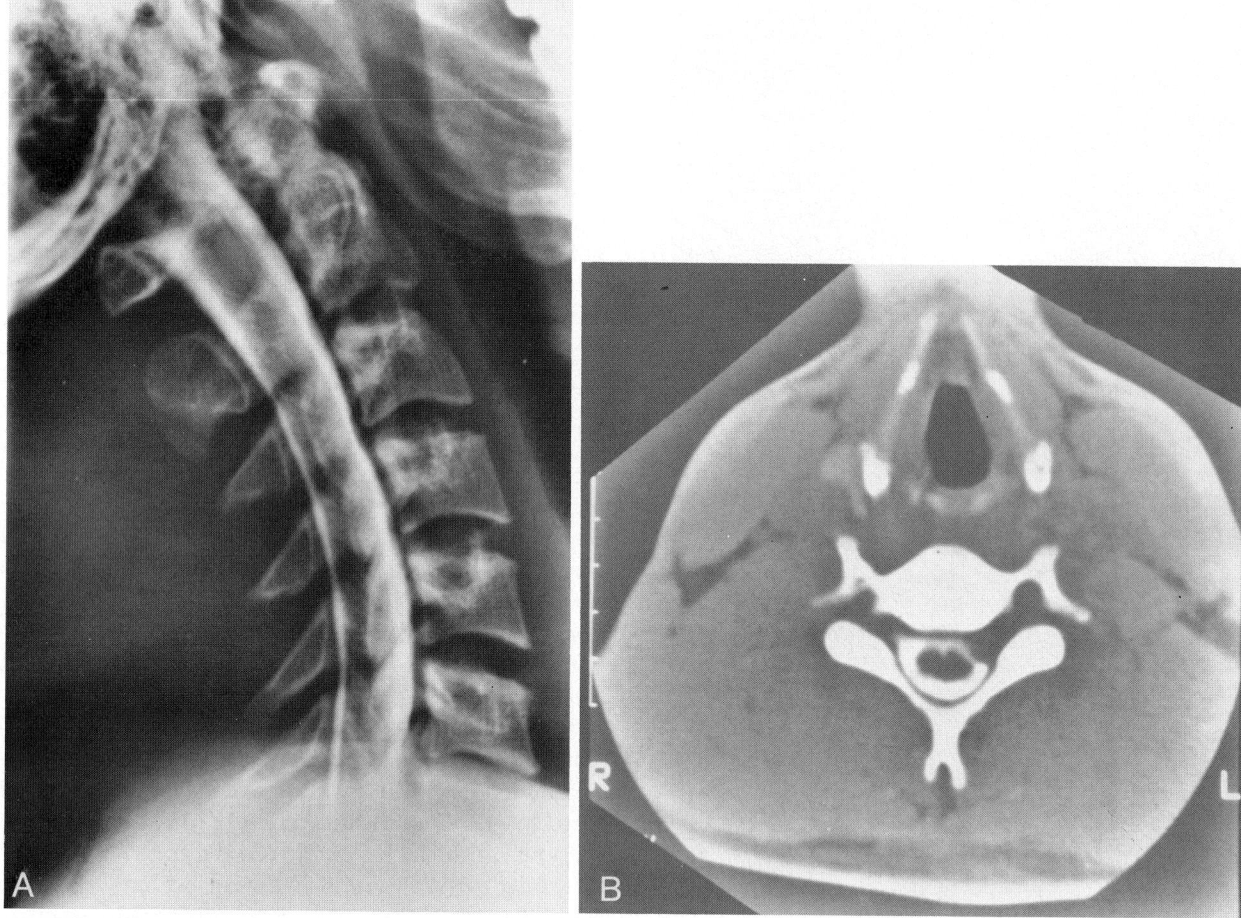

Figure 34.3. **A,** AP and lateral views of cervical spine myelogram showing herniated nucleus pulposis at C6–7 left side. **B,** Postmyelogram CT scan of cervical spine demonstrating a left-sided posterolateral disc herniation.

to verify position of the graft, and the traction may be discontinued. A small Penrose drain is placed into the depths of the wound. The skin and subcutaneous tissues are closed. Postoperatively, a Philadelphia collar is used for 4 to 6 weeks, and then a soft collar is worn for another 6 weeks. The progress of the graft incorporation can be followed with lateral cervical spine films. If pseudarthrosis is suspected at 6 months, a lateral flexion/extension lateral film should be performed.

Results

Modification of Odom et al.'s (16) criteria for evaluating the results for surgery for radiculopathy in cervical spondylosis and disc herniation can be used to analyze this group of patients. To briefly summarize, with an excellent result the patient has no cervical complaints, no pain, and the patient is able to return to work. With a good result the patient has intermittent cervical discomfort which does not interfere with work, and a satisfactory result meant improvement from the preoperative state, but the patient still had some work limitation. A patient with a poor result was unimproved or worse from their preoperative state.

Robinson, using this criteria, had 72% good or excellent results in relieving neck or arm pain. Adding-in the satisfactory results, he had 94% of patients that improved after the procedure (19). Gore (9) reported 96% of patients improved by surgery. Multiple other reviews [6, 12, 14, 18, 21, 25] in intervening years closely approximate these results, validating the basic premise of the surgery: removal of the disc and spurs if present, distraction of the disc space, and insertion of a graft to maintain distraction and promote fusion. These series did not address cervical myelopathy and frequently did not distinguish between absolute radiculopathy and referred discogenic pain. Pressing controversies in anterior cervical surgery are several, most predominantly the type of bone graft to be used and whether bone graft is actually needed or not. With bone bank capabilities proliferating, many surgeons have been using bone allograft, especially fibula, for interbody fusion. Brown, in 1976 (2), reviewed roentgenographically the fusions in 53 patients in whom a frozen allograft ilium was

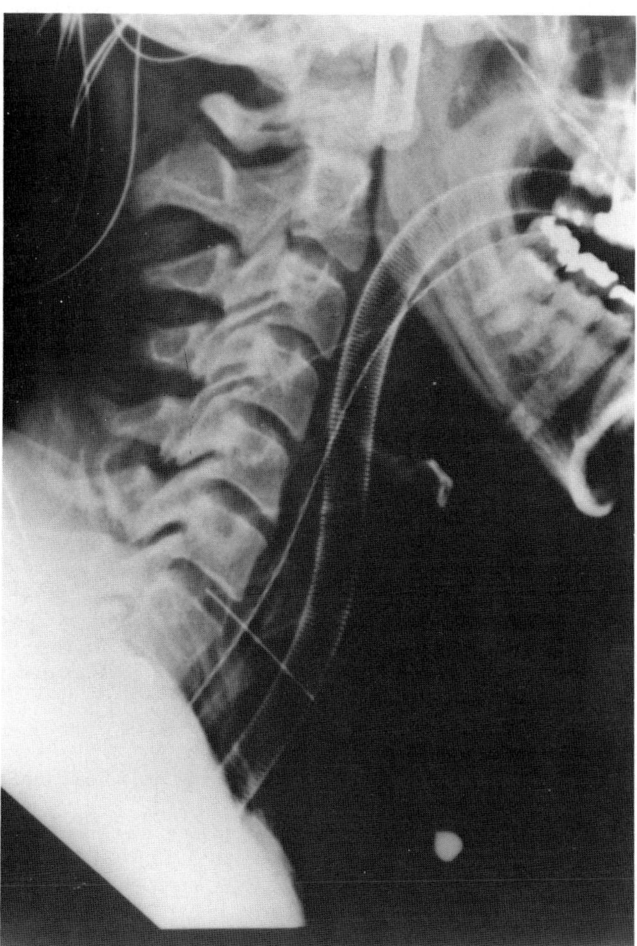

Figure 34.4. Lateral view of cervical spine in operating room demonstrating placement of needle for checking position.

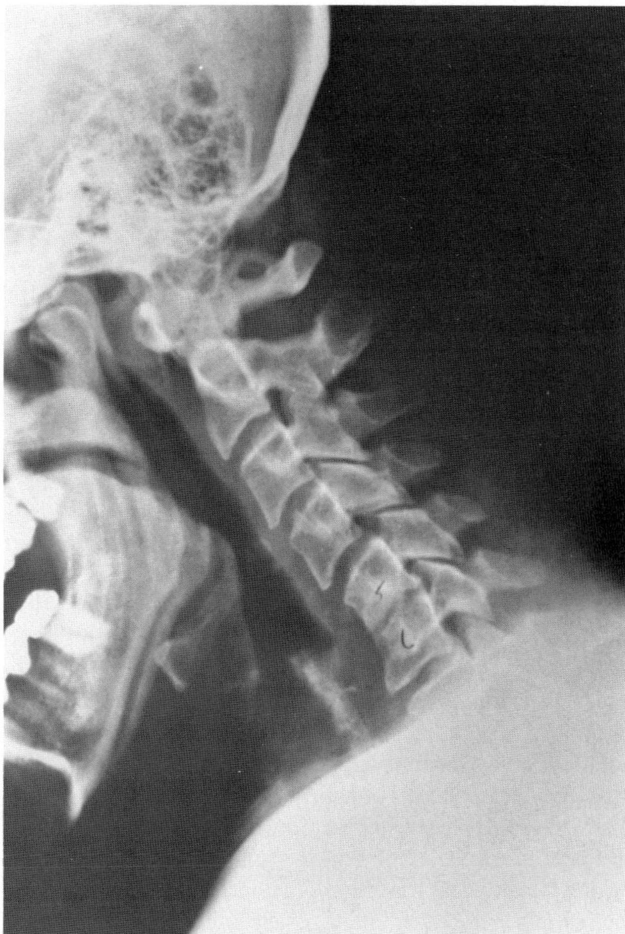

Figure 34.5. Flexion-extension lateral views of a solid C5–6 fusion at 6 months.

used. He found no statistical significance in nonunion or delayed union between the groups; however, extrusion and collapse were more common in the allograft group. This study suggested that the problem of graft site morbidity may be resolved by using donor bone.

Four differently shaped grafts have been advocated, each with its own particular advantages (1, 2, 21, 22). A biomechanical study by White and Hirsch (24) of the horseshoe graft of Smith-Robinson, the dowel type of Cloward, and the modified strut graft of Bailey and Badgely demonstrated that all three types were able to tolerate high vertical loads but that the horse-shoe graft had a significantly higher load tolerance than the other two. The Simmons Keystone technique was developed to add stability, especially when multiple levels are fused. A fibular strut graft has been recommended by Whitecloud and LaRocca (27) for multiple level fusions, with partial vertebrectomies being performed to accept the graft which is notched at both ends. Once again, some have considered bone allograft fibula in this procedure to reduce the donor site morbidity.

Although anterior cervical discectomy without fusion has been recommended the original principles of interbody fusion afford distraction across the disc space in addition to stabilization by fusion. A prospective study by Rosenorn (20) which compared discectomy with and without fusion for herniated cervical discs showed better results for discectomy alone only when the majority of the patients (40 of 60) had single level involvement. Murphy and Gado (15) reported a small series (26 patients) who only underwent discectomy with 92% good or excellent results and a 72% spontaneous fusion rate in single level procedures. He noted on the postoperative x-ray that there was always a loss of disc height, and in 4 of 20 cases a kyphosis of 5° to 15° developed in single level procedures, and a 25° kyphosis occurred in a single two-level procedure. Dunsker (7), when reporting his series of anterior cervical discectomy patients, pointed out that if large amounts of bone are removed in spondylotic ridge removal and discectomy, then interbody fusion should be performed. He advocated removing the posterior longitudinal ligament if no fusion is performed to prevent buckling when the disc space collapsed. Although the possibility of avoiding the morbidity of procuring iliac autograft and shortening the operative time are attractive, the authors believe that distraction and fusion are intregral parts of the procedure which contribute to the high number of good or excellent results characteristic of this procedure.

COMPLICATIONS

Complications can be divided into those occurring at the operative site and the donor site (26). The most frequent complications consist of dysphagia or hoarseness which usually resolve in several weeks. Perforation of the large vessels adjacent to the operative site can occur if sharp pointed retractors are used. Similarly, the trachea or esophagus may be perforated during the dissection if not protected by dull retractors. The recurrent laryngeal nerve may be injured with a right-sided approach. The thoracic duct may be injured during an approach on the left side with resultant chylothorax. Spinal cord injury is the most devastating complication which can occur, but Flynn reported the risk to be less than 2/1000 (8). The most common neurologic injury reported to be 0.9% in a large series (8), was iatrogenic radiculopathy, followed by permanent myelopathy, and recurrent laryngeal nerve palsy. Graft migration may occur and contribute to collapse at the fusion site; however, this is uncommon.

Complications at the donor site include incisional pain which lasts longer than the cervical incisional pain, a wound hematoma, serious drainage, or an infection. The surgical morbidity can be minimized by paying strict attention to hemostasis and by placing a drain at the donor and graft sites.

In summary, anterior cervical discectomy and fusion is a procedure which is relatively safe with only minor complications when performed by a surgeon well trained in the approach. It is a procedure with a high percent of surgical success and has stood the test of time, having initially been performed more than 30 years ago.

REFERENCES

1. Bailey RW, Badgley CG. Stabilization of the cervical spine by anterior fusion. J Bone Joint Surg 1960;42-A:565–594.

2. Brown MD, Malinin TJ, Davis PB. A roentgenographic evaluation of frozen allografts versus autografts in anterior cervical spine fusions. Clin Orthop 1976;119:231–236.

3. Clements DH, O'Leary PF. Anterior cervical discectomy and fusion. Presented at Cervical Spine Research Society Annual Meeting, December 1989.

4. Cloward RB. The anterior approach for removal of ruptured cervical discs. J Neurosurg 1958;15:602–617.

5. Cloward RB. Cervical diskography. Ann Surg 1959;150:1052–1064.

6. DePalma AF, Rothman RH, Lewinek GG, Canale ST. Anterior interbody fusion for severe cervical disc degeneration. Surg Gynecol Obstet 1972;134:755–758.

7. Dunsker SB. Anterior cervical discectomy with and without fusion. Clin Neurosurg 1977;24:516–520.

8. Flynn T. Neurologic complications of anterior cervical fusion spine. 1982;7:535.

9. Gore DR, Sepic SB. Anterior cervical fusion for degenerated or protruded discs. Spine 1984;9:667–671.

10. Horwitz T. Degenerative lesions in the cervical portion of the spine. Arch Intern Med 1940;55:1178–1187.

11. Herkowitz HN. The surgical management of cervical spondylotic radiculopathy and myelopathy. Clin Orthop 1989;239:94–107.

12. Jacobs B, Krueger EG, Leivy DM. Cervical spondylosis with radiculopathy. JAMA 1970;211:2135–2139.

13. Kelsey JL, et al. An epidemiological study of acute prolapsed cervical intervertebral disc. J Bone Joint Surg 1984;66-A:907–914.

14. Lunsford LD, et al. Anterior surgery for cervical disc disease. J Neurosurg 1980;53:1–11.

15. Murphy MG, Gado M. Anterior cervical discectomy without interbody bone graft. J Neurosurg 1972;37:71–74.

16. Odom GL, Finney W, Woodhall B. Cervical disc lesions. JAMA 1958;166:23–28.

17. O'Laoire SA, Thomas DGT. Spinal cord compression due to prolapse of cervical intervertebral disc. J Neurosurg 1983;59:847–853.

18. Riley LH, et al. The results of anterior interbody fusion of the cervical spine. J Bone Joint Surg 1962;44-A:1569–1587.

20. Rosenorn J, et al. Anterior cervical discectomy with and without fusion. J Neurosurg 1983;59:252–255.

21. Simmons GH, Bhalla SK. Anterior cervical discectomy and fusion. J Bone Joint Surg 1969;51B:225–237.

22. Smith GW, Robinson RA. The treatment of certain cervical spine disorders by anterior removal of the intervertebral disc and interbody fusion. J Bone Joint Surg 1958;40-A:607–623.

23. Stookey B. Compression of the spinal cord due to ventral extradural cervical chondromas. Arch Neurol 1928;20:275–291.

24. White AA, Hirsch CC. An experimental study of the immediate load bearing capacity of some commonly used iliac bone grafts. Acta Orthop Scand 1971;42:482–490.

25. White AA, et al. Relief of pain by anterior cervical spine fusion for spondylosis. J Bone Joint Surg 1973;55-A:525–534.

26. Whitecloud TS. Complications of anterior cervical fusion. AAOS Instructional Course Lectures 1986;27:223–227.

27. Whitecloud TS, LaRocca RH. Fibular strut grafting in reconstructive surgery of the cervical spine. Spine 1976;1:33.

28. Whitecloud TS, Scago RA. Cervical discogenic syndrome. Spine 1987;12:313–316.

35

Anterior Decompression and Fusion for Cervical Myelopathy Associated with Cervical Spondylosis and Deformity

Sanford E. Emery and Henry H. Bohlman

Introduction

Cervical cord compression associated with cervical spondylosis was described as early as 1911 by Bailey and Kasamajor (3) and later, in 1928, by Stookey (17). A better understanding of the pathophysiology and treatment of this condition has really taken place only in the last three decades with significant contributions by Brain (7, 8), Nurick (14), Robinson (16), and others. Although cervical spondylosis is the most common cause of cervical myelopathy, other conditions such as acute soft disc herniations, vertebral subluxations, ossification of the posterior longitudinal ligament, and kyphotic deformities can cause anterior cord compression.

Pathophysiology

The underlying etiology of cervical spondylitic changes in the neck is progressive disc and joint degeneration. Aging intervertebral discs lose water content and undergo proteoglycan alterations. There is loss of elasticity in the disc with desiccation and fissuring of the cartilage end-plates. Clefts form in the disc, and the disc space collapses, producing narrowing that is seen radiographically. Once the disc space has become degenerate and collapsed, the biomechanics of the segment are altered. Chondro-osseous spurs form at the insertion of the ligament structures to bone. The uncovertebral joints are also affected by degenerative disease, and osteophytes grow by enchondral ossification. Spurring at the annulus and uncovertebral joints together may form a transverse bar across the anterior spinal canal. If large enough, or in association with another factor such as soft disc protrusion or kyphosis, spinal cord compression may occur, resulting in myelopathy. This often becomes clinically manifest in patients with a congenitally narrow spinal canal (1, 2).

Robinson in 1977 emphasized the importance of abnormal intervertebral motion in the development and maintenance of chrondro-osseous spurs (16). Motion may also exacerbate the problem by intermittent dynamic compression of the spinal cord between anterior spurs and hypertrophied posterior ligamentum flavum. Experimental and clinical studies suggest flattening of the cord causes interruption of blood supply via the transverse arterioles within the cord tissue itself, leading to central ischemia (10, 18). Blocking of axoplasmic flow most certainly occurs as well, with demyelinization, neuronal cell death, and gliosis, the sequential end-stages of cord compression (11, 12, 15).

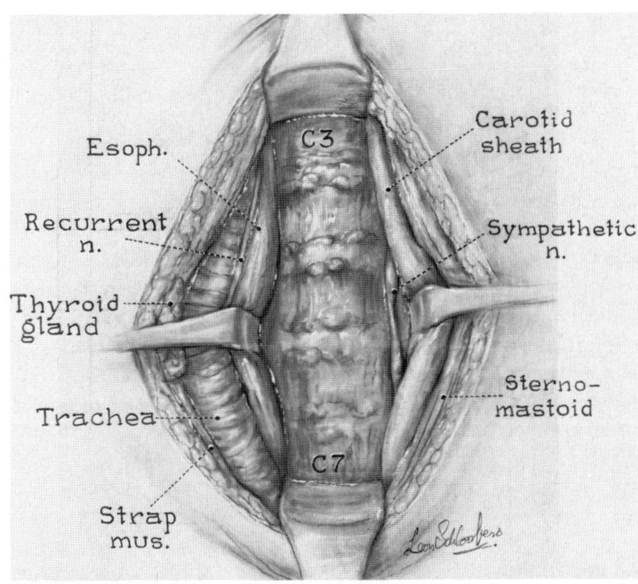

Figure 35.1. The operative approach includes an anterior transverse incision and dissection between the carotid sheath and the trachea and esophagus to expose the anterior aspect of the spine. (Reprinted with permission J Bone Joint Surg 1989;71-A:170–182.) A longitudinal incision of the deep cervical fascia is important to facilitate sliding blunt retractors superiorly and inferiorly to allow exposure from C3 to C7.

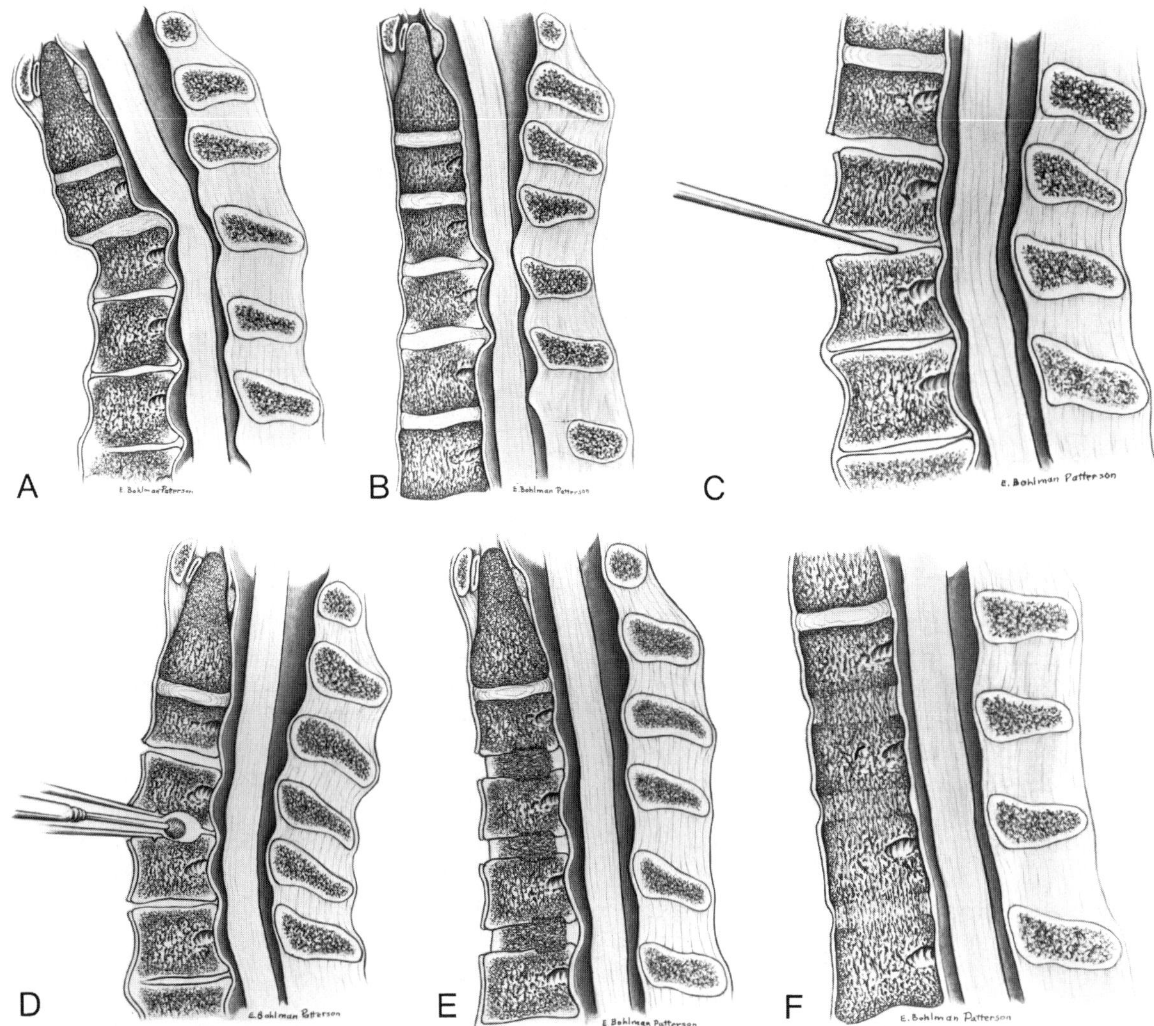

Figure 35.2. **A,** Diagrammatic illustration of compensatory anterior subluxation of the third on fourth cervical vertebrae above the stiff spondylotic segments. Cord compression occurs anteriorly. **B,** Illustration of a cervical spondylotic spine demonstrating a narrow canal, decreased height of the disc spaces, posterior osteophytes, and disk protrusions with buckled posterior longitudinal ligament and ligamentum flavum. **C,** Illustration of technique used to pry apart the narrowed disk space to allow acceptance of a graft 5 mm in height. Smaller grafts resorb and collapse. **D,** Illustration demonstrates technique of removing posterior aspect of sclerotic end-plates with a power burr without violating any posterior osteophytes. **E,** Illustration demonstrates the bone blocks in place and properly countersunk. The entire disk has been removed at each level without violating the posterior longitudinal ligament. Distraction straightens the redundant posterior longitudinal ligament and ligamentum flavum, and immediate stability is achieved. **F,** Illustration demonstrating incorporation of the bone grafts, loss of osteophytes by normal bone remodeling, and no further redundancy of the ligamentous structures. The pathologic segments have been stabilized. (Reprinted with permission from Spine 1977;2:151–162.)

CLINICAL PRESENTATION

Clinical evidence of myelopathy may occur before these irreversible cellular changes. The spondylitic process and clinical course is generally slow, but, as shown by Clark and Robinson (9), it is usually progressive and rarely spontaneously improves. Often patients initially complain of gait abnormalities or balance difficulty. Neck pain with or without radicular arm pain is common; however, some patients may have no neck complaints at all. Symptoms may progress to upper or lower extremity weakness and eventually sphincter disturbance. Evidence of sphincter or posterior column dysfunction on physical examination is a poor prognostic sign, but it does not preclude some spinal cord recovery with appropriate surgical intervention. Sensory changes may or may not be present and are often a mixed dermatomal pattern. Spinal cord and local nerve root compression at the level of the pathology often produces a mixture of upper and lower motor neuron signs in the extremities, with specific root weakness or diminished reflex in the face of generalized long tract signs.

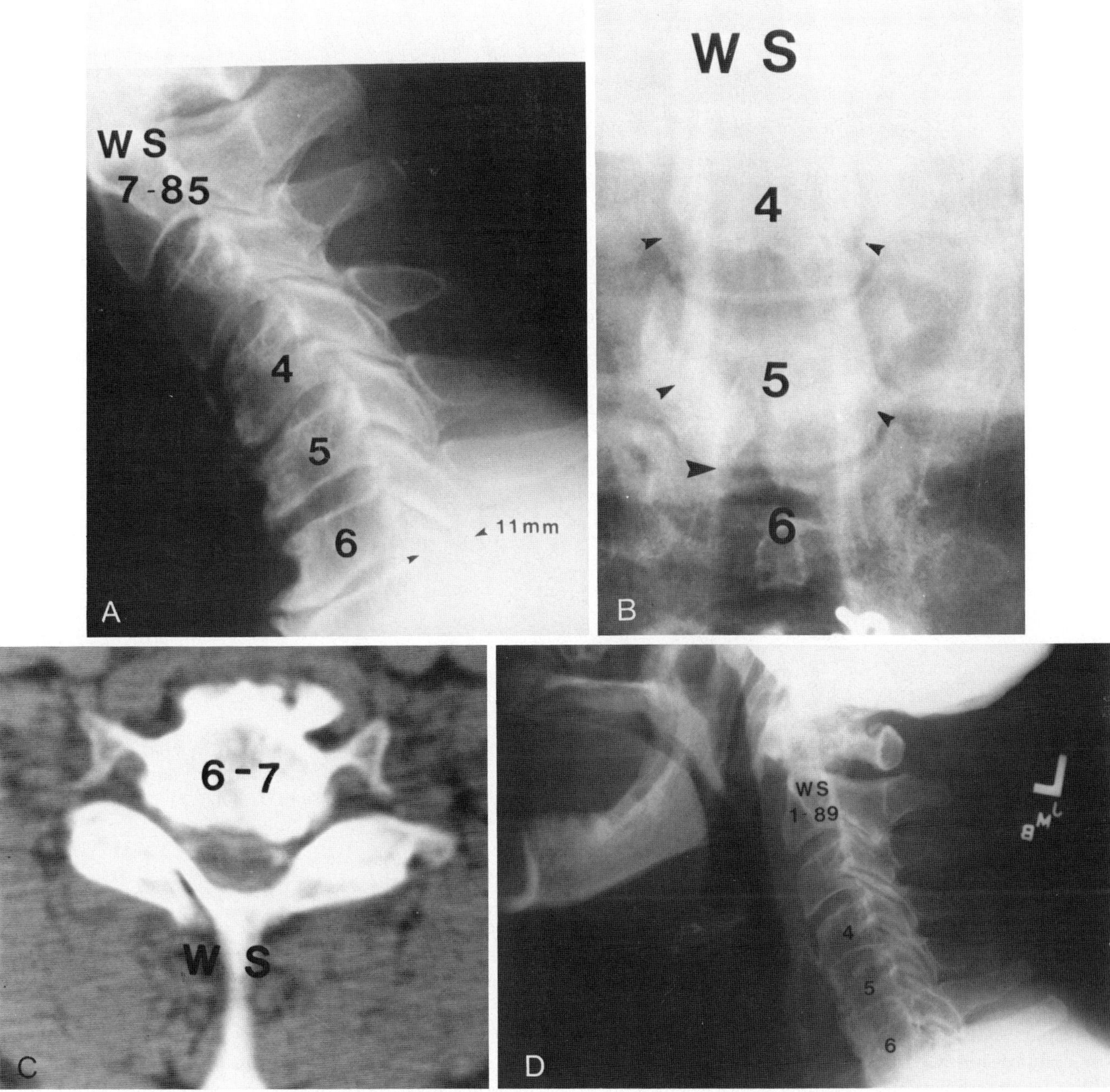

Figure 35.3. This 67-year-old male presented with neck pain, bilateral shoulder pain, upper extremity weakness, and an abnormal gait. His lateral x-ray (**A**) shows a kyphotic deformity with spondylotic changes and a narrow cervical canal. The AP myelogram (**B**) shows a complete block at C5–C6 (*large arrow*) and an anterior bar at C4–C5. The smaller arrows show root cut-off at multiple levels. His CT-myelogram (**C**) shows a kidney-bean-shaped spinal cord from anterior compression at C6–C7. He underwent a three-level anterior cervical discectomy and fusion with resolution of his pain and gait abnormality. His lateral x-ray 3.5 years after surgery (**D**) shows a solid fusion.

Diagnostic Evaluation

The diagnosis of myelopathy is generally evident on physical examination; however, thorough radiographic investigation is mandatory to confirm a cervical etiology and to determine the extent of the disease for preoperative planning. The number of levels involved, size and location of chondro-osseous spurs, and presence of ossification of the posterior longitudinal ligament or kyphosis will directly influence the type and extent of the decompression procedure. Plain roentgenograms provide much information regarding spinal canal size, posterior spurs, and foraminal encroachment. Flexion-extension views are performed to rule out vertebral subluxation since dynamic cord compression can occur as well. Magnetic resonance imaging can be helpful to rule out other causes of myelopathy and has

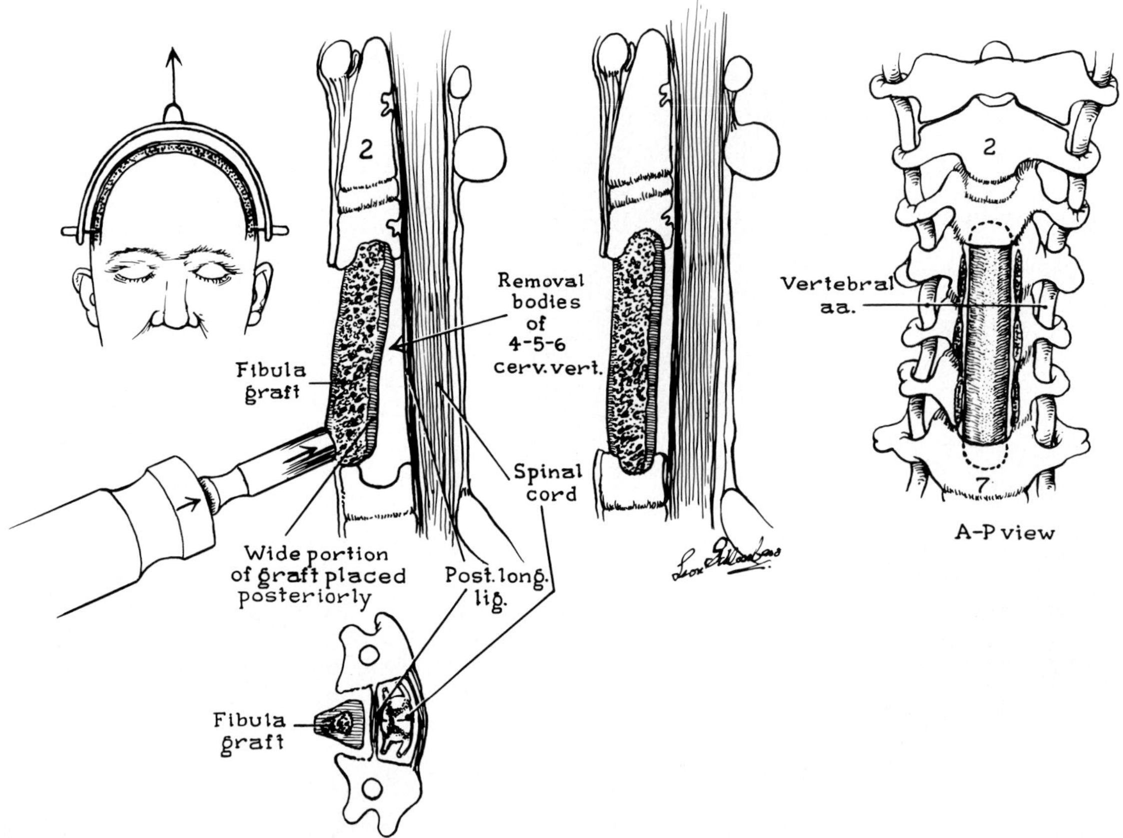

Figure 35.4. The steps of the procedure that are performed after anterior corpectomy and decompression. Skeletal traction is increased to reduce the kyphosis. Extension of the neck may also be needed. Seating holes are made in the end-plates of the superior and inferior intact vertebral bodies with a burr. The ends of the graft are then rounded, and the graft is impacted into place. When the traction is released the graft is locked in place. (Reprinted with permission, J Bone Joint Sur 1989;71-A: 170–182.)

improved in resolution since its early use. However, we believe myelography with water soluble contrast and CT are essential for accurate and complete evaluation. These two studies provide anatomic detail of cord compression, bony spurs and ridges, soft disc protrusions, and nerve root compression. Cystometrograms are useful for establishing baseline function in the presence of sphincter abnormalities. Somatosensory evoked potentials may be compared preoperatively and postoperatively and are used intraoperatively for some cases; however, their diagnostic and prognostic value has yet to be fully determined. We do not believe electromyography or nerve conduction velocity studies alone add significantly to the work-up of a patient with cervical myelopathy.

TREATMENT

Patients with cervical myelopathy will occasionally improve with a cervical collar or even bed rest, as any dynamic compression of the cord secondary to abnormal motion is minimized with these measures. This is of transient benefit, however, and because the disease process is progressive, unless major contraindications to general anesthesia exist, we recommend surgical treatment for patients with myelopathy.

Our goal is to address the two primary factors responsible for spondylitic myelopathy, i.e., spinal cord compression secondary to bone and/or disc protrusions and abnormal motion. Since the majority of compressive pathology is anterior to the spinal cord, we have utilized the Smith-Robinson anterior approach for both decompression and fusion. This method allows direct visualization and removal of the pathology without manipulation of the spinal cord. Multiple level discectomies and fusions or multi-level corpectomies can easily be done through a transverse incision (6) (Fig. 35.1).

Most patients with cervical spondylitic myelopathy have compression at the level of the disc space; therefore, we recommend the Robinson anterior discectomy and fusion technique using tricortical autogenous iliac crest graft (Fig. 35.2a through 2f; Fig. 35.3). High powered loupe magnification and a headlight are critical for visualization. No attempt is made to remove spurs with a curette if they are small to moderate in size. These will remodel with time,

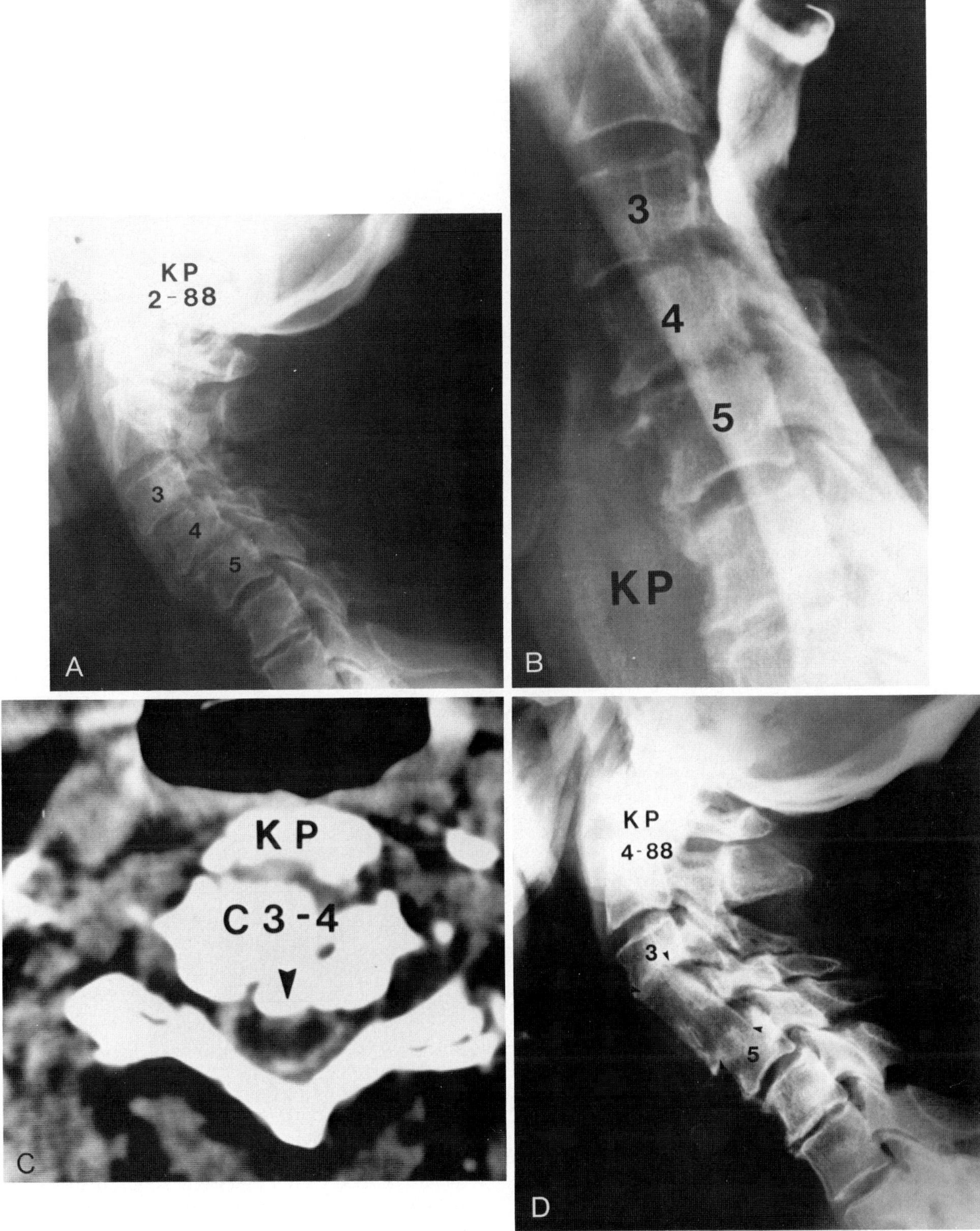

Figure 35.5. K.P. is a 75-year-old male with a history of progressive neck pain, difficulty walking, and numbness in his hands. On examination he had upper extremity weakness, a wide-based gait, and pathologic reflexes in both the upper and lower extremities. His preoperative lateral x-ray (**A**) shows anterior subluxation at C3–C4 as well as C4–C5, with associated spondylosis. His lateral myelogram (**B**) shows obstruction of the dye column at C3–C4. His CT-myelogram (**C**) shows severe flattening of the cord at the superior aspect of the body of C4. He underwent a corpectomy of C4 to totally decompress the spinal cord with placement of an iliac crest strut graft from C3 to C5 (**D**). He had significant resolution of his pain and myelopathy, and died approximately 1 year later of unrelated causes.

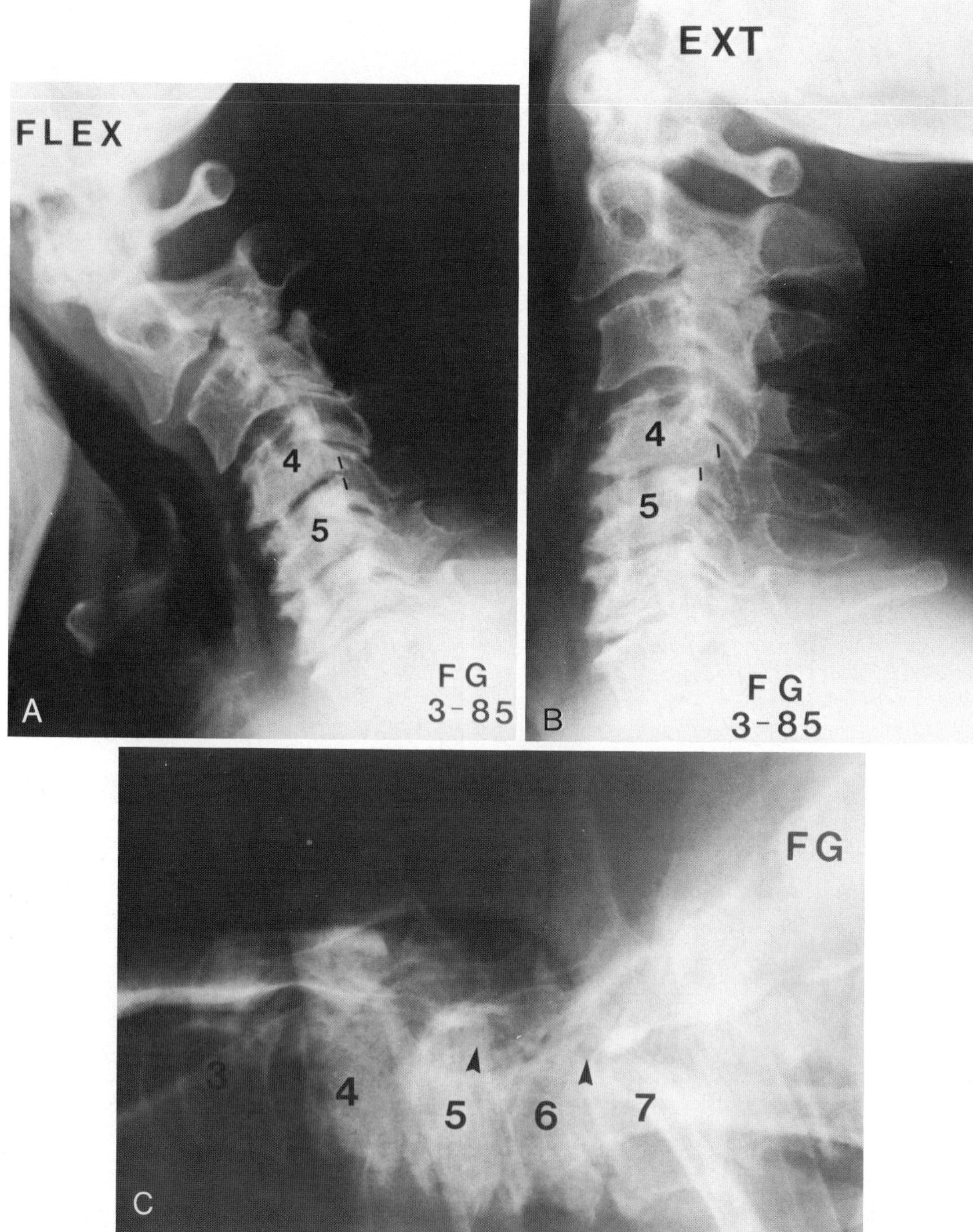

Figure 35.6. This 68-year-old white male presented with a chief complaint of right arm weakness and neck pain. He had a mild kyphotic deformity on exam as well as bilateral upper extremity weakness and bilateral Hoffmann reflexes. His lateral flexion (**A**) and extension (**B**) radiographs show significant cervical spondylosis with a narrow canal and retrolisthesis of C4 on C5 in extension. His lateral myelogram (**C**) shows a large extradural defect at C3–C4 with severe wasting of the dye column and suspected anterior compression at C5–C6 and C6–C7 (*arrows*).

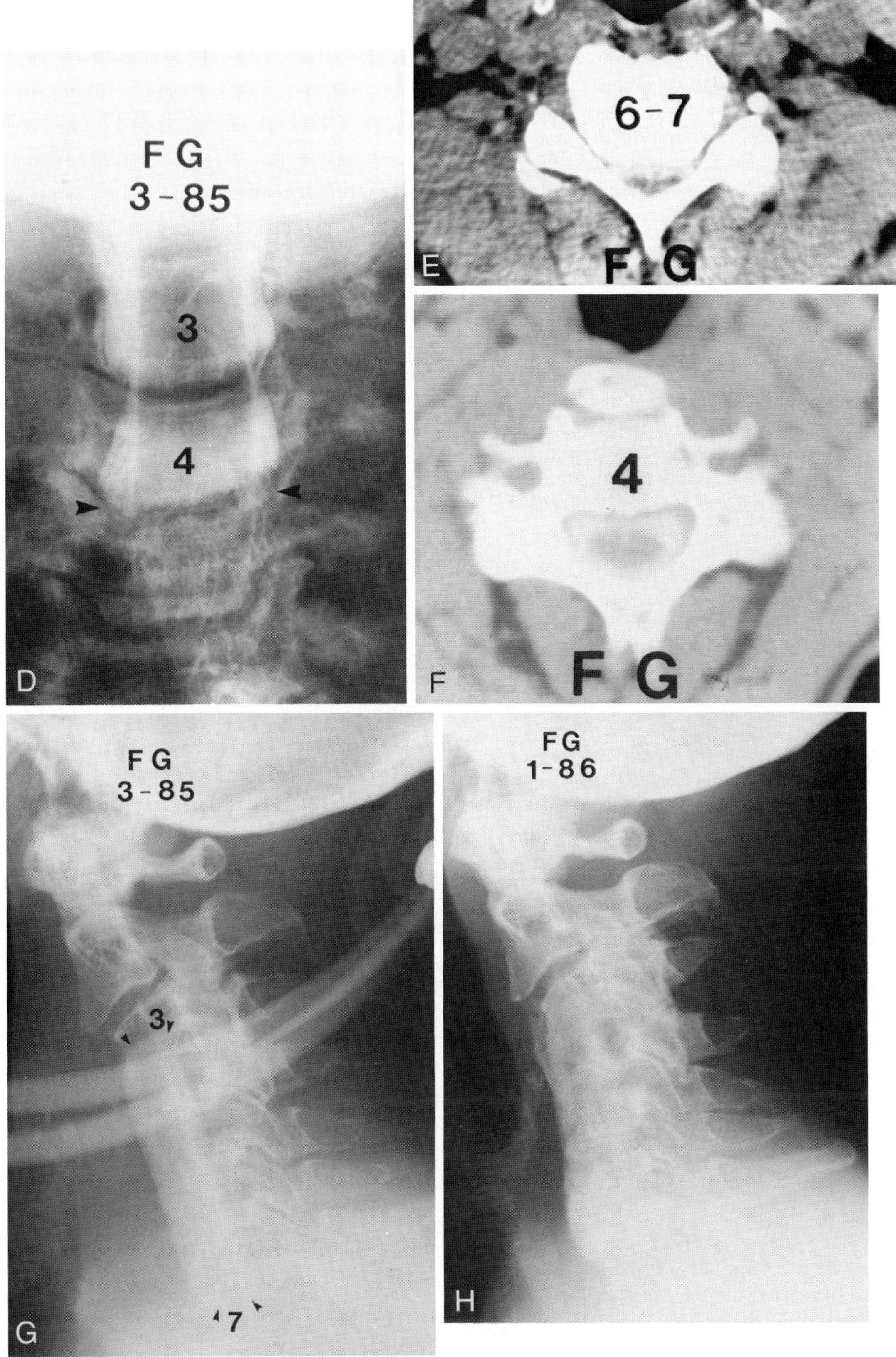

Figure 35.6D-H. His AP myelogram (**D**) shows a transverse bar at C3–C4 and a block at C4–C5. The CT-myelogram (**E**) shows severe spinal cord compression, here at the C6–C7 level. A normal CT slice behind the body of C4 (**F**) is included for comparison. He underwent a three-level anterior corpectomy with a fibular strut fusion from C3 to C7, with his immediate post-operative lateral x-ray shown (**G**). The follow-up films 10 months later show a solid fusion with extensive bony remodeling (**H**). His motor strength returned to normal and he was eventually able to resume downhill skiing.

provided solid fusion is obtained. Larger spurs or ossification of the posterior longitudinal ligament should be removed if compressing the cord in association with severe myelopathy. This is done through a complete or partial vertebrectomy using high speed diamond burrs. This is safer than reaching posteriorly through the disc space behind the vertebra with angled curettes, endangering the spinal cord. All areas of compression must be addressed based on preoperative studies. After decompression is completed, concavities are made in the end-plates of the bodies above and below, and a graft of the appropriate size is tapped into place (Fig. 35.4). A posterior lip of bone is usually left on the vertebral bodies with the posterior longitudinal ligament to prevent the graft from slipping into the canal. For one- or two-level corpectomies, we generally use an iliac strut graft (Fig. 35.5). For three- and four-level corpectomies an autogenous fibular strut is utilized (Fig. 35.6). Traction with Gardner-Wells tongs and spinal cord monitoring are used for corpectomy procedures, but neither are necessary for a standard Robinson anterior discectomy and fusion.

RESULTS

Bohlman in 1977 reported on 17 patients with moderate to severe myelopathy secondary to cervical spondylosis (5). Preoperatively, 14 of these patients required walking aids and three were bedridden with severe quadriparesis. Robinson anterior discectomies and iliac crest grafts were performed without attempting removal of posterior osteophytes. Most patients had multiple levels of pathology addressed. All 14 ambulatory patients improved to walking without aid within 6 months of their decompression and fusion. Two of the three bedridden patients became ambulatory with aid. No patient lost neural function. A more recent review with 2–14 year follow-up of patients with cervical myelopathy treated with this technique has yielded similar gratifying results with minimal complications. Spinal cord recovery can occur to varying degrees depending on the amount and duration of compression. Other clinical studies report favorable results with anterior decompression and fusion for spondylitic myelopathy (4, 13, 19).

CERVICAL KYPHOSIS AND MYELOPATHY

Cervical kyphosis and myelopathy can result from degenerative, traumatic, iatrogenic, or neoplastic conditions. The spinal cord is flattened and stretched over the anterior kyphus with resultant long tract dysfunction. Vertebral corpectomies are nearly always needed to adequately decompress the cord and correct the deformity. Iliac or fibular strut grafts are used, depending on the length of the decompression to provide postoperative stability and obtain fusion. Posterior arthrodesis is recommended as well for remote posttraumatic kyphotic deformities with torn posterior ligamentous structures. Post laminectomy kyphosis is also especially difficult to treat, given the relative lack of posterior stability. Zdeblick and Bohlman reported on 14 patients with cervical kyphosis and myelopathy treated by anterior corpectomy and strut grafting with good results (20). No patient lost neural function, and 13 improved. Solid fusion occurred in all 14 patients, and the average correction in kyphosis was 28°. Three grafts dislodged in the early postoperative period, two of which involved post laminectomy kyphosis patients. This experience suggests a halo vest be used in managing these patients if posterior instability coexists.

In general, cervical myelopathy secondary to spondylosis or deformity can be treated in most instances by an anterior decompression and fusion with significant recovery of neurologic function and without great risk.

REFERENCES

1. Adams CBT, Logue V. Studies in cervical spondylotic myelopathy: II. The movement and contour of the spine in relation to the neural complications of cervical spondylosis. Brain 1971;94:569.

2. Arnold JG Jr. The clinical manifestations of spondylochondrosis (spondylosis) of the cervical spine. Ann Surg 1955;141:872–889.

3. Bailey P, Casamajor L. Osteoarthritis of the spine as a cause of compression of the spinal cord and its roots, with reports of 5 cases. J Nerv Ment Dis 1911;38:588–609.

4. Bernard TN Jr, Whitecloud TS III. Cervical spondylotic myelopathy and myeloradiculopathy: anterior decompression and stabilization with autogenous fibula strut graft. Clin Orthop 1987;221:149.

5. Bohlman HH. Cervical spondylosis with moderate to severe myelopathy. A report of seventeen cases treated by Robinson anterior cervical discectomy and fusion. Spine 1977;2:151–161.

6. Bohlman HH. Degenerative arthrosis of the lower cervical spine. In: Evarts CM, ed. Surgery of the musculoskeletal system, Vol II. London: Churchill Livingstone, 1983.

7. Brain RW, Northfield D, Wilkinson M. The neurologic manifestations of cervical spondylosis. Brain 1952;75:187–225.

8. Brain L, Wilkinson M. Cervical spondylosis and other disorders of the cervical spine. First edition. Philadelphia: WB Saunders, 1967.

9. Clarke E, Robinson PK. Cervical myelopathy: a complication of cervical spondylosis. Brain 1956;79:483.

10. Doppman JL. The mechanism of ischemia in anteroposterior compression of the spinal cord. Invest Radiol 1975;10:543.

11. Gledhill RF, Harrison BM, McDonald NI. Demyelination and remyelination after acute spinal cord compression. Exp Neurol 1973;38:472.

12. Gooding MR, Wilson CB, Hoff JT. Experimental cervical myelopathy: effect of ischemia and compression of the canine cervical spinal cord. J Neurosurg 1975;43:9.

13. Hanai K, Fujiyoshi F, Kamei K. Subtotal vertebrectomy and spinal fusion for cervical spondylotic myelopathy. Spine 1986;11:310.

14. Nurick S. The pathogenesis of the spinal cord disorder associated with cervical spondylosis. Brain 1972;95:87.

15. Ono K, Ota H, Tada K, Yamamoto T. Cervical myelopathy secondary to multiple spondylotic protrusions: a clinico-pathologic study. Spine 1977;2:109–125.

16. Robinson RA, Afeiche N, Dunn EJ, Northrup BE. Cervical spondylotic myelopathy: etiology and treatment concepts. Spine 1977;2: 89–99.

17. Stookey B. Compression of the spinal cord due to ventral extradural cervical chondromas. Arch Neurol Psychiatry 1928;20:275–291.

18. Taylor AR. Vascular factors in the myelopathy associated with cervical spondylosis. Neurology 1964;14:62.

19. Yonenobu K, Fugi T, Ono K, Okada K, Yamamoto T, Harada N. Choice of surgical treatment for multisegmental cervical spondylotic myelopathy. Spine 1985;10:710.

20. Zdeblick TA, Bohlman HH. Cervical kyphosis and myelopathy: treatment by anterior corpectomy and strut-grafting. J Bone Joint Surg 1989;71A:170–182.

36

Anterior Decompression and Fusion for Cervical Myelopathy

George W. Sypert

Introduction

Cervical myelopathy is the most serious consequence of cervical spine degenerative disease. Degenerative spine disease causing cervical myelopathy is associated with spinal stenosis due to spondylotic changes (intervertebral disc protrusion, bone bars, osteophytes, and laminar, ligamentous, and hypophyseal joint hypertrophy) and ossification of the posterior longitudinal ligament (OPLL) (2, 7, 26–28, 39–42, 45, 49). Although the pathology of typical cases and pathogenesis of spondylosis and OPLL appear to be different, modern high resolution thin-section computed tomographic (CT) imaging reveals that these two degenerative processes appear to overlap and are frequently found in the same patient (52). At the present time, compression of the spinal cord or its blood vessels appears to be one of the most important causes of cervical myelopathy secondary to degenerative spondylosis and/or OPLL (6, 7, 18, 19, 27, 30, 39). Moreover, the effects of direct neural compression and ischemia appear to be additive, each separately having less effect on neurological deficit and pathology than both acting together (18). Another significant causal variable appears to be repeated dynamic trauma to the spinal cord from neck motion and minor injuries (6, 7, 59).

Medical therapies do not appear to favorably alter the natural history of the cervical myelopathies related to degenerative spine disease. Therefore, a variety of surgical strategies in various combinations have been advocated for the treatment of the cervical myelopathies related to degenerative spine disease (1–3, 5, 10, 14, 15, 17, 26, 34, 37, 46, 47, 50, 56). Unfortunately, there remains no general consensus or scientific evidence to prove the superiority of one surgical procedure over another. Given the observations that the principal mass lesions compressing the spinal cord lie anterior to the neural elements (6, 7, 18, 19, 27, 39) and that dynamic factors play a role in the pathogenesis of the myelopathies (6, 7, 59), a prospective study was initiated by the author in 1983 to examine the clinical role of single-stage anterior radical decompressive operative procedures with allograft bone fusion in the management of cervical myelopathy. The patients were graded on a myelopathy scale (26) preoperatively and at follow-up. The data presented here is preliminary, based on patient chart review by the author. The final results will be forthcoming after a detailed follow-up of the patients and final grading by an investigator independent of the operating surgeon. Hence, the present data should be considered somewhat biased in favor of good results as they are derived, in part, from personal interactions between the patients and their operating surgeon.

Clinical Material

This series includes 60 consecutive patients (9/26/83 to 7/14/88) that were thought to represent cervical myelopathy and myeloradiculopathy secondary to degenerative spinal stenosis (i.e., spondylosis, OPLL, or combined spondylosis/OPLL) treated surgically via an extensive anterior microsurgical decompression and arthrodesis by the author. All such patients were included who exhibited signs of myelopathy, including those who had simple spasticity. They consisted of 20 patients with cervical spondylosis, 17 patients with OPLL, and 23 patients with combined neural compression from both spondylosis and OPLL. There were 14 women and 56 men, ranging in age from 22–75 years, with an average age of 54 years. Forty-nine were Caucasians, 10 Black, and 1 Asian.

Three additional patients were excluded from this study as they proved to suffer from primary motor neuron disease. They were treated with uncomplicated anterior intervertebral decompression and interbody arthrodesis and failed to show any improvement in symptoms or signs.

Clinical Presentation

A steady progressive cervical myeloradiculopathy or a myelopathy were the most common clinical presentation. Weakness or clumsiness of the upper extremity (60), numbness (54) or paresthesia (18) of the upper extremity, difficulty with walking (52), leg weakness (49), and neck pain (45) were the most common symptoms. Leg numbness (23) or paresthesia (13), upper-extremity radicular pain (31), urinary incontinence (9), and impotence (6) were less regularly mentioned. The duration of interval between onset of symptoms and radical anterior microsurgical decompression ranged from 1 month to 23 years (mean 14.3 months). Trauma to the neck precipitated symptoms in 18 patients and was mentioned as a remote occurrence in another 8 patients. A history of repeated minor trauma was present in 6 patients. Twelve patients had previously undergone surgery on the cervical spine for compressive myeloradiculopathy; five had received multiple-level laminectomies, one a posterior cervical fusion, and seven had undergone anterior cervical discectomy with or without fusion (one patient on three separate occasions).

At presentation, the following physical findings were prevalent: limitation of neck motion (54), upper-extremity sensory loss (54), myelopathic sensory loss (21), upper-extremity weakness (60), lower extremity weakness (52), lower extremity spasticity (60), and Babinski sign (56). Upper extremity atrophy and hypertonia or hypotonia and Hoffmann sign were also common findings.

METHODS

Clinical Grading

As mentioned, all patients presented with symptoms and objective signs of myelopathy or myeloradiculopathy. Because of great difficulties with grading, quantifying, and classifying the upper extremity myeloradiculopathy, an established myelopathy grading scale (Harsh et al., 1987) familiar to the author was used to evaluate the results in these patients. Each patient was allotted to one of the following eight disability grades, preoperatively, at discharge, and at follow-up. The grading system is based on clinical involvement of the spinal cord and impairment of physical performance:

Grade O : No evidence of myelopathy
Grade I : Able to run, but abnormal strength, tone, or reflexes on examination.
Grade II : Difficulty in running or climbing stairs.
Grade III : Difficulty in walking.
  A: Independent but unsteady.
  B: Requires cane.
  C: Requires walker or assistance.
Grade IV : Difficulty standing.
Grade V : Paraplegia.
  Subscript 0 : Continent of urine and stool, voids spontaneously.
  Subscript 1 : Minor sphincter disturbance.
  Subscript 2 : Requires catheterization.

Neurodiagnostic Imaging

Conventional cervical spine radiographs and water-soluble contrast myelography followed by axial thin-section CT myelography (including vertebral bodies) were obtained in each patient. Conventional spine radiographic series generally demonstrated the typical findings associated with cervical spondylosis in most patients. OPLL was only recognized as being present prior to CT myelography in six patients. The spine films were read as normal in eight patients. Conventional myelography showed widening of the spinal cord shadow in the anteroposterior projection in 46 patients with an anterior epidural defect seen in 54 patients. The abnormalities on conventional myelography appear to be localized to the disc space regions in the majority of patients despite CT myelography demonstrating retrovertebral midline ventral mass (OPLL) in 40 patients. Thin-section, high-resolution CT myelography definitively demonstrated the sites of spinal cord and nerve root compression in all cases (Figs. 36.1 and 36.2). Magnetic resonance imaging performed in 14 cases often failed to demonstrate ventral spinal cord compression or the extent and location of the ventral extradural neural compressive lesion. Hence, CT myelography was used to define the extent of ventral neural compression and guide the microsurgical decompressive procedure (Table 36.1).

Surgical Procedures

Prior to induction of anesthesia the patient is positioned supine on the operating table with either cervical halter or halo traction initiated. Normal cervical lordosis is maintained by a small sandbag placed beneath the neck. Gentle endotracheal intubation and anesthetic induction are accomplished. In patients with neck deformities or potential instability, an awake, fiber-optic nasotracheal intubation may be necessary. The head is rotated slightly to the side opposite that planned for the surgery. If only two interspaces are to be exposed, a transverse, skin-fold incision is made from the midline across the anterior border of the sternocleidomastoid muscle. When more than two interspaces or vertebrae must be exposed, a vertical incision along the anterior border of the sternocleidomastoid muscle is preferred. The rostral-caudal position of the incision is determined by reviewing the patient's radiographic anatomy.

Skin flaps are elevated over the platysma muscle, and the muscle is incised in the direction of its fibers. The cervical fascia bridging the sternocleidomastoid and laryngeal strap muscles is incised longitudinally. Blunt dissection is used to separate the tracheo-pharyngo-esophageal structures medially from the sternocleidomastoid muscle and carotid sheath laterally. Using blunt dissection, the tracheo-pharyngo-esophageal structures are mobilized medially exposing the deep cervical fascia overlying the longus colli muscles and the anterior longitudinal ligament of the cervical spine.

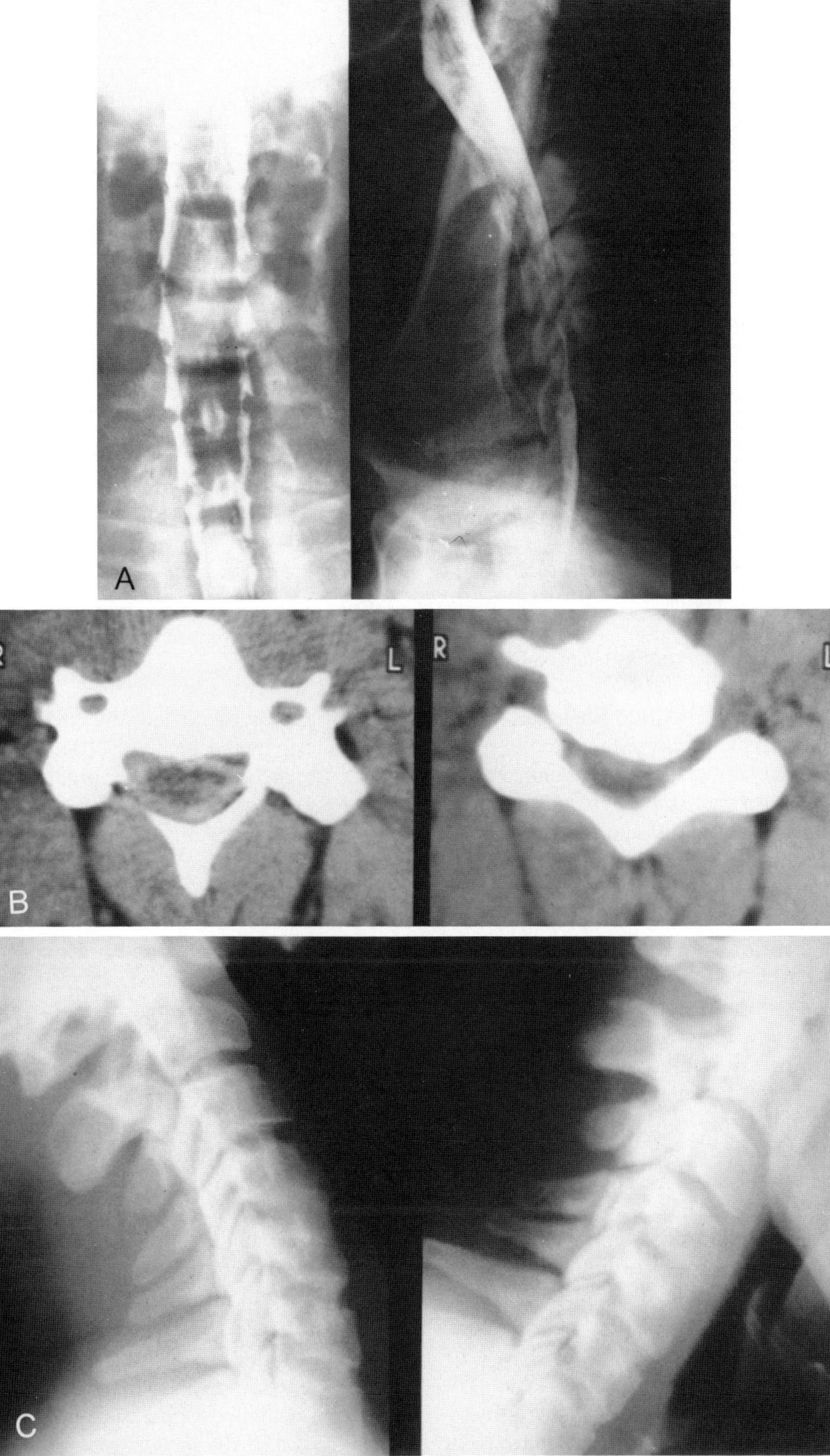

Figure 36.1. Fifty-four-year-old male with progressive spastic quadriparesis and left cervical-brachial pain. **A,** AP and lateral convention water soluble contrast myelogram. **B,** CT myelogram demonstrating that neural compressive lesions were located adjacent to the disc interspace. **C,** Postoperative lateral flexion-extension radiographs demonstrating stable spine after anterior interspace microsurgical decompression and fusion at C4–C5, C5–C6, and C6–C7 using fibular allograft wedges. The patient is now 5 years postoperative and is neurologically normal, pain-free, and working full-time.

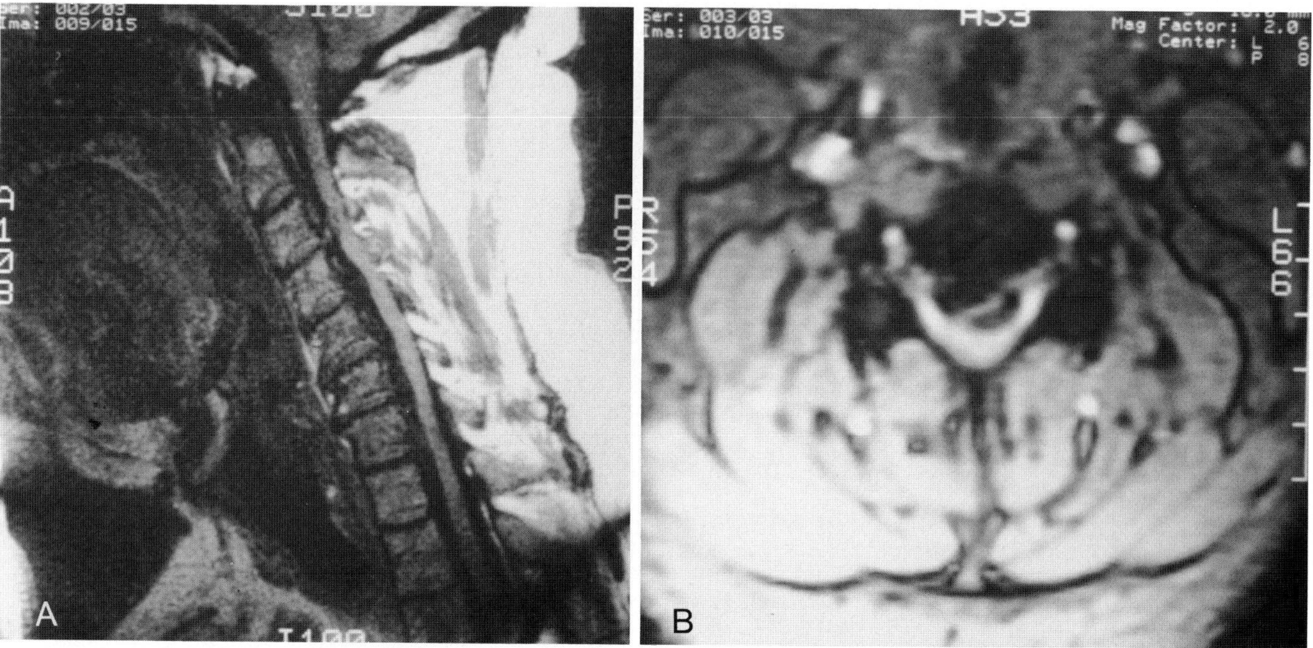

Figure 36.2. Fifty-six-year-old male with severe progressive spastic quadriparesis (Grade IV, limited to wheelchair). **A,** Sagittal MRI demonstrating severe spinal cord compression from ventral bone mass extending from C3 to T1 consistent with OPLL. **B,** Axial MRI demonstrating severe spinal cord compression.

The prevertebral fascia is incised longitudinally in the midline. A short blunt needle is inserted into a disc space, and an intraoperative lateral radiograph is obtained to establish the level of the cervical spine that is exposed. If necessary, additional soft-tissue dissection is performed. The longus colli muscles are elevated from the medial anterior vertral surface. Self-retaining anterior cervical retractors are placed (e.g., Caspar, Cloward). Toothed retractor blades are carefully placed beneath the dissected margins of the longus colli muscles.

The operating microscope is draped and brought into position for the cervical decompression and reconstruction.

Interspace Decompression/Arthrodesis. If the anterior neurocompressive lesion is adjacent to the disc (spondylosis) and the decompression is to be accomplished via the disc intervertebral space, the appropriate annulus(i) is incised and the nucleus radically removed with straight and angled curettes. When the posterior margin of the disc is exposed, the cartilaginous end-plate is removed with curettes or a burr, using a high speed drill. Additional exposure is obtained at this stage with a disc space spreader. Under careful microsurgical control, the anterior compressive lesions (osteophyte, soft disc material) are removed with a burr or small microsurgical curettes. The posterior longitudinal ligament is opened with a microsurgical nerve hook and excised with angled curettes. The neuroforamina are enlarged with angled curettes. The decompression is not considered complete until the dura has migrated anteriorly and bulges into the decompression site. A small pledget of gel-foam is generally sufficient for epidural hemostasis. The bony end-plate is perforated, and a small cup measuring about 10 mm is made for acceptance of a fibula bone allograft, preserving at least 3 mm of anterior and posterior shelf of end-plate to prevent graft migration. Under cervical traction by the anesthesiologist, the bone graft, measuring 10 mm depth, 10 mm width, and 6–7 mm height is gently impacted into the interspace and countersunk 3 mm.

Medial Decompressive Corpectomy/Arthrodesis. When the ventral mass extends behind the vertebral body(s) as with OPLL, a medial partial or complete corpectomy will be necessary to achieve adequate neural decompression. Discectomies are performed at all levels adjacent to the vertebral body that is to be excised. Under careful microsurgical control, a high speed drill with a cutting burr attached is used to drill a trench 12–14 mm in width through the medial portion of the involved vertebral bodies. As the corpectomy proceeds posteriorly, the surgeon must guard against migrating toward the opposite vertebral artery by continually reorienting. Moreover, the surgeon must make the decompression wide enough to ensure adequate access to the lateral margins of the mass; that is, the full width of the ventral spinal canal. After the rostral, caudal, and lateral borders of the ventral mass are exposed, ossified or hypertrophied posterior longitudinal ligament is removed. If the ligament is solidly calcified, it is drilled down with a small burr to a very thin shell of bone. A small sharp microsurgical nerve type hook is used to elevate and incise the ligament. Small angled microcurettes are then used to elevate and excise the remaining ligament and

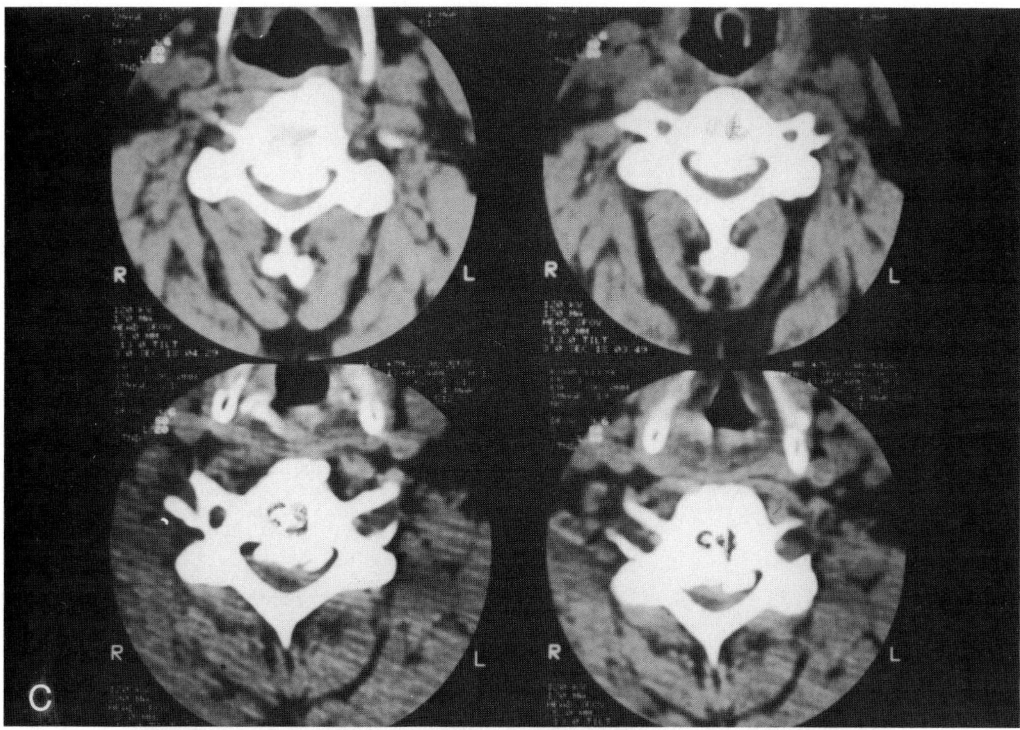

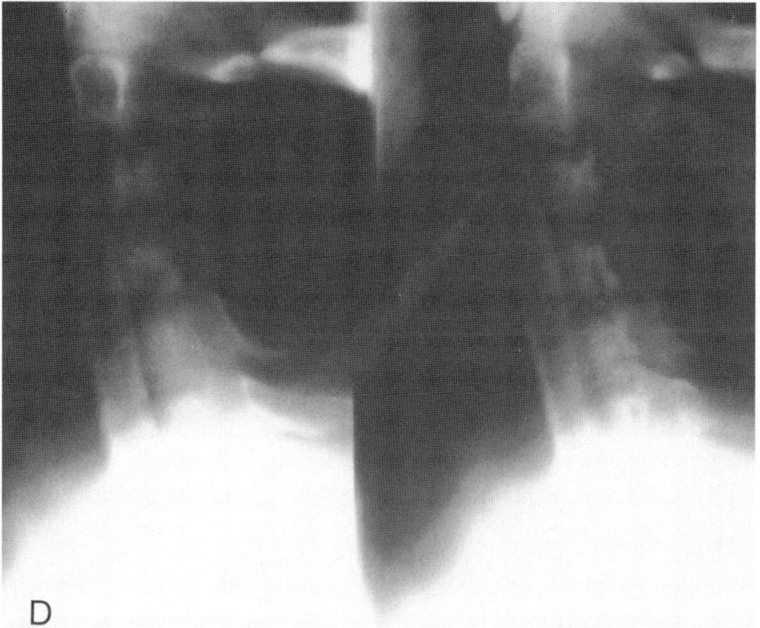

Figure 36.2.C-D. **C,** Axial CT myelogram images demonstrating OPLL compressing spinal cord over multiple vertebral segments. **D,** Lateral tomogram 6 months postoperative demonstrating graft healing extending from C2 to T1. The patient is now 2 years postoperative and has shown a remarkable recovery (Grade II, independent and ambulatory).

mineralized material. In most cases, the ligament is incompletely ossified and can be peeled from the anterior surface of the dura with microcurettes and micro-punches. In some cases, however, there is continuity of bone from the vertebral body through the ligament and into the dura such that removal of the mass results in simultaneous dural excision and cerebrospinal fluid leakage. In these instances the dural opening is occluded with gelfoam. Once the medial portion of the spinal canal is widely decompressed, angled curettes or micro-punches are used to remove any additional mass behind the lateral aspect of the vertebral body and to perform foraminotomies at each disc level. The dura is then covered with gelfoam. Slots are drilled into the end-plates of the rostral and caudal vertebral bod-

Table 36.1. Analysis of CT Myelography Data and Operative Procedures in 60 Cases*

	No. of IVC sites	No. of VBC sites	No. of cases	No. of IVD/ cases	No. of VBD/ cases
Spondylosis	1		8	1	
	2		7	2	1
	3		3	3	
	4		2	4	
OPLL	2	1	6	2	1
	3	2	7	3	2
	4	3	3	4	3
	7	6	1	7	6
Combined Spondylosis	2	1	15	2	1
+	3	2	7	3	2
OPLL	4	3	1	4	3

*Abbreviations: IVC = compressive lesion at intervertebral space; VBC = compressive lesion at retro-vertebral body; IVD = decompression via interspace; VBD = decompression via mesial corpectomy and adjacent interspace.

ies. A fibular allograft bone strut is cut to the appropriate length to slightly distract the decompressed levels. It is fashioned to lock about the anterior cortex of the rostral and caudal vertebral bodies. Under substantial halter or halo traction by the anesthetist, the bone graft is impacted and locked in place.

Upon insertion of the bone graft(s), an intraoperative lateral radiograph is obtained to verify optimal graft position prior to wound closure. If there is residual bone bleeding, a drain may be brought out through a stab wound for closed, suction drainage. The platysma is then closed with 3–0 absorbable suture. A 4–0 subcuticular absorbable suture is used to close the subcutaneous tissues. The skin may be closed with steri-strips or a fine nylon suture.

The author generally prefers to use a Philadelphia collar for 8 weeks of immobilization in those patients with one- or two-level interspace fusions or single vertebral body reconstruction. A Guilford type or cervicothoracic orthosis is prefered for three or more level interspace fusions. In patients who undergo two or more vertebral body corpectomies or those patients with softened bone secondary to osteoporosis, the author prefers to use a halo-vest for 8 weeks, followed by 4 weeks in a Philadelphia collar prior to obtaining flexion-extension radiographic verification of graft bonding and stability (see Complications).

RESULTS

The immediate postoperative neurological condition was unchanged or improved in all but two of the 60 patients. In these two patients, a transient increase in their spastic quadriparesis was observed followed by a rather dramatic recovery of neurological function compared to their preoperative grade (IV2→IIIA1 and IIIA2→I). In both patients, extensive ossified mass over multiple vertebral bodies extended through the posterior longitudinal ligament into the dura necessitating very difficult microsurgical dissection.

Table 36.2. Possible Clinical Myelopathy Grade Permutations*

	0	I	II	IIIA	IIIB	IIIC	IV
I	8	0					
II	5	3	1				
IIIA	6	9	1	1			
IIIB		3			0		
IIIC	1		3	4	1	1	
IV		1	2	6	2	2	0

*Clinical myelopathy grade: vertical axis = preoperative grade; horizontal axis = follow-up grade. Numbers in the plot correspond to number of patients with the given preoperative:postoperative grade combinations. All grades within the heavily lined squares of the plot show unchanged postoperative clinical myelopathy status. Those patients lying to the left or right of these squares show improvement or deterioration, respectively. Since all patients either stabilized or improved, there are no numbers to the right of the squares.

The 60 patients treated surgically by wide anterior microsurgical decompression have been followed for a mean period of 27 months (range 3 months to 5 years). There was a clinical myelopathic improvement at the most recent follow-up visit in all but 3 patients who were unchanged by the surgery (Table 36.2). No patient showed any permanent loss of neurological function. The improvement was observed to occur progressively over 6 months. No patient demonstrated improvement after that time interval. In the 57/60 patients who improved, improvement was observed in all categories of symptoms and signs. The least likely to improve were complaints of paresthesias and longstanding upper extremity atrophy. With respect to improvement, no significant relationship was found between the patient's age, number of levels involved, or type of anterior pathology (spondylosis versus OPLL) and the outcome of the surgical results. Two variables did appear to carry a negative prognosis for recovery of function: the severity of the preoperative myelopathy ($p < 0.01$) and the duration of symptoms prior to surgical decompression ($p<0.01$). In other words, the greater the deficit and/or the longer the duration of preoperative symptoms, the less improvement likely to be achieved. It should be noted, however, that one patient (1/10) improved from grade IIIC to normal and another patient (1/17) improved from grade IV to grade I. All arthrodeses proceeded to solid stable bony fusions at follow-up.

Complications

Nineteen patients suffered from one or more postoperative complications. In the majority of patients, these complications were considered minor. Nine patients complained of mild dysphagia (temporary in seven and permanent in two). Hoarseness of voice occurred in 10 patients (transient in eight) with non-disabling permanent recurrent laryngeal nerve pareses in two patients. Halo pin site infections occurred in two patients.

There were no deaths, but 10 major complications were encountered in eight patients. Four patients suffered respiratory obstruction postoperatively within 48 hours of surgery and required intubation and observation and management in the surgical intensive care unit for 2 days. One of these patients underwent wound exploration, but no hematoma was observed. All of these patients fully recovered. Seven patients suffered bone graft-related complications. Six of these latter patients, all with fibular strut grafts initially managed postoperatively in a Philadelphia collar orthosis, suffered dislodgement of the graft which fractured forward out of the vertebral bodies. One graft dislodgement was partial and successfully managed in the collar for 4 months. The other five patients required surgical replacement of the graft or insertion of a new fibula allograft strut followed by 8 weeks in a halo-vest orthosis. There were no graft dislodgements in patients with interspace grafts or patients managed with halo-vest orthoses. One patient with osteoporosis and rheumatoid arthritis suffered a kyphotic deformity related to telescoping of the fibular strut graft and required posterior internal fixation and fusion. All of the graft-related complications were managed successfully without compromising the patient's neurological function.

Discussion

Since the aim of this study was to assess the effect of radical anterior microsurgical decompression and reconstruction, only those patients who demonstrated evidence of spinal cord dysfunction (myelopathy) and degenerative cervical spine anterior spinal cord compression on neurodiagnostic imaging were included. The symptoms and signs of these cases were similar to those cases previously reported in the literature (1, 13, 14, 22, 26, 36, 37, 39, 46). The demographic, clinical, and pathophysiological characteristics in the present series are also similar to those previously reported for both spondylosis and OPLL: male predominance; more frequent involvement of mid-cervical vertebrae; and involvement of multiple vertebrae in most cases. The majority of patients in this and other series of cervical myelopathy secondary to degenerative spinal disease also presented with a slowly progressive myelopathy. Although neck pain and arm radicular pain and sensory loss were common, the most prevalent feature at presentation was a spastic quadriparesis. There were no distinguishing clinical features to differentiate patients suffering myelopathy or myeloradiculopathy secondary to spondylosis, OPLL, or combined spondylosis/OPLL. When graded according to extent of lower extremity dysfunction, at the time of presentation 43% of patients were severely impaired (Grades IIIB, IIIC, and IV): see Table 36.2, 43% were moderately impaired (Grades II and IIIA), and 14% were only mildly impaired (Grade I).

The following differential diagnosis should be considered in patients with this clinical presentation: structural spinal disease; neoplastic disease of the spine or spinal cord; vascular spinal cord disease (insufficiency or malformation); infectious disease of the spine or spinal cord (osteomyelitis, discitis, epidural or intramedullary abscess); myelitis, multiple sclerosis, motor neuron disease (amyotrophic lateral sclerosis, primary lateral sclerosis), or other inherited or primary degenerative myelopathic disease. The structural spinal diseases include: congenital canal stenosis or deformity and/or instability; traumatic deformity and/or instablity; disc herniation; cervical spondylosis; OPLL; diffuse idiopathic spinal hyperostosis; ossification of the ligamentum flavum; and ankylosing spondylitis. These various disease processes may present in the same patient simultaneously. In the author's experience, the most frequent difficult differential diagnostic problem has been between motor neuron disease and spinal cord compression from degenerative cervical spine disease (spondylosis/OPLL).

Clinical localization and conventional cervical spine radiology have been shown to be unreliable from a diagnostic standpoint (31, 38, 43). Although myelography has been considered as essential to localize the offending neural compressive lesions and to rule out other causes of myelopathy and myeloradiculopathy (13, 37, 45), recent evidence including the present study found that conventional myelography is unreliable in demonstrating the full extent of the spinal cord compression. (26) High-resolution, thin-section CT myelographic images with serial transverse section taken not only at the level of the disc spaces but also at the level of the vertebral bodies permit an accurate analysis of the degree of encroachment on the spinal canal and compression of the spinal cord that is superior to that obtained from conventional myelography (12, 26, 32). The ultimate role of magnetic resonance imaging (MRI) in the evaluation of patient's suffering cervical myelography is in evolution. In the present series, MRI was found to be very unreliable. Its only useful role was in ruling-out intramedullary lesions. MRI frequently failed to demonstrate ossified ventral neural compressive lesions.

In the author's practice, CT myelography is obtained whenever cervical myelography is indicated. In all cases of cervical spine stenosis, CT myelography is considered essential to fully delineate the extent of the spinal cord compression, particularly to rule out or diagnose OPLL. Even when this technique is used, however, significant spinal cord compression by a retrovertebral body mass (OPLL) can be missed if the images are limited to the level of the disc space. To ensure that an adequate study is obtained, scans must be taken at 3 mm intervals throughout each vertebral body. Otherwise, retrocorporeal mass lesions may be missed entirely, and the neural compressive lesion may be misdiagnosed as a spondylotic bar confined to the level of the disc space.

Although a trial of conservative therapy consisting of bed rest, cervical traction, and cervical collar may be attempted in cases of cervical myelopathy secondary to cervical spine degenerative disease (23, 55), recent evidence indicates that early, appropriate surgical decompression affords the patient the best chance of achieving a good long-term result (1, 4, 5, 15, 20, 24–26, 35, 37, 47, present series). The cervical spine degenerative diseases, spondylosis and OPLL, are progressive conditions (7, 41, 42, 57–59). The changes in the cervical spine may damage one or more nerve roots, the spinal cord at one or more levels, or may cause simultaneous injury to the nerve roots and spinal cord (58).

Surgical management is indicated for those patients with persistent or progression of a neurological deficit, intractable pain, and neurodiagnostic imaging demonstrating compression of the spinal cord with the risk of further spinal cord damage. In the 1960s and 1970s, posterior decompression (laminectomy) was the preferred treatment (3, 4, 14, 15, 22, 49). The benefits of laminectomy, however, are limited by the following factors. First, the ventral compressive lesions remain and continue to enlarge such that disruption of the circulation and spinal cord compression may persist. Second, the extensive decompressive laminectomy frequently required for adequate posterior decompression carries the risk of instability, deformity, loss of osseous protection, aggravation of the progression of the degenerative spine disease, and delayed neurological deterioration. Third, because the nerve roots remain stretched over the ventral mass, radiculopathy often persists. Dissatisfaction with the results of laminectomy have led some surgeons to advocate various methods of laminoplasty or a combination of laminectomy with anterior cervical fusion (48, 54). Anterior cervical discectomy combined with fusion has also been used as a sole treatment (16, 24, 29, 36). Unless stability contributes substantially to spinal cord injury, or the ventral mass is exclusively limited to the level of the disc space, cord compression will persist, especially when underlying developmental stenosis is present. Similarly, corpectomy and discectomy with release but not removal of the anterior spinal canal mass may permit regrowth of the mass with persistent or recurrent spinal cord compression; for instance, one group using this technique reported incomplete decompression in 7 of 15 patients so treated (24). All of the preceding factors may account, in part, for the limited results of the various surgical strategies that have been designed to treat the cervical myelopathies secondary to spinal degenerative disease (approximately ⅓ improved; ⅓ stabilized; and ⅓ deteriorate, acutely or delayed).

Radical anterior microsurgical cervical spine decompression and bone graft reconstruction appears to be the most direct and rational approach to the problem for most patients (1, 33, 35, 37). In 11 of the present patients and in other series, this approach has proven successful when others have failed. With proper technique, the offending ventral mass can be removed in its entirely without injuring the spinal cord. Regrowth is precluded, lateral and posterior structural elements remain intact, and nerve root compromise is relieved by the combination of removal of the central mass and foraminotomies. The anterior approach does require bony arthrodesis, and, if more than a single vertebral body and disc pair are removed or if the patient suffers osteoporosis, external fixation in the halo-vest or other orthosis for 8–12 weeks is recommended (26). In all patients so treated in this series, there have been no deaths or deterioration of neurological function. Most complications of anterior surgery are minor and transient (53), but an overall risk of serious morbidity of 2/1000 has been suggested (51). In the present series, 30% of cases had one or more complications. This is consistent with the referenced literature (11, 13, 36, 37). A higher incidence of bone graft related complications appear in the present series (17% of corpectomy patients). This can be attributed to a learning curve regarding the necessity of using halo-vest orthoses in the postoperative management of patients undergoing medial decompressive cervical corpectomies. All bone graft complications occurred in this group and should be substantially reduced by the application of an appropriate orthosis. For instance, there were no graft-related complications in the 18 patients managed postoperatively in a halo-vest orthosis.

Assessment of the postoperative results is often difficult due to several variable factors (36). Therefore, the author has attempted to quantify the disability depending upon the patient's functional capacity. This was done using the Harsh et al. (26) scale which is a combination and modification of the available methods of assessment (6, 37, 41, 43, 56). This method appears to give a better overall description of the disability rather than the individual systems which were based upon symptoms, work status, or ability to walk alone. Moreover, the present system is simple and permits reasonably straightforward comparison between different groups of patients and progress in individual patients. Using this method, the author observed an improvement of one clear grade in 15 cases (25%), including eight patients improving from Grade I to 0. Improvement of two clear grades was observed in 20 cases (33%), of three grades in 18 cases (30%), of four grades in two cases (3%) and of five grades in two cases (3%). Three patients failed to improve their myelopathy grade following surgery (5%). Hence, 95% of patients demonstrated some recovery of spinal cord function following radical anterior microsurgical decompression and reconstruction. Similar results have been reported by others approaching the problem in a similar fashion (1, 11, 26, 33, 35, 37).

In an attempt to summarize the present data in another manner, the postoperative condition of the patients may be classified as excellent (Grades 0, I) in 36 cases (60%), good (Grades II, IIIA) in 18 cases (30%), satisfactory (Grade IIIB) in 3 cases (5%), and poor (Grades III, IV, V) in 3 cases (5%). Since the severity of the preexisting myelopathy definitely influences the ultimate outcome for the patient, it is important to consider the degree of myelopathy relative to the results of surgical management. Of those patients who presented with a myelopathy grade of good or excellent, 34 of 34 cases were classified as excellent or good postoperative results (100%). In contrast, only 20 of 26 cases who presented with a poor myelopathy grade (IIIB, IIIC, IV) were classified as excellent or good results (77%).

Conclusions

Cervical myelopathy secondary to degenerative cervical spine disease is a diverse disease caused by many complex pathogenic factors (6–9, 17–19, 21, 27, 30, 39, 44, 58). The two principal pathological processes, spondylosis and OPLL, frequently overlap and may be found in the same patient. Appropriate radical anterior excision of all compressing elements appears to be successful in reversing and arresting the signs of spinal cord dysfunction in most cases (1, 26, 33, 35, 37). Not all patients will fully recover neurological function if their disease is severe and permanent pathological alterations have developed in the spinal cord prior to surgical management. Earlier recognition and application of appropriate surgical decompressive procedures may decrease the number of patients who suffer irreversible spinal cord damage.

References

1. Abe H, Tsuru M, Ito T, et al. Anterior decompression for ossification of the posterior longitudinal ligament of the cervical spine. J Neurosurg 1981;55:108–116.

2. Allen KL. Neuropathies caused by bony spurs in the cervical spine with special reference to surgical treatment. J Neurol Neurosurg Psychiatry 1952;15:20–36.

3. Bakay L, Cares HL, Smith RJ. Ossification in the region of the posterior longitudinal ligament as a cause of cervical myelopathy. J Neurol Neurosurg Psychiatry 1970;33:263–268.

4. Bishara SN. The posterior operation in treatment of cervical spondylosis with myelopathy: a long-term follow-up study. J Neurol Neurosurg Psychiatry 1971;34:393–398.

5. Boni M, Cherubino P, Denaro V, et al. Multiple subtotal somatectomy. Technique and evaluation of a series of 39 cases. Spine 1984;9:358–362.

6. Bradshaw P. Some aspects of cervical spondylosis. Q J Med 1957;41:509–516.

7. Brain W, Northfield D, Wilkinson M. Effects of mechanical stresses on the cervical spondylosis. Brain 1952;75:187–225.

8. Breig A, Turnbull I, Hassler O. Effects of mechanical stresses on the spinal cord in cervical spondylosis. A study on fresh cadaver material. J Neurosurg 1966;25:45–56.

9. Bull J, El Gammal T, Popham M. A possible genetic factor in cervical spondylosis. Br J Radiol 1969;42:9–16.

10. Cloward RB. The anterior approach for removal of ruptured cervical disks. J Neurosurg 1958;15:602–617.

11. Connonlly ES, Seymour RJ, Adams JE. Clinical evaluation of anterior cervical fusion for degenerative cervical disc disease. J Neurosurg 1965;23:431–437.

12. Cooper PR, Cohen W. Evaluation of cervical spinal cord injuries with metrizimide myelography-CT scanning. J Neurosurg 1984;61:281–289.

13. Crandall PH, Batzdorf U. Cervical spondylotic myelopathy. J Neurosurg 1966;25:57–66.

14. Epstein JA, Carras R, Lavine LS, et al. The importance of removing osteophytes as part of the surgical treatment of myeloradiculopathy in cervical spondylosis. J Neurosurg 1969;30:219–226.

15. Fager CA. Results of adequate posterior decompression in the relief of spondylotic cervical myelopathy. J Neurosurg 1973;38:684–692.

16. Galera GR, Tovi R. Anterior disc excision with interbody fusion in cervical spondylotic myelopathy and rhizopathy. J Neurosurg 1968;28:305–310.

17. Gonzalez-Feria L. The effect of surgical immobilization after laminectomy in the treatment of advanced cases of cervical spondylotic myelopathy. Acta Neurochir 1975;31:185–193.

18. Gooding MR, Wilson CB, Hoff JT. Experimental cervical myelopathy. Effects of ischemia and compression of the canine cervical spinal cord. J Neurosurg 1975;43:9–17.

19. Gooding MR, Wilson CB, Hoff JT. Experimental cervical myelopathy: autoradiographic studies of spinal cord blood flow patterns. Surg Neurol 1976;5:233–239.

20. Gorter K. Influence of laminectomy on the course of cervical myelopathy. Acta Neurochir 1976;33:265–281.

21. Gower WE, Pedrini V. Age related variations in protein polysaccharides from human nucleus pulposus, annulus fibrosus, and costal cartilage. J Bone Joint Surg 1969;51A:1154–1162.

22. Gregorius FK, Estrin T, Crandall PH. Cervical spondylotic radiculopathy and myelopathy. A long-term followup study. Arch Neurol 1976;33:618–625.

23. Gruninger W, Gruss P. Stenosis and movement of the cervical spine in cervical myelopathy. Paraplegia 1982;20:121–130.

24. Hanai K, Inouye Y, Kawai K, et al. Anterior decompression for myelopathy resulting from ossification of the posterior longitudinal ligament. J Bone Joint Surg 1982;64B:561–564.

25. Hanai K, Fujiyoshi F, Kamei K. Subtotal vertebrectomy and spinal fusion for cervical spondylotic myelopathy. Spine 1986;11:310–315.

26. Harsh GR IV, Sypert GW, Weinstein PR, et al. Cervical spine stenosis secondary to ossification of the posterior longitudinal ligament. J Neurosurg 1987;67:349–357.

27. Hashizume Y, Iijima S, Kishimoto H, et al. Pathology of spinal cord lesions caused by ossification of the posterior longitudinal ligament. Acta Neuropathol 1984;63:123–130.

28. Hinck VC, Sachdev NS. Developmental stenosis of the cervical spinal canal. Brain 1966;89:27–36.

29. Hirsch C. Cervical disk rupture: diagnosis and therapy. Acta Orthop Scand 1960;30:172–186.

30. Hukuda S, Wilson CB. Experimental cervical myelopathy: effects of compression and ischemia on the canine cervical cord. J Neurosurg 1972;37:631–652.

31. Irvine DH, Foster JB, Newell DJ, et al. Prevalence of cervical spondylosis in a general practice. Lancet 1965;1:1089–1092.

32. Isu T, Ito T, Iwasaki Y, et al. computed tomography in the diagnosis of spinal disease. No Shinkei Geka 1979;7:1171–1178.

33. Kadoya S, Nakamura T, Kwak R. A microsurgical anterior osteophytectomy for cervical spondylotic myelopathy. Spine 1984;9:437–441.

34. Kahn EA. The role of the dentate ligaments in spinal cord compression and the syndrome of lateral sclerosis. J Neurosurg 1947;4:191–199.

35. Kojima T, Waga S, Kubo Y. Anterior subtotal somatectomy for multilevel spondylosis and OPLL. No Shinkei Geka 1987;15:117–123.

36. Lunsford LD, Bissonette DJ, Zorub DS. Anterior surgery for cervical disc disease. Part 2: treatment of cervical spondylotic myelopathy in 32 cases. J Neurosurg 1980;53:12–19.

37. Mann KS, Khosla VK, Gulati DR. Cervical spondylotic myelopathy by single-stage multilevel anterior decompression. J Neurosurg 1984;60:81–87.

38. McRae DL. The significance of abnormalities of the cervical spine. AJR 1959;84:3–25.

39. Murakami N, Muroga T, Sobue I. Cervical myelopathy due to ossification of the posterior longitudinal ligament. A clinicopathologic study. Arch Neurol 1978;35:33–36.

40. Nugent GR. Clinicopathologic correlations in cervical spondylosis. Neurology 1959;9:273–281.

41. Nurick S. The natural history and the results of surgical treatment of the spinal cord disorder associated with cervical spondylosis. Brain 1972;95:101–108.

42. Nurick S. The pathogenesis of the spinal cord disorder associated with cervical spondylosis. Brain 1972;95:87–100.

43. Pallis C, Jones AM, Spillane JD. Cervical spondylosis. Incidence and implications. Brain 1954;77:274–289.

44. Payne EE, Spillane JD. The cervical spine. An anatomicopathological study of 70 specimens (using a special technique) with particular reference to the problem of cervical spondylosis. Brain 1957;80:571–596.

45. Penning L, van der Zwagg P. Biomechanical aspects of spondylotic myelopathy. Acta Radiol (Diagn) 1966;5:1090–1103.

46. Phillips DG. Surgical treatment of myelopathy with cervical spondylosis. J Neurol Neurosurg Psychiatry 1973;36:879–884.

47. Piepgras DG. Posterior decompression for myelopathy due to cervical spondylosis: laminectomy versus laminectomy with dental ligament section. Clin Neurosurg 1977;24:508–515.

48. Rappaport ZH, Rovit R. Ossification of the posterior longitudinal spinal ligament in association with anterior longitudinal ligament ankylosing hyperostosis: case report. Neurosurgery 1979;4:175–177.

49. Rozario RA, Levine H, Stein BM. Cervical myelopathy and radiculopathy secondary to ossification of the posterior longitudinal ligament. Surg Neurol 1978;10:17–20.

50. Scoville WB. Cervical spondylosis treated by bilateral facetectomy and laminectomy. J Neurosurg 1961;18:423–428.

51. Sugar O. Spinal cord malfunction after anterior cervical discectomy. Surg Neurol 1980;15:4–8.

52. Sypert GW. Cervical myelopathy: spondylosis versus OPLL. Cervical Spine Research Soc 1987;15:22.

53. Tew JM Jr, Mayfield FH. Complications of surgery of the anterior cervical spine. Clin Neurosurg 1976;23:424–434.

54. Tominaga S. The effects of intervertebral fusion in patients with myelopathy due to ossification of the posterior longitudinal ligament of the cervical spine. Int Orthop 1980;4:183–191.

55. Tsuyama N, Terayama K, Ohtani K, et al. The ossification of the posterior longitudinal ligament of the spine. J Jap Orthop Assoc 1981;55:425–440.

56. Verbiest H, Paz Y, Geuse HD. Anterolateral surgery for cervical spondylosis in cases of myelopathy or nerve root compression. J Neurosurg 1966;25:611–622.

57. Wilkinson HA, Lemay ML, Ferris EJ. Roentgenographic correlations in cervical spondylosis. AJR 1969;105:370–382.

58. Wilkinson M. Cervical Spondylosis: its early diagnosis and treatment. Philadelphia: WB Saunders, 1971:35–57.

59. Wilkinson M. The morbid anatomy of cervical spondylosis and myelopathy. Brain 1960;83:589–617.

37

Posterior Approach to Cervical Disc Disease and Cervical Spondylosis

Thomas A. Sweasey and Julian T. Hoff

Even though the anterior approach to the cervical spine has received much attention in recent years, the posterior approach to the cervical spine for disc and spondylosis remains an important part of the neurosurgeon's armamentarium. In some instances the approach, whether anterior or posterior, is dictated by the lesion itself. In other circumstances, the choice of approach is based on the expertise of the neurosurgeon with the approach. Importantly, the procedure with the lowest risk to the patient and the highest likelihood of success is preferable.

This chapter reviews the posterior approach for cervical disc disease and cervical spondylosis. Although comparisons of the anterior and posterior approaches are made, this chapter is not intended to promote the posterior approach as the "best" or "only" surgical approach to the cervical spine.

History

The first reported operation for herniated disc in the cervical spine was presented by Taylor and Collier in 1901 when they described an operation performed by Horsley in 1892 (1). In that instance the disc herniation was secondary to trauma. Subsequently, simple disc herniation was discussed by Semmes and Murphey in 1943 and by Chenault a year later. The first pathological description of spondylosis was made by Key in 1838 (2). In 1888 Strumpell and, later, Marie were the first to refer to cervical spondylitis as a cause of paraplegia. Gowers was probably the first to describe cervical spondylosis in 1892 when he reported cases of "exostoses" which were characterized by osteophytes arising from vertebral bodies. In 1911, Bailey and Casamajor presented cases of compression of the spinal cord and its roots secondary to osteoarthritis (3). They defined cervical spondylosis as narrowing of discs and subsequent vertebral body injury with osteophytic growth. Elliot then reported narrowing of the intervertebral foramina by osteoarthritis and resultant radicular symptoms (4). Anterior osteophytes were first described by Stookey in 1928 as cervical chondromas (5). Peet and Echols later showed that these "chondromas" were actually osteophytes caused by disc protrusion (6). Finally, Brian described the neurological syndromes of cervical spondylosis in 1950.

Anatomy

Important to the posterior approach to the cervical spine is a thorough understanding of surgical anatomy. The skin incision is based on the spinous processes of the vertebrae. Palpation superiorly in the midline reveals the occipital protuberance. Directing palpation inferiorly, the surgeon encounters the sloping of the skull to the foramen magnum. The ring of the first cervical vertebra, often difficult to palpate, is felt as a gap with the first palpable vertebra actually being the process of the second cervical vertebra. Cervical vertebrae three through six are usually bifid. The seventh cervical vertebra is not bifid, but is most prominent. Often the first thoracic vertebral spinous process cannot be distinguished from the seventh cervical spinous process. A lateral cervical radiograph, taken during the operation, confirms the correct levels.

The ligamentum nuchae (extending from the external occipital protuberance to the spinous process of the seventh cervical vertebra) and supraspinal and interspinal ligaments are in the midline. They provide an essentially bloodless plane for the posterior approach. The cervical laminae are directed laterally and inferiorly from the bases of the spinous process to the facet joints. The laminae generally overlap slightly with the superior lamina over the inferior lamina. The ligamentum flava extends from the inferior surface of the superior lamina to the superior surface of the inferior lamina. This structure is consistently present from the second cervical vertebra caudally, but may be absent between the first and second cervical vertebrae. The superior articular facets face posteriorly while the inferior facets face anteriorly, allowing the superior facet to overhang the inferior facet. The interverbral foramina are formed by the intervertebral discs anteriorly and the joints between the articular processes posteriorly.

The spinal canal varies in dimension throughout the

cervical spine. For example, minimum normal height of the spinal canal of the fifth cervical vertebrae is 14 mm. The canal is generally oval to triangular in shape. Arnold demonstrated the normal range of cervical spinal canals (7). The height of the canal can be measured on a lateral cervical radiograph. A measurement of 13 mm or less is often clinically significant, depending on other pathology present. The breadth of the spinal canal generally is not significant unless there is a laterally placed mass such as a tumor or herniated disc large enough to compress the spinal cord.

The spinal cord is fusiform in the neck with the maximum width at the cervical enlargement in the region of the fifth cervical vertebra. The anteroposterior dimension of the cord is approximately 8 mm at that level with the lateral dimension being approximately 13 mm. Surrounding the normal cord are spinal fluid, dura, fat, and veins. The spinal cord is attached laterally by the dentate ligaments which limit rostral-caudal movement of the cord. The nerve roots themselves exit the cord and descend slightly to reach the intervertebral foramina. There are 8 cervical roots with the first cervical root exiting above the first cervical vertebra and the eighth cervical root exiting below the seventh cervical vertebra.

The blood supply to the spinal cord is derived from one anterior and two posterior spinal arteries. These vessels are formed by radicular arteries coursing intradurally in the intervertebral foramina from the vertebral, thyrocervical, and deep cervical arteries. The anterior spinal artery subserves the anterior two-thirds of the cord while the smaller posterior spinal arteries provide blood supply to the posterior one-third of the spinal cord. Veins accompany the arteries, in general, exiting the spinal canal through the neural foramen and foramen magnum.

PATHOLOGY

The pathologic anatomy of cervical spondylosis and cervical disc disease are related. There is a reduced water content and fragmentation of the nuclear portion of the disc with aging (8). As a result, disc height is lessened from the normal disc height of approximately one-half the height of the vertebral body. Decreased disc height allows increased motion in the cervical spine. Osteophytes form which limit motion by stabilization of the joint. Osteophytes also increase the weight-bearing surface of the vertebral endplates. The actual morphology of each osteophyte is determined by the ligamental integrity and the disc herniation adjacent to it. It has been found that osteophytes which are in a horizontal plane are associated with disk herniation, while those that project upward and/or downward are not (9). Herniated cervical discs are not always accompanied by osteophytes; however, they usually develop over time at this site or at the site of removal of a herniated disc.

In addition to compression which occurs secondary to osteophytes, the ligamentum flavum thickens and loses elasticity with aging. The ligament folds inward with extension. There is a slight increase in the height of the spinal canal with extension, but folding of the ligament with the narrowing caused by the osteophytes causes maximum compression in this position.

The spinal cord itself shows various changes secondary to compression. The cord may flatten depending upon the severity of stenosis. Microscopically the spinal cord shows demyelination, worst at the levels of osteophytic compression in the lateral columns. The dorsal columns are not as severely affected. There may also be loss of anterior horn cells and loss of substance in the grey matter (10). Whether the changes in the cord or root are due directly to compression or secondarily to ischemia has not been resolved (11). It is important to note that, despite the fact that cervical spondylosis is a chronic condition, once symptoms of spinal cord compression are present the cord can sustain irreversible damage in a short time (12).

With flexion and extension of the cervical spine the nerve roots move slightly within their neural foramina. As the process of bone spur formation occurs the roots develop adhesions in the dura-arachnoid space causing relative entrapment (13). The dura may also be adherent to the neural canal. Pathologically, the nerve root may show loss of axons and myelin along with fibrotic changes. Myelin sheaths tend to be more susceptible to damage via compression than axons.

POSITIONING FOR SURGERY

Positioning for surgery generally depends on the surgeon's preference. Arguments for or against both the prone and the sitting position can be made. Specifically in favor of the prone position is the decreased risk of air embolus. Because air embolism is the major risk associated with the sitting position, placement of a central venous catheter for both monitoring and treatment of air embolus is required. Doppler monitoring of heart sounds and end-tidal carbon dioxide measurements are necessary monitoring devices for air embolism. The sitting position, on the other hand, allows the field to remain clear throughout the operation because blood drains from the field naturally. Proponents of the sitting position also feel that gravity opens the lamina slightly, allowing better access to the nerve roots.

We perform most of our posterior approach operations with the patient in the prone position because of the risks noted above. We have not had difficulty with access to nerve roots with this position. Extension and flexion should be minimized since either can cause compression of the spinal cord when the canal is narrowed from cervical spondylosis. A study by Taylor, using Pantopaque myelography in cadavers, showed the importance of avoiding hyperextension since the ligamentum flavum narrows the canal by almost 30% in this position (14).

For patients with cervical spondylosis, the anesthesiologist must be aware of the potential for spinal cord injury during intubation. For this reason, intubation should be monitored by the surgeon so that both hyperextension and hyperflexion are avoided. Depending on the skills of the anesthesiologist, either an awake intubation or fiberoptic intubation are preferred. In either case, the safe range of motion of the neck needs to be demonstrated to the anesthesiologist while the patient is awake.

Regardless of the position, the head must be firmly fixed during the procedure. For cervical disc and spondylosis operations, the Mayfield head holder provides appropriate fixation. The pins of the head holder are placed with the single pin just above the ear on the one side with two pins centered just above the ear on the opposite side. The anterior-most pin of the two is forward enough so that when the patient is turned prone the patient "rests" on this pin. The forehead and nose are checked to make sure they are not in contact with the transverse bar of the head holder. Once properly positioned in the head holder, the patient is turned prone. The head is positioned in the neutral or slightly flexed position.

Symptoms and Signs of Cervical Disc Disease

Symptomatic cervical disc herniation is uncommon, accounting for only 15% of all herniated discs in the spine. Cervical disc disease can be divided into two forms: soft disk herniation and foraminal spondylosis. The syndrome of soft disk herniation tends to be an acute process. Often the patient awakens with pain in the neck and arm. Persons in the fourth decade of life are affected most frequently, with men outnumbering women 1.4 to 1 (15). Herniation of a soft disk implies displacement of nucleus pulposus through the surrounding annulus fibrosis. Herniation tends to occur in a posterolateral direction towards the axilla of the adjacent nerve root in its foramen. The disks between the fifth and sixth and the sixth and seventh cervical vertebrae are most frequently affected.

The pain of foraminal stenosis is often intermittent, allowing periods of normal function between episodes of pain. The usual presentation of cervical radiculopathy is pain in the neck and arm in the appropriate dermatome. Additionally, pain may radiate into the medial scapular area or upper chest. Paresthesia may be present, tending to be distal in the extremity. Asymmetry of reflexes may also be of diagnostic value. With compression of a root over time, weakness and atrophy of upper extremity musculature may develop. Extension of the neck toward the side of the lesion usually causes pain in a radicular distribution (Scoville-Spurling test).

Diagnostic Studies

Plain radiographs of the cervical spine, including oblique views, should be obtained in all patients. Specific conditions including posterior spurring, abnormal fusions, and decreased disc height should be noted. The width between the posterior vertebral body and the lamina should be measured. Canal width less than 13 mm is considered to be stenotic, a measurement that may influence the choice of approach. Osteophyte formation anteriorly may also give a clue to the level of increased motion. Finally, an osteophyte at the margin of a foramen on the oblique view sometimes indicates the level of nerve root compression.

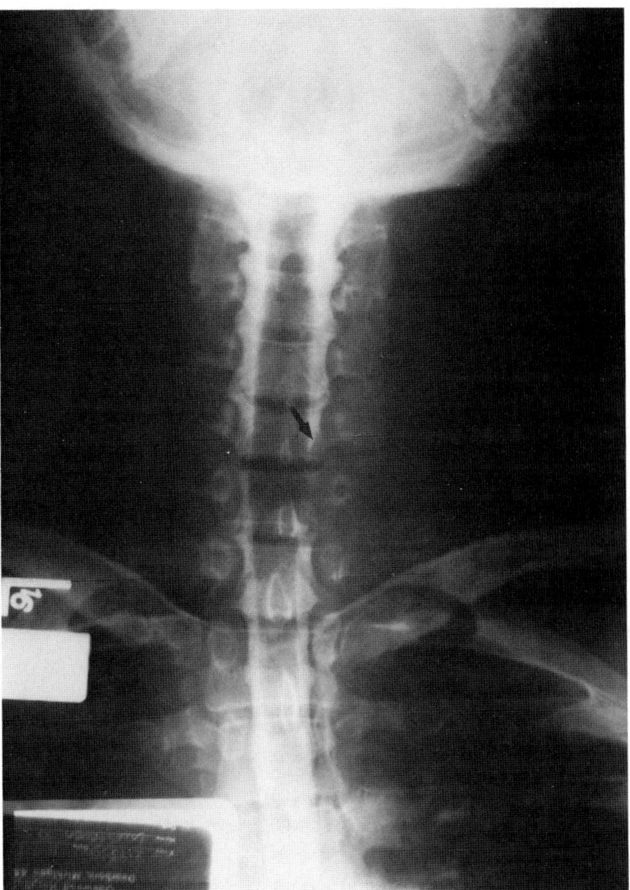

Figure 37.1. Water soluble contrast myelogram showing asymmetry of nerve root contrast at the C6–7 level on the right (*arrow*).

Myelography with water soluble contrast and postmyelography computed tomography have been the most useful studies for preoperative evaluation in our experience. The myelographic dye may be injected either in the cervical or lumbar region. We prefer a cervical injection. The myelographic views (anteroposterior, lateral, and oblique) provide information about nerve roots and the dimensions of the spinal canal (Fig. 37.1). Computed tomography compliments this procedure with additional information about the lateral recesses and shape of the canal (Figure 37.2). Extreme lateral disc herniations, which would ordinarily be missed on myelography, can be seen clearly with computed tomography. There is a 92% concurrence rate with surgical findings using these radiographic techniques (16). These studies must be carefully correlated with the patient's

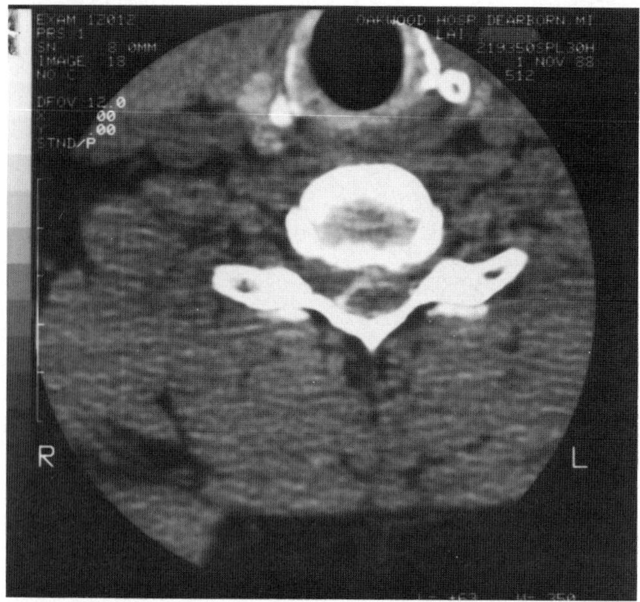

Figure 37.2. Post-myelographic computed tomography scan in the same patient as in Figure 37.1 showing the disc protruding into the spinal canal.

symptoms, since a significant percentage of patients with abnormal myelograms are asymptomatic (17).

The magnetic resonance scan is also useful in cervical disc disease although it is too early to judge its role. MRI provides excellent information in the sagittal plane (Fig. 37.3). At this time, though, roots are not as well visualized in the axial plane. Correlation with pathologic specimens is necessary to evaluate MRI's impact on evaluation of cervical disc disease. MRI may replace myelography and CT as the technique is used more. One distinct disadvantage of MRI is the lack of bone detail it provides. Often, bony compression can only be inferred by deviation of neural tissue from its normal course with MRI alone.

Electromyography is helpful in differentiating the compression neuropathies, such as carpal tunnel syndrome or ulnar neuropathy, which may confuse the diagnosis. This test, when combined with the physical examination, can be very specific for root compression. On the other hand, the EMG can be normal in patients with true radiculopathy. Consequently, the EMG is generally used only as a confirmatory test.

PATIENT SELECTION FOR SURGERY

Those patients selected for surgery should have signs and symptoms consistent with cervical radiculopathy. Unless symptoms are unusually severe or there is a significant neurological deficit, patients should initially be treated without operation. Initial treatment should involve rest, analgesics, a cervical collar, and often cervical traction. The radiological workup should correlate with the clinical symptoms. Patients treated without operation for nerve root compression may demonstrate a myelographic defect even many years after resolution of symptoms (17).

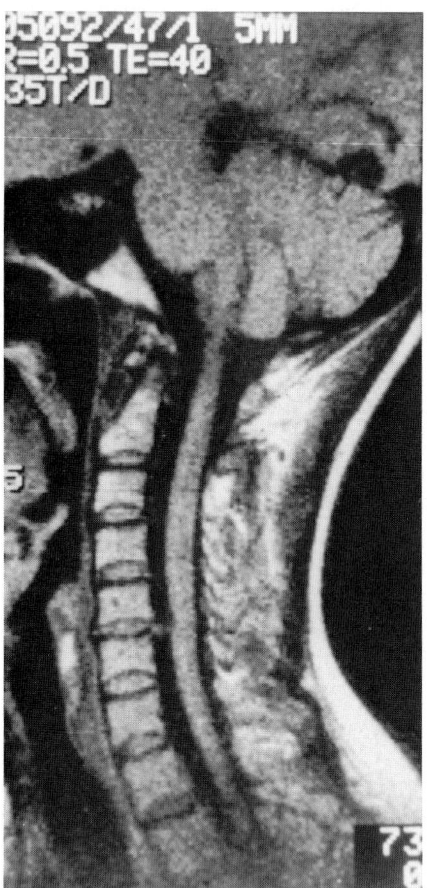

Figure 37.3. Magnetic resonance imaging scan showing a herniated disc at the C5–6 level.

It is important to remember that surgery is not indicated for neck pain alone. Additionally, patients involved in litigation should not undergo a surgical procedure until the litigation is settled or there is evidence of progressive neurological deficit.

SURGICAL PROCEDURES

The general approach for a one-level cervical laminectomy with foraminotomy requires an incision centered over the symptomatic level. Dissection is carried along the ligamentum nuchae which provides a bloodless plane. The cervical muscles are dissected subperiosteally from the spinous processes working from inferior to superior. Dissection from inferiorly to superiorly allows the surgeon to work in the direction of insertion of the muscle fibers. The muscles must be reflected laterally over the facets (Fig. 37.4). Dissection subperiosteally in the midline controls the amount of blood loss in this procedure.

The laminotomy is initiated once the appropriate level is confirmed with a lateral cervical spine radiograph. A small "keyhole" is made at the medial one-third of the superior facet (18). This opening can be made using either the air drill or a narrow foot plate Kerrison punch (Fig. 37.5). The lateral aspect of the foraminotomy is then extended into the facet joint. For this portion of the procedure the air drill is preferable. The bone is drilled away until only a thin cortical margin remains over the neural foramen. The cortical margin is then removed using a small curette. The foraminotomy should be about 1 cm in length from the lateral edge of the dural sac. Liagmentum flava which extends over the medial aspect of the nerve root is removed.

The nerve root is gently retracted superiorly. The disc fragment can usually be seen near the axilla of the root (Fig. 37.6). The herniated disc can be removed with either a small pituitary ronguer or an Epstein curette (Fig. 37.7). Occasionally, the disc does not rupture completely through the annulus. The annulus, then, is sharply incised and the disc extracted. Once the major portion of the disc is removed, gentle retraction is used to be sure the nerve root is entirely decompressed. The disc space does not have to be entered nor are the cartilaginous end-plates removed with a curette. Spur removal is best accomplished with Epstein curettes. The microscope can be used for this procedure but is not necessary when an adequate foraminotomy is performed. Hemostasis at the lateral aspect of the foraminotomy is accomplished with small bits of Gelfoam. The bone edges are covered with bone wax. The wound is then closed in layers.

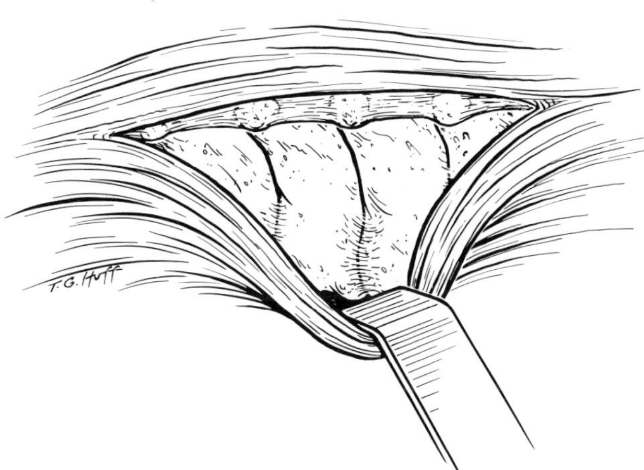

Figure 37.4. The drawing shows the retraction of the muscle laterally over the facets at the level for the laminectomy.

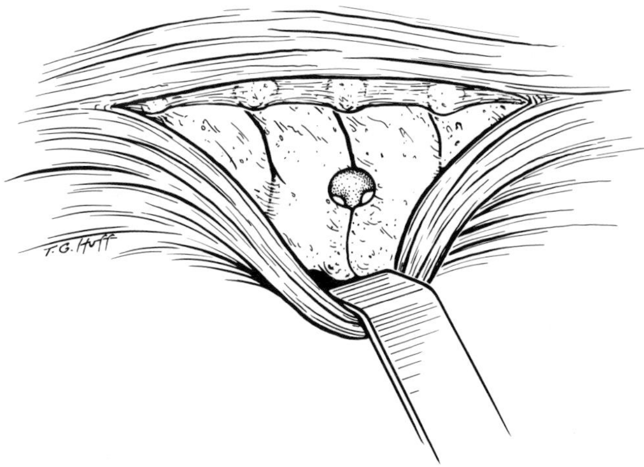

Figure 37.5. The drawing shows the initiation of the laminotomy and foraminotomy via the "keyhole."

RESULTS AND COMPLICATIONS

The posterior approach for cervical disc disease was associated with 96% good to excellent results in a study by Roberts and Collias (19). Murphey's patients had a 96% success rate in 653 cases (20). Recently, Henderson re-

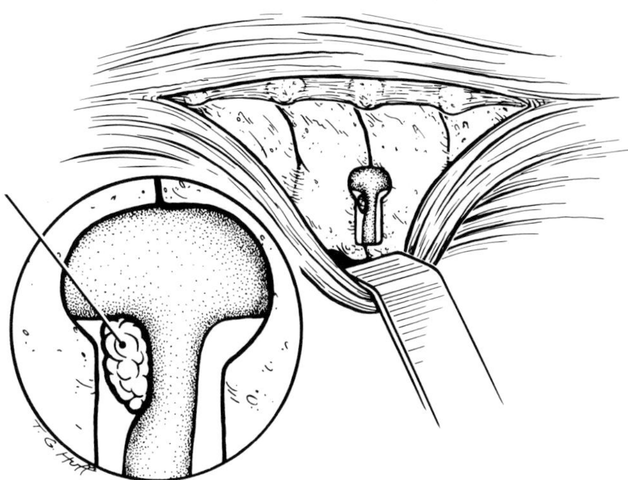

Figure 37.6. The drawing shows the completed laminotomy and foraminotomy with the disc evident below the nerve root near the axilla.

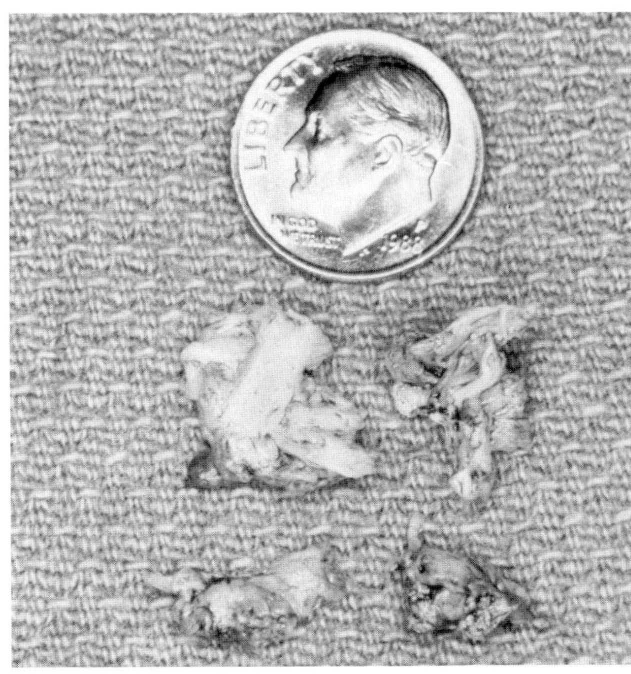

Figure 37.7. Demonstration of disc fragments removed via a posterior approach for disc on the patient with the myelogram shown in Figure 37.1.

ported 92% good to excellent results in his series of 846 cases with a posterolateral foraminotomy for acute cervical disc (21). In all these series most patients were mobilized immediately without the aid of a cervical collar.

Immediate relief of symptoms and improvement of neurologic deficit in many patients is remarkable. The complication rate is generally 1–2%; infection tends to occur most frequently. Technical operative failures are usually due to missed disc fragments. Most overall failures with this procedure are due to poor patient selection.

COMPARISON TO ANTERIOR APPROACH

Exposure of the cervical roots from the posterior approach provides the advantage of direct visualization of the root along with the dural sac (22). After the posterior approach for cervical disc there can be immediate mobilization of the neck without need for a brace. Additionally, there is no fusion involved so that increased motion at a level above or below the operative site does not create additional spurring later on. Finally, decompression of nerve roots at different levels can be performed without disruption of the disc structure at each level.

SYMPTOMS AND SIGNS OF CERVICAL SPONDYLOSIS

The symptoms of cervical spondylosis may be insidious, progressive, or associated with remissions and exacerbations (23). The first description of these symptoms was by Brain et al. in 1952 (24). Patient complaints generally include cramping in both lower extremities and a loss of coordination in the lower extremities. Younger patients with cervical stenosis often note a decrease in the ability to run. Patients may have spasticity of the lower extremities, clonus, and pathologic reflexes including hyperactivity, Babinski reflexes, and reflex spread. When stenosis is severe or has been present for a prolonged time, weakness of the lower extremities may be a prominent presenting feature. Ataxis is noted at times, as is a scissoring gait. Upper extremities are also involved, depending on the level of stenosis. Weakness and atrophy of the hands may occur. Clumsiness of fine motor movements can be an early clue to cervical myelopathy and myeloradiculopathy. Bowel and bladder function are generally spared, but when involved, are a predictor of poor outcome.

Although cervical myelopathy from cervical stenosis is thought by many to be due to cord ischemia, Hughes showed no stenosis or occlusion of cord vessels in an autopsy study of patients with cervical spondylotic myelopathy (25). As patients age, the ligamentum flavum becomes inelastic, buckling inward with extension of the neck and narrowing the spinal canal further. The diagnosis of cervical myelopathy may be complicated by the fact that amyotrophic lateral sclerosis, spinal cord tumor, combined systems disease, syringomyelia (occasionally associated with cervical stenosis), and demyelinating disease may present with many of the same symptoms. Approximately 20% of patients initially suspected to have cervical myelopathy from spondylosis will later be shown to have one of these other diseases. As with cervical disc disease, the fifth and sixth cervical vertebrae are the most commonly involved levels in cervical spondylosis. Stenosis over two levels is more common than stenosis at a single level. Often multilevel stenosis is present.

DIAGNOSTIC STUDIES

As with the evaluation of soft herniated disc, plain cervical radiographs should be obtained in all patients undergoing evaluation for cervical stenosis. The initial suspicion of stenosis as the cause for the patient's symptoms may come from a narrow canal noted on these plain films. It must be remembered that many asymptomatic individuals have narrow canals and multiple osteophytes (9). Flexion-extension cervical spine films should be obtained to determine stability. Computed tomography of the cervical spine without intrathecal contrast can confirm the presence of a narrowed canal but usually does not provide sufficient information about spinal cord and nerve root compression to allow decisions regarding specific treatment.

Currently, cervical myelography with postmyelography computed tomography provides the most useful information for surgical planning. The lateral views on the myelogram show the levels which require decompression (Fig. 37.8). Many patients show a complete block of dye movement at the level of the most severe stenosis. These patients are at risk for deterioration of their neurologic status both during the myelogram and after. The anteroposterior view may show a widened and flattened spinal cord at the levels of stenosis. The roots are often not well visualized in the cervical myelograms of patients with cervical stenosis. Postmyelographic computed tomography gives exquisite detail regarding these roots.

Magnetic resonance imaging (MRI) is becoming an important tool in the evaluation of cervical stenosis. Currently, it helps to limit the differential diagnosis by showing spinal cord tumors, plaques of multiple sclerosis, and syringomyelia. Additionally, at areas of severe stenosis, the MRI scan may show signal change in areas of cord damage (Fig. 31.9). However, the usefulness of this technique to evaluate bony cervical stenosis has not been determined. As noted above, the MRI does not demonstrate bone, so the actual compression of the spinal cord is only inferred from this study.

Electromyography can be more useful for cervical spondylosis than for simple cervical radiculopathy since it can determine which nerve roots require foraminotomy for decompression. The EMG also is helpful in differentiating amyotrophic lateral sclerosis from cervical myelopathy. For this reason, the lower extremities should be included with

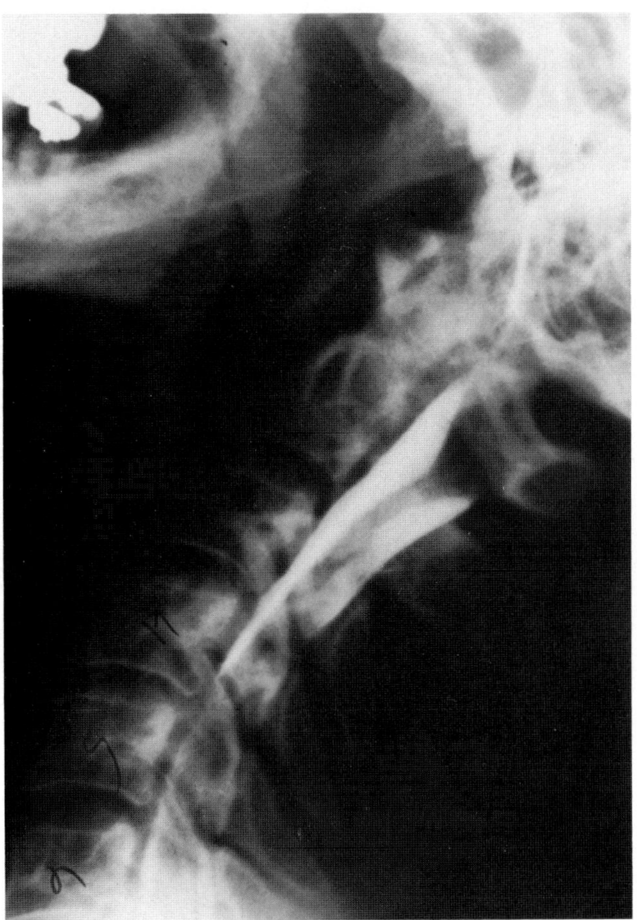

Figure 37.8. Water soluble contrast myelogram showing cervical stenosis over the lower C3, C4, C5 levels. In this instance there is minimal anterior extradural compression.

the upper extremity EMG exam to aid in differentiation of amyotrophic lateral sclerosis from cervical spondylotic myelopathy.

PATIENT SELECTION FOR SURGERY

Patients with cervical spondylosis on the whole tend to be older than patients with soft disc disease. The majority of patients are male and are in their sixth and seventh decades of life. Patients with congenital anomalies such as fusion of one or more vertebrae, surgical fusion, trauma, or malformed cervical vertebrae usually present with cervical stenosis at a much younger age.

Those patients with symptomatic cervical stenosis may present with the Brown-Sequard syndrome, anterior spinal artery syndrome, or a transverse myelopathy. A study by Guidetti and Fortuna attached more prognostic significance to the preoperative duration of myelopathy than either the age of the patient or the severity of symptoms (26). Verbiest suggested that operations should not be performed on patients with an acute onset of symptoms or with rapid deterioration of myelopathy (27).

Since the course of cervical myelopathy may be static or progressive, initial therapy is often nonoperative. Patients may respond well to treatment with analgesics, exercise, a cervical collar, and, in some instances, traction. Those who stabilize or improve may be simply followed. Patients who do not improve with medical therapy or who have increasing neurologic deficits may be candidates for surgery. Since these patients generally are older, attention needs to be directed toward the patient's general health status first. Often these patients have significant cardiovascular or pulmonary disease which may make the surgical risk prohibitive. As mentioned with cervical radiculopathy, patients who are involved with litigation should have surgical treatment deferred until the litigation is settled if possible. An exception to this treatment plan is progression of a neurologic deficit.

Patients with ossification of the posterior longitudinal ligament can be grouped separately. These patients present with symptoms of myeloradiculopathy. This condition may be better treated by the anterior approach, though the best procedure remains to be determined (28). The posterior approach should be considered in those instances where stenosis secondary to ossification of the ligament exists over multiple levels. It may be necessary to approach these lesions both anteriorly and posteriorly.

SURGICAL PROCEDURES

In our view, there are three specific indications for a posterior approach to the cervical spine for cervical spondylosis: **A,** Spinal cord compression at three or more levels; **B,** Multilevel stenosis of the cervical canal with an AP diameter less than 13 mm; and **C,** Compression of the neural foramina by lateral osteophytes.

As with the approach for cervical radiculopathy the incision is made in the midline. The bloodless plane along the ligamentous nuchae is followed to the spinous processes. The muscles inserting on the spinous processes course in a superomedial direction. Thus, working from inferior to superior on the muscle, dissection is easier, resulting in less blood loss. Once the laminae are exposed laterally to the facets, decompression of the spinal cord can be accomplished. Attention to hemostasis must be diligent throughout.

Different criteria for the length of laminectomy have been offered. Scoville reported that laminectomy one level above and one level below the area of stenosis is sufficient. Another author depends upon observance of dural pulsation for the rostral limit of the laminectomy and the beginning of normal dural-epidural relationships as the caudal limit (19). We perform a laminectomy which is at least one level above and below the area of stenosis, based on the preoperative myelogram. If there is concern during operation that compression still exists, ultrasonography is used to determine if additional decompression is required

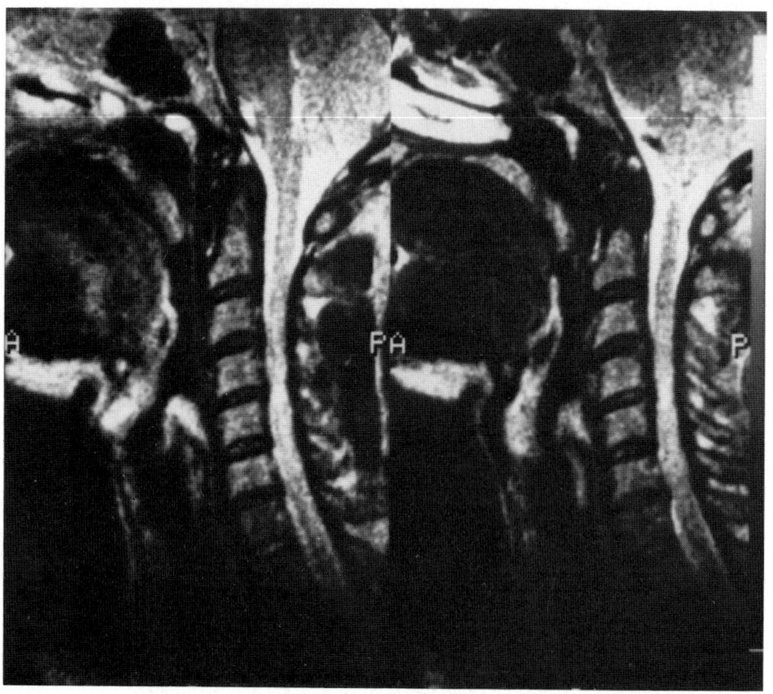

Figure 37.9. Magnetic resonance imaging in a patient with cervical stenosis. There is increased signal within the spinal cord indicating cord pathology at the level of stenosis.

(29). Pulsation of the dura is not a reliable sign of decompression in many surgeons' experience (30).

Curvature of the spine must also be considered in the decision of approach and the length of laminectomy (31). Batzdorf and Batzdorff showed that patients with a lordotic spine improved most with decompressive cervical laminectomy. They also suggested that patients with reduced cervical lordosis should undergo a more extensive laminectomy.

The width of the laminectomy defect should allow the lateral margin of the dura to be seen readily. Epidural veins are often encountered at the lateral edge of the laminectomy. Hemostasis is best accomplished by bipolar cautery and tamponade. The laminectomy itself can be performed using either rongeurs or an air drill or both. When using Kerrison rongeurs, the safest procedure is creation of a channel bilaterally from inferior to superior, adjacent to the facets (32). Once this is complete the lamina can be lifted free. The spinous processes should be removed initially before the channels are developed (Fig. 37.10).

The air drill may be used to create bony channels along the lateral gutters and also to thin the laminae over the entire extent of the laminectomy. The thin layer of bone remaining can then be removed with curettes. If the ligamentum flavum was not removed during the laminectomy it is incised and removed at this point. For patients with myeloradiculopathy, the foraminotomy can be performed before or after the laminectomy. It is generally easier to perform foraminotomies after the laminectomy, since the roots can be identified and followed into their respective foramina either with a Kerrison rongeur or with the air drill (Fig. 37.11). Care needs to be taken to protect

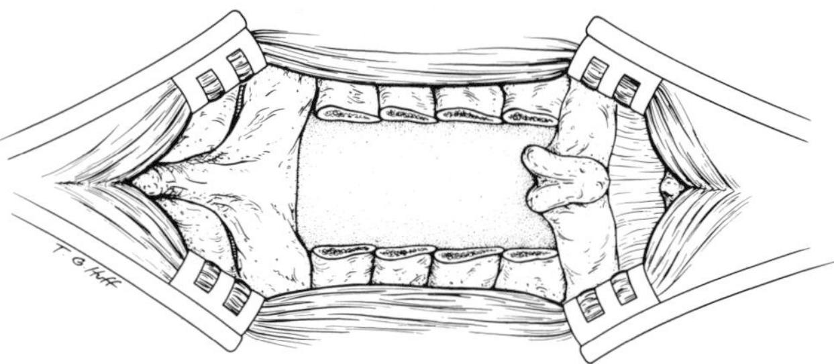

Figure 37.10. Drawing shows the completed laminectomy for cervical stenosis.

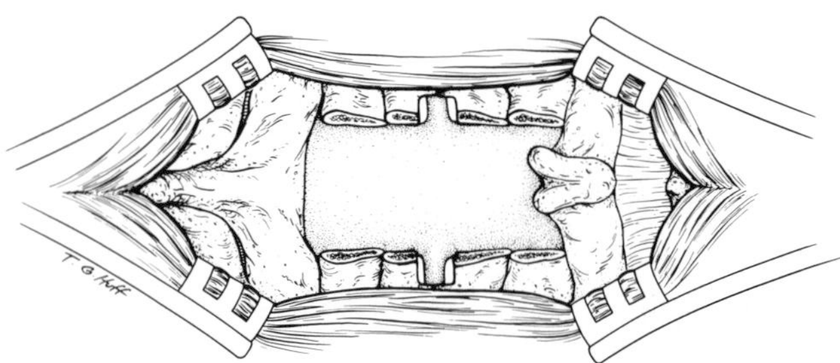

Figure 37.11. Drawing shows a completed laminectomy with bilateral foraminotomies performed for root decompression.

the dural sac in both instances. A foraminotomy should extend laterally about 1 cm from the lateral edge of the dura.

RESULTS AND COMPLICATIONS

A study by Casotto and Buoncristiani showed that 46% of patients with cervical spondylotic myelopathy had full recovery while arrest of natural progression occurred in 89% (33). Only 11% of adult patients showed kyphotic deformity after decompressive laminectomy. The large majority of patients with postoperative kyphosis had ossification of the posterior longitudinal ligament, not cervical spondylosis (34). In Symon's study of decompressive laminectomy significant improvement was documented in 29 of 41 or 70% of cases with an operative mortality rate of 2% (35). The most common causes of failure of surgery was related to patient selection, errors in diagnosis, and inadequate decompression.

Mortality rate is higher in the posterior cervical decompression group than for simple posterior disc excision. This is most likely due to age and extent of the procedure. The posterior approach should not be used if there is kyphosis or straightening of the cervical spine, since these deformities are worsened by extensive laminectomy (36).

COMPARISON TO ANTERIOR APPROACH

The posterior approach to cervical stenosis is valuable in those patients with marked narrowing throughout the cervical spinal cord. Patients with multilevel stenosis are also candidates for a posterior approach, since the number of levels which can be decompressed anteriorly becomes impractical. Both approaches may be necessary in some instances; an example is the patient with severe stenosis over multiple levels and a significant anterior defect. We currently believe these patients should initially be decompressed posteriorly to allow room for the spinal cord and then anteriorly if their symptoms are not completely relieved by the posterior approach.

CONCLUSION

The posterior surgical approach remains a valuable procedure for the treatment of cervical disc disease and cervical spondylosis. Prompt mobilization of patients after surgery without external cervical support is a distinct advantage of this approach. The posterior approach also allows access to the spinal cord from the first cervical vertebrae to the first thoracic vertebrae. Finally, nerve roots can be readily seen during operation, so that sites of compression and deformity can be corrected under direct vision.

REFERENCES

1. Taylor AR, Collier J. The occurrence of optic neuritis in lesions of the spinal cord. Injury, tumor, myelitis. Brain 1901;24:533–552.
2. Key CA. On paraplegia depending on disease of the ligaments of the spine. Guy's Hosp Rep 1838;3:17–34.
3. Bailey P, Casamajor L. Osteoarthritis of the spine as a cause of compression of the spinal cord and its contents. J Nerv Ment Dis 1911;38:588–609.
4. Elliot GR. Contribution to spinal osteoarthritis involving the cervical region. J Bone Joint Surg 1926;8:42.
5. Stookey B. Compression of the spinal cord due to ventral extradural cervical chondromas. Diagnosis and surgical treatment. Arch Neurol Psychiatry 1928;20:275–291.
6. Peet MM, Echols DH. Herniation of the nucleus pulposus. A cause of compression of the spinal cord. Arch Neurol Psychiatry 1934;32:924.
7. Arnold JG. The clinical manifestations of spondylochondrosis (spondylosis) of the cervical spine. Ann Surg 1955;141:872–889.
8. Coventry MB, Ghormley RK, Kernohan JW. The intervertebral disc: its microscopic anatomy and pathology. Part I. Anatomy, development, and physiology. J Bone Joint Surg 1945;27A:105–112.
9. McRae DL. The significance of abnormalities of the cervical spine. AJR 1960;84:3–25.
10. Hughes JT. Pathology of the spinal cord. London: Lloyd-Luke Medical Books Ltd., 1966.
11. Hoff JT, Wilson CB. The pathophysiology of cervical spondylotic radiculopathy and myelopathy. Clin Neurosurg 1977;24:474–487.
12. Okazaki H. Fundamentals of neuropathology. New York: Igaku-Shoin Ltd., 1983.
13. Frykholm R. Cervical nerve root compression resulting from disc degeneration and root-sleeve fibrosis. A clinical investigation. Acta Chir Scand Suppl 1951;160:1–149.
14. Taylor AR. The mechanism of injury to the spinal cord in the neck without damage to the vertebral column. J Bone Joint Surg 1951;33B:543–547.
15. Kelsey JL, Githens PB, Walter SD, et al. An epidemiological study of acute prolapsed cervical intervertebral disc. J Bone Joint Surg 1984;66A:907–913.
16. Modic MT, Masaryk TJ, Mulopulos GP, et al. Cervical radiculopathy: prospective evaluation with surface coil MR imaging, CT with metrizamide and metrizamide myelography. Radiology 1986;161:753–759.
17. Fager CA. Failed neck syndrome: an ounce of prevention. Clin Neurosurg 1979;27:450–465.
18. Scoville WB. Cervical disc: classification, indications and approaches with special reference to posterior keyhole operation. In: Dunsker SB ed. Cervical spondylosis. New York: Raven Press, 1981.
19. Collias JC, Roberts MP. Posterior operations for cervical disc herniation and spondylotic myelopathy. In: Schmidek and Sweet, Operative neurosurgical techniques. Orlando: Grune and Stratton, 1988:1347–1358.
20. Murphey F, Simmons J, Brunson B. Ruptured cervical discs 1939–1972. Clin Neurosurg 1973;20:9–17.
21. Henderson CM, Hennessy RG, Shuey HM, Shackelford EG. Posterior-lateral foraminotomy as an exclusive operative technique for cervical radiculopathy: a review of 846 consecutively operated cases. Neurosurgery 1983;13:504–512.
22. Raynor RB. Anterior or posterior approach to the cervical spine: an anatomical and radiographic evaluation and comparison. Neurosurgery 1983;12:7–13.
23. Lees F, Aldren-Turner JW. Natural history and prognosis of cervical spondylosis. Br Med J 1963;92:1607–1610.
24. Brain WR, Northfield D, Wilkinson M. The neurological manifestations of cervical spondylosis. Brain 1952;75:187–225.
25. Jeffreys RV. The surgical treatment of cervical myelopathy due to spondylosis and disc degeneration. J Neurol Neurosurg Psychiatry 1986;49:353–361.
26. Guidetti B, Fortuna A. Long-term results of surgical treatment of myelopathy due to cervical spondylosis. J Neurosurg 1969;30:714–21.

27. Verbiest H. The management of cervical spondylosis. Clin Neurosurg 1973;20:262–294.

28. Harsh GR, Sypert GW, Weinstein PR, et al. Cervical spine stenosis secondary to ossification of the posterior longitudinal ligament. J Neurosurg 1987;67:349–357.

29. Knake JE, Gabrielson TO, Chandler WF, et al. Real time sonography during spinal surgery. Radiology 1984;151:461–465.

30. Dohrmann GJ, Rubin JM. Cervical spondylosis and syringomyelia: suboptimal results, incomplete treatment, and the role of intraoperative ultrasound. Clin Neurosurg 1986;34:378–388.

31. Batzdorf U, Batzdorff A. Analysis of cervical spine curvature in patients with cervical spondylosis. Neurosurgery 1988;22:827–836.

32. Fager CA. Results of adequate posterior decompression in the relief of spondylotic cervical myelopathy. J Neurosurg 1973;38:684–692.

33. Casotto A, Buoncristiani P. Posterior approach in cervical spondylotic myeloradiculopathy. Acta Neurochir 1981;57:275–285.

34. Mikawa M, Shikata J, Yamamuro T. Spinal deformity and instability after multilevel cervical laminectomy. Spine 1987;12:6–11.

35. Symon L. The surgical treatment of cervical spondylotic myelopathy. Neurology 1967;17:117–127.

36. Epstein J, Janin Y. Management of cervical spondylitic myeloradiculopathy by the posterior approach. In: Bailey RW, ed. The cervical spine. Philadelphia: JB Lippincott, 1983.

38

LAMINOPLASTY

Sohei Ebara and Keiro Ono

INTRODUCTION

Laminectomy has long been a standard procedure used world-wide to decompress the spinal cord secondary to pressure from a tumor, spondylosis, intraspinal ligamentous ossification, or even trauma.

A long-term follow-up study of postoperative patients, however, showed a high incidence of swan-neck deformity and/or instability of the cervical spine. Occasional late deterioration of spinal cord function and postoperative vulnerability to acute neck trauma have also been reported (1–4). Multiple studies (1–4) attributed these disadvantages and instability to loss of the posterior bone elements and compression of the spinal cord from subsequent growth of scar tissue—the so called "laminectomy membrane" (Fig. 38.1).

In order to avoid these postlaminectomy hazards and at the same time to accomplish posterior decompression, a few Japanese surgeons developed an operation in which decompression of the spinal cord was feasible, and yet the posterior elements were saved. In 1972, Hattori (5) first introduced "expansive lamina Z-plasty" and then, in 1977, expansive open door laminoplasty was devised by Hirabayashi (6). These procedures were modified and refined by Kurokawa (7) and Tuji (8) et al. The purpose of this article is to define the indications, describe the procedure, and summarize the surgical results utilizing the technique of laminoplasty.

INDICATION

Indications for this procedure are similar to those for ordinary cervical laminectomy: multiple spondylotic lesions compressing the spinal cord or root over a distance of three intervertebral spaces, continuous type of ossified posterior longitudinal ligament (OPLL), and spinal canal stenosis under 13 mm of the AP spinal canal diameters as estimated in lateral roentgenograms. Unlike an ordinary laminectomy, laminoplasty can be indicated in cervical spondylosis accompanying instability or kyphotic deformity, provided an additional stabilization by bone grafting is feasible with the laminoplasty procedure. Laminectomy, particularly over three segments and in young adults, is often apt to enhance instability or to increase kyphosis which reduces the decompression effect of laminectomy or can worsen neurological function (1–4, 20).

SURGICAL PROCEDURE OF LAMINOPLASTY

Principally we have adopted Ito's method (9) in which the resected spinous process was utilized for strengthening the divided and elevated lamina [Hirabayashi's open door laminectomy (6)]. Surgery is performed through a midposterior approach as in an ordinary laminectomy. The patient is in a prone position on Hall's surgical frame with his head firmly fixed with a head holder (generally Mayfield tongs). In order to hold the neck as straight and horizontal as possible, the patient is positioned in a "neck neutral" and then in a "head up" position by tilting the surgical table more than 10°. The spinous processes, laminae, and articular facets are exposed with an electrocautery in the usual way from C3 to T1. Next, the spinous processes from C3 to T1 are resected, while the tip of the C2 spinous process is split with the paraspinal muscles, as shown in Fig. 38.2. At the end of surgery, these bone fragments with the spinal erector muscles are fixed onto their original position with a thin wire (Fig. 38.2), because the C2 spinous process and the inserting erector spinal muscles are key structures to rendering the neck stable. Two lateral gutters have to be made on the lamina-facet border. The lines of excision are shown in Fig. 38.3. A lateral gutter has to be deepened near the internal plate of the lamina on one side, which is not to be resected (Fig. 38.4-**A**) and has to be made into a hinge during expansion of the lamina (Fig. 38.4-**B**). The internal plate on the other side is then removed (Fig. 38.4-**A**) so that the laminae is divided on that side (Fig. 38.4-**B**). Then, the yellow ligaments are divided carefully with a small L-figured hook and a knife as the laminae are split and elevated on the side of division (Fig. 38.4-**B**). Usually the C3–C7 laminae are elevated as one flap, and partial laminectomies for C2 and T1 are performed to augment decompression (Fig. 38.3). Bleeding from the epidural vein can be controlled with a bipolar coagulator and/or hemostatic materials, if necessary. Dur-

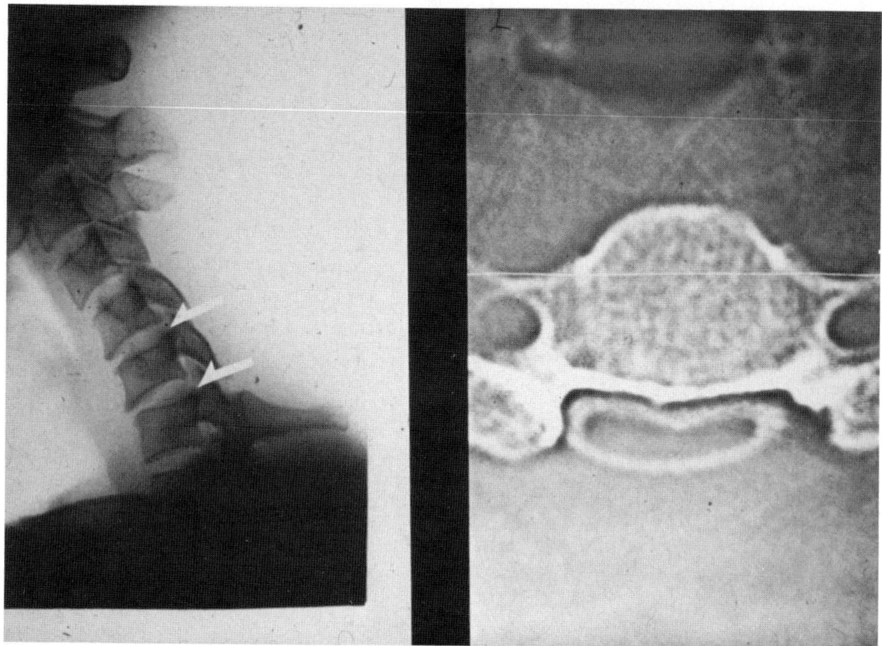

Figure 38.1. Compression of the spinal cord due to the subsequent growth of scar tissue—so-called "laminectomy membrane" and postlaminectomy kyphotic deformity.

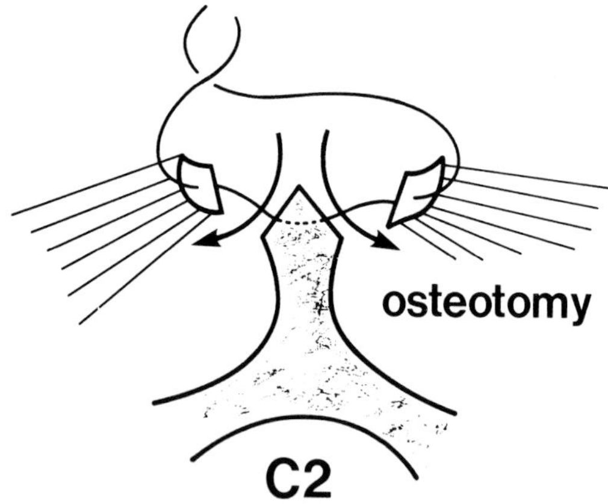

Figure 38.2. The tip of the C2 spinous process is split with the paraspinal muscles. At the end of surgery, these bone fragments with the spinal erector muscles are fixed onto their original position with a thin wire because the C2 spinous process and inserted erector spinal muscles are key structures to rendering the neck stable.

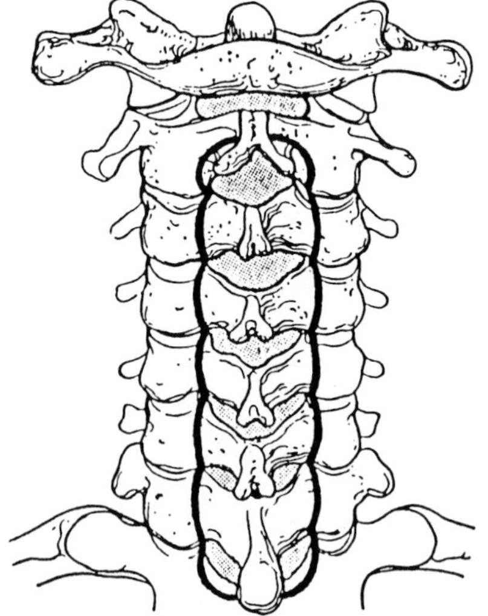

Figure 38.3. Two lateral gutters have to be made on the lamina-facet border. The lines of excision are shown in this figure. Partial laminectomy for C2 and T1 is added to augment decompression.

ing the elevation of the laminae, mild fibrous adhesions between the dura and the inner surfaces of the yellow ligament are gently separated with scissors and dissectors. The laminae is elevated, in an open door fashion, to approximately 60° or more, enough to obtain "spinal canal expansion" which results in a sufficient space between the dura and the laminae to cause a revival of dural pulsation. After the spinal canal is expanded, elevated laminae should be stabilized with bone blocks which have been harvested from the C7 and T1 spinous processes and trimmed to be fitted in the space created by the "open door lamina." Tunnels for the passage of wire are made in the inferior articular process at the C4 and C6 levels or all cervical levels when a diffuse cervical instability exists, on the side where the laminae were divided (Fig. 38.4–**C**). A small starting hole should be made at first with a surgical air drill with a small bit, after which the tunnel is opened with a small bone perforator (Fig. 38.4–**C**). A tunnel is also made through the elevated laminae (Fig. 38.4–**C**). Two pieces of bone from spinous process (C7, T1) are inserted

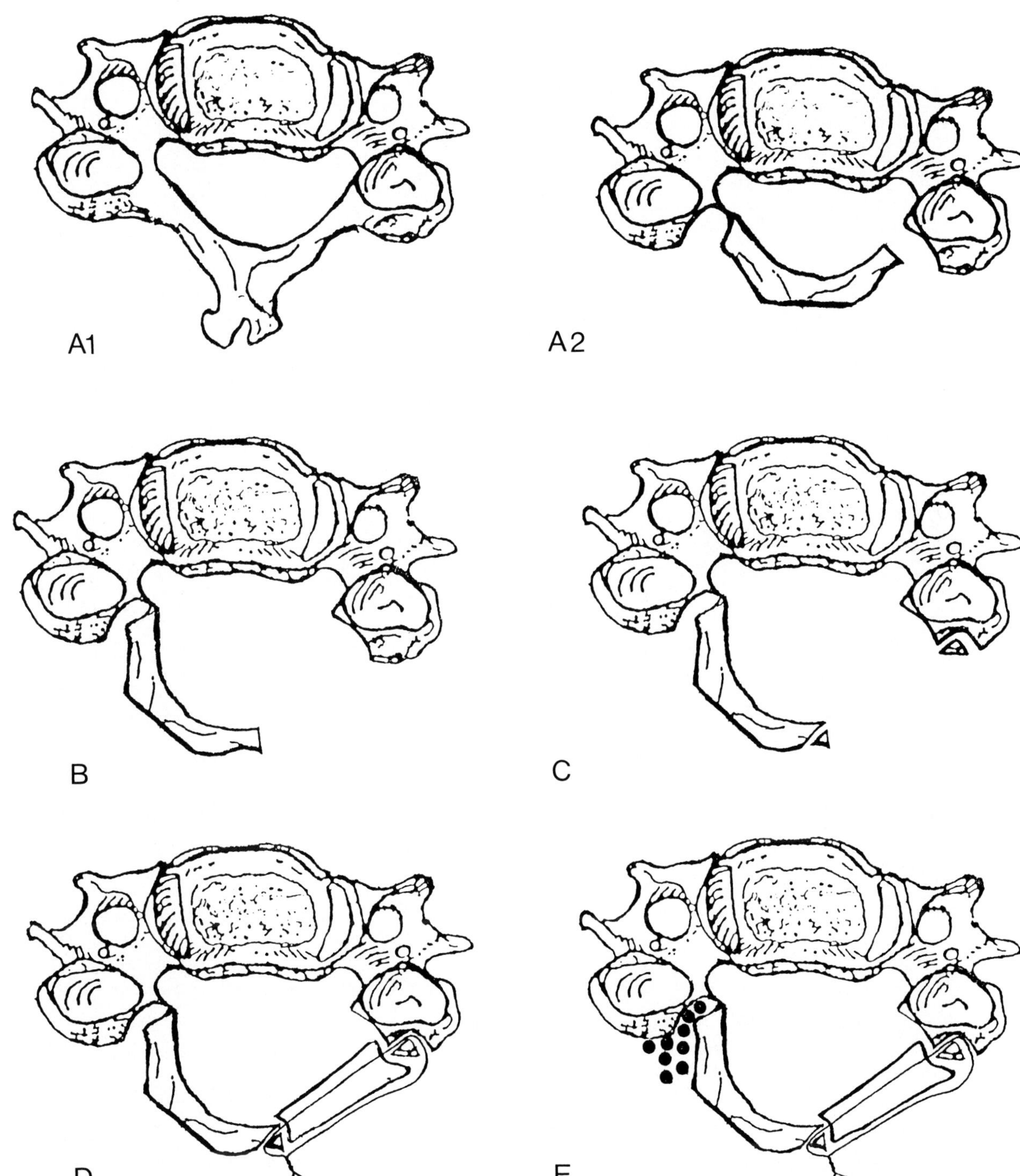

Figure 38.4. **A1, A2,** A lateral gutter has to be deepened near the internal plate of the lamina on one side, which is not to be resected and has to be made into a hinge during expansion of the lamina. The internal plate on the other side is then removed **B**, so that the laminae is divided on that side. The yellow ligaments are divided carefully with a small L-figured hook and a knife as the laminae are split and elevated on the side of division in an open door fashion, to approximately 60° or more, enough to obtain "spinal canal expansion." **C**, Tunnels for the passage of wire are made within the inferior articular process at the C4 and C6 levels or all cervical levels when a diffuse cervical instability exists, on the side where the laminae were divided. A tunnel is also made through the elevated laminae. **D,** Two pieces of bone from spinous processes (C7, T1) are inserted into the gaps between the laminae and the articular facets of C4 and C6 on the open door side. A very thin wire is threaded first through the C4 and C6 or all articular facets, through the pieces of bone, and finally through the lamina. The pieces of bone and the lamina are fixed together by tightening the wire to stabilize the laminae. **E,** Bone chips from the other spinous processes already resected are put into the gutter on the hinged side.

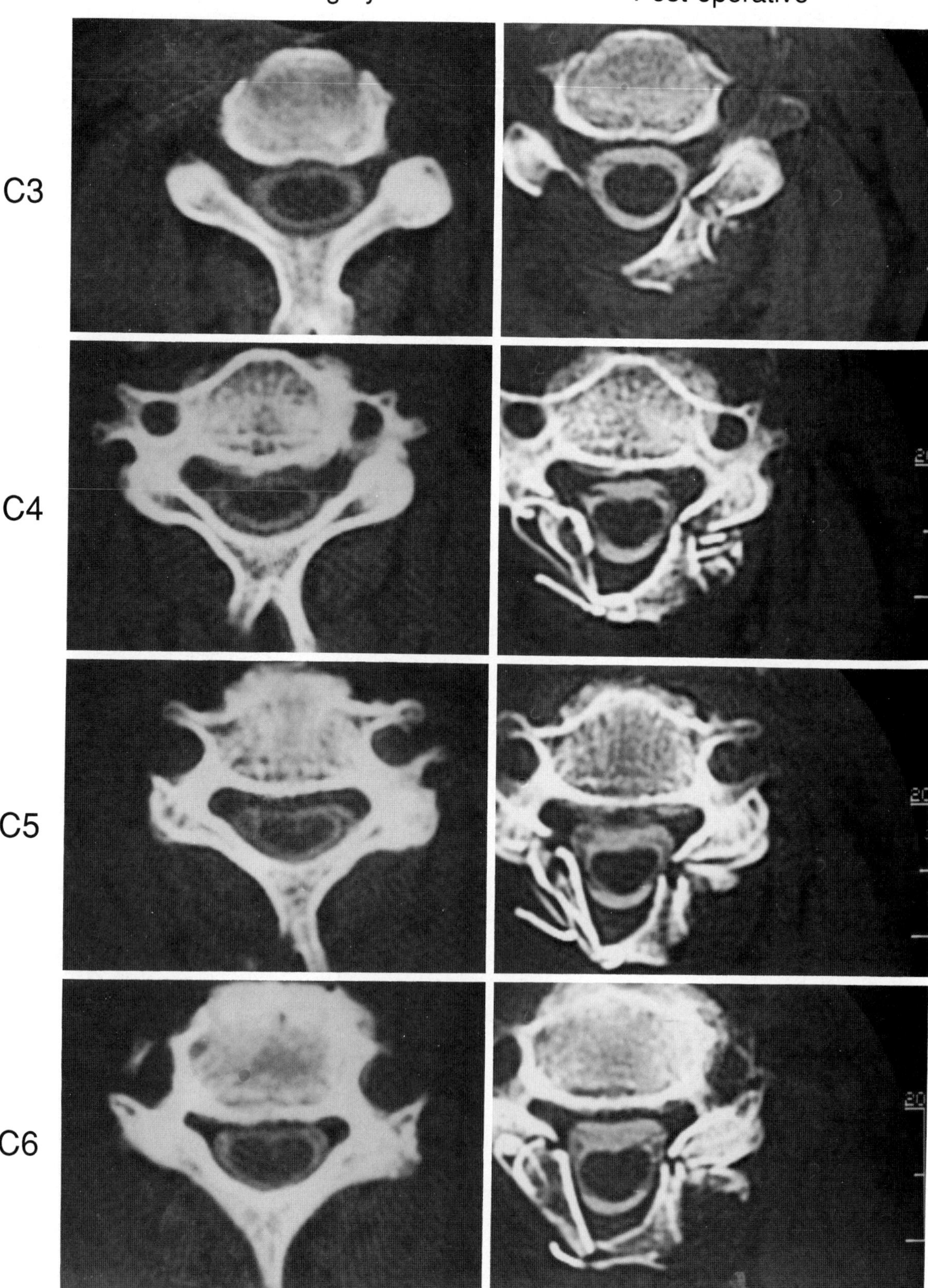

Figure 38.5. A 43-year-old female with cervical spondylotic myelopathy. Distortion and flattening of the spinal cord as visualized in CTM before surgery (left) were often satisfactorily restored to normal appearance in the postoperative images (right). Three weeks after the operation, the spinal cord often recovered its size at all levels of the cervical spine. The dural tube, which appeared to be flat before operation, became nearly circular postoperatively, and no constriction by spondylotic protrusions, scar tissues, adhesions, or calluses was observed. Such a recovery of size and shape was accompanied by a postoperative shift of the dural sac and spinal cord.

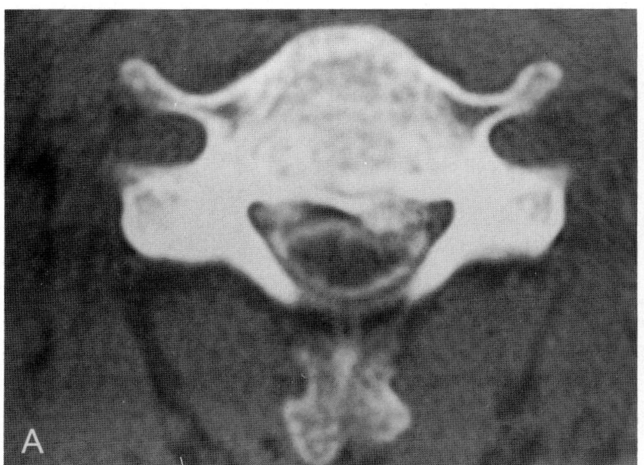

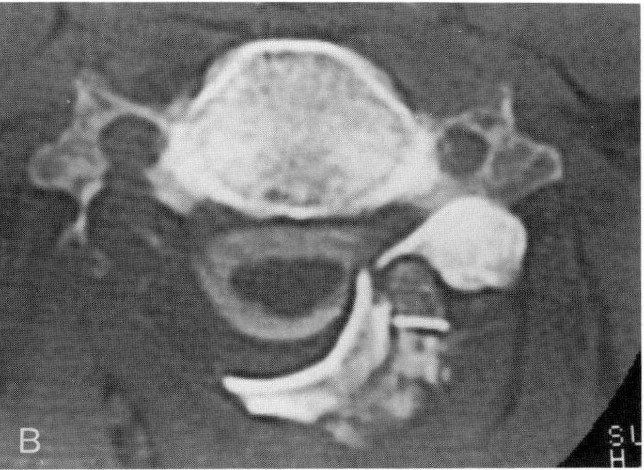

Figure 38.6. A 48-year-old man with cervical spondylotic radiculopathy and amyotrophy. A decompression facetectomy can easily be accomplished along with the laminoplasty, if radiculopathy in conjunction with myelopathy must be treated on either one or both sides. A—before surgery. B—after surgery.

into the gaps between the laminae and the articular facets of C4 and C6 on the open door side. A very thin wire is threaded first through the C4 and C6 or all articular facets, through the pieces of bone, and finally through the lamina. The pieces of bone and the lamina are fixed together by tightening the wire to stabilize the laminae (Fig. 38.4–**D**). Bone chips from the other spinous processes already resected are put into the gutter on the hinged side (Fig. 38.4–**E**). The wound is closed with a suction drain.

After the operation, the patient is kept recumbent with his neck in a neutral position but is urged to change positions in bed and 2 weeks later is allowed to stand and walk wearing a front-occipital-zygomatic brace. This brace is recommended to be worn for 2 months after the operation.

RESULTS

The operation was performed on 45 patients, 35 with cervical spondylotic myelopathy (CSM) and 10 with OPLL (ossified posterior longitudinal ligaments), among whom 28 were accompanied with spinal canal stenosis. The series was composed of 30 men and 15 women. Their age ranged from 39 to 81, with an average age of 58.2 years. The follow-up ranged from 12 to 60 months (average: 27.3 months).

Patient's ADL level before and after surgery was assessed according to the Japan Orthopedic Association score system for CSM (Table 38.1), and the recovery rate by Hirabayashi (6) was calculated as follows.

$$\text{recovery rate (\%)} = \frac{\text{post-op. score} - \text{pre-op. score}}{\text{17 (full)} - \text{pre-op. score}} \times 100$$

The neurological recovery after the operation can be estimated on the basis of this recovery rate, in which excellent means 75–100%, good 50–74%, fair 25–49%, and poor 0–24%.

Table 38.1. Criteria adopted by the Japanese Orthopedic Association for evaluation of the surgical results for cervical myelopathy

I. *Motor dysfunction of the upper extremity*	
Unable to feed oneself	0
Unable to handle chopsticks, able to eat with a spoon	1
Able to handle chopsticks with much difficulty	2
Able to handle chopsticks with slight difficulty	3
None	4
II. *Motor dysfunction of the lower extremity*	
Unable to walk	0
Can walk on flat floor with walking aid	1
Can walk up and/or down stairs with handrail	2
Lack of stability and smooth gait	3
None	4
III. *Sensory deficit*	
Upper extremity	
Severe sensory loss or pain	0
Mild sensory loss	1
None	2
Lower extremity	0–2
Trunk	0–2
IV. *Sphincter dysfunction*	
Unable to void	0
Marked difficulty in micturition (retention)	1
Difficulty in micturition (frequency, hesitation)	2
None	3

*A normal patient scores 17 points

According to this evaluation, the average ADL score was 8.5 points before operation and 13.2 points after operation. The clinical results were excellent for 12 patients (27%), good for 23 patients (51%), fair for 4 patients (9%), and poor for 6 patients (13%). Laminoplasty seemed, therefore, to provide good and stable results.

The width of the spinal canal increased as measured in the pre- and postoperative anterior-posterior (AP) diam-

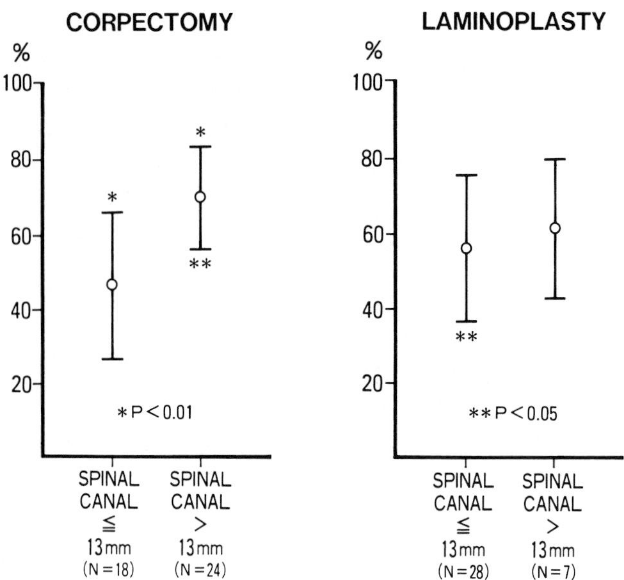

Figure 38.7. In cases with spinal canal stenosis (anterior-posterior diameter less than 13 mm) the postoperative outcome of subtotal spondylectomy was significantly inferior to that of laminoplasty.

eter on a lateral roentgenogram. The mean preoperative and postoperative measurements of the narrowest part of the spinal canal were 9.0 and 16.3 mm, respectively. The average increase in AP canal diameter at each level was as follows: 9.7 mm before and 13.7 mm after operation at the C5 vertebral level, 10.8–13.7 at C2, 10.8–14.4 at C3, 9.9–16.8 at C4, 9.4–17.2 at C6, 10.8–17.3 at C7. The enlargement of the canal was well maintained with the supporting pieces of bone to prevent collapsing of the elevated laminae.

Recent advances in imaging techniques, such as computed tomographic myelography (CTM) have made it possible to visualize the cross-sectional size and shape of the spinal canal, the arachnoid space, and the spinal cord (10–12). Distortion and flattening of the spinal cord as visualized in CTM before surgery were often satisfactorily restored to normal appearance in the postoperative images. Three weeks after the operation, the spinal cord often recovered its normal size at all levels of the cervical spine (Fig. 38.5). The dural tube, which appeared to be flat before the operation, became nearly circular postoperatively, with no constriction by spondylotic protrusions, scar tissues, and adhesions (Fig. 38.5). Such a recovery of size and shape was accompanied by a postoperative shift of the dural sac and spinal cord (Fig. 38.5).

The range of motion in the operated area decreased soon after surgery. Within 12 months after surgery, it was reduced, on average, from 42.2° to 19.7° between C3 and C7 in a total flexion-extension. Flexion was more limited than extension in 28 cases. Extension was more limited than flexion in 17 cases. This might have been caused in part by osseous ankylosis of the facets on the hinged side and bone union of grafted spinous process on the open door side. The range of cervical motion gradually improved as time elapsed, but the final follow-up still revealed a slight degree of limitation in all directions compared with the preoperative range, although patients' daily activities were not markedly restricted by this stiffness. Motion at the uppermost cervical spine may compensate for the restriction of motion in the middle and lower cervical area.

The average operation time was approximately 176 minutes, and the average blood-loss was 612 ml.

The postoperative complication to be noted in this surgery is C5 root irritation which was occasionally encountered in association with or without a transient weakness in C5 innervated muscles, such as the deltoid and the biceps brachii. C5 root irritation usually appears immediately after surgery in the form of severe shoulder pain on one side, accompanying numbness in the affected shoulder area, and occasionally weakness of the deltoid and biceps brachii. This was thought due to a tethering effect on the C5 root secondary to a large backward shift of the spinal cord (the largest shift was confirmed at C5 root level) after laminoplasty (13). Analgesics, corticosteroids, or, sometimes, traction of the neck should be utilized for relief of pain. In our series, postoperative complications of the C5 root irritation as mentioned above were as follows: shoulder pain was evident in 7 patients (severe, 4; mild, 3) and muscle weakness of the C5, C6 segments appeared within 48 hours after operation in 6 cases. However, shoulder pain disappeared within a week, and all 6 cases who showed muscle weakness recovered to normal within 3–6 months after surgery.

Twenty-nine percent of the patients who had laminoplasty complained of neck pain, which often appeared after standing, with gradual relief within 1 or 2 years.

None of the cases having undergone this procedure showed postoperative development of kyphosis in the cervical spine, but a decrease of cervical lordosis appeared in 6 cases (13%).

No infection was encountered in this series.

DISCUSSION

Laminoplasty has several advantages over an ordinary laminectomy: (**A**) postoperative instability in the cervical spine is avoidable, and the cervical spine can be further strengthened by additional bone grafting if necessary; (**B**) since a laminectomy membrane can be prevented, the decompression effect can be maintained; (**C**) a decompression facetectomy can easily be accomplished along with the laminoplasty, if radiculopathy in conjunction with myelopathy must be treated on either one or both sides (Fig. 38.6). In these cases, an iliac bone graft of a larger size is obtained and transplanted onto the split lamina over a few segments.

As for indication, the anterior procedure would be better

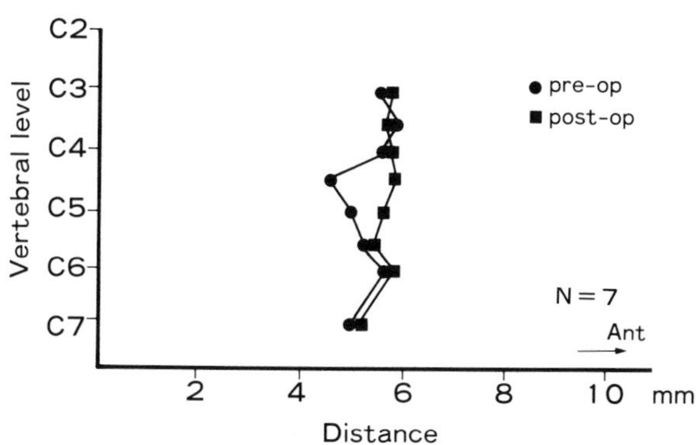

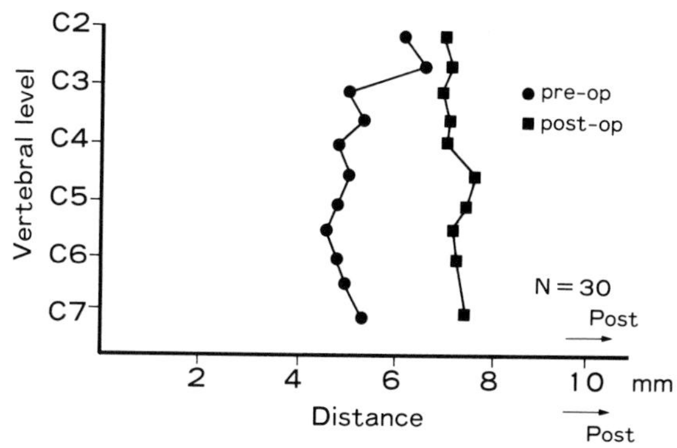

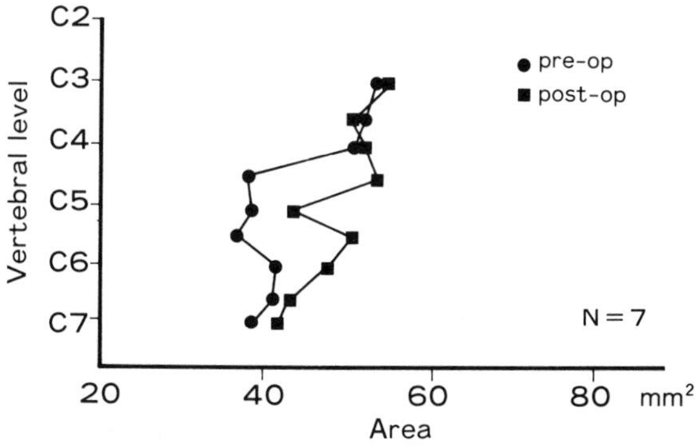

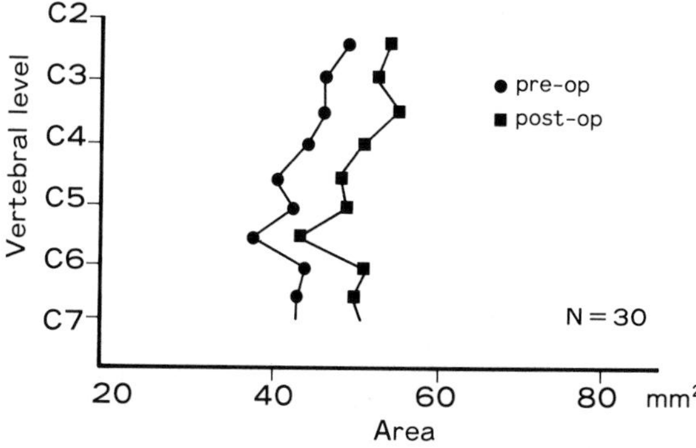

Figures 38.8 & 9. In the cases of C5 subtotal spondylectomy shift of the spinal cord and recovery of the transectional area of the spinal cord took place within the vertebral segment where subtotal resection was performed. Outside the segment no increase in these sizes was noted. On the other hand, after laminoplasty from C3 to C7, both were recognized throughout all the cervical area, not only at the compression levels, but also at levels without compression.

for patients without accompanying developmental canal stenosis and suffering from cord compression by spondylotic protrusion or disc herniation at one or two levels. The existence of spinal canal stenosis is the most important factor for deciding the choice of the surgical approach. Today, we can use various anterior decompression and stabilization techniques for cervical spondylotic myelopathy, such as anterior-interbody fusion or subtotal spondylectomy and strut graft transplantation, and good functional recovery can generally be obtained (14–16). However, in cases with spinal canal stenosis (anterior-posterior diameter less than 13mm), the postoperative outcome of subtotal spondylectomy was significantly inferior to that of laminoplasty (Fig. 38.7) (17). The spinal canal stenosis, thus, should be appreciated as the greatest contributing factor in the development of cervical compression myelopathy and therefore should be dealt with appropriately (18–19).

Fig. 38.8 and Fig. 38.9 verify the surgical decompression effects by means of CT myelography. Shift of the spinal cord and recovery of the transectional area of the spinal cord were depicted respectively in the cases of C5 subtotal resection (Fig. 38.8) and those in laminoplasty from C3 to C7 (Fig. 38.9). In subtotal spondylectomy, anterior shift of the spinal cord, recovery of the transectional area of the spinal cord, and expansion of the dural sac also took place within the vertebral segment where subtotal resection was performed. Outside the segment no increase in these sizes was noted. On the other hand, after laminoplasty, posterior shift of the spinal cord, recovery of the transectional area of the spinal cord, and expansion of the dural sac were recognized throughout the cervical area, not only at the decompression levels but also at levels without decompression. There was no difference in recovery of the transectional area of the spinal cord at the maximum compression level between subtotal spondylectomy and laminoplasty; however, a diffuse recovery from compression of the spinal cord occurred only after the laminoplasty. This means that the effect of decompression expanded over the entire cervical area. From these findings, it would be apparent that in the cases with spinal canal stenosis, only laminoplasty has a sufficient effect of decompression on the spinal cord. On the other hand, it is considered that the posterior shift of the spinal cord and expansion of the dura cause a tethering effect on a nerve root (13). This might explain an occasional C5 root irritation which was often subjected to the largest elongation in conjunction with the foregoing spinal cord shift.

Considering surgical complications in CSM, various complications were encountered with anterior intervention to multisegmental compression of the spinal cord (16). In spondylectomy, dislodging or anterior displacement of the grafted bone was not an uncommon complication. Nonunion of grafted bone was another complication, particularly in multiple interbody fusion series. The rate of these complications increased as the number of disc spaces operated-on increased. Because the risk of spinal cord injury during anterior and posterior decompression procedures was not identical, laminoplasty was considered a safer procedure. Anterior approach using subtotal resection is technically difficult, especially in cases of multisegmental compression and does not necessarily lead to results as good as those obtained with laminoplasty. Compromising the esophagus or major blood vessels in the neck is another risk that should not be ignored, particularly among elderly persons.

Furthermore, if one or two abnormal discs adjacent to the fused segment were left untreated in anterior surgery, there is a high potential of the later progression of spondylosis in the untreated levels, which might produce a recurrence of compression myelopathy (20).

Patients with cervical kyphosis or evident instability require particular consideration before indication of posterior decompression surgery, including laminoplasty. How can we treat or correct the malalignment of the cervical spine? Do we have to treat malalignment cases with an anterior approach?

Of the 45 patients operated on, three cases showed kyphotic scoliotic deformity which were included in an S-shaped deformity in their cervical spine prior to surgery. No increase of the deformity was evident after laminectomy despite the fact that no particular correction or augmentation of stabilization was attempted. Table 38.2 summarizes the results obtained in these three patients that showed cervical deformity prior to surgery. The average ADL score of these patients was 10 points before operation and 14.7 points after operation. The clinical results were excellent for 1, good for 2. The width of the spinal canal increased, to the

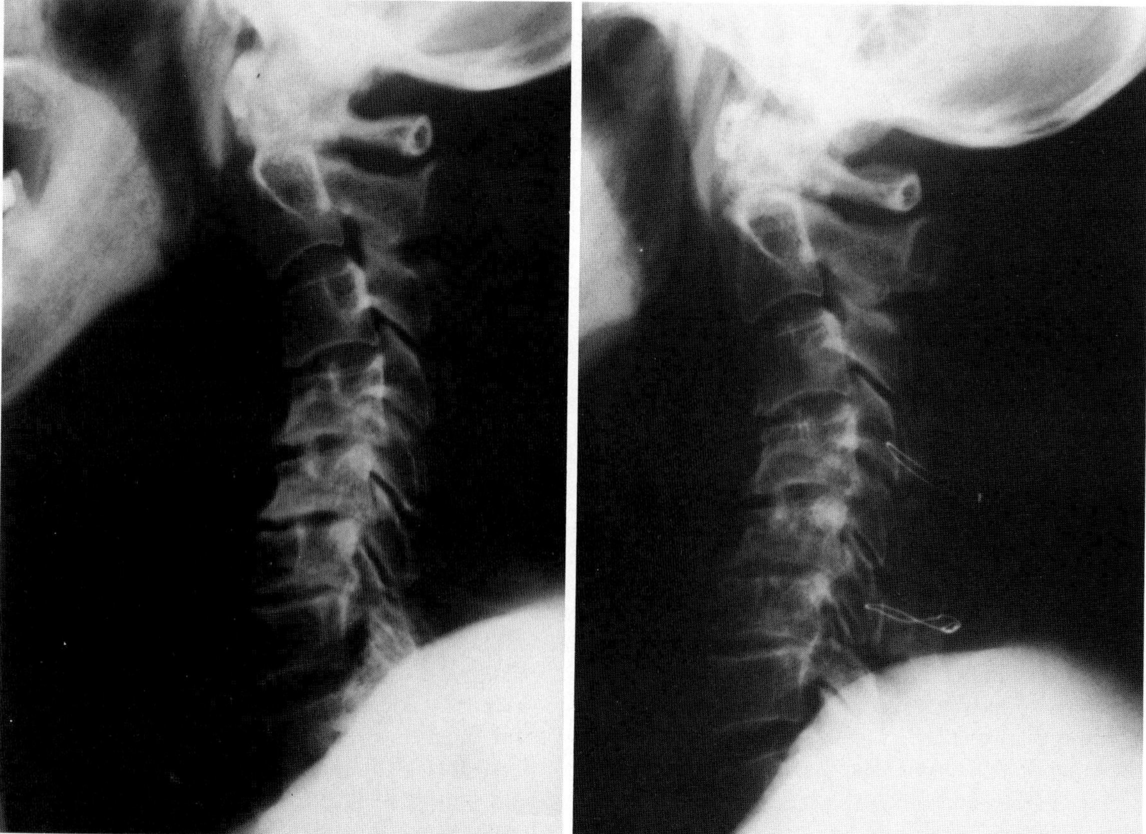

Figure 38.10. A 56-year-old man with cervical spondylotic myelopathy and kyphotic deformity. The width of the spinal canal increased to the same amount as in those without kyphosis.

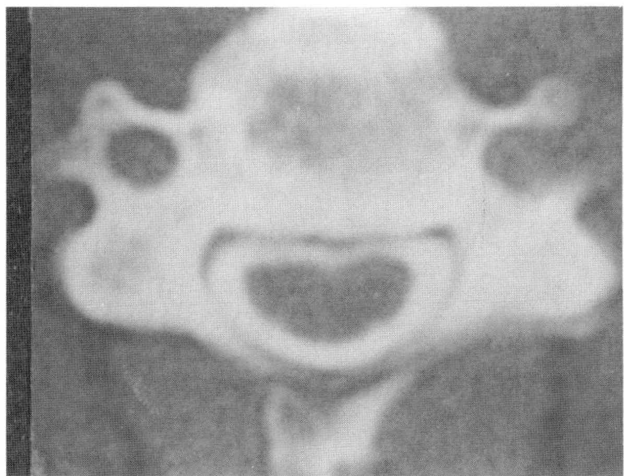

Figure 38.11. The transectional area of the spinal cord in the patient of Fig. 38.10 showed increase in the kyphotic segments as well as the lordotic segments, although shift of the midpoint of the dural sac and the spinal cord was smaller at the apex of the kyphosis as compared with the other cervical segments and flattening of the spinal cord as visualized in CTM prior to surgery remains after surgery at the apex of kyphosis.

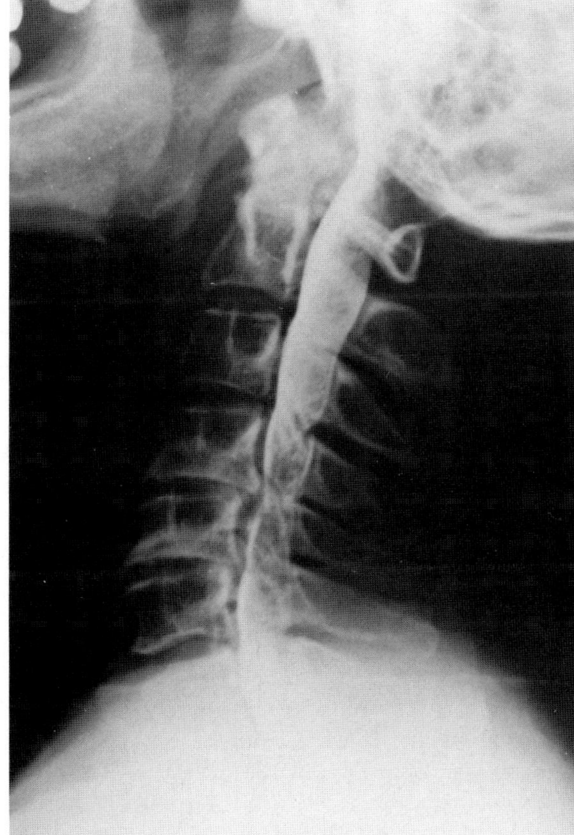

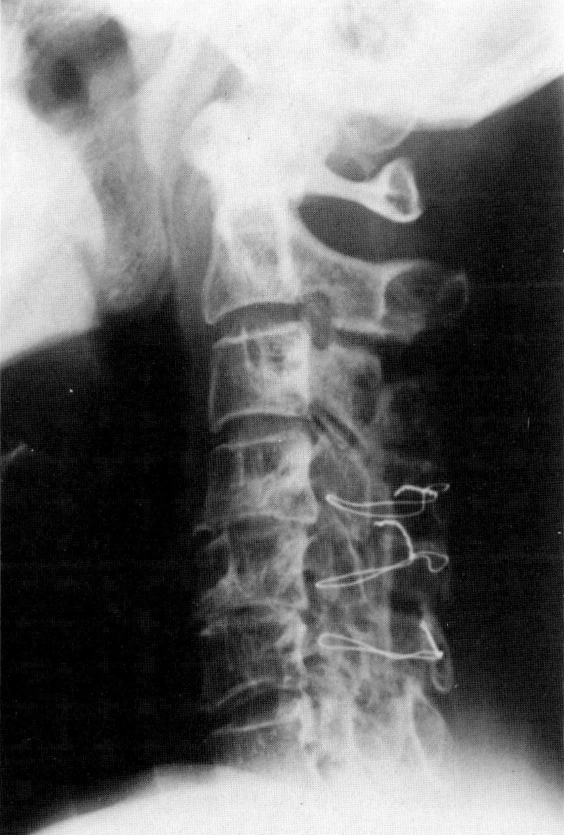

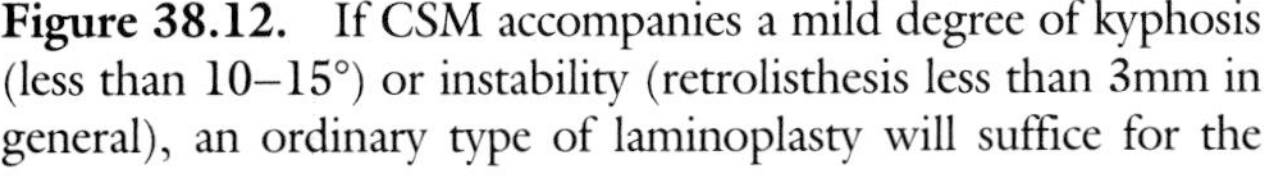

Figure 38.12. If CSM accompanies a mild degree of kyphosis (less than 10–15°) or instability (retrolisthesis less than 3mm in general), an ordinary type of laminoplasty will suffice for the condition. But if the deformity or the instability are beyond that grade, it is necessary to maintain spinal stability as well by means of a long iliac bone graft.

Table 38.2. 3 cases of Kypho-lordotic cervical spine

	Kyphotic region					Lordotic region				
				Increase					Increase	
Patient	Apex	Angle	Shift	Cord area	Dura area	Apex	Angle	Shift	Cord area	Dura area
EM	C3	−12	0.1	8	13	C6/7	10	1.4	43	75
RU	C3/4	−5	0.4	21	26	C5/6	5	1.4	11	58
YH	C4	−28	0	15	18	C6	13	3.7	35	37
		degree	m	mm	mm					

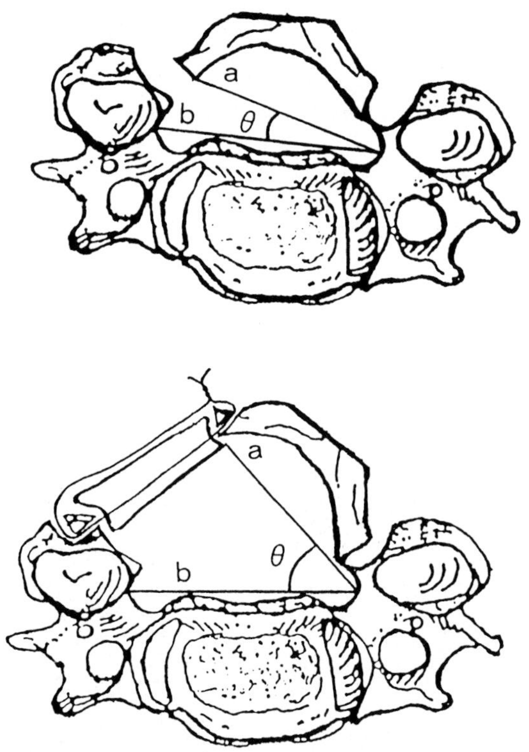

Figure 38.13. If we regard the cervical spinal canal as triangular, the area of the spinal canal is accomplished by 1/2absin0.

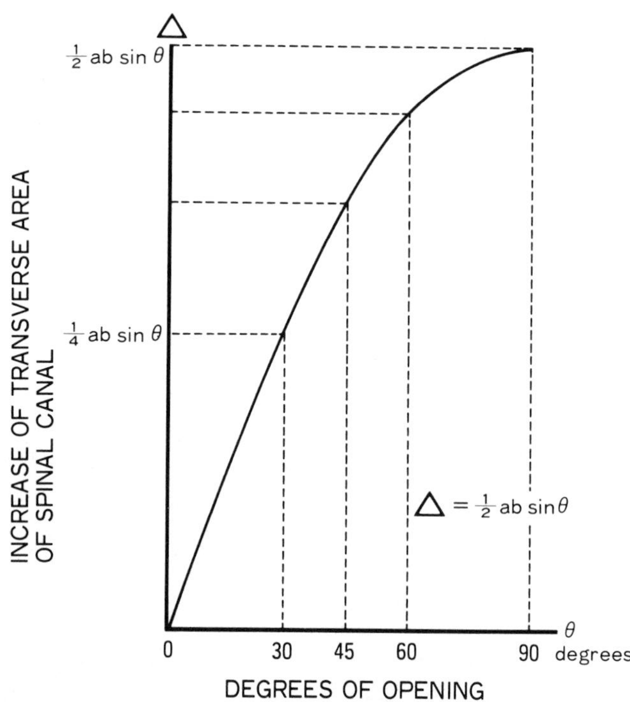

Figure 38.14. This figure shows the area of the spinal canal varying with the degrees of elevation of laminae. When the lamina is elevated to 60°, the transectional area of the spinal canal attains its near-maximum size.

same amount as in those without kyphosis (Fig. 38.10). But shift of the midpoint of the dural sac and the spinal cord is smaller at the apex of the kyphosis as compared with the other cervical segments, and flattening of the spinal cord as visualized in CTM before surgery continued after surgery at the apex of kyphosis, although the transectional area of the spinal cord showed increase in the kyphotic segments as well as the lordotic segments (Fig. 38.11). Thus, operative results of these kyphotic patients are as good as those of the patients without cervical deformity (with normal lordosis). However, it should be born in mind that there exists a critical grade of kyphosis, beyond which the effect of posterior decompression surgery is not guaranteed. This limit is unknown and remains for future studies to determine. At present we did not experience a progression of kyphosis or S-shaped deformity after laminoplasty. Conclusively, if CSM accompanies a mild degree of kyphosis (less than 10–15°) or instability (retrolisthesis less than 3mm in general), an ordinary type of laminoplasty will suffice for the condition. If the deformity or the instability are beyond this, however, it is necessary to maintain spinal stability as well by means of a long iliac bone graft (Fig. 38.12).

How much the laminae must be widened for sufficient decompression of the spinal cord and dural sac is one of the most important factors to consider in securing the best clinical results. If we regard the cervical spinal canal as trianglular, as in Fig. 38.13, the area of the spinal canal is approximated by 1/2 ab sin0. Fig. 38.14 shows the area of the spinal canal varying with the degree of elevation of the laminae. When the laminae is elevated to 60°, the transectional area of the spinal canal attains its near-maximum size. From this calculation, we can recommend that the laminae be elevated to about 60° in order to maximize the decompression effect on the spinal cord. Upon elevation of the hinged laminae to about 60°, the dural sac was markedly expanded to its maximum size, and pulsation was restored.

REFERENCES

1. Crandall PH, Gregorius FK. Long-term follow-up of surgical treatment of cervical spondylotic myelopathy. Spine 1977;2:139–146.

2. Gregorius FK, Estrin T, Grandall PH. Cervical spondylotic radiculopathy and myelopathy. Arch Neurol 1976;33:618–625.

3. Guidetti B, Fortuna A. Long-term results of surgical treatment of myelopathy due to cervical spondylosis. J Neurosurg 1969;30:714–721.

4. Sim FH, Svien HJ, Bickel WH, Janes JM. Swan-neck deformity following extensive cervical laminectomy. A review of twenty-one cases. J Bone Joint Surg 1974;56A:564–580.

5. Hattori S. Cervical myelopathy. J Japanese Orthop Assn 1978;52:581–593.

6. Hirabayashi K, Miyakawa J, Satomi K, Maruyama T, Wakano K. Operative results and postoperative progression of ossification among patients with of cervical posterior longitudinal ligament. Spine 1981;6:354–364.

7. Kurokawa K, Tanaka H, Tyuyama N, et al. Double door laminoplasty through longitudinal slitting of the spinous process for cervical spondylotic myelopathy. Clin Orthop (Jpn) 1984;19:483–490.

8. Tsuji H. Laminoplasty for patients with compressive myelopathy due to so-called spinal canal stenosis in cervical and thoracic regions. Spine 1982;7:28–34.

9. Itoh T, Tsuji H. Technical improvements and results of laminoplasty for compressive myelopathy in the cervical spine. Spine 1985;10:729–736.

10. Thijssen HOM, Keyser A, Horstink MWM, Meijer E. Morphology of the cervical spinal cord on computed myelography. Neuroradiology 1979;18:57–62.

11. Fujiwara K, Yonenobu K, Hiroshima K, Ebara S, Yamashita K, Ono K. Morphometry of the cervical spinal cord and its relation to pathology in cases with compression myelopathy. Spine 1988;13:1212–1216.

12. Fujiwara K, Yonenobu K, Ebara S, Yamashita K, Ono K. The prognosis of surgery for cervical compression myelopathy. J Bone Joint Surg 1989;71B:393–398.

13. Ebara S, Yonenobu K, Fujiwara K, Yamashita K, Ono K. Neurological complications after surgical treatment for cervical radiculopathy and myelopathy. Clin Orthop (Jpn) 1987;22:802–810.

14. Cloward RB. The anterior approach of removal of ruptured disks. J Neurosurg 1958;15:602.

15. Smith GW, Robimson RA. The treatment of certain cervical spine disorders by anterior removal of the intervertevral disc and interbody fusion. J Bone Joint Surg 1958;40A:607–624.

16. Yonenobu K, Fuji T, Ono K, Okada K, Yamamoto T, Harada N. Choice of surgical treatment for multisegmental cervical spondylotic myelopathy. Spine 1985;10:710–716.

17. Fujiwara K, Yonenobu K, Ebara S, Ono K. Choice of treatment for multisegmental cervical spondylotic myelopathy. 6th Cervical Spine Research Society (European Edition). Switzerland: St Gallen, 1989.

18. Ogino H, Tada K, Okada K, et al. Canal diameter, anteroposterior compression ratio, and spondylotic myelopathy of the cervical spine. Spine 1983;8:1–15.

19. Ono K, Ota H, Tada K, Yamamoto T. Cervical myelopathy secondary to multiple spondylotic protrusions. A clinicopathologic study. Spine 1977;2:109–125.

20. Yonenobu K, Okada K, Fuji T, Fujiwara K, Yamashita K, Ono K. Causes of neurologic deterioration following surgical treatment of cervical myelopathy. Spine 1986;11:818–823.

39

Ossification of Posterior Longitudinal Ligament

Juji Takeuchi and Yoshihiro Takebe

Introduction

The spinal vertebral column is supported by six ligaments; anterior longitudinal ligament (ALL), posterior longitudinal ligament (PLL), ligamentum flavum or yellow ligament (YL), capsular ligaments, supraspinous ligament (SSL), and interspinous capsular ligament. Ossification may occur in any ligament. Ossification of the posterior longitudinal ligament (OPLL), however, is frequently accompanied by severe and devastating neurological deficits.

OPLL was reported as early as 1838 by Key in the Guy's Hospital Report (1); however, reports thereafter of Caucasians have been very few (2).

In 1960, Tsukimoto reported the autopsy findings of a 47-year-old Japanese male with OPLL extending between C3 and C4 vertebral bodies (3). Since then many reports have appeared in Japan, enabling some understanding of the disease more profoundly and clearly, and establishing it as a disease entity (4–20). Further, the Ministry of Public Health and Welfare of Japan organized the Investigation Committee for OPLL, and many cases have been collected and analyzed (21–23). Features of this disease which have been distinguished are as follows: (*a*) it seems to be rare in Caucasians but is common in Asians (24–27), particularly the Japanese; (*b*) it is estimated that 3–5% of Japanese over the age of 40 years have OPLL; (*c*) it is definitely hereditary in origin; (*d*) it tends to develop in the cervical region, but there are a few occurrences in the thoracic or lumbar region; (*e*) it is frequently associated with ossification of the anterior longitudinal ligament, yellow ligament, or supraspinous ligament (diffuse idiopathic skeletal hyperostosis); and (*f*) it can be asymptomatic in the early stages, but in later stages it is accompanied either by radiculopathy, myelopathy, or by both; (*g*) it is slightly more common in males.

Heredity

Investigation by the Committee on large numbers of patients and their immediate relatives (fathers, mothers, brothers, sisters, or children) disclosed that heredity is one of the important pathogenetic factors.

Terayama, who analyzed the collected cases, reported that among patients' relatives there was a higher incidence of OPLL; as many as 30–40% of them showed OPLL on radiographs. This was especially notable if relatives of the age between 40–70 years were selected (Fig. 39.1). The figure was quite high comparing the same age control group, in which 3–5% of people had OPLL on radiographs. Those relatives also had a high incidence of ossification of yellow ligament (31.4%) and ossification of anterior longitudinal ligament (41.1%). On the other hand, the rate of OPLL involvement of spouses of patients was found to be within the normal range (Tables 39.1, 39.2, 39.3).

Accordingly, the hereditary incidence of OPLL was as much as 10 times higher in afflicted family lines than in control groups. However, factors other than heredity may also be involved. For example, it is usual that a family eats the same food. If the food, especially that habitually taken in the early, formative years, might have some influence on OPLL development, then a patient's family could have developed OPLL more frequently than other groups based on dietary factors. Accordingly, the question of heredity investigated by the Committee was not a simple one, and the pathogenesis of OPLL may involve several factors (28).

Epidemiology

In 1982, Otsuka et al. picked a small village (Yachiho village) in Nagano prefecture of Japan and performed an epidemiological investigation (29, 30). People over the age 50 were adopted for the study, as it was necessary to take radiographs. The result is now considered to be representative and to express the average epidemiological aspect in Japan (Table 39.4).

A total of 404 men (50.9% of residents) and 569 women (51.5% of residents) cooperated in the study. Mean age was 62.9 years old.

It was disclosed that OPLL was found in the x-rays of 20 men (5.0%) and in 18 women (3.2%) totaling 38 persons (3.9%) of all subjects investigated (Fig. 39.2).

As for ossification of YL (OYL), 25 men (6.2%) and 23 women (4.0%) showed it in radiographs. These figures

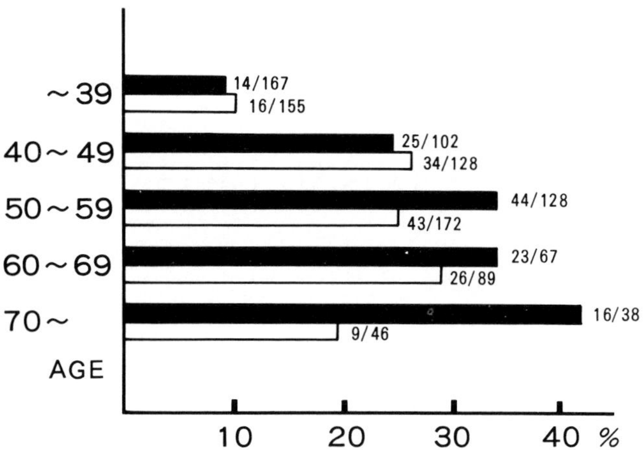

Figure 39.1. Incidence of OPLL in patient's relatives (The Committee). Notice the high incidence of OPLL; (solid bar: male; empty bar: female).

Table 39.1. No. of Cases Investigated by the Committee

	No. of probands	No. of relatives	Total
1981–1983	152	456	608
1984	100	317	417
1985	95	341	436
Total	347	1114	1461

Table 39.2. Frequency of OPLL in 347 Families (The Committee)

	No.	OPLL(+)	%
Parents	69	17	24.6
Brothers	636	192	30.2
Children	304	33	10.9
Others	104	12	11.5
Total	1113	254	22.8

may be somewhat high, even among the Japanese people. However, considering the age of the subjects investigated, many consider the figures to be reasonably acceptable (Tables 39.5, 39.6).

In 1984, Merlini and Terayama investigated cervical radiographs of 1258 patients taken and stored in Instituto Ortopedico Rizzoli and Centro Traumatologi Ortopedico, Bologna, Italy (31). Twenty-one patients had cervical symptoms, but the other 1237 patients had no symptoms. The study was considered useful as an estimate of epidemiology of OPLL in Italy, since the subjects were over the age of 35 years and age distribution was even.

Twenty-two out of 1258 patients had OPLL on x-rays (1.7%); 12 were male (1.9%), and 10 were female (1.6%). There were 3 patients with thoraco-lumbar OPLL. Of the 22 cases having OPLL, 7 had symptoms due to OPLL.

These figures may be unexpectedly high but may be instructive that even in Caucasians, OPLL may be more frequent than hitherto considered.

Table 39.3. Frequency of OPLL in Relatives of 347 Probands (The Committee)

Age	Male	Female	Total	%
–39	14/167	16/155	30/322	9.3
40–49	25/102	34/128	59/230	25.7
50–59	44/128	43/172	87/300	29.0
60–69	23/67	26/89	49/156	31.4
70–	16/38	9/46	25/84	29.8
unknown	3/9	1/12	4/21	19.0
Total	125/511	129/602	254/1113	22.8
(%	24.5	21.4	22.8	)

Table 39.4. Frequency of OPLL in Yachiho village (The Committee)

	Male	(404)	Female	(569)	Total	(973)
A. Cervical OPLL	18	(4.5%)	15	(2.6%)	33	(3.4%)
B. Thoracic OPLL	4	(1.0%)	4	(0.7%)	8	(0.8%)
C. OPLL of both levels	2		1		3	
Total (A+B−C)	20	(5.0%)	18	(3.2%)	38	(3.9%)

Wan and Sakou investigated residents in 12 villages in the Southwest region of Taiwan. The subjects were 406 men and 598 women, ranging from 36–88 years old with the mean age being 56.2 years old. Out of 1004 persons, 12 had OPLL (1.2%).

Likewise, Lie investigated cervical x-rays of 1093 patients in Taiwan University and found 14 persons having OPLL (1.3%) (Table 39.7).

Hereditary and epidemiological studies performed by the Committee disclosed that OPLL is frequently associated with OALL, OYL, or OSSL, and vice versa. For instance OALL and OPLL are commonly associated. The Committee has the view that, essentially, ossification of each of the four ligaments is merely a different aspect of one and the same disease (6, 32–34). Although OPLL has rarely been found in Caucasians, OALL is not rare.

In 1971, Forestier and Lagier reported a condition based upon a study of 245 cases under the name of "ankylosing hyperostosis of the spine" (35). They reported that "the disorder is characterized by the appearance of large osteophytic spurs or bony proliferation in the form of anterior osseous bridges with a thickening of the corresponding vertebral cortex. Ossification occurs in the connective tissue surrounding the spine, including the ligamentum longitudinale anterius and the peripheral part of the disc." They noticed, accordingly, the ossification along the anterolateral aspect of the vertebral bodies, but they did not pay much attention to the ossification of the posterior longitudinal ligament. Later, in 1975, Resnick et al. called the condition diffuse idiopathic skeletal hyperostosis (DISH) (36, 37). However, in 1978, they first stressed that DISH was frequently associated with OPLL (38). They reviewed

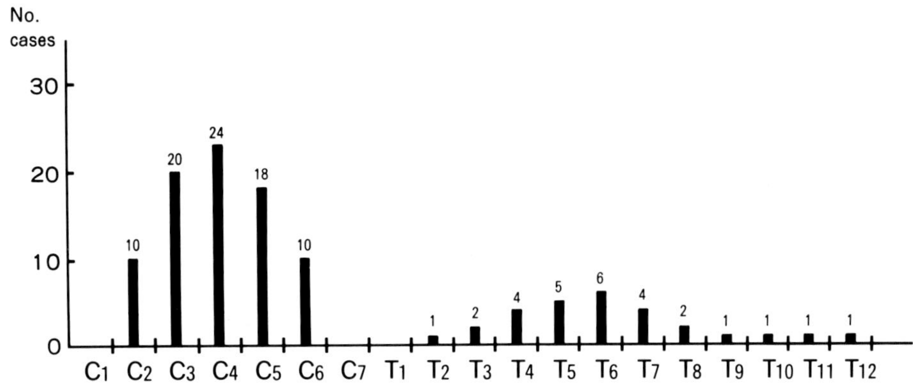

Figure 39.2. Distribution of OPLL in the spine (Epidemiology survey of Yachiho village).

Table 39.5. Frequency of OALL Associated with OPLL (The Committee)

Stage	I (mild)	II (moderate)	III (severe)	II + III
Cervical	180 (18.5%)	109 (11.2%)	29 (3.0%)	138 (14.2%)
Thoracic	74 (7.6%)	118 (12.1%)	123 (12.6%)	241 (24.8%)

Table 39.6. Frequency of OSSL Associated with OPLL (The Committee)

Male	Female	Total
111 (27.5%)	54 (9.5%)	165 (17.0%)

cervical spine radiographs in 74 patients with DISH and found OPLL in 37 patients (50%). From their experience, they concluded that "if DISH is considered a frequent disease in this country with an incidence that may reach 12% of middle-aged and elderly patients, calcification and ossification of the posterior longitudinal ligament should no longer be regarded as findings almost confined to Japanese individuals."

Investigation in Bologna, Italy, showed that OPLL is not rare even in Caucasians. Often a disease becomes prevalent as soon as many doctors take an interest in that disease. OPLL may be such a one.

Very recently, several reports appeared from Europe, United States, and Canada describing experiences of OPLL (39–55). Among them, the reports of McAfee et al. and of Harsh et al. are interesting (56, 57) because both of them unexpectedly treated so many cases. Bozman et al. reported that OPLL is far more frequent than hitherto considered even among Caucasians. They postulated, but without showing any clinical data, that OPLL may be found in 1.5% of the population, the figure being very near to the Japanese figure.

McAfee et al.'s report is important from another aspect, because it stated that many cases had been misdiagnosed and mistreated by other doctors before a correct diagnosis was made.

PROGRESS OF OPLL

The Committee investigated whether surgery had any effect on the progress of ossification of the ligament.

In the early days, the type of surgery preferred in Japan was posterior laminectomy of appropriate cervical levels. The Committee followed 295 patients who underwent this type of surgery more than 5 years ago. Three hundred and thirty-eight nonsurgical patients with the same diagnosis made more than 5 years ago were also investigated as a control group.

About 60% of the patients either with or without surgery showed progress of OPLL along the cranio-caudal direction. The extent of the progression varied from case to case, from limited progress to remarkable extension over one vertebra in some cases. The disease has, accordingly, a feature of worsening, irrespective of any treatment (58).

Furthermore, the thickness of ossification increased as well in about 50% of the patients after surgery. The increment of thickness was no different between conservative and surgical groups. Accordingly, posterior laminectomy was found to have no effect on stopping the progress of the disease.

METABOLISM OF CALCIUM

The cause of OPLL is not yet known. Speculating that calcium metabolism might be abnormal, calcium metabolites as well as related substances were investigated. Kasahara et al. reported that serum concentration of 25 (OH) vitamin D and 1.25 (OH)2 vitamin D showed wider range than normal but was not statistically significant. In 30% of their cases, serum parathyroid hormone was below normal range. Serum calcium was within normal range, whereas

Table 39.7. Frequency of OPLL on X-ray Photos Investigated by Japanese Doctors

	Author	Year	Country	OPLL/ person	OPLL (%)
Southeast Asia	Kurokawa	1978	Taiwan	12/496	2.4
	Yamaura	1978	Philippines	5/332	1.5
	Kurokawa	1978	Singapore	2/253	0.8
	Isawa	1980	Korea	5/529	0.95
	Committee	1984	6 countries	46/3053	1.53
Europe & U.S.A.	Yamauchi	1977	Hawaii	3/490	0.6
	Yamauchi	1977	U.S.A. (Mayo)	2/854	0.23
	Isawa	1980	U.S.A.	1/840	0.12
	Isawa	1980	West Germany	1/981	0.10

serum phosphate was abnormally low in 15% of cases. Serum magnesium and serum alkaline-phosphatase activity was normal. Other routine laboratory data showed normal values. They concluded that some cases were due to hypoparathyroid activity, but the majority of cases showed normal calcium metabolism (59, 60).

Other investigators have studied diabetes mellitus in order to determine whether OPLL had any relationship to abnormal glucose metabolism. They failed, however, to demonstrate any etiological relationship.

SIGNS AND SYMPTOMS

In our series, the initial signs were (*a*) numbness, (*b*) motor weakness, (*c*) pain, (*d*) gait disturbance, or (*e*) dizziness. When patients complained of "numbness" of any extremity, detailed examination would disclose slight motor weakness usually accompanying the numbness. Gait disturbance was caused by a mixture of motor weakness and mild sensory disturbance of bilateralism, which was especially exaggerated by a feeling of unsteadiness when walking. Dizziness was complained of when walking or moving the body, especially the neck.

As initial signs of 103 patients, 46 patients complained of numbness (=44.8%), 14 patients complained of gait disturbance (=13.6%), 10 complained of motor weakness of one to four extremities (=10.0%), and 8 complained of pain in one to four extremities (=7.8%). Pain in the neck was complained of by 14 patients (=13.6%), and dizziness was complained of by 8 (=7.8%) (Table 39.8).

Symptoms appeared in upper extremities in 42 cases (=40.8%), in lower extremities in 31 cases (=30.0%), and in both upper and lower extremities in 7 (=6.8%). It is noteworthy that some of the patients whose symptoms first appeared in the lower extremities were misdiagnosed as having lumbar disc herniation or lumbar spinal canal stenosis.

In 13 cases (=12.6%), trauma caused by such incidents as bicycle accidents, simple stumbling, and motor vehicle rear-end collision triggered the symptoms. In 2 cases, paraplegia or quadriplegia followed the trauma. Once para- or quadriplegia had occurred, the patient was miserable thereafter, because at present no treatment has been able to ameliorate this condition. However, paraparesis can be improved by surgical treatment and should be treated aggressively.

Table 39.8. Initial Signs of 103 Cases of OPLL (Takeuchi & Takebe)

A. Upper limbs	(42)
Numbness in one limb	16
Pain in one limb	3
Motor weakness in one limb	2
Numbness in both limbs	18
Pain in both limbs	2
Motor weakness in both limbs	1
B. Lower limbs	(31)
Pain in one limb	1
Weakness in one limb	2
Numbness in both limbs	5
Pain in both limbs	2
Motor weakness in both limbs	5
Rigidity in both limbs	1
Muscle cramp in both limbs	1
Gait disturbance	14
C. Numbness in upper and lower limbs of one side	1
Numbness in four limbs	6
D. Dizziness	8
E. Bladder and bowel dysfunction	1*

*The figure may be more frequent.

Neurological findings on admission have not been complex. Sensory or motor disturbances, corresponding to the compressed nerve roots in upper extremities, or due to myelopathy in lower extremities are common findings.

Progress of Symptoms

Although the disease is chronic, the speed with which the symptoms progress varies considerably between cases. For example, the duration of symptoms before admission in our cases was usually between 2–6 months. However, there is a wide range from several days to over 10 years (Table 39.9, Fig. 39.3).

If some trauma triggered symptoms, they developed fully soon after the trauma and showed little or no progress

Table 39.9. Duration from Initial Signs to Admission (Takeuchi & Takebe)

– 1 week	8
– 1 month	18
– 6 months	26
– 1 year	16
– 2 years	17
– 5 years	9
– 10 years	7
over 10 years	2
Total	103 cases

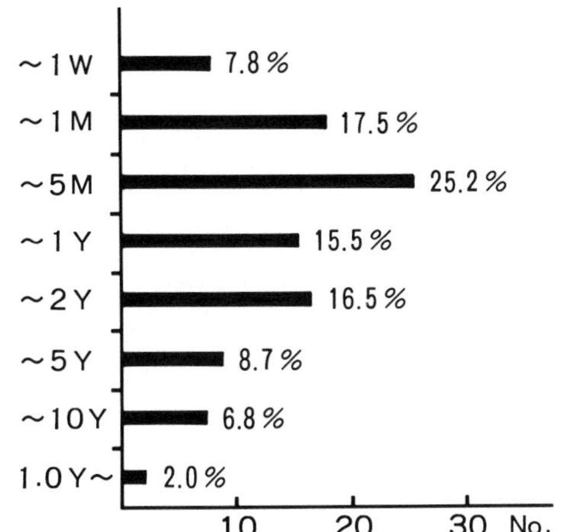

Figure 39.3. The duration of symptoms before admission in our 103 cases.

thereafter. Symptoms triggered by traumas were unexpectedly moderate in most cases, but in a few cases they were severe.

Symptoms on Admission

It is rare that patients complained of only one symptom at admission. Symptoms which prompted patients to consult their physicians were: sensory disturbance of upper extremities, 57.5%; sensory disturbance of lower extremities, 12%; motor weakness of upper extremities, 19.2%; motor weakness of lower extremities, 15.0%; pain in the neck, back, shoulder, arm, or hand, 38.3%; gait disturbance, 24.7%; dysuria, 11%; and others.

Neurological Findings on Admission

Neurological abnormalities presented were radiculopathy and/or myelopathy. Distribution of sensory impairment, such as paresthesia, hypesthesia, or hypalgesia, was usually strictly in accordance with the compressed nerve roots in the upper extremities. Brachial, triceps, or brachioradial reflexes were exaggerated in 60% and abolished in 10% of cases. When the lower extremities were involved, patellar or achilles tendon reflexes were exaggerated, although ankle clonus was rare. Deep sensation was also involved. Romberg's test was useful, as the test examines deep sensation and motor weakness of the lower extremities. Abnormal reflexes such as Babinski were elicited only by paraplegia or quadriplegia. Motor weakness of the upper limbs was roughly detected by ring formation between thumb and other fingers or by dynamometric examination. Also, weakness of the lower limbs was easily tested by dorsiflexion of the big toes when supine on an examination table.

Even when dizziness was the chief complaint, otological tests revealed no abnormalities in the labyrinth.

Neuroradiological Findings

Simple cervical roentgenograms were very important in detecting OPLL. Examining physicians who suspect OPLL have a higher chance of determining the existence of even early calcification in the ligament. Whenever diagnosis is questionable, 2 or 3 cervical tomograms should be taken without hesitation. Tomography has proven superior to simple roentgenography, especially when patients have thick necks.

Neuroradiologically, OPLL is classified as (*a*) localized, (*b*) segmental, (*c*) continuous, and (*d*) mixed type (Figs. 39.4, 39.5, 39.6). In our cases, mixed type occurred in 30.5% of the cases; localized type, 25.6%; segmental type, 23.2%; and continuous type, 20.7%.

Myelographical findings were compatible with those of an extradural mass. As ossification did not always progress along the midline; shadow defect was frequently asymmetrical. When a complete block was anticipated, myelography was performed after setting up for emergency surgery, if necessary. But actually, we have had to perform no emergency operation so far. The cisterna magna has frequently been selected as the site of needle puncture for contrast material.

Introduction of high resolution CT scanning was truly epochmaking (61–65). For example, Metrizamide or other water-soluble contrast myelography followed by CT is now commonly performed as one examination. On axial CT myelograms, it is quite clear to what degree the spinal cord has been compressed or distorted or how the nerve roots are compressed by OPLL (Fig. 39.7). We can define canal stenosis (CS) ratio as follows;

$$\text{Canal Stenosis Ratio} = \frac{\text{maximum thickness of OPLL}}{\text{A–P diameter of spinal canal at the same level}}$$

This ratio may practically indicate the degree of spinal cord compression. In 97 cases we examined, 58 (=59.8%) showed CS ratios of over 50%. Eleven cases (=11.3%) showed 80% ratio. Among them, 8 cases showed a complete block to metrizamide. Among them, 3 cases showed a 70% ratio, and the other 8 cases showed an 80% ratio.

On the other hand, MRI has shown no superior diagnostic value over CT myelography, although it is a noninvasive procedure, and the sagittal section of T1-weighted

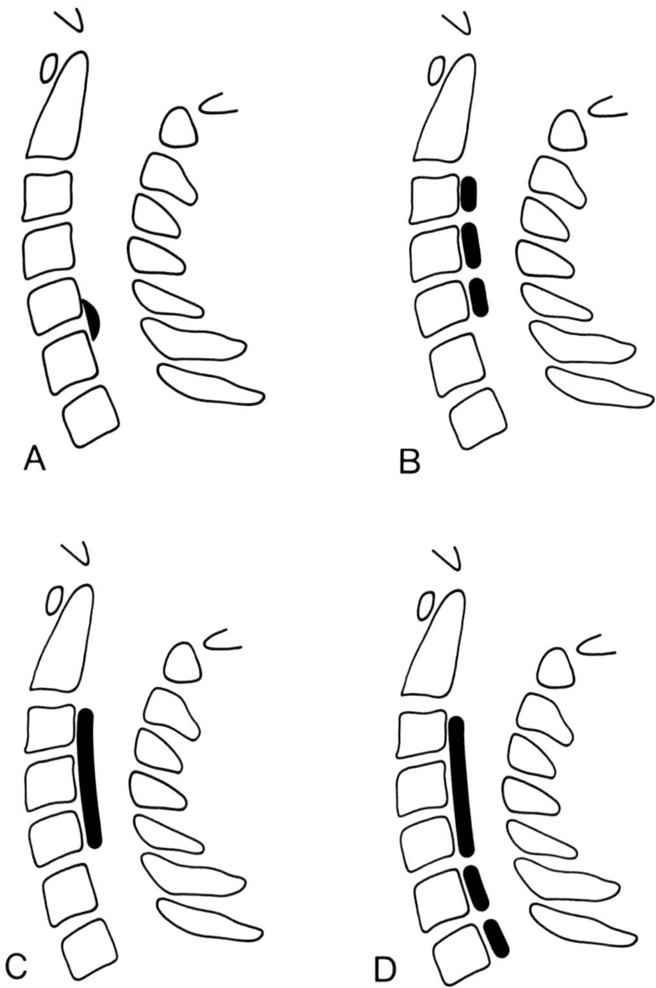

Figure 39.4. Schematic illustration of OPLL: **A,** Localized, **B,** segmental, **C,** continuous, and **D,** mixed type.

figures are of value to diagnose whether or not there is spinal cord compression (Fig. 39.8) (66). Because ossification is positively revealed on CT, while it is negatively outlined on MRI, CT myelography gives the most information. MRI is extremely useful to discriminate OPLL from a soft disc.

PATHOLOGY

One of the typical histological changes in the ligament is not calcification, but ossification itself (20, 23, 67, 68). The process of ossification occurs as follows; an early change in the ligament may be a proliferation of connective tissues, accompanied by sporadic neovascularization. Connective tissue fibers gradually form thick bundles. Then, osteoblast-like "OPLL cells" appear and ossification starts, and gradually connective tissue fibers are replaced. At the border of ossification, three layers are usually observed; connective tissue layer, ossifying layer, and layer of the os (Fig. 39.9). "OPLL cells," which have round nuclei with a moderately dense chromatin network, and round but shrunk cytoplasm due to fixation, are most frequently seen in the ossifying layer (Fig. 39.10). The layer of the os is usually clearly demarcated from the ossifying layer by darker staining with hematoxylin and eosin. Eventually, ossification proceeds dorsally and craniocaudally. Since connective tissue merges into the dura, ossification also involves the dura. This is the cause of CSF leakage from dural tears during surgery.

As has been pointed-out by Tsukimoto, the spinal cord, at the level of the compressed portion, shows various degenerative changes. Demyelination in anterior, lateral, or dorsal columns and loss of anterior horn cells is observed according to the degree of compression. Demyelinated nerve fibers are replaced by fat accumulation. Gliosis also occurs. Below the level of compression, lateral tract fiber degeneration occurs (69).

TREATMENT

Conservative Treatment

Before surgical treatment, bed rest, cervical fixation with a soft collar, or skeletal traction is first tried to correct cervical instability. Intense neurological observation of the

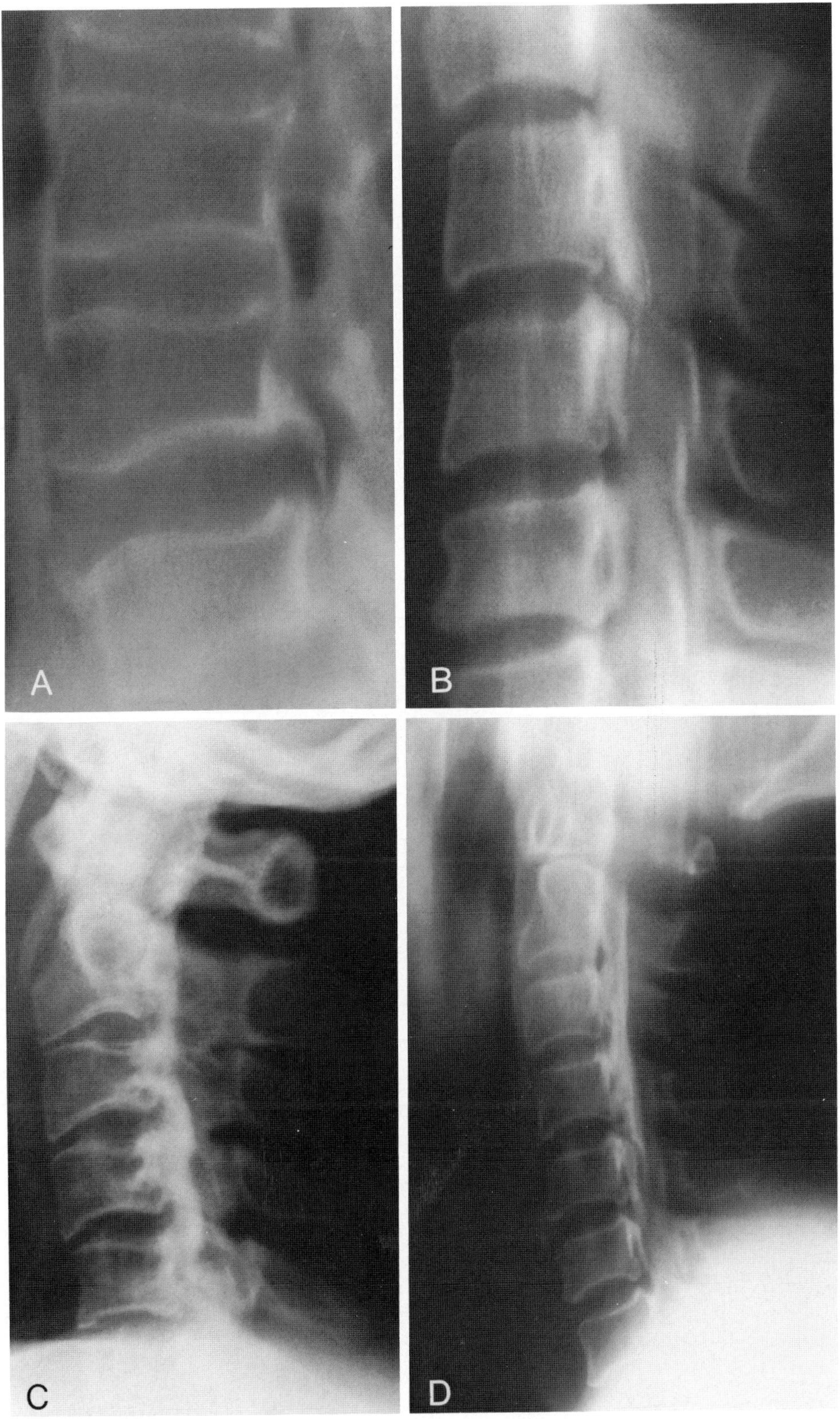

Figure 39.5. Roentgenograms of OPLL: **A,** Localized, **B,** segmental, **C,** continuous, and **D,** mixed type.

patient is essential to avoid any delay in making the decision for surgical treatment.

Surgical Treatment

For the relief of spinal compression by OPLL, either anterior approach such as extirpation of OPLL with anterior fusion (22, 70), or a posterior approach such as laminectomy or laminoplasty is used (71). We prefer extirpation of OPLL and anterior fusion because this procedure can remove the OPLL itself with a good long-term prognosis. Another advantage of the anterior approach is that it can provide good cervical stability by vertebral fusion. However, the operation should be performed very carefully to avoid either injury to the spinal cord or nerve roots which are close to OPLL sites, or to prolapse of the transplanted bone for fusion. These complications occur more frequently when the operative field is wide.

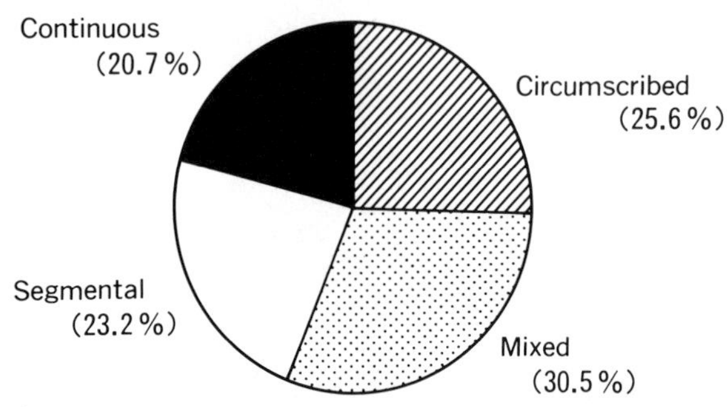

Figure 39.6. Frequency of OPLL type in our 103 cases.

On the other hand, the posterior approach is utilized when the extent of OPLL is so long that an anterior approach cannot cover it. Whether the approach should be anterior or posterior should be carefully decided, considering such factors as the length, level and type of OPLL, the patient's age, symptoms, general condition, or familial backgrounds.

Some insist that posterior decompression should be initially attempted before an anterior approach, especially in cases where OPLL is extremely long and spinal compression is severe; however, we have no such experience.

Anterior Approach

Prior to surgery, the surgeons must comprehend the three-dimensional shape and extent of OPLL from plain roentgenograms, tomograms, or CT. The anesthesiologist should carefully perform intubation so as not to over-extend the patient's neck. Before induction of anesthesia, the safe range of mobility of the neck should be tested.

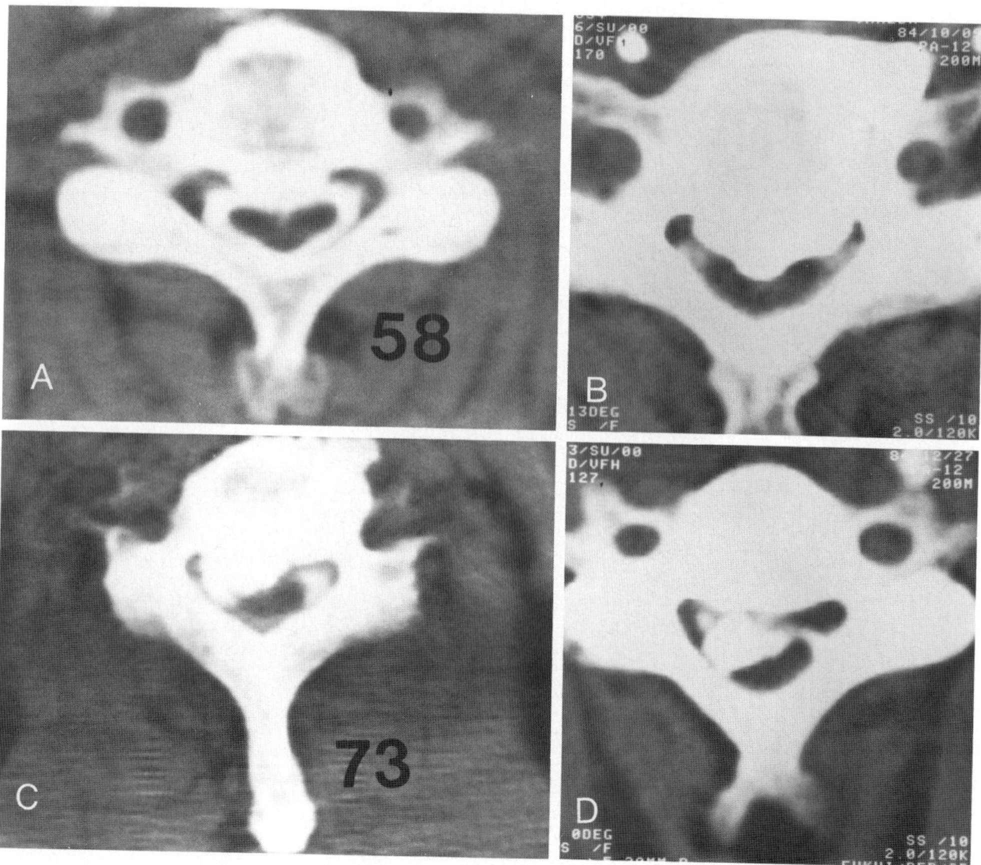

Figure 39.7. CT myelography. (**A**, **B**) OPLL in the midline, (**C**, **D**) OPLL off midline. Distortion of the spinal cord is clearly demonstrated.

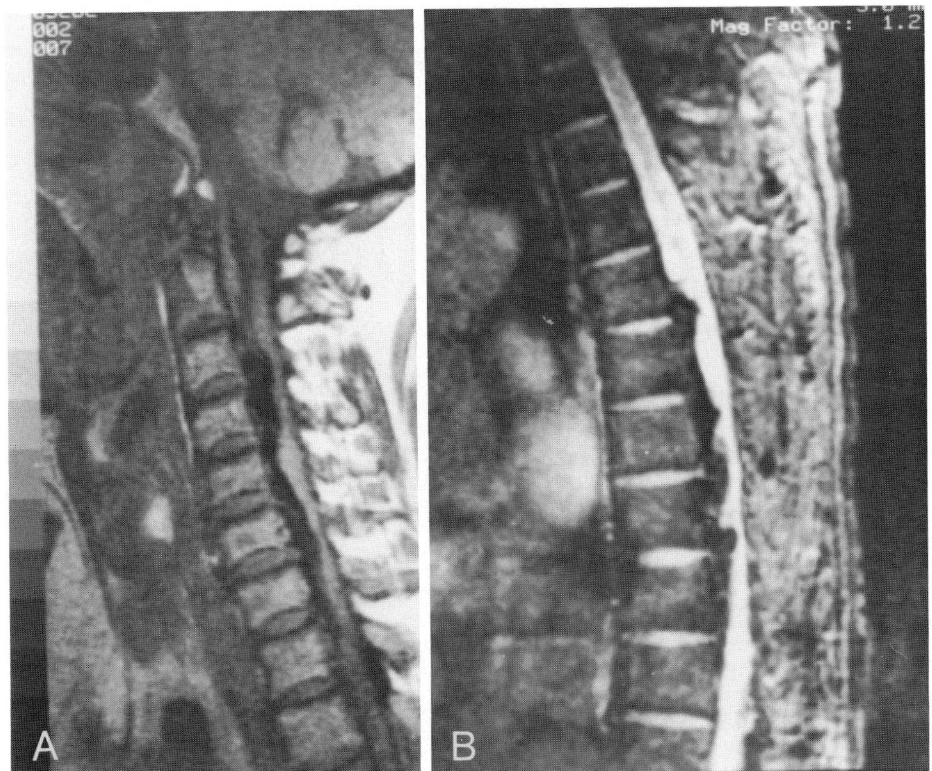

Figure 39.8. MRI CT (600/25). **A**, Cervical and **B**, thoracic OPLL. OPLL has low intensity. (Courtesy of Dr. S. Minami.)

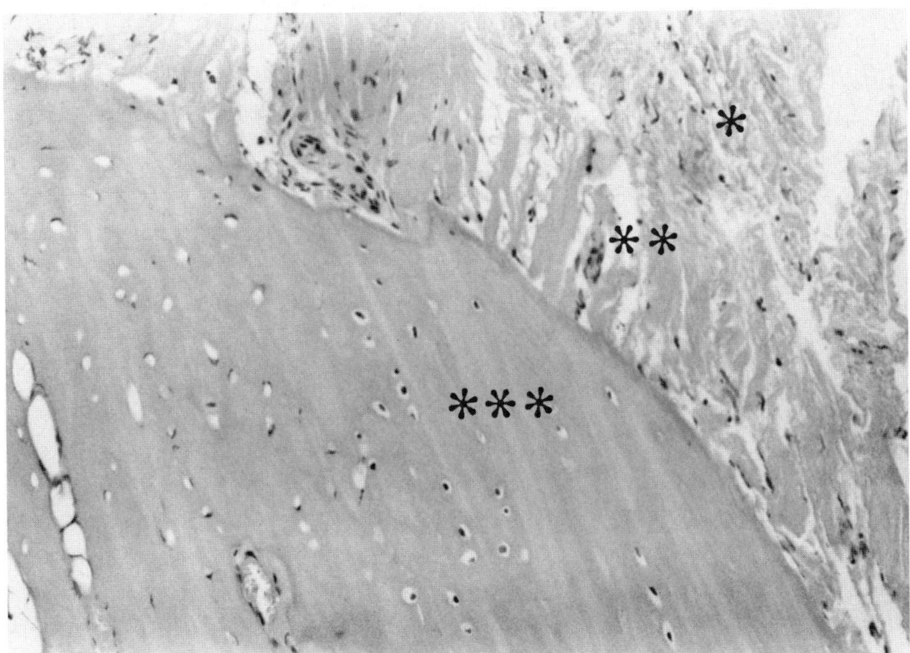

Figure 39.9. Histology of ossifying zone; (*) layer of connective tissue; (**) ossifying layer; and (***) layer of os.

The procedure from skin to vertebral body is the same as that of Smith-Robinson or Cloward and is not described here (72, 73). The upper limit of this procedure is C2–3 and the lower limit is C7–T1. When the vertebral surface is exposed, the level is confirmed by a portable radiograph.

The appropriate vertebral body is initially drilled cautiously with a 15 mm drill width transversely, not in the midline, but very slightly proximal to the surgeon. Water irrigation should be carried out continuously during the drilling procedure. The operating microscope is then introduced, and a diamond burr is attached to the drill when drilling approaches the posterior surface of the vertebral body. Drilling must be sufficiently deep for complete removal of OPLL.

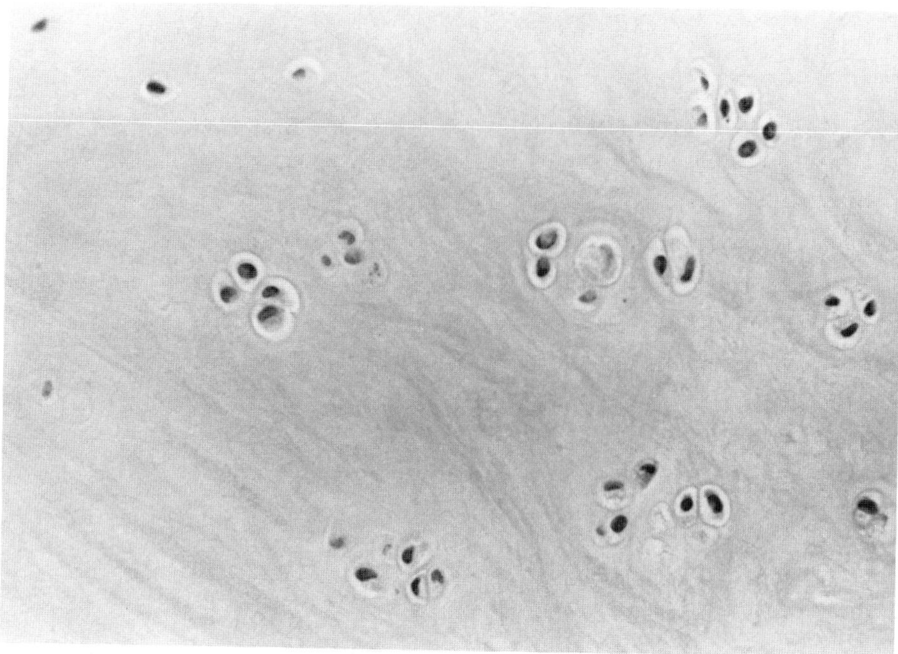

Figure 39.10. Osteoblast-like 'OPLL cells', which are most frequently seen in the ossifying layer but which are also observed in connective tissue layer.

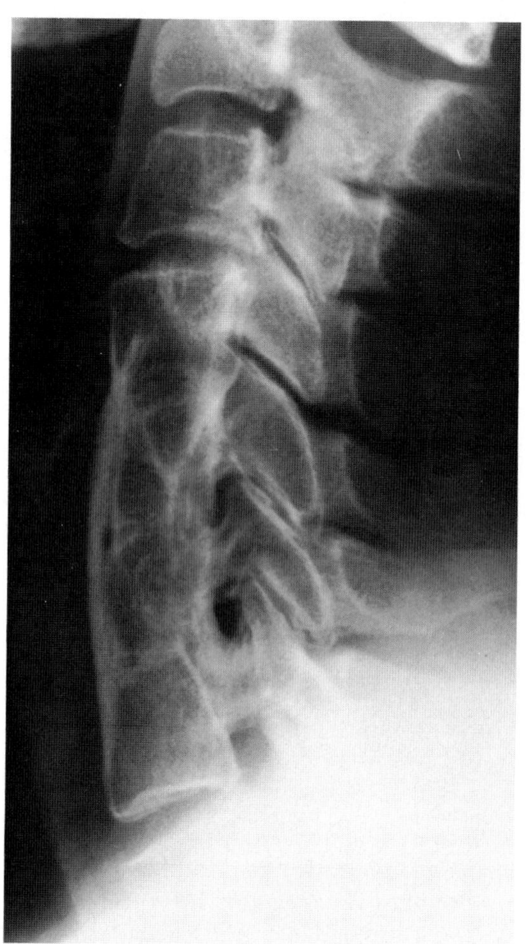

Figure 39.11. Iliac bone graft after C4–7 vertebrotomy.

There is usually no definite demarcation between the posterior surface of the vertebral body and OPLL. To avoid spinal cord damage during the procedure, normal dura cranial and caudal to the OPLL should be exposed. Then OPLL is shaved with a new diamond burr from both cranial and caudal ends. The lateral edge of OPLL should not be freed until OPLL becomes paper-thin. The last step is to remove OPLL from center to lateral border. It is advisable not to free OPLL from surrounding bone at the beginning. This is likely to cause spinal cord damage.

If an attempt is made to remove dural ossification, the dura easily tears and CSF leakage occurs. It has actually occurred in 13 cases out of 43 anterior approaches we attempted. In such cases, muscle patch soaked with Biobond is useful. CSF leakage is sometimes very troublesome, and, accordingly, dural calcification is frequently unremoved (in 8 out of our 43 cases). Bleeding from an old ossified ligament is minimal, but that from nonossified thick ligament is troublesome. Sometimes, bleeding from venous plexus between dura and OPLL is profuse. Small-angled bipolar forceps designed for this purpose are very useful.

Harvest of Iliac Bone

Iliac bone of appropriate length beginning from 2 cm posterior to the superior anterior iliac spina is cut and removed. A small amount of muscle and fascia is left attached, which is then sutured to the longus coli muscle. We anticipate collateral blood supply will develop to the transplanted bone from the longus colli muscle. When the iliac bone flap is wider than necessary, one side of the bone is shaved. Both sides should not be shaved to preserve the

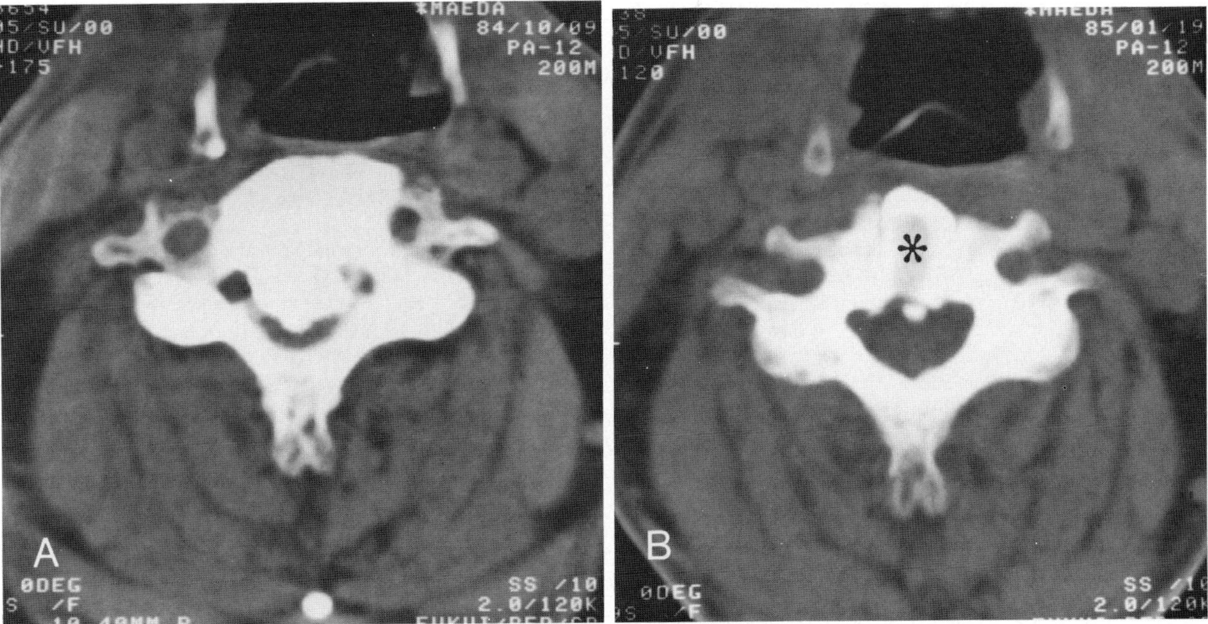

Figure 39.12. CT before (**A**) and after (**B**) surgery. Small fragment of ossification in the dura was left unremoved. (*) Iliac bone graft.

strength of transplant. Before anesthesia, Gardner-Wells traction is applied. At the time of insertion of the transplant, the patient's head is retracted. To prevent prolapse of the transplant, the bony edge of the recipient should be 1 mm–2 mm higher (Figs. 39.11, 39.12).

Postoperative Management

At the time of extubation, bucking must be avoided to prevent prolapse of the transplant. On the 2nd postoperative day the patient is allowed to sit. After the third day, walking to the toilet with a supporting walker is allowed. If a halo-vest is applied, walking is best delayed till 5 days postoperatively (74). Check of the transplant is necessary once a week by radiographs.

Even if CSF leakage occurs, it usually heals in 3 weeks with aspiration. Infection should be prevented by prophylactic antibiotics.

Posterior Approach

Indications for a posterior approach have been described above. Laminoplasty is preferable to laminectomy for decompression of the spinal cord and for avoiding deformity of the spinal canal, which is frequently observed in wide laminectomy (75). As for laminoplasty, a detailed description can be found in Chapter 38 of this textbook, by Dr. Ono.

Result of Operation

Motor weakness and urinary disturbance are usually greatly improved, numbness and sensory disturbance are not improved as much as patients expect.

OSSIFICATION OF YELLOW LIGAMENT (OYL)

OYL, which is rare even among Japanese, usually occurs in the thoracic vertebra (76–79). Half of the cases are associated with OPLL. Symptoms are confined to the lower half of the body. Gait disturbance, intermittent claudication, lumbago, subjective and objective sensory disturbance of lower limbs, or urinary disturbance are cardinal manifestations. Those symptoms are relieved only by surgery. Diagnosis must be carefully made from neurological and electrophysiological findings, myelograms, or positive contrast CT myelograms. As for treatment, conservative management is of no use, and surgery is recommended. Laminectomy and removal of OYL is the most effective treatment. Mild or moderate symptoms improve with surgery, but severe symptoms such as paraplegia are not benefited even by surgery.

REFERENCES

1. Key CA. On paraplegia depending on disease of the ligaments of the spine. Guys Hosp Rep (Series 1) 1938;3:17–34.

2. Bakay L, Cares HL, Smith RJ. Ossification in the region of the posterior longitudinal ligament as a cause of cervical myelopathy. J Neurol Neurosurg Psychiatry 1970;33:263–268.

3. Tsukimoto H. A case report: autopsy of syndrome of compression of spinal cord owing to ossification within spinal canal of cervical spine. Arch Jpn Chir 1960;29:1003–1007.

4. Hiramatsu Y, Nobechi T. Calcification of the posterior longitudinal ligament of the spine among Japanese. Radiology 1971;100:307–312.

5. Murakami N, Muroga T, Sobue I. Cervical myelopathy due to ossification of the posterior longitudinal ligament. A clinicopathologic study. Arch Neurol 1978;35:33–36.

6. Hukuda S, Mochizuki T, Ogata M, Shichikawa K. The pattern

of spinal and extraspinal hyperostosis in patients with ossification of the posterior longitudinal ligament and the ligamentum flavum causing myelopathy. Skeletal Radiol 1983;10:79–85.

7. Nagashima C. Cervical myelopathy due to ossification of the posterior longitudinal ligament. J Neurosurg 1972;37:653–660.

8. Nakanishi T, Mannen T, Toyokura Y, Sakaguchi R, Tsuyama N. Symptomatic ossification of the posterior longitudinal ligament of the cervical spine. Neurology 1974;24:1139–1143.

9. Nose T, Egashira T, Enomoto T, Maki Y. Ossification of the posterior longitudinal ligament: a clinico-radiological study of 74 cases. J Neurol Neurosurg Psychiatry 1987;50:321–326.

10. Okamoto Y. Ossification of the posterior longitudinal ligament of cervical spine with or without myelopathy. J Jpn Orthop Assoc 1967;40:1349–1360.

11. Ono K, Ota H, Tada K, Hamada H, Takaoka K. Ossified posterior longitudinal ligament. A clinicopathologic study. Spine 1977;2:126–138.

12. Onji Y, Akiyama H, Shimomura Y, Ono K, Hukuda S, Mizuno S. Posterior paravertebral ossification causing cervical myelopathy: a report of eighteen cases. J Bone Joint Surg 1967;49:1314–1328.

13. Sato M, Tsuru M, Yada K. The antero-posterior diameter of the cervical spinal canal in the ossification of the posterior longitudinal ligament. No Shinkei Geka 1977;5:511–517.

14. Suzuki K, Udagawa E, Nagano M, Takada S. Clinical significance of the calcification in the cervical epidural space. J Jpn Orthop Assoc 1962;36:256.

15. Nakanishi T, Mannen T, Toyokura Y. Asymptomatic ossification of the posterior longitudinal ligament of the cervical spine. Incidence and roentgenographic findings. J Neurol Sci 1973;19:375–381.

16. Yanagi T. Ossification of the posterior longitudinal ligament. A clinical and radiological analysis of forty-six cases. Brain Nerve 1987;22:909–921.

17. Tsuyama N: Ossification of the posterior longitudinal ligament of the spine. Clin Orthop 1984;184:71–84.

18. Takahashi M, Kawanami H, Tomonaga M, Kitamura K. Ossification of the posterior longitudinal ligament. A roentgenologic and clinical investigation. Acta Radiol 1972;13:25–36.

19. Yamaura I, Kurasa Y. Anterior floating method for cervical myelopathy caused by ossification of the posterior longitudinal ligament. Seikeigeka 1985;36:1031–1041.

20. Yasui N, Ono K, Yamaura I, Konomi H, Nagai Y. Immunohistochemical localization of types I, II, and III collagens in the ossified posterior longitudinal ligament of the human cervical spine. Calcif Tissue Int 1983;35:159–163.

21. Terayama K, Maruyama S, Miyashita R, et al. Ossification of the posterior longitudinal ligament in the cervical spine. Seikagaku 1964;15:1083–1095.

22. Tominaga S. The effects of intervertebral fusion in patients with myelopathy due to ossification of the posterior longitudinal ligament of the cervical spine. Int Orthop 1980;4:183–191.

23. Tsuzuki N, Imai T, Hatta Y. Histopathological findings of the ossification of the posterior longitudinal ligament of the cervical spine and their significance. Nippon Seikeigeka Gakkai Zasshi 1981;55:387–397.

24. Chin WS, Oon CL. Ossification of the posterior longitudinal ligament of the spine. Br J Radiol 1979;52:865–869.

25. Howng SL, Chui C. Ossification of the posterior longitudinal spinal ligament in association with anterior longitudinal ligament ankylosing hyperostosis: report of two cases. Kaoshung J Med Sci 1987;3:684–688.

26. Izawa K. Comparative roentgenographical study on the incidence of ossification of the posterior longitudinal ligament and other degenerative changes of the cervical spine among Japanese, Koreans, Americans and Germans. Nippon Seikeigeka Gakkai Zasshi 1980;54:461–474.

27. Yu YL, Leong JCY, Fang D, Woo E, Huang CY, Lau HK. Cervical myelopathy due to ossification of the posterior longitudinal ligament. Brain 1988;111:769–783.

28. Tanikawa E, Furuya K, Nakajima H. Genetic study on ossification of posterior longitudinal ligament. Bull Tokyo Med Dent Univ 1986;33:117–128.

29. Ohtsuka K, Terayama K, Yanagihara M, Wada K, Kasuga K. An epidemiological survey on ossification of ligaments in the cervical and thoracic spine in individuals over 50 years of age. J Jpn Orthop Assoc 1986;60:1087–1098.

30. Ohtsuka K, Terayama K, Yanagihara M, Wada K, Kasuga K, Machida T, Matsushima S. A radiological population study on the ossification of the posterior longitudinal ligament in the spine. Arch Orthop Trauma Surg 1987;106:89–93.

31. Terayama K, Ohtsuka K, Merlini L, Albisinni U, Gui L. Ossification of the spinal ligament: A radiographic revaluation in Bologna, Italy. J Jpn Orthop Assoc 1987;61:1373–1378.

32. Barsony T, Winkler K. Calcinosis circumscripta ligamenti nuchae. Fortschr Geb Rontgenstr 1936;54:39–49.

33. Mitsui H, Sonozaki H, Juji T, Kobata K. Ankylosing spinal hyperostosis (ASH) and ossification of the posterior longitudinal ligament (OPLL). Arch Orthop Trauma Surg 1979;94:21–23.

34. Nozaki H, Nagai T, Miura Y, Suzuki Y, Nasu T. On the clinical findings of the ossification of the posterior longitudinal ligament, especially its combination with the ossification of the anterior longitudinal ligament. J West Pacific Orthop Assoc 1969;6:127–136.

35. Forestier J, Lagier R. Ankylosing hyperostosis of the spine. Clin Orthop 1971;74:65–83.

36. Resnick D, Shaul SR, Robin JM. Diffuse idiopathic skeletal hyperostosis (DISH): Forestier's disease with extraspinal manifestations. Radiology 1975;115:513–524.

37. Resnick D, Niwayama G. Radiographic and pathologic features of spinal involvement in diffuse idiopathic skeletal hyperostosis (DISH). Radiology 1976;119:559–568.

38. Resnick D, Guerra J, Robinson CA, Vint VC. Association of diffuse idiopathic skeletal hyperostosis (DISH) and calcification and ossification of the posterior longitudinal ligament. AJR 1978;131:1049–1053.

39. Alenghat JP, Hallett M, Kido DK. Spinal cord compression in diffuse idiopathic skeletal hyperostosis. Radiology 1982;142:119–120.

40. Becker DH, Conley FK, Anderson ME. Quadriplegia associated with narrow cervical canal, ligamentous calcification and ankylosing hyperostosis. Surg Neurol 1979;17–19.

41. Bozman RE, Downey EF, Brower AC. Diffuse idiopathic skeletal hyperostosis and ossification of the posterior longitudinal ligament in the thoracic spine. Comput Radiol 1985;9:243–246.

42. Correa AV, Beasley BAL. Ossification of posterior longitudinal ligament. N Y State J Med 1980;80:1972–1984.

43. Dietmann JL, Dirheimer Y, Babin E, Edel L, Dosch JC, Hirsch E, Wackenheim A. Ossification of the posterior longitudinal ligament (Japanese disease). A radiological study in 112 cases. J Neuroradiol 1985;12:212–222.

44. Firooznia H, Benjamin VM, Pinto RS, et al. Calcification and ossification of posterior longitudinal ligament of spine. Its role in secondary narrowing of spinal canal and cord compression. N Y State J Med 1982;82:1193–1198.

45. Gui L, Merlini L, Savini R, Davidovits P. Cervical myelopathy due to ossification of the posterior longitudinal ligament. Ital J Orthop Traumatol 1983;9:269–280.

46. Minagi H, Gronner AT. Calcification of the posterior longitudinal ligament: a cause of cervical myelopathy. AJR 1969;105:365–369.

47. Palacios E, Brackett CE, Leary DJ. Ossification of the posterior longitudinal ligament associated with a herniated intervertebral disc. Radiology 1971;100:313–314.

48. Portha C, Coche G, Moussa K, et al. Ossification of the posterior longitudinal ligament after cervical irradiation. Neuroradiology 1982;24:111–113.

49. Pouchot J, Watts GS, Esdaile JM, Hill RO. Sudden quadriplegia complicating ossification of the posterior longitudinal ligament and diffuse idiopathic skeletal hyperostosis. Arthritis Rheum 1987;30:1069–1072.

50. Rappaport ZH, Rovit R. Ossification of the posterior longitudinal spinal ligament in association with anterior longitudinal ligament ankylosing hyperostosis: case report. Neurosurgery 1979;4:175–177.

51. Rozario RA, Levine H, Stein BM. Cervical myelopathy and radiculopathy secondary to ossification of the posterior longitudinal ligament. Surg Neurol 1978;10:17–20.

52. Soo YS, Sachdev AS. Calcification in the posterior longitudinal ligament as a cause of cervical myelopathy. Med J Aust 1971;1:743–744.

53. Yagan R, Khan MA, Bellon EM. Spondylitis and posterior longitudinal ligament ossification in the cervical spine. Arthritis Rheum 1983;26:226–230.

54. Hyman RA, Merten CW, Liebeskind AL, Naidich JB, Stein HL. Computed tomography in ossification of the posterior longitudinal spinal ligament. Neuroradiology 1977;13:227–228.

55. Johnsson KE, Peterson H, Wollheim FA, Saveland H. Diffuse idiopathic skeletal hyperostosis (DISH) causing spinal stenosis and sudden paraplegia. J Rheumatol 1983;10:784–789.

56. Harsh GR, Sypert GW, Weinstein PR, Ross DA, Wilson CB. Cervical spine stenosis secondary to ossification of the posterior longitudinal ligament. J Neurosurg 1987;67:349–357.

57. McAfee PC, Regan JJ, Bohlman HH. Cervical cord compression from ossification of the posterior longitudinal ligament in non-Orientals. J Bone Joint Surg 1987;69:569–575.

58. Hirabayashi K, Miyakawa J, Satomi K, Maruyama T, Wakano K. Operative results and postoperative progression of ossification among patients with ossification of cervical posterior longitudinal ligament. Spine 1981;6:354–364.

59. Adams JE, Davis M. Paravertebral and peripheral ligamentous ossification: an unusual association of hypoparathyroidism. Postgrad Med 1977;53:167–172.

60. Nichols JN, Tehranzadeh J, Vaccarino F. Posterior longitudinal ligament ossification myelopathy and hypothyroidism. J Comput Assist Tomogr 1987;11:61–65.

61. Hanai K, Adachi H, Ogasawara H. Axial transverse tomography of the cervical spine narrowed by ossification of the posterior longitudinal ligament. J Bone Joint Surg (Br) 1977;59:481–484.

62. Isu T, Ito T, Iwasaki Y, Tsuru M, Nakagawa T, Miyasaka K. Computed tomography in the diagnosis of spinal disease. No Shinkei Geka 1979;7:1171–1178.

63. Kadoya S, Nakamura T, Tada A. Neuroradiology of ossification of the posterior longitudinal spinal ligament. Comparative studies with computer tomography. Neuroradiology 1978;16:357–358.

64. Murakami J, Russell WJ, Hayabuchi N, Kimura S. Computed tomography of posterior longitudinal ligament ossification: its appearance and diagnostic value with special reference to thoracic lesions. J Comput Assist Tomogr 1982;6:41–50.

65. Yamamoto I, Kageyama N, Nakamura K, Takahashi T. Computed tomography in ossification of the posterior longitudinal ligament in the cervical spine. Surg Neurol 1979;12:414–418.

66. Takahashi M, Sakamoto Y, Miyawaki M, Bussaka H. Increased MR signal intensity secondary to chronic cervical cord compression. Neuroradiology 1987;29:550–556.

67. Goto S. Studies of ossification of the posterior longitudinal ligament in the cervical spine using microradiography and histochemistry. Nippon Seikeigeka Gakkai Zasshi 1981;55:451–466.

68. Yokoi K. Ectopic calcification in the epidural space. Report of three cases. Orthop Surg 1963;14:1262.

69. Hashizume Y, Iijima S, Kishimoto H, Yanagi T. Pathology of spinal cord lesions caused by ossification of the posterior longitudinal ligament. Acta Neuropathol 1984;63:123–130.

70. Manabe S, Nomura S. Anterior decompression for ossification of the posterior longitudinal ligament of the cervical spine. No Shinkei Geka 1977;5:1253–1259.

71. Kimura I, Ouhama M, Shingu H. Cervical myelopathy treated by canal-expansive laminoplasty. Computed tomographic and myelographic findings. J Bone Joint Surg (Am) 1984;66:914–920.

72. Abe H, Tsuru M, Ito T, Iwasaki Y, Koiwa M. Anterior decompression for ossification of the posterior longitudinal ligament of the cervical spine. J Neurosurg 1981;55:108–116.

73. Hanai K, Inouye Y, Kawai K, Tago K, Itoh Y. Anterior decompression for myelopathy resulting from ossification of the posterior longitudinal ligament. J Bone Joint Surg (Br) 1982;64:561–564.

74. Koyanagi I, Isu T, Iwasaki Y, et al. Experimental immobilization of cervical spine with a halo vest—experience with 31 cases. No Shinkei Geka 1985;13:615–621.

75. Mikawa Y, Shikata J, Yamamuro T. Spinal deformity and instability after multilevel cervical laminectomy. Spine 1987;12:6–11.

76. Hattori A, Endoh H, Suzuki K, et al. Ossification of the thoracic ligamentum flavum with compression of the spinal cord. A report of six cases. J Jpn Orthop Assoc 1976;50:1141–1146.

77. Koizumi M. Three cases of spinal cord paralysis proved by ligamenta flava ossification. Rinsho Geka 1962;17:1181–1188.

78. Yamaguchi H, Tamakake S, Hujita S. A case of ossification of the ligamentum flavum with myelopathy. Seikagaku 1960;11:951–956.

79. Yonenobu K, Ebara S, Fujiwara K, et al. Thoracic myelopathy secondary to ossification of the spinal ligament. J Neurosurg 1987;66:511–518.

40

Lateral Approaches to the Cervical Spine

William A. Shucart and Robin Koeleveld

Introduction

Lesions of the cervical spine may be thought of as two groups—those involving primarily the bony structures with alignment and stabilization as the major goals of treatment and those compromising neural or vascular structures with decompression of the normal structures and removal of a mass as the goals. Occasionally, these problems overlap, but one is usually dominant.

In any situation the best surgical approach would be that which allowed maximum exposure, avoided injury to adjacent structures, required the least manipulation of neural elements, and allowed visualization of normal structures early in the dissection.

History

The oldest and still most commonly used surgical approach to the cervical spine is from the back. For abnormalities involving the spinous processes, laminae, and pedicles as well as lesions within the canal situated dorsally or laterally this remains an excellent route. The obvious limitations of the posterior approach for lesions involving the vertebral bodies and ventral and ventrolateral portions of the spinal canal led surgeons to devise a variety of operations using anterior, anterolateral, and lateral approaches. Nearly 100 years ago the direct anterior transoral route to the upper cervical spine was described primarily for the treatment of tuberculous lesions and has since 1950 been utilized increasingly for the treatment of bony craniocervical anomalies (1–5) and rarely for the treatment of lesions within the upper spinal canal (6, 7) and bony tumors (8). Many of the surgical problems associated with the anterior transoral approach in the past have been lessened with the use of antibiotics, and most importantly, with the introduction of the operating microscope which affords excellent illumination and magnification. The role of this exposure for extradural upper cervical spine abnormalities is now well established but it remains problematical if the lesion is intradural. The major complications in dealing with the intradural masses are cerebrospinal fluid (CSF) leakage and infection, primarily because of the technical difficulty of closing or replacing the dura; the great depth of the operating field which limits instrumentation; and the hazard of working through a tumor toward the spinal cord without being able to visualize normal tissue.

The lateral approach to the cervical spine was developed initially to deal with traumatic lesions of the vertebral artery (9) and somewhat later used to remove osteophytes compressing the vertebral arteries or cervical nerve roots (10). The basic surgical anatomy and operative technique for the lateral cervical approach were most clearly defined by Henry in his extraordinary textbook *Extensile Exposure* (11); subsequent reports have generally been modifications of this basic work (12). Verbiest extended this technique to remove some cervical disc protrusions, certain spinal tumors, and to treat traumatic lesions of the anterior rami of the brachial plexus. Orthopaedic surgeons have used this method for anterior cervical fusion of C1–C2 and to expose the facet joints of C1 and C2 for arthrodesis with screw fixation for fractures of the odontoid process (8, 13). Neurosurgeons have used this approach for the removal of high cervical ventral intradural tumors (12).

Indications and Evaluation

The indications for using the lateral cervical approach are limited. In the upper cervical spine (from the mid-portion of C3 cephalad) the major uses would be for intradural lesions such as meningiomas or neurofibromas which are primarily ventral or ventrolateral to the spinal cord, abnormalities involving the vertebral artery from C3 to the foramen magnum, and for fusion of C1 to C2 when anterior and posterior approaches have either failed or are not feasible. The lateral approach to the lower cervical spine would be best used for lesions involving the vertebral artery. There is little need for the lateral approach for lesions of the bony spine or spinal canal from C3 through C7, for these can more easily be dealt with using standard anterior or posterior techniques.

Evaluation of the patient for spinal column problems is done in the usual fashion with plain x-rays, including motion views and now frequently supplemented with MRI or cervical myelogram followed by high resolution computerized tomography. Imaging of abnormalities within the spinal canal is best done using MRI with images in several planes and in some instances three dimensional reconstructions. Vertebral angiography is often helpful in defining intraspinal lesions both for determining tumor blood supply and displacement of the vessels, and it is, of course, essential for defining lesions of the vertebral arteries (14, 15). If the lesion is vascular or has a rich blood supply, endovascular intervention may facilitate surgery or, rarely, be curative.

SURGICAL TECHNIQUE

Upper Cervical Spine

The technique for removing a ventral intraspinal tumor will be given in detail, since prior to removing the laminae the approach is essentially the same for dealing with any lesion. References for the special techniques required for fusions are given (8, 13, 16). For those attempting this operation for the first time a careful review of the anatomy is essential, and a trial run in the anatomy laboratory would be preferable. The operating microscope is essential for the intraspinal portion of the operation and extremely helpful in all of the operation after the large muscles have been reflected. The Cavitron and laser can facilitate tumor removal, and bipolar cautery is preferable throughout the procedure.

Procedure

Nasotracheal intubation is preferable, as it allows the mouth to be nearly closed so the angle of the mandible is forward and does not compromise the operative field. Further anterior displacement of the mandible can be accomplished by pulling it forward with adhesive tape. It is also helpful to place a suture through the skin of the back of the ear or ear lobe and pull it forward.

The patient is placed in the true lateral position. The neck is extended and the chin is turned 10° toward the down side (Fig. 40.1). The skin incision is made along the anterior border of the sternocleidomastoid muscle, beginning about 1 cm below the level of the cricoid cartilage and is extended up to the base of the mastoid process, where it is curved back across the base of the skull for approximately 6–8 cm. The platysma muscle and the deep fascia are divided in the neck, and the insertions of the sternocleidomastoid muscle and part of the splenius capitis muscle are divided at the base of the skull. The muscles are mobilized inferiorly and posteriorly until the spinal accessory nerve is identified entering the deep surface of the sternocleidomastoid muscle about 3 or 4 cm below the mastoid tip. At this point the tip of the transverse process of C1 can be identified by palpation 1 cm below and 1 cm in front of the mastoid tip. The transverse process of C2 is shorter and more difficult to palpate; it can be confused

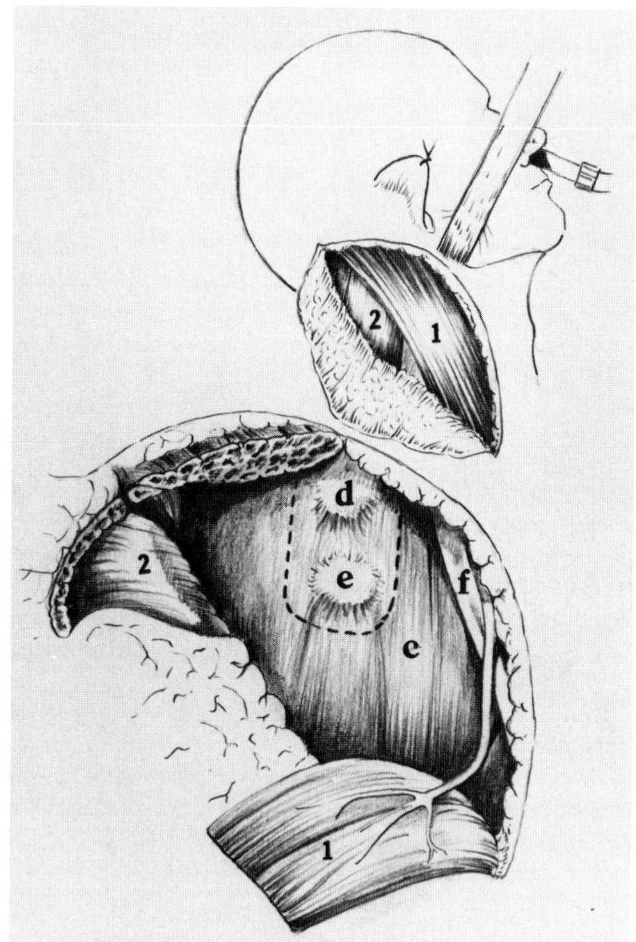

Figure 40.1. Extent of incision and head position. Note the nasotracheal intubation, the ear sewn forward, and the angle of the jaw pulled forward with tape. The sternomastoid (*1*) and splenius capitis (*2*) have been divided and reflected. The spinal accessory nerve is shown entering the undersurface of the sternomastoid; the internal jugular vein (*f*) is seen. The tips of the transverse processes of C-1 and C-2 (*d* & *e*) can be partially seen and palpated beneath the thick fascia overlying the levator scapulae. The distance between the internal jugular vein and the tips of the transverse processes is exaggerated in the diagram. Dissection should be kept posterior in order to avoid injury to the jugular vein.

with the C2–3 facet joint, which lies slightly posterior and inferior (Fig. 40.2).

The deep fascia is incised from the tip of the C1 transverse process obliquely downward parallel to the course of the spinal accessory nerve. The attachments of the thick levator scapulae muscle and the slender splenius cervicis muscle to the C1 transverse process are then seen; they are picked-up and divided, remembering that the vertebral artery is just beneath them. The vertebral artery then comes clearly into view, and the remaining muscle fibers running between the transverse processes of C1 and C2 are divided (Fig. 40.3). The muscle attachments to the tip of the transverse process of C2 are divided. The lateral aspect of the

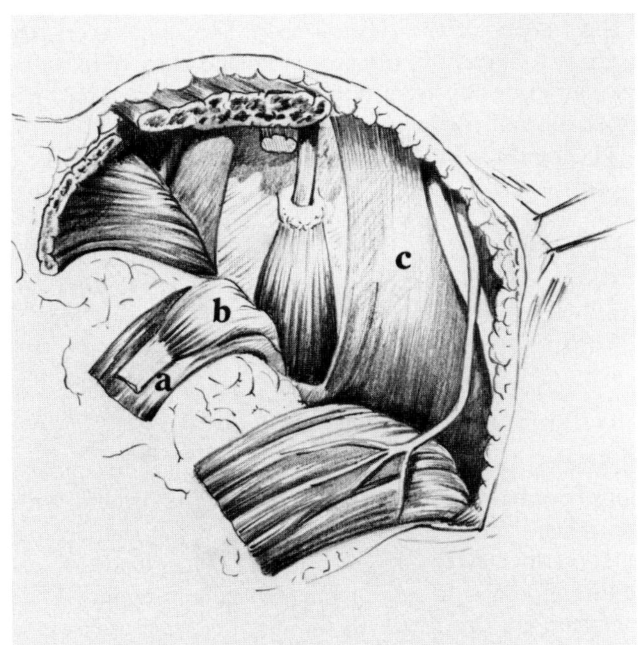

Figure 40.2. The fascia over the levator scapulae has been incised, and the divided levator scapulae (*a*) and small underlying splenius cervicis (*b*) reflected. The vertebral artery can be seen between the foramina at C-1 and C-2.

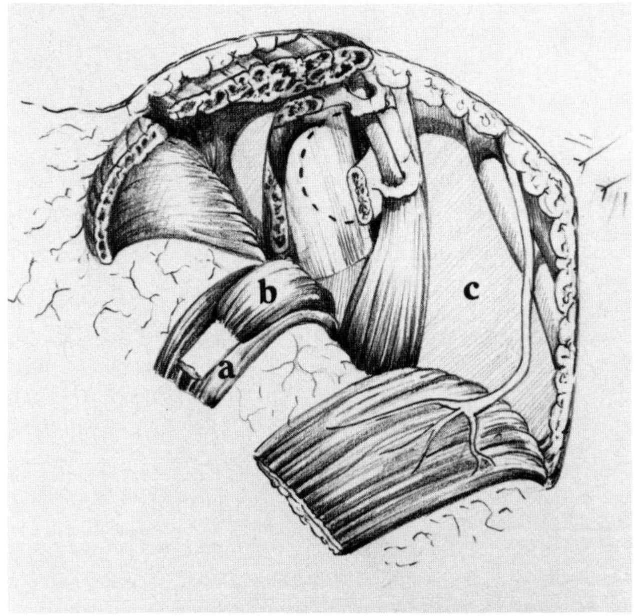

Figure 40.3. The muscles have been reflected from the lamina of C-2 and the arch of C-1 and bone removal performed. The underlying dotted line shows the area of dural incision.

arch of C1 and the C2 lamina can then be palpated and partially seen.

Curettes are used to reflect the muscle attachments from the lamina of C2 and the inferior portion of C1. The muscle attachments to the superior portion of the C1 arch can be removed using an angled curette, keeping the plane of dissection subperiosteal to avoid injuring the vertebral artery. The muscle attachments are removed almost to the midline posteriorly.

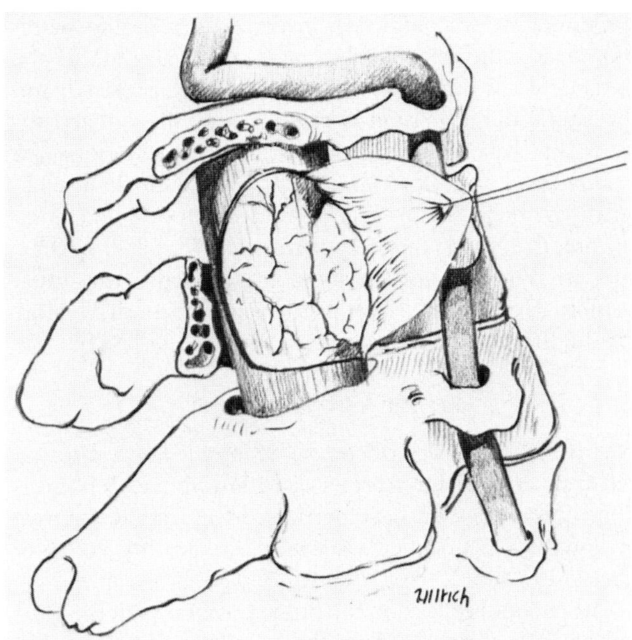

Figure 40.4. Extent of removal of C-1 and C-2 shown, dura opened to show view of tumor ventral to spinal cord.

With the use of a high speed drill with diamond burrs, the exposed arch of C1 and the lamina of C2 are removed. The lamina of C2 is removed to within a few millimeters of the foramen transversarium, but the C2–3 facet joint and a portion of the pedicle are spared. The arch of C1 is removed to the point where the vertebral artery is on the superior surface. From that point laterally to the transverse foramen the bone is undercut but not removed totally (Fig. 40.4).

There is usually little epidural fat present, and the dura is easily exposed from the foramen magnum to the superior portion of the C3. The dura is best opened using a curved incision beginning at the anterior-superior portion of the exposed dura and creating a convex backward incision which ends coming back to the anterior-inferior portion of the exposed dura. This allows the dura to be flapped anteriorly. For tumors which are ventral to the spinal cord this opening will expose both the compressed cord and the tumor. For ventrolateral tumors this opening should expose at least a small portion of the normal cord in its posterior extent. The tumor is best removed in a piecemeal fashion, and little or no manipulation of the spinal cord should be done. The Cavitron may be helpful in debulking the central portion of the lesion if standard suction and gentle curetting are not effective. The variety of curettes and forceps used for transsphenoidal pituitary surgery are particularly appropriate for this part of the operation. The laser and bipolar cautery are both good for shrinking the tumor. If the tumor is a meningioma, involved dura should be removed and the dura patched with a fascial graft. If the dural defect is purely ventral, then no graft is placed, and the lateral dural incision is closed. Ventrally-situated tumors that have displaced the spinal cord posteriorly are readily seen, and more laterally placed tumor lie just beneath the dural incision. After tumor removal and dural closure, the muscles are reapproximated with 2–0 sutures, and the remainder of the incision is closed in the usual fashion. A cervical collar helps to lessen patient discomfort for the first few postoperative weeks.

Lower Cervical Spine

This technique is described only to provide access to the vertebral arteries for reasons discussed above. Modifications of this method have been used to facilitate removal of dumbbell neurofibromas which displace the vertebral artery (17, 18).

The patient is placed in the prone position with the head turned 20°–30° away from the operative side. The skin incision used is the same used to expose the carotid artery in the neck, that is, paralleling the anterior border of the sternomastoid muscle from approximately C2 down to the clavicle. Clearly, this exposure is more properly considered an anterior approach to the lateral aspect of the spine rather than a true lateral approach. After dividing the platysma, the plane separating the sternomastoid muscle, carotid artery, and jugular vein laterally from the trachea and esophagus medially is developed. The dissection is carried down to the anterolateral aspect of the vertebral bodies, and the longus colli muscle is identified. The midline raphe separating the two longus colli muscles is easily identified. The longus colli on the side of the surgery is then displaced from lateral to medial. In the lower portion of the cervical spine adequate exposure will require division of the omohyoid muscle. At this stage, the muscles arising from the transverse processes are encountered and can either be retracted or dissected free from their origin. The anterior scalene muscle arises from the transverse processes of C3, C4, C5, and C6, and the levator scapulae also arises from C3 and C4. The vertebral artery transverses the transverse foramina from C6 through C1 but is anterior to the transverse process of C7. Unless a tumor has eroded bone, further exposure of the vertebral artery, bone spurs, disc material, or nerve roots will require removal of part or all of the transverse process and uncinate process.

DISCUSSION

Potential complications with this procedure include injury to the spinal accessory nerve and the vertebral artery. The landmarks for locating the vertebral artery before it is seen are so prominent that untoward injury is unlikely. Once the artery is identified, it is easy to avoid and remains at the periphery of the surgical area. The spinal accessory nerve is seen early in the procedure and is more likely to be injured during retraction by excessive stretching than by division of the nerve itself.

The jugular vein lies anterior to the tips of the transverse processes of C1 and C2, well removed from the operative area. The risks of spine instability and spinal cord injury seem less with this approach than with others.

CSF leakage is not usually a problem, as the dura can usually be closed primarily or grafted, and there are several soft tissue layers between the dura and the skin.

SUMMARY

The lateral approach to the cervical spine and its applications have been presented. Its major use is in dealing with ventral and ventrolateral masses in the upper spinal canal and occasionally for C1–C2 fusions. The major advantages of this approach are: **A**) there is no spine instability if the joints are not disturbed; **B**) the surgeon's line of vision is truly lateral; **C**) little or no spinal cord retraction is necessary; and **D**) the surgical exposure is wide enough and superficial enough to not be confining. The lateral approach throughout the cervical spine is good for dealing with vertebral artery problems, and these are probably the only distances in which the lateral approach in the lower cervical spine is appropriate.

REFERENCES

1. Apuzzo MLJ, Weiss MH, Heiden JS. Transoral exposure of the atlantoaxial region. Neurosurgery 1978;3:201–207.

2. DiLorenzo N. Transoral approach to extradural lesions of the lower clivus and upper cervical spine: an experience of 19 cases. Neurosurgery 1989;24:37–42.

3. Fang HSY, Ong GB. Direct anterior approach to the upper cervical spine. J Bone Joint Surg [Am] 1962;44A:1588–1604.

4. Menezes AH, VanGilder JC. Transoral-transpharyngeal approach to the anterior craniocervical junction. J Neurosurg 1988;69:895–903.

5. Pasztor E, Vajda J, Piffko P, Horvath M, Gador I. Transoral surgery for craniocervical space-occupying processes. J Neurosurg 1984;60:276–281.

6. Crockard HA, Bradford R. Transoral transclival removal of schwannoma anterior to the craniocervical junction. J Neurosurg 1985;62:293–295.

7. Mullan S, Naunton R, Herkmat-Panah J, Vailati G. The use of an anterior approach to ventrally placed tumors in the foramen magnum and vertebral column. J Neurosurg 1966;24:536–543.

8. Southwick WO, Robinson RA. Surgical approaches to the vertebral bodies in the cervical and lumbar regions. J Bone Joint Surg [Am] 1957;39A:631–643.

9. Elkin DC, Harris MH. Arteriovenous aneurysm of the vertebral vessels. Ann Surg 1946;124:934–950.

10. Verbiest H. A lateral approach to the cervical spine: technique and indications. J Neurosurg 1968;28:191–203.

11. Henry AK. Extensile exposure. 2nd ed. Edinburgh: Churchill Livingstone, 1973.

12. Shucart WA, Kleriga E. A lateral approach to the upper cervical spine. Neurosurgery 1980;6:278–281.

13. Whitesides TE, Kelly RP. Lateral approach to the upper cervical spine for anterior fusion. South Med J 1966;59:879–883.

14. George B, Laurian C, Keravel Y, Cophignon J. Neurosurg 1985;16:591–594.

15. Rinaldi I. The value of preoperative angiography in the surgical management of cervical hourglass neurofibroma. J Neurosurg 1972;36:97–101.

16. Simmons EH, Toit G Jr. Lateral atlantoaxial arthrodesis. Orthop Clin North Am 1978;9:1101–1114.

17. Habal MB, McComb JG, Shillito J Jr., Eisenberg HM, Murray JE. Combined posteroanterior approach to a tumor of the cervical spinal foramen. J Neurosurg 1972;37:113–116.

18. Love JG, Dodge HW Jr. Dumbell (hourglass) neurofibromas affecting the spinal cord. Surg Gynecol Orthop 1952;94:161–172.

41

Management of Cervical Spine Facet Fracture-Dislocations

Volker K. H. Sonntag and Mark N. Hadley

Introduction

The management of facet fracture-dislocation injuries of the cervical spine is controversial. Their initial treatment, methods of reduction, and methods of spinal stabilization are issues of considerable debate (1–5). This monograph reviews 68 patients with acute traumatic cervical spine facet fracture-dislocations. The management algorithm employed in their evaluation and treatment will be presented, and the long-term outcome from specific therapies will be reviewed. The issues of controversy as outlined above will be discussed.

Overview

The cervical spine is the most vulnerable and the most commonly injured spinal segment following a trauma. It is estimated that approximately 200,000 traumatic spinal column injuries occur each year in the United States, roughly 70% of which involve the cervical spine (1). Traumatic injuries of sufficient force associated with flexion of the head and neck with respect to the torso (with or without rotation of the head and neck) may result in facet fracture-dislocation injuries. Although facet fracture-dislocations are uncommon, they are associated with a high incidence of severe neurological morbidity and represent difficult patient management problems (1, 4, 5). Our experience with 68 patients with cervical spine facet injuries and our approach to their evaluation and treatment is reported.

Patient Population

Sixty-eight consecutive patients with cervical facet fracture-dislocations are included in this review. These patients represented 7% of our total acute traumatic cervical spine injured population treated over a 12-year period. Thirty-seven patients had bilateral locked facet dislocations (+/− fracture) (Fig. 41.1) and 31 patients presented with unilateral facet fracture-dislocation injuries (Fig. 41.2). Males outnumbered females four to one (median age, 29 years; range, 14–63 years). Motor vehicle accidents, diving injuries, and falls were the most common causes of traumatic injury. Thirteen patients presented with evidence of spinal shock. All had complete neurological injuries at the level of the facet fracture-dislocation.

Unilateral Injuries

The most common level of unilateral facet fracture-dislocation was C6–7 (Table 41.1). Of the 31 patients with this injury type, 24 presented with neurological injuries referable to their cervical spine trauma. Seven patients had root deficits only, 10 had incomplete spinal cord injuries, and 7 patients had complete neurological deficits. Six patients were neurologically intact and presented with pain only. One patient presented with a combination of severe head injury and cervical fracture-dislocation and was difficult to assess neurologically (Table 41.2).

All patients but two were treated with prompt attempts to achieve closed reduction in the emergency room upon presentation. Typically, this involved the placement of Gardner-Wells tongs or the application of the halo cranial ring followed by rapid employment of cervical traction. The two exceptions to rapid, progressive cervical traction presented in a delayed fashion following cervical trauma (3 weeks and 8 weeks, respectively). Eighteen patients were reduced with closed cervical traction and required an average weight of 9.8 pounds per superior level. Sixteen of these patients were subsequently treated with external fixation in a halo immobilization device. Two patients were treated with internal fixation followed by halo vest application.

Of the 11 patients who failed closed reduction in the emergency room, 8 were taken to the operating room for open reduction and internal fixation. Three complete patients with severe head injuries or other concomitant diseases were treated with external stabilization only (halo vest) without reduction.

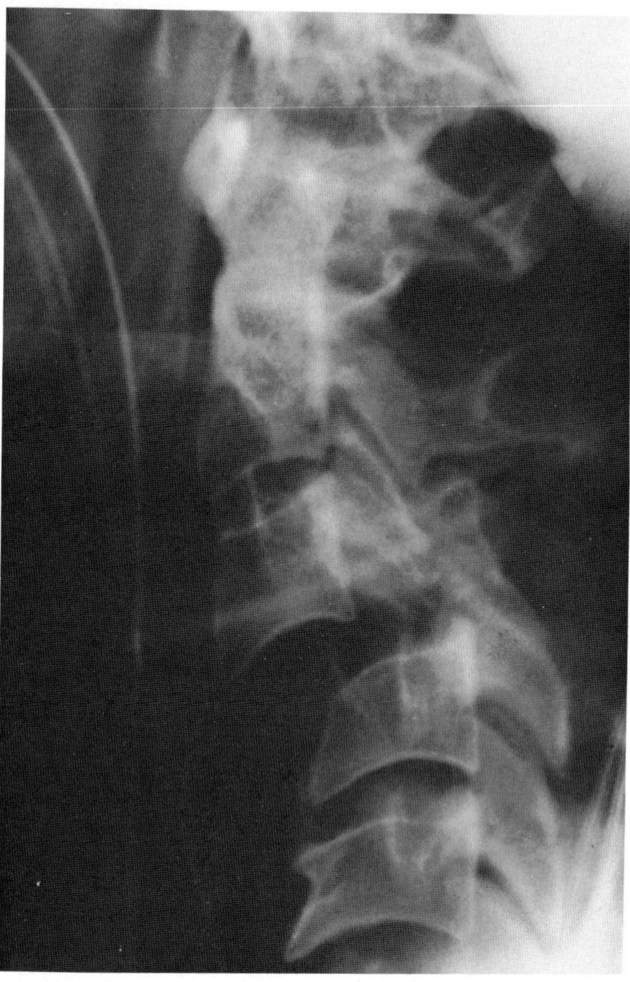

Figure 41.1. Lateral radiograph revealing bilateral C3–4 facet dislocation.

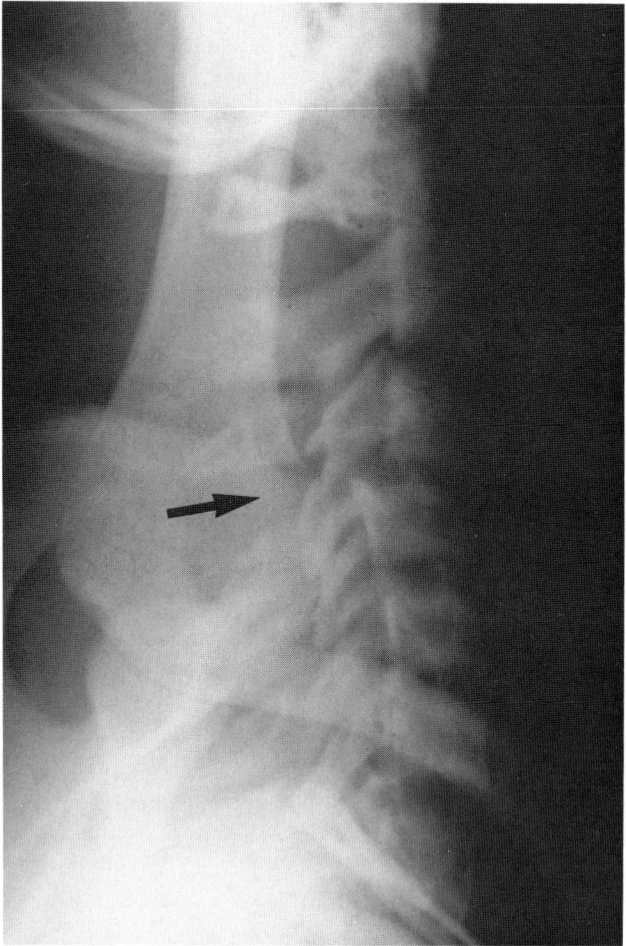

Figure 41.2. Lateral radiograph (swimmer's view) of unilateral C3–4 facet dislocation injury (*arrow*).

BILATERAL INJURIES

Similar to unilateral fracture-dislocations, the most common level of bilateral facet injuries was C6–7 (Table 41.1). All patients in this injury subgroup presented with neurological injuries: 6 with incomplete injuries, and 31 with complete spinal cord injuries (Table 41.2). All patients were treated with early and aggressive attempts at closed reduction of their fracture-dislocations with the use of cervical spine traction. These attempts were successful in 20 patients (average, 9.4 pounds per superior level), 15 of whom were subsequently treated with external stabilization alone (halo vest), and 5 of whom were treated with internal fixation followed by external stabilization.

Of the 17 patients who failed closed reduction, 2 had associated cervical spine fractures of a higher, noncontiguous cervical head; 5 had worsening of neurological deficits; 6 had facet fractures at the subluxed level that hindered reduction and realignment; and 4 were thought to be overly distracted at cervical levels distinct from the level of fracture-subluxation or had a marked increase in pain symptoms. All 17 of these patients underwent open reduction and internal fixation.

OPERATIVE TECHNIQUE

Patients who are operative candidates for the indications outlined (failure of closed reduction, failure of external stabilization or neural compression from bone, disk, or hematoma) are immobilized in the halo-vest or Gardner-Wells tong traction in the prone position on the operating room table. Our standard approach is a posterior one with far lateral exposure of the posterior elements and facet joints at the levels of injury. In those that are not reduced, reduction is first achieved by gentle manipulation and/or by removing part of the facet involved. Offending compressive components (e.g., lamina, disk, hematoma) are removed, often with the aid of a microscope. We typically perform a posterior wiring and fusion procedure utilizing 24-gauge twisted, stainless steel wire (3 turns per centi-

Table 41.1. Facet Dislocation

Level	Unilateral	Bilateral
C2–3	1	0
C3–4	8	2
C4–5	5	4
C5–6	7	11
C6–7	10	15
C7–T1	0	5
Total	31	37

Table 41.2. Facet Dislocation

Neurological Injury	Unilateral	Bilateral
None	6	0
Root	7	0
Incomplete	10	6
Complete	7	31
Total	30*	37

*One patient with severe head injury could not be assessed for level of spinal cord injury.

meter) and autologous iliac crest bone for fusion. A single loop of wire is placed in a sublaminar fashion under the lamina of the intact posterior elements of the superior vertebral segment and is then looped under and affixed to the intact spinous process of the inferior vertebra. The exposed bony surfaces and injured facet joints are decorticated with curettes and a high speed drill, and iliac crest bone is used to provide the fusion materal. Postoperatively, the patient is immobilized in a halo-vest for 10–12 weeks (Fig. 41.4).

Less frequently, we have used a spinous-process-to-spinous-process wiring technique. This approach is considered for patients who have incomplete neurological deficits and preoperative evidence of spinal canal stenosis. The spinous-process-to-spinous-process wiring technique obviates the need to place a wire in the sublaminar space at the superior level of injury. This wiring procedure is accompanied by the bone fusion as described above.

For both of these procedures to be effective, the posterior elements of the superior and inferior vertebral segments must be intact. For individuals without intact posterior elements, we have utilized posterior lateral mass plates and bicortical screws to achieve internal stabilization. An autologous iliac crest bone fusion accompanies this procedure to provide long-term stability.

Any patient with nerve root compromise, either clinically or radiographically, at the level of injury should receive a posterior root decompression and foraminotomy in an attempt to improve neurological function at that level. We do not advocate the use of methyl methacrylate for these procedures. In our experience acrylic does not add to the strength of the temporary internal stability provided by the wires or plates, and it does not enhance the long-term effectiveness of the bony fusion mass.

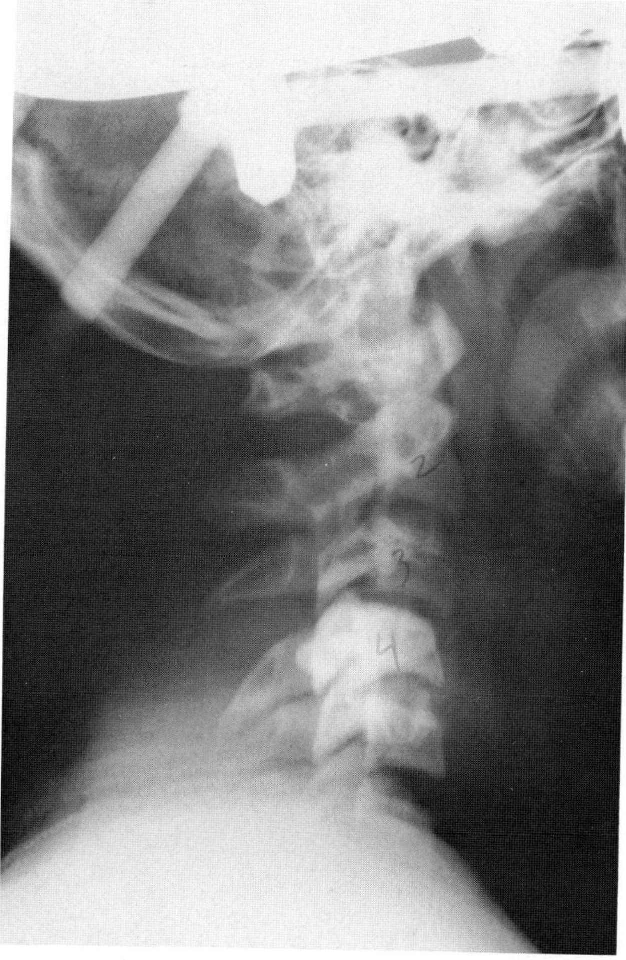

Figure 41.3. Patient with unstable unilateral C3–4 facet dislocation despite halo immobilization.

Outcome from Treatment

Follow-up was achieved in 20 of 31 patients (65%) with unilateral facet injuries (one patient with a severe head injury died early in his hospital course) for a mean duration of 18 months (range, 4–94 months). Of 37 patients with bilateral facet injuries, 33 (89%) were available for follow-up (mean duration, 25 months; range, 12–87 months).

Method of Stabilization

Of 16 patients with unilateral facet injuries who were treated with closed reduction and external fixation, 3 patients (19%) were unstable in the halo device despite repeated attempts at proper alignment (Fig. 41.3) and ultimately required open reduction with internal fixation (Figs. 41.4 and 41.5). Fifteen patients with bilateral injuries were treated with closed reduction and external fixation, only 4 of which

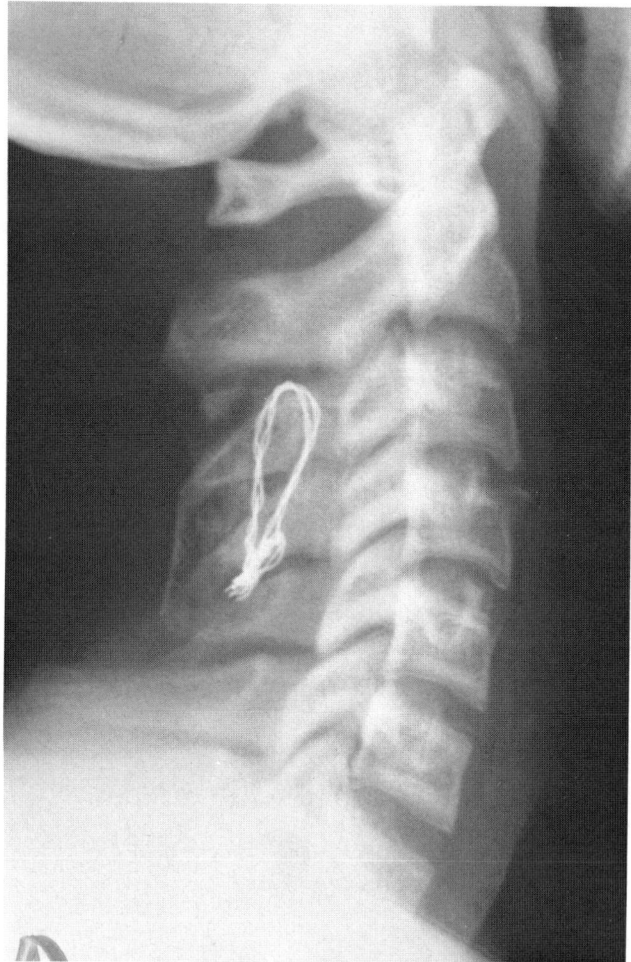

Figure 41.4. Postoperative lateral x-ray revealing wiring and fusion at C3–4 level following open reduction and internal fixation for unstable C3–4 facet dislocation. NOTE: Sublaminar twisted stainless steel wires are used only at the superior level. They are affixed around the spinous process at the inferior level.

were unstable in the halo device (27%) (Fig. 41.6). All 4 patients were markedly unstable in the halo vest such that alignment could not be maintained when the patient was placed in the upright position. All 4 underwent successful open reduction and internal fixation.

Eight patients with unilateral injuries were treated with open reduction, seven of which included internal fixation. Six of 7 patients with unilateral injuries in whom open reduction with internal fixation was performed were stable on long-term follow-up. One patient treated with open reduction and internal fixation developed progressive kyphosis at the level of injury that required subsequent surgical corpectomy and strut graft fusion 6 years after his initial injury. The single patient treated with open reduction and external fixation had evidence of resubluxation after surgery. This patient had a neurologically complete injury; therefore, the redislocation was not subsequently treated.

Seventeen patients with bilateral facet fracture-disloca-

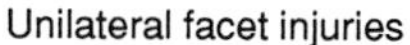

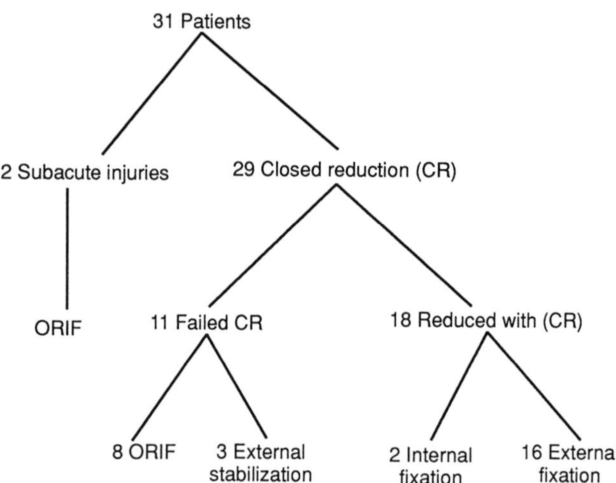

ORIF= Open reduction and internal fixation

Figure 41.5. Graphic representation of treatment of patients with unilateral facet injuries.

Bilateral facet injuries

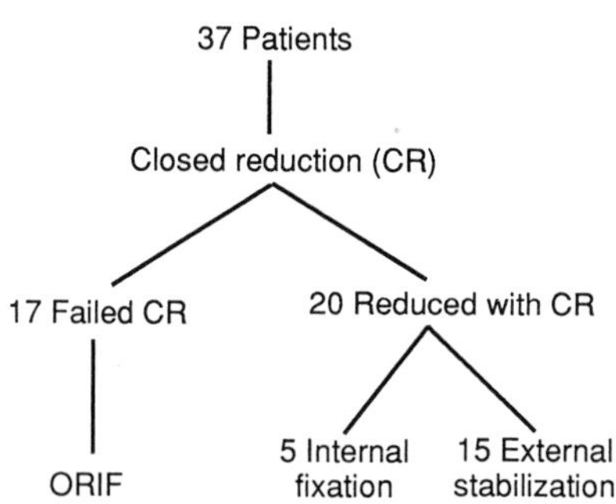

ORIF = Open reduction and internal fixation

Figure 41.6. Graphic representation of treatment of bilateral facet dislocation injuries.

tions were treated with open reduction and internal fixation. All were stable at follow-up as were the five patients who had successful closed reduction and who were subsequently treated with internal fixation.

Neurologic Recovery

Of the 31 patients with unilateral facet injuries, one died early in his hospital course. All six patients who presented neurologically intact but with severe neck and arm pain improved. Of seven patients who presented with radicular signs, five improved (four intact); two did not. Only seven patients in the unilateral facet injury subgroup with spinal cord injuries were available for neurologic follow-up. Of five patients with *incomplete* motor and sensory deficits, two were neurologically intact at last examination (8 and 20 months). Three of the five had significant but incomplete recoveries; two of the three were ambulatory. One of two *complete* patients was improved at last evaluation (94 months). While he still had residual motor and sensory deficits, he was ambulatory with arm braces. One C5-level complete patient was worse following failed open reduction and subsequent stabilization in a halo vest. He developed a posterior fossa infarction despite a normal vertebral artery angiogram. He survived but lost bicep function bilaterally (11 months).

Four patients with incomplete spinal cord injuries and 29 patients with complete injuries who had bilateral facet fracture-dislocation injuries were available for follow-up. Of these, 13 improved neurologically. One patient with a complete injury who was reduced within 6 hours of injury was neurologically intact at last follow-up (54 months). One complete injury patient regained modest motor and sensory function in both lower extremities following surgical reduction and internal fixation (10 hours postinjury), but he remains profoundly impaired at the C6 level (40 months follow-up). One complete patient gained a cervical root level of function, and 5 complete patients had improvements in existing root function after therapy.

Of four patients with incomplete injuries, two had marked improvement in both motor and sensory function and were able to ambulate independently. One incomplete patient regained sensory function only below the level of injury, and one incomplete-injury patient gained a cervical root level of function but had persistent and severe motor and sensory deficits below the level of fracture-subluxation at last evaluation.

Of the 5 patients whose neurological deficits worsened during closed reduction, 4 improved beyond baseline after open reduction and internal fixation. One patient with a complete injury who lost a cervical root level during attempts at closed reduction did not improve. One patient deteriorated after open reduction and internal fixation. He was a C5-level complete-injury patient who lost bilateral bicep function postoperatively.

Discussion

While facet-fracture dislocations of the cervical spine are relatively uncommon after spinal column trauma, they represent devastating injuries to the victims involved. Seven percent of a large population of cervical spine-injured patients had either unilateral or bilateral facet dislocations; of these, 90% sustained neurological injuries. This high incidence of neurological morbidity was particularly apparent in the bilateral facet dislocation group, of which 31 of 37 patients had complete spinal cord deficits.

Most investigators favor rapid and aggressive reduction of the fracture-dislocation; however, some clinicians question this practice, particularly for patients who present with complete neurological injuries (1–6). Among those who agree on an aggressive approach to these injuries, controversy exists regarding the methods of initial reduction. From our review of 68 consecutive cervical spine facet-dislocation patients, several conclusions may be drawn.

Early, rapid closed reduction of facet dislocation injuries has merit. Thirty-eight of 66 patients (58%) on whom this practice was employed had successful closed reduction with realignment of the cervical spine using Gardner-Wells tongs and cervical traction. After reduction most of these patients demonstrated improvements in neurological function that ranged from alleviation of pain and improved root function to complete or near complete resolution of spinal cord deficits (including one complete-injury patient who had a full recovery after reduction).

Closed reduction is not without liability, however. Forty-two percent of facet-dislocation injuries could not be reduced with closed techniques, and seven patients (11%) had worsening of neurological deficits, although six of the seven subsequently recovered.

Factors that inhibited our ability to effectively reduce fracture-dislocation injuries of the cervical spine included worsening pain, fractures at another cervical segment, fracture of the facet at the level of subluxation, overdistraction at cervical levels distinct from the level of injury, and the aforementioned patients who had exacerbation of their neurological injuries. Successful closed reduction was achieved with patients placed in a slightly flexed position and with progressive application of cervical weight traction beginning at 3 pounds per superior injury level and increasing to 12 pounds per superior level in certain cases (average, 9.4 pounds per superior level). Patients who failed closed reduction were easily reduced with open reduction, performed with the patient in tongs and traction in the operating room.

The issue of stabilization following reduction, either open or closed, remains controversial (1–6). Of 31 patients treated with closed reduction and external stabilization, 24 (77%) were stable at long-term follow-up. Seven patients (23%) failed external stabilization and required internal fixation. External stabilization was most effective if a fracture was identified at the level of injury (22 of 24 patients = 92%), thus requiring bone-healing to play a major role in long-term spinal column stability. Of those patients who failed external stabilization despite good alignment with closed reduction, all, in our experience, had ligamentous disruption only without evidence of fractures at the facet-dislocation injury site.

In general, if open reduction is required, we believe internal fixation at the same operative setting is the most efficacious treatment plan for these patients. All but one patient in our series treated with open reduction, internal fixation, and fusion was stable at last examination (96%). Only one patient deteriorated neurologically after this procedure (4% morbidity).

Treatment Recommendations

Patients with facet-fracture dislocations of the cervical spine should immediately be immobilized in the field. This strategy must be rigidly enforced and continued throughout the patient's course of treatment. Serial neurological examinations will document the extent of injury and monitor improvement or deterioration with therapy. After resuscitation and treatment of spinal shock (as necessary), lateral cervical radiographs will document the facet-dislocation injury. Other evidence of cervical trauma or noncontiguous fractures must be identified.

Cervical traction should be implemented immediately unless cranial trauma precludes its application. Once the facet dislocation injury is identified, reduction and realignment becomes the most important goal. Transfer to the radiology suite for computerized tomography (CT) is not indicated in the acute setting (1, 5). Close attention to the patient's examination and the serial radiographs is essential. As stated, a deterioration in the clinical examination or overdistraction of the cervical spine at levels distinct from the facet-dislocation are criteria for discontinuing attempts at closed reduction.

If closed reduction can be accomplished, placement in a halo immobilization device provides the best available protection and immobilization. A CT scan at this point will identify fracture fragments in or around the facet injury and is more safely obtained with the halo immobilization device in place (1, 5, 7, 8). If a fracture is identified on the CT images and alignment can be maintained with the halo vest, this form of therapy is continued for 12 weeks.

Patients who cannot be effectively realigned with closed reduction techniques and those patients, once reduced, who do not have CT evidence of a cervical fracture should be offered surgical therapy for reduction and/or internal fixation with fusion as required.

After proceeding as rapidly as possible with the diagnostic assessment and reduction, keeping the cervical spine aligned is of the utmost importance. While facet-dislocation injuries of the cervical spine are associated with a high incidence of neurological compromise, a select percentage of these injuries can be reversed with aggressive and compulsive early management and treatment.

REFERENCES

1. Sonntag VKH, Hadley MN. Nonoperative management of cervical spine injuries. Clin Neurosurg 1988;34:630–649.

2. Cloward RB. Reduction of traumatic dislocation of the cervical spine with locked facets. Technical note. J Neurosurg 1973;38:527–531.

3. Hollin SA, Hayashi H, Gross SW. Management of cervical spine dislocations with locked facets. Surg Gynecol Obstet 1967;124:521–524.

4. De Oliveira JC. Anterior reduction of interlocking facets in the lower cervical spine. Spine 1979;4:195–202.

5. Sonntag VKH. Management of bilateral locked facets of the cervical spine. Neurosurgery 1981;8:150–152.

6. Bucholz RD, Cheung KC. Halo vest versus spinal fusion for cervical injury: evidence from an outcome study. J Neurosurg 1989;70:884–892.

7. Yetkin Z, Osborn AG, Giles DS, et al. Uncovertebral and facet joint dislocations in cervical articular pillar fractures: CT evaluation. AJNR 1985;6:633–637.

8. Scher AT. Unilateral locked facet in cervical spine injuries. AJR 1977;129:45–48.

42

Cervical Spine Infections

R. Geoffrey Wilber and Nancy Ann Frantz

Introduction

Infection of the cervical spine is a relatively rare but extremely serious disorder. Recognition and appropriate management are essential in the care of these often quite ill patients. The potential catastrophic consequences of untreated spinal infection can be avoided by early diagnosis and comprehensive care.

The problem of spinal infection is not new, in fact, prehistoric evidence of spinal involvement with tuberculosis has been found. It was also described in the early Egyptian as well as Greek civilizations. Percival Pott described cervical spine involvement with tuberculosis and discussed its poor prognosis with upper spinal involvement (1). Death or paralysis were the usual sequelae.

Spinal infections may present as discitis, osteomyelitis or as epidural abscesses. Three hundred eighteen cases of spinal pyogenic infections have been recorded in the recent literature (2–7). Vertebral osteomyelitis represents only approximately 1% of all skeletal osteomyelitis. Cervical involvement occurs in only 8% of the total cases of pyogenic spinal infections. Sepsis of the cervical spine carries the highest rate of neurologic sequelae, compared to other areas of spinal involvement.

Infection of the spine usually is seen in the extradural space. Associated meningeal processes can occur with direct extension or breakdown of the blood-brain barrier. Classically, infection is thought to begin as a peridiscal lesion of septic loci (Fig. 42.1). Spread then occurs with involvement of the disc, vertebral body, epidural space, or combination of the three. Mycotic and pyogenic processes have different presentations, courses, and treatment. A separate discussion of mycotic spinal infections is included later.

Pathogenesis of Pyogenic Infections

Batson's venous plexus and the rich venous plexuses surrounding the spine are thought to be associated with venous spread of infection to the spine (8). Probably of more importance for pyogenic processes is the arterial route, as demonstrated by Wiley and Trueta (9). Direct sludging of bacteria in the tortuous capillary loop adjacent to the disc space is thought to be the most common mechanism for initiation of infection. Crock clearly showed the microanatomy of the subchondral postcapillary venous network where this sludging is thought to occur (10).

Infection can also occur by direct extension. This can happen in the neck from infections in the pretracheal space or mediastium. Penetrating wounds of the neck (i.e., gunshot wounds and knife wounds) can cause direct inoculation of organisms into the cervical spine. Seeding of the discs can also be seen after surgical procedures.

Once infection gains a foot-hold, spread occurs to the adjacent structures, and the disc can be involved. Discs are avascular structures that receive their nutrition by diffusion from the vertebral end-plate vessels. Once inoculated by bacteria, rapid deterioration and destruction of the disc space is common. The poor vascularity of the disc also inhibits penetration of antibiotics during treatment. Spread of infection into the vertebrae can induce osteomyelitis with its typical histopathologic sequelae. The epidural and subdural spaces can be involved either by direct extension of pus or by vertebral body and/or disc collapse with resultant spinal kyphosis and retropulsion of bone, disc, and granulation tissue. Extension into tissue adjacent to the spine can induce abscess formation in the prevertebral space (Fig. 42.2).

Bacteriology

In the classic review of osteomyelitis, Waldvogel et al. (5) found approximately 66% of all cases were caused by *Staphylococcus aureus*. Spacio and Montgomerie (7) compiled bacteriologic data from 222 patients with pyogenic vertebral osteomyelitis, of which gram positive cocci were responsible for 67% of the cases reviewed. The majority of these were due to *Staphylococcus aureus*. This was followed by *Streptococcus viridans*, *Streptococcus pneumoniae* and *Enterococcus*. It was felt that the high incidence of *Staphylococcus* was due to bacteremia.

Cases of gram negative bacterial vertebral osteomyelitis accounted for less than one-half the total number of gram positive. Among the gram negative organisms, *Escherichia coli* was the most frequent. Historically, gram negative infections were usually associated with infection or manip-

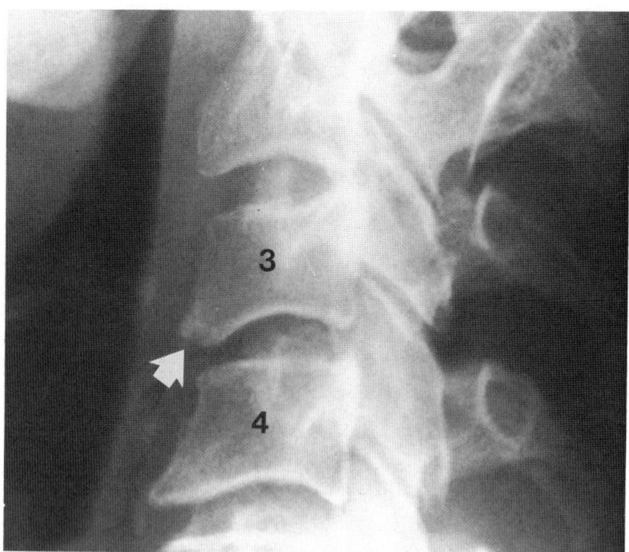

Figure 42.1. Peridiscal lesion (*arrow*) in patient with early vertebral osteomyelitis (staphylococcal). This was noted in retrospect on serial review of radiographs.

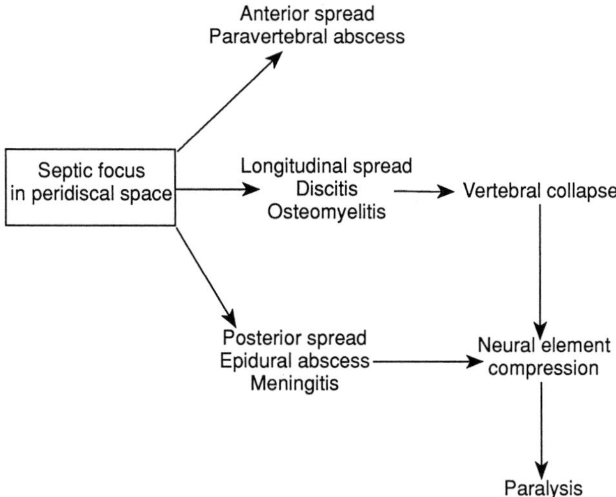

Figure 42.2. Paraspinal abscess located in the prevertebral space.

ulation of the genital urinary tract or previous spinal surgery (11). Gram negative bacteria have played an increasing role recently, especially in intravenous drug abusers. In a review of 67 cases of vertebral osteomyelitis in drug abusers (12), *Pseudomonas* was the organism recovered in 65.5% of cases. *Staphylococcus aureus* was next in frequency, with 15.5% of cases, followed by *Serratia* (8%) *Klebsiella* (6%) *Enterobacter* (3%); *Streptococcus, Candida*, and *Mycobacterium tuberculosis* combined comprised 1.5% of the total. It should be noted that the distribution of the site of infection in the intravenous drug abusers varies from the previous literature, with a higher incidence of cervical and a lower incidence of thoracolumbar involvement.

Anaerobes appear to be a rare cause of vertebral osteomyelitis and are exceedingly rare in the cervical spine (13). Two cases of *Propionibacterium acnes* have been reported (14). Both patients had skin lesions present, and this was felt to be the source of infection.

Fungal vertebral osteomyelitis is also quite uncommon. In a review by Friedman and Simon (15) of vertebral osteomyelitis caused by *Candida*, only one case was cervical.

Tuberculous infection of the spine is still seen today. The overall incidence of bone and joint tuberculosis has declined dramatically since 1950. Vertebral tuberculous infection represents 50–60% of all cases of skeletal involvement (16). Farer et al. (17), in a retrospective review of records from 1969–1973 in 26 cities in the United States, found 676 cases of bone and joint tuberculosis, of which 40% were spinal. Cervical spine infection due to *Mycobacterial tuberculosis* is the least common site of involvement. It comprises only about 3–5% of cases (18). The necessity of proper culture techniques must be emphasized in tuberculous infection due to the usual low number of viable organisms in bone disease. Allen et al. (19) reviewed 62 operative specimens for culture and found only 75% yielded growth. The specimens most likely to yield the organisms are those appearing caseous or puslike and involved bone. Twenty-four per cent of the patients yielded positive cultures from the tissue lining the abscess or from the involved bone alone (20).

The tuberculin skin test (PPD) still remains one of the most valuable diagnostic tools and is usually positive in skeletal tuberculosis. However, a negative skin test does not absolutely rule out the diagnosis.

The bacteriology of spinal epidural abscess is similar to osteomyelitis; *Staphylococcus aureus* is the most common agent. In a review (21) of 166 cases of spinal epidural abscess at any level 78% were due to gram positive organisms. *Staphylococcus aureus* accounted for approximately 60% of the cases. Gram negative rods were the next most frequent, comprising 30% of the cases. Isolation of coagulase negative staphylococcus, pneumococcus, *Actinomyces israelii*, and gram negative anaerobes has been reported.

Lasker and Harler (22) reviewed 15 cases of cervical epidural abscess. As in other reviews, *Staphylococcus aureus* was the overwhelming causative bacteria in 10 of the 15 cases. There were also single cases of Beta streptococcus, *Pseudomonas aeruginosa*, and Enterococcus.

DIAGNOSIS

The initial diagnostic management of suspected spinal infection should include a thorough history and physical examination. Classically, a previous history of a septic episode or of possible transient bacteremia (i.e., urologic manipulation) can be elicited. Risk factors include diabetes, hemodialysis, furunculosis, oral surgery, i.v. drug abuse, and immunocompromised conditions (e.g., HIV positive). Severe neck pain is common in this condition and is seen in approximately 90% of patients with spinal infections. This is usually *not* activity related. Fever may or may not be present and is seen in only approximately 52% of patients. General malaise is common, as is weight loss. Vague pain referred to the occipital or trapezial region is not uncommon. Neurologic loss is seen in approximately 17% of patients with vertebral infections (4). Meningitis is present in only 1% of patients. It is very common for symptoms to be present for protracted periods with approximately half of patients having symptoms for 3 months or greater.

Laboratory Studies

The most predictive laboratory study in spinal infection is the erythrocyte sedimentation rate (E.S.R.) In a literature review, 92% of the patients have an elevated E.S.R. with pyogenic vertebral osteomyelitis. It is also seen to have a predictive value in monitoring the success of the treatment regimen (4).

The leukocyte count is less accurate in predicting spinal sepsis. Only 43% of patients in one series had white blood counts of greater than 10,000/mm (3, 4). The presence of a normal white blood count by no means excludes the possibility of spinal sepsis.

Bacteriologic data are essential in the successful treatment of cervical spine infections. Shotgun approaches to antibiotic coverage are generally not appropriate. Attempts at gathering bacteriologic data are essential for patient management. Bacteriologic isolates should be considered significant only when cultured from the bone, abscess adjacent to bone, or the blood. Blood cultures alone are positive approximately 25% of the time. Needle biopsy is positive 70% of the time (Fig. 42.3). Open biopsy is positive 86% of the time. Reasons for negative culture results are previous antibiotic treatment, poor culture techniques, inaccurate timing of blood cultures, or placement of the biopsy needle. Urine cultures and sensitivity may have some value in diagnosing sources of spinal infection.

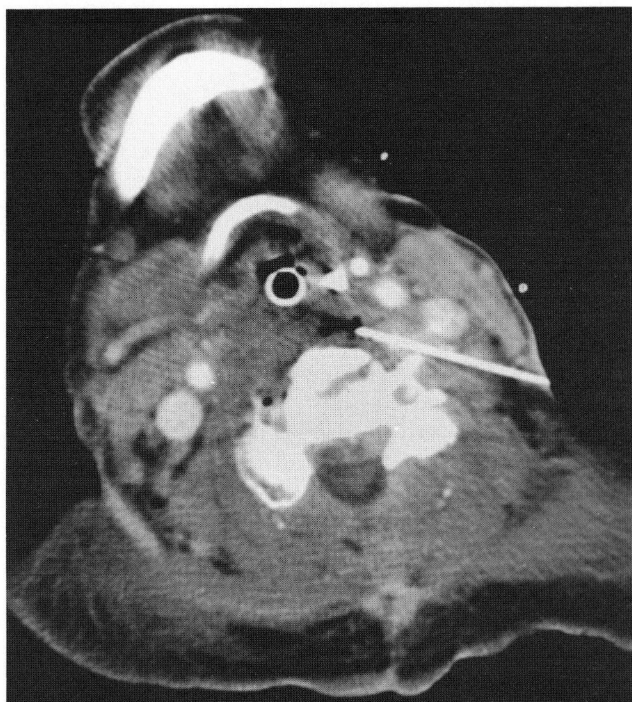

Figure 42.3. CT-guided biopsy of soft tissue abscess in prevertebral space. Note air density at tip of needle which represents the abscess cavity.

Imaging Techniques

Plain radiographic evidence of early spinal infections is usually not present. Changes in bone and disc spaces evolve over weeks to months (23). The earliest changes occur with a focal lesion in the vertebral end-plate. This is often followed by the more typical changes of disc space narrowing and bony sclerosis. Late changes can show severe instability with listhesis or spontaneous fusion (Fig. 42.4). Occasionally soft tissue swelling and abscess formation can be seen on plain radiographic studies.

Bone scanning is an excellent tool in localizing vertebral infectious processes. Technetium 99 diphosphonate bone scanning is the most common study and is usually very good at identifying evidence of infections and inflammatory processes involving the vertebrae. The

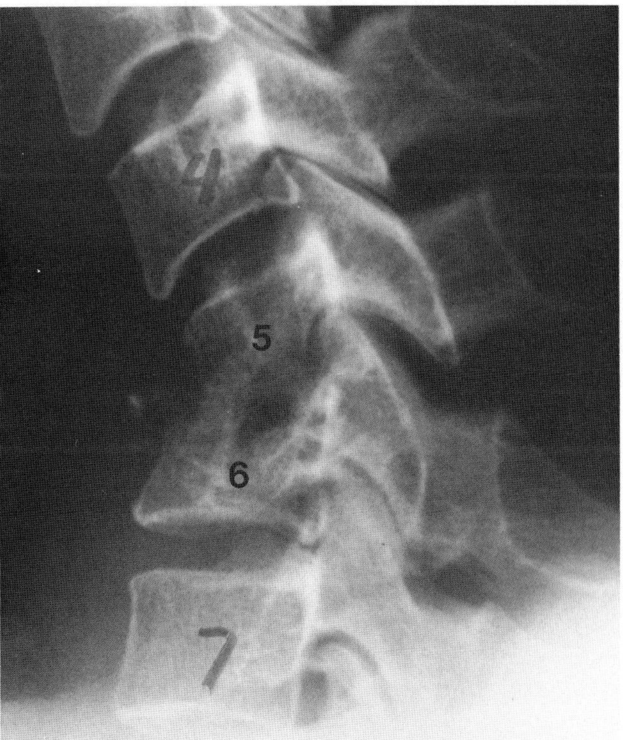

Figure 42.4. Kyphotic collapse in a patient with disc space and subchondral bone destruction. This patient presented with quadriparesis and vertebral osteomyelitis.

early scan studies with TC-99m show diffuse increased uptake. The delayed views show more localized involvement (24) (Fig. 42.5).

Gallium 67 scanning is more specific for infections and can be used in conjunction with other scanning techniques. Indium-labeled white blood cell scans are quite specific for both acute and chronic infectious processes (25).

Plain tomography may be useful in defining exact changes in bone morphology in both the sagittal and coronal planes. It is generally poor at looking at soft tissue involvement. Computed tomography (CT) is especially helpful in defining involvement in the axial plane. Changes in perivertebral tissues can be seen and abscess cavities. Identified disc hypointensity as well as bony changes in spinal infections are well described with CT studies. Sagittal reformatting and contrast studies with intrathecal dye are quite useful in detecting epidural spread as well as dural compression (Fig. 42.6).

Magnetic resonance imaging (MRI) has been applied to osteomyelitis and discitis of the spine by Modic (24). He described the classic changes in pyogenic infections of the disc space and subchondral bone. Marked hypointensity of the disc and adjacent bone on T1 weighted images and increased intensity of the disc space and bone on T2 weighted images are pathognomonic. MRI also is excellent in identifying dural compression in both the axial and sagittal planes and useful in predicting the extent of the infection including skin lesions and epidural spread (Figs. 42.7, 42.8).

MEDICAL TREATMENT

Once the suspicion of spinal infection has been raised, accurate identification of the causative organism is essential. This should be done before antibiotic administration. As discussed earlier, blood cultures may often be helpful. Sources of septic loci must be excluded (i.e., subacute bacterial endocarditis). Needle biopsy under fluoroscopy or computerized tomography is very accurate in organism identification. Open biopsy, usually through an anterior approach, also has a high success rate. Decompressive surgical procedures can be used to obtain appropriate biopsy specimens for culture and histology.

In general, most spinal infections can be handled in their early stages with appropriate antibiotic administration. Table 42.1 shows current protocols for antibiotic choice in these patients. Antibiotic regimens of 6 weeks or greater are standard. The sedimentation rate is usually reliable in demonstrating patient response to antibiotic treatment.

There are some patients with poor response to antibiotic administration alone. Reasons for this are multifactorial. Either inappropriate antibiotic coverage or poor penetration of antibiotics into the site of infection (i.e., disc space) can be causes. Abscesses usually do not respond to medication alone, and surgical drainage should be strongly considered.

Immobilization of infected spinal elements has been a recognized treatment mainstay for years. The neck should be held in an appropriate orthosis to allow for healing of the infectious process. In cases of severe instability, halo

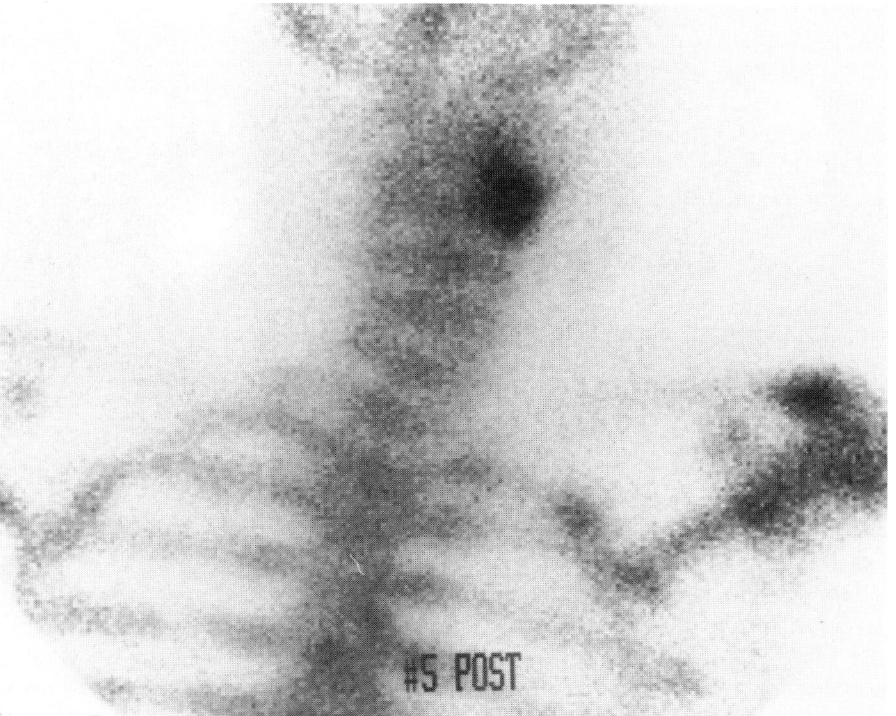

Figure 42.5. Bone scan showing increased uptake in a patient with C3–4 vertebral osteomyelitis. This process was present unilaterally and also involved the lateral mss.

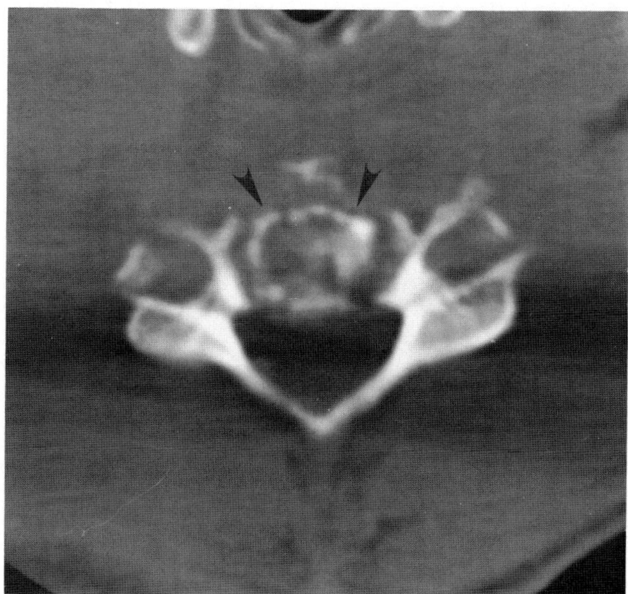

Figure 42.6. Destructive changes due to infection in the vertebral end-plate including cystic change visible on CT scan.

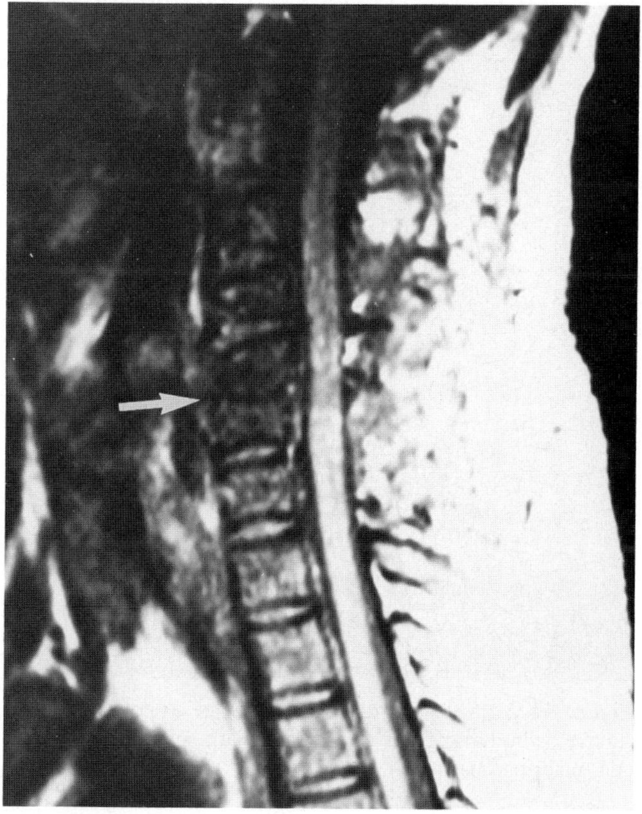

Figure 42.7. T1 weighted magnetic resonance image of C5–6 disc space showing decreased signal intensity as well as mild kyphosis. This patient had *Staphylococcus aureus* spinal osteomyelitis.

immobilization is appropriate. Less rigid orthotics are the 2-poster and Somi braces. The latter is best applied to upper cervical lesions. The Philadelphia collar does provide some degree of immobilization. The soft cervical collar only acts to remind the patient that he has a neck problem and should voluntarily avoid using his neck. Orthotic protection should be continued until there is evidence of resolution of infection with bony stability.

SURGICAL MANAGEMENT

There are general indications for surgical approaches to the infected spine. As mentioned earlier, open biopsy techniques have the highest success rate in organism identification. These should be applied when other noninvasive techniques for culture have failed.

Abscess cavities should be drained. This can occasionally be done with CT-guided needle drainage procedures. This may, however, not provide adequate drainage, and debridement is not possible. Open drainage historically has been very successful in managing perivertebral abscesses. These are best approached from the anterior route in the cervical spine. Success rates of obtaining the correct organism approaches 90% or better with good surgical and culture technique (4).

Open anterior procedures are indicated when there is poor response to antibiotic therapy with continuing high sedimentation rates. This can be manifested by continuing bony destruction and kyphosis. These patients are best managed by open debridement. Chronically infected devascularized tissue is removed, and the stage is set for better potential healing. Eismont (26) has demonstrated that autogenous iliac crest bone graft can be used anteriorally after appropriate debridement of infected tissue. This provides an anterior strut graft with a high likelihood of healing. Other autogenous cortical bone and allograft are probably not appropriate for use in the face of infection. Appropriate antibiotic therapy is essential for the success of these procedures.

In the case of spinal cord compression with neurologic deficit, the anterior surgical route is the best treatment (Fig. 42.9). The literature abounds with cases of poor results from decompressive laminectomies for basically anterior spinal pathology. Laminectomy in these cases often removes the last normal stabilizing structures: lamina interspinous ligaments, and facet joints and sets the stage for severe instability. Revision surgery in these patients can be exasperating. Gaining stability in an infected bed with a kyphotic, unstable spine is especially challenging if not impossible.

Anterior decompression with iliac crest bone graft seems to provide the highest likelihood of success. The compressive pathology is addressed, and debridement of the infected structures is facilitated. Immobilization can be accomplished with a halo vest as necessary.

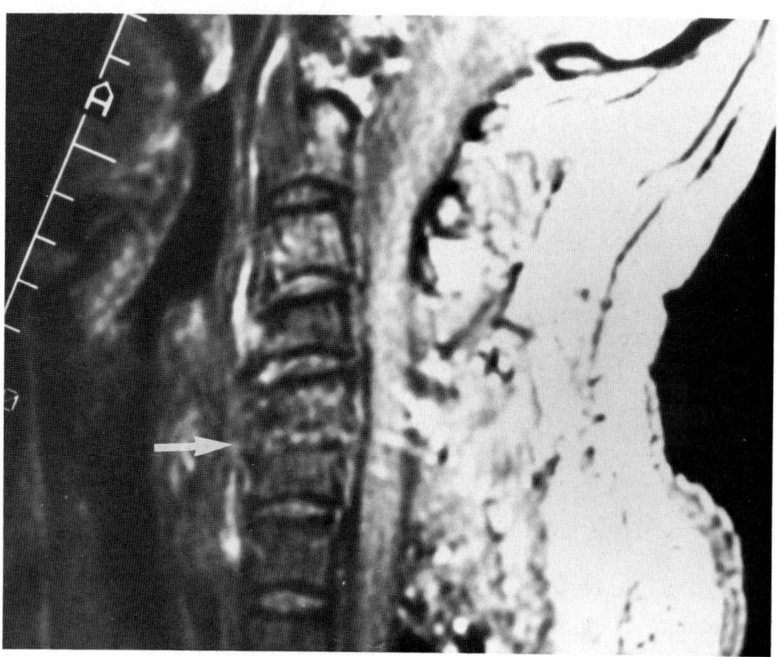

Figure 42.8. T2 weighted image of same cervical spine as in Figure 42.7 with increased signal intensity in the disc space. These are classic changes for osteomyelitis according to Modic.

Table 42.1. Recommended Drug of Choice

Organism	Antibiotic
Staphylococcus aureaus	
Methicillin sens.	— Penicillinase-resistant penicillin
Methicillin resist.	— Vancomycin
Streptococcus	
Viridans	— Penicillin
Pneumococcus	— Penicillin
Enterococcus	— Penicillin or Ampicillin + Aminoglycoside
Gram negatives	
E. coli	— Ampicillin or Third Generation Cephalosporin
Pseudomonas	— Aminoglycoside + Anti-pseudomonal Penicillin
Mycobacterium tuberculosis	— Isoniazid + Rifampin + Pyrazinamide

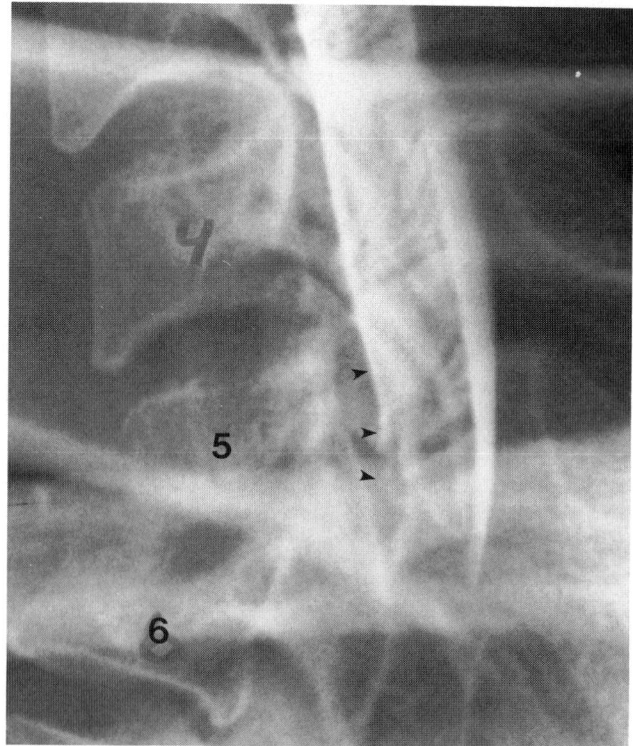

Figure 42.9. Spinal cord compression due to both soft tissue as well as bony kyphosis in a patient with spinal osteomyelitis and quadriparesis.

In the high cervical spine, there are two options for the surgical approach. The anterior transoral route allows for excellent visualization of the occiput to the C3 region (27). There is significant morbidity associated with this procedure. The wound itself is only semi-sterile with the route through the open oral mucosa. The anterior retropharyngeal approach as described by McAffee (28) provides adequate exposure of the upper cervical spine, allowing decompression and bone grafting in a sterile extraoral route.

In the lower cervical spine (C3–T1), the traditional approach described by Sothwicke and Robinson is used (29). This provides excellent exposure and is very reliable. Debridement can then be accomplished under a controlled environment, and bone grafting is facilitated.

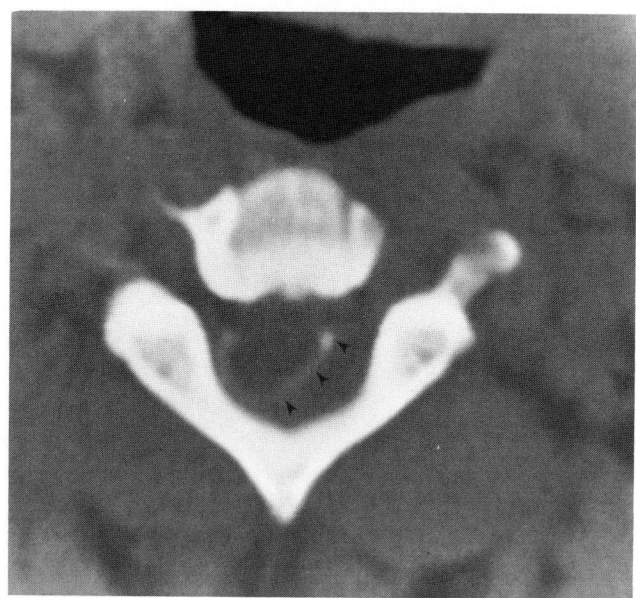

Figure 42.10. Epidural abscess causing spinal cord displacement. This is mainly a dorsal process in this patient. The offending organism was *E. coli.*

The posterior approach does have a place in managing cervical spine infection. It is best applied for pure epidural abscesses without significant anterior involvement (Fig. 42.10). In these cases, posterior exposure does not destabilize and provides the best surgical exposure as well as drainage of an epidural abscess cavity. In pure epidural or subdural abscesses, there is a standard sequence of clinical progression. The onset of spinal pain is followed by pain along the nerve roots. The third stage of sensory, motor, and sphincter disturbance culminates in paraplegia. Recognition of epidural abscesses is often difficult with insidious onset in some cases and rapid progression in others. Paralysis, once it has occurred, has a poor prognosis for recovery.

While metal implants should be avoided in the face of active infection, they may have a role in the late management of spinal instability and kyphosis. Extended antibiotic coverage may be needed when using metal fixation late, even after the infection is considered cured.

REFERENCES

1. Pott P. Medical classics. Vol. 1. Baltimore: Williams & Wilkins, 1937.
2. Bonfiglio M, Lange TA, Kim YM. Pyogenic vertebral osteomyelitis. Clin Orthop 1973;96:234–247.
3. Ross PM, Fleming JL. Vertebral body osteomyelitis, spectum and natural history. Clin Orthop 1976;118:190.
4. Griffiths HED, Jones PM. Pyogenic infections of the spine. J Bone Joint Surg 1971;53B:383.
5. Waldvogel FA, Medoff G, Swartz MN. Osteomyelitis: a review of clinical features, therapeutic considerations and unusual features. N Engl J Med 1970;282:198.
6. Sapico FL, Montgomerie JL. Pyogenic vertebral osteomyelitis: report of nine cases and review of the literature. Rev Infect Dis 1979;1:754.
7. Sapico FL, Montgomerie JL. Vertebral osteomyelitis in intravenous drug abusers: report of three cases and review of the literature. Rev Infect Dis 1980;2:196.
8. Batson OU. The function of vertebral veins and their rule in the spread of metastasis. Ann Surg 1940;112:138.
9. Wiley AM, Trueta J. The vascular anatomy of the spine and its relationship to pyogenic vertebral osteomyelitis. J Bone Joint Surg 1959;41B:796.
10. Crock HV, Yoshizawa H, Kame SK. Observations on the venous drainage of the human vertebral body. J Bone Joint Surg 1973;55B:528.
11. Henson SW Jr., Coventry MB. Osteomyelitis of the vertebrae as the result of infection of the urinary tract. Surg Gynecol Obstet 1956;102:207.
12. Sapico FL, Montgomerie JL. Vertebrae osteomyelitis in intravenous drug abusers. Rev Infect Dis 1980;2:196.
13. Raff MJ, Nelo JC. Anaerobic osteomyelitis. Medicine 1978;57:83.
14. Noble RC, Overman SB. Propionibacter acnes osteomyelitis: case report and review of the literature. J Clin Microbiol 1987;25:251–254.
15. Friedman BC, Simon GL. Candida vertebral osteomyelitis: report of three cases and a review of the literature. Diagn Microbiol Infect Dis 1987;8:31.
16. Gorse GJ, Pais MJ, Kusske JA, et al. Tuberculosis spondylitis. Medicine 1983;62:178.
17. Farer S, Lowell AM, Meador MP. Extrapulmonary tuberculosis in the United States. Am J Epidemiol 1979;109:205.
18. Martin NS. Tuberculosis of the spine: a study of the results of treatment during the last twenty-five years. J Bone Joint Surg (Br) 1970;53-B:613.
19. Allen BW, Mitchison DA, Darbyshire J, et al. Examination of operation specimens from patients with spinal tuberculosis for tubercle bacilli. J Clin Pathol 1983;36:662–666.
20. Davidson PT, Fernandez E. Bone and joint tuberculosis. In: Schlossberg D, ed. Tuberculosis. New York: Springer-Verlag, 1987.
21. Danner RL, Hartman BJ. Update on spinal epidural abscess, 35 cases and review of literature. Rev Infect Dis 1987;9:265.
22. Lasker BR, Harter DH. Cervical epidural abscess. Neurology 1987;37:1747.
23. Onofrio BM. Intervertebral discitis: incidence, diagnosis and management. Clin Neurosurg 1980;27:481.
24. Modic MT, Feighlin OH, Piraino DW. Vertebral osteomyelitis: assessment using MR. Radiology 1985;157:157.
25. Al-Sheikh W, Sfakianakas GN, Mnaymeh W. Subacute and chronic bone infections: diagnosis using IN-111, GA-67 and Tc-99m MDP bone scintigraphy and radiology. Radiology 1985;155:501.
26. Eismont FJ, Bohlman HH, Prasanna LS, Goldberg VM, Freehafer AA. Pyogenic and fungal vertebral osteomyelitis with paralysis. J Bone Joint Surg 1983;65-A:19.
27. Spetzler RF. Transoral approach to the upper cervical spine. In: Evarts CM. ed. Surgery of the musculoskeletal system. Vol 4. New York: Churchill Livingston, 1983: 99–34.
28. McAfee RC, Bohlman HH, Riley LH Jr. The anterior retropharyangeal approach to the upper part of the cervical spine. J Bone Joint Surg 1987;691:1931.
29. Riley LH. Surgical approaches to the anterior structures of the cervical spine. Clin Orthop 1973;91:16.

43

Complications of Cervical Spine Surgery

Ensor E. Transfeldt

The complication rate reported for cervical spine surgery is relatively low. However, the variety of complications that can occur are high, and many of these can be quite devastating. This diversity of complications is due to the wide range of anatomic structures including vascular, respiratory, intestinal, and neural which traverse the neck. It is important, therefore, for the surgeon to be familiar with the anatomic relationships of these structures in order to avoid damage to any one of them at the time of surgery. In addition to an understanding of the anatomy for the surgical exposure, the surgeon also needs to pay attention to careful technique, including the handling of soft tissue structures, appropriate placement of retractors, and hemostasis.

Complications in cervical spine surgery may occur preoperatively, intraoperatively, or postoperatively.

There are numerous intraoperative complications which are peculiar to the specific surgical approach. The incidence of reported complications is considerably higher and more serious with anterior exposures than posterior exposures, due to the increased number of vital anatomical structures at risk with this exposure. There are also complications such as infections, hematomas, and neurologic injuries which are common to both approaches.

In systematically considering the complications for these approaches, one can classify them into, *a*) soft tissue, *b*) bony, and *c*) neurologic involvement. There are also certain complications which are peculiar to different diagnostic categories.

Preoperative Complications

Preoperative complications may be due to poor patient selection, be associated with the investigative procedures, or may be related to the anatomic diagnosis itself.

Patient Selection

An incorrect diagnosis will lead to the incorrect operation, and it is, therefore, important that the appropriate history and physical examinations and investigations be carried out in order to make the correct diagnosis. The findings in each of these categories should all be consistent with the diagnosis. The timing of the surgery is also important. It is possible that the surgery may be performed too soon or too late. Sometimes a failure to operate may also result in old complications which could have been avoided by the surgery itself. Anesthesia itself poses a risk to any patient who has general systemic problems and is physiologically unstable. These problems need to be addressed and stabilized prior to surgery.

Investigations

The risks associated with most of the investigations for cervical conditions are extremely low, but there are numerous invasive, investigative techniques which do carry the risk of complications such as infection. These include myelograms and discograms. In additions, myelograms have the risk of producing severe postural hypotension, headaches, or spinal cord damage. Cisternal puncture requires good anatomical understanding and careful technique in experienced hands to avoid penetration of the spinal cord. Adherence to the correct tissue planes are important in needle placement for discograms. Failure to do so and to retract the esophagus can easily result in penetration of the esophagus and thus result in introduction of bacteria into the disc space, producing a discitis.

Anatomic Diagnosis

It is important that the patient's symptoms, the physical findings, and the investigations all correlate with each other in arriving at the correct pathological as well as anatomical level of diagnosis. In planning the surgery, the surgeon should be aware of any anatomical variations and ensure operating at the correct level. The surgeon also needs to plan the correct approach. Whether he operates from the left side or the right side or whether he operates from the front or the back may depend on his or her own level of comfort and experience. However, the exact site of the pathology needs also to be considered. If a patient with a traumatic spinal injury has significant disruption of the posterior ligamentous structures and is operated on from the front, further destabilization of the spine occurs, and the altered biomechanics may result in devastating complications. In these types of instances, a specific posterior approach may be indicated. Individual judgment needs to be considered in the preoperative planning of all specific surgeries.

Multiple pathology or additional levels of injury or pathology may exist, and these missed diagnoses may result in significant complications. This may be due to poor or inadequate x-rays or failure to do certain radiologic investigations. It is important, therefore, to be aware of specific x-ray techniques or other investigative procedures which may rule out specific pathology or levels of injury which could exist.

INTRAOPERATIVE COMPLICATIONS

Careful attention to the positioning of the patient immediately prior to surgery is important. In posterior exposures, hyperextension of the neck should be avoided. If the patient has a residual spinal stenosis with hypertrophy of the ligamentum flavum, hyperextension may result in a further narrowing of the spinal canal due to a buckling of the ligamentum flavum, and during prolonged surgery, local pressure on the spinal cord may result in ischemia and a profound neurologic deficit. It may be necessary to place the patient in traction for the duration of the surgery. Immediately before surgery the surgeon should routinely check the position of the head, the neck, as well as the limbs to ensure that there is no pressure on any vital structures. Pressure on the eyes, for example, particularly in the prone position for posterior exposures, may result in increased intraocular pressure, with retinal artery thrombosis and blindness. The use of a horseshoe-shaped rest or Mayfield tongs to support the head is of considerable help in the patient placed in the prone position.

Anterior Surgical Exposures

Complications are said to be more common following the use of anterior surgical exposures and may frequently be more serious due to the anatomical structures at risk. However, the incidence of complications are fortunately quite low. They are usually transient and more frequently involve dysphagia, a sore throat, hoarseness, or neck pain. They appear to be related to both the surgical approach as well as to the retraction required for exposure during the operation. The basic pathology for these is usually associated with the edema. Many of these symptoms may also occur simply from endotracheal intubation when general anesthesia is used. More serious perforating injuries of the trachea, esophagus, or pharynx are significantly more serious and are usually related to improper retraction during the surgical procedure. It is important that retractors be released frequently during the procedure and to ensure that they are appropriately placed throughout the procedure. The use of sharp or pointed retractor blades should be avoided. Retractors should be placed under the elevated medial borders of the longus colli muscles. Perforation of the carotid artery or jugular vein may also occur. This can be avoided, however, by careful dissection by appropriate placement of dull retractors. Thrombosis of the carotid artery with cerebral ischemia may also occur with prolonged pressure against the carotid artery. In patients with significant arteriosclerosis and plaques they may have embolization from inappropriate manipulation or retraction. Perforation of the vertebral vessels has also been reported. Tears of the vertebral artery are associated with dissection too far lateral from the vertebral bodies. This is best handled by initially controlling the hemorrhage by packing the intervertebral space and then obtaining both proximal and distal control prior to repair or ligation of the damaged vessel. Prior to ligation, however, an attempt should be made to ascertain the presence of an intact vertebral artery on the opposite side. Anomalies of vertebral arteries do include a vessel on one side. If the only vertebral artery is ligated, then clearly this may result in devastating neurologic complications.

Pneumothorax and mediastinitis have also been reported. This is fortunately quite rare but should be considered in low cervical exposures. Treatment for this would include chest tube drainage. Low cervical exposures below C6 on the left side may also place the thoracic duct in jeopardy.

Postoperative hematomas may result in early postoperative problems. This may result in tracheal obstruction and respiratory insufficiency. It is avoided by ensuring meticulous hemostasis at the time of surgery, and the use of a drain such as a Penrose drain or Jackson-Pratt drain is recommended. The condition is treated by removing any restrictive bandages or collars and evacuation of the clot. The respiratory problems may be due to a combination of the edema as well as the hematoma, and it may be necessary to intubate the patient immediately.

Wound infections in anterior spinal surgery are rare, and reported incidents are usually less than 1%. Infections should be drained early and treated with intravenous antibiotics for a few weeks.

Neural complications may involve the spinal cord, the nerve roots, the peripheral nerves, the cranial nerves, or the sympathetic chain. Spinal cord deficits are usually related to intraoperative manipulation of the cord. It should be noted, however, that certain conditions, such as patients with existing myelopathies due to spinal stenosis or patients with recent fracture dislocations with cord swelling and edema or the presence of a cord that has been previously damaged, are at risk for developing neurologic spinal cord deficits. More careful attention to detail and meticulous surgery is required in these situations. Epidural hematomas occur more frequently with posterior exposures but have also been reported following anterior cervical exposures.

Spinal cord injuries may also be a result of vascular damage. Injury to the anterior spinal artery has been reported by Kraus. The blood supply to the spinal cord is critical, particularly on the anterior aspect, and it relies on specific feeder vessels. There may be a watershed phenomenon occurring if there is anomalous blood supply.

In certain conditions such as long-standing cervical spondylotic myelopathy, the dura may be adherent to the posterior cortex of the vertebral body, and following decompression and removal of the vertebral body, a significant dural leak may be produced. It is usually impossible to repair dural leaks under these circumstances, but a draining dural catheter should be placed at a distant site to decompress the cerebral spinal fluid pressure and allow spontaneous healing. Failure to do so will result in a persistent cerebral fluid leak and fistula. Nerve root deficits are more likely to occur with foraminotomies and surgery related to the uncinate processes or neurocentral joints. The recurrent laryngeal nerve may be damaged due to improper retraction and results in hoarseness. If the injury occurs bilaterally or occurs unilaterally in a patient with a previous recurrent laryngeal nerve injury on the opposite side, approximation of the vocal cords may result in severe respiratory insufficiency, requiring persistent endotracheal intubation and possibly tracheostomies. Fortunately most recurrent laryngeal nerve injuries from retraction are neuropraxias and resolve within a few days after the surgery. The nerve is at greater risk through exposures on the right side when exposing below the C6 level. On the left side, the nerve has a longer course and lies fairly well protected in the tracheoesophageal groove. On the right side, the nerve may course with the inferior thyroid artery or may be accompanied by a venous plexus. Care should therefore be exercised when attempting to obtain hemostasis for profuse bleeding at this level. Exposures of the upper levels of the cervical spine place the glossopharyngeal, the hypoglossal, and the facial nerves at risk. A Horner's syndrome which includes ptosis, enophthalmos, and myosis may be due to damage of the sympathetic trunk. This may also result in differences in temperature gradients on the two sides of the body. This is usually the result of damage to the sympathetic trunk if dissection or retraction lateral to the longus colli muscles has occurred. It is more likely to occur with lower cervical exposures. It is fortunately a transient phenomenon and does not result in any significant clinical deficit.

Neurologic complications, especially those of the spinal cord and nerve roots, are best avoided by paying attention to meticulous dissection, applying a thorough knowledge of the anatomy, and using appropriate illumination and magnification where necessary. The reported incidence of neurologic damage to the spinal cord or nerve roots is low and generally reported as below 1%. This complication is thought by many to be best avoided by preserving the posterior longitudinal ligament which will act as a "barrier to cord injury." However, a disc fragment may herniate through a rent in the posterior longitudinal ligament, or osteophytes to which the posterior longitudinal ligament is attached may need to be removed in order to provide adequate decompression.

Complications Related to Grafting Techniques

These complications are again more common with anterior exposure. They include graft extrusion, collapse, resorption, or pseudarthrosis. Late degenerative changes may occur at the adjacent segments, that is, above or below the fused segments. This particular complication is again more common with anterior fusions. The incidence of grafting techniques varies from 0% to 13%. The incidence of graft displacement and collapse has been reported more frequently with the use of the Cloward technique. The rate of graft complications including pseudarthrosis appears to increase when two or more levels are fused. The reported incidence of pseudarthrosis is between 0% and 21%. Graft displacement does have the potential to produce injuries to the spinal cord if there is retropulsion, or to the esophagus and trachea if there is anterior displacement. This complication appears to be more common with dowel type grafts. It is valuable to leave a small anterior and posterior cortical ledge of bone and to carefully recess the graft between these ledges in order to avoid dislodgement. If a graft does become extruded, it should be immediately replaced.

Complications Associated with a Posterior Approach

There appears to be very little risk to the soft tissues from a posterior surgical approach to the neck because of the local anatomical structures. There is generally a much lower complication rate from posterior exposures. The sitting position for posterior exposures is said to increase the risk for air embolism. The incidence of neurologic damage to the spinal cord or nerve roots varies in different centers, and while some centers report a higher incidence of neurologic damage from anterior exposures, there are other centers that report a higher incidence of neurologic damage from posterior exposures. This incidence of neurologic damage from posterior exposure varies between 1% and 14%. The vertebral artery may also be at risk if the dissection is carried too far laterally. The incidence of infection is extremely low. More recently, there has been a great interest in fixation of the spine. Pedicle and lateral mass screws have been used in association with plates to provide stabilization. An understanding of the precise anatomical relationships to these structures is important. Improper placement of the screws can result in damage to the vertebral arteries, nerve roots, or spinal cord. Wiring techniques are generally much safer, and the reported results appear to be as satisfactory as those with plate and screw fixation. However, the risk of bone pull-out from wire fixation also exists. It may be necessary if the posterior fixation is tenuous to use appropriate external bracing to protect the internal fixation until fusion has occurred.

Extensive laminectomies may result in instabilities with residual kyphosis. The development of postoperative cervical kyphosis is a serious risk factor in extensive laminectomies in the pediatric population.

Complications from the Donor Site

Patients will more frequently complain of pain from the donor site than from the major surgical site in the neck itself. The donor site may be prolonged for many months. Other complications from the donor site may include hematoma, which is minimized by the use of appropriate drains for 24–48 hours. Careful attention should be paid to hemostasis, and it is often useful to place gelfoam over the raw bony surface prior to wound closure. Meticulous water type closure of the muscle and fascial layers is also useful. The lateral femoral cutaneous nerve may be damaged during the exposure of the anterior crest and can result in a meralgia paresthetica. In posterior exposures of the crest, the superficial gluteal nerve may be damaged during the exposure or be compressed in scar tissue. This is more likely to occur if the surgical incision over the iliac crest is made more than 2–3 inches from the midline. Incisions for the anterior exposure of the iliac crest should be made approximately 1 inch below the level of the crest by retracting the skin upward at the time of the incision to avoid irritation by belts or clothing.

POSTOPERATIVE COMPLICATIONS

The major postoperative complications have been discussed under the sections on anterior and posterior exposures. The major soft tissue complications occurring in the postoperative period include edema, particularly of the trachea and esophagus. In addition, the development of CSF fistulae, meningitis, infections, and wound problems may occur. Graft dislodgement, fractures of the bone graft, pseudarthrosis, aseptic necrosis, and discitis are late bony complications. Neurologic complications occurring in the postoperative period are usually related to instability but may be due to progressive epidural hematoma formation.

COMPLICATIONS RELATED TO TRACTION AND HALO FIXATION

The prolonged use of halos in the pre- or postoperative management of patients undergoing spinal surgery can result in complications. The halos may be used for traction or in conjunction with vests to provide additional stabilization and protection of the cervical spine. Pin site complications are the most frequent and include infection, loosening, or penetration. Prolonged traction in a halo or other device may result in cranial nerve damage, and frequent examination of the cranial nerves, especially of the ocular muscles, should be performed on a routine basis. Excessive traction may, in fact, result in displacement of unstable spinal fractures. The direction of pull is obviously also important in preventing sagittal plane displacements.

CONCLUSIONS

The complications from cervical spinal surgery are generally quite low, but this surgery does demand attention to detail before, during, and after surgery. The incidence of soft tissue problems and graft complications appears to be higher with the anterior approach, while the posterior approach appears to have neurologic complications equal to or slightly higher than those from an anterior approach. A good understanding of the potential complications as well as of the surgical anatomy and the use of good surgical technique with appropriate and satisfactory exposure, illumination, and magnification are all crucial in preventing or reducing these complications.

44

Problems and Complications of Craniocervical Junction and Upper Cervical Spine Surgery

Arnold H. Menezes

The craniovertebral junction refers to the occipital bone surrounding the foramen magnum and the atlas and axis vertebrae. These bones, together with their ligamentous complex, form a funnel-shaped enclosure through which the medulla oblongata continues into the cervical spinal cord. There are numerous congenital, developmental, and acquired conditions of the bony craniovertebral junction that have been recognized since the early nineteenth century (1). The surgical treatment of these conditions affecting the craniovertebral junction was generally a posterior decompression by enlargement of the foramen magnum and removal of the posterior arch of the atlas and axis vertebrae (Figs. 44.1 and 44.2). However, the morbidity and mortality associated with such treatment in irreducible lesions with cervicomedullary compression was high. A surgical physiological approach based on the understanding of craniocervical dynamics, the site of encroachment, and stability of the craniovertebral junction was adopted at the University of Iowa by the author in 1977 (2). Since then, 870 patients with abnormalities of the craniovertebral junction have undergone surgical therapy for their lesions in this manner.

The factors that influence specific treatment are whether the bone abnormality can be reduced to its normal position, the etiology of the lesion, and the direction and mechanics of compression (2). The primary treatment for craniovertebral junction (CVJ) lesions that can be reduced is stabilization (Fig. 44.3). An external immobilization is accomplished in those conditions such as ligamentous relaxation and inflammatory states to allow for reconstitution of bone and ligament. In other irreducible pathological conditions with persistent instability, a dorsal fixation is necessary. Surgical decompression of the cervicomedullary junction is required in patients with irreducible pathology. This disorder is divided into ventral and dorsal catagories. In the former, the operative procedure of choice in our hands is a transoral-transpharyngeal decompression, and the latter requires posterior decompression. If instability is present following either the ventral or dorsal decompression, posterior fixation is required. Preoperative neuroradiological investigations have been previously outlined (3, 4). These studies comprise plain radiographs of the CVJ with dynamic pleuridirectional polytomography in the flexed and extended positions, magnetic resonance imaging in the flexed and extended midsagittal planes, as well as axial visualization of the abnormality. CT myelography compliments the neuroradiological armamentarium as required (3).

To understand the problems and complications of craniovertebral surgery, this will be divided into the anterior approach, the posterior approach, and the anterolateral approaches.

Anterior Approaches to the Craniovertebral Junction

A. Midline— (*a*) transoral-transpharyngeal and (b) median labial mandibular glossotomy combined with transoral-transpharyngeal.

B. Anterolateral:— transcervical extrapharyngeal

C. Lateral:— (*a*) subtemporal extrapharyngeal and (b) transcervical mandibular ramus rotation.

It is felt that the operative procedure of choice is a transoral-transpharyngeal decompression for ventral abnormalities (3). The indications for this operation are *a*, irreducible ventral compression on the cervicomedullary junction caused by osseous abnormality, granulation tissue, or abscess formation; *b*, tumors which are extradural, such as bony tumors, chordomas, and rarely, an intradural meningioma or schwannoma.

The operative procedure for the transoral-transpharyngeal approach to the anterior craniocervical junction has been previously described in detail (1, 2). A transoral approach is not essential to tackle problems below the C2 and C3 vertebral bodies which can easily be approached via an extrapharyngeal manner as described by McAfee, et al. (5) and DeAndrade (6). Identification of a ventral abnormality at the craniovertebral junction such as in rheumatoid cranial settling, does not by itself form an indication for a transoral operation (7). Unless the irreducibility of

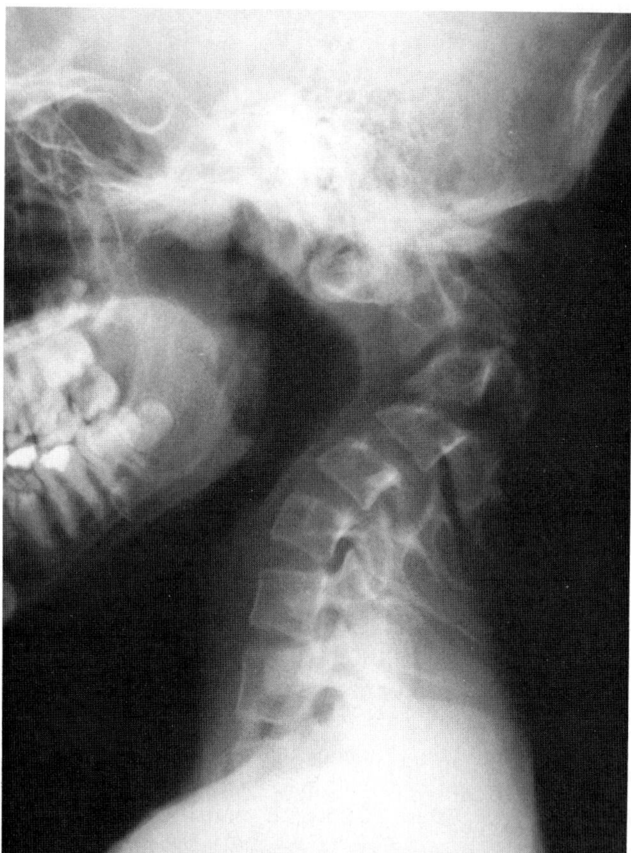

Figure 44.1. Lateral radiograph of craniovertebral junction and cervical spine in a 9-year-old male. This radiograph was made 1 year following posterior fossa decompression and upper cervical laminectomies for mild quadriparesis associated with basilar invagination and atlas assimilation. He presented with sleep apnea, difficulty swallowing, absent gag response, and severe spastic quadriparesis. Note the swan-neck deformity and basilar invagination.

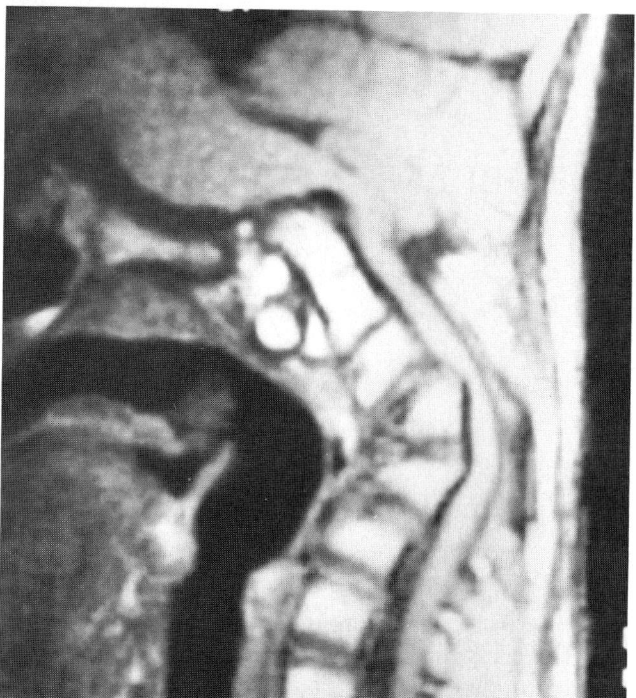

Figure 44.2. Same patient as in Figure 44.1. Midsagittal T1-weighted MRI of the craniovertebral junction and cervical spine. There is odontoid invagination into the ventral cervicomedullary junction, sagging of the cerebellum into the posterior fossa bony defect, and cervical kyphosis from C3–C6 with cervical spinal cord compression.

the lesion has been attempted by cervical traction, a ventral operative decompression is of questionable value. Thus, of 89 patients with severe cranial settling and odontoid upward migration and rheumatoid arthritis, only 19 had irreducible ventral lesions requiring transoral decompression with subsequent dorsal fixation (8). The remaining 70 underwent dorsal occipitocervical arthrodesis with excellent results.

The salient features of the ventral transoral operation are performance of the operative procedure in skeletal traction with the head in mild extension. This prevents impingement of the medulla by the bony abnormality. If no pathological flora are found on nasopharyngeal culture, Penicillin G is given intravenously during the operation and for 24 hours postoperatively. We feel that an operative procedure at the craniovertebral junction requires incision of the soft palate and maximum exposure of the high nasopharynx and clivus for excision of the offending pathology. A tracheostomy serves to prevent respiratory embarrassment should there be tongue swelling postoperatively. This is also important in patients who have medullary dysfunction for which a craniocervical operation is essential. Both these steps are unessential if surgery is limited only to the upper cervical spine. Following removal of the offending ventral pathology, closure of the operative site requires careful attention. Of the 128 patients who have undergone a ventral transoral operative procedure at our institution, 116 had an extradural lesion, and in 12 there was both an extradural and an intradural lesion. Of these 12, 7 had a sequestered odontoid process which invaginated into the pons; 3 had clivus chordoma; and in 2 there was an abnormal location of the odontoid process due to previous trauma and occipito-atlanto-axial rotatory dislocation. If an intradural exposure is required, a cruciate incision is made in the dura caudal to foramen magnum and extended cranially. Both leaves of the marginal sinus are cauterized, and cerebral spinal fluid must be drained by previously placed lumbar subarachnoid drain. Dural closure with 4–0 vicryl sutures is made as complete as possible and must be reinforced by placing fascia harvested from the external oblique aponeurosis adjacent to the dural closure. A fat pad then reinforces the fascia. The closure of the longus colli muscles and the pharyngeal musculature must be in layers. The mucosa is then individually approximated with dyed 3–0 vicryl sutures so as to allow

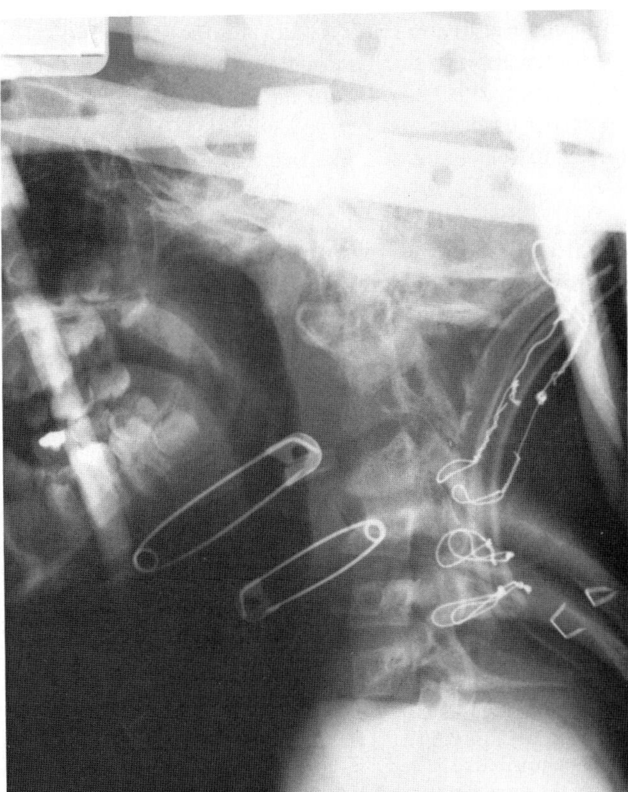

Figure 44.3. Same patient as in Figure 44.1. Lateral cervical roentgenogram made in halo-vest immobilization; 10 days after posterior occipito-cervical fusion. Note the reduction of basilar invagination and normal cervical realignment. The patient recovered neurological function.

identification of the suture line postoperatively. Soft palate closure is made in two layers, and the pharyngeal pack is removed at the end of the procedure. Intraoperative median nerve evoked responses are recorded to check for the brain stem latencies and thus act as neurophysiological monitors (3).

Dexamethasone, 4 mg every 6 hours for the first 24-hours, reduces postoperative lingual swelling. Intravenous hyperalimentation should be continued for the first 4–5 days with no oral intake permitted. Following this, an external stabilizing device, such as a Philadelphia collar, may be utilized to keep the patient in a more upright position for respiratory care as well as aspiration of secretions.

Subsequent to the ventral operative procedure, craniovertebral postoperative stability is investigated with pleuridirectional lateral tomography extending from facet to facet. This is done in the flexed and extended positions. Should there be instability, a dorsal fixation must be accomplished between the occiput and the upper cervical spine.

Of the 128 patients who underwent a ventral operative procedure, 28 had severe basilar invagination presenting with sleep apnea and compressive brain stem signs with a Chiari malformation and in various degrees of mechanical ventilator dependency. These patients underwent a primary ventral procedure with complete resolution of their symptoms.

There were two mortalities in this series, one a patient who was admitted with septicemia and improved after ventral decompression but succumbed to urinary tract sepsis. The second patient was a 79-year-old male with rheumatoid arthritis who had undergone both a ventral and dorsal procedure and expired from myocardial infarction 4 weeks after discharge (3). The main morbidity is wound dehiscence. This occurred in two patients. In one this was iatrogenic and brought about by a Yankow suction that the patient had utilized against the posterior pharyngeal wall. It was recognized on the sixth postoperative day. The treatment for this was hyperalimentation and keeping the oral cavity cleansed. There was no evidence of meningitis. One patient had a retropharyngeal abscess with secondary epistaxis felt to be due to osteomyelitis of the vertebral body that responded to intravenous antibiotics and drainage.

If no instance was a pharyngeal flap or a septomucoperiosteal flap needed for closure of the dura of the posterior pharyngeal wall, nor did we have to utilize fibrin glue (9, 10). Other complications from a ventral procedure that have been brought to our attention are meningitis (bacterial and fungal), persistent CSF fistula, and pharyngeal incompetence. This is easily prevented by a careful operative closure of the wound.

ANTEROLATERAL PROCEDURES

The anterior occipitocervical fusion described by De-Andrade, utilizing an extrapharyngeal exposure, is feasible and has been used by ourselves (6). The disadvantage is the limited extent of the exposure, as well as the required head tilt. A similar exposure has been utilized by Barbour (11) for screw fixation of fractures of the odontoid process, and also by Borne (12). The disadvantage in the latter procedure is the necessity for an angled approach to the facet joints of the atlas-axis complex and migration of the pedicle screws.

POSTERIOR DECOMPRESSION AND OCCIPITO-ATLANTO-AXIAL FUSION

In 1979, Sherk and Snyder reviewed the literature dealing with craniovertebral junction fusions for trauma and found 386 posterior fusions which had been reported (13). There was a failure rate of fusion for posterior atlanto-axial arthrodesis of 10%, and a 20% failure rate when the occiput was incorporated. The main complications, apart from failure of bone union, were the increased brainstem and spinal cord deficit, evidence of nonunion, and infection. There are several important points to be recognized with the various forms of fusion techniques. Larsson et al. reviewed

32 patients who underwent atlanto-axial fusion for rheumatoid arthritis between 1976 and 1980 (14). This operation was performed under local anesthesia without skull traction. The operative technique utilized was a modified "Brooks fusion" with wire and iliac crest. The postoperative immobilization was in a plastic brace. Fourteen patients had a nonunion; a wire breakage occurred in four; spasticity persisted in three of four patients; and there were three operative deaths. Subaxial subluxation was noted in several other patients. In another review, Conaty's concern was to obtain "improvement of neurological deficit and achieve fusion in the subluxed and osteoporotic spine" (15). Of 21 patients who underwent occipital and atlanto-axial decompression, 8 patients showed no improvement. There was one operative death, and two patients expired at the end of 2 years. Atlanto-axial instability was recognized in 12 patients of Ferlic's series of 550 rheumatoid patients admitted for surgical procedures (16). Only 6 had a solid union, and in 6 others a nonunion or death occurred. In a subsequent series by Bohlman, only 10 patients had solid fusion after 17 atlanto-axial procedures, and in 7 of 9 occipital fusions, complete bony fusion was achieved (17). However, it was Fielding et al. who showed precisely that identification of the type of abnormality required careful placement of the bone graft and of 46 Gallie-type fusions, there was only 1 nonunion (18). Most patients achieved solid bony union with an average follow-up of 4.2 years. We feel that the key to the success of the operative procedure is preoperative traction and realignment of the craniovertebral junction, maintaining the alignment intraoperatively with traction, and subsequently postoperatively with prolonged external fixation (1).

Surgical fusion at the craniovertebral junction has two aims, the first being immediate stability and the latter long-term. Immediate stability is achieved by incorporation of bone, wire, at times metallic rods, and poly methyl methacrylate. However, the long-term stability can only be achieved by an osseous bony "construct" (1, 19). Clinically, one needs to achieve a solid bony fusion before fixation construction fatigue occurs. The term "fatigue stress" reflects strength of the material while undergoing repeated cycles of loading and unloading that take place with the everyday stress of life. The stress concentration usually takes place at the sites of fixation. These are the most prone to show abnormalities such as nonunion, fibrous union, and pseudoarthrosis. Hence, it is a race between stress fatigue and achievement of a clinical bony union which is long-term.

Should bony fusion be incorporated with the immediate stabilization provided by the contoured rods, or Luque fixation devices, then our purpose is achieved (20, 21). Recently a new altanto-axial arthrodesis device, as proposed by Mitsui (22), shows poor construct value since it only increases the problem of cranial settling, as with patients with rheumatoid arthritis. On the other hand, occipitocervical fusion reinforced by Luque segmental spinal instrumentation or that used with a Knodt rod, have proved to be efficacious (22). In our hands we have found that a construct of bone and braided wire with methyl methacrylate, in selected cases, has been to our advantage with great success (1, 24).

Postoperative immobilization for bony fusion at the atlanto-axial joint, with posterior arthrodesis, requires 3 months of immobilization, while at the occipito-atlantal region a minimum of 5–6 months is essential.

REFERENCES

1. Menezes AH, VanGilder JC. Abnormalities of the craniovertebral junction. In: Youmans J, ed. Neurological surgery, Chapter 45. Philadelphia: WB Saunders, 1989.
2. Menezes AH, VanGilder JC, Graf CJ, McDonnell DE. Craniocervical abnormalities. A comprehensive surgical approach. J Neurosurg 1980;53:445–455.
3. Menezes AH, VanGuilder JC. Transoral-transpharyngeal approach to the anterior craniocervical junction. J Neurosurg 1988;69:895–903.
4. Smoker WRK, Keyes WD, Dunn VD, Menezes AH. MRI versus conventional radiology examinations in the evaluation of the craniovertebral and cervicomedullary junction. Radiographics 1986; 6:953–994.
5. McAfee PC, Bohlman HH, Riley LH, Robinson RA, Southwick WO, Nachlas NE. The anterior retropharyngeal approach to the upper part of the cervical spine. J Bone Joint Surg 1987;69A:1371–1383.
6. DeAndrade JR, MacNab I. Anterior occipito-cervical fusion using an extra-pharyngeal exposure. J Bone Joint Surg 1969;51A:1621–1626.
7. Crockard HA, Pozo JL, Ransford AO, Stevens JM, Kendall BE, Essigman WK. Transoral decompression and posterior fusion for rheumatoid atlanto-axial subluxation. J Bone Joint Surg 1986;68B:350–356.
8. Menezes AH, Clark CA. Cranial settling: odontoid upward migration in rheumatoid arthritis—management and long-term results. Paper No. 41. Scientific Manuscripts of Annual Meeting of American Association of Neurological Surgery 1989;138–140.
9. Hadley MN, Spetzler RF, Sonntag VK. The transoral approach to the superior cervical spine. A review of 53 cases of extradural cervicomedullary compression. J Neurosurg 1989;71:16–23.
10. Yamaura A, Makino H, Isobe K, Takashima T, Nakamura T, Takemiya S. Repair of cerebrospinal fluid fistula following transoral transclival approach to a basilar aneurysm. Technical Note. J Neurosurg 1979;50:834–836.
11. Barbour JR. Screw fixation and fractures of the odontoid process. S Australian Clin 1971;5:20–24.
12. Borne GM, Bedou GL, Pinaudeau M, Cristino G, Hussein A. Odontoid process fracture osteosynthesis with a direct screw fixation technique in nine consecutive cases. J Neurosurg 1988;68:223–226.
13. Sherk HH, Snyder B. Posterior fusions of the upper cervical spine: indications, techniques and prognosis. Orthop Clin North Am 1979;9:1091–1099.
14. Larsson SE, Toolanen G. Posterior fusion for atlanto-axial subluxation in rheumatoid arthritis. Spine 1986;11:525–530.
15. Conaty JP, Mongan ES. Cervical fusion in rheumatoid arthritis. J Bone Joint Surg 1981;63A:1218–1227.
16. Ferlic DC, Clayton ML, Leidholt JD, Gamble WE. Surgical treatment of the symptomatic unstable cervical spine in rheumatoid arthritis. J Bone Joint Surg 1975;57A:349–354.
17. Bohlman HH. Atlantoaxial dislocations in the arthritic patient. A report of 45 cases. Orthop Trans 1978;2:197.
18. Fielding JW, Hawkins RJ, Ratzan SA. Spine fusion for atlanto-axial instability. J Bone Joint Surg 1976;58A:400–407.
19. Taitsman JP, Saha S. Tensile strength of wire-reinforced bone

cement and twisted stainless steel wire. J Bone Joint Surg 1977;59A:419–425.

20. Flint GA, Hockley AD. Internal fixation for atlanto-axial instability in children. Childs Nerv Syst 1987;3:368–370.

21. Ransford AO, Crockard HA, Pozo JL, Thomas NP, Nelson IW. Craniocervical instability treated with contoured loop fixation. J Bone Joint Surg 1986; 68B:173–177.

22. Mitsui H. A new operation for atlanto-axial arthrodesis. J Bone Joint Surg 1986;66B:422–425.

23. Itoh T, Tsuji H, Katoh Y, Yonezawa T, Kitagawa H. Occipito-cervical fusion reinforced by Luque's segmental spinal instrumentation for rheumatoid disease. Spine 1988;13:1234–1238.

24. Menezes AH, VanGilder JC, Clark CR, El-Khoury G. Odontoid upward migration in rheumatoid arthritis. J Neurosurg 1985;63:500–509.

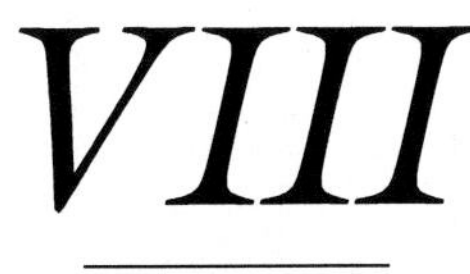

Surgical Instrumentation

45

Surgical Management Approaches and Techniques: Power Tools

Fremont P. Wirth

Power Tools

Power instrumentation has been utilized in surgery for over a century. George F. Greene, an English dentist, is credited with the development of the first power instrument in 1889. This foot powered device preceded the development of an air powered drill and osteotome first used in neurosurgery by Dr. Ogilvie at Guys Hospital, London in 1928. In the United States, a drill developed by Dr. Hall, a Pittsburgh oral surgeon, was used originally for dental surgery in 1959. This drill was adapted for bone work in 1963. Subsequently a number of drills have become available. A vane-type motor was developed in 1967 by Dr. Forest Barber and is marketed as the Midas Rex drill. Subsequently, the Hall and Anspach Companies have developed similar vane-type pneumatic powered drills. A variety of electrical drills, some of which are reversible, are also available. Since the author has had the most experience with the Midas Rex drill, the discussion which follows will be referable primarily to this instrument. It should be noted, however, that many of the techniques discussed can be performed with other drills. It is clear that most of the drills on the market at this time are of high quality. The selection of a specific model may depend more on personal preference than clearly defined technical differences in many instances. The author has used the Midas Rex drill for over 10 years and has been quite satisfied with its performance and quality. This drill, with its many hand pieces, appears to have the greatest versatility in application to spine surgery and for this reason remains the author's primary choice.

High speed drills operate in the range of 75,000 to 100,000 RPM. These motors have very little torque when in use, thus minimizing a tendency to shift in position when starting, stopping, or changing speed. This allows greater control and therefore enhances the safety of application in areas where great precision is required. The high speed also produces very rapid bone removal. Most of these drill motors are small and weigh in the range of 3–4 ounces. The drills are controlled by hand or foot switches, and it is the author's preference to utilize the foot switch. This allows the operator's hand to be dedicated to control of the motor itself.

There are three basic applications of power tools to surgery in the cervical spine. The first of these is the use of the high speed burr. The second is the use of a cutting tool similar to the craniotome. The third is the use of large drills and hole saws for anterior cervical discectomy and fusion.

High Speed Burr

This application of a power instrument is probably the most widely used and familiar technique to neurosurgeons (1). The high speed burr has been used to remove the posterior aspect of the neural foramen and adjacent lamina for approaching cervical discs, and for decompressing nerve roots compressed by bone spurs (Fig. 45.1). During initial removal of the inferior aspect of the superior lamina and superior aspect of the inferior lamina the underlying ligamentum flavum separates neural structures from the bone. As dissection of bone is carried further laterally, superiorly, or inferiorly beyond the ligamentum flavum, greater care must be utilized to avoid potential damage to the underlying dura. All high speed drills, whether employing a cutting or diamond burr, have the potential to damage dura and underlying nervous tissue by either heat or direct trauma. Especially in instances where the nerve root is compressed by bone or disc and cannot easily move away from the drill, it is advisable to remove only the outer layer of the bone with the high speed drill. Once the bone is thinned, the inner aspect of the bone overlying neural elements can be broken and removed with a fine curette. This technique has the advantage of avoiding compression of the nerve root which is unavoidable if the bone is removed with a rongeur. Since bony hypertrophy is frequently the etiologic factor requiring surgical decompression, this technique is both rapid and safe.

From the anterior approach, the high speed burr has similar advantages in removing bony bars which often constitute the offending element of degenerative disc disease

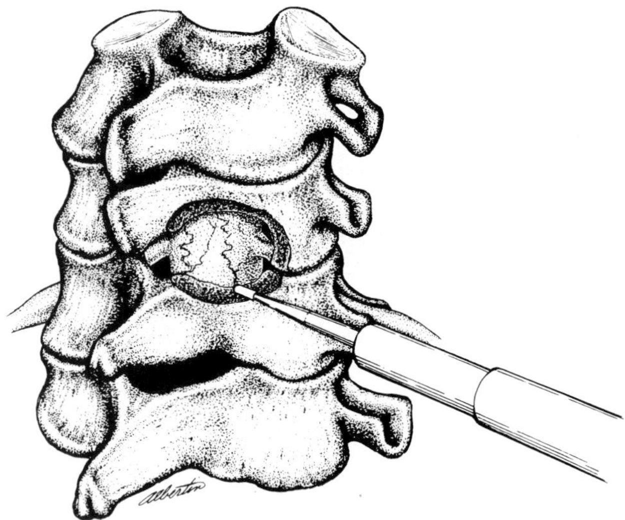

© Neurological Institute of Savannah, 1989

Figure 45.1. The high speed burr is used to remove portions of the lateral lamina and medial facet joint to expose the cervical nerve root as it exits the dural sac. Depicted here is the M-8 burr of the Midas Rex Drill which is the author's preference.

and spondylosis (2). It is often impossible in the degenerative joint to remove the posterior inferior aspect of the superior vertebra and the superior posterior aspect of the inferior vertebra through the disc space with rongeurs or curettes. In these instances, the high speed drill with a long, small drill bit can be very helpful in removing the posterior aspect of the vertebra. Use of the operating microscope with its additional light provides greater control in this instance. It is also frequently necessary to drill out the anterior aspect of the interspace to allow room to approach the posterior bars. It is important in so doing not to drill so deeply as to produce heavy bleeding from the cancellous portion of the vertebral body which can obscure vision and slow the procedure.

It is more difficult in the author's experience to safely approach the lateral aspect of these spondylotic bars from anteriorly with the power drill. Once the interspace is open centrally, however, it is often possible to remove the residual lateral spur and open the foramen with a variety of small rongeurs. Always when using the power drill, it is the author's strong recommendation that both hands be employed for control of the drill when working in the depths of the interspace or when approaching the spine posteriorly.

The high speed burr may also be used to "rough up" the vertebrae prior to fusion and to drill the necessary holes in spinous processes and/or facet joints if necessary for the placement of wires for immobilization with various fusion techniques. Right angle attachments are available with most of the drills to allow placement of wires through spinous processes.

Another use of the high speed burr is in corpectomy for various conditions. Removal of vertebral bodies for resection of the ossified posterior longitudinal ligament, removal of tumors involving vertebrae, and removal of crushed vertebrae may be facilitated with the drill. The high speed drill removes the bone rapidly with minimal blood loss, often sealing vascular channels in the bone. Because very little pressure is needed to remove bone with the high speed drill, greater control is possible increasing the safety and speed of this technique as compared, for instance, with use of rongeurs for bone removal. Furthermore, the discs and cartilaginous plates can be removed simultaneously, simplifying the approach and greatly speeding the process.

LAMINECTOMY

Laminectomy, whether for decompression or for wide exposure to remove intraspinal lesions such as tumors, is greatly facilitated by use of power instruments. Various techniques have been employed. One of these uses the high speed burr to cut through lamina on each side so that the entire lamina and spinous process may be reflected to one side or the other or may be removed. The lamina can then be replaced after the intraspinal surgery has been completed. This technique has been reported to be particularly important in children (3).

An alternative and much faster technique for removing the lamina is one employing a cutting tool such as the Midas Rex craniotome. In the cervical spine the craniotome cutting tool (The B1 attachment of the Midas Rex drill) is quite reliable. This instrument cuts the lamina and ligamentum flavum on either side, preserving most of the lamina and all of the spinous processes which can, if necessary, be replaced. Because of the small size of the footplate, compression of neural elements is minimal, even in the presence of severe spinal stenosis and spinal cord compression. Indeed, the placement of the small footplate is probably significantly less traumatic than the multiple introductions of the footplate of a rongeur necessary to remove the bone with manual techniques. The cut is made from inferiorly to superiorly, introducing the footplate through a small laminotomy (Fig. 45.2). The anatomy of the spine is such that even with a vigorous attempt to be as far lateral as possible it is not possible to expose the nerve roots themselves with this technique. For this reason, injury to a nerve root by catching it on the footplate of the drill has not occurred. Slight upward pressure on the drill to hold the footplate against the undersurface of the spine is sufficient to prevent compression of underlying elements. This technique has been employed by the author in over 100 cases in the cervical and lumbar spine without complications attributable to the technique.

A note of caution is necessary, however. This technique is not applicable in all cases. It should not be employed in dysraphic states or in patients who have had spinal surgery at the levels to be operated. This is due to the possibility

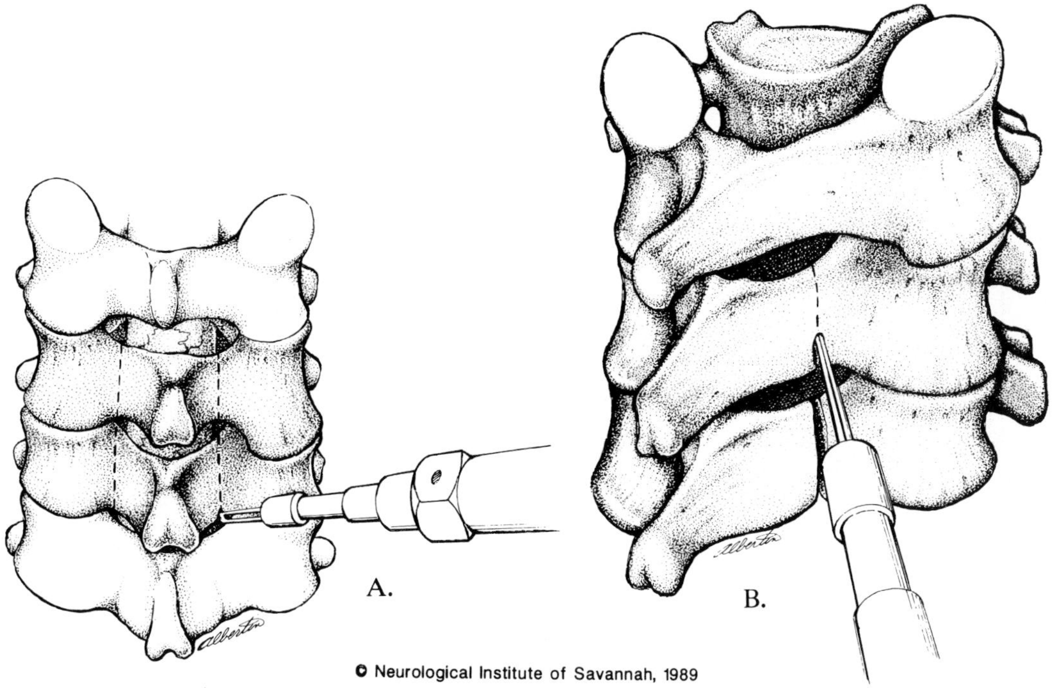

A.

B.

© Neurological Institute of Savannah, 1989

Figure 45.2. The craniotome attachment of the drill is used to cut the lamina on either side prior to removal. The cut is made in a caudal to rostral direction. Depicted here is the B1 cutting tool of the Midas Rex Drill which is the author's preference.

of adhesions between the dura and scar. Abnormal bony structures may also render the dura susceptible to laceration. Likewise, when dural penetration or laceration from trauma is anticipated this technique is not suitable. It is also recommended that the technique not be employed above the level of C3 because of the medial course of the vertebral artery at C1–C2 which makes this structure susceptible to injury.

ANTERIOR CERVICAL FUSION

The anterior approach to the cervical spine was developed by Cloward, Dereymaeker and Mulier, and Smith and Robinson (4–6). The techniques they described have changed little since their introduction, although power instruments have been used to shape graft materials in selected Smith-Robinson procedures. Working with design personnel at the Midas Rex Company in 1979, the author developed a set of tools for performance of the Cloward type of anterior cervical fusion with the high speed drill. These have been modified over the last several years to their present design which has proven very reliable in over 200 fusions.

These special tools with the power drill can greatly facilitate anterior cervical fusion and can decrease operating time. The disc and bone spur removal is carried out in the standard fashion as has been described. Various smaller burrs may be utilized to remove spurs or enlarge the disc space when necessary. To accomplish anterior cervical fusion, a hole saw has been developed which allows removal of an iliac crest bone plug. The high speed drill is much less cumbersome and much faster than the hand drill for this task. This is particularly true in obese patients where the approach to the iliac crest may be deep. The iliacus muscle on the inner surface of the iliac crest protects the underlying structures, although this is probably not necessary since with the power drill it is easy in most instances to feel the penetration of the inner table of bone itself. The bone plug is usually removed in the drill. If not, it is easily extracted using nerve hooks and various clamps. The inevitable heating associated with cutting a bone dowel with the high speed drill results in decreased bleeding from the donor site. The scorching of the bone plug which frequently occurs does not appear, however, to impair function as a satisfactory bone graft.

The interspace is drilled with a matching drill designed as a mate to the hole saw (Fig. 45.3). This produces a cavity into which the bone plug can be fitted nicely. Minimum trimming may be necessary in those individuals whose interspaces are relatively fixed and will not open easily with traction on the cervical spine. Use of the high speed drill for drilling out the interspace offers a number of advantages over the hand held drill. Since no guide is necessary, direct inspection of the depth of the drilled hole is possible. The angle of the hole can be changed if necessary and when fusing adjacent interspaces it is possible to offset the holes so that the majority of the central vertebral body may be preserved. Measurement of the depth of the interspace is not necessary prior to drilling. This is determined from direct observation by inserting and removing the drill on

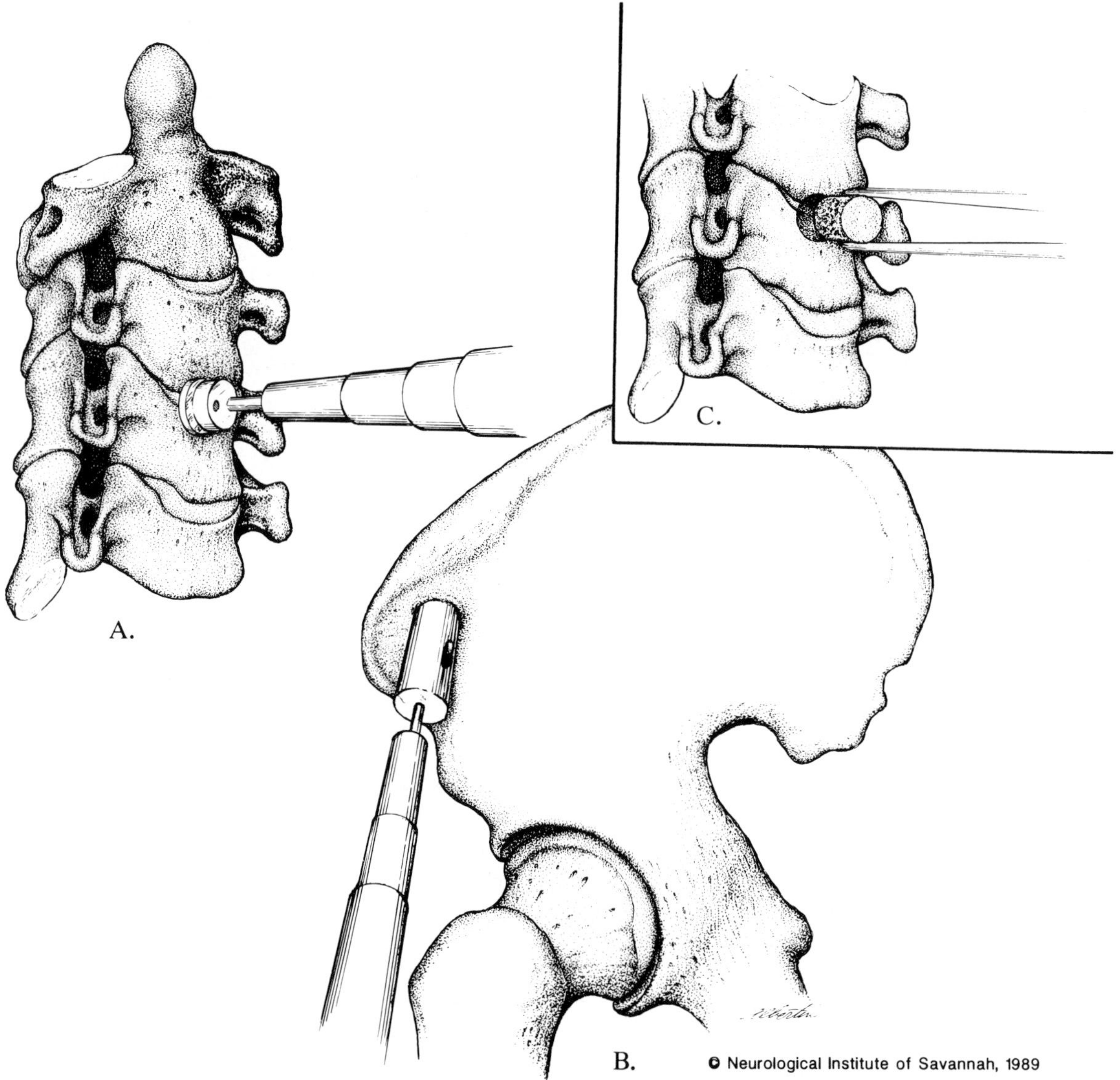

Figure 45.3. After removal of the cervical disc the interspace is drilled out with an appropriate sized drill. **A,** Three sizes are available; M-17, 13 mm, for single level operations; M-18, 9.5 mm, for multiple level operations; and M-19, 16 mm, for situations where a limited anterior approach to the spinal canal is desired. A hole saw of matching size is used to cut a bone dowel from the iliac crest. **B,** Occasionally minor trimming of the bone dowel is necessary to allow seating of the dowel in the prepared interspace without the use of force. **C,** Depicted here are the HS-17 and M-17 tools of the Midas Rex Drill designed by the author for this procedure.

a number of occasions. It is possible to carefully observe the preservation of bone posterior to the drill hole to prevent posterior migration of the bone plug or otherwise inadvertent injury of neural elements. In addition to being more hemostatic than the manual technique for drilling the interspace, the procedure is much quicker and, in the author's opinion, is inherently safer than the blind technique employed with the hand drill.

From a technical point of view, it is important when using the power drill in the neck to place four quadrant retractors to protect delicate deep cervical structures from inadvertent lateral movement of the drill as the initial portion of the hole is being created. At the same time, use of two hands is mandatory, as in other areas where the drill is used near delicate structures.

The author has had the opportunity to perform anterior cervical discectomy and fusion using this technique in over 150 patients at over 200 levels. Of the first 101 patients operated upon with this technique, 142 of the 150 levels fused as determined by follow-up lateral cervical spine films. This 95% rate of fusion compares favorably with that reported for manual techniques. In single level operations, the rate of fusion was 97%; 94% of levels in double level operations fused; and 93% of joints at triple level operations fused. With the exception of extrusion of one bone plug in a patient with an unstable cervical fracture who required reoperation for replacement, there have been no other complications associated with the technique. Infection, wound hematoma, and new neurologic deficit have not occurred. The technique thus provides a safe, rapid, and effective alternative to manual techniques for anterior cervical discectomy and fusion. Because of the cutting nature of the high speed drill, it is also possible to use this technique in patients with an unstable cervical spine. In such unstable cervical spines the pressure necessary to drill an interspace with manual techniques would not be tolerated. The use of a small dowel resulting in minimal removal of the vertebral body also allows the use of this technique for fusion with Caspar plates.

REFERENCES

1. Scoville WB, Dohrmann GJ, Corkill G. Late results of cervical disc surgery. J Neurosurg 1976;45:203–210.
2. Clark, K. Anterior operative approach for benign extradural cervical lesion. In: Youmans J, ed. Neurological surgery. 2nd ed. Philadelphia: WB Saunders, 1982.
3. Raimondi AJ, Gutierrez FA, DiRocco C. Laminectomy and total reconstruction of posterior spinal arch for spinal canal surgery in childhood. J Neurosurg 1976;45:555–560.
4. Cloward RB. The anterior approach for removal of ruptured cervical discs. J Neurosurg 1958;15:602–617.
5. Dereymaeker A, Muelier J. La fusion vertebrale par voie ventrale dans la discopathie cervicale. Rev Neurol 1958;99:597–616.
6. Smith GW, Robinson RA. The treatment of certain cervical spine disorders by anterior removal of the intervertebral disc and interbody fusion. J Bone and Joint Surg 1958;40A:607–624.

46

Laser and the Cervical Spine

Charles R. Neblett

Introduction

For no good reason, or for no reason, a debate evolves about the virtue, value, need, or even the wisdom of laser application in spinal surgery. Splitting of camps into the "do's" and the "don't's" occurs. Allowing this division to take place is counterproductive because of its polarizing effects. Resultant is a "schizophrenic" split concerning varying technical approaches. This is unwarranted because it is unnecessary.

The laser is a sophisticated instrument providing technical advantages that are universally recognized. Benefits include precision, delicateness, minimal tissue manipulation, less trauma, less blood loss, etc.—all of which lend to making laser usage desirable. Application of these favorable features can make the laser most efficacious in spinal surgery. The duality of opinions thus becomes a moot point, and the individual surgeon's choice of cervical spinal surgery technique remains uniquely his/hers. The issue of with or without the laser should not be a point of conjecture or criticism.

In the operating room the surgeon is decisionally alone—The term, "schizophrenia," describes one aspect of the dilemma because it illustrates that there is not just one single technical approach utilized in the performance of any one procedure. The fact that choices are available is a distinct positive. When petty controversy arises over one's sound choice, however, the illness suggested by "schizophrenia" is applicable because it describes the unwanted, unnecessary intrusion and diversion.

The practitioners of the art of cervical spinal surgery may use whatever instrumentation is available to them and establish its use at their discretion. This chapter outlines some ways the laser can be applied. It will be repetitive only because the desirable laser qualities are constantly and consistently the same.

"Cookbook" surgery this is not. Currently medicine is experiencing an increasing intrusion of "checklist" procedures as if a certain formula can be universally applied. This mechanism is not rationally adaptable to our topic of laser use in cervical spinal surgery because of the uniqueness of each patient and the requirement that the patient's physician customize the surgical procedure. Notwithstanding, general rules or guidelines can be provided and are here forthcoming.

Rationale

The precision provided by the laser is the quality that lends itself to cervical spinal surgery almost regardless of the pathologic process. If the laser is desirable because of the finesse offered in the removal of a spinal cord tumor, then why is it not reasonable to apply the same desirable physical properties against other pathologic processes? Is it admirable to desire special delicateness in tumor surgery and not to desire the same special benefit for the spinal cord when it battles the compression of the long-term neurologic devastation of spondylosis? Are the nerve roots or the long tracks different when at risk from an arteriovenous malformation (AVM) than from a ruptured disk? Is it bravado to utilize specialized equipment for the glamourous disease but unnecessary in a majority of cervical spinal surgeries simply because it represents "just another old routine pinched nerve"? A nerve is a nerve is a nerve—and preservation is the ultimate goal. Is it a gimmick in one case and miraculous in another?

Is it essential? Is it really necessary? Can't surgery be done without it? No—no—yes. It is applicable today in part because it is available today. This same surgery was done many years ago when it was not available. So indeed perspective is required. But perhaps an alternative question is, "Why not?" If it is good enough for the worst of problems, why is it not good enough for the ordinary problems?

The Thermal Scale

Degrees of thermal force introduced by the CO_2 laser determine its effect on organic tissue. 100°C—ablative—is the primary attraction. Most pathologic processes which today we know how to surgically treat, require ablation, the destruction of the offending agent. Seventy-five degrees centigrade—reparative—is usury for vascular coaptation. This process may be applied to vascular anomalies and epidural veins. Seventy degrees centigrade—reconstructive—is the fusion of tissue. Dural—arachnoidal—

pial fusion can be useful. Less than 70°C—stimulation/inhibition—is the exciting unknown arena. Possibly not the thermal but the less defined nonthermal forces that are generated at this range of thermal energy may have a most significant future.

The thermal range varies, the therapeutic form is dependent, and the applicability extends from almost always (ablation) to not now (stimulation/inhibition) the mode of need. Thus, the overview of the treatment of the cervical spinal cord and nerve roots by the CO_2 laser will be framed by the level of energy force as represented in this thermal scale. Not included is the less than 70°C field because it is nonsurgical therapy and because it remains inconclusively defined.

LASER PROPERTIES

The CO_2 laser provides the wavelength which will be discussed. The Nd:Yag can be applied for vascular anomalies and for vascular tumors. The Argon laser as well as other wavelengths currently demonstrate few if any appreciable advantages.

More specifically, the CO_2 instrumentation described in this chapter relates to the parameters provided by the Bioquantum milliwatt CO_2 microlaser. Although none of these qualities are essential for ablation, all represent the personal preference of this author. It is essential for reparation and reconstruction. Others have different experiences and different recommendations.

The microscopic mode has two advantages which make it most attractive. The enhanced visualization afforded by the increased magnification and the more intense light simply allows a better view of the interface between the good, "the neural, the vascular, the dural structures" and the bad, "the pathologic processes." The micromanipulator with its bias control helps minimize variances in movement of the laser beam that are more likely to be present in the hand held mode.

The spot size is 350 μm. The small spot size lends to the precision of the application of the laser energy where preciseness is most critical in the interface between the vital structures and the disease process.

The power is low (between 50 mW and 5W). The necessity to achieve temperatures far in excess of 100°C is nil, and the power density with these properties is conducive to fine control in that delicate surgical borderline zone. The time mode is not machine dependent and may be continuous or intermittent. Super-pulse may be desired. Super-pulsing minimizes thermal spread. The advantages of the continuous mode is the sustained effect provided and the repetitivity of constant ablation. The intermittent mode is less applicable; it allows less thermal buildup, but it is slower and in some situations lends to more tissue dehydration.

The focal distance is 400 mm. This distance allows sufficient room between the undersurface of the laser/microscope and the surgical field for passage of hand held instruments.

The summation of these qualities is a smaller zone of destruction (450 μm, including thermal spread devitalizing force of about 50 μm on either side) and lesser thermal spread of nondevitalizing forces. Whether ablating, fusing, or repairing, this is of value.

THE OPERATION

To pore over a litany of pathologic processes describing the technique for each would be redundant. Specifics are well described in the other chapters. Since the principles are the same, a single operation will be presented from skin to skin including variations. Anterior approaches to the cervical spine will not be discussed.

The opening is with a skin knife. At 100°C, the incised skin edges take slightly longer to heal. (There is building evidence that wound healing can be enhanced with special low energy laser application.) Cutting through subcutaneous tissues is routine; the laser is slow when applied to fat. Its first use is on the fascia. The fascia is incised, and the paraspinous muscles are dissected laterally. Some lesser degree of postoperative scarring appears to result with this technique.

Bony removal is possible. The laser at 5W penetrates the outer table of the bone extending into the diploic channels. This serves to "etch" the lamina at the desired site of removal. The inner-table of the bone is not entered; therefore, there is no risk to underlying structures. That section of bone is then removed with standard instruments. The advantage is better hemostasis because the diploic channels are significantly sealed and the bone pops out with minimal force required.

If bone is the offender, as in spondylosis, then the laser may be of benefit through the vaporization of visualizable spondylotic ridges. This is most helpful in the very tightly squeezed area of the medial surface of the pedicle against the exiting nerve root. The laser can vaporize that bone which otherwise is manually tedious to remove. A nice decompression is accomplished.

The disk-complex pathology is amenable to laser treatment. Using the posterior cervical approach, the posterior longitudinal ligament requires opening to gain access to extruded disk fragments, and this opening can be accomplished by the laser. Visible fragments can be vaporized and fragments tucked under the nerve root or spinal cord require some mechanical manipulation for accessibility through the posterior longitudinal ligament window. Neural tissue compression by annular bulging, laminar leaves, or other irregularities are readily vaporizable. Herniated nucleus pulposi also are thermally removed. Degenerated disk material within the interspace can be removed by the laser, but this author prefers the usual application of the pituitary rongeurs. Any materials remaining which might create current or future encroachment, ligamentum flavum, fragmented annulus, adhesions, etc., and which represent manually difficult tissues to remove using standard instruments, can be vaporized.

Extradural tumors are compressive type pathology that are ideal for CO_2 laser treatment. The literature is replete with definitions and illustrations of this application. Also, as described before, tissue creating a damaging or potentially damaging force, if visible, is vaporizable.

The interface between the dura and the tumor mass can be developed to initiate the alleviation of the compression. The direct thermal force is to the tumor; the thermal spread is present but insufficient to produce adverse affects on the surrounding viable tissues. This is particularly true with use of a power of about 5W and a spot size of 350 μm in the micro-mode. Upon freeing the sensitive, vital structures, the remainder of the tumor can be removed with the laser or hand held instruments. However, the laser is preferred because of the limited space, better hemostasis, and precision not afforded by mechanical manipulation, or tumor removal may begin with opening the tumor at a distance from the dura and debulking it. Extra room is obtained and then the interface is easier to develop. Most tumor removal benefits from a combination of both methods.

Undesired vascular structures can be treated. Epidural varicosities as well as arterial and/or venous malformations can be shrunk by thermal force of about 75°C. At 400 mm with a spot size of 350 μm and a wattage of 90–100 mW, the veins, arteries, or arteriovenous malformations can be shrunk, co-opted, sealed, or ablated. This is the reparative mode.

Intradural pathology obviously requires opening of the dura, which is easily achieved with the laser. Shrinkage of the dura is minimized using a wattage of two. Extraarachnoid or subarachnoid planes may be developed with the laser. It is beneficial should removal of arachnoidal veils or adhesions be present. Cicatrix is more delicately removed by thermal force than by mechanical force.

Tumor removal, because of its intimate relationship with the spinal cord, rootlets, and vital vascularity, is enhanced with the CO_2 laser. Principles are the same; finesse is available where it is most desirable.

Approaching intramedullary abnormalities means opening of the spinal cord. Opening at the site of maximum pathology, at the least vascular area, and as interfascicularly as possible are the desirable goals. Again the milliwatt, micro-mode CO_2 laser approach is helpful, and this can be achieved in the least traumatic manner. One watt helps to divide the tough pia, less than one watt can be applied to the developing interfascicular plane. Less mechanical manipulation, better hemostasis, and minimal nonharmful thermal spread are the important features.

The syrinx of syringomyelia, hydromyelia, cystic neoplasms, etc. can be fenestrated. A clean opening of the syrinx is accomplished. Whether there are other beneficial gains is to be established.

Intramedullary tumors are considered by most spinal cord surgeons to be a well-established indication for the laser. Debulking can be provided. The ever critical meeting of the tumor with the viable neural tissues, if a discernible plane does exist, can be gently developed and extended by the laser.

DREZ lesions can easily and predictably be produced with the laser.

The reconstruction applies to the fusion of tissues including pia, arachnoid, and dura to itself or to other component tissues.

Conclusion

The Mount Everest mentality—"I climbed it because it was there"—is not the reason for laser application in cervical spinal surgery. It is not used just because it is there. The average spinal surgery set-up has about 300 instruments, yet on the average only about 20 are used per case. No one feels guilty that they did not use one, much less all, of the hemostats available. They were there should a need arise.

The laser is a large capital expense item, but today almost every hospital has one or more lasers. Expense, therefore, is not the issue; it is not a mountain too high to climb.

Again, when needed, the amount of time applied should reflect the amount of time required to achieve the desired specific goals, whether 2 minutes or 2 hours. Pituitary rongeurs of which there are usually eight in a set are most important in many surgeries. Yet, the total time of their usage is only a few minutes. This does not negate their importance.

These are neither rationalizations nor justifications. The milliwatt CO_2 laser affords the user a surgical technique which possesses the advantages of precision and finesse in vital areas. The laser has a place in the armamentarium of the spinal surgeon.

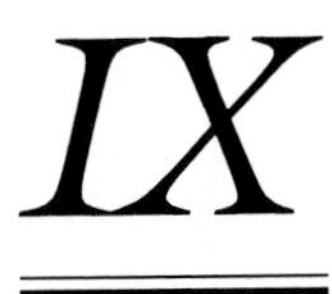

Cervical Tumors/Vascular Disorders

47

The Diagnosis and Surgical Treatment of Craniocervical Junction Tumors

Martin J. Buckingham, John M. Tew, Jr., and J. Geoffrey Wiot

"To err in the diagnosis of a relievable disorder is a tradegy. A readily missed and usually eminently relievable lesion of the nervous system is one about the junction of the medulla and cervical spinal cord (a junction lesion)."

C.D. Aring

Six decades have passed since Elsberg and Strauss described the clinical features of the lesion at the junction of the medulla and spinal cord (8, 9). Others have elucidated the oftentimes confusing syndrome which may delay accurate diagnosis for years from the onset of symptoms (1–3, 10, 14, 16, 19, 20, 23, 24, 26). In a recent report by Meyer of 102 benign extramedullary tumors of the foramen magnum, the mean elapsed time from onset of symptoms to diagnosis was 2¼ years (18). Before the availability of imaging techniques, radiological diagnosis depended upon posterior fossa myelography and pneumoencephalography. Computed tomography facilitated discovery of junction lesions. MR imaging provides a noninvasive method to evaluate this region which permits the most accurate anatomic diagnosis.

Numerous surgical approaches have been used in the treatment of craniocervical junction tumors (4–8, 11, 17, 21, 22, 25). Elsberg described a posterior approach *via* a suboccipital craniectomy and cervical laminectomy which proved inadequate for tumors extending anterior to the neuraxis (8). In 1966 Mullan et al. reported a transoral approach to an intradural foramen magnum sarcoma and a chordoma of the clivus axis (21). This approach had been limited to extradural tumors because of the risk of postoperative CSF leak and meningitis.

Stevenson described a transcervical transclival approach to remove a clivus chordoma (25). Crockard, Hadley, Hayakawa, Yamaura, and others have improved the transoral approach to intradural tumors and vascular lesions by developing techniques for dural closure which permit a safe approach to intradural lesions (4, 12, 13, 27).

Most craniocervical junction tumors can be removed via a posterolateral approach. A suboccipital craniectomy carried laterally to the sigmoid sinus and an extreme lateral upper cervical laminectomy and facetectomy facilitates removal of tumor posterior, lateral, and anterior to the brain stem and spinal cord. Tumors that cannot be totally removed by this approach can be resected *via* the transoral approach or a combination of both approaches.

The goal of this chapter is to present a comprehensive review of the diagnosis and surgical treatment of extraaxial tumors of the craniocervical junction. Preoperative assessment, operative positioning, intraoperative monitoring, surgical management, and postoperative care will be discussed. A review of our experience and presentation of illustrative cases will demonstrate the approach to lesions of the craniocervical junction.

Clinical Material

Fourteen extraaxial intradural tumors of the craniocervical junction form the basis of this study. Nontumorous lesions, such as aneurysms and congenital abnormalities, and extradural lesions are excluded. There are 11 meningiomas, 1 schwannoma, 1 chordoma, and 1 osteoblastoma. The age ranges from 16–85 years and the male-to-female ratio is 2:12. The clinical features are summarized in Table 47.1. Prior to 1976, diagnosis was established with myelography and pneumoencephalography. Myelography with CT has been used from 1976 through 1986. MR imaging with contrast enhancement is now the preferred diagnostic study.

Symptoms and Signs

The clinical diagnosis of a craniocervical junction lesion is difficult to make for several reasons. No single symptom or neurologic finding is pathognomonic of this lesion. A lesion below the medulla yet above the cervical plexus produces no cranial nerve or radicular findings to help identify the level of neural involvement. The spinal canal is wide in this region, enabling a tumor to become very large before neurologic signs are produced. Patients with junction lesions often have a fluctuating course, mimicking multiple sclerosis and brainstem glioma. Junction tumors have several common features which should lead to diagnosis.

Table 47.1 Clinical Summary and Results of 14 Patients with CCJ Tumors

Case	Age	Sex	Histology	Symptoms and Signs: Pain	Paralysis	Paresthesia	C.N. Palsy	Approach	Extent of Resection	Outcome	Complications
S.W.	50	F	meningioma	+	+	+	–	PL	CR	good	none
L.L.	37	F	meningioma	–	–	–	+	PL	NCR	exc.	none
P.F.	25	F	meningioma	+	+	+	–	PL	CR	exc.	none
Y.D.	50	F	meningioma	+	+	–	–	PL	CR	exc.	transient VIth nerve paresis
D.J.	26	M	meningioma	–	+	–	–	PL	CR	fair	hydrocephalus
R.B.	75	F	meningioma	–	–	–	+	PL	STR	fair	none
M.H.	85	F	meningioma	–	–	–	+	PL	STR	fair	partial Wallenberg's syndrome
G.B.	69	F	chordoma	+	+	+	–	PL	STR	good	none
F.U.	68	F	meningioma	+	–	–	–	PL	CR	exc.	transient XIth nerve paresis
M.R.	41	F	meningioma	+	+	+	+	PL & ANT	NCR	good	none
D.H.	42	F	schwannoma	–	+	+	–	PL	CR	exc.	none
J.G.	16	M	osteoblastoma	–	–	–	+	PL	CR	good	none
M.B.	63	F	meningioma	–	+	+	–	PL	NCR	exc.	none
V.E.	34	F	meningioma	+	+	+	+	PL	CR	fair	delayed brain stem infarct

KEY: ANT – anterior
CR – complete removal
Exc – excellent
NCR – near complete removal
PL – posterolateral
STR – subtotal removal

Symptoms can be remembered as the 4 P's: pain, paralysis, paresthesias, and palsies of cranial nerves.

Occipital headache or neck pain exacerbated by neck motion is usually present. Patients may hold their heads in a tilted or fixed position, partially due to irritation of the upper cervical rootlets. Neck pain was present in 66% of patients in a large series of patients reported by Meyer et al (18).

Spastic paralysis is repeatedly seen. Weakness usually involves one upper limb followed by involvement of both lower limbs, and finally, the contralateral upper limb as well. Signs of pyramidal tract involvement include gait disturbance, hypertonicity, and extensor plantar responses. Atrophy of intrinsic hand muscles may cause confusion with a lesion of the cervical roots. In the past, the diagnosis was frequently overlooked because a complete myelogram was not performed.

Paresthesias or dysesthesias of the hands, limbs, and face occur frequently. The complaint of a cold sensation in the lower limbs is often elicited. A dissociated sensory and motor loss may be associated with a Brown-Sequard or a partial medullary syndrome.

Cranial nerve palsies and nuclear involvement in the brainstem can be present. The spinal accessory nerve is most often involved as manifested by torticollis and weakness of the trapezius and sternocleidomastoid muscles. A few patients will develop hearing loss, vertigo, dysphagia, or dysarthria indicating involvement of the VIIIth, IXth, Xth, or XIIth cranial nerves. Awareness of all the varied features of junction lesions is required to avoid unnecessary delay in diagnosis.

RADIOLOGIC EVALUATION

The complex anatomy of the craniocervical junction makes accurate imaging an essential part of preoperative evaluation. Depiction of tumor extent and its relationship to the brainstem, cranial nerves, and vital vascular structures requires a multi-modality approach utilizing CT, MR, and angiography.

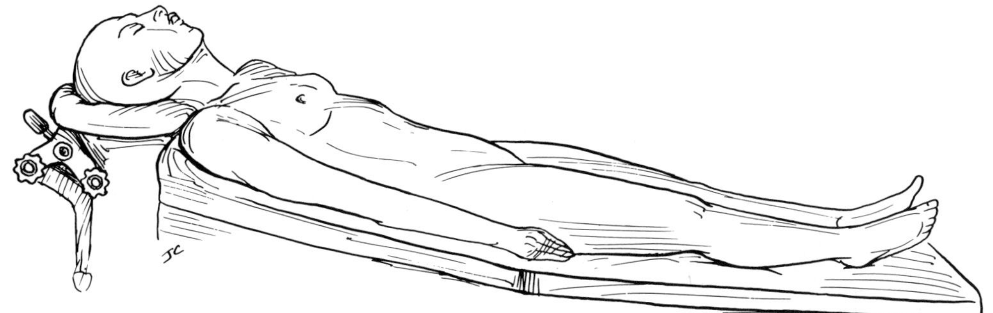

Figure 47.1. Position used for transoral approach. Table is flexed 10° for head elevation.

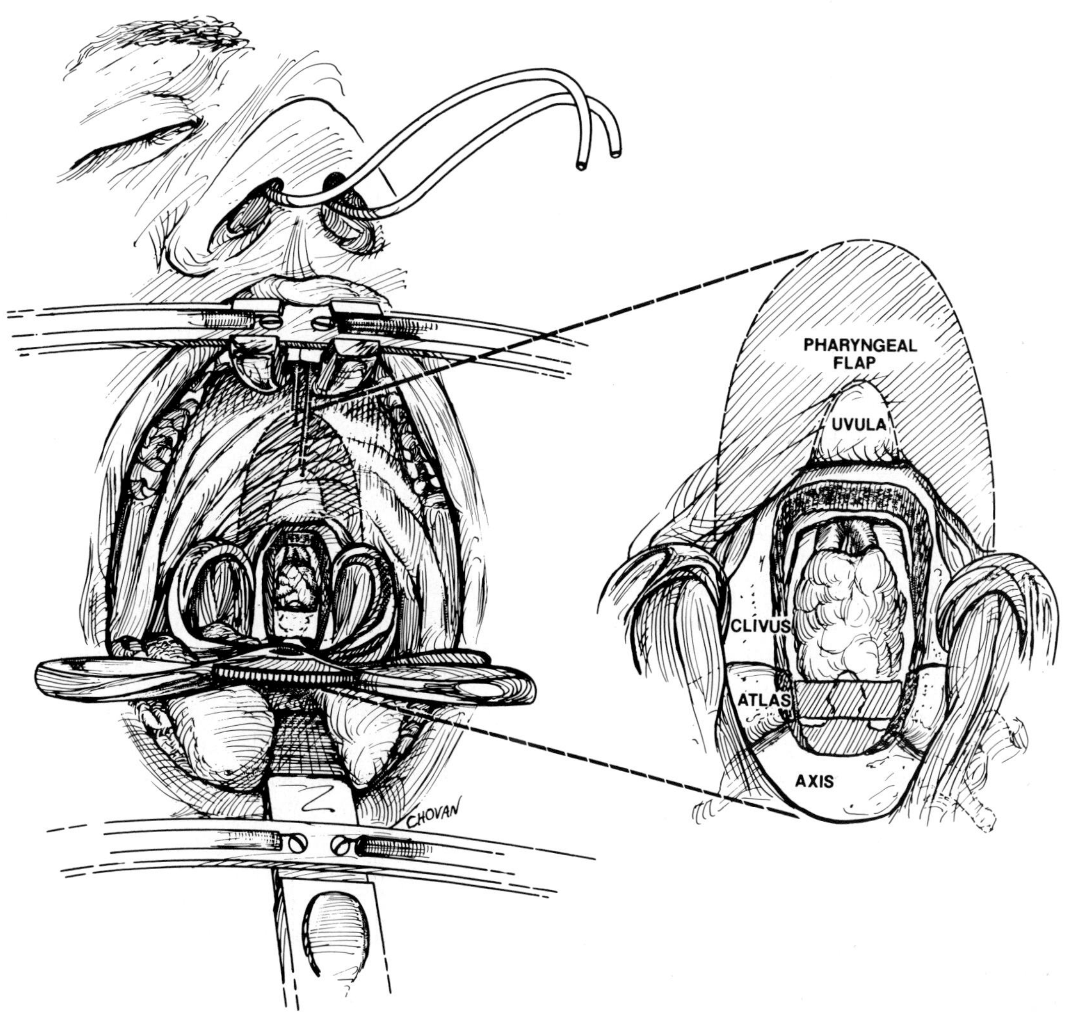

Figure 47.2. Surgeon's view of exposure obtained in transoral approach. The uvula and pharyngeal wall flaps are retracted superiorly with catheters passed through the nasopharynx. A Gelpe retractor provides lateral exposure. Inset shows detail of intradural tumor anterior to vertebral arteries.

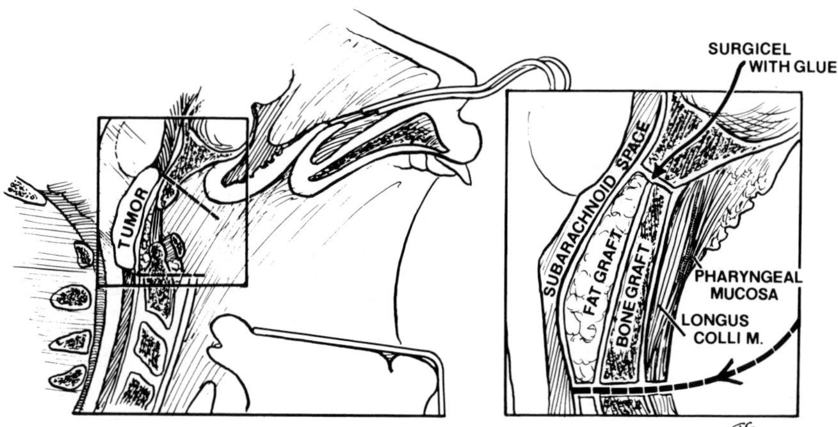

Figure 47.3. Artist's representation of sagittal view of transoral exposure (left) and extent of bone removal required (*dotted lines*). Detail (right) demonstrates repair of surgical defect with fat graft, fascia with surgical glue, bone graft, and soft tissue closure.

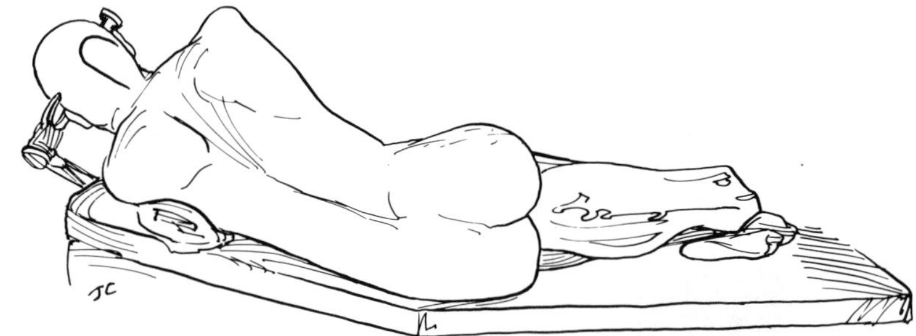

Figure 47.4. Position and incision used for right posterolateral approach using the lateral oblique position.

Computed tomography has proven its value in the evaluation of the skull base and neural foramina. High resolution scanning with bone algorithms accurately depicts bone involvement, but the technique is limited by artifact caused by the dense bone of the skull base.

MR imaging, unhampered by bony artifact, is superior in revealing anatomic relationships at the base. Demonstration of tumor extent and anatomic relationships is possible in multiple planes. Sagittal imaging displays the tumor's relationship to the brainstem and its rostrocaudal extent.

High resolution techniques consistently identify cranial nerves V, VII, VIII, and XII as they pass through the basilar cisterns. The low signal intensity appearance of flowing blood within major vessels is distinct from adjacent brain, tumor, and CSF, permitting identification of patent vessels.

Occasionally, the MR signal of a lesion is sufficiently characteristic to allow prediction of histology. More commonly, the shape, location, and presence or absence of bone involvement are better predictors of tumor type. Gd-Dtpa (Gadopentetate dimeglumine or gadolinium) enhancement increases the sensitivity of MR imaging in the evaluation of small tumors and the examination of the postoperative surgical bed for residual or recurrent tumor.

Cerebral angiography is of limited value in the initial evaluation of foramen magnum lesions. Vascular encasement or displacement is more easily seen with MR imaging. However, angiography does play an important role in determining tumor vascularity and the dynamics of collateral circulation. Temporary balloon occlusion techniques provide a means of gauging tolerance to vascular occlusion prior to surgery. Permanent balloon occlusion of major arteries encased in tumor will reduce operative hemorrhage and permit total resection of difficult lesions.

Meningiomas are the most common benign intracranial neoplasm and craniocervical junction tumor. They develop as dural based lesions that intensely enhance on contrast CT or MR studies. MRI of meningiomas image a hypointense (40%) to isointense (60%) mass relative to brain tissue on T1-weighted images. T2-weighted images demonstrate more variability with approximately 50% of meningiomas isointense to cortex, 40% hyperintense, and 10% hypointense. Considerable signal heterogenicity of unknown etiology produces a speckled or mottled appearance on T1-weighted images that is characteristic of meningioma.

Neuromas of cranial and spinal nerves comprise the second most common junction tumor and are readily seen with MR imaging. They tend to be hypointense on T1-weighted images, isointense on T2 images, and to enhance greatly with Gd-Dtpa. Multiplanar, high resolution enhanced imaging consistently demonstrates small (<1 cm) lesions.

Chordomas are uncommon tumors that arise from the

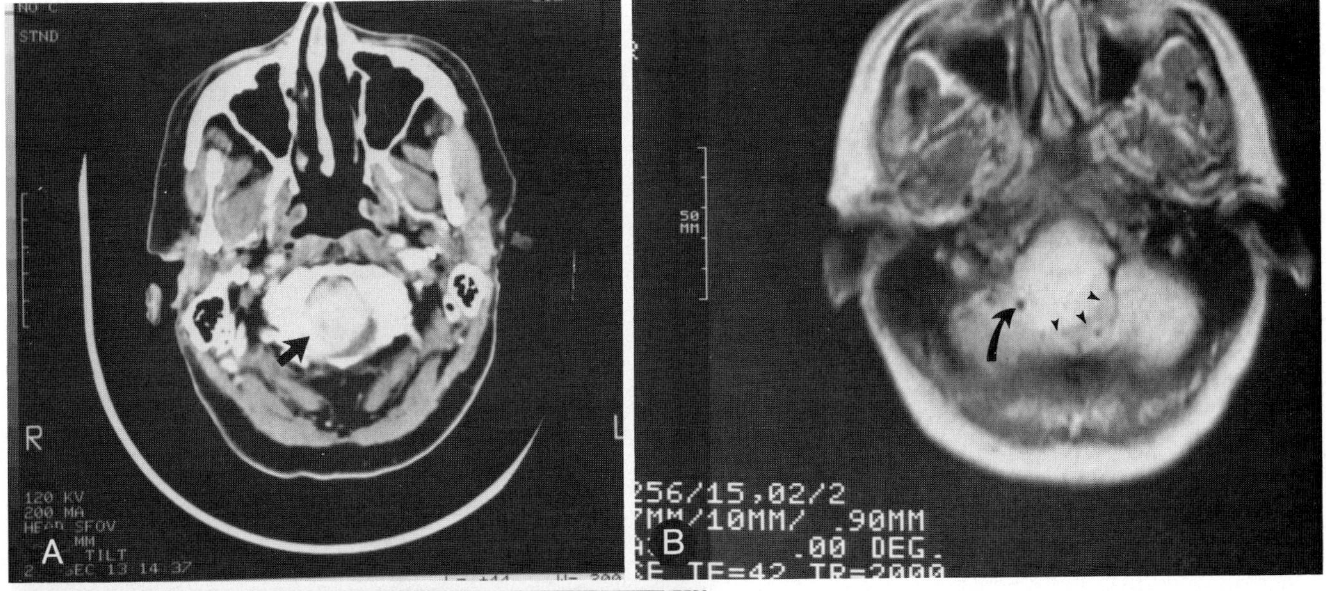

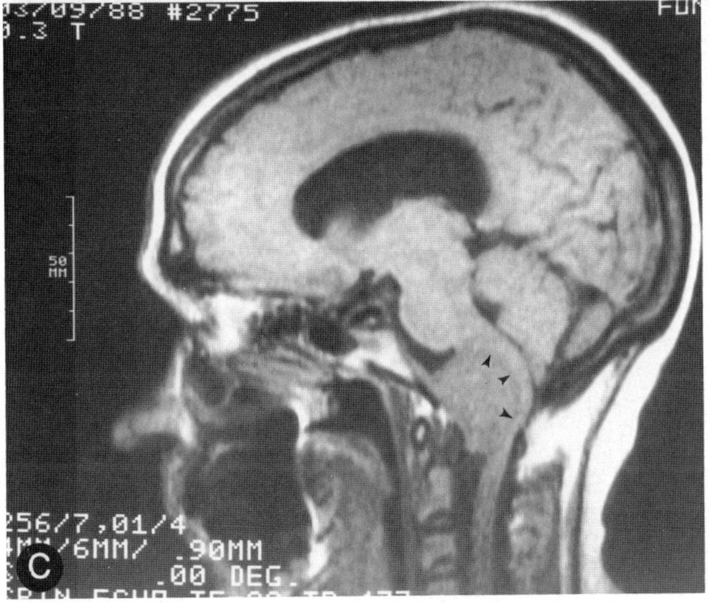

Figure 47.5. Contrast enhanced CT **A**, demonstrates an enhancing mass within the foramen magnum (*arrow*). Axial, proton weighted (TR 2000, TE42) **B**, and sagittal T1 weighted (TR 477, TE 28) **C**, MR images reveal an extraaxial foramen magnum mass, compressing the brain stem (*arrow heads*) and displacing the vertebral artery (*arrow*).

primitive notochord. Approximately one-third are intracranial, where they typically arise from the clivus near the spheno-occipital synchondrosis. CT and MR imaging are equally sensitive in the detection of chordomas. However, the multiplanar capabilities of MR imaging are superior to CT in defining extent and vascular relationships. MR signal characteristics of chordoma are nonspecific; variable low signal on T1 and high signal on T2-weighted images are common.

PREOPERATIVE EVALUATION AND PERIOPERATIVE MANAGEMENT

Preoperative and intraoperative somatosensory and brainstem evoked potentials are obtained in all patients. When a tumor extends to the cerebellopontine angle, facial EMGs are monitored. Perioperative antibiotics and dexamethasone are administered in all cases. External pneumatic compression boots are placed preoperatively and remain operational until the patient is ambulatory. All patients receive postoperative care in the neurosurgical intensive care unit (NSICU).

SURGICAL MANAGEMENT

The goals of surgery of craniocervical junction tumors are to preserve or restore neurologic function, to resect as much of the tumor as is safely possible, and to avoid the complications attendant to intradural surgery. The following protocol has evolved through extensive experience over 20 years. Two surgical approaches are used: anterior (transoral) and posterolateral (suboccipital). Most tumors can be removed via the latter approach. Occasionally both ap-

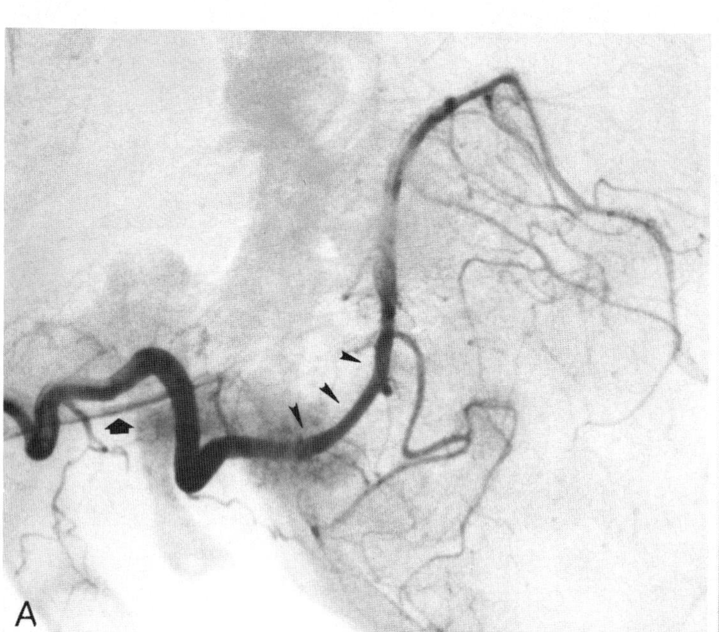

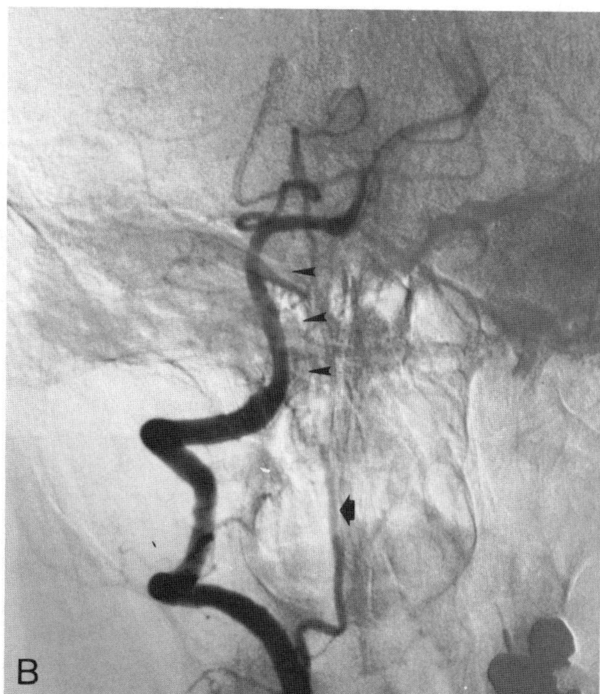

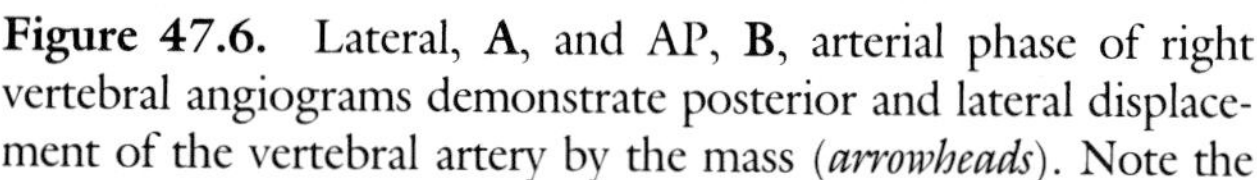
Figure 47.6. Lateral, **A**, and AP, **B**, arterial phase of right vertebral angiograms demonstrate posterior and lateral displacement of the vertebral artery by the mass (*arrowheads*). Note the prominent anterior spinal artery blood supply to the tumor (*large arrowhead*).

proaches are necessary in staged procedures. Stability of the craniocervical junction must be evaluated by pleuridirectional tomography after an anterior procedure. Preservation of the lower half of the odontoid, the transverse atlantal ligament, and a portion of the anterior arch of C1 will usually maintain stability.

The best surgical approach depends upon the relationship of the mass of the tumor to the neuraxis. If the tumor is directly anterior to the medulla and spinal cord and extradural in location, an anterior approach is preferred. If the tumor is anterior and intradural, or if the bulk of the tumor is not directly anterior to the neuraxis, then an extreme posterolateral approach is indicated. A second stage anterior approach may be necessary for resection of residual tumor invading the dura, clivus, or dens.

Complete resection is our goal, but never at the expense of creating a major neurologic deficit. The morbidity associated with sacrifice of the VIIth, IXth and Xth nerves, is particularly unacceptable. Meningiomas, the most common tumors of the region, often involve C.N. IX, X, and XI. We prefer to leave residual tumor in the jugular foramen dura unless IXth and Xth nerve function has already been lost. A similar decision may be made about VIIth and VIIIth nerve involvement at the porus acusticus. Occasionally, the vertebral artery will be encased in tumor, but it can be sacrificed if the posterior inferior cerebellar artery is preserved and the other vertebral artery is functionally well-formed.

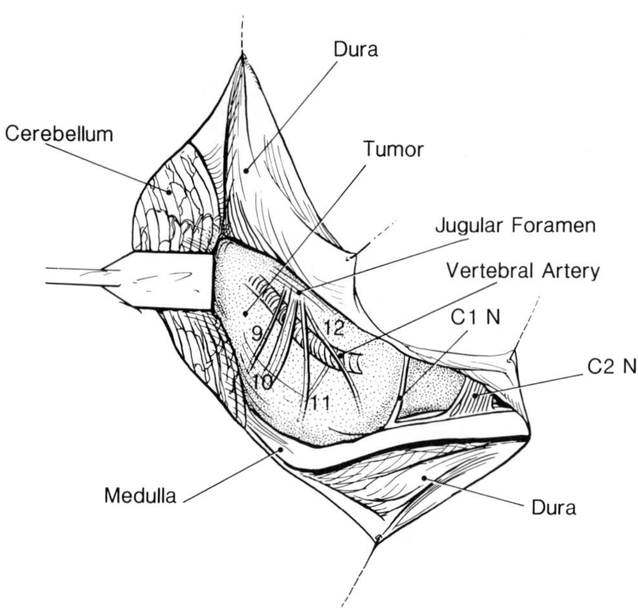

Figure 47.7. Artist's representation of tumor compressing spinal cord and medulla. Cranial nerves 9–12 and the vertebral artery are deep to the tumor.

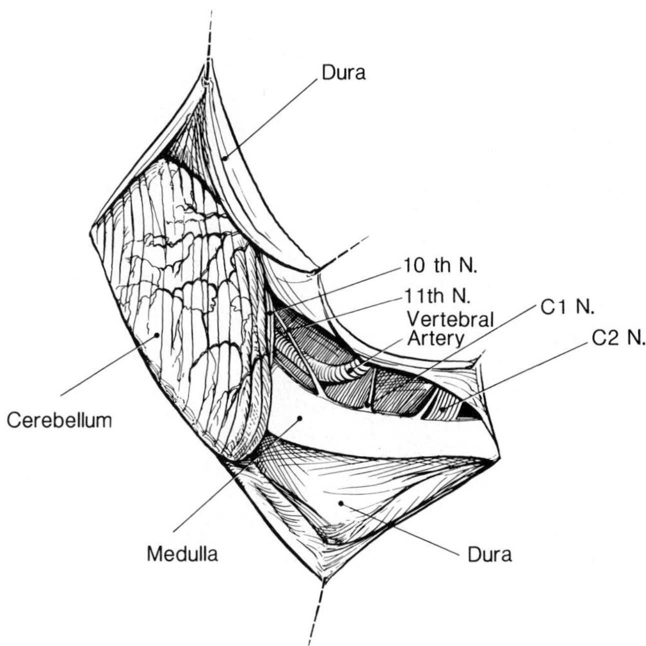

Figure 47.8. After tumor resection the medulla and spinal cord are decompressed and the cranial nerves and vertebral artery spared.

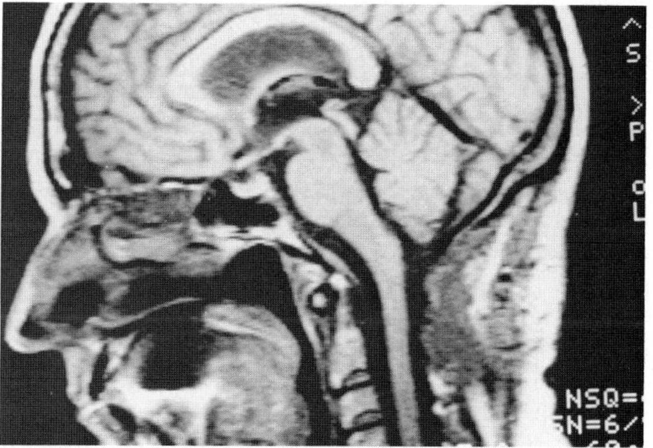

Figure 47.9. Postoperative sagittal proton weighted MR image reveals decompression of cervicomedullary junction and no evidence of tumor.

The patient's age and neurologic status and the tumor histopathology must be given careful attention in determining the benefits of global resection of meningiomas and chordomas. Other neoplastic lesions that occur in this region are likely to be resected with acceptable deficit.

TRANSORAL-TRANSPHARYNGEAL TECHNIQUE

The patient is placed supine with his head on a cerebellar headrest or in skeletal traction (Fig. 47.1). After orotracheal intubation with a reinforced tube and placement of a Dingman mouth retractor, the uvula is sewn to a catheter which is passed through the nasopharynx for retraction. It may be necessary to split the soft palate and partially excise the hard palate to gain access to lesions which extend more cephalad. The posterior pharyngeal wall is opened using a U-shaped flap based superiorly and is retracted in a manner similar to the uvula (Fig. 47.2). The operative microscope (Zeiss Microscope on Contraves stand, manufactured by Zeiss Company, Ober Kochen, Germany) and CO_2 laser (Sharplan CO_2 laser manufactured by Sharplan Company, Tel Aviv, Israel) are used to expose and remove the anterior longitudinal ligament. The laser is very effective in removing this tough tissue in a bloodless fashion. The lower clivus, a portion of the anterior arch of C1, and the upper half of the dens are removed with a high-speed pneumatic drill (high speed pneumatic drill manufactured by Midas Rex, Ft. Worth, TX). Intraoperative fluoroscopy helps determine the level of bone removal. The transverse atlantal ligament is spared unless exposure below C2 is required. Intradural lesions require removal of the tectorial membrane prior to opening the dura. A lumbar drain is maintained for 6 days postoperatively if the dura is opened. The limits of exposure are the hypoglossal canals laterally, the hard palate superiorly, which can be partially removed, and the body of C2 inferiorly. The dura and tumor are removed with the CO_2 laser and bipolar cautery.

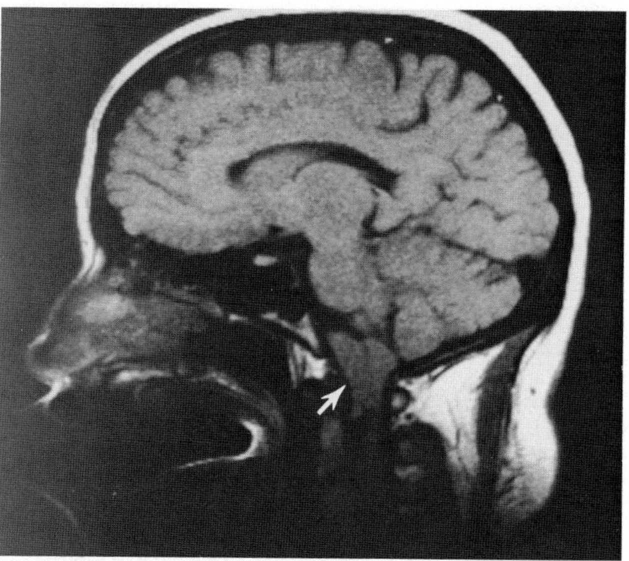

Figure 47.10. Sagittal, T1 weighted (TR 500, TE 40) image demonstrates an extraaxial, foramen magnum mass (*arrow*) compressing the cervicomedullary junction.

Closure is as follows: An autogenous fascia lata graft is secured to the dural edges with a biological adhesive after a free fat graft is placed in the tumor bed (Fig. 47.3). A fitted autogenous iliac crest bone graft is manipulated into place and secured by adhesive. The longus colli muscle and posterior pharyngeal mucosa are closed in two layers with interrupted absorbable sutures. The patient's neck is stabilized in a four-poster brace until craniocervical stability

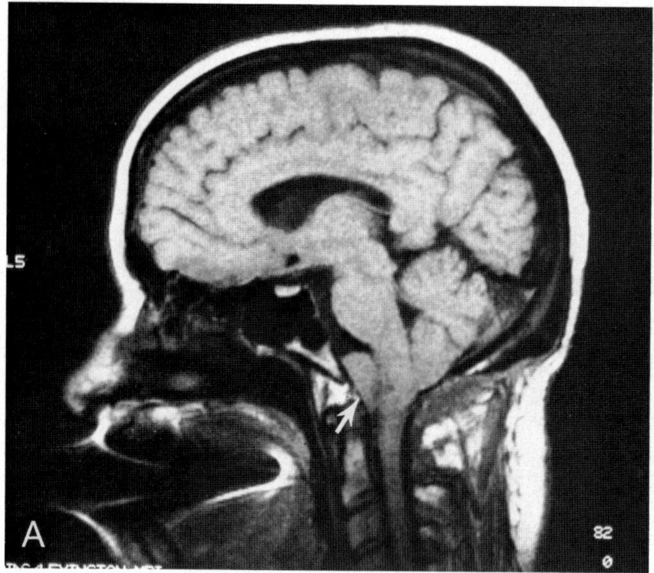

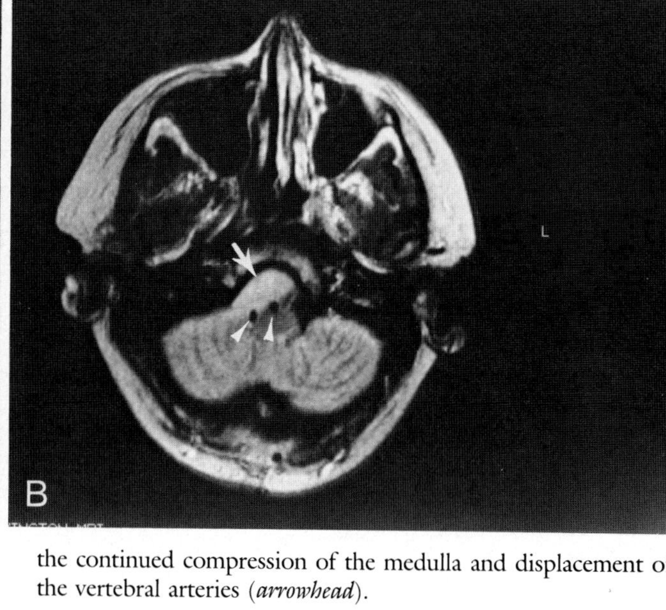

Figure 47.11. Sagittal, T1 weighted (TR 500, TE 40) **(A)** and axial, proton weighted (TR 3000, TE 40) **(B)** images, following the first operation, reveal a reduction in tumor size (*arrow*). Note the continued compression of the medulla and displacement of the vertebral arteries (*arrowhead*).

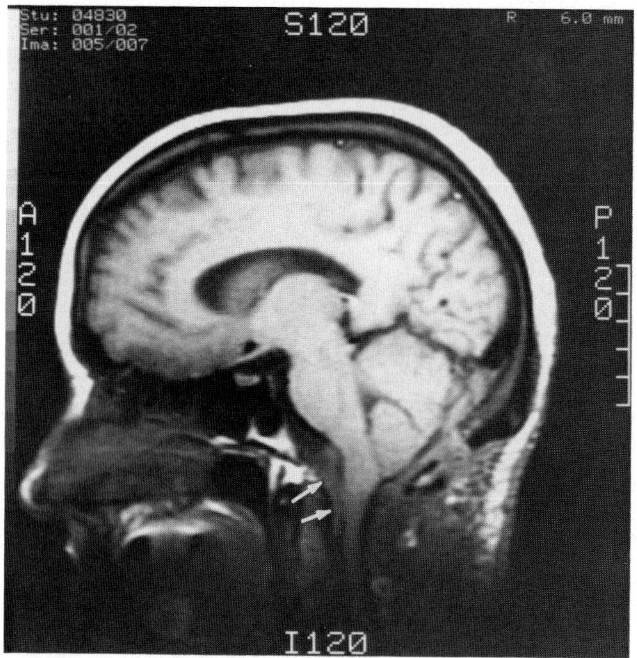

Figure 47.12. Sagittal, T2 weighted (TR 500, TE 20) image, following the second operation, demonstrates further reduction in tumor mass (*arrows*).

is documented with flexion-extension tomography. Continuous lumbar drainage is maintained for 6 days.

POSTEROLATERAL TECHNIQUE

The patient is secured in the lateral oblique position with the approach side placed superior (Fig. 47.4). This position provides excellent exposure, is comfortable for the surgeon and patient, and does not carry a significant risk for air embolus. The table is flexed to give 15° of head elevation. The head is secured with a skeletal fixation head holder (Mayfield skeletal fixation device manufactured by Ohio Medical Instrument Company, Cincinnati, Ohio), slightly flexed, and turned inferiorly to a position which has been demonstrated to be well tolerated in the awake patient. A midline suboccipital incision is made, curved laterally above the inion, and carried inferiorly over the mastoid. A high speed pneumatic craniotome is used to perform a suboccipital craniotomy with exposure of the sigmoid sinus. A cervical laminectomy and radical facetectomy are performed in order to expose the lowest extent of tumor and the vertebral artery if necessary. After the dura is opened, the Budde flexible halo retraction system (Budde retractor system manufactured by Ohio Medical Instrument Company, Cincinnati, Ohio), operative microscope, and CO_2 laser are positioned, and the tumor is progressively resected. As tumor mass is vaporized increasing room is provided, allowing retraction of the tumor away from the brainstem and medulla. A water-tight dural closure is obtained, the bone flap replaced, and the incision closed in layers.

Case Report A: (M.B.)

A 63-year-old woman presented with a 1-year history of dysesthesias in all four limbs. Right-sided spasticity and hand weakness was documented. CT and MRI scans demonstrated a massive intradural extramedullary foramen magnum tumor (Fig. 47.5). Angiography revealed marked displacement of the right vertebral artery (Fig. 47.6). The patient was placed in the right lateral oblique position, and monitoring devices were prepared. The operative microscope and CO_2 laser were used to remove the

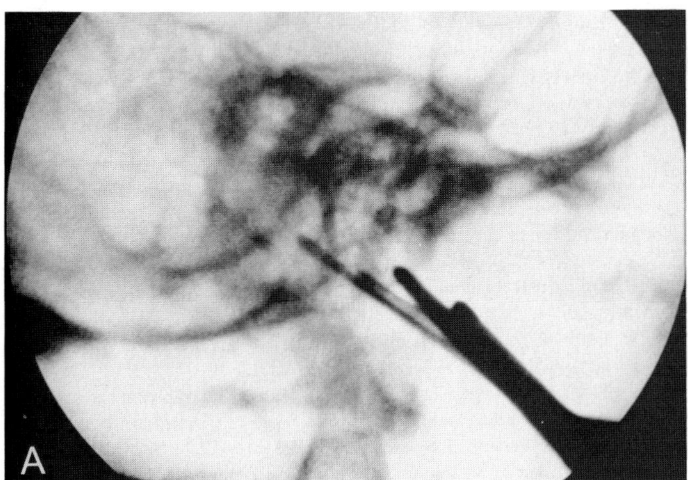

Figure 47.13. Intraoperative right lateral fluoroscopic image **(A)** demonstrates the tip of drill at the superior extent of exposure along the clivus (*arrow*). Postoperative sagittal proton weighted MR image **(B)** reveals fat graft in the tumor bed (*arrowheads*) and no evidence of residual tumor.

tumor (Fig. 47.7). A small volume of tumor, which enveloped the dura of the jugular foramen, was left in order to avoid cranial nerve deficit (Fig. 47.8). Postoperatively, her dysesthesias and neurologic findings resolved (Fig. 47.9).

Case Report B: (M.R.)

A 41-year-old woman presented with a 1-year history of left-sided numbness. Over the ensuing 7 months she developed progressive weakness leading to quadriplegia and respirator dependency before diagnosis was made and treatment implemented (Fig. 47.10). A posterior approach with subtotal removal of a large foramen magnum meningioma was performed. She gradually improved over several months, became ambulatory with a moderate spastic quadriparesis, and tolerated removal of her tracheostomy. She was referred to us for further treatment. Repeat MR imaging demonstrated residual tumor anterior to the medulla (Fig. 47.11). A right posterolateral approach was used, as in Case A, but the tumor could not be completely removed from the basal dura and proximal basilar artery (Fig. 47.12). Two weeks later a transoral approach was used to remove the remaining tumor (Fig. 47.13). A secure dural closure and bone graft was achieved. Continuous lumbar drainage was maintained for 6 days. A mild spastic quadriparesis was the only residual deficit. Tomography demonstrated no evidence of craniocervical instability.

Results

The results are summarized in Table 47.1. There have been no deaths, and persistent deficit occurred in only 2 of 14 patients (14%). Both complications were related to vascular injuries. The delay in onset of symptoms seen in one patient suggests that vasospasm was a significant causative factor. All cranial nerve palsies were transient. One patient required a shunt for hydrocephalus. Microscopic total removal was possible in eight patients, near complete removal in three, and subtotal removal in three patients. Long-term follow-up at yearly intervals is essential, since skull base tumors are characterized by delayed recurrence, and thus, none of the patients can presume to be cured. Outcome is defined as excellent if the patient's neurological status returned to normal or if the deficit did not interfere with normal activity, good if a mild deficit persisted which did not prevent the patient from returning to work, fair if the deficit persisted preventing return to work, and poor if the patient required assistance in the activities of daily life.

Discussion

Craniocervical junction tumors continue to pose diagnostic and surgical challenges. If these challenges are met, the results are excellent, but if not, inexorable deterioration of the patient will follow. MR imaging provides the opportunity for precise diagnosis of junction lesions. The clinician must consider the possibility of a lesion early because symptoms may be overlooked until the tumor has reached great proportions and invaded critical structures of the skull base.

An aggressive surgical approach, tempered with good judgement, is needed. Most of these tumors can be removed *via* a posterolateral approach. The lateral oblique position provides excellent exposure and allows the surgeon to operate in a position of comfort during the lengthy procedure required. Evoked potential monitoring provides a constant reminder of the status of the brainstem, spinal cord, and cranial nerves during tumor manipulation. A self-retaining retractor system allows gentle retraction of the cerebellum, medulla, cranial nerves, and tumor. The CO_2 laser permits tumor removal through a very narrow exposure in a bloodless field with minimal manipulation of normal tissue.

The refinement of the transoral approach for intradural pathology offers great promise in the treatment of craniocervical junction lesions and is appropriate for tumors directly anterior to the lower brainstem and upper cervical spinal cord. Mullan first described this approach in 1966, but it was subsequently abandoned because most surgeons felt that the risk of CSF leakage and meningitis was too great (21). Recently, the problem of CSF leakage has been largely solved (4, 12, 13, 27). Closure of the dura with adhesive and CSF diversion with continuous lumbar drainage appear to be the keys to prevention of CSF leakage. We have found that 6 days of continuous drainage is adequate. Placement of an LP shunt may be required in order to discontinue external drainage.

CONCLUSION

The description of the signs and symptoms of craniocervical junction lesions over 6 decades ago has been documented. The development of MR imaging provides an undeniable picture of the pathologic anatomy. There is no reason for needless delay in diagnosis of junction lesions. Surgical resection is the treatment of choice for extraaxial junction tumors. Optimal results depend upon the use of a number of recent advances in technology. Complete resection of these tumors is the goal, even if staged procedures are required, but not at the expense of sacrificing important neural and vascular structures.

REFERENCES

1. Abrahamson I, Grossman M. Tumors of the upper cervical cord. Trans Am Neurol Assoc 1921;47:149–168.

2. Blom S, Ekbom KA. Early clinical signs of meningiomas of the foramen magnum. J Neurosurg 1962;19:661–664.

3. Cohen L, Macrae D. Tumors in the region of the foramen magnum. J Neurosurg 1962;19:462–469.

4. Crockard HA, Bradford R. Transoral transclival removal of a schwannoma anterior to the craniocervical junction. J Neurosurg 1985;62:293–295.

5. Delgado TE, Garrido E, Harwick RD. Labiomandibular, transoral approach to chordomas in the clivus and upper cervical spine. Neurosurgery 1981;8:675–679.

6. Dodge HW Jr, Love JG, Gottlieb CM. Benign tumors at the foramen magnum. Surgical considerations. J Neurosurg 1956;13:603–617.

7. Fang HSY, Ong GB. Direct anterior approach to the upper cervical spine. J Bone Joint Surg 1962;44A:1588–1604.

8. Elsberg CA. Tumors of the spinal cord. Problems in their diagnosis and localization; procedures for their exposure and removal. Arch Neurol Psychiatry 1929;22:949–965.

9. Elsberg CA, Strauss I. Tumors of the spinal cord which project into the posterior cranial fossa. Report of a case in which a growth was removed from the ventral and lateral aspects of the medulla oblongata and upper cervical cord. Arch Neurol Psychiatry 1929;21:261–273.

10. Guidetti B, Spallone A. Benigh extramedullary tumors of the foramen magnum. Surg Neurol 1980;13:9–17.

11. Guthkelch AN, Williams RG. Anterior approach to recurrent chordomas of the clivus. J Neurosurg 1972;36:670–672.

12. Hadley MN, Spetzler RF, Sonntag VKH. The transoral approach to the superior cervical spine. A review of 53 cases of extradural cervicomedullary compression. J Neurosurg 1989;71:16–23.

13. Hayakawa T, Kamikawa K, Ohnishi T, Yoshime T. Prevention of postoperative complications after a transoral transclival approach to basilar aneurysms. J Neurosurg 1981;54:699–703.

14. Howe JR, Taren JA. Foramen magnum tumors. Pitfalls in diagnosis. JAMA 1973;225:1061–1066.

15. Lee BCP, Deck MDF, Kneeland JB, Cahill PT. MR imaging of the craniocervical junction. AJNR 1985;6:209–213.

16. Love JG, Thelen EP, Dodge HW Jr. Tumors of the foramen magnum. J Int Coll Surg 1954;22:1–17.

17. Menezes AH, VanGilder JC. Transoral-transpharyngeal approach to the anterior craniocervical junction. J Neurosurg 1988;69:895–903.

18. Meyers FB, Ebersold MJ, Reese DF. Benign tumors of the foramen magnum. J Neurosurg 1984;61:136–142.

19. Michael WF. Posterior fossa aneurysms simulating tumors. J Neurol Neurosurg Psychiatry 1974;37:218–223.

20. Missed foramen magnum tumours. (Editorial) Lancet 1973;2:1482.

21. Mullan S, Naunton R, Hekmat-Panah J, et al. The use of an anterior approach to ventrally placed tumors in the foramen magnum and vertebral column. J Neurosurg 1966;24:536–543.

22. Pasztor E, Vajda J, Piffko P, et al. Transoral surgery for craniocervical space-occupying processes. J Neurosurg 1984;60:276–281.

23. Smolik EA, Sachs E. Tumors of the foramen magnum of spinal origin. J Neurosurg 1954;11:161–172.

24. Stein BM, Leeds NE, Taveras JM, et al. Meningiomas of the foramen magnum. J Neurosurg 1963;20:740–751.

25. Stevenson GC, Stoney RJ, Perkins RK, et al. A transcervical transclival approach to the ventral surface of the brainstem for removal of a clivus chordoma. J Neurosurg 1966;24:544–551.

26. Symonds CP, Meadows SP. Compression of the spinal cord in the neighbourhood of the foramen magnum. Brain 1937;60:52–84.

27. Yamaura A, Makino H, Isobe K, et al. Repair of cerebrospinal fluid fistula following transoral transclival approach to a basilar aneurysm. J Neurosurg 1979;50:834–836.

48

Intramedullary Spinal Cord Tumors

Paul R. Cooper

Intramedullary spinal cord tumors (IMSCT) are uncommon lesions; few neurosurgeons have treated more than a handful of these neoplasms, and the reports of this entity in the literature have been anecdotal, based on small series of patients, or patients operated on by multiple surgeons over a long period of time (12, 15, 18). Many of the patients reported in the literature were treated before the advent of the operating microscope, ultrasound, laser, the ultrasonic tissue aspirator, or MRI, all of which have made surgery safer and more likely to result in significant tumor removal (3, 6, 15, 24, 26, 27, 29). Thus results achieved in the past have been inferior to those which may be obtained in the modern era. Moreover, the dangers of treating these tumors without these technical adjuncts has led some authors to conclude that IMSCT are best managed with biopsy and radiation and that an aggressive attempt at removal should not be undertaken (18).

In the past 8–10 years this author has had an extensive experience with these lesions and has taken a more aggressive approach in their management. While some of the initial optimism regarding the efficacy of operative treatment in curing IMSCT has been tempered by long-term outcome, to a large extent operative treatment has been safe, palliative in patients with malignant or unresectable lesions, and curative in certain others.

Epidemiology

Approximately 15% of all primary intradural tumors are intramedullary in location. The most common lesions are astrocytomas and ependymomas. In children astrocytomas predominate (24). However, in adults there is a nearly equal incidence of these lesions which together comprise one-half to two-thirds of all IMSCT (3, 15, 19, 28, 29). About one-third of the astrocytomas seen in adults are histologically malignant in our experience, although others (15) have reported a lower incidence. Other less common lesions include, but are not limited to, oligodendrogliomas, hemangioblastomas, lipomas, dermoids, epidermoids, and metastatic lesions.

The mean age in a recent series of adult patients treated by this author was 38 years (4). Females represented just over 60% of the total number of patients in this author's series. Others have found an equal incidence in males and females (29) and a similar mean age (3, 28). IMSCT occur over the entire length of the spinal cord from the cervicomedullary junction to the conus medullaris. Over one-half are located in the cervical or cervico-thoracic region (4, 5, 15).

Clinical Presentation

The clinical manifestations of IMSCT are not specific and may be confused with other conditions which result in myelopathic signs and symptoms. In patients with malignant tumors, the clinical course is rapid, and in a recently published series there was less than a 10-month interval from the time of the first clinical manifestations until operation (5). More often, the symptoms are subtle and slow in onset and develop over a period of years (3, 24, 29), suggesting a more benign process. The mean duration of symptoms in all patients in our series who had not received prior treatment was just over 3 years. Indeed it is not unusual for some patients to recall mild clumsiness, weakness, or sensory symptoms dating back many years.

Sensory Signs and Symptoms

Neck or back pain is often the first and most common manifestation of IMSCT (23, 24). Sensory symptoms frequently antedate motor symptoms and are consistent with the central location of the lesion within the spinal cord. This is especially true in patients with ependymomas which infiltrate the adjacent spinal cord little or not at all and tend to be located centrally in the spinal cord. Astrocytomas, on the other hand, usually infiltrate the adjacent spinal cord and are frequently located in an eccentric position in relation to the center of the spinal cord. Thus, patients with astrocytomas are more likely to present with motor findings which are more severe than sensory ones.

A suspended sensory loss involving the upper extremities or trunk may be present and is indistinguishable from that seen with syringomyelia. Lesions of the cervical spinal cord may present with sensory symptoms radiating to one or both upper extremities with paresthesias, dysesthesias, and areas of sensory loss (29). Thoracic lesions will present with mid-back pain and radicular symptoms of the trunk and a thoracic sensory level consistent with the location of the tumor. Deficits of joint position sense are unusual because of the central location of most of these tumors.

Motor Signs and Symptoms

Patients with tumors involving the cervical spinal cord will frequently present with upper extremity weakness prior to the onset of symptoms in the legs consistent with the central location of the tumor. In the cervical spinal cord, the central location of IMSCT may result in invasion or compression of anterior horn cells. Physical examination may demonstrate lower motor neuron dysfunction with muscular wasting and weakness and decreased deep tendon reflexes in the upper extremities. Involvement of the more peripherally located corticospinal tracts occurs later and will produce spasticity and weakness in the lower extremities and a combination of upper and lower motor signs in the upper extremities.

Thoracic spinal cord lesions will produce a spastic paraparesis and bladder dysfunction consistent with corticospinal tract dysfunction. Lesions of the conus medullaris will characteristically result in a hypotonic bladder and fecal incontinence. Lower extremity motor weakness is uncommon with lesions at this level, but rostral extension to involve the spinal cord at the level of the L5 or S1 nerve roots may produce foot weakness.

Hydrocephalus

Hydrocephalus occurs in 1–12.5% of patients with spinal cord tumors (1, 21). In some patients dissemination of tumor cells from malignant astrocytomas or ependymomas into the subarachnoid space or ventricular system will cause obstruction of the cerebrospinal fluid pathways with ventriculomegaly and signs of elevated intracranial pressure. A markedly elevated cerebrospinal fluid protein produced by the tumor may also result in impaired absorption of cerebrospinal fluid.

DIAGNOSTIC IMAGING

Magnetic Resonance Imaging

Magnetic resonance imaging (MRI) is the modality of choice for the diagnosis of IMSCT. It is generally the only examination necessary for the diagnosis of this entity because it is capable of imaging the pathologic anatomy of the spinal cord as well as the relationship of the spinal cord to surrounding bone and soft tissue structures.

We begin the evaluation of the spinal cord in the sagittal plane with T1- and T2-weighted images. Axial views are then obtained at the levels of suspected pathology. Gadolinium enhanced scans are useful to define the exact configuration and extent of the lesion and associated cysts.

Intense enhancement with gadolinium and the presence of areas of signal void caused by rapidly flowing blood should strongly suggest the diagnosis of a hemangioblastoma (Fig. 48.1). Lipomas will have a characteristic signal intensity that should suggest their diagnosis (Fig. 48.2).

Astrocytomas and ependymomas are the most common intramedullary spinal cord tumors. The length of these lesions is similar (5.3 spinal segments for astrocytomas and 4.7 for ependymomas) and there is no consistent way in which they may be distinguished from one another (Fig. 48.3). However, the enhancement of ependymomas after the administration of gadolinium contrast tends to be more intense and homogeneous than is the case for astrocytomas (Fig. 48.4). Ependymomas are almost always central in location and symmetrical, whereas astrocytomas are frequently irregular and paracentral.

Other Diagnostic Modalities

Myelography and CT/Myelography. The advent of water soluble contrast agents with subsequent imaging using CT represented an important advance in the diagnosis of IMSCT. For the first time the spinal cord and its relationship to the spine could be viewed in an axial projection. Subtle enlargement of the spinal cord could be more easily appreciated than was the case using routine myelography, and the nature of lesions such as lipomas or epidermoids which differed significantly in radiodensity from the spinal cord could be ascertained. Some cystic lesions of the spinal cord could be identified by their tendency to take up the contrast material after a delay of several hours, but it was frequently difficult to distinguish tumor-associated cysts from non-neoplastic cystic lesions with absolute certainty.

Plain Films. Plain films of the spine still have a certain usefulness as a screening examination in the patient who presents with pain or myelopathy. Widening of the pedicles on the frontal projection will suggest an intraspinal mass, but the compartment that the mass occupies and the nature of the mass itself cannot be determined. Overall, less than 20% of patients with IMSCT will have abnormal plain films (29).

Spinal Cord Angiography. Angiography of the spinal cord is usually not indicated in the evaluation of IMSCT. However, if there is suspicion from the clinical history or MRI appearance that a lesion may represent an arteriovenous malformation (AVM) or a hemangioblastoma, spinal angiography will clarify the diagnosis and define the anatomy of the lesion (Fig. 48.5).

DIFFERENTIAL DIAGNOSIS

Multiple Sclerosis

When multiple sclerosis (MS) involves the spinal cord the signs and symptoms may resemble those seen with IMSCT. In general, however, the onset of neurological deficit is more rapid in onset in patients with MS, and remissions

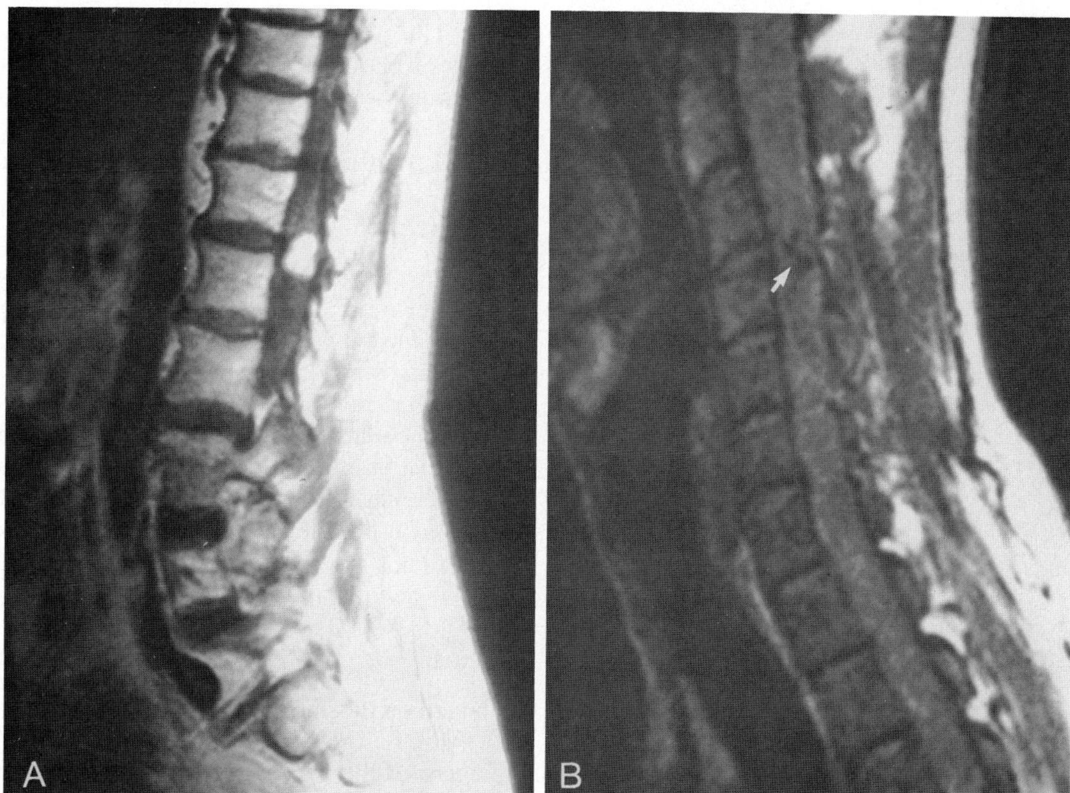

Figure 48.1. **A,** Gadolinium enhanced MRI (T1-weighted image) of a patient with a documented hemangioblastoma of the conus medullaris at the L1–2 level. **B,** T1-weighted image of another patient with a hemangioblastoma showing characteristic signal void (*arrow*) from blood flowing in large vessels supplying the tumor.

and exacerbations are a common part of the clinical picture. Although the rapidity of the clinical course in patients with spinal cord tumors may vary from patient to patient and even in the same patient, relentless progression is the rule, and remissions and exacerbations are unusual except in rare instances of intratumoral hemorrhage.

In MS, the cerebrospinal fluid will usually test positive for oligoclonal bands, and visual evoked responses will frequently be abnormal. MRI of the brain will often identify lesions consistent with plaques. To the inexperienced observer of MRI scans lesions of the spinal cord caused by demyelination of MS may bear a superficial resemblance to IMSCT. The spinal cord lesions of MS will almost always be limited to one or two spinal segments in their rostral-caudal extent. Although the signal intensity of the acute lesions of MS may be similar to that seen with IMSCT and may enhance following the administration of gadolinium, the spinal cord is minimally widened in distinction to IMSCT.

Syringomyelia

The clinical course of syringomyelia tends to be more indolent than IMSCT, but in all other respects the manifestations of the two conditions may be indistinguishable. The administration of gadolinium is essential to rule out a small enhancing tumor adjacent to an apparent syringomyelic cavity. Visualization of the cervicomedullary junction in the sagittal plane will also identify tonsillar herniation, an almost invariable accompaniment of the syrinxes associated with the Chiari malformation.

Operative Decision Making

The decision to operate on patients with far advanced neurological deficit must be made with realistic expectations. These include a desire to preserve residual sensory function in bed-ridden patients who are likely to suffer skin breakdown in anesthetic areas or preservation of residual sphincter function. However, patients who are unable to stand are unlikely to regain enough motor function to ambulate as a result of tumor resection. Nevertheless, operation may maintain the quality of a patient's life by preserving the ability to transfer or to turn in bed. Patients with complete motor and sensory deficit will not regain function with surgery and are not operative candidates.

Patients with progressive neurological deficit who are still able to walk represent the ideal operative candidates. In most, operation provides an opportunity to arrest the progression of neurological deterioration and improve motor and sensory function. Although the risks of increasing the patient's neurological deficit as a result of operation

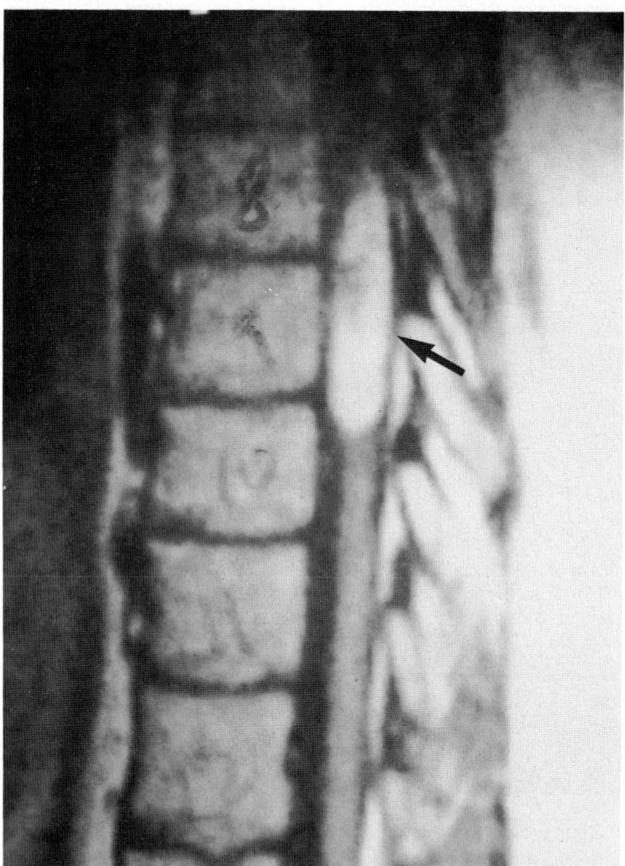

Figure 48.2. T1-weighted sagittal MRI at T8 level shows hyperintense lesion (*arrow*) which was found to be a lipoma at operation.

are real, they are more than outweighed by the natural history of the disease process.

Decision making in the patient who presents with neck or back pain and mild sensory symptoms and a paucity of objective deficits is more difficult. Many patients are unwilling to risk neurological deterioration when their symptoms are minor and they have minimal or no functional impairment. In this situation it is not unreasonable to closely follow the patient for the appearance of additional symptoms or the appearance of objective deficit. Frequently once patients realize that their symptoms have progressed as predicted, they are more prepared psychologically to face the risks of operative treatment.

OPERATIVE MANAGEMENT

All patients are treated with high dose corticosteroids for 48 hours prior to operation. We administer methyl prednisolone 125 mg every 6 hours, although comparable doses of dexamethasone are also satisfactory. Prophylactic antibiotics (usually appropriate doses of vancomycin) are given just prior to operation.

The extent of the tumor is marked on the patient's skin after x-rays are taken localizing the appropriate vertebral level. This may be done in the x-ray department the day before operation or using portable x-ray equipment in the operating theatre after the patient is positioned.

Technical Adjuncts to Tumor Removal

ULTRASONIC ASPIRATOR

The ultrasonic aspirator utilizes high-frequency sound waves to fragment tumor which is simultaneously aspirated by a suction apparatus in the tip of the device. This instrument represents a major technical advance in the removal of spinal cord tumors. By placing it into contact with the tumor the lesion may be removed atraumatically without manipulation of the adjacent spinal cord. This is a particular advantage in resecting hard tumors which cannot be removed using the suction. Without the ultrasonic aspirator tumor removal necessitates sharp dissection using a scissors and manipulation of the spinal cord.

LASER

The carbon dioxide laser is occasionally useful in resection of IMSCT. The pinpoint laser beam is directed through the lens of the operating microscope and vaporizes neoplastic tissue. It is hemostatic for vessels the size of capillaries and slightly larger but will cut through small arteries and veins without obtaining hemostasis. It offers no particular advantage over the ultrasonic aspirator for soft tumors but is very helpful in resecting scirrhus tumors which cannot be removed with the ultrasonic aspirator.

Intraoperative Management

EVOKED POTENTIAL MONITORING

The efficacy of evoked potential monitoring in improving outcome after operation for intramedullary lesions of the spinal cord is unproven. In spite of this, however, intraoperative monitoring during intramedullary spinal cord surgery is widely practiced in the United States where monitoring is most commonly performed by recording and analyzing somatosensory evoked potentials. Sensory nerves in the extremities (the median or ulnar in the arms, and the posterior tibial or peroneal in the lowers) are stimulated using low voltage electrical current, and the evoked responses in the sensory cortex are recorded using scalp electrodes, and multiple responses are averaged using a computer.

In theory any injury to the dorsal columns and spinothalamic tracts which serve as the pathways for the transmission of the evoked potentials should be reflected in changes in the amplitude or latency of the recorded wave forms. Unfortunately, currently available evoked potential monitoring techniques are not always useful in guiding the surgeon during the course of the operation. Patients with profound sensory deficits will have evoked responses that

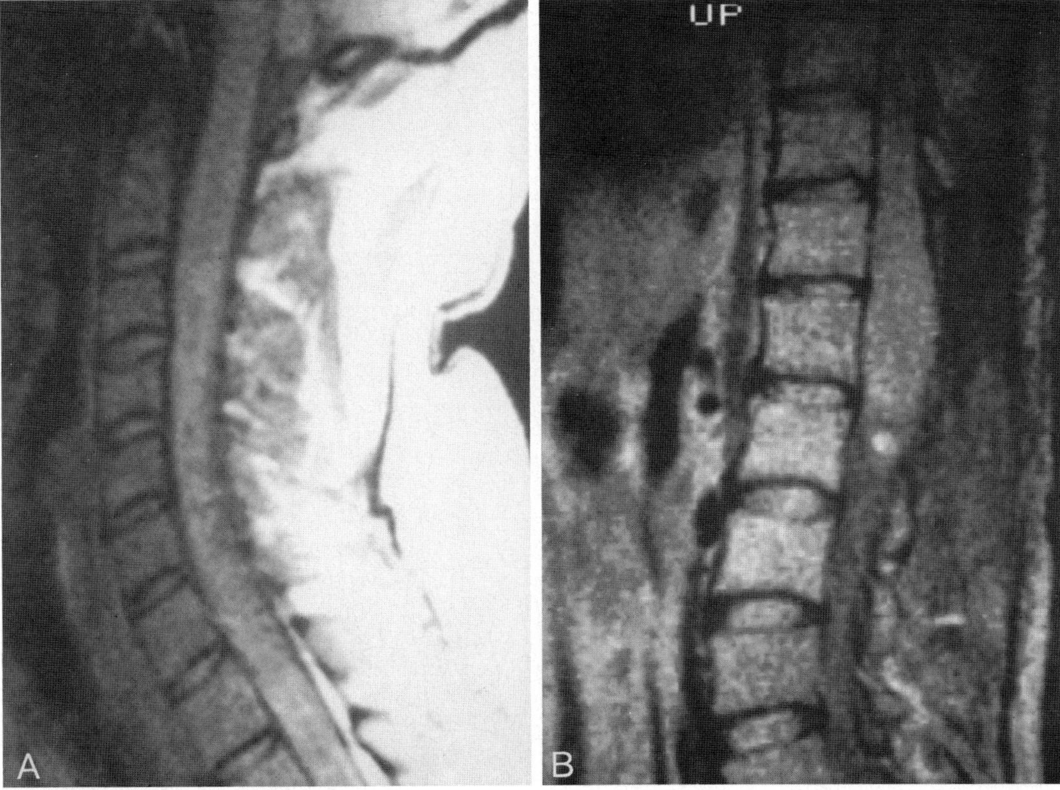

Figure 48.3. **A,** Sagittal MRI (T1-weighted image) shows diffuse spinal cord widening from C1–T1 in a patient with an ependymoma. No cyst is seen, nor was one found at operation. **B,** T1-weighted MRI of a grade II astrocytoma of the conus medullaris. Without gadolinium enhancement there is no way that the ependymoma in **A** can be distinguished from the astrocytoma in **B**.

are either absent or of such low amplitude that meaningful recordings cannot be obtained. Depending on the computer averaging techniques used there is a delay of 10–60 seconds from the time that an injury to spinal cord sensory pathways occurs until changes in the evoked potential wave form is observed. Because the surgery entails operating on structures within the spinal cord, irreversible damage may occur as the surgeon proceeds with his dissection during this period of time.

Although knowledge of injury to sensory pathways is important, monitoring of sensory pathways gives no direct information regarding the integrity of the corticospinal tract. Thus injury may occur to the motor pathways without any change in the somatosensory evoked potentials. In practice the proximity of the corticospinal and the spinothalamic tracts is such that injury to motor pathways will usually be reflected in changes of the sensory evoked potentials. However, this is not invariably the case.

There have been several new approaches which have been employed recently in an attempt to obviate some of the disadvantages of standard evoked potential monitoring techniques. Stimulation of motor pathways in an attempt to gain information about spinal cord function is an increasingly popular technique that is being used in a number of clinical centers. Stimulation of the motor cortex using scalp electrodes may be used to evoke motor responses in the upper or lower extremities which may be recorded by EMG techniques. Alternatively, direct epidural recording of spinal cord motor pathways may be used to assess the integrity of spinal cord motor pathways. Stimulation and recording of both sensory and motor pathways may be used for a more complete assessment of spinal cord function.

In brief, it must be emphasized that at this time there is no statistically valid evidence that the use of any electrophysiological monitoring technique improves outcome of patients undergoing surgery for IMSCT. The efficacy of these techniques must await a randomized prospective study comparing neurological outcome in monitored and unmonitored patients.

OPERATIVE TECHNIQUE

Regardless of the location of the tumor, patients are positioned prone on the operating table. For tumors below T2, the patient's head is turned to one side and placed on a soft cushion. When dealing with tumors at T2 and higher the patient should be placed in the three pin head holder with the head in the neutral and unrotated position. We no longer use the horseshoe head rest for these procedures,

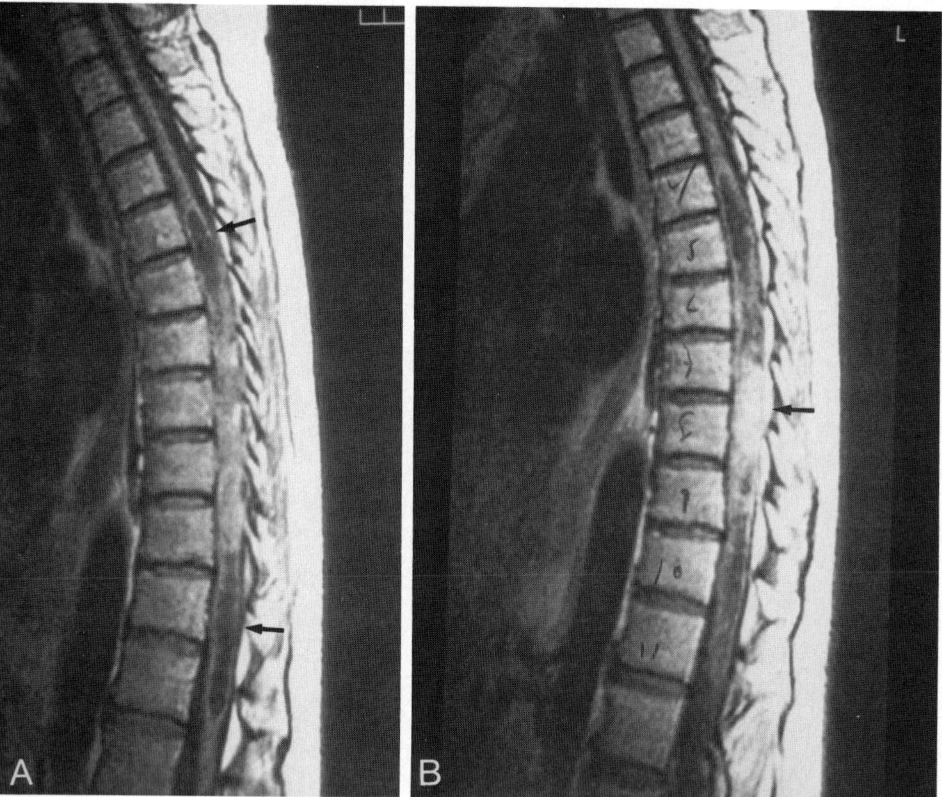

Figure 48.4. **A,** Sagittal MRI of a thoracic ependymoma before administration of contrast. Cysts (*small arrows*) are identified above and below the tumor which is poorly distinguished from the spinal cord. **B,** Following the administration of gadolinium the tumor enhances and is well-defined (*arrow*).

as skin breakdown over the face and forehead is common after prolonged operative procedure. After the head is fixed the position of the table is adjusted so that the area of the laminectomy is horizontal to prevent irrigating fluid from running out of the wound when ultrasonography is performed.

Laminectomy is performed at the site of the solid tumor. Tumor-associated cysts are present in 40–50% of patients (5, 22) and are frequently more extensive than the tumor itself, but it is unnecessary to extend the laminectomy rostrally or caudally to areas of cystic enlargement of the spinal cord (7). The cyst fluid is produced by the tumor and will disappear with total tumor removal. The walls of the cyst are composed of nonneoplastic glial tissue which should not be resected.

After the laminectomy is performed the intraoperative ultrasound is brought into the field to confirm the location of solid tumor and any cysts located rostral or caudal to the tumor (25) (Fig. 48.6). The dura mater is then opened, and from this point until tumor resection is complete the operating microscope is utilized.

A dorsal myelotomy is performed in the midline over the area of solid tumor (Fig. 48.7). It is essential that both the left and right dorsal roots be identified, as the midline will be located midway between the left and right dorsal roots. The pia-arachnoid and dorsal surface of the spinal cord are then incised sharply to a depth of 2–3 mm over the length of the spinal cord occupied by the solid tumor. Alternatively, the carbon dioxide laser co-axial to the operating microscope and sharply focused at a setting of less than 5 W can be used to perform the myelotomy.

The pia-arachnoid and dorsal surface of the spinal cord are held apart by passing a 6–0 atraumatic suture through the pia-arachnoid at intervals of 1 cm on either side of the midline. Traction is placed on the ends of the sutures with light hemostats to open the center of the spinal cord for further dissection. If the tumor is not immediately visible the dissection in the spinal cord is continued sharply in a ventral direction until the tumor is encountered. Specific details of tumor removal are determined by the nature of the tumor encountered and will be discussed in the subsequent section.

After the tumor resection is terminated, the dura is tightly closed with interrupted or running locked sutures. If residual tumor is present or the spinal cord remains swollen, a dural graft should be placed to preclude constricting the spinal cord. The remainder of the closure is done in a standard fashion.

Ependymomas. Along with astrocytomas these are the most common tumors found within the spinal cord. Although the central canal is normally closed before birth in humans, nests of ependymal cells remain in the center of the spinal cord. Ependymomas presumably take origin from these cells and are located centrally, although their major blood supply is ventral. As they grow from their point of origin they push the adjacent spinal cord aside.

Ependymomas are thus distinct from the surrounding

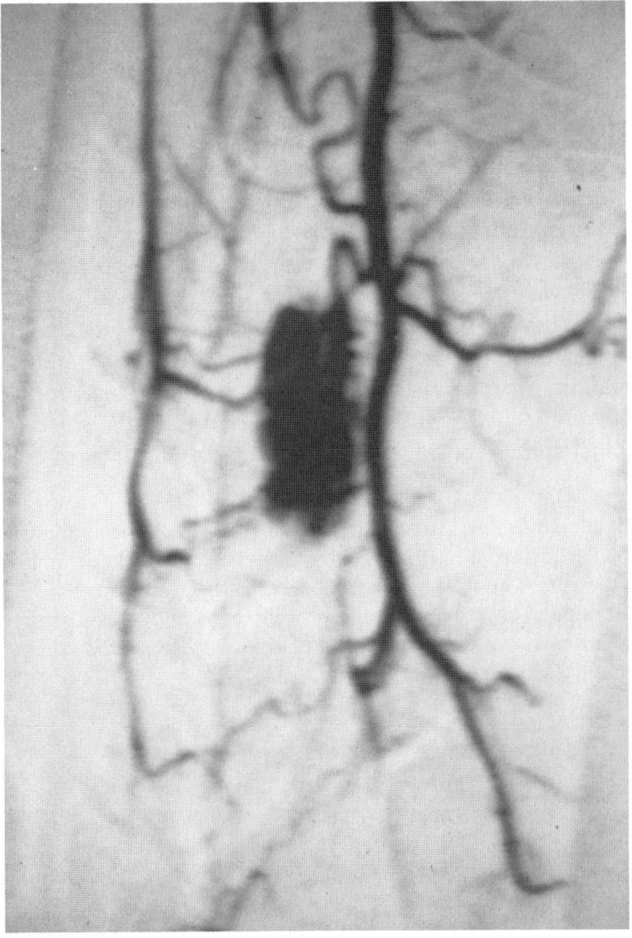

Figure 48.5. Spinal cord angiogram showing intensely vascular hemangioblastoma at the C2 level.

spinal cord and may be dissected from it. They are firm in consistency and reddish, gray, or yellow in color. The myelotomy should be extended ventrally and in a rostral-caudal direction so that the upper and lower tumor margins as well as the entire dorsal surface of the tumor can be seen. Cysts are frequently found at either or both ends of the tumor.

Although smaller lesions may often be removed in one piece, it is generally wiser to first reduce the bulk of the tumor. If the tumor is highly vascular this can be accomplished by grasping its surface with the bipolar cautery and shrinking it with the cautery at a low setting. If the lesion is avascular or relatively so, it may be gutted with the ultrasonic aspirator. As the tumor is reduced in size it is rolled in on itself and sharply dissected from the surrounding spinal cord. As the tumor is rotated out of the spinal cord, its ventral vascular supply is cauterized and cut and the tumor is removed from its bed (Fig. 48.8). In most patients a total resection is possible. However, in some patients the resection must be stopped when the interface between the tumor and normal spinal cord becomes indiscernible.

Astrocytomas. Spinal cord astrocytomas in adults are infiltrating tumors which are histologically identical to intracranial astrocytomas. They are located several millimeters beneath the dorsal surface of the spinal cord, and although they may be distinguished from the surrounding spinal cord they blend imperceptibly with the spinal cord at their margins. The lower grade lesions are relatively avascular and lend themselves to resection using the ultrasonic aspirator. Resection is continued until the interface with the spinal cord at the tumor margins becomes indistinguishable or if resection produces changes in the evoked potential signals.

In children it is possible that these tumors behave in a fashion similar to low grade posterior fossa astrocytomas where total resection may be achieved. Indeed Garrido and Stein (10) found astrocytomas no more difficult to resect than ependymomas. However, theirs is a minority opinion, and most authors believe that total resection of these tumors

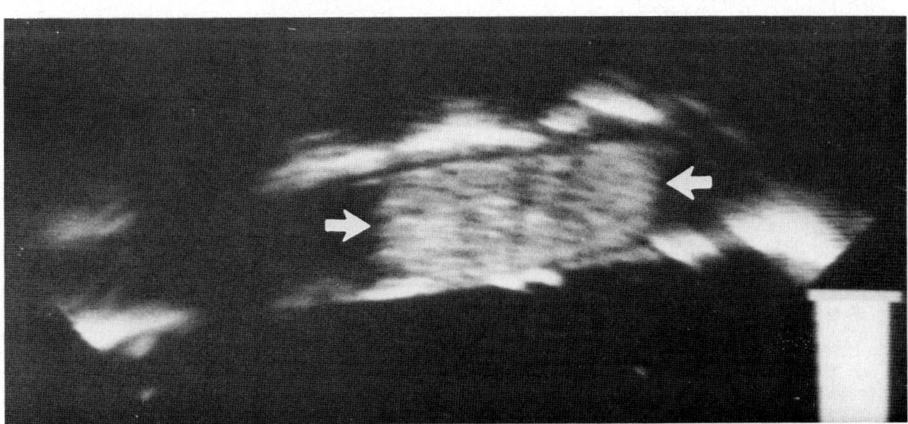

Figure 48.6. Intraoperative ultrasound performed in the sagittal plane shows solid tumor (*large arrows*). Dark areas of decreased echogenicity above and below the tumor represent tumor-associated cysts.

in adults is infrequently possible as they infiltrate the normal spinal cord beyond the point of grossly or microscopically visible tumor (15, 29). These tumors may also infiltrate viable functioning spinal cord pathways at the periphery of the tumor resulting in postoperative exacerbation of neurological deficit even when the surgeon was confident that resection was strictly confined to grossly apparent tumor (19).

By dint of their location and tendency to infiltrate, even small tumors can produce severe neurological deficit; recurrence after incomplete removal is common; and transformation to histologically malignant tumors occurs. The malignant tumors (Kernohan grades III and IV) behave in a fashion analogous to the same tumors located intracranially. If complete resection is impossible, they recur rapidly after surgery, metastasize through the subarachnoid space, and inevitably result in the death of the patient (15, 17).

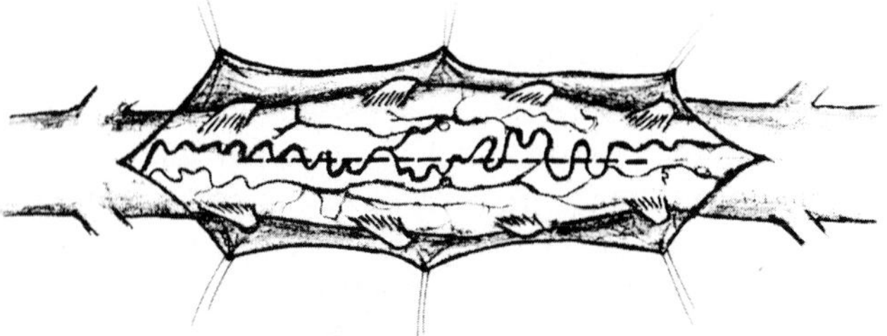

Figure 48.7. Artist's drawing shows location of myelotomy (*dotted line*) midway between the posterior roots.

Hemangioblastomas. Hemangioblastomas occur as isolated lesions or in association with other hemangioblastomas in the posterior cranial fossa or elsewhere in the spinal cord. They are immediately apparent on the dorsal surface of the spinal cord along with a profusion of vessels which supply and drain the lesion. They range in size from a few millimeters in diameter to the size of a large grape and are well-defined from the surrounding spinal cord.

No attempt should be made to enter the tumor until its vascular supply is totally interrupted, as these tumors are highly vascular. The arterial supply, part of which is visible on the dorsal surface of the spinal cord, is coagulated and cut, and the tumor is very slowly reduced in size by coagulating it with the bipolar cautery. When this is done the tumor may be more easily dissected from the adjacent spinal cord, exposing additional vascular supply which is

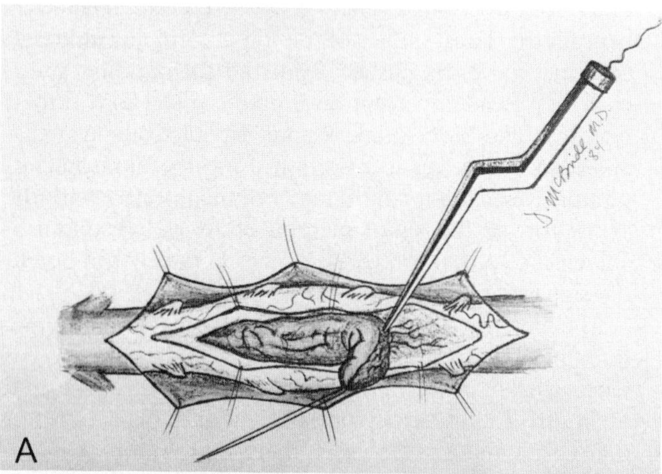

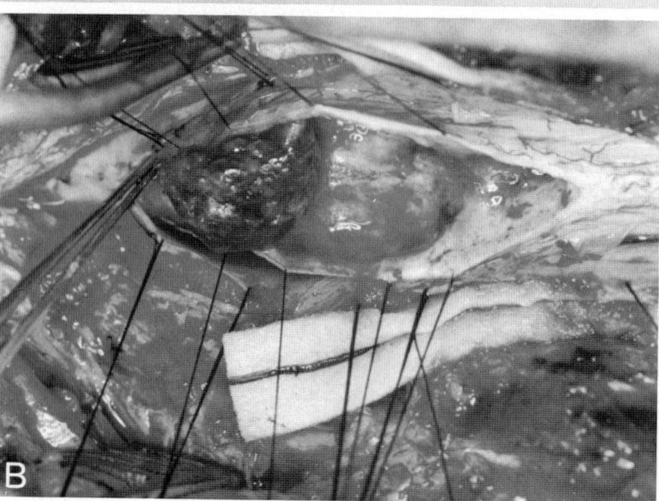

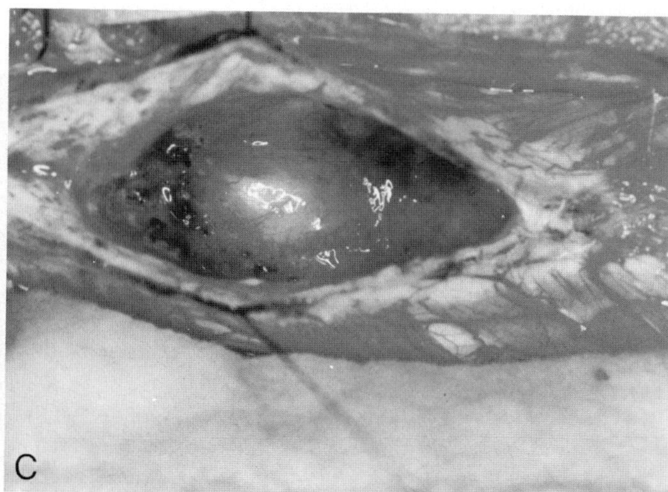

Figure 48.8. **A,** Artist's drawing of removal of ependymoma. Bipolar forceps are shown cauterizing the ventral blood supply as traction is applied to the tumor in a dorsal direction. **B,** Corresponding operative photograph showing removal of ependymoma from its tumor bed. **C,** Operative photograph shows total tumor resection.

progressively interrupted allowing total removal. Hemangioblastomas are curable tumors but may recur as a result of the growth of residual tumor or, as is more commonly the case, growth of additional tumors which were clinically silent or radiographically unapparent at the time of the first surgery.

Lipomas. Lipomas of the spinal cord are most commonly seen at the level of the conus medullaris in association with spina bifida occulta, cutaneous lumbar or sacral lipoma, and a tethered spinal cord. Less commonly, isolated lipomas occur more rostrally in the thoracic and cervical spinal cord. Histologically identical to normal fat, these tumors are located on the dorsal surface of the spinal cord covered by little or no neural tissue.

Although distinct from adjacent spinal cord and noninvasive, they are densely adherent to normal spinal cord, and total removal is not possible without incurring unacceptable neurological deficit (12). The most effective operative strategy consists of subtotal removal, leaving a rim of tumor at the interface with the spinal cord. The laser is ideal for removal of lipomas, as the fibrous interstices of the lesion make removal with the ultrasonic aspirator difficult. These are slowly growing lesions, but recurrence may take place as a result of continued growth of residual tumor.

Intramedullary Metastatic Tumors. Although metastases to the brain from systemic malignancies are common, metastases to the spinal cord are rare and represent less than 8% of all IMSCT (3). Chason et al. (2) were able to find only ten cases in 200 patients with central nervous system metastases who were autopsied. The lung and the breast are the most common primary sites (13). In one-third of cases the intramedullary lesion is the presenting sign of the primary tumor. Progression of neurologic signs is rapid, and complete neurologic deficit develops within 1 month in over 70% of patients (13) who are not treated. Over 80% of patients die within 3 months after seeking medical attention.

These lesions tend to be vascular and well-defined from the adjacent spinal cord. The most effective operative strategy consists of slow bipolar coagulation of the tumor, visualization and section of the vascular supply, and total removal.

Other Tumors. Other tumors include gangliogliomas, oligodendrogliomas, epidermoids, and intramedullary neurofibromas. These tumors are rare, and the problems they present to the surgeon are similar in nature to the tumors discussed above.

POSTOPERATIVE COMPLICATIONS

Exacerbation of Neurological Deficit

Patients with the most severe preoperative motor deficit have the greatest chances of sustaining a permanent increase in neurological deficit. Neurological deterioration does not seem to be related to the histological type of tumor or the extent of surgical resection. Overall, approximately 20% of patients will have a permanent increase in their deficit.

Loss of joint position may occur as a result of injury to the dorsal columns as the myelotomy is made. The spinothalamic tracts may also be injured during dissection at the lateral aspect of a centrally located tumor. Abnormalities of intraoperative somatosensory evoked potentials may provide early warning of disturbance to these pathways.

Dysesthesias, hyperesthesias, and hyperpathia are dreaded complications of surgery. Their presence may render an otherwise functional extremity useless and prevent a patient with minimal or no motor deficit from returning to a former occupation or resuming a normal social life. Frequently these symptoms will be present preoperatively from tumor invasion of sensory pathways and will persist or be exacerbated as a result of tumor removal.

Operative Wound Breakdown

In patients who have had a previous operation and irradiation, there is a high incidence of wound dehiscence (7, 10), cerebrospinal fluid fistula, and meningitis regardless of how meticulous a closure is performed. For this reason in all patients who have had previous operation and irradiation the incision is closed with the assistance of plastic surgical colleagues who utilize rotational flaps of the trapezius or latissimus dorsi muscles from outside the irradiated field (30).

Spinal Deformities

The development of kyphoscoliosis of the thoracic or lumbar spine and swan neck deformity of the cervical spine are frequently seen in children following surgery for IMSCT (24). Its appearance in adults is unusual if it has not been present preoperatively.

In children deformities of the thoracic and lumbar spine are frequently seen in association with IMSCT and may represent the initial manifestation of this condition months or years before the appearance of neurological signs and symptoms. It is not clear whether the appearance or exacerbation of these deformities in the postoperative period results from the effect of the tumor or laminectomy. In the cervical spine, however, it is likely that laminectomy and denervation of the paraspinous muscles lead to flexion deformity. Severe untreated flexion deformity may result in spinal cord compression and progressive neurological deficit which may be mistaken for tumor recurrence. Because the incidence of postoperative deformities of the spine in children is high, frequent follow-up is essential. In the cervical spine early fusion at the first sign of flexion deformity is indicated. In the thoracic and lumbar spine orthopaedic instrumentation and fusion are also indicated when progressive deformity is recognized.

ADJUNCTIVE TREATMENT

Radiation Therapy

No study has been performed demonstrating a beneficial effect of radiation therapy on neurological function or survival in patients with glial tumors of the spinal cord. Guidetti et al. (15) did not find any consistent benefit from radiation therapy. Others (18, 26–28) have reported improvement or disappearance of deficits after irradiation, but none of these studies were controlled and there is no proof that the radiation treatment itself resulted in improvement. Moreover, the efficacy of radiation therapy is difficult to determine, as the natural history of low grade astrocytomas is unpredictable, and long-term survival without radiation may occur (24). Nevertheless, it has been our policy to irradiate all adult patients with spinal cord astrocytomas regardless of the surgeon's impression of the completeness of removal or the histologic grade of the tumor. The treatment consists of 4500 Gys given in divided doses to the region of the tumor. Marsa et al. (20) used doses greater than 5000 Gy, but such treatment is not recommended because of the risk of radiation myelopathy.

Because of the detrimental effect of radiation therapy on development in children and the possibility that low grade astrocytomas in children are potentially curable by surgery, treatment is deferred in pediatric patients who are thought to have had a gross total resection of their tumors. These patients should be followed with MRI to detect any evidence of tumor recurrence.

Patients with ependymomas who are thought to have had a complete removal are not irradiated (8, 12). They are followed with MRI and treated with reoperation or radiation if recurrence becomes apparent. When removal of ependymomas is incomplete patients should be treated with local radiation to the area of residual tumor.

Chemotherapy

For the past decade chemotherapeutic agents such as 1-3-bis-2-chloroethyl-*l*-nitrosourea (BCNU) have been a standard part of the management protocol for treatment of patients with astrocytomas of the brain. However, the usefulness of BCNU and other chemotherapy for the management of astrocytomas of the spinal cord is unknown, and they have not been used by this author.

LONG-TERM OUTCOME

Long-term survival and neurological function are related to tumor histology, the patient's preoperative neurological status, and extent of tumor resection.

Survival

The prognosis for patients with malignant astrocytomas is remarkably similar to that of patients with the same tumors located intracranially, and no patient in this author's series survived longer than 1 year. Others hve reported similar survival statistics (3, 16, 17, 24). Although the outlook for patients with low grade astrocytomas is better, slow progression of tumors in the cervical region can result in death from respiratory paralysis. Other complications of quadriplegia such as pulmonary embolus, sepsis, and pneumonia will also shorten the lives of these patients and make this anything but a benign lesion. Degeneration of low grade tumors into malignant ones occurs with time and will further adversely affect outcome. Twelve of 18 of our patients with astrocytomas of all grades in this author's series have died after a mean follow-up of just over 3 years.

Fortunately the long-term survival of patients with ependymomas is less bleak than is the case for patients with astrocytomas. Unlike astrocytomas, the outcome of patients with ependymomas does not appear to be related to histologic grade (23). Although ependymomas can seed in the subarachnoid space, this method of spread seems to be the exception rather than the rule. Of 24 patients with ependymomas only one has died as a result of tumor growth.

Hemangioblastomas are benign tumors which are curable if totally removed. As such they should have little effect on long-term survival. In practice hemangioblastomas are frequently found in multiple locations, and outcome is determined by the behavior of tumors located elsewhere in the nervous system. Other varieties of tumors found within the spinal cord are encountered too infrequently to make a definitive statement regarding their effect on longevity.

Neurological Function

PREOPERATIVE NEUROLOGICAL FUNCTION

Neurological outcome in the immediate postoperative period is most closely related to the patient's immediate preoperative neurological state (7, 8, 15). Patients who have no motor function may on rare occasions regain some movement after operation, but it is unlikely that they will be able to walk or stand as a result of tumor resection. Similarly, patients who cannot stand are unlikely to be able to walk in the postoperative period.

The combination of increased neurological deficit from operation and progressive growth of residual tumor leaves a high percentage of patients with considerable neurological impairment in the years following operation. Almost one-half of all patients available for follow-up examination were worse than they were prior to the time of operation by one or more neurological grades (4).

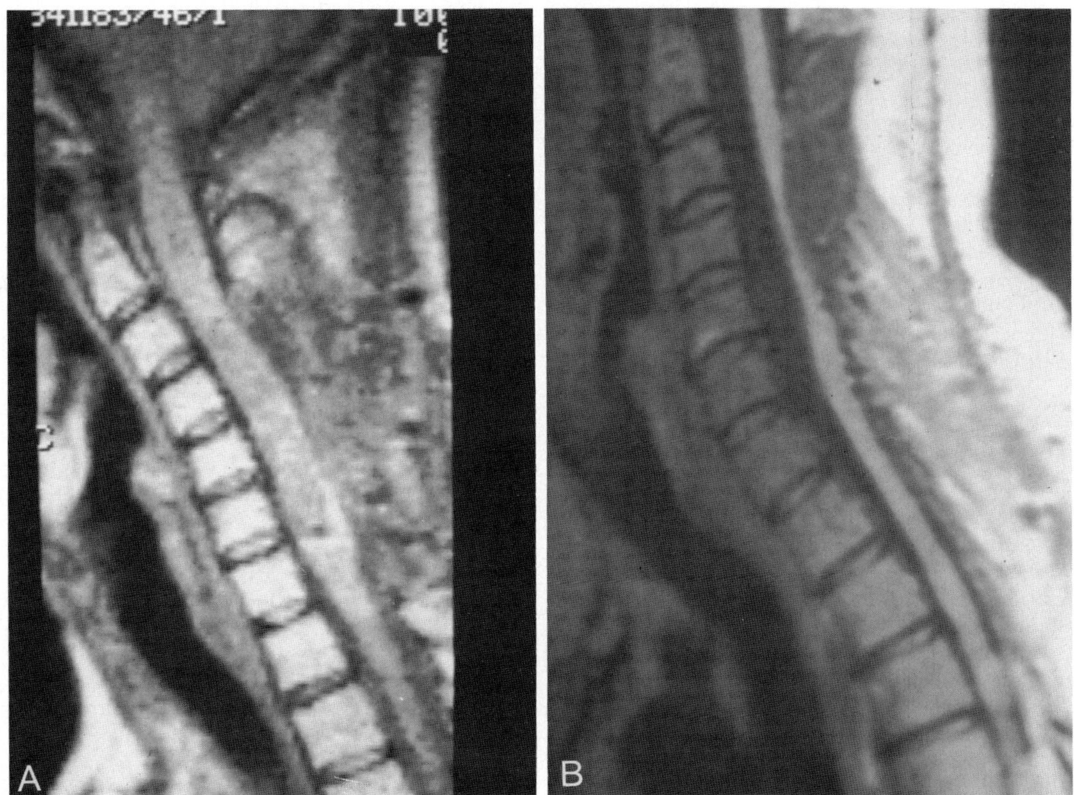

Figure 48.9. **A,** Preopertive MRI of a patient with an extensive cervical ependymoma. **B,** Postoperative MRI with gadolinium enhancement 2 years following operation shows an atrophic spinal cord and no evidence of recurrence.

EXTENT OF TUMOR RESECTION

Spinal cord tumors usually grow slowly, and the relationship between outcome and extent of tumor resection must be examined after a sufficiently long period has elapsed from the time of operation. Unfortunately, this has not been done in a systematic way in series reported in the literature. Because the extent of tumor resection is estimated by the operating surgeon it is subject to inaccuracy and bias.

In the case of astrocytomas the surgeon's estimate of the extent and completeness of resection is most suspect. Because these are infiltrating tumors, "total removal" is probably achieved less frequently than has been thought in the past. In reviewing the outcome of patients with astrocytomas who had total or 99% removal the high frequency of tumor recurrence and progression of neurological deficit strongly suggests that complete or nearly complete removal is infrequently achieved (4). Indeed the extent of resection correlates poorly with survival and neurological outcome (16). On the other hand, the extent of resection of ependymomas correlates well with outcome. Of patients with ependymomas who had total tumor resection only one person in our series was made worse by operation, and none has had recurrence (Fig. 48.9). Others have reported similar results (19, 23).

CONCLUSIONS

In spite of a number of advances in the last decade, tumors of the spinal cord continue to present a challenge to neurosurgeons. While advances in imaging and, in particular, the advent of the MRI, have eliminated much of the uncertainty in diagnosis, they remain a particularly difficult entity to treat surgically.

It has become clear that radical removal of IMSCT can be achieved by experienced surgeons with minimal morbidity. However, most spinal cord astrocytomas in adults are infiltrative and not totally resectable, and recurrence is frequent. This is especially true for the malignant astrocytomas which behave in a fashion similar to such tumors located intracranially where early neurological deterioration and death are the rule. For many ependymomas surgical cure is possible, but for infiltrating ependymomas and other spinal cord tumors of glial origin improved management awaits a greater understanding of the biology of these lesions.

REFERENCES

1. Ammerman BJ, Smith DR. Papilledema and spinal cord tumors. Surg Neurol 1975;3:55–57.

2. Chason JL, Walker FB, Landers JW. Metastatic carcinoma in the

central nervous system and dorsal root ganglia. Cancer 1963;16:781–787.

3. Chigasaki H, Pennybacker JB. A long follow-up study of 128 cases of intramedullary spinal cord tumours. Neurol Med Chir 1968;10:25–66.

4. Cooper PR. Outcome after operative treatment of intramedullary spinal cord tumors in adults. Intermediate and long-term results in 51 patients. Neurosurgery 1989;25:855–859.

5. Cooper PR, Epstein F. Radical resection of intramedullary spinal cord tumors in adults. Recent experience in 29 patients. J Neurosurg 1985;63:492–499.

6. Elsberg CA. Tumors of the spinal cord and the symptoms of irritation and compression of the spinal cord and nerve roots. Pathology, Symptomatology, Diagnosis and Treatment. New York: Paul B. Hoeber, 1924.

7. Epstein F, Epstein N. Surgical treatment of spinal cord astrocytomas of children. A series of 19 patients. J Neurosurg 1982;57:685–689.

8. Fischer G, Mansuy L. Total removal of intramedullary ependymomas: follow-up study of 16 cases. Surg Neurol 1980;14:243–249.

9. Garcia DM. Primary spinal cord tumors treated with surgery and postoperative irradiation. Radiat Oncol Biol Phys 1985;11:1933–1939.

10. Garrido E, Stein BM. Microsurgical removal of intramedullary spinal cord tumors. Surg Neurol 1977;7:215–219.

11. Goy AMC, Pinto RS, Raghavendra BN, Epstein FJ, and Kricheff II. Intramedullary spinal cord tumors. MR imaging with emphasis on associated cysts. Radiology 1986;161:381–386.

12. Greenwood J. Intramedullary tumors of spinal cord. A follow-up study after total surgical removal. J Neurosurg 1963;20:665–668.

13. Grem JL, Burgess J, Trump DL. Clinical features and natural history of intramedullary spinal cord metastasis. Cancer 1985;56:2305–2314.

14. Grisold W, Pernetzky G, Jellinger K. Giant-cell glioblastoma of the thoracic cord. Acta Neurochir 1981;58:121–126.

15. Guidetti B, Mercuri S, Vagnozzi R. Long-term results of the surgical treatment of 129 intramedullary spinal gliomas. J Neurosurg 1981;54:323–330.

16. Hardison HH, Packer RJ, Rorke LB, Schut L, Sutton LN. Outcome of children with primary intramedullary spinal cord tumors. Childs Nerv Syst 1987;3:89–92.

17. Kopelson G, Linggood RM. Intramedullary spinal cord astrocytoma versus glioblastoma. Cancer 1982;50:732–735.

18. Kopelson G, Linggood RM, Kleinman GM, Doucette J, Wang CC. Management of intramedullary spinal cord tumors. Radiology 1980;135:473–479.

19. Malis LI. Intramedullary spinal cord tumors. Clin Neurosurg 1978;25:512–539.

20. Marsa GW, Goffinet DR, Rubinstein LJ, Bagshaw MA. Megavoltage irradiation in the treatment of gliomas of the brain and spinal cord. Cancer 1975;36:1681–1689.

21. Neau JP, Roualdes G, Bataille B, et al. Hypertension intracranienne et hydrocephalie par tumeurs medullaires. A propos de trolis observations. Neurochirurgie 1987;33:216–219.

22. Okazaki H. Fundamentals of neuropathology. New York/Tokyo: Igaku-Shoin, 1983.

23. Rawlings CE, Giangaspero F, Burger PC, Bullard DE. Ependymomas: a clinicopathologic study. Surg Neurol 1988;29:271–281.

24. Reimer R, Onofrio BM. Astrocytomas of the spinal cord in children and adolescents. J Neurosurg 1985;63:669–675.

25. Rubin JM, Dohrmann GJ. Work in progress: intraoperative ultrasonography of the spine. Radiology 1983;146:173–175.

26. Stein BM. Surgery of intramedullary spinal cord tumors. Clin Neurosurg 1979;26:529–542.

27. Woltman HW, Kernohan JW, Adson AW, Craig WM. Intramedullary tumors of spinal cord and gliomas of intradural portion of filum terminale. Fate of patients who have these tumors. Arch Neurol Psychiatry 1951;65:378–395.

28. Wood EH, Berne AS, Taveras JM. The value of radiation therapy in the management of intrinsic tumors of the spinal cord. Radiology 1954;63:11–24.

29. Woods WW, Pimenta AA. Intramedullary lesions of the spinal cord. Study of sixty-eight consecutive cases. Arch Neurol Psych 1944;52:383–399.

30. Zide BM, Wisoff JH, Epstein FJ. Closure of extensive and complicated laminectomy wounds. Operative technique. J Neurosurg 1987;67:59–64.

49

Bony Lesions of the Cervical Spine

Bruce R. Rosenblum and Martin B. Camins

Introduction

A small subset of patients with pain emanating from the cervical spine, most of whom additionally demonstrate evidence of underlying spondylolytic changes or post-traumatic injury, may have osseous neoplasms. The majority of these primary neoplasms are benign, and the ratio of benign to malignant primary lesions is reversed in the cervical region as compared to the remainder of the spinal column (42). Primary osseous neoplasms usually occur in patients less than 30 years of age, as do primary unicentric malignant masses, while solitary metastases and plasmacytomas exist in an older population (3, 13, 41). Solitary metastases most frequently compromise the spinal cord in the thoracic region but do occur in the cervical spine (23). In the cervical column, metastatic lesions are more common than primary masses with the most common bony tumor being a plasmacytoma (15). Infectious or inflammatory masses involving the cervical axis also occur infrequently. Atlanto-axial subluxation with the development of pannus is the most common manifestation of rheumatoid involvement of the cervical spine (19). This occurs in close to 25% of patients with rheumatoid arthritis (10).

Irrespective of the type of mass, neck pain is the most common presenting complaint. Plain radiographs of the cervical spine are essential in the initial evaluation to determine whether a mass lesion is responsible for the neck pain. In one series, 99% of cervical spine tumors were detected by routine radiographs alone (42). Subsequent CT and MR imaging with and without contrast are useful to delineate the degree of encroachment upon the spinal cord, nerve roots, vertebral arteries, or adjacent soft tissues. Angiography should be utilized to demonstrate the vascular pattern, involvement or compression of the vertebral arteries, and as a route for embolization of tumors such as hemangiomas, or extremely vascular metastatic lesions. Radionuclide scans are regarded as a general determinant of malignancy (40).

Since primary tumors, either benign or malignant, metastatic lesions, or infectious processes carry such differing prognoses, and require different therapeutic approaches, the initial objective in the management of these patients should be to establish a tissue diagnosis. This can be performed via either an open surgical procedure or by a skinny needle biopsy under radiographic guidance. The goals of surgical and adjuvant therapy include improvement in and prevention of further neurologic impairment, correction of mechanical instability created either by the pathologic process or surgical intervention, and eradication of the tumor when possible.

Benign Tumors

Hemangiomas

Hemangiomas are the most frequent benign tumor in the cervical spine, arising from newly formed blood vessels. They occur in the spine in approximately 10% of the cases in large autopsy series (25). Hemangiomas account for 2–3% of all spinal tumors, with young females being predominantly affected. Cervical lesions are decidedly rare (22, 36).

Although usually asymptomatic, they may present as a cervical myeloradiculopathy secondary to either an epidural tumor, bleeding into the epidural space, or expansion of the involved vertebral body. The radiographic fingerprint of hemangiomas is the vertical trabeculation predominantly present in the vertebral body (Fig. 49.1). Up to one-third of these lesions may have a second hemangioma located elsewhere in the spine, usually in either the thoracic or lumbar region (25). Upon histological examination, these tumors demonstrate vascular channels either capillary, cavernous, venous, or mixed types, in a fibrous and connective tissue background.

Treatment of painful tumors consists of simple irradiation, while those patients presenting with a neurological deficit require more aggressive therapy (18). Vertebral angiography should be performed prior to any surgical procedure. Preoperative embolization may be necessary and will help to significantly diminish intraoperative blood loss and the possible need for a transfusion. The surgical approach to these lesions is similar to the exposure for an anterior cervical discectomy. Vertebrectomy of the involved body can be carried out with subsequent stabili-

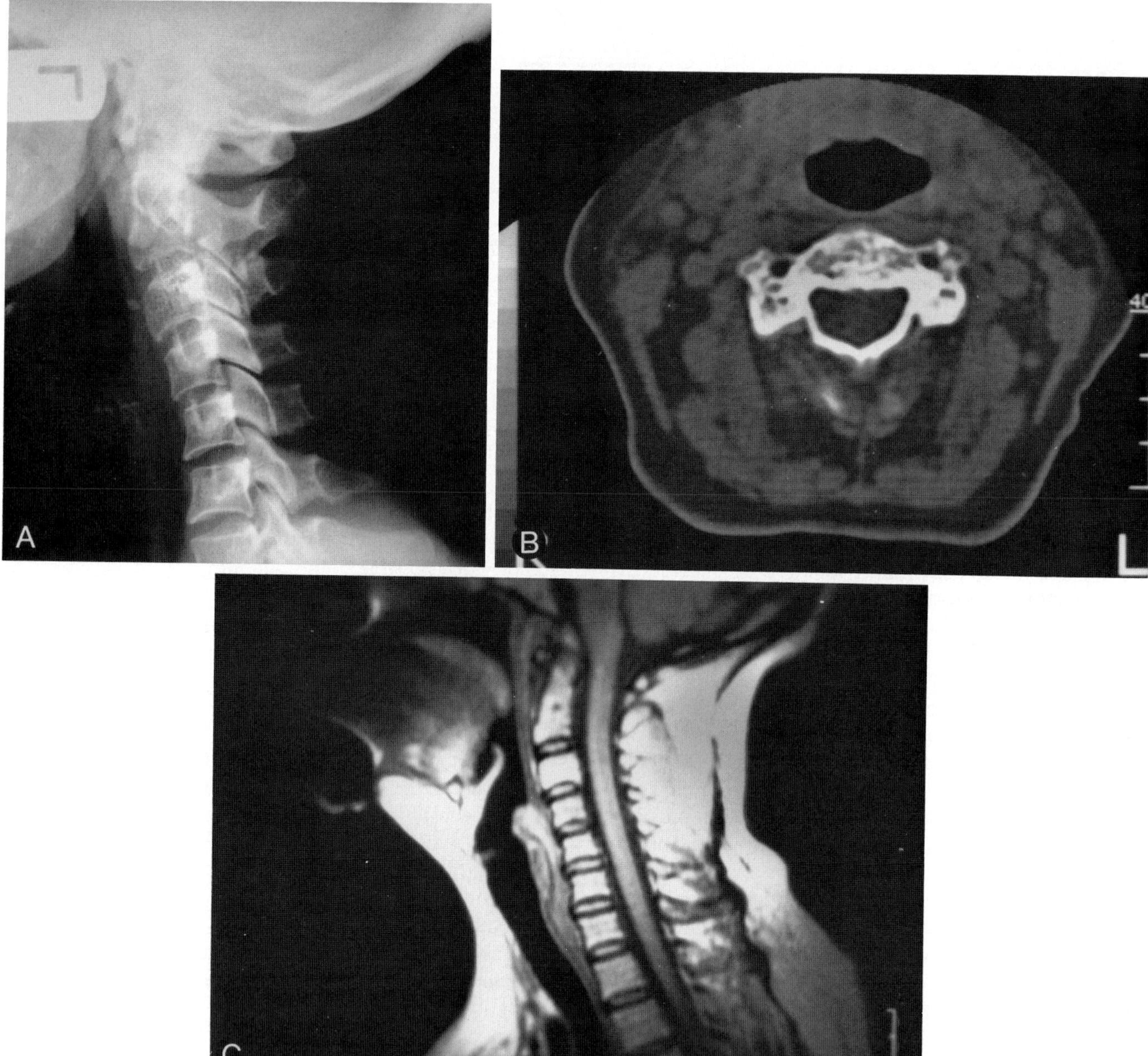

Figure 49.1. **A**, Vertical striations characteristic of a vertebral hemangioma are seen on this lateral radiograph of the C3 vertebral body. **B**, A CT scan through the C3 vertebral body reveals the pathognomic vertical trabeculations surrounding the dilated vascular spaces. **C**, A sagittal MRI in the same patient reveals a hyperintense signal in the C3 vertebra.

zation utilizing either autogenous bone from the iliac crest, fibula strut, or prosthetic devices such as Steinman pins, Caspar plates, or acrylic.

Giant Cell Tumor

This primary osseous tumor is composed of a dimorphic population of cells. Histologically, multinucleated giant cells are mixed with a stroma of mononuclear cells. Occurring in a young female population, these tumors are frequently seen in the sacrum. It has been suggested that those occurring along the remainder of the spinal axis, including the cervical spine, carry a better prognosis. Neurologic findings are the consequence of bony destruction or enlargement of the tumor itself. Preoperative embolization of these vascular tumors may allow more radical curettage, which may be followed by bone grafting, stabilization procedures, or radiotherapy to diminish the chances of recurrence and metastasis.

Aneurysmal Bone Cyst

Accounting for 12% of all aneurysmal bone cysts (6), those which occur along the vertebral axis may produce

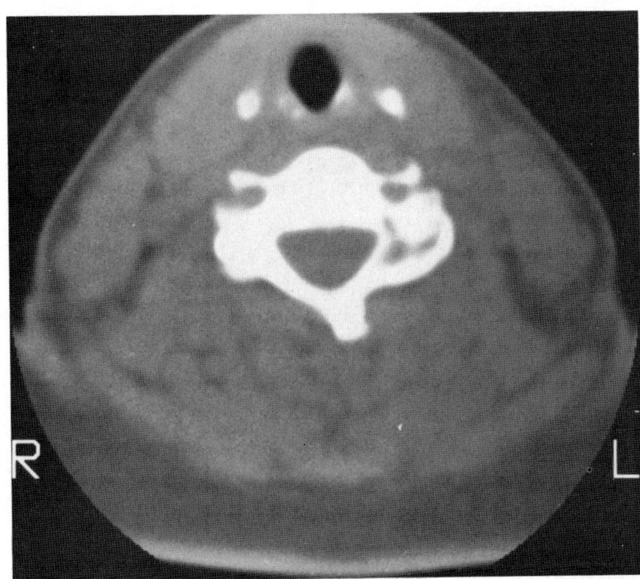

Figure 49.2. CT scan of the osteoid osteoma shows a sclerotic rim around the lucent lesion within the vertebral arch.

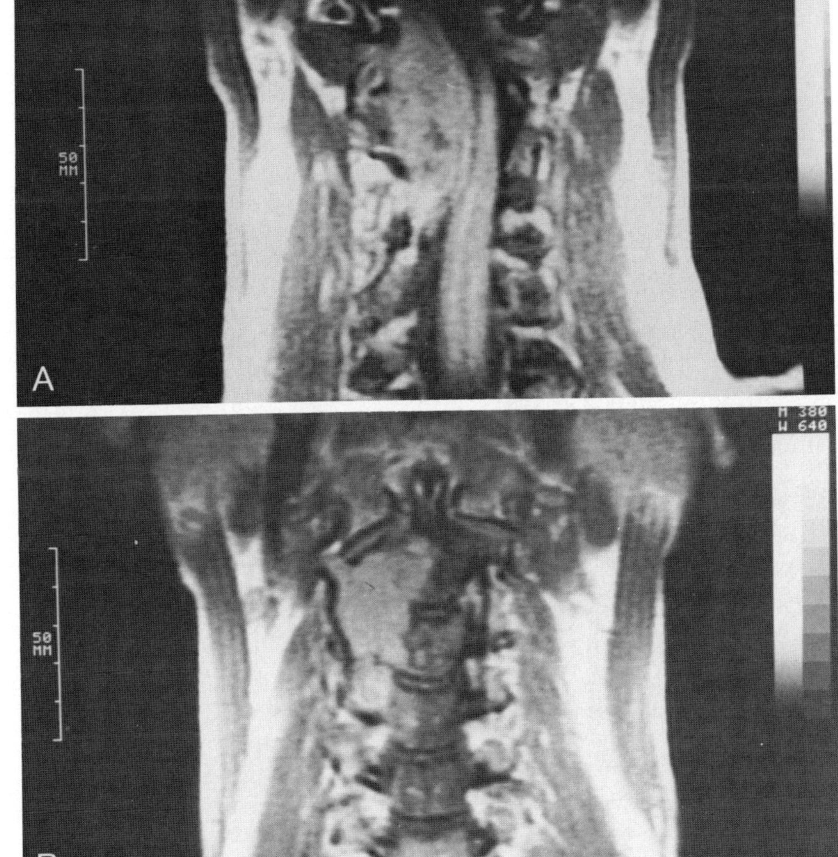

Figure 49.3. **A**, A coronal MRI scan demonstrating a high intensity signal of a smooth bordered epidural mass extending from C2–C4 displacing the spinal cord. Surgical pathology confirmed a chordoma. **B**, This coronal MRI image in the same patient shows involvement of the articular processes and bodies of C2–C4.

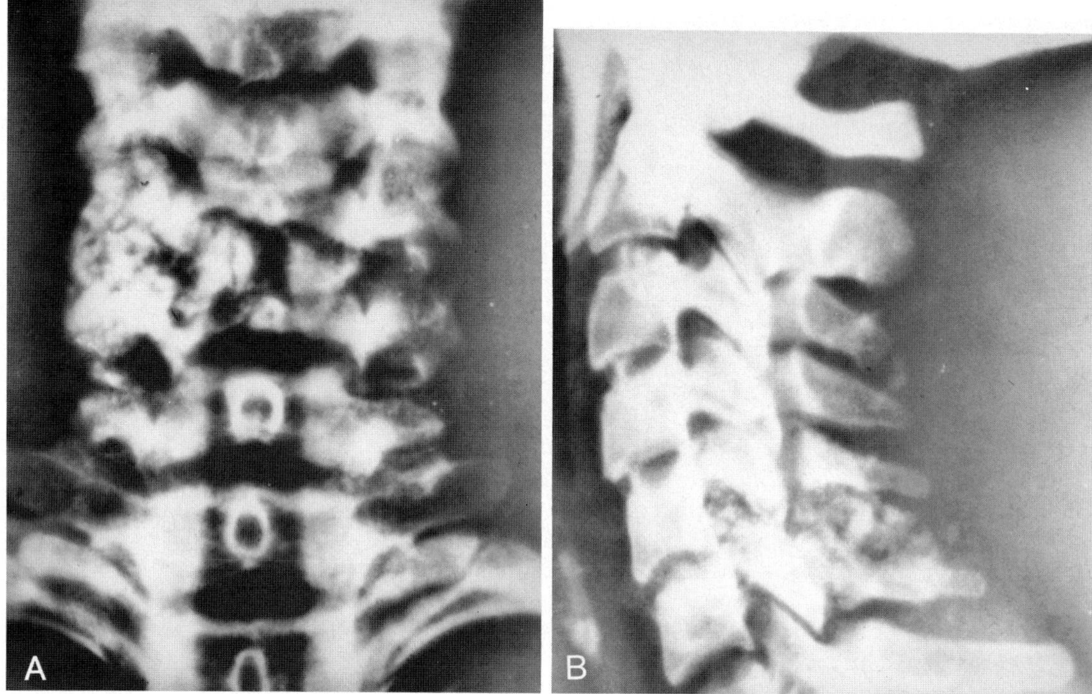

Figure 49.4. Artero-posterior and lateral radiographs show a chondrosarcoma arising in the C5–C6 articular process and characterized by fluffy radiodensities interspersed with adjacent areas of radiolucency.

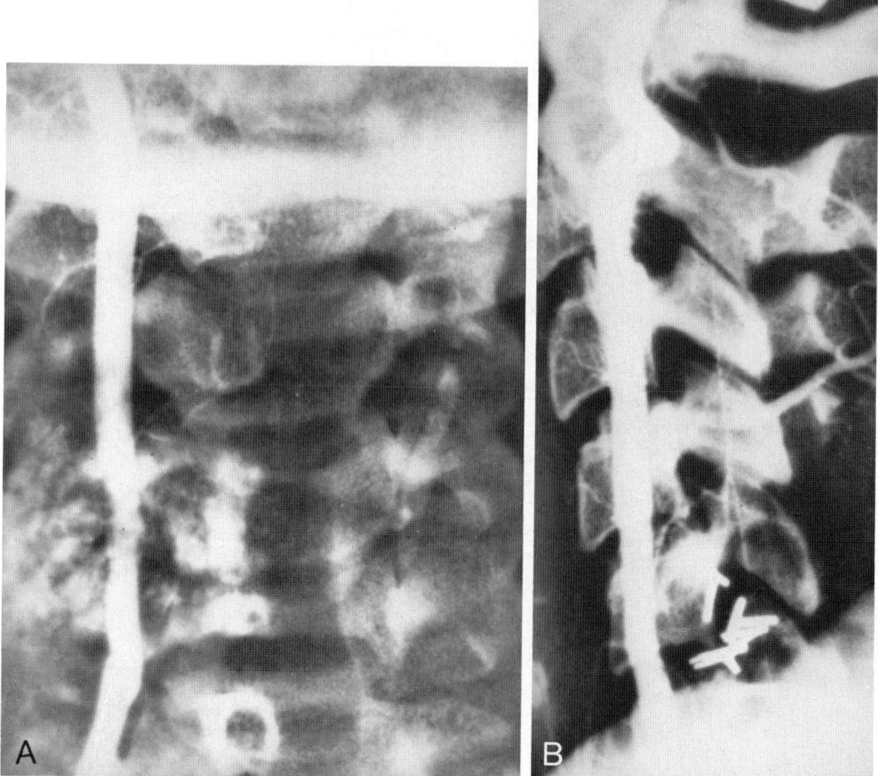

Figure 49.5. A pre- and post-operative angiogram demonstrating irregular narrowing of the vertebral artery by the surrounding neoplasm preoperatively. The post-operative study shows preservation of the spinal branch of the vertebral artery.

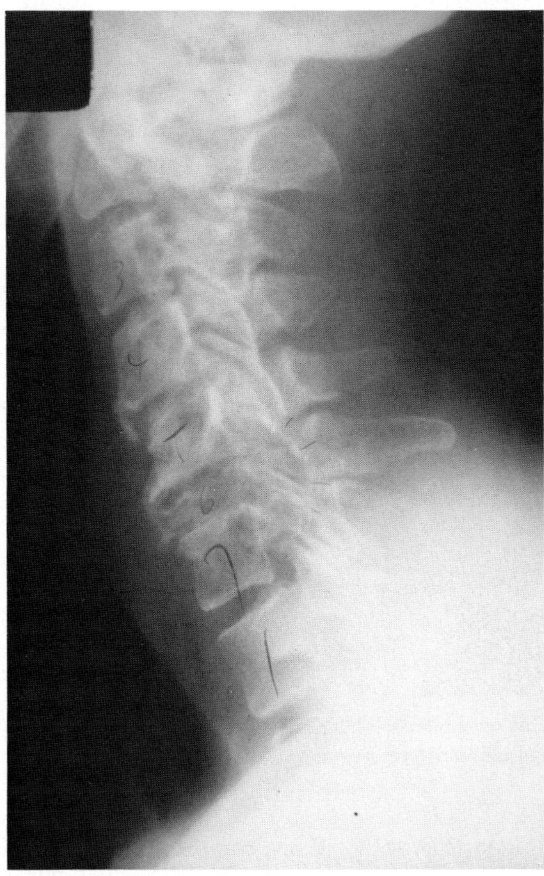

Figure 49.6. There is collapse of the C6 vertebral body with relative preservation of the adjacent disc spaces in this patient with metastatic disease.

radicular pain or myelopathy as they destroy the vertebral arches of predominantly young patients. Neuroradiologic investigations reveal a thin cortical shell with a trabeculated honeycombed inner appearance containing lakes of blood. Embolization may allow more radical resection, and the masses may be amenable to low dose irradiation.

Osteoblastomas

In a large series of these primary bone tumors, 13% occurred in the cervical spine (33). Seen in young men, these tumors involve the posterior elements as well as the transverse processes. A central lytic area surrounded by a rim of sclerosis is usually greater than 2 cm in diameter. The pain is usually described as a dull ache but may be responsible for torticollis, reversal of the cervical lordosis, and cervical myeloradiculopathy. Radiographically, a zone of sclerosis usually surrounds a large central lucent area. Radionuclide scans demonstrate an intense uptake, and computerized scans with bone windows help in planning "en bloc" complete excision, which is the only curative technique.

Osteoid Osteoma

These benign bone-forming tumors occur in young males and are generally smaller than osteoblastomas (24). The nidus is usually less than 1.5 cm. The cervical spine is involved second most frequently and commonly in the region of the posterior elements (Fig. 49.2). The pain may be intense and is most common during activity and at night. The radiologic and radionuclide appearance of these lesions are similar to that of the larger osteoblastomas. Similarly, complete surgical excision is the recommended curative therapy. The chances of this are enhanced with preoperative and intraoperative localization utilizing radioactive technetium diphosphonate and a scintillation probe or administering oral tetracycline preoperative and fluorescing the surgical specimen with a Wood's light to confirm complete tumor resection.

MALIGNANT TUMORS

Chordomas

Chordomas are slow growing tumors that arise from embryonic remnants of the notochord. More than half occur in the sacrum, with 35% arising at the skull base, and the remaining 15% occupying the remainder of the axial column, including the cervical spine (31, 35). The latter is the most frequent site of occurrence after the sacrum and basicranium. The frequency of chordomas occurring in the cervical region, predominantly upper, has been estimated to be between 9% and 15% (3, 34, 35). Metastasis is rarely associated with cervical chordomas (15).

Slightly more prevalent in males in the fifth to seventh decades of life, cervical chordomas may present with neck pain, neural compressive syndromes, or as a retropharyngeal mass. Chordomas of the cervical spine demonstrate a ballooning mass with flecks of bone predominantly involving the pedicle, lamina, and spinous process (Fig. 49.3). There may be associated osteosclerosis of the disc with loss of disc height or ivory vertebra with vertebral body collapse. An associated soft tissue component may fill the epidural space. These soft grey tumors histologically demonstrate the presence of foamy physaliphorous cells arranged in sheets.

To gain access to the involved posterior elements, these tumors should be exposed and surgically resected through a posterior cervical laminectomy approach. Treatment consists of radical excision of the osseous and epidural tumor. Great care should be taken since these tumors frequently are quite adherent to the dura of the cervical cord. These procedures should be performed in the lateral position rather than sitting when stabilization is anticipated at the time of the initial posterior procedure, especially if the atlas is involved. Local recurrence has necessitated the admin-

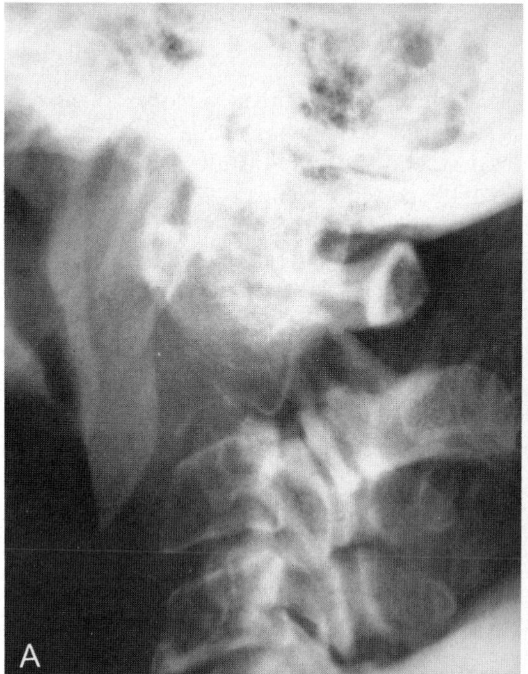

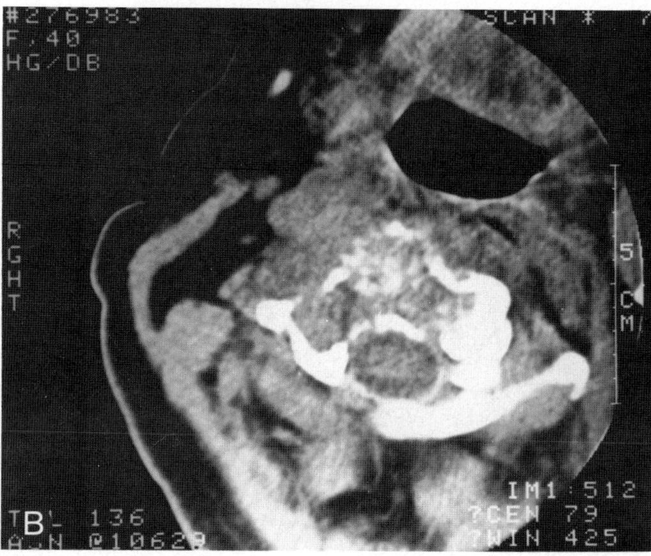

Figure 49.7. **A**, Lytic destruction of the body of C2 and the odontoid process are seen on this lateral radiograph in a patient with metastatic breast carcinoma. **B**, A post-intrathecal contrast CT scan reveals massive lytic destruction and expansion of the body of C2 with preservation of the subarachnoid space.

istration of high dose postoperative radiotherapy. In view of decreasing mortality rates associated with aggressive treatment and chemotherapy regimens, alternative forms of radiotherapy should be investigated as well (15).

Multiple Myeloma

This is the most common primary malignant tumor in the adult cervical spine, occurring most frequently in males between the ages of 50 and 70. Laboratory evaluation reveals anemia, elevated ESR, hypercalcemia, a monoclonal gammopathy, and Bence-Jones proteinuria. Radiographs reveal punched-out lytic lesions that may eventually coalesce and cause collapse of a cervical vertebra. CT scans and MR imaging can demonstrate extension of the plasmacytoma into the epidural space with the possible compression of the cervical cord and myelopathy. Without evidence of neurologic impairment, the treatment of choice is systemic chemotherapy and irradiation.

Chondrosarcoma

Those occurring in the spine constitute 6% of all chondrosarcomas and are evenly distributed along the vertebral axis (40). This malignant cartilage-forming tumor may appear in either the vertebral body or the cervical neural arch. Patients initially complain of a persistent dull neckache. Associated soft tissue components may extend into the neck or spinal canal. Radiographs reveal irregular lobular opacities due to calcification (Fig. 49.4). While computerized scans help to plan surgery, angiography may be useful to embolize these vascular tumors (Fig. 49.5). Spinal cord decompression and debulking should be followed by spinal stabilization to prevent pain and instability of the spinal axis.

Secondary Tumors

Metastatic tumors of the cervical spine are more frequent than primary osseous lesions (15). Commonly, they may be the first manifestation of a malignant process, with more than 50% of vertebral metastasis originating from the breast, lung, prostate, thyroid, or colon (7). Spread to the cervical region is less common than to other areas of the spine. In adults, the most common cervical tumor is multiple myeloma (15). Lymphomas present as a solitary ivory vertebral body in the cervical spine.

Metastatic lesions commonly occur in patients in their fourth to sixth decade. The skeleton is the most common site of distant metastases with the spine being most frequently affected. The diagnosis of spinal metastases should be suspected when a radionuclide scan detects multiple lesions, Bence-Jones proteinuria is present, a bone marrow biopsy is positive, or a primary lesion is detected on metastatic evaluation. Although the vertebral body is initially involved, it is not until there is disappearance of a pedicle that there is radiographic confirmation of metastatic disease (23) (Figs. 49.6, 49.7). Pain or a cervical myeloradiculopathy develops secondary to entrapment of cervical nerve roots, compression fractures, cervical instability, or epidural spinal cord compression. Secondary spinal cord ischemia accounts for the development of neurologic symptoms (38).

Radiation therapy, possibly in conjunction with chemotherapeutic agents, is usually the initial form of treatment. In patients with lytic lesions confined to the osseous spine, a halo orthosis may be all that is necessary while medical treatment is carried out. Yet when there is a question as to the histologic diagnosis or the tumor has known radioresistance, a biopsy or surgical decompression with stabilization may be necessary. Simple posterior decompression is an inadequate solution for the patient with metastatic disease originating anteriorly in the body. For these patients, the procedure of choice is a vertebrectomy via an anterior cervical approach followed by fusion, usually with implantable metallic devices, bone grafts, or methylmethacrylate (Fig. 49.8). Preoperative embolization may make tumors such as thyroid carcinoma or hypernephroma less formidable (23).

Although these are frequently not curative procedures,

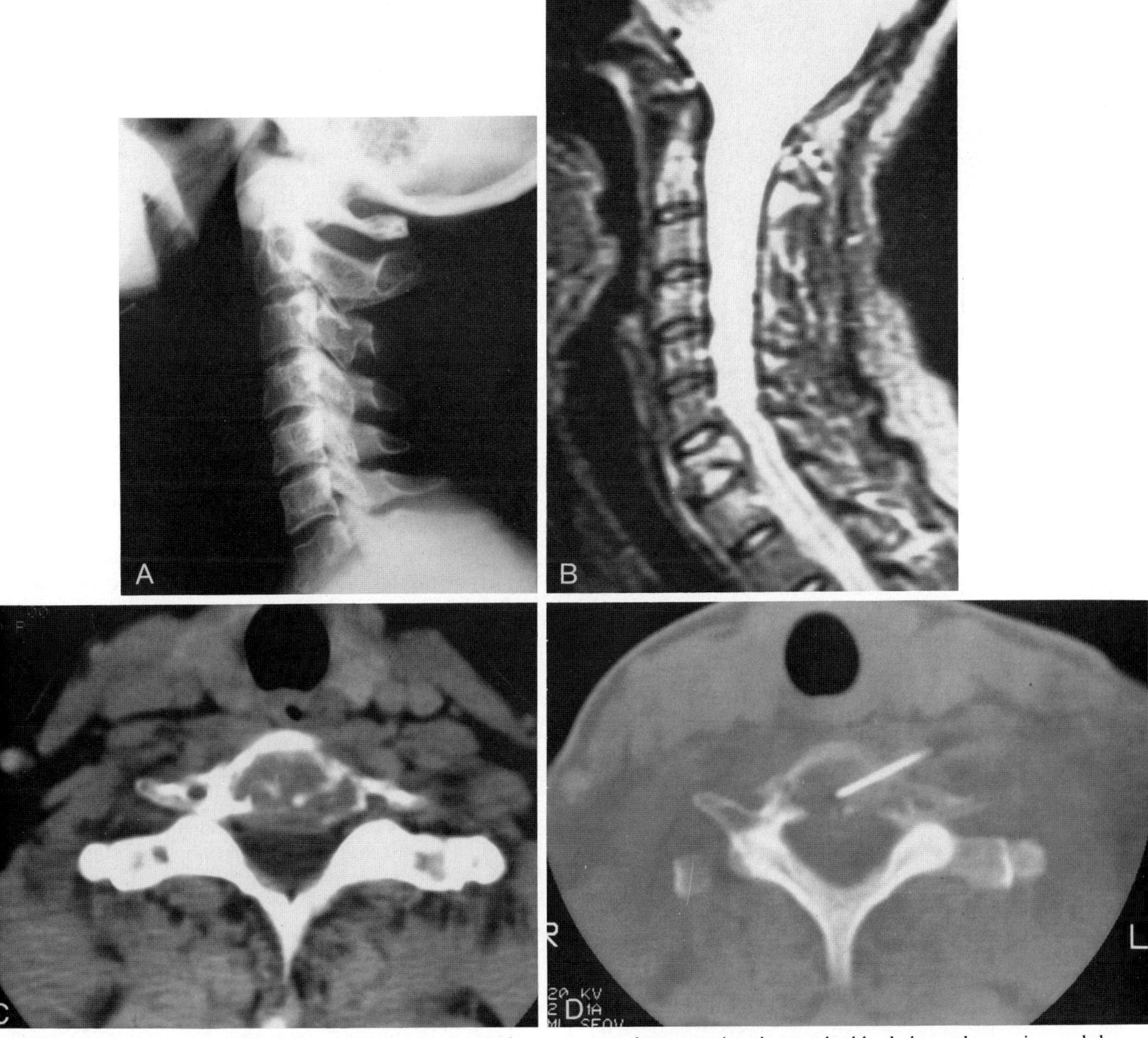

Figure 49.8. **A**, A lateral cervical radiograph demonstrating collapse of the C-7 vertebral body; **B**, A sagittal MRI scan in the same patient demonstrating the C-7 vertebral body collapse as well as the epidural spinal cord compression; **C**, An axial CT scan demonstrating the vertebral body bone destruction and the epidural component; **D**, An axial CT scan demonstrating the needle placement in attempts at obtaining a tissue biopsy.

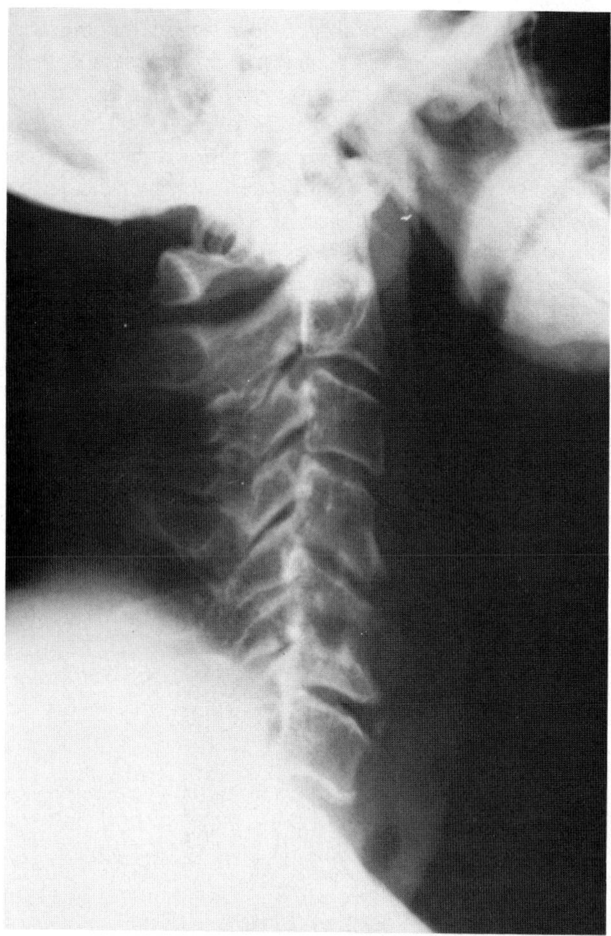

Figure 49.9. Lateral cervical radiograph in a patient with osteomyelitis demonstrating destruction of the C5–C6 disc space.

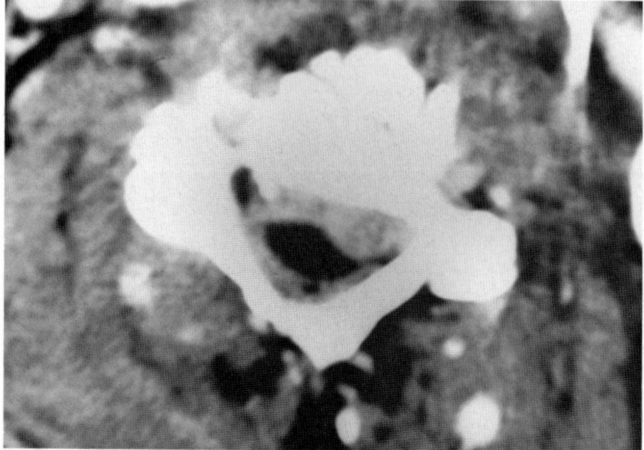

Figure 49.10. A CT scan in the same patient confirms an epidural abscess circumferentially surrounding the thecal sac.

the short term prognosis is excellent in those patients with good preoperative neurologic function. Most patients unfortunately ultimately succumb to their primary tumor.

Miscellaneous

Although fibrous, mesenchymal, and desmoid tumors do occur in the cervical region, they are distinctly more uncommon than the previously discussed tumors. Their diagnosis is generally not entertained unless suggested by skinny needle biopsy results or the presence of a syndrome of which they are a component.

INFLAMMATORY

Osteomyelitis

Although not a tumor, osteomyelitis may occasionally mimic the appearance of a mass lesion involving the vertebral axis. With the advent of effective treatment for tuberculosis, infectious processes involving the spine are now predominantly bacterial in nature (8). Unusual pathogens are now appearing among HIV positive intravenous drug abusers with spinal osteomyelitis. Severe localized pain, weight loss, and a low grade fever are the most common presenting symptoms. When the infectious process involves the epidural space, myelopathic and radicular findings occur. The incidence of neurologic complications varies from 3 to 40% (21). The infection may be from a distant source transported to the spinal column via hematogenous spread or a local phenomenon within contiguous neck structures in conjunction with previous neck surgery, spinal surgery, or after a tracheostomy.

Routine cervical spine radiographs frequently demonstrate osteomyelitis. Compression fractures of the vertebral bodies, with loss of height and destructive involvement of the intervening disc space are seen initially (Fig. 49.9). Later, kyphotic deformities may develop. With appropriate treatment, healing is represented by sclerosis and new bone formation at the end-plates. CT scanning and an MRI, particularly with contrast, may be useful, especially if granulation tissue is present or abscesses involve the epidural space (Fig. 49.10). A lumbar puncture rarely yields purulent matter from the subarachnoid space and should be avoided if there is the possibility of spinal cord compression by the infectious process. Technetium- and indium-labelled WBC bone scans are uniformly positive in cases of cervical osteomyelitis. Erythrocyte sedimentation rate is more sensitive than a WBC count and is a good indicator of the progression of the disease.

Detection of a bacterial or fungal etiologic agent may be made either by positive blood cultures or skinny needle aspiration of the disc space under fluoroscopic control. An open biopsy is preferably carried out through an anterior cervical discectomy approach since the vertebral bodies and disc space are the major focus of involvement. Alterna-

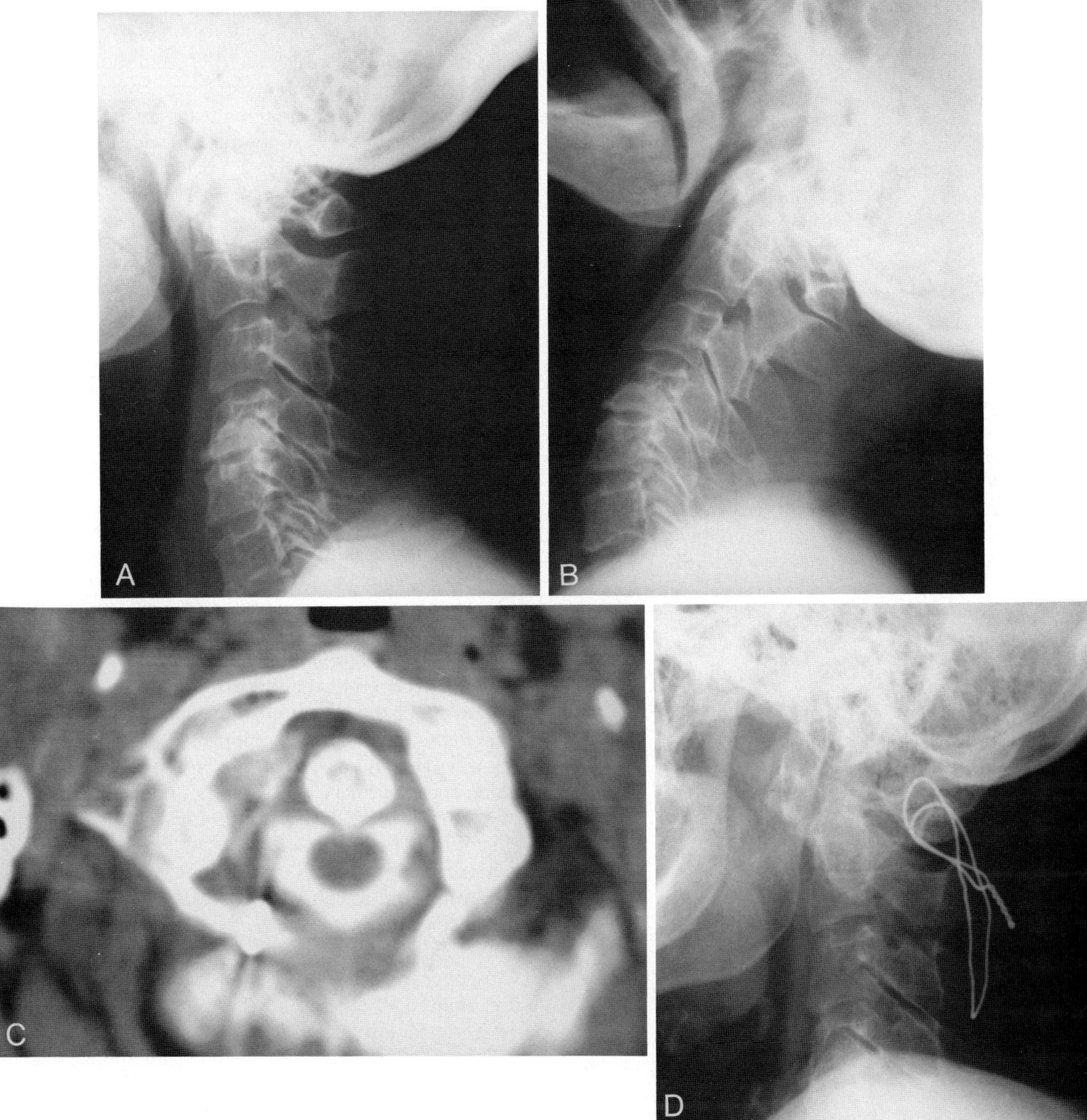

Figure 49.11. **A**, A lateral cervical radiograph demonstrates a widened predental space and erosion of the apex of the odontoid peg. **B**, A lateral cervical radiograph in extension illustrates that the predental space has returned to a normal distance. **C**, A post-contrast CT scan reveals impingement of the odontoid process upon the ventral subarachnoid space. **D**, A post-operative lateral cervical radiograph demonstrates fusion from C1 to C3 with acrylic and stainless steel wire.

tively, surgical procedures are designed primarily to relieve spinal cord compression due to epidural abscesses, kyphotic deformity, or secondarily to provide adequate stabilization when nonoperative therapy fails (1, 14). Epidural abscesses are reported in 5–18% of patients with vertebral osteomyelitis (2). True abscesses may develop dorsal to the cord and spread over several levels (2). The incidence of kyphosis complicating vertebral osteomyelitis has been estimated between 2 and 28% (17).

Whether or not neurologic compromise is present, long-term intravenous antibiotics are the mainstay of therapy. Throughout treatment, it is best to immobilize the cervical spine with an external orthosis. When a spinal deformity progresses despite healing of the infectious process, fusion

Table 49.1. Organization of Commonly Occurring Cervical Spine Tumors

VASCULAR Hemangioma	OSSEOUS Giant cell tumor Aneurysmal Osteoblastoma Osteoid osteoma
INFLAMMATORY Tuberculosis Rheumatoid arthritis Osteomyelitis	CARTILAGINOUS Chondrosarcoma
EMBRYONIC Chordoma	MARROW ELEMENTS Multiple myeloma
SECONDARY TUMORS Metastatic	

with bone grafting and a halo orthosis, or occasionally internal fixation with Caspar plates may be required (28). The latter is infrequently required, as bony healing usually provides adequate fusion.

With early detection and aggressive antibiotic therapy, good result are seen in patients with vertebral osteomyelitis so that an incidence of permanent neurologic deficits as low as 6% is reported in some large series (37).

Tuberculosis

Although skeletal tuberculosis most commonly affects the vertebral column (50% of all affected), Pott's disease involving the cervical spine is relatively uncommon (26, 29). Recently, though, it has assumed increasing importance due to its resurgence in the HIV-afflicted population. In a series of 1000 cases of spinal tuberculosis, cervical involvement was demonstrated in 3.5% of cases (27). When tuberculosis involves the cervical spine, it most commonly is found in the lower vertebrae. On an average, two vertebral bodies and one disc space are involved at the time of identification of the disease (32).

Pain and stiffness are the most common presenting complaints (18, 19, 32). Subsequent sequelae may include torticollis, kyphotic deformity or subluxation, draining sinus tracts into the posterior triangle of the neck, compression of adjacent soft tissue and vascular structures, and, ultimately, quadriparesis or quadriplegia. The latter results from either the epidural spread of the granuloma, or it may be secondary to subluxation from ligamentous laxity and spinal column deformities.

Since a tuberculous lesion is disseminated to the spine via hematogenous spread along Batson's vertebral plexus the cervical spine is infrequently involved. The typical sequestrum and caseating granuloma initially spread along the longitudinal ligaments and then involve the vertebral body. Eventually, the infectious process crosses the disc space. Long-term bony changes associated with healing include end-plate sclerosis and tuberculous spondylitis with fusion of the facet joints.

The sedimentation rate is routinely elevated, and tests for the tubercle bacilli are positive in almost all cases (32). Bone scans are positive in two-thirds of patients with spinal lesions. CT and T2-weighted images on MRI can demonstrate granulation tissue and epidural or paraspinal abscesses.

Although the antituberculous drugs are the mainstay of therapy, anterior cervical approaches with thorough debridement and bone grafting are mandatory in the face of neurologic deficit, failure of medical therapy, or spinal instability. A posterior fusion may be required secondarily. When therapy is instituted early, the prognosis for recovery is excellent.

Rheumatoid Arthritis

Atlanto-axial subluxation is the most common manifestation of rheumatoid involvement of the cervical spine, occurring in more than half of patients with rhematoid arthritis (19). Although this type of lesion is not influenced by the age of the patient nor duration of the disease, another common finding, upward migration of the odontoid, most definitely is (39). While most of the patients with cervical involvement are asymptomatic, others present with pain or occipital neuralgia that is worsened by movement (11, 12). In the most severe cases, compression of the brainstem, spinal cord, nerve roots, and vertebral artery may develop. Synovial proliferation, inflammatory ligamentous laxity, destruction of the synovial joints, and pannus formation about the odontoid peg all contribute to atlanto-axial instability and cord compression (11). Palpation of the cervical spine may actually reveal atlanto-axial crepitation and movement which can be confirmed with carefully monitored flexion and extension radiographs (Fig. 49.11).

Most patients do well with simple external immobilization in a Philadelphia collar. Those with a neurologic deficit or greater than 8 mm of predental space should be considered candidates for posterior cervical fusion with wire, bone, or acrylic (31). In an attempt to limit further immobilization, the occiput is not included in the fusion. To avoid the use of a halo vest in an already debilitated patient, methylmethacrylate may be incorporated in the fusion to obtain immediate stability. Others advocate approaching the pathology directly via a transoral route to resect the odontoid peg and pannus (11, 12).

CONCLUSIONS

Although tumors of the cervical vertebral column are rare, they remain as difficult problems to both diagnose and treat. The organization of these tumors, which has been presented, into vascular, embryonic, inflammatory, metastatic, infectious, osseous, and chondroid categories, presents a logical method for organizing these osseous masses of the cervical spine (Table 49.1). Emphasis should be placed on the early recognition of a cervical spinal tumor with confirmation of a diagnosis via neuroradiologic testing and open or closed biopsy. This should be followed by aggressive treatment of the lesion and secondary stabilization of the vertebral axis.

REFERENCES

1. Abramowitz JN, Batson RA, Yablon JS. Vertebral osteomyelitis. The surgical management of neurologic complications. Spine 1986;11:418–420.
2. Baker AS, Ojemann RG, Swartz MN, Richardson EP. Spinal epidural abscess. N Engl J Med 1975;293:463–468.
3. Bohlman HH, Sachs BL, Carter JR, Riley L, Robinson RA. Primary neoplasms of the cervical spine. J Bone Joint Surg (Am) 1986;68:483–494.
4. Camins MB, Duncan AW, Smith J, Marcove RC. Chondrosarcoma of the spine. Spine 1978;3:202–209.
5. Camins MB, Rosenblum BR. Osseous lesions of the vertebral axis. In: Lewis MM, ed. Musculoskeletal oncology. Philadelphia: W.B. Saunders (in press).
6. Campanacci M, Capanna R, Picci P. Unicameral and aneurysmal bone cysts. Clin Orthop 1987;204:25–36.
7. Cohen D, Dahlin D, Maccarthy C. Apparently solitary tumors of the vertebral column. Proceedings of the Mayo Clinic 1964;39:509–518.
8. Collert S. Osteomyelitis of the spine. Acta Orthop Scand 1977;48:283–290.
9. Compere EL. Vertebra plana due to eosinophilic granuloma. J Bone Joint Surg (Am) 1954;36:969.
10. Conlon PW, Isdale IC, Rose BS. Rheumatoid arthritis of the cervical spine. An analysis of 333 cases. Ann Rheum Dis 1966;25:120–125.
11. Crockard HA. Anterior approaches to lesions of the upper cervical spine. Clin Neurosurg 1988;34:389–416.
12. Crockard HA, Pozo JL, Ransford AU, Stevens JM, Kendall BE, Essigman WK. Tansoral decompression and posterior fusion for rheumatoid atlantoaxial subluxation. J Bone Joint Surg (Am) 1986;68:350–356.
13. Dahlin DC. Bone tumors: general aspects and data on 6221 cases. 3rd ed. Springfield, IL: Charles C. Thomas, 1978.
14. Digby JM, Kersley JB. Pyogenic nontuberculous spinal infection. An analysis of thirty cases. J Bone Joint Surg (Br) 1979;61:47–55.
15. Dunn EJ, Davidson RI, Desai S. Diagnosis and management of tumors of the cervical spine. In: Sherk HH, ed. The cervical spine. Philadelphia: J.B. Lippincott Co., 1989:693–722.
16. Enneking WF, Conrad EV. Common bone tumors. Clin Symp 1989;41:1–32.
17. Fredericson B, Yuan H, Olans R. Management and outcome of vertebral osteomyelitis. Clin Orthop 1978;131:160–167.
18. Graham JJ, Yang WC. Vertebral hemangioma with compression fracture and paraparesis treated with preoperative embolization and vertebral resection. Spine 1984;9:97–101.
19. Grantham SA. Atlantoaxial instability. In: Sherk HH, ed. The cervical spine. Philadelphia: J.B. Lippincott Co., 1989:356–361.
20. Grantham SA, Lipson SJ. Rheumatoid arthritis and other noninfectious inflammatory diseases. In: Sherk HH, ed. The cervical spine. Philadelphia: J.B. Lippincott Co., 1989:564–598.
21. Griffiths HED, Jones DM. Pyogenic infections of the spine. J Bone Joint Surg (Br) 1971;55:383–391.
22. Greenspan A, Klein MJ, Bennett AJ, Lewis MM, Neuwirth M, Camins MB. Hemangioma of the T6 vertebra with a compression fracture, extradural block and spinal cord compression. Skeletal Radiol 1983;10:183–188.
23. Harrington KD. Metastatic disease of the spine. J Bone Joint Surg (Am) 1986;68:1110–1117.
24. Healey JH, Ghelman B. Osteoid osteoma and osteoblastomas. Clin Orthop 1986;204:76–85.
25. Healey M, Herz DA, Pearl L. Spinal hemangiomas. Neurosurgery 1983;13:689–691.
26. Hsu LCS, Leong JCY. Tuberculosis of the lower cervical spine (C2 to C7). J Bone Joint Surg (Br) 1984;66:1–5.
27. Hsu LCS, Yau ACMC. Infections. In: Sherk HH, ed. The cervical spine. Philadelphia: J.B. Lippincott Co., 1989:544–563.
28. Kemp HBS, Jackson JW, Jeremiah JD, Hall AJ. Pyogenic infections and anterior fusion of the spine for infective lesions in adults. J Bone Joint Surg (Br) 1973;55:715–734.
29. Krol G, Sundaresan N, Deck M. Computed tomography of axial chordomas. J Comput Assist Tomogr 1983:286–289.
30. Lee CK, Rosa R, Fernand R. Surgical treatment of tumors of the spine. Spine 1986;11:201–208.
31. Lesoin F, Duquesnoy B, Destee A, Leys D, Rousseaux M, Carini S, Verier A, Jomin M. Cervical neurological complications of rheumatoid arthritis. Surgical treatment techniques and indications. Acta Neurochir 1985;78:91–97.
32. Lifeso RM, Weaver P, Harder EH. Tuberculous spondylitis in adults. J Bone Joint Surg (Am) 1985;67A:1405–1413.
33. Mirra J. Bone tumors. Philadelphia: J.B. Lippincott Co., 1980.
34. O'Neill P, Bell BA, Miller JD, Jacobson I, Guthrie W. Fifty years of experience with chordomas in southeast Scotland. Neurosurgery 1985;16:166–170.
35. Rich TA, Schiller A, Suit HD, Mank HJ. Clinical and pathologic review of 48 cases of chordoma. Cancer 1985;56:182–187.
36. Richardson RR, Cerullo JL. Spinal epidural cavernous hemangioma. Surg Neurol 1979;12:266–268.
37. Sapico FL, Montogomerie J. Pyogenic vertebral osteomyelitis: Report of nine cases and review of the literature. Rev Infect Dis 1976;1:754–776.
38. Shibasaki K, Harper CG, Bedbrook GM, Kakulas BA. Vertebral metastases and spinal cord compression. Paraplegia 1983;21:47–61.
39. Smith PH, Benn RT, Sharp J. Natural history of rheumatoid cervical subluxations. Ann Rheum Dis 1972;31:431–435.
40. Vanzanten TEG, Tevle GJJ, Golding RP, Heidndal GAK. CT and nuclear medicine imaging in vertebral metastases. Clin Nucl Med 1985;14:334–336.
41. Verbiest H. Benign cervical spine tumors. In: Sherk HH, ed. The cervical spine. Philadelphia: J.B. Lippincott Co., 1989:723–774.
42. Weinstein JN, Mclain RF. Primary tumors of the spine. Spine 1987;12:843–851.

50

METASTATIC TUMORS OF THE CERVICAL SPINE

R.G. Perrin and R.J. McBroom

Metastatic tumors of the spine are the most common spinal tumors. It is estimated that 5% to 10% of cancer patients will develop symptoms and signs of spinal cord and nerve root compromise due to spinal secondaries (3, 6, 12, 21, 22). Symptomatic spinal secondaries represent an ominous complication of systemic cancer, the treatment of which remain controversial. Metastases involving the cervical segments exemplify the challenges and dilemmas posed by the management of symptomatic spinal secondaries.

CLASSIFICATION

Spinal metastases are classified anatomically, according to the site of involvement (Fig. 50.1) (3, 11, 18, 31, 36). The vast majority of secondary spinal tumors are extradural (ED)—and remain so, since the dura poses a formidable barrier to metastatic tumor penetration. Intradural extramedullary (ID/EM) metastases are uncommon. ID/EM metastases usually represent tertiary spread via the cerebral spinal fluid (CSF) from intracranial sites of secondary involvement ("drop metastases"). Intramedullary (IM) metastases are rarely encountered.

PATHOLOGY

Spinal metastases most often arise from breast, prostate, and lung, reflecting both the prevalence of tumors at these primary sites as well as their propensity to spread to bone (2, 3, 17, 23, 28). The red marrow of the vertebrae is considered an especially fertile soil for metastatic tumor seeding. Secondary spinal involvement occurs as a result of blood-borne metastases (via Batson's plexus) (4), by direct extension (especially carcinoma of lung), and through CSF spread ("drop metastases").

The distribution of spinal metastases along the vertebral column closely parallels the bulk or volume of the vertebral bodies (46). Autopsy studies show that spinal secondaries most commonly target the lumbar spine followed by the thoracic and then the cervical segments. Clinically, however, symptomatic spinal metastases most frequently involve the thoracic region followed by the lumbar spine (3, 10, 11, 17, 28, 43, 45). Cervical secondaries account for 10% of symptomatic spinal metastases.

SYMPTOMS AND SIGNS

The characteristic clinical syndrome begins with local neck pain followed by weakness, sensory loss, and sphincter dysfunction (Fig. 50.2) (8). Pain is the earliest and most prominent feature in 90% of patients. Local neckache may be associated with a radicular pain syndrome, for example, when an apical lung tumor involves the cervical nerve roots and brachial plexus by direct extension. A burning, dysesthetic pain syndrome raises the probability that the involved nerve roots are strangled by encasing tumor or that the roots are irritated by ID/EM metastases.

When the cervical pain is aggravated by movement and relieved by immobility, then spinal instability should be suspected, and the risk of pathological fracture dislocation must be considered.

The insidious onset of local neck pain is often initially dismissed as "arthritis," "muscle strain," or "disc disease," and the correct diagnosis is then delayed until more blatant manifestations of spinal cord or nerve root compromise are evident (3, 28). It is axiomatic that NECK PAIN IN A CANCER PATIENT MEANS SPINAL METASTASES UNTIL PROVEN OTHERWISE.

Weakness develops in the majority of patients following the onset of neck pain and, if ignored, will progress relentlessly to complete and irreversible paralysis. When weakness occurs abruptly, then pathologic fracture and spinal mal-alignment must be suspected (30).

Sensory abnormality may be manifest as an ascending numbness, a radicular deficit affecting the arm and hand, or a combination of these patterns.

CLASSIFICATION

Extradural	(ED)	95%
Intradural / Extramedullary	(ID / EM)	4.5%
Intramedullary	(IM)	.5%

Figure 50.1. Classification of spinal metastases according to site of involvement.

Sphincter dysfunction is a late and more ominous clinical feature.

INVESTIGATIONS

Plain x-rays of the neck provide the simplest and most useful screening test for symptomatic spinal secondaries (3, 35, 40). Metastatic bone involvement is most often lytic, but sclerotic secondaries may occur—particularly from breast and prostatic primary sites. The routine plain film findings include pedicle erosion (or sclerosis), paravertebral soft tissue shadow, vertebral collapse, and frank pathologic fracture dislocation (Fig. 50.3).

Pedicle erosion is the earliest and most common abnormality seen on plain films (25, 28). A vertebral body with an eroded pedicle produces the "winking owl" sign on a plain AP radiograph (and which is best seen in the thoracolumbar segments). A paravertebral soft tissue shadow often occurs at the site of pedicle erosion (3, 25, 37). More advanced bony destruction can result in vertebral collapse causing wedge compression, and which may progress to frank pathological fracture dislocation (Fig. 50.4) (30). The cervical segments are particularly prone to pathological fracture dislocation. The dependent weight of the head, superimposed on the wide range of neck movements and lack of ribcage supporting structure, all render the cervical segments particularly vulnerable to pathologic fracture dislocation.

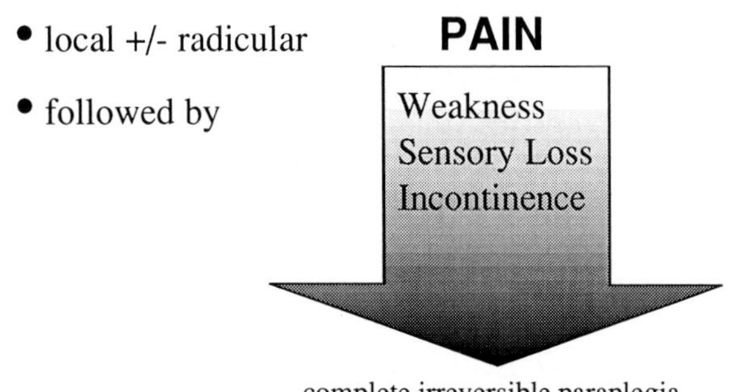

Figure 50.2. Characteristic clinical syndrome associated with symptomatic cervical metastases. Local neck pain (with or without radicular syndrome) is followed by weakness, numbness, and sphincter dysfunction—and all of which will progress to complete and irreversible paralysis.

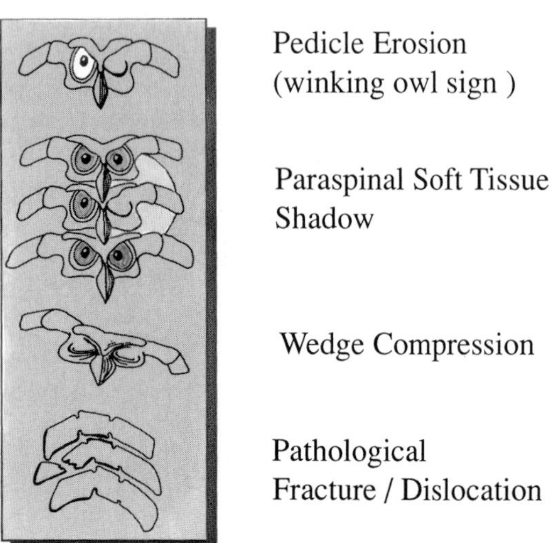

Figure 50.3. Common plain film findings due to spinal metastases.

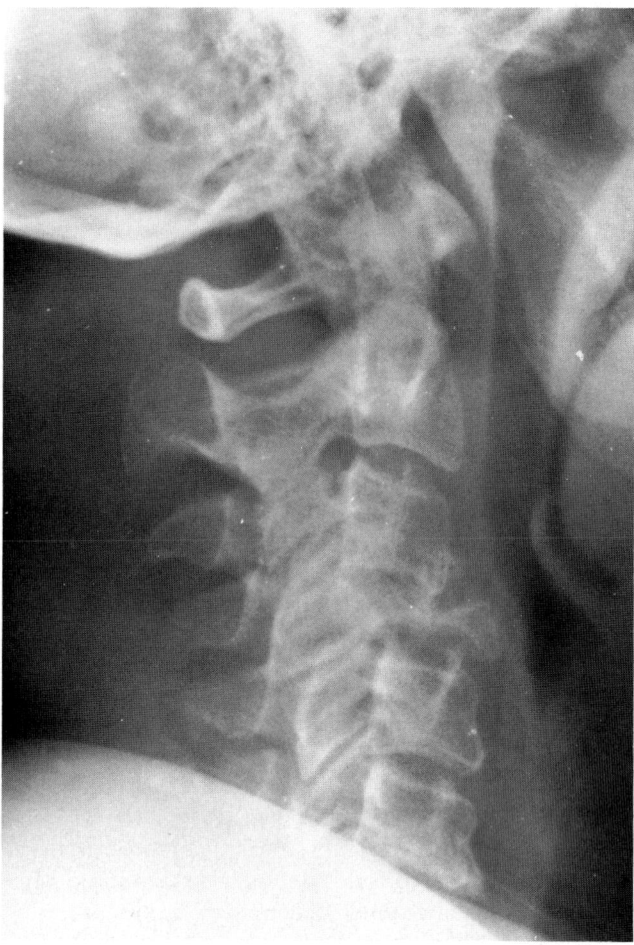

Figure 50.4. Lateral x-ray showing pathologic fracture dislocation at C4.

Myelography is useful to accurately localize the compressing lesion. The majority of patients with symptomatic spinal metastases coming to surgery will show a complete myelographic block to the flow of contrast at the level of cord compression. A cisternal myelography may also be indicated to define the extent of the compressing lesion—especially when the anatomic level of a complete lumbar myelographic block does not correspond to the clinical localization, or when multiple levels of involvement are suspected. As well as demonstrating the segmental limits

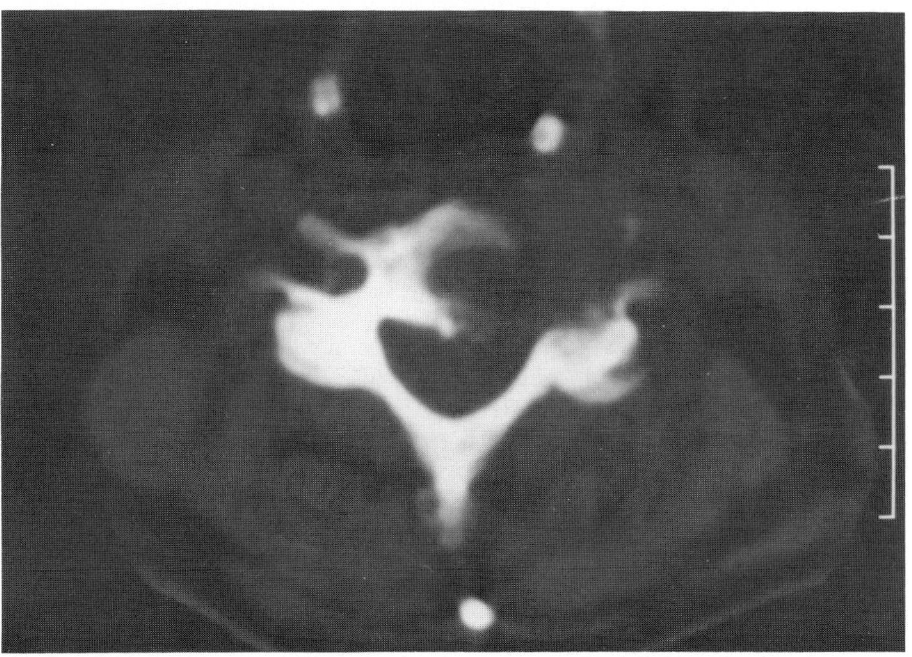

Figure 50.5. CAT showing lateral ED spinal metastasis.

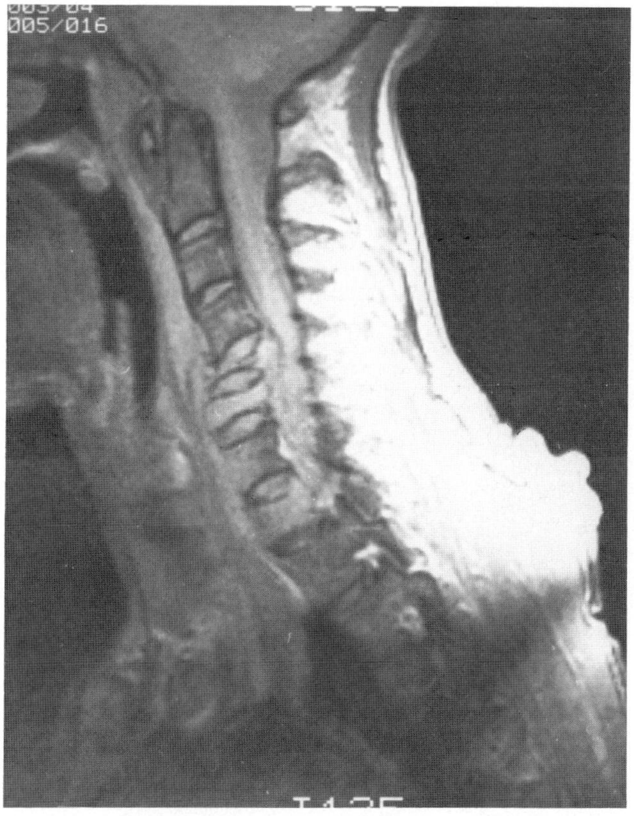

Figure 50.6. MRI showing multiple levels of bony metastasis.

INDICATIONS for SURGERY

- Radiation Failure
- Diagnosis in Doubt
- Pathologic Fracture / Dislocation
- Paralysis - rapid onset / far advanced

Figure 50.7. Indications for surgery.

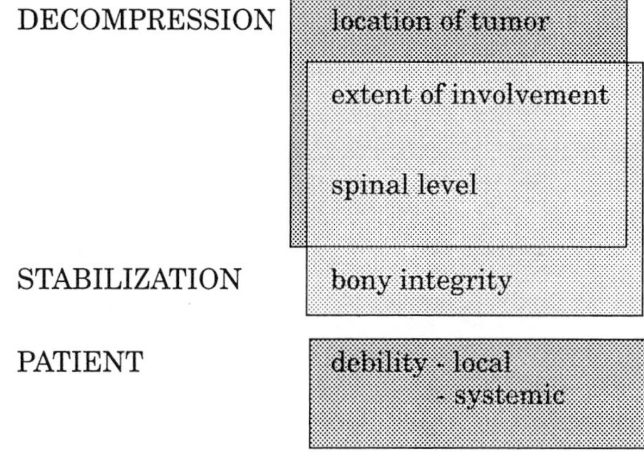

Figure 50.8. Factors to be considered in determining the optimal surgical strategy.

of a compressing lesion, myelography can help to distinguish ED, ID/EM, IM tumors, and whether the lesion is primarily anterior, lateral, or posterior to the spinal cord.

Computerized axial tomography (CAT) can demonstrate the disposition of spinal metastases in the horizontal plane (Fig. 50.5). CAT scan may also provide information concerning the extent of vertebral destruction about the symptomatic site, and which intelligence is essential in anticipating possible stabilization procedures (32, 33).

Magnetic resonance imaging (MRI) has become the radiographic investigation of choice (Fig. 50.6). MRI will show multiple levels of local, contiguous, or remote involvement through sagittal planes extending the length of the spine. The extent of vertebral destruction demonstrated by MRI at segments adjacent to the intended decompression site also provides important information to determine the feasibility of the decompression and stabilization alternatives.

MANAGEMENT

Rationale

The characteristic clinical syndrome caused by cervical spine metastases includes local neck pain (with or without radicular pain syndrome), followed by weakness, sensory loss, and sphincter dysfunction—and all of which will progress relentlessly to complete and irreversible paralysis unless timely treatment is undertaken. The goals of treatment are pain relief and preservation or restoration of neurologic function. Management of symptomatic spinal metastases in a patient with systemic cancer is generally palliative. Nevertheless, relief from pain and restoration or preservation of neurologic function contributes immeasurably to the quality of remaining life and may alleviate the burden of care for a cancer patient in the terminal stages of disease.

Radiation versus Surgery

The relative merits of therapeutic irradiation and surgical intervention for symptomatic spinal metastases have been the focus of considerable debate (1, 5–9, 17, 20, 23, 28–30, 42, 45, 47, 48). Therapeutic irradiation is generally considered to be the initial treatment of choice. The specific indications for surgical intervention are depicted in Figure 50.7.

Indications for Surgery

Radiation failure is the most common reason for referral of a patient with symptomatic spinal metastasis for surgical decompression. This group includes patients with persisting or recurring tumor causing spinal cord and

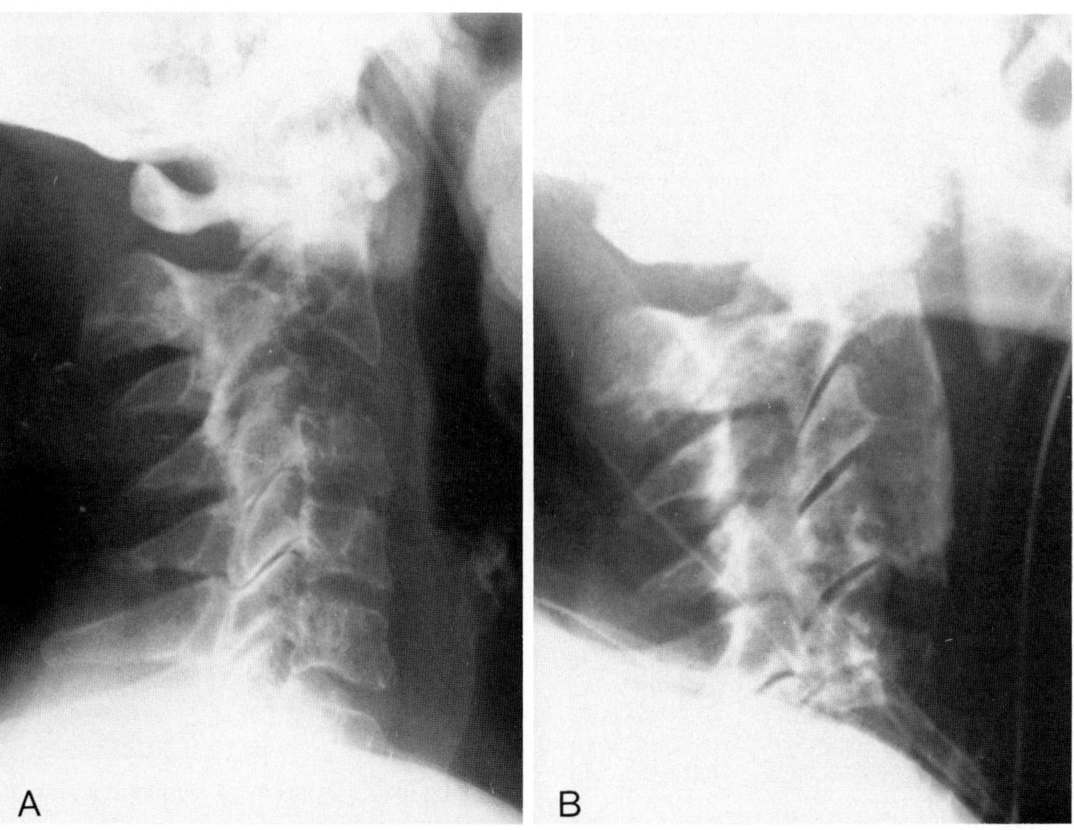

Figure 50.9. Anterior cervical decompression and bone graft interpositions.

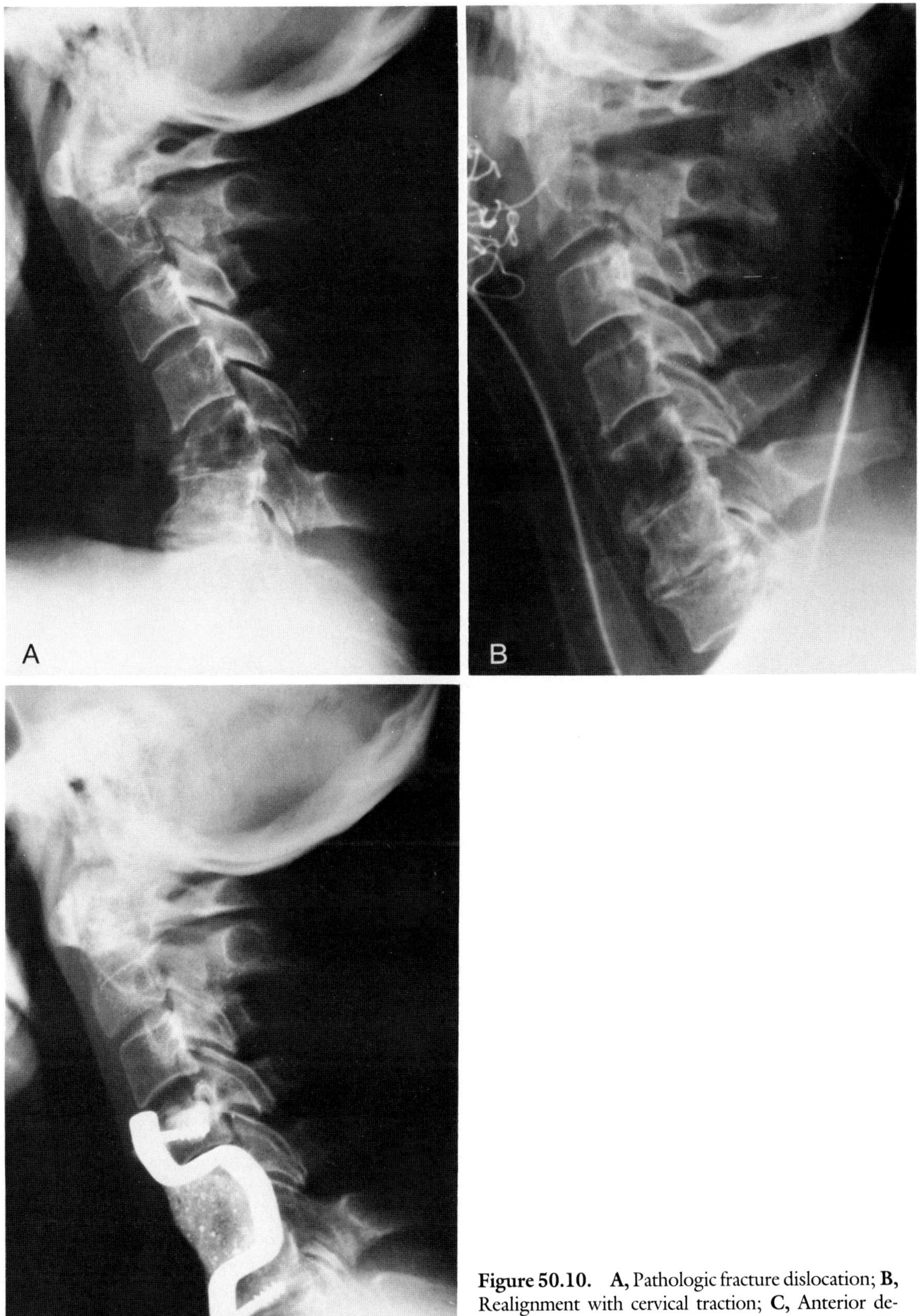

Figure 50.10. **A,** Pathologic fracture dislocation; **B,** Realignment with cervical traction; **C,** Anterior decompression followed by "Wellesley Wedge" stabilization.

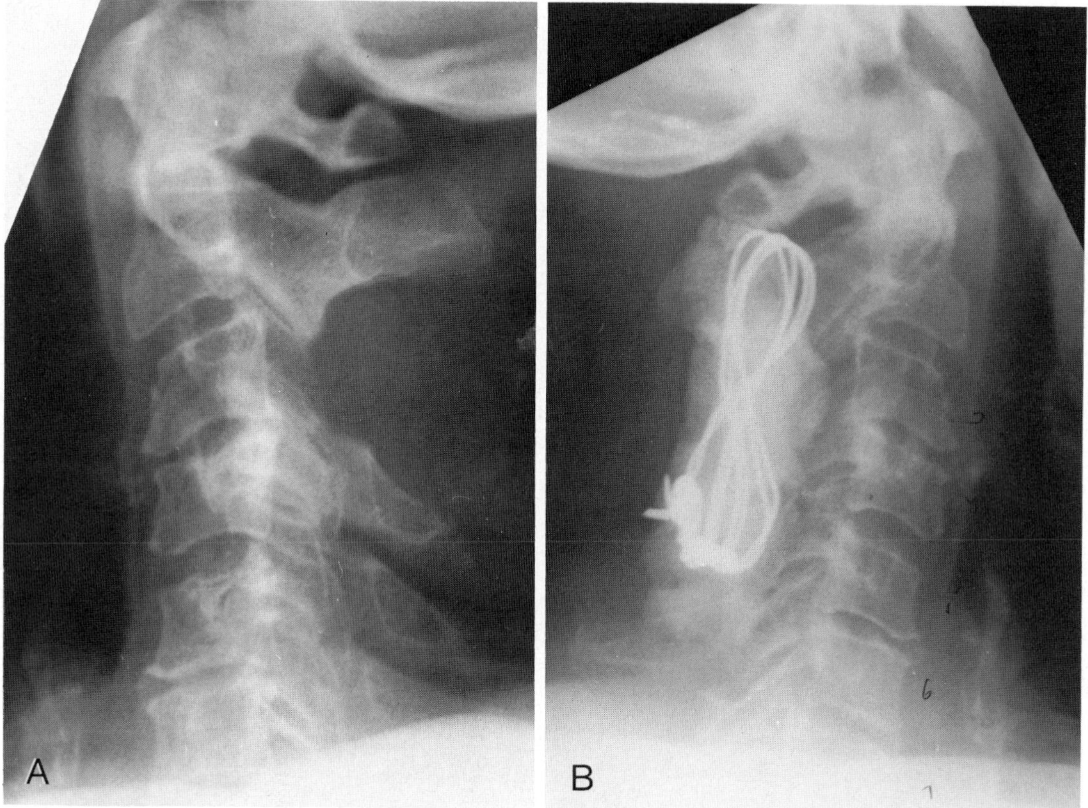

Figure 50.11. **A,** Posterior elements at C3 destroyed by spinal metastasis; **B,** Posterior decompression followed by sublaminar wires and methylmethacrylate struts stabilization.

PROGNOSTIC FACTORS

- Primary Tumor
- Secondary Site
- Speed of Onset
- Degree of Deficit
- Patient Debility

Figure 50.12. Prognostic factors for surgical treatment of symptomatic cervical metastases.

nerve root compromise after the maximum tolerable therapeutic irradiation dose has been administered to the affected area.

Surgical intervention is indicated when the diagnosis is in doubt. Some 10% of patients with symptomatic spinal metastases present with no known underlying primary. Surgical decompression may then be diagnostic as well as therapeutic. The same applies when pathology other than spinal metastases (i.e., degenerative disc disease, infection, hematoma, etc.) is suspected as the cause for spinal cord and nerve root compromise in a cancer patient (24).

Pathologic fracture dislocation of the neck produces neurologic compromise caused by: (*a*) distortion of the dural sac and contents due to spinal mal-alignment and (*b*) compression of the spinal cord and nerve roots produced by extradural tumor (30). Surgical intervention is then necessary to reduce the dislocation, to relieve compression of the dural sac and its contents, and to secure stabilization of the spinal column.

Patients with rapidly progressing or far advanced paraplegia require urgent surgical decompression. In such circumstances, complete and irreversible paraplegia may supervene before the potential benefits of therapeutic irradiation can be effective.

SURGICAL STRATEGIES

Surgical treatment for cervical spine metastases must provide for both decompression of the spinal cord and nerve roots as well as stabilization of the spinal column—and in selected patients who are sufficiently fit to withstand the necessary operative interventions.

Anterior versus Posterior Approach

The surgical approach may be anterior or posterior. A number of factors must be considered in determining the optimum surgical strategy for a given patient (Fig. 50.8) (32).

Tumor Location. Extradural spinal metastases most often originate laterally (or anterolaterally) along the spinal canal (Fig. 50.5)—and may extend circumferentially about the dural sac. It is uncommon for symptomatic ED metastases to occur exclusively anterior, and rarely is the lesion exclusively posterior to the dural sac. A posterior (posterolateral) approach will permit a very thorough spinal decompression, allowing tumor removal circumferentially about the dural sac and nerve roots bilaterally (34). Such radical resection and circumferential decompression is less likely to be achieved through an anterior approach.

Intradural spinal metastases are rarely encountered in the cervical region. Nevertheless, if surgical exploration is to be undertaken for intradural spinal metastases, a posterior decompression is most suitable to provide adequate transdural exposure.

Tumor Extent. Destruction of one or two adjacent vertebral bodies (with or without fracture dislocation) can be effectively decompressed from in front (vertebral corpectomy) (33). While it may be technically possible to extend the anterior decompression for additional segments, stabilization is less likely to be secured with currently available anterior spinal constructs. It may then be necessary to reinforce the anterior stabilization with a posteriorly applied apparatus.

Spinal Level. Anterior decompression procedures are difficult to perform at the highest cervical segments (C1, 2). Furthermore, the problems imposed by an anterior approach for decompression at the craniocervical junction are compounded by the technical challenge associated with anterior spinal stabilization in this region. Consequently, decompression and stabilization of symptomatic spinal metastases involving the atlantoaxial segments are best dealt with from a posterior approach.

Bony Integrity. The application of stabilization devices depends upon the integrity of the bony elements adjacent to a decompression site which is sufficient to accept the fixation apparatus.

Patient Debility. Local or systemic factors may preclude surgical management. Surgical approach through a previously irradiated field should, if possible, be avoided to minimize wound complications (26). Needless to say, the patient must be systemically fit to withstand an operation.

Anterior Approach

The anterior approach between the carotid sheath (laterally) and the trachea esophagus (medially) permits excellent access to the vertebral bodies (and anterior spinal canal) from C3 through C7 (27). Cervical traction (10 pounds) is maintained intraoperatively with skull tongs or halo device. Surgical decompression is performed using the operating microscope to facilitate precise technique. Adequate anterior spinal decompression involves excising the tumor-destroyed vertebral body (corpectomy). The diseased vertebra is often identified by gross paraspinal tumor extension, causing deformity and discoloration of the anterior longitudinal ligament.

Localization is confirmed with intraoperative x-ray. Decompression of the symptomatic segment is begun by excising the intervertebral disc above and below the area of involvement, followed by removal of the tumor-destroyed vertebral body. Care must be taken to avoid injuring the vertebral arteries which may be buried in tumor or tethered to lateral bony fragments. The posterior longitudinal ligament is divided to permit removal of epidural tumor extension. Finally, end-plates at the upper and lower ends of the decompressed segment are cleaned of residual disc material to provide a suitable surface for apposition of the spinal stabilization device.

Spinal stabilization may be achieved with a variety of methods and materials (13, 14, 16, 17, 19, 39, 42). Axial support can be provided with inter-position bone grafts from iliac crest, tibia, or fibula. A bone graft is appropriate when the patient's prognosis is judged to be good and a prolonged survival is anticipated (Fig. 50.9). However, bone grafts are less likely to incorporate in a milieu characterized by radiation saturation, residual tumor, and severe osteoporosis.

Immediate stabilization can be achieved with methylmethacrylate inter-position incorporated about a fixation device that bridges the decompression defect. The "Wellesley Wedge" method has proven to be a simple and effective means of spinal stabilization following anterior decompression for symptomatic spinal metastases (Fig. 50.10) (33).

Posterior Approach

The posterior approach provides easy access to the posterior and lateral spine elements and posterior spinal canal, as well as the dural sac and nerve roots from C1 through C7 (and along the entire spinal column). Adequate decompression from behind involves a wide laminectomy extending for half a level above to half a level below the compressing lesion, and with exposure of the dural sac to beyond its equator. The tumor-destroyed lateral elements may be resected posterolaterally to permit access to the vertebral body. More anteriorly situated tumor can then be removed until circumferential decompression of the dural sac and nerve roots is achieved.

Spinal stabilization can be carried out using sublaminar wires fixed to Luque rods or methylmethacrylate struts. It is essential to secure multiple levels of fixation to the spine, including a minimum of two levels above and two levels below the decompressed segment (Fig. 50.11).

PROGNOSIS

The results of treatment for symptomatic cervical metastases are highly variable. The outcome depends on a number of factors (Fig. 50.12).

The degree of neurologic deficit at the time of treatment is generally considered the most reliable prognostic factor.

Patients who are ambulatory at the time of treatment do best; patients with complete paralysis below the level of spinal cord compression stand a poor chance of recovering motor function.

Optimum outcome for the treatment of patients with symptomatic spinal metastases requires proper patient selection, strategic operative planning, and effective surgical execution.

REFERENCES

1. Alexander E, Davis CH, Field CH. Metastatic lesions of the vertebral column causing cord compression. Neurology 1956;6:103–107.
2. Auld AW, Buerman A. Metastatic spinal epidural tumors. Arch Neurol 1966;15:100–108.
3. Barron KD, Hirano A, Araki S, Terry RD. Experiences with metastatic neoplasms involving the spinal cord. Neurology 1959;9:91–106.
4. Batson OV. Role of vertebral veins in metastatic processes. Ann Intern Med 1942;16:38–45.
5. Benson WJ, Scarffe JH, Todd IDH, Palmer M, Crowther D. Spinal cord compression in myeloma. Br Med J 1979;1:1541–1544.
6. Black P. Spinal metastasis: current status and recommended guidelines for management. Neurosurgery 1979;5:726–745.
7. Bogoch ER, English E, Perrin RG, Tator CH. Successful surgical decompression of spinal extradural metastases of liposarcoma. Spine 1983;8:228–235.
8. Brady LW, Antoniades J, Prasasvinichai S, et al. The treatment of metastatic disease of the nervous system by radiation therapy. In: Seydel HG, ed. Tumors of the nervous system. New York: John Wiley & Sons, 1975:177–188.
9. Brice J, McKissock W. Surgical treatment of malignant extradural spinal tumors. Br Med J 1965;1:1341–1344.
10. Bruckman JE, Bloomer WD. Management of spinal cord compression. Semin Oncol 1978;5:135–140.
11. Chade HO. Metastatic tumors of the spine and spinal cord. In: Vinken PJ, Bruyn GW, eds. Handbook of clinical neurology Vol. 20. Amsterdam: North-Holland Publishing Co., 1976:415–433.
12. Clarke E. Spinal cord involvement in multiple myelomatosis. Brain 1986;79:332–348.
13. Cloward RB. The anterior approach for ruptured cervical discs. J Neurosurg 1958;15:602–614.
14. Conley FK, Britt RH, Hanberry JW, Silverberg GD. Anterior fibular strut graft in neoplastic disease of the cervical spine. J Neurosurg 1979;51:677–684.
15. Cross GO, White HL, White LP. Acrylic prosthesis of the fifth vertebra in multiple myeloma. Technical note. J Neurosurg 1971;35:112–114.
16. Dunn EJ. The role of methylmethacrylate in the stabilization and replacement of tumors of the cervical spine. Spine 1977;2:15–24.
17. Dunn RC Jr, Kelly WA, Wohns RN, Howe JF. Spinal epidural neoplasia: a 15-year review of the results of surgical therapy. J Neurosurg 1980;52:47–51.
18. Edelson RN, Deck MDF, Posner JB. Intramedullary spinal cord metastases: clinical and radiographic findings in nine cases. Neurology 1972;22:1222-1231.
19. Fisher RG, Acker S, Day RW. Extension of cervical carcinoma to lumbar spine. Obstet Gynecol 1975;45:101–105.
20. Fielding JW, Pyle RN, Fietti VG. Anterior cervical vertebral body resection and bone-grafting for benign and malignant tumors. J Bone Joint Surg (Am) 1979;61:251.
21. Friedman M, Kim TH, Panahon AM. Spinal cord compression in malignant lymphoma: treatment and results. Cancer 1976;37:1485–1491.
22. Galasko CSB. Pathological fracture secondary to metastatic cancer. J R Coll Surg Edinb 1974;19:351–362.
23. Gilbert RW, Kim JH, Posner JB. Epidural spinal cord compression from metastatic tumor: diagnosis and treatment. Ann Neurol 1978;3:40–51.
24. Goodkin R, Carr BI, Perrin RG. Herniated lumbar disc disease in patients with malignancy. J Clin Oncol 1987;5:667–671.
25. Hall AJ, Mackay NNS. The results of laminectomy for compression of the cord or cauda equina by extradural malignant tumor. J Bone Joint Surg (Br) 1973;55:497–505.
26. Heller M, McBroom RJ, MacNab T, Perrin RG. Treatment of metastatic disease of the spine with posterolateral decompression and Luque instrumentation. Neuro-Orthopedics 1986;2:70–74.
27. Hoff JF, Wilson CB. Microsurgical approach to the anterior cervical spine and spinal cord. Clin Neurosurg 1978;26:513–528.
28. Livingston KE, Perrin RG. Neurosurgical management of spinal metastases. J Neurosurg 1978;49:839–843.
29. Marshall LF, Langfitt TW. Combined therapy for metastatic extradural tumors of the spine. Cancer 1977;40:2067–2070.
30. Perrin RG, Livingston KE. Neurosurgical treatment of pathological fracture-dislocation of the spine. J Neurosurg 1980;52:330–334.
31. Perrin RG, Livingston KE, Aarabi B. Intradural extramedullary spinal metastasis. J Neurosurg 1982;56:835–837.
32. Perrin RG, McBroom RJ. Anterior versus posterior decompression for symptomatic spinal metastasis. Can J Neurol Sci 1987;14:75–80.
33. Perrin RG, McBroom RJ. Spinal fixation after anterior decompression for symptomatic spinal metastasis. Neurosurgery 1988;22:324–327.
34. Perrin RG, McBroom RJ. Surgical treatment for spinal metastasis: the posterolateral approach. In: Sundaresen N, Schmidek HH, Schiller AL, Rosenthal DI, eds. Tumors of the spine. Philadelphia: W.B. Saunders Co., 1990:305–318.
35. Rodichok LD, Harper GR, Ruckdeschel JC, Price A, Robertson G, Barron KD, Horton J. Early diagnosis of spinal epidural metastases. Am J Med 1981;70:1181–1188.
36. Rogers L, Heard G. Intrathecal spinal metastases (rare tumors). Br J Surg 1958;45:317–320.
37. Rome RM, Nelson JH. Compression of the spinal cord or auda equina complicating gynecological malignancy. Gynecol Oncol 1977;5:273–290.
38. Roscoe MW, McBroom RJ, St. Louis E, Grossman H, Perrin RG. Preoperative embolization in the treatment of osseous metastases from renal cell carcinoma. Clin Orthop 1989;238:302–307.
39. Scoville WB, Palmer AH, Samra K, Chong G. The use of acrylic plastic for vertebral replacement or fixation in metastatic disease of the spine. J Neurosurg 1967;27:274–279.
40. Sellwood RB. The radiological approach to metastatic cancer of the brain and spine. Br J Radiol 1972;45:647–651.
41. Shoskes DA, Perrin RG. The role of surgical management for symptomatic spinal cord compression in patients with metastatic prostate cancer. J Urol 1989;142:337–339.
42. Sundareson N, Galicich J, Bains M, Martini N, Beattie EJ. Vertebral body resection in the treatment of cancer involving the spine. Cancer 1984;53:1393–1396.
43. Vieth RG, Odom GL. Extradural spinal metastases and their neurosurgical treatment. J Neurosurg 1965;23:501–508.
44. White WA, Patterson RH Jr, Bergland RM. Role of surgery in the treatment of spinal cord compression by metastatic neoplasm. Cancer 1971;27:558–561.
45. Wild WO, Porter RW. Metastatic epidural tumor of the spine. Arch Surg 1963;87:825–830.
46. Willis RA. The spread of tumors in the human body. 3rd ed. London: Butterworths, 1973.
47. Wilson CB, Fewer D. Role of neurosurgery in the management of patients with carcinoma of the breast. Cancer 1971;28:1681–1685.
48. Wright RI. Malignant tumors in the spinal extradural space. Ann Surg 1963;157:227–231.

51

Radiation Therapy in the Treatment of Cervical Spine Malignancies

Shalom Kalnicki and Roy Buchsbaum

Introduction

X-rays were first described by William C. Röentgen in 1895 (168). Henri Becquerel and the Curies discovered natural radioactivity 1 year later (23). It was soon recognized that cellular damage and death were among the biological effects of these newly discovered radiations, leading to their utilization in the treatment of malignant neoplasms, with the first tumor responses being described at the turn of the century (155).

Ionizing radiation causes cellular death by formation of highly reactive intracellular free radicals with resultant nuclear DNA damage (63). For slow turnover cell systems, such as muscle and nerve, radiation damage may lead to loss of a specific cellular function (194). For rapidly dividing cell populations such as bone marrow or gastrointestinal tract, it results in loss of reproductive potential. Although some cells may still undergo several mitoses after being exposed to radiation, they are considered "clonogenically dead" if they ultimately lose their potential to undergo indefinite divisions (31).

Survival curves for cultured cells exposed to single hit conventional, low linear energy transfer (LET) radiation have two components—an initial bend or "shoulder" region at low doses followed by a linear slope at higher dose levels (93, 163). The shoulder region, where increasing doses cause little additional damage, reflects the cells' ability to repair sublethal radiation injury; the width of the shoulder varies, according to the cell system repair capacity and type of radiation utilized (64).

The straight slope of the survival curve represents exponential cell killing at higher dose levels; linearity implies no repair of radiation damage in this region (31). The slope of this portion of the survival curve is a measure of cellular radiosensitivity. The therapeutic ratio of radiation therapy is based, at least to some extent, on the assumption that normal cell systems repair sublethal or potentially lethal damage better than neoplastic ones (162). In central nervous system tumors, attempts at measuring radiation response in vitro showed highly individualized patterns of sensitivity in glioblastomas and astrocytomas, translated by widely different survival curve patterns (69).

The sensitivity of individual cells to radiation also varies with their position in the cell cycle, being greatest at mitosis and early synthesis (94). Following a single exposure to ionizing radiation, a higher proportion of cells in the most sensitive phases of the cycle will be killed and the population will cycle in a partially synchronized manner. Within tumor masses containing hypoxic centers with dormant neoplastic cells, serial reduction in tumor cell numbers may lead to their reoxygenation, recruiting them into active cycling again and rendering them more radiosensitive. Reoxygenation and repopulation are part of the rationale upon which the utilization of multiple treatment fractions in clinical radiotherapy regimens is based (113).

The radiosensitivity of most cell systems can be enhanced as much as threefold in the presence of oxygen (85). The free radicals generated through the radiation-induced intracellular ionization events undergo an irreversible oxygen fixation reaction (7). Under hypoxic conditions, ionization events can be reversible, facilitating repair of radiation damage, with radiosensitivity being consequently reduced (44). The ratio of the radiation doses necessary to achieve the same biological effect is called the oxygen enhancement ratio (OER). There is a steep rise in the OER as oxygen tension increases from 0 to 33 mm Hg, beyond which the OER remains constant at approximately three, regardless of oxygen tension (95).

Thomlinson and Gray described the histological pattern of hypoxia in malignant tumors, where cords of healthy tumor cells surrounded necrotic appearing ones and central areas of overt necrosis (196). As neoplastic cells outgrow their blood supply, areas of central hypoxia, rich in relatively radioresistant cells, develop in many large solid tumors (57). Central hypoxia is a major limiting factor for radiocurability; it may be difficult to eradicate bulky tumor masses with clinically tolerable levels of irradiation, while the same doses can be extremely effective for sterilization of microscopic, well-oxygenated tumor deposits in a surgical field, after debulking has been performed (70, 71).

As early as 1934, Coutard observed that fractionated radiation therapy regimens led to improved tumor control with lower complication rates (50). Utilizing relatively small daily increments of radiation in protracted treatment regimens, reoxygenation of previously hypoxic tumor tissue may occur, leading to increased cell killing. In mouse RIF-1 sarcomas, almost 100% of tumor cells surviving a single dose of 1.5 Gy were hypoxic, but only 50% remained hypoxic within 1 hour after irradiation (61), anesthesia-induced hypotension and hypoxia had radioprotective effects in these tumors (51).

There is experimental data to support the relevance of the oxygen effect in central nervous system tumors and in radiation tolerance of brain and spinal cord (59). Clinical evidence for the importance of hypoxia has been established for carcinomas of the uterine cervix and other sites (102, 210).

The hypoxic cell fraction of a tumor mass is directly affected by its circulatory pattern; this tumor bed effect (TBE) influences response to radiation and chemotherapy (108). Tumors transplanted into previous irradiated, poorly oxygenated tissues, become less radiosensitive (141, 142); radiation-induced injury to the tumor bed stroma can play an important role in radiocurability (140).

Radiation dose is measured in Grays, one Gray (Gy) defined as one joule of absorbed energy per kilogram of tissue. The Gray has replaced the rad and equals 100 rad; for convenience, the term centiGray (cGy) is commonly used as it equals one rad. The biological effect of a fractionated radiation therapy regimen depends upon the total dose delivered, the number and size of each individual fraction and on the total treatment time (65). This time-dose relationship is one of the cornerstones of clinical radiation therapy, affecting not only tumor control but also normal tissue tolerance. Mathematical formulas have been derived in order to compare both effects of different treatment schedules, originating the "nominal standard dose" (NSD) (148), "time-dose factor" (TDF) (66), and the Linear Quadratic (LQ) model concepts (190, 202).

According to those models, protracted treatment regimens strive for daily doses within the shoulder or repair region of normal tissues while in the exponential killing region for tumor cells; reoxygenation of hypoxic neoplastic cells with their recruitment into active cycling increases tumor cell killing in multi-fraction regimens (152). Radiation-induced cell division delay and cycling synchronization also occur in fractionated schedules (11). Care must be taken so tumor repopulation does not exceed radiation-induced cell killing if treatment regimens become too protracted. In most radiation therapy schedules, daily doses range from 150 to 200 cGy, delivering 900 to 1000 cGy per week.

The radiation tolerance of the spinal cord, a late responding tissue, strongly depends upon the size of the dose fraction and is relatively unaffected by total treatment time (9, 206). In the rat cervical spinal cord, normal tissue sparing markedly increases as the daily dose is lowered to 200 cGy, after which it plateaus, except for some additional sparing at 100 cGy, a fraction size generally too low for achieving tumor control (209). Mathematical models, such as the local stem cell depletion, have been proposed in order to predict spinal cord tolerance in different treatment regimens (224).

Clinical trials in humans have traditionally considered spinal cord tolerance as the dose-fractionation regimen that carries a 5% risk of radiation myelitis; daily doses of 180 to 200 cGy to a total of 4500 cGy are recommended by many, while others believe that 5000 cGy in 5 weeks may be tolerated (156, 214). Emphasizing fraction size, some authors have delivered even higher doses, up to 5500–6000 cGy at less than 180 cGy per day (114, 136). One must exercise caution, as there is evidence that if the blood supply to the cord is altered by the presence of tumor and or previous surgery, radiation injury could be manifest at tolerance doses (134); cervical cord myelitis has been described after 5040 cGy following subtotal resection of ependymomas (123, 133).

When irradiated cells are prevented from progressing through the cell cycle, their surviving fraction increases, due to repair of "potentially lethal damage" (158). This phenomenon is particularly important in situations where tumor bed conditions affect cell cycling times. In the rat cervical cord, the rate if sublethal and potentially lethal damage repair is exponential, becomes faster with decreasing dose fractions; the time to complete cellular repair following 110 to 150 cGy was estimated at 8 hours (10).

Relatively radioresistant tumors may contain a higher proportion of cells capable of repairing "potentially lethal damage." Survival curve analysis of cultured tumor cells may lead to response predictive assays (154, 216). Care must be taken, however, in interpreting the in vitro data; experimental studies showed very little difference in radiosensitivity between cultured glioblastoma and medulloblastoma cells, although the latter are far more radiocurable (81, 217); the radically different clinical outcome could be secondary to repair and other cell kinetic mechanisms rather than cellular radiosensitivity, and this would not become apparent in the laboratory setting.

The characterization of radiation-induced nuclear damage as a chemical reaction prompted the search for substances that would act as modifiers of radiation response. Oxygen was the obvious initial choice, in the form of hyperbaric oxygen breathing (138). Some benefit was reported in advanced head and neck and uterine cervix cancers, but in general, results of clinical trials were not encouraging. The use of hyperbaric oxygen is cumbersome, with the bulky chambers interfering with daily treatment reproduction; normal tissue reactions were also enhanced. Furthermore, the inhalation of hyperbaric oxygen does not always translate into a decreased tumor hypoxic cell fraction (100).

Emphasis has recently shifted to chemical modifiers of radiation response. Electron-affinic radiosensitizing compounds, such as metronidazole (Flagyl) and misonidazole (RO-07-0582), have been tested, albeit with little clinical impact, because of their dose-limiting neurotoxicity (68, 157). Whole body autoradiography showed presence of misonidazole in the central nervous system in the first hours after intravenous administration (4). Other nitroimidazole derivatives, RO-03-8799 (103) and RSU-1069 (211), showed some therapeutic advantage, with less neurotoxic side effects and are currently being evaluated in clinical trials.

Chemotherapeutic agents may have radiosensitizing effects (124). This effect can be of extreme clinical usefulness in treatment of pediatric tumors, where reducing the total radiation dose while maintaining tumor control rates significantly decreases severe radiation morbidity (115). Some chemotherapeutic agents may also enhance adverse normal tissue reactions, especially on bone marrow, skin, and small bowel (46, 164).

Pyrimidine analogues have radiomimetic mechanisms of action. Among those, BUdR and IUdR are subjects of intensive investigation. BUdR is not incorporated by normal neurons and glial cells but penetrates malignant gliomas. Greenberg (86) treated 18 patients with malignant astrocytomas utilizing a continuous 8-week intra-arterial BUdR infusion during radiation therapy, with 11 being alive after 22 months. Jackson, at the National Cancer Institute (109) combined a 14-day intravenous infusion with 65–70 Gy of radiation in 60 patients with unresectable high grade gliomas; median survival was increased to 14 months in the 48 patients who completed treatment.

Studies with cisplatinum have also shown reduced hypoxic cell fractions and increased tumor response to irradiation (58). Carboplatinum may have similar properties and is the subject of several ongoing experimental and clinical trials (48).

Nitrosoureas (CCNU, BCNU) cross the blood-brain barrier and are being increasingly studied as radiosensitizers, alone or combined with misonidazole (184, 185). Deutsch reported on the Brain Tumor Cooperative Group Study 77–02 (55), where 557 patients received several combinations of radiation, misonidazole, streptozotocin and BCNU; the group treated with BCNU or streptozotocin had a slightly better control rate, although no statistically significant survival difference was observed; peripheral neuropathy was a major dose limiting factor in patients receiving misonidazole. ACNU, another nitrosourea, is currently being tested in Japan, so far without significant clinical impact (203).

Methotrexate and cytosine arabinoside (Ara-C) are the antineoplastic agents most commonly injected into the subarachnoid space. Being the agents of choice for treatment of leukemias and meningeal carcinomatosis, they are frequently combined with craniospinal irradiation. Appropriate sequence and dosage in combining these drugs with radiation is crucial, as central nervous system injury, mostly leukoencephalopathy, has been reported in patients who received methotrexate after irradiation, but far less frequently if the drug is administered only prior to radiation therapy (29, 82). Intrathecal Ara-C impairs central nervous system regeneration in the rat spinal cord, while this effect can be observed with both systemic and intrathecal methotrexate (126, 205).

Most radioprotectors are sulfhydril compounds. WR-2721 was initially shown to reduce experimental radiation injury to normal lung and colonic mucosa (107, 199); studies in the rat cervical spinal cord revealed radioprotective effects for nervous tissue, but only when the compound was administered through a route that bypassed the blood-brain barrier (187, 188). The effects of other compounds such as picibanil are being studied and results are forthcoming (12).

The interaction of biologic response modifiers with radiation is currently under investigation. Radioresponsiveness can be increased by pretreatment of tumor cells with tumor necrosis factor (TNF) while maintaining it's protective effect on normal bone marrow cells (181). Ongoing studies are addressing the simultaneous use of interferon, interleukin-2, and radiation (110, 143).

Steroids are routinely administered during irradiation of central nervous system neoplasms, in order to decrease edema secondary to tumor and/or irradiation. Concern has arisen from a hypothesized radioprotective effect of steroids in some cell lines. Studies with cultured C6 astrocytoma cells, however, failed to demonstrate any influence of dexamethasone on their radiosensitivity (125).

The use of heat as an antineoplastic agent can be traced to early in the century, when fever induced by injected bacterial toxins produced tumor regressions. The development of sophisticated heat delivery and thermometry equipment, allied to the recognition of the chemical nature of radiation induced cell killing, led to research combining hyperthermia and radiation (191). Heat affects hypoxic cells in the S-phase, at their most radioresistant state; it also causes greater cell cycle delay than ionizing radiation, further affecting the cell population distribution (56). Malignant cells seem to be more sensitive to thermal damage than normal ones. Temperatures between 42° and 43°C provide the highest tumor cell kill while still within the range of normal tissue tolerance (83). Thermal enhancement ratios of 3.4–3.9 were reported with interstitial implantation of iridium-192 and hyperthermia (144).

Radiation response and normal tissue tolerance can be greatly modified by altering therapy fractionation. Most radiation therapy schedules call for one treatment session a day, 5 days per week (conventional fractionation). Alternatively, large weekly doses (hypofractionation) or several fractions per day (hyperfractionation) can be administered. Twice a day radiation regimens yielded some therapeutic advantage in advanced head and neck cancers (212). There is experimental evidence that decreasing fraction size further improves spinal cord tolerance when multiple daily fractions are delivered (225). In treating central nervous system structures, one should choose the longest possible delay between the two daily sessions, as repair of spinal cord sublethal damage is relatively slow, taking at least 4 hours (8, 195).

In the Pediatric Oncology Group, Freeman and coworkers studied the effects of hyperfractionated irradiation in children with brain stem gliomas (74). Doses of 110 cGy were delivered twice daily to a total of 6600 cGy; although 24 of 34 patients (71%) sustained clinical improvement, there were no CT or MRI proven complete responders. As no patient developed symptoms suggestive of radiation induced central nervous system damage, a higher total dose of 7200 cGy is currently being studied. Wara has previously reported on a group of both pediatric and adult brainstem glioma patients treated to this dose with hyperfractionation, with no cases of radiation myelitis being recorded (215). The addition of sensitizers such as misonidazole to hyperfractionated radiation did not result in increased tumor control (78).

Radiation therapy can be delivered by means of external beams such as cobalt-60 or linear accelerators (teletherapy), as well as by the placement of radioactive sources into the tumor or tumor bed (brachytherapy). External beams of photon radiation have different energies, increasing from orthovoltage (100–300 kV) to megavoltage irradiation from linear accelerators (generally four to 25 MV). Advantages of high energy irradiation include greater percentage depth doses (better penetration into deep tissues), skin sparing (maximal energy deposition at depths between 0.5 to 5 cm below the skin), and precise beam definition with minimal scatter of radiation outside the desired treatment field.

High energy electron beams are produced by some linear accelerators. Electrons are physically stopped in tissue, and thus provide sparing of deep-seated structures, particularly useful when treating superficial targets. In some centers, 15 MV electrons are being utilized to deliver whole spine irradiation in leukemia and medulloblastoma; tolerance is improved and the potential decrease in late effects is currently under investigation (132).

Neutrons are densely ionizing particles that have higher linear energy transfer (LET) than X-rays or photons. The OER for neutrons decreases from three to one, probably because of direct formation of molecular oxygen from neutron induced radiolysis of water (22). In a review of the literature, Cohen (42) concluded that local control with neutrons alone is comparable or better than with high energy x-rays, but at the expense of significantly higher complication rates. Mixed beams of photons and neutrons usually show marginally better results than conventional photon irradiation, but complications can be kept at acceptable levels. Due to the relatively poor neutron depth dose distribution, severe morbidity was described after treatment of deep-seated tumors (21, 73), including cervical spinal cord injury after neutron irradiation of head and neck tumors (119).

Lower numerical doses of neutron radiation are given because neutrons have a higher relative biological effectiveness (RBE) than conventional irradiation. Cohen (41) delivered cord doses between 10 and 17 neutron Gy to 76 patients; there were no cases of myelopathy with follow-up ranging from one to 5 years. In a review of the literature, he concluded that the spinal cord tolerance dose for high energy neutrons is 15 neutron Gy in 4 weeks.

Budach (33) delivered fast neutron irradiation to 10 patients with spinal cord ependymomas, utilizing doses equivalent to 7400–10400 cGy of conventional photon irradiation, well above photon cord tolerance levels. There were two complete and two partial remissions, with no severe late effects. Despite some promising studies, the role of neutron therapy in the treatment of central nervous system tumors is not yet established, as randomized studies comparing neutron and photon irradiation are unavailable (88). Further radiobiological studies and technical refinements are necessary in order to reduce neutron irradiation morbidity (153).

Heavy charged particles, such as protons, alpha particles (helium nuclei) and negative pi-mesons (pions), are characterized by high linear energy transfer (LET), high relative biological effectiveness (RBE), and low oxygen enhancement ratios (OER). Their energy is preferentially deposited at a certain depth in their path, the Bragg peak, allowing for better normal tissue sparing than neutrons, and making them especially suitable for irradiation of small tumor volumes in the cervical spine and brainstem (40). The depth of the Bragg peak is a function of the energy of the particle; its width can be customized by utilizing mixed energy heavy particle beams.

Negative pi-mesons are currently being evaluated at the Los Alamos (United States), Vancouver (Canada), and Villigen (Switzerland) particle accelerators. Experimental studies in the rat spinal cord have shown the RBE for pions to be less than 1.5, in contrast to the higher RBE values for neutrons, which reaches a value close to 4.0, especially for late effects (207, 208).

Encouraging proton beam results are being reported by the Harvard Cyclotron group, with 89% 3-year actuarial local control in 67 patients with chordomas and chondrosarcomas of the base of skull and cervical spine (16). At the Lawrence Berkeley Laboratories, Berson et al. delivered alpha particle doses equivalent to 8000 cGy of conventional irradiation to 45 patients with chordomas, meningiomas, and low grade chondrosarcomas of the cervical spine and base of skull. Outside of the Bragg peak distribution, there was a precipitous fall in dose toward the adjacent central nervous system, where tolerance is 4500 to 5000 cGy; the actuarial survival and local control rates at 5 years were 62% and 59%, respectively; complications occurred in 13% of patients, four of whom sustained radiation induced brainstem injury (28). Treatment planning is extremely complex, including division of the tumor volume in two or more portions and utilization of multiple energy ion beams (39).

The rapid decrease of energy deposited by alpha particles (175) allowed for successful attempts at stereotactic helium beam irradiation of intracranial arteriovenous malformations (AVM) (67, 130); after two years follow-up, 14 of 18 patients irradiated at the Lawrence Berkeley Synchrocyclotron had complete AVM obliteration, with three treatment-related complications being described (122).

External beam irradiation can be given pre- or postoperatively, or as the sole treatment modality. In most cervical cord and brainstem tumors, therapy is delivered after incomplete resection or stereotactic biopsy only; doses between 4500 and 5500 cGy in 5–7 weeks are utilized, at or close to normal tissue tolerance. The addition of interstitial implants, radiation sensitizers or fractionation changes are being tested in an attempt to improve the therapeutic ratio.

Treatment planning for external beam irradiation starts with close interaction between the neurosurgeon, diagnostic radiologist, pathologist, and radiation oncologist (89). Through this team effort, the target volume for the radiation is identified; this includes the tumor or tumor bed, with all potential areas of spread. The target volume is obtained by combining data from clinical examination, x-rays, angiograms, contrast-enhanced computerized tomography (39, 106), and gadolinium-enhanced magnetic resonance imaging, which currently provides the most accurate tumor localization (37, 99, 197). Treatment volume is defined as the target volume plus a margin of safety; it should include peritumoral edema and, in lesions with potential for cerebrospinal fluid seeding, the entire subarachnoid space.

Radiation oncologist, physicist, and dosimetrist then proceed to study the appropriate radiation field arrangement to treat the target volume, attempting at maximal normal tissue sparing (197). This is done with the aid of a therapy simulator, a fluoroscopic x-ray device that mimics all movements and physical characteristics of a linear accelerator or cobalt-60 teletherapy unit. Localizing precision within less than 2 mm can be optically obtained with modern simulator techniques (43). Multiple portals, arc therapy, and multileaf collimating devices are often utilized to minimize normal tissue irradiation.

Treatment devices are custom built for each patient. Head and neck immobilization supports are built for precise day-to-day repositioning; these may include stereotactic frames. Wedge filters and tissue compensators can be inserted into the beam in order to homogenize the dose along irregular surfaces such as sloping edges of the neck, or to compensate for the increasing width above the foramen magnum when neck and brainstem are irradiated. Custom lead-alloy blocks are used to shape the beams in any form needed to cover the target volume, while preventing unnecessary irradiation of critical structures. Careful immobilization and optimal conditions for daily treatment setup reproduction are mandatory; minimal variations may lead to underdosing or overdosing in multiple field junctions, as in craniospinal irradiation for medulloblastoma and leukemias (192, 193, 222).

Precise calculation of the dose delivered from each treatment portal is then performed utilizing treatment planning computers where all beam data for the treatment unit have been entered. These provide accurate dose mapping throughout the treatment field and precise setting of the linear accelerator monitor unit counter to provide the desired daily dose.

Verification x-rays (or portal films) are then obtained on the treatment unit and compared with simulator films to assure precise beam reproduction (120). Linear accelerators typically deliver 250 to 500 cGy/min in air, so daily fractions of 180 to 200 cGy can be delivered in seconds, minimizing the possibility of significant patient motion.

Special external beam techniques may be employed for irradiation of small central nervous system targets. The "Leksell Stereotactic Gamma-knife" is a unit (35, 128), where over 200 small Cobalt-60 sources are arranged into a multicollimator stereotactic helmet that directs irradiation from all sources toward a small target. In "arc stereotactic radiosurgery," several tridimensional arcs are described by the linear accelerator, again centered on a target volume secured by a stereotactic frame (161). Both techniques allow for the delivery of high doses to a small volume in one single fraction (60), with excellent normal tissue sparing; they are being increasingly utilized for the irradiation of arteriovenous malformations (45), meningiomas, craniopharyngiomas, acoustic neuromas, and for boosts in malignant gliomas and metastatic sites after wide field conventional irradiation (204).

Interstitial implantation of radioactive isotopes can deliver high doses of radiation to a small target volume. The most commonly utilized isotopes for central nervous system implantation are iridium-192 and iodine-125 (92). Due to the physical characteristics of these and other interstitially applied radionuclides, radiation doses fall off rapidly at the edge of the implant volume, with consequent normal tissue sparing. Modern "afterloading" techniques allow for placement of hollow guide catheters and radiographic documentation of their positioning before loading them with the radioactive sources. Computer calculations determine the duration of radiation exposure, depending upon the dose rate and total dose desired. Implants can deliver radiation boosts to small treatment volumes, such as areas of gross residual disease or tight resection margins after surgical resection, or treat recurrent tumors after external irradiation (127).

The most common acute side effect of radiation is skin reaction. Glancing fields over sloped surfaces of the neck and occipital areas tend to increase the risk of radiation-induced skin damage. The initial erythema may develop into dry and, later, moist desquamation. Decreasing the daily fraction size may be all that is necessary to minimize skin reactions. Occasionally, rest periods may be required for healing of moist desquamation (49). Care must be taken not to extend rest periods unnecessarily, so as not to decrease the regimen's biologic effectiveness.

Alopecia is another common side effect, apparent at doses above 2000 cGy in 2 weeks. Regrowth of hair can be seen 2–6 months following irradiation, although in many instances hair loss may be permanent.

Dysphagia is a common side effect of cervical spine irradiation, as the posterior pharyngeal and laryngeal walls have to be included in the treatment volume. It is more pronounced in patients undergoing simultaneous chemotherapy and irradiation, as many antineoplastic agents enhance radiation-induced mucositis (52). Additional acute side effects may include mild fatigue, anorexia and, in cases where the salivary or lacrimal glands are included in the radiation portals, xerostomia and xerophthalmia.

Radiation-induced acute central nervous system changes are relatively unusual; brain and spinal cord edema have been described, although its existence and nature are controversial. It can be prevented or treated with steroids, which are usually required for edema secondary to the underlining tumor. L'Hermitte's syndrome, or electrical paresthesias in the extremities upon neck flexion, has been attributed to transient subacute radiation myelopathy; it appears 1–3 months after radiation, in approximately 25% of patients receiving more than 3500 cGy to the cord. It is a self-limited phenomenon, usually regressing in 1–9 months, without leaving neurological sequelae; its presence is not related to late progressive radiation myelopathy (112).

Late effects of radiation therapy of cervical spine lesions are mostly secondary to central nervous system, bone, and connective tissue changes. Epilation and mild subcutaneous fibrosis are also common late sequelae; bone growth abnormalities and radiation-induced carcinogenesis are of special concern in the younger patient population.

Documented instances of radiation-induced central nervous system necrosis are fortunately very rare (118), as radiation myelitis is one of the most feared complications of radiotherapy. Latent periods can vary from 3–18 months, with an experimental median of 165 +/− 14 days (54). Latency decreases with increasing radiation dose (178). The clinical picture can mimic a Brown-Sequard syndrome or transverse myelitis, with abnormalities depending upon the affected cord levels (26, 27). Radiation myelopathy may be difficult to differentiate from recurrent disease and paraneoplastic neurologic abnormalities. Imaging techniques may show cord edema initially, to be followed by atrophy (201), and myelin basic protein can be elevated in the cerebrospinal fluid, although those findings are nonspecific (172). Stereotactic biopsies have been proposed when diagnosis between recurrence and radionecrosis cannot be made using noninvasive methods (227).

Among the multiple factors that determine the tolerance of the spinal cord to irradiation are the total dose and the fractionation regimen utilized, length of cord irradiated, and the patient's age (2, 104, 223). Experimental evidence points to the size of the dose per fraction as being the prime determinant of spinal cord radiation tolerance (25). Safe doses for spinal cord tolerance are 4500 to 5000 cGy, at 175 to 180 per day. Fractions exceeding 200 cGy are not recommended, except for treatment of metastatic disease (14). Yamada (226), utilizing the life-table method, estimated the 5-year cumulative risk of radiation myelitis to be 0% at 4000 cGy, 5% at 5000 cGy, 10% at 6000 cGy, and 20% at 7000 cGy, establishing the radiation tolerance of the cervical cord at 5000 cGy in 25 fractions. The association of chemotherapy can lead to increased incidence of myelitis, especially when methotrexate is administered concurrently or after irradiation (15).

Radiation myelopathy is usually attributed to delayed vascular changes, with obliteration of the end-arterial supply of portions of the spinal cord causing ischemia and necrosis (36, 150). Morphologically, the initial asymptomatic period is characterized by increased capillary permeability and myelin vacuolation which is evident at 30 days and peaks at 60 days. There is no progression until approximately 150 days, when one observes endothelial damage and capillary obliteration, with consequent necrosis of the posterior and lateral columns, preserving the grey matter (54). White matter damage has been described without any evidence of blood vessel obliteration (145). Schultheiss has classified radiation injury to the spinal cord into three types: primary white matter parenchymal lesions (type 1), primary vascular lesions (type 2), and combination of vascular and white matter lesions (type 3) (177). Limiting the cord's total and daily doses and avoiding areas of potential overlap when treating adjoining brain and cervical cord fields are essential steps in preventing irreversible myelopathy (34).

Because neuronal division and myelinization are completed only between 1 and 2 years of age, high doses of irradiation prior to that time are likely to produce significant morbidity (176). For children under 2, doses are routinely reduced by 10%, and the fraction sizes are also decreased; some pediatric patients are maintained on chemotherapy until they reach an age at which radiation is deemed to be safer (121). Neuropsychiatric abnormalities have been occasionally described in children following craniospinal irradiation (24).

Bone growth retardation is another major concern in irradiation of pediatric patients (3). This effect is more pronounced in the younger age groups (182) and is directly correlated with total radiation doses (53, 84). When growing vertebral bodies are irradiated, both pedicles should be included in the treatment portals in order to avoid severe spinal curvatures (147). Most pediatric patients treated with spinal irradiation suffer little overall height loss but have significant reduction of sitting height (101). There is experimental evidence that hyperfractionation may increase the radiation tolerance of growing bones (62, 98).

Fromm (76) reported on late effects in 20 children treated for soft tissue sarcomas of the head and neck, most of them with combined radiotherapy and chemotherapy. Findings included xerophthalmia, cataracts, hearing loss, dental caries, and maleruption, hypopituitarism, and craniofacial bone deformities. Attentive follow-up is necessary for prompt recognition and therapy of treatable abnormalities.

Osteonecrosis is a rare complication in patients treated with megavoltage radiation. It generally occurs at doses in excess of 5000–6000 cGy (105), no evidence of osteocyte death being found below 4000 cGy (111). The widespread use of megavoltage beams, which lack the preferential bone absorption of orthovoltage x-rays, has resulted in a marked decrease in the incidence of this complication (189).

Radiation-induced neoplasms have been described in heavily irradiated tissues of long-term survivors. Although extremely rare, they are usually diagnosed at advanced stages, or at sites beyond surgical resectability. Their prognosis is generally poor, and only early detection may improve the patient's survival (167). A 4% incidence of second primary tumors has been reported in children followed for 25 years after irradiation (99). Second malignancies have been seen after successful irradiation of several central nervous system tumors and other primaries (38, 146, 149). Thyroid carcinoma has been reported after cervical spine irradiation for medulloblastoma (169), and a retroperitoneal sarcoma has been described at the edge of a whole spine radiation portal for a high grade ependymoma (80). Associated chemotherapy increases the chance for developing sarcomas and other neoplasms in previously irradiated areas (200).

Radiation Therapy in Tumors of the Spinal Cord

Early diagnosis and prompt therapeutic intervention are mandatory in the treatment of intramedullary spinal cord tumors. Neurologic symptoms appear early even with small tumors, as there is very little room for expansion in the cervical canal. Surgery is usually the initial approach, in order to provide tissue diagnosis and to microscopically resect as much tumor as feasible without undue neurological deficit (47). Postoperative irradiation is usually indicated in patients with gross or microscopic residual disease (221). An interval of 1–2 weeks is necessary to allow for neurologic stabilization and wound healing. For most localized spinal cord tumors, general local fields encompassing the tumor volume plus two vertebral bodies in both directions are utilized (72, 213). In cases where cerebrospinal fluid seeding is present or likely, craniospinal irradiation may be utilized to cover the entire neuraxis.

Garcia and co-workers (80) studied the radiation dose-response levels for spinal cord tumors. Nine of 10 patients treated to 4000 cGy or less failed locally, while doses greater than 4000 cGy yielded a 75% local control rate. Doses close to or at spinal cord tolerance level, i.e., 5000 cGy at standard fractionation, are recommended. Hyperfractionated regimens may allow for delivery of higher radiation doses.

Astrocytoma

Spinal cord astrocytomas may have varied histological patterns, ranging from benign encapsulated ones, amenable to complete surgical removal, to aggressive infiltrative lesions, usually unresectable and with the potential for cerebrospinal fluid dissemination (116, 220). Most intramedullary astrocytomas in children are low grade, and 10-year survival rates of 62% have been reported (220).

Radiation therapy can produce long-term symptomatic improvement, lasting for 5 years or more. Tumor doses of 5000 cGy in 6 week are generally utilized (134, 180, 221). Attempts at increasing the dose have been hampered by the threat of radiation myelitis (214). Marsa treated 15 patients with spinal cord gliomas to a mean dose of 5700 cGy (range 5000–6700 cGy), with three cases of myelitis being observed (134).

The group at the University of California, San Francisco (123) reported on 15 patients with primary spinal cord astrocytomas, three anaplastic and 12 low grade ones. No patient underwent gross total excision, with surgery limited to biopsy only in 10 patients, and the radiation doses ranged between 3250 and 5180 cGy. Acutarial disease-specific survival rates were 91% at 10 and 74% at 15 years. Three patients with glioblastoma multiforme died within 8 months of diagnosis, two of them developing diffuse craniospinal disease. Similar results were observed by Guidetti (91) on 19 patients irradiated after incomplete resection, with only one tumor related death and 14 patients alive at 2 years. Five patients were treated with surgery only, with three disease related deaths.

Chondrosarcoma

These tumors often present as large lesions located in sites where surgical resection is not feasible. Conventional irradiation regimens can increase symptom-free survival. Innovative approaches utilizing hyperfractionation, radiation sensitizers, particle beams, and chemotherapy, either by systemic or intra-arterial infusion, may improve cure rates.

Particle beam studies show particularly encouraging results. McNaney irradiated 20 unresectable patients with a combination of neutrons and photons (4000–7000 cGy), with a 65% 5-year survival (137). Two patients who recurred were salvaged by surgery. Austin-Seymour (17) reported on 68 patients with skull base lesions treated with the proton beam, achieving an 82% actuarial 5-year local control, while complications were kept at very low levels. Berson, with the Lawrence Berkeley Laboratories alpha particle beam, obtained a 62% local control rate, with four of 45 patients suffering radiation-induced brainstem injury (28).

Chordoma

These notochordal remnant tumors are slow growing but may be highly invasive, eroding into adjacent bone. Radical surgical resection is extremely difficult. Palliative results can be obtained with postoperative conventional radiotherapy, as the high doses needed for cure would carry an undue risk of myelitis (18).

Rich (165) reported encouraging results with a combination of photon and 160 MV proton beams, achieving tumor doses of 6500 cGy or higher, while keeping spinal cord dose at tolerance levels. Castro and co-workers (39) irradiated 15 patients with heavy charged particles (helium ions) to total doses equivalent to 6000–7500 cGy, while restricting the spinal cord and brainstem doses to a maximum of 5000 and 6000 cGy-equivalent, respectively. The local control rate was 62%, with very low complication rates.

Ependymoma

These rare tumors originate from the ependymal lining of the central medullary canal, making their complete surgical resection difficult, but possible. For the same reason, drop metastasis is common, and sometimes the entire spinal canal or entire central nervous system has to be included in the radiation treatment volume (123). If no cerebrospinal fluid contamination is present, generous local fields treated to 5000 cGy in 150–180 cGy fractions will yield excellent local control (179).

Ependymomas are radiosensitive and radiocurable tumors. A dose response curve for ependymomas has been established by Kopelson (117), although others have not been able to duplicate these findings (133).

Utilizing sophisticated microneurosurgical techniques, some intramedullary ependymomas can be completely excised. Guidetti (91) reported on 16 such patients with ony one recurrence observed during a follow-up period of 2 to 21 years. The role of postoperative irradiation in those patients is unclear, as patient numbers are small and local control is usually quite good (87). Shaw and co-workers (183) reviewed 22 patients treated with laminectomy, partial resection, and postoperative irradiation at the Mayo Clinic, two of whom had cervical spine lesions. Ten-year survival was 95%; seven patients failed locally, including all three with high grade lesions. The authors recommend a total dose of 5500 cGy at 180 cGy per fraction, with 5000 cGy delivered to the tumor with a margin of two vertebral bodies on each side, followed by a 500 cGy boost to the lesion.

Linstadt reviewed the experience with 21 patients treated at the University of California San Francisco (123). Three patients with multifocal disease received craniospinal irradiation. The others were treated to generous local fields to doses between 4500 and 5470 cGy, 160 cGy per fraction. The actuarial disease specific survival was 93% at 10 years and 46% at 15 years. Six patients failed locally, but only two died of uncontrolled disease. Late recurrences were observed, developing between 7 and 12 years after therapy. Barone (20) reported on seven incompletely excised intramedullary ependymomas, with all three nonirradiated patients experiencing local recurrence within 3 years, while no recurrences were observed in the irradiation group.

Bone Metastasis

Palliation of symptomatic bone metastasis is one of the most frequently encountered problems in oncology. It is estimated that over 30% of metastatic bone sites will require radiation therapy (77). Lesions in weight bearing areas presenting with greater than 50% cortical destruction should be initially submitted to surgical stabilization, in an attempt to prevent pathological fracture. Post operative radiotherapy should be delivered, in order to prevent tumor regrowth and prosthetic displacement (79).

Multiple radiation regimens have been proposed for the treatment of bone metastasis, ranging from single doses of 800–1000 cGy to 5000 cGy in 5 weeks (151). The Radiation Therapy Oncology Group conducted a prospective randomized trial of several dose schedules, initially concluding that short courses were equally effective to the more protracted ones (198). Analysis of long-term palliation data from the same study suggested that 3000 cGy in ten sessions provided the best results, with lasting pain relief being obtained in 80% of patients so treated (30). For terminal patients, 1000 cGy in one or two fractions can provide excellent short-term palliation (6).

Half body irradiation (HBI) can be utilized for patients with extensive disease suffering from multiple painful sites. In the Radiation Therapy Oncology Group study, single doses of 600 cGy upper HBI and 800 cGy lower HBI were followed by pain relief within 48 hours in 80% of 168 irradiated patients, with 30% not needing any additional pain treatment measures (174).

Spinal Cord Compression

Metastatic disease in the epidural space develops in 5% of all cancer patients (166). In most instances, these are extensions of vertebral metastasis from lung, breast, prostate, and renal cell carcinomas (13). Lymphomas (75), leukemias (139), and sarcomas can also metastasize into the epidural space. Spinal cord compression can be the first manifestation of an unknown primary neoplasm (32).

Recovery of neurologic function after treatment is intimately associated with prompt diagnosis and early intervention, prior to the onset of irreversible nerve damage. Over 50% of patients who are not completely paralyzed at the time of diagnosis remain ambulatory, while almost no recovery is seen in patients who have been paralyzed for 48 hours or more (32).

The diagnosis of spinal cord compression prior to paralysis or loss of sphincter control may be difficult to differentiate from paraneoplastic syndromes, chemotherapy side effects, and from compression due to benign disorders (5, 96, 97). Early diagnostic imaging studies of bone metastasis are mandatory, as vertebral collapse can be predictive of an epidural lesion (159). Makin (131), reviewing 87 patients treated at the Christie Hospital, observed that although patients were irradiated immediately upon referral, only 38% were treated less than 48 hours after onset of weakness. In the Cleveland Veterans Administration Hospital series, 19 of 20 patients who could walk at diagnosis remained ambulatory, while only 11 of 21 paralyzed patients regained some motor strength at the completion of therapy (173).

Radiation therapy is the initial treatment modality for patients with cord compression, with decompressive laminectomy, vertebrectomy and stabilization being reserved for patients who fail to show prompt neurologic response to irradiation or in whom there is no histological proof of malignancy (19, 32). Surgery may be the only therapeutic alternative when compression occurs in an area previously irradiated to spinal cord tolerance (160, 219). High dose dexamethasone, at least 16 mg per day, is usually administered to decrease spinal cord edema (218).

Most radiation regimens call for a total dose in the range of 3000–4000 cGy, depending upon fractionation (32). High doses per fraction (400–500 cGy) can be initially administered, followed by 300 cGy to total doses of 3000 cGy, at cord tolerance levels (170, 171). Some prefer to continue at 400–500 cGy fractions with a lower total dose of 2000 cGy with lymphomas. This regimen yields the same results as more protracted fractionation ones (1). The radiation portal usually includes the compression level as determined by myelogram, CT or MRI scanning, plus a two vertebral body margin superiorly and inferiorly (228).

Satisfactory treatment outcome is usually measured by the patient's ability to ambulate and to retain sphincter control for at least 3 months following irradiation. Such results can be obtained in up to 90% of Hodgkin's and non-Hodgkin's lymphoma patients (1, 129) and in approximately one-third of breast and prostate primaries. Results with lung carcinoma, hypernephroma, and sarcomas are generally discouraging (32). As mentioned above, pretreatment motor function seems to be the single most important factor in predicting neurological outcome (135, 186).

References

1. Aabo K, Walbom-Jorgensen S. Central nervous system complications by malignant lymphomas: radiation schedule and treatment results. Int J Radiat Oncol Biol Phys 1986;12:197–202.
2. Abbatucci JS, Delozier T, Quint R, Roussel A, Brune D. Radiation myelopathy of the cervical spinal cord: time, dose and volume factors. Int J Radiat Oncol Biol Phys 1978;4:239–248.
3. Ackman JD, Rouse L, Johnston CE 2nd. Radiation induced physeal injury. Orthopedics 1988;11:343–349.
4. Akel G, Benard P, Canal P, Soula G. Distribution and tumor penetration properties of a radiosensitizer 2-[14C] misonidazole (Ro 07-0582), in mice and rats as studied by whole-body autoradiography. Cancer Chemother Pharmacol 1986;17:121–6.
5. Akman SA, Block JB. Neurologic complications of systemic cancer. Prim Care 1984;11:597–623.
6. Allen KL, Johnson TW, Hibbs GG. Effective bone palliation as related to various treatment regimens. Cancer 1976;37:984–987.
7. Alper T, Howard-Flanders P. Role of oxygen in modifying the radiosensitivity of E. coli B. Nature 1956;178:978–979.
8. Ang KK, Thames HD Jr, van der Kogel AJ, van der Schueren E. Is the rate of repair of radiation-induced sublethal damage in rat spinal cord dependent on the size of dose per fraction? Int J Radiat Oncol Biol Phys 1987;13:557–562.
9. Ang KK, van der Kogel AJ, van der Schueren E. Lack of evidence for increased tolerance of rat spinal cord with decreasing fraction doses below 2 Gy. Int J Radiat Oncol Biol Phys 1985;11:105–110.
10. Ang KK, van der Kogel AJ, Van Dam J, van der Schueren E. The kinetics of repair of sublethal damage in the rat cervical spinal cord during fractionated irradiations. Radiother Oncol 1984;1:247–253.
11. Ang KK, Thames HD, Jones SD, et al. Proliferation kinetics of a murine fibrosarcoma during fractionated irradiation. Radiat Res 1988;116:327–336.
12. Aoki V. Radiotherapy of medulloblastoma combined with OK-432 (picibanil): utilization of its alleviating action on radiation induced myelosupression. Nippon Gan Chiryo Gakkai Shi 1986;21:1376–1385.
13. Arguello F, Baggs RB, Duerst RE, Johnstone L, McQueen K, Frantz CN. Pathogenesis of vertebral metastasis and epidural spinal cord compression. Cancer 1990;65:98–106.
14. Aristizabal S, Caldwell WL, Avila J, et al. Relationship of time dose factors to tumor control and complications in the treatment of Cushing's disease by irradiation. Int J Radiat Oncol Biol Phys 1977;2:47–54.
15. Aur R, Hustu HO, Simone J. Leukoencephalopathy in children with acute lymphocytic leukemia receiving preventive contral nervous system therapy. Proc Am Soc Clin Oncol 1976;17:97.
16. Austin-Seymour MM, Munzenrider JE, Goitein M, et al. Progress in low-LET heavy particle therapy: intracranial and paracranial tumors and uveal melanomas. Radiat Res 1985;104(suppl):S219–226.
17. Austin-Seymour M, Munzenrider J, Goitein M, et al. Fractionated proton radiation therapy of chordoma and low-grade chondrosarcoma of the base of skull. J Neurosurg 1989;70:13–17.
18. Azzarelli A, Quagliuolo V, Cerasoli S, Zucali R, Bignami P, Mazzaferro V, Dossena G, Gennari L. Chordoma: natural history and treatment results in 33 cases. J Surg Oncol 1988;37:185–191.
19. Barcena A, Lobato RD, Rivas JJ, Cordobes F, de Castro S, Cabrera A, Lamas E. Spinal metastatic disease: analysis of factors determining functional prognosis and the choice of treatment. Neurosurgery 1984;15:820–827.

20. Barone BM, Elvidge AR. Ependymomas. A clinical survey. J Neurosurg 1970;33:428–438.

21. Battermann JJ, Mijnheer BJ. The Amsterdam fast neutron therapy project: a final report. Int J Radiat Oncol Biol Phys 1986;12:2093–2099.

22. Baverstock KF, Burns WG. Primary production of oxygen from irradiated water as an explanation for decreased radiobiological enhancement at high LET. Nature 1976;260:316–318.

23. Becquerel H, Curie P. Action physiologique des rayons du radium. C R Acad Sci (III) 1901;132:1289–1291.

24. Bendersky M, Lewis M, Mandelbaum DE, Stanger C. Serial neuropsychological follow-up of a child following craniospinal irradiation. Dev Med Child Neurol 1988;30:816–820.

25. Bentzen SM, Thames HD, Travis EL, Ang KK, van der Schueren E, Dewit L, Dixon DO. Direct estimation of latent time for radiation injury in late-responding normal tissues: gut, lung, and spinal cord. Int J Radiat Biol 1989;55:27–43.

26. Berlit P, Harle M, Johann A. Cervical radiation myelopathy with spastic paraparesis of the arms. Case report and a review of the literature. Nervenarzt 1987;58:40–46.

27. Berlit P. Radiation myelopathy. Clinical analysis of the disease picture. Schriftenr Neurol 1987;27:1–116.

28. Berson AM, Castro JR, Petti P, et al. Charged particle irradiation of chordoma and chondrosarcoma of the base of skull and cervical spine: the Lawrence Berkeley Laboratory experience. Int J Radiat Oncol Biol Phys 1988;15:559–565.

29. Bleyer WA, Griffin TW. White matter necrosis, mineralizing microangiopathy, and intellectual abilities in survivors of childhood leukemia: associations with central nervous system irradiation and methotrexate therapy. In: Gilbert HA, Kagan AR, eds. Radiation damage to the nervous system. NY: Raven Press, 1980:155–174.

30. Blitzer P. Reanalysis of the RTOG study of the palliation of symptomatic bone metastasis. Cancer 1985;55:1468–1472.

31. Bloomer WD, Adelstein SJ. The mammalian radiation survival curve. J Nucl Med 1982;23:259–265.

32. Bruckman JE, Bloomer WD. Management of spinal cord compression. Semin Oncol 1978;5:135–140.

33. Budach V, Bamberg M, Sack H, Rauhut F, Rassow J. Neutron therapy of low grade "pencil" gliomas of the spinal cord: a review of ten cases. Strahlenther Onkol 1989;165:315–319.

34. Bukovitz AG, Deutsch M, Slayton R. Orthogonal fields: variations in dose vs gap size for treatment of the central nervous system. Radiology 1978;126:795–798.

35. Burini G, Cassinari V, Giuliani G, et al. Theoretical study for use of Leksell's stereotactic frame in radiosurgery. J Neurosurg Sci 1989;33:131–133.

36. Burns RJ, Jones AN, Robertson JS. Pathology of radiation myelopathy. J Neurol Neurosurg Psychiatry 1972;35:888–898.

37. Bydder GM, Brown J, Niendorf HP, Young IR. Enhancement of cervical intraspinal tumors in MR imaging with intravenous gadolinium-DTPA. J Comput Assist Tomogr 1985;9:847–851.

38. Casentini L, Visona A, Colombo F, et al. Osteogenic sarcoma of the calvaria following radiotherapy for cerebellar astrocytoma: report of a case in childhood. Tumori 1985;71:391–396.

39. Castro JR, Collier JM, Petti PL, et al. Charged particle radiotherapy for lesions encircling the brain stem or spinal cord. Int J Radiat Oncol Biol Phys 1989;17:477–484.

40. Castro JR, Reimers MM. Charged particle radiotherapy of selected tumors in the head and neck. Int J Radiat Oncol Biol Phys 1988;14:711–720.

41. Cohen L, Ten Haken RK, Mansell J, Yalavarthi SD, Hendrickson FR, Awschalom M. Tolerance of the human spinal cord to high energy p(66)Be(49) neutrons. Int J Radiat Oncol Biol Phys 1985;11:743–749.

42. Cohen L, Hendrickson F, Kurup PD, et al. Clinical evaluation of neutron beam therapy. Current results and prospects. Cancer 1985;55:10–17.

43. Coia L, Chu J, Larsen R, Myerson R. Spinal cord protection during radiation therapy. Int J Radiat Oncol Biol Phys 1986;12:1697–1705.

44. Coleman CN. Hypoxia in tumors: a paradigm for the approach to biochemical and physiologic heterogeneity. J Natl Cancer Inst 1988;80:310–317.

45. Colombo F, Benedetti A, Pozza F, Marchetti C, Chierego G. Linear accelerator radiosurgery of cerebral arteriovenous malformations. Neurosurgery 1989;24:833–840.

46. Concannon JP, Summers RE, King J, et al. Enhancement of x-ray effects on the small intestinal epithelium of dogs by Actinomycin D. Radiology 1969:105:126–134.

47. Cooper PR, Epstein F. Radical resection of intramedullary spinal cord tumors in adults. Recent experience in 29 patients. J Neurosurg 1985;63:492–449.

48. Coughlin CT, Richmond RC. Biologic and clinical developments of cisplatin combined with radiation: concepts, utility, projections for new trials and the emergence of carboplatin. Seminars Oncol 1989;16(suppl 6):31–43.

49. Coutard H. Roentgentherapy of epitheliomas of the tonsillar fossa, hypopharynx and larynx from 1920 to 1926. Am J Roentgenol 1932;28:313–331.

50. Coutard H. Principles of x ray therapy of malignant diseases. Lancet 1934;ii:1–8.

51. Cullen BM, Walker HC. The effect of several different anesthetics on the blood pressure and heart rate of the mouse and on the radiation response of the mouse sarcoma RIF-1. Int J Radiat Biol 1985;48:761–71.

52. D'Angio GJ, Farber S, Maddock CL. Potentiation of x-ray effect of Actinomycin D. Radiology 1975;73:175–177.

53. D'Angio GJ. The late consequences of successful treatment given children and adolescents. Radiology 1975;114:145.

54. Delattre JY, Rosenblum MK, Thaler HT, Mandell L, Shapiro WR, Posner JB. A model of radiation myelopathy in the rat. Pathology, regional capillary permeability changes and treatment with dexamethasone. Brain 1988;111:1319–1336.

55. Deutsch M, Green SB, Strike TA, et al. Results of a randomized trial comparing BCNU plus radiotherapy, streptozotocin plus radiotherapy, BCNU plus hyperfractionated radiotherapy, and BCNU following misonidazole plus radiotherapy in the postoperative treatment of malignant glioma. Int J Radiat Oncol Biol Phys 1989;16:1389–96.

56. Dewey WC, Hopwood LE, Sapareto, SA et al. Cellular responses to combinations of hyperthermia and radiation. Radiology 1977;123:463.

57. Dewhirst MW, Tso CY, Oliver R, et al. Morphologic and hemodynamic comparison of tumor and healing normal tissue microvasculature. Int J Radiat Oncol Biol Phys 1989;17:91–99.

58. Dewit L. Combined treatment of radiation and cisdiaminedicholoroplatinum (II): a review of experimental and clinical data. Int J Radiat Oncol Biol Phys 1987;13:403–426.

59. Dische S, Saunders MI, Warburton MF. Hemoglobin, radiation, morbidity and survival. Int J Radiat Oncol Biol Phys 1986;12:1335–1337.

60. Dixon-Brown A, Hopewell JW. The calculation of absorbed doses for radiobiological studies involving the use of small irradiation fields. Br J Radiol 1988;61:261–263.

61. Dorie MJ, Kallman RF. Reoxygenation in the RIF-1 tumor. Int J Radiat Oncol Biol Phys 1984;10:687–693.

62. Eifel PJ. Decreased bone growth arrest in weanling rats with multiple radiation fractions per day. Int J Radiat Oncol Biol Phys 1988;15:141–145.

63. Elkind MM. DNA damage and cell killing: cause and effect? Cancer 1985;56:2351–2363.

64. Elkind MM, Sutton H. Radiation response of mammalian cells

grown in culture. I. Repair of x-ray damage in surviving Chinese hamster cells. Radiat Res 1960;13:556–593.

65. Ellis F. Dose, time and fractionation: A clinical hypothesis. Clin Radiol 1969;20:1–7.

66. Ellis F. Is NSD-TDF useful to radiotherapy? Int J Radiat Oncol Biol Phys 1985;11:1685–1697.

67. Fabrikant JI, Lyman JT, Frankel KA. Heavy charged-particle Bragg peak radiosurgery for intracranial vascular disorders. Radiat Res (Suppl) 1985;8:S244–58.

68. Fazekas J, Pajak TF, Wasserman T, et al. Failure of misonidazole sensitized radiotherapy to impact upon outcome among stage III-IV squamous cancers of the head and neck. Int J Radiat Oncol Biol Phys 1987;13:1155–1160.

69. Fischer H, Hartmann GH, Sturm V, et al. In vitro model for the response to irradiation of different types of human intracranial tumours. Acta Neurochir (Wien) 1987;85:46–9.

70. Fletcher GH. Implications of the density of clonogenic infestation in radiotherapy. Int J Radiat Oncol Biol Phys 1986;12:1675–1680.

71. Fletcher GH. Subclinical disease. Cancer 1984;53:1274–1284.

72. Forbes AR, Goldberg ID. Radiation therapy in the treatment of meningioma: the Joint Center for Radiation Therapy experience 1970 to 1982. J Clin Oncol 1984;2:1139–43.

73. Franke HD, Schmidt R. Clinical results with fast neutrons (DT, 14 MV). Radiat Med 1985;3:151–160.

74. Freeman CR, Krischer J, Sanford RA, Burger PC, Cohen M, Norris D. Hyperfractionated radiotherapy in brain stem tumors: results of a Pediatric Oncology Group study. Int J Radiat Oncol Biol Phys 1988;15:311–8.

75. Friedman M, Kim TH, Panahon AM. Spinal cord compression in malignant lymphoma. Cancer 1976;37:1485–1491.

76. Fromm M, Littman P, Raney RB, Nelson L, Handler S, Diamond G, Stanley C. Late effects after treatment of twenty children with soft tissue sarcomas of the head and neck. Experience at a single institution with review of the literature. Cancer 1986;57:2070–2076.

77. Front D, Scheneck SO, Frankel A, et al. Bone metastases and bone pain in breast cancer. JAMA 1979;42:1747–1748.

78. Fulton DS, Urtasun RC, Shin KH, et al. Misonidazole combined with hyperfractionation in the management of malignant glioma. Int J Radiat Oncol Biol Phys 1984;10:1709–12.

79. Galasko CSB. The management of skeletal metastases. J R Coll Surg Edinb 1980;3:148–151.

80. Garcia DM. Primary spinal cord tumors treated with surgery and postoperative irradiation. Int J Radiat Oncol Biol Phys 1985;11:1933–1939.

81. Gerweck LE, Kornblith PL, Burlett P et al. Radiation sensitivity of cultured human glioblastoma cells. Radiology 1977;125:231–234.

82. Geyer JR, Taylor EM, Milstein JM, et al. Radiation, methotrexate, and white matter necrosis: laboratory evidence for neural radioprotection with preirradiation methotrexate. Int J Radiat Oncol Biol Phys 1988;15:373–5.

83. Giovanella BC, Stehlin JS, Morgan AC. Selective lethal effect of supranormal temperatures on human neoplastic cells. Cancer Res 1976;36:3944.

84. Gonzalez DG, Breuer K. Clinical data from irradiated growing long bones in children. Int J Radiat Oncol Biol Phys 1985;9:841–846.

85. Gray LH, Conger AD, Ebert M, et al. The concentration of oxygen dissolved in tissues at the time of irradiation as a factor in radiotherapy. Br J Radiol 1953;26:638.

86. Greenberg HS, Chandler WF, Diaz RF, et al. Intra-arterial bromodeoxyuridine radiosensitization and radiation in treatment of malignant astrocytomas. J Neurosurg 1988;69:500–5.

87. Greenwood J. Intramedullary tumors of the spinal cord. J Neurosurg 1963;20:665–668.

88. Griem ML. Treatment of malignant gliomas with neutron radiation. Neurol Clin 1985;3:895–900.

89. Griem ML. Radiation therapy treatment planning for tumors of the central nervous system. Front Radiat Ther Oncol 1987;21:221–35.

90. Griffin BR, Shuman WP, Wisbeck W, Berger M, Spence A. Improved localization of infratentorial ependymoma by magnetic resonance imaging: implications for radiation treatment planning. J Neurooncol 1988;6:147–155.

91. Guidetti B. Intramedullary tumors of the spinal cord. Acta Neurochir 1967;17:7–23.

92. Gutin PH, Leibel SA, Wara WM, et al. Recurrent malignant gliomas: survival following interstitial brachytherapy with high-activity iodine-125 sources. J Neurosurg 1987;67:864–873.

93. Hall EJ. Radiobiology for the radiologist. Chapter 2: Cell survival curves. 3rd ed. Philadelphia: J.B. Lippincott Co., 1988.

94. Hall EJ. Radiobiology for the radiologist. Chapter 5: Radiosensitivity and cell age in the mitotic cycle. 3rd ed. Philadelphia: J.B. Lippincott Co., 1988.

95. Hall EJ. Radiobiology for the radiologist. Chapter 7: The oxygen effect and reoxygenation. 3rd ed. Philadelphia: J.B. Lippincott Co., 1988.

96. Harries B. Spinal cord compression. Br Med J 1970;1:611–614.

97. Harries B. Spinal cord compression II. Br Med J 1970;1:673–676.

98. Hartsell WF, Hanson WR, Conterato DJ, Hendrickson FR. Hyperfractionation decreases the deleterious effects of conventional radiation fractionation on vertebral growth in animals. Cancer 1989;63:2452–2455.

99. Hawkins MM, Draper GJ, Kingston E. Incidence of second primary tumors among childhood cancer survivors. Br J Cancer 1987;56:339–347.

100. Henk JM. Does hyperbaric oxygen have a future in radiation therapy? Int J Radiat Oncol Biol Phys 1981;7:1125.

101. Herber SM, Kay R, May R, Milner RD. Growth of long term survivors of childhood malignancy. Acta Paediatr Scand 1985;74:438–41.

102. Hirst DG. Anemia: a problem or an opportunity in radiotherapy? Int J Radiat Oncol Biol Phys 1986;12:2009–2017.

103. Hofer KG, Lakkis M, Hofer MG. Cytocidal effects of misonidazole, RO-03-8799 and RSU-1164 on euoxic and hypoxic BP-8 murine sarcoma cells at normal and elevated temperatures. Cancer 1989;63:1501–1508.

104. Hopewell JW, Morris AD, Dixon-Brown A. The influence of field size on the late tolerance of the rat spinal cord to single doses of X-rays. Br J Radiol 1987;60:1099–108.

105. Howland WJ, Loeffler RK, Starchman DE, Johnson RB. Post irradiation atrophic changes of bone and related complications. Radiology 1975;117:677–685.

106. Ishikawa T, Iwasaki Y, Isu T, et al. Spinal intramedullary tumor with exophytic growth. No Shinkei Geka 1988;16:1339–1345.

107. Ito H, Meistrich ML, Barkley T Jr, Thames HD, Milas L. Protection of acute and late radiation damage of the gastrointestinal tract by WR-2721. Int J Radiat Oncol Biol Phys 1986;12:211–219.

108. Ito H, Barkely T Jr, Peters LJ, Milas L. Modification of tumor response to cyclophosphamide and irradiation by preirradiation of the tumor bed. Prolonged growth delay but reduced curability. Int J Radiat Oncol Biol Phys 1985;11:547–553.

109. Jackson D, Kinsella T, Rowland J, et al. Halogenated pyrimidines as radiosensitizers in the treatment of glioblastoma multiforme. Am J Clin Oncol 1987;10:437–43.

110. Jacobs SK, Kornblith PL, Wilson DT et al. *In vitro* killing of human glioblastoma by interleukin-2 activiated autologous lymphocytes. J Neurosurg 1986;64:114–117.

111. Jacobsson M, Kalebo P, Tjellstrom A, Turesson I. Bone cell viability after irradiation. An enzyme histochemical study. Acta Oncol 1987;26:463–465.

112. Jones A. Transient radiation myelopathy—reference to L'Hermitte's sign of electrical paresthesia. Br J Radiol 1964;37:727–744.

113. Kallman RF. The phenomenon of reoxygenation and its implications for fractionated radiotherapy. Radiology 1972;105:135–142.

114. Kim YH, Fayos JV. Radiation tolerance of the cervical cord. Radiology 1981;139:473–478.

115. Knerich R, Butti G, Pezzotta S, et al. Chemotherapy of malignant brain tumors in childhood. Minerva Med 1984;75:1441–4.

116. Kopelson G, Linggood RM. Intramedullary spinal cord astrocytoma versus glioblastoma. The prognostic importance of histologic grade. Cancer 1982;50:732–735.

117. Kopelson G, Linggood RM, Kleinman GM, Doucette J, Wang CC. Management of intramedullary spinal cord tumors. Radiology 1980;135:473–479.

118. Kramer S, Southard MF, Mansfield CM. Radiation effect and tolerance of the central nervous system. Front Radiat Ther Oncol 1972;6:322–345.

119. Laramore GE, Blasko JC, Griffin TW, Groudine MT, Parker RG. Fast neutron teletherapy for advanced carcinomas of the oropharynx. Int J Radiat Oncol Biol Phys 1979;5:1821–1827.

120. Leong J, Shimm D. A method for consistent precision radiation therapy. Radiother Oncol 1985;3:89–92.

121. Levin VA, Rodriguez LA, Edwards MS, et al. Treatment of medulloblastoma with procarbazine, hydroxyurea, and reduced radiation doses to whole brain and spine. J Neurosurg 1988;68:383–387.

122. Levy RP, Fabrikant JI, Frankel KA, Phillips MH, Lyman JT: Stereotactic heavy-charged-particle Bragg peak radiosurgery for the treatment of intracranial arteriovenous malformations in childhood and adolescence. Neurosurgery 1989;24:841–852.

123. Linstadt DE, Wara WM, Leibel SA, Gutin PH, Wilson CB, Sheline GE. Postoperative radiotherapy of primary spinal cord tumors. Int J Radiat Oncol Biol Phys 1989;16:1397–1403.

124. Looney WB, Hopkins HA, Carter WH. Solid tumor models for the assessment of different treatment modalities. XXII. The alternate utilization of radiotherapy and chemotherapy. Cancer 1984;54:416–425.

125. Lordo CD. Stroude EC, Del Maestro RF. The effects of dexamethasone on C6 astrocytoma radiosensitivity. J Neurosurg 1989;70:767–73.

126. Lund E, Hamborg-Pedersen B. Computed tomography of the brain following prophylactic treatment with irradiation therapy and intraspinal methotrexate in children with acute lymphoblastic leukemia. Neuroradiology 1984;26:351–358.

127. Lunsford LD, Deutsch M, Yoder V. Stereotactic interstitial brachytherapy—current concepts and concerns in twenty patients. Appl Neurophysiol 1985;48:117–120.

128. Lunsford LD, Flickinger J, Lindner G, Maitz A. Stereotactic radiosurgery of the brain using the first United States 201 cobalt-60 source gamma knife. Neurosurgery 1989;24:151–9.

129. Lyding JM, Tseng A, Newman A, Collins S, Shea W. Intramedullary spinal cord metastasis in Hodgkin's disease. Rapid diagnosis and treatment resulting in neurologic recovery. Cancer 1987;60:1741–4.

130. Lyman JT, Kanstein L, Yeater F, Fabrikant JI, Frankel KA. A helium-ion beam for stereotactic radiosurgery of central nervous system disorders. Med Phys 1986;13:695–699.

131. Makin WP. Treatment of spinal cord compression due to malignant disease. Proc Br Inst Radiol 1989;61:715.

132. Maor MH, Fields RS, Hogstrom KR, van Eys J. Improving the therapeutic ratio of craniospinal irradiation in medulloblastoma. Int J Radiat Oncol Biol Phys 1985;11:687–697.

133. Marks JE, Adler SJ. A comparative study of ependymomas by site of origin. Int J Radiat Oncol Biol Phys 1982;8:37–43.

134. Marsa GW, Goffinet DR, Rubinstein LR, et al. Megavoltage irradiation in the treatment of gliomas of the brain and spinal cord. Cancer 1975;36:1681–1689.

135. Martenson JA Jr, Evans RG, Lie MR, et al. Treatment outcome and complications in patients treated for malignant epidural spinal cord compression (SCC). J Neurooncol 1985;3:77–84.

136. McCunniff AJ, Liang MJ. Radiation tolerance of the cervical spinal cord. Int J Radiat Oncol Biol Phys 1989;16:675–8.

137. McNaney D, Lindberg RD, Ayala A, et al. Fifteen year radiotherapy experience with chondrosarcoma of bone. Int J Radiat Oncol Biol Phys 1982;8:187–190.

138. Medical Research Council Working Party. Radiotherapy and hyperbaric oxygen. Lancet 1978;2:881–884.

139. Michalevicz R, Burnstein A, Razon N, Reider I, Ilie B. Spinal epidural compression in chronic lymphocytic leukemia. Cancer 1989;64:1961–1964.

140. Milas L, Ito H , Hunter N, Jones S, Peters LJ. Retardation of tumor growth in mice caused by radiation induced injury of tumor bed stroma: dependency on tumor type. Cancer Res 1986;46:723–727.

141. Milas L, Hunter N, Peters LJ. Tumor bed effect: induced reduction of tumor radiocurability through the increase ion hypoxic cell fraction. Int J Radiat Oncol Biol Phys 1989;16:139–142.

142. Milas L, Hunter N, Peters LJ. The tumor bed effect: dependence of tumor take, growth rate and metastasis on the time interval between irradiation and tumor cell transplantation. Int J Radiat Oncol Biol Phys 1987;13:379–383.

143. Miyoshi T, Saito M, Arimizu N, Akiyama S. Modifying effects of interferon on the growth of irradiated sarcoma 180 cells in vitro. Nippon Igaku Hoshasen Gakki Zasshi 1984;44:88–92.

144. Moorthy CR, Hahn EW, Kim JH, et al. Improved response of a murine fibrosarcoma (Meth-A) to interstitial radiation when combined with hyperthermia. Int J Radiat Oncol Biol Phys 1984;10:2145–2148.

145. Munro P, Mair WGP. Radiation effects on human central nervous system fourteen weeks after x-radiation. Acta Neuropath (Berlin) 1968;11:267–274.

146. Nagatani M, Ikeda T, Otsuki H, et al. Sellar fibrosarcoma following radiotherapy for prolactinoma. No Shinkei Geka 1984;12:339–346.

147. Neuhauser EBD, Wittenborg MH, Bergman CZ, Cohen J. Irradiation effects of roentgen therapy in the growing spine. Radiology 1952;59:637–650.

148. Orton CG, Ellis F. A simplification in the use of the NSD concept in practical radiotherapy. Br J Radiol 1973;46:529–537.

149. Pages A, Pages M, Ramos J, Benezech J. Radiation-induced intracranial fibrochondrosarcoma. J Neurol 1986;233:309–310.

150. Palmer JJ. Radiation myelopathy. Brain 1972;95:109–122.

151. Penn CRH. Single dose and fractionated palliative irradiation for osseous metastasis. Clin Radiol 1976;27:405–408.

152. Peschel RE, Fischer JJ. Optimization of the time-dose relationship. Semin Oncol 1981;8:38–48.

153. Peters LJ, Schultheiss T, Maor MH. Tolerance of human spinal cord to high energy neutrons [letter]. Int J Radiat Oncol Biol Phys 1986;12:292–293.

154. Peters LJ, Brock WA, Johnson T, et al. Potential methods for predicting tumor radiocurability. Int J Radiat Oncol Biol Phys 1986;12:459–467.

155. Pfahler G. The treatment of skin cancers with x-rays. Am X-ray J 1901;9:980–983.

156. Phillips TL, Buschke F. Radiation tolerance of the spinal cord. Am J Roentgenol 1969;105:659–664.

157. Phillips TL, Wasserman TH, Johnson RJ, et al. Final report on the United States Phase I trial of the hypoxic cell radiosensitizer misonidazole. Cancer 1981;48:1697.

158. Phillips TL, Rolmach RJ. Repair of potentially lethal damage in x-irradiated HeLa cells. Radiat Res 1966;29:413.

159. Portenoy RK, Galer BS, Salamon O, et al. Identification of epidural neoplasm. Radiography and bone scintigraphy in the symptomatic and asymptomatic spine. Cancer 1989;64:2207–2213.

160. Posner J. Management of spinal cord compression. Clin Bull 1971;1:65–71.

161. Pozza F, Colombo F, Chierego G, et al. Low-grade astrocytomas:

treatment with unconventionally fractionated external beam stereotactic radiation therapy. Radiology 1989;171:565–9.

162. Puck TT, Morkovin D, Marcus PI, et al. Action of x-rays on mammalian cells. II. Survival curves of cells from normal human tissues. J Exp Med 1957;106:483–500.

163. Puck TT, Marcus PI. Action of X-rays on mammalian cells. J Exp Med 1956;103:653.

164. Redpath JL, Colman M. The effect of Adriamycin and Actinomycin D on radiation-induced skin reactions in mouse feet. Int J Radiat Oncol Biol Phys 1979;5:483–486.

165. Rich TA, Schiller A, Suit HD, Mankin JH. Clinical and pathologic review of 48 cases of chordoma. Cancer 1985;56:182–187.

166. Richter MP, Coia LR. Palliative radiation therapy. Semin Oncol 1985;12:375–383.

167. Robinson E, Neugut AI, Wylie P. Clinical aspects of postirradiation sarcomas. J Natl Cancer Inst 1988;80:233–240.

168. Roentgen WC. On a new kind of rays (preliminary communication). Physikalische-medicinischen Gesellshaft of Wurzburg, December 28, 1985.

169. Roggli VL, Estraka R, Fechner RE. Thyroid neoplasia following irradiation for medulloblastoma. Cancer 1979;43:2232–2238.

170. Rubin P. Extradural spinal cord compression by tumor. Part I: experimental production and treatment trials. Radiology 1969;93:1243–1248.

171. Rubin P, Mayer E, Poulter C. Extradural spinal cord compression by tumor. Part II: high dose experience without laminectomy. Radiology 1969:93:1248–1260.

172. Rubin P, Whitaker JN, Ceckler TL, et al. Myelin basic protein and magnetic resonance imaging for diagnosing radiation myelopathy. Int J Radiat Oncol Biol Phys 1988;15:1371–81.

173. Ruff RL, Lanska DJ. Epidural metastases in prospectively evaluated veterans with cancer and back pain. Cancer 1989;63:2234–2241.

174. Salazar OM, Rubin P, Hendrickson FR, et al. Single-dose half-body irradiation for palliation of multiple bone metastases from solid tumor. Final Radiation Therapy Oncology Group Report. Cancer 1986;58:29–36.

175. Saunders WM, Chen GT, Austin-Seymour M, et al. Precision high dose radiotherapy. II. Helium ion treatment of tumors adjacent to critical central nervous system structures. Int J Radiat Oncol Biol Phys 1985;11:1399–1347.

176. Schjeide OA, Yamazaki J, Haack K, Ciminelli E, Clemente CD. Biochemical and morphological aspects of radiation inhibition of myelin formation. Acta Radiol Ther Phys Biol 1966;5:185–203.

177. Schultheiss TE, Stephens LC, Maor MH. Analysis of the histopathology of radiation myelopathy. Int J Radiat Oncol Biol Phys 1988;14:27–32.

178. Schultheiss TE, Higgins EM, El-Mahdi AM. The latent period in clinical radiation myelopathy. Int J Radiat Oncol Biol Phys 1984;10:1109–1115.

179. Schwade JG, Wara WM, Sheline GE et al. Management of primary spinal cord tumors. Int J Radiat Oncol Biol Phys 1978;4:389–393.

180. Schwade JG, Wara WM, Sheline GE et al. Management of primary spinal cord tumors. Int J Radiat Oncol Biol Phys 1978;4:389–393.

181. Sersa G, Willingham V, Milas L. Anti-tumor effects of tumor necrosis factor alone or combined with radiotherapy. Int J Cancer 1988;42:129–34.

182. Shalet SM, Gibson B, Swindell R, Pearson D. Effect of spinal irradiation on growth. Arch Dis Child 1987;62:461–4.

183. Shaw EG, Evans RG, Scheithauer BW, Ilstrup DM, Earle JD. Radiotherapeutic management of adult intraspinal ependymomas. Int J Radiat Oncol Biol Phys 1990;12:323–327.

184. Siemann DW, Alliet KL. Combinations of CCNU, MISO and fractionated radiotherapy. Int J Radiat Oncol Biol Phys 1986;12:1379–1382.

185. Siemann DW, Hill SA. Enhanced tumor responses through therapies combining CCNU, Misonidazole and radiation. Int J Radiat Oncol Biol Phys 1984;10:1623–1626.

186. Sorensen PS, Borgensen SE, Rohde K, et al. Metastatic epidural spinal cord compression. Results of treatment and survival. Cancer 1990;65:1502–1508.

187. Spence AM, Krohn KA, Steele JE, Edmondson SE, Rasey JS. WR-2721, WR-77913 and WR-3689 radioprotection in the rat spinal cord. Pharmacol Ther 1988;39:89–91.

188. Spence AM, Krohn KA, Edmondson SE, Steele JE, Rasey JS. Radioprotection in rat spinal cord with WR-2721 following cerebral lateral interventricular injection. Int J Radiat Oncol Biol Phys 1986;12:1479–82.

189. Spiers FW. A review of the theoretical and experimental methods of determining radiation dose in bone. Br J Radiol 1966;39:216–221.

190. Streffer C. Radiobiological bases of time and dose distribution in radiotherapy. Strahlenther Onkol 1988;164:648–52.

191. Suit HD, Gerweck LE. Potential for hyperthermia and radiation therapy. Cancer Res 1979;39:2290–2298.

192. Tatcher M, Glicksman AS. Field matching considerations in craniospinal irradiation. Int J Radiat Oncol Biol Phys 1989;17:865–9.

193. Tate T, Shentall G. Conformation therapy to improve the irradiation of the spinal axis. Int J Radiat Oncol Biol Phys 1989;16:505–10.

194. Thames HD, Hendry JH, Moore JV, Ang KK, Travis EL. The high steepness of dose-response curves for late-responding normal tissues. Radiother Oncol 1989;15:49–53.

195. Thames HD, Ang KK, Stewart FA, van der Schueren E. Does incomplete repair explain the apparent failure of the basic LQ model to predict spinal cord and kidney responses to low doses per fraction? Int J Radiat Biol 1988;54:13–9.

196. Thomlinson RH, Gray LH. The histological structure of some human lung cancers and the possible implications for radiotherapy. Br J Cancer 1955;9:539–549.

197. Tiver K. Treatment of CNS tumours with conventional radiotherapy: the importance of dose & volume factors in tumour control & CNS radiation tolerance. Australas Radiol 1989;33:15–22.

198. Tong D, et al. The palliation of symptomatic osseous metastases—final results of the study by the Radiation Therapy Oncology Group. Cancer 1982;50:893–899.

199. Travis EL, Meistrich ML, Finch-Neimeyer M, et al. Protection by WR-2721 of late functional and biochemical changes in mouse lung after irradiation. Radiat Res 1983;103:219–231.

200. Tucker MA, D'Angio GJ, Boice JD Jr, et al. Bone sarcomas linked to radiotherapy and chemotherapy in children. N Engl J Med 1987;317:588–593.

201. Tugendhaft P, Baleriaux D, Gerard JM, Hildebrand J. Sequential CT scanning in radiation myelopathy. J Neurooncol 1984;2:249–252.

202. Ulmer W. Aspects of the volume effect in the linear-quadratic and cubic model. Strahlenther Onkol 1987;163:123–9.

203. Ushio Y, Abe H, Suzuki J, et al. Evaluation of ACNU alone and combined with tegafur as additions to radiotherapy of the treatment of malignant gliomas—a cooperative clinical trial. No To Shinkei 1985;37:999–1006.

204. Valentino V. Radiosurgery in cerebral tumours and AVM. Acta Neurochir Suppl (Wien) 1988;42:193–197.

205. van der Kogel AJ, Sissingh HA. Effects of intrathecal methotrexate and cytosine arabinoside on the radiation tolerance of the rat spinal cord. Radiother Oncol 1985;4:239–251.

206. van der Kogel AJ. Radiation tolerance of the rat spinal cord—time dose relationships. Radiology 1977;122:505–509.

207. van der Kogel AJ, Raju MR. Tolerance of spinal cord, lung and rectum after fractionated pions and X-rays. Strahlenther Onkol 1989;165:286–289.

208. van der Kogel AJ. Chronic effects of neutrons and charged particles on spinal cord, lung, and rectum. Radiat Res (Suppl) 1985;8:S208–216.

209. van der Schueren E, Landuyt W. Ang KK, van der Kogel AJ. From 2 Gy to 1 Gy per fraction: sparing effect in rat spinal cord? Int J Radiat Oncol Biol Phys 1988;14:297–300.

210. Vuigario G, Kurohara SS, George FW. Association of hemoglobin levels before and during radiotherapy with prognosis in uterine cervix cancer. Radiology 1973;106:649–652.

211. Walton MI, Workman P. Pharmacokinetics and metabolism of the mixed-function hypoxic cell sensitizer prototype RSU 1069 in mice. Cancer Chemother Pharmacol 1988;22:275–281.

212. Wang CC, Blitzer PH, Suit HD. Twice-a-day radiation therapy for cancer of the head and neck. Cancer 1985;55:2100.

213. Wara WM, Sheline GE, Newman H et al. Radiation therapy of meningiomas. Am J Roentgenol 1975;123:1558–1562.

214. Wara WM, Phillips TL, Sheline GE, Schwade JG. Radiation tolerance of the spinal cord. Cancer 1975;35:1558–1562.

215. Wara WM, Edwards MSB, Levin VA, et al. A new treatment regimen for brainstem glioma: a pilot study of the brain tumor research center and children's cancer study group (Abstr). Int J Radiat Oncol Biol Phys 1986;(Suppl 1):143–144.

216. Weichselbaum RR, Beckett M. The maximum recovery potential of human tumor cells may predict clinical outcome in radiotherapy. Int J Radiat Oncol Biol Phys 1987;13:709–713.

217. Weishselbaum RR, Epstein J, Little JB et al. Inherent cellular radiosensitivity of human tumors of varying clinical curability. Am J Roentgenol 1976;172:1027–1032.

218. Weissman DE. Glucocorticoid treatment for brain metastasis and epidural spinal cord compression. A review. J Clin Oncol 1988;6:543–551.

219. White WA, Patterson RH, Bergland RM. Role of surgery in the treatment of spinal cord compression by metastatic neoplasm. Cancer 1971;27:558–561.

220. Woo SY, Donaldson SS, Cox RS. Astrocytoma in children: 14 years' experience at Stanford University Medical Center. J Clin Oncol 1988;6:1001–1007.

221. Wood EH, Berne AS, Traveras JM. The value of radiation therapy in the management of intrinsic tumors of the spinal cord. Radiology 1954;63:11–22.

222. Wu A, Sternick ES, Shahabi S, Zwicker RD. A technique for delivering uniform dose at the junction of two spinal fields. Br J Radiol 1986;59:929–930.

223. Yaes RJ, Kalend A. Local stem cell depletion model for radiation myelitis. Int J Radiat Oncol Biol Phys 1988;14:1247–1259.

224. Yaes RJ, Kalend A. Local stem cell depletion model for radiation myelitis. Mathl Comput Modelling 1988;11:1041–1046.

225. Yaes RJ. Linear-quadratic model isoeffect relations for proliferating tumor cells for treatment with multiple fractions per day. Int J Radiat Oncol Biol Phys 1989;17:901–905.

226. Yamada S, Hoshi A, Takai Y, et al. Radiation tolerance dose of the spinal cord following conventionally fractionated irradiation. Gan No Rinsho 1987;33:1189–1192.

227. Zamorano L, Katanick D, Dujovny M, Yaker D, Malik G, Ausman JI. Tumour recurrence vs radionecrosis: an indication for multitrajectory serial stereotactic biopsies. Acta Neurochir Suppl (Wien) 1989;46:90–93.

228. Zevallos M, Chan PYM, Munoz L, Wagner J, Kagan AR. Epidural spinal cord compression from metastatic tumor. Int J Radiat Oncol Biol Phys 1987;13:875–878.

52

Cervical Spinal Arteriovenous Malformations

Van V. Halbach, Grant B. Hieshima and Charles B. Wilson

Arteriovenous malformations (AVMs) located in the region of the cervical spinal can be subdivided into several anatomic categories and can present with a wide variety of signs and symptoms that may be manifested distant to the site of the vascular pathology. Recent advances in imaging technology and neurosurgical technique have greatly improved the diagnosis and treatment of these complicated lesions. Although several imaging modalities have been used to detect arteriovenous malformations and fistulas in this region, no single modality has emerged as the screening modality for all of these disorders.

Intramedullary Vascular Malformations

These malformations are located partially or totally within the spinal cord substance and are generally supplied by enlarged anterior spinal arteries, posterior spinal arteries, and medullary vessels. AVMs in the cervical region constitute 5–13% of all spinal cord AVMs (1). Compared with thoracic and lumbar region AVMs, cervical AVMs tend to occur in younger patients and to have a higher incidence of subarachnoid hemorrhage. In a recent review of spinal cord AVMs, it was reported that the mean age at the onset of symptoms was between the second and third decade and that the majority of patients presented with hemorrhage (2). Nearly half of the patients had associated aneurysms in either the feeding spinal arteries or the draining veins (2). The hemorrhage can involve the spinal cord substance and produce abrupt neurologic decline and even complete spinal cord transection; less commonly, a ruptured arterial or venous aneurysm can produce subarachnoid hemorrhage without hemorrhage into the spinal cord substance. Clinically, these hemorrhages can be differentiated from those caused by rupture of an intracerebral aneurysm by the localized onset of neck or back pain. Patients suffering repeat episodes of hemorrhage have a much poorer prognosis (3, 4). The nidus of the AVM can be compact within the spinal cord substance and is generally referred to as a glomus-type; if the nidus is diffusely infiltrated within the spinal cord parenchyma, it is referred to as a juvenile-type (2).

Radiologic Evaluation

Plain Films

These studies are generally unremarkable unless a large arteriovenous fistula has caused local bone erosion.

Magnetic Resonance Imaging

Because the malformation is surrounded by the spinal cord substance, magnetic resonance (MR) imaging is an excellent screening modality (5). On both T1 and T2 images, the nidus of the malformation can be identified within the spinal cord substance as an area of signal void (decreased signal). Adjacent hemorrhage and myelomalacia can be seen as well. Both thin sections and cardiac-gated scans should be obtained for optimum delineation of the malformation. Chronic hemorrhage can be visualized optimally with gradient refocusing techniques.

Computerized Tomography

Computerized tomography (CT) performed with intravenous iodinated contrast material can often show enhancement within the cord at the level of the malformation. There is a report of spinal myoclonus and clinical deterioration after the intravenous administration of contrast material in a patient with a spinal cord AVM, presumably caused by leakage of contrast material into the surrounding cord parenchyma through a defective spinal cord-blood barrier (6).

Myelography

Myelography has been used in the past to evaluate spinal cord AVMs and commonly shows a focal cord enlargement, enlarged feeding arteries, and dilated medullary veins draining the fistula.

Arteriography

Although MR imaging is now the screening method of choice in this disease, selective spinal angiography remains essential for complete evaluation (7). It is important to use selective injections involving multiple spinal arteries to delineate the entire extent of the malformation. Oblique and lateral projections are useful to establish the relation of the vascular supply to the spinal cord; angiotomography can also be used to locate the feeding arteries in relationship to the spinal cord. Rapid filming is imperative to identify feeding arterial aneurysms and draining venous aneurysms (8).

Several groups have reported that intraarterial digital subtraction angiography is an effective modality for the evaluation of spinal cord AVMs (9–11). On arteriograms, the feeding arteries have an increased diameter and tortuosity. The majority of the arterial supply generally arises from the anterior spinal artery and only rarely arises from the posterior spinal arteries. In the cervical spinal region it is important to inject selectively both vertebral arteries and the costocervical and thyrocervical trunks. If the malformation is located in the lower cervical spine, recruitment from supreme intercostal and upper thoracic intercostal arteries can also occur. Venous drainage occurs through dilated medullary veins to radicular veins and sometimes to the epidural plexus. It is occasionally difficult to distinguish hemangioblastoma from intramedullary AVMs.

Treatment

Treatment of these complex malformations falls into three categories: neurosurgical clipping of the feeding arteries or excision of the malformations, endovascular embolization, and combined therapies. While advances in microsurgical technique have greatly facilitated the excision of these malformations, the location of the lesion within the spinal cord substance sometimes makes surgical excision a formidable task (12). There have been rare reports in which the feeding arteries were ligated or cauterized (13, 14), but the desired goal of surgery remains complete excision of the malformation (15). Intraoperative ultrasonography can be used to localize the nidus (16), and spinal cord evoked potentials have also been used as an adjunct during neurosurgical procedures (17).

EMBOLIZATION AND SURGICAL EXCISION

Combined preoperative embolization followed by neurosurgical excision has been reported (18). Preoperative embolization can reduce the pressure within the nidus and can also occlude surgically inaccessible arterial supply to the malformation (18). Embolization has also been advocated as a sole treatment (19–21). Because the supply to the malformation generally arises from spinal arteries, it is imperative that the embolic agent passes through the anterior or posterior spinal cord supply and lodges within the malformation itself without occluding draining veins or important medullary perforators. The majority of embolizations in the region of the cervical cord have been performed with particulate emboli, primarily polyvinyl alcohol of a known particle size (22–24). In humans the normal anterior spinal artery diameter is in the range 340–1100μ and the diameter of the normal central spinal artery varies between 60–72μ (25). Therefore, calibrated polyvinyl alcohol sponge particles with diameters of 150–250μ should pass through a normal spinal artery without lodging in the central spinal arteries. In most cases the feeding anterior spinal and posterior spinal arteries have hypertrophied in size to supply the malformation, and even larger particles can be flow-directed into the nidus if necessary. There are several reports (20, 21) of the use of nondetachable balloons to occlude the vertebral artery transiently, which allows the safe embolization of a small feeding spinal artery proximal to the site of occlusion. With the development of newer microcatheters and soft guidewires, superselective embolization of these spinal cord arteries can usually be performed. In rare instances the microcatheter can be navigated to the malformation or an associated arterial aneurysm, and platinum coils or particles deposited at this site. The majority of these procedures are performed in an awake patient under local anesthesia to allow continuous monitoring of neurologic status. Amytal or lidocaine can be injected selectively to assess the functional territory to be embolized. Evoked potentials can also be obtained during these provocative tests.

Figure 52.1 is an MR image of a 24-year-old female who had two episodes of severe quadriparesis secondary to hemorrhage from a cervical intramedullary AVM (**A**). Subsequently she had an almost complete neurologic recovery but suffered severe right neck pain. Selective spinal angiography showed that the primary arterial supply arose from radicular branches of the left and right vertebral artery with venous drainage to medullary and radicular veins (**B** and **C**). After subselective catheterization and embolization of these branches with polyvinyl alcohol particles, the malformation was almost completely obliterated (**D** and **E**). At a 6-month follow-up examination, there was approximately 10% recanalization of the malformation, coincident with symptoms of increasing radiculopathy. A second embolization procedure was performed; complete angiographic obliteration was obtained, and the patient remains symptom-free 1 year after the procedure. It is important to follow these patients clinically and to obtain follow-up angiograms to rule out recanalization of the malformation.

Cavernous hemangiomas are collections of sinusoidal vascular spaces. The caliber of the feeding arteries and draining veins is normal and no arteriovenous shunting can be seen on an angiogram. These lesions, which can produce hemorrhage and neurologic deficit, are commonly missed on myelography, CT scanning, and spinal arteriography. They can be seen on MR images, however, and are being recognized as a cause of cervical myelopathy with increasing frequency. In our limited experience, the MR image shows an area of subacute and chronic hemorrhage. The margins of the cavernous hemangioma are fusiform,

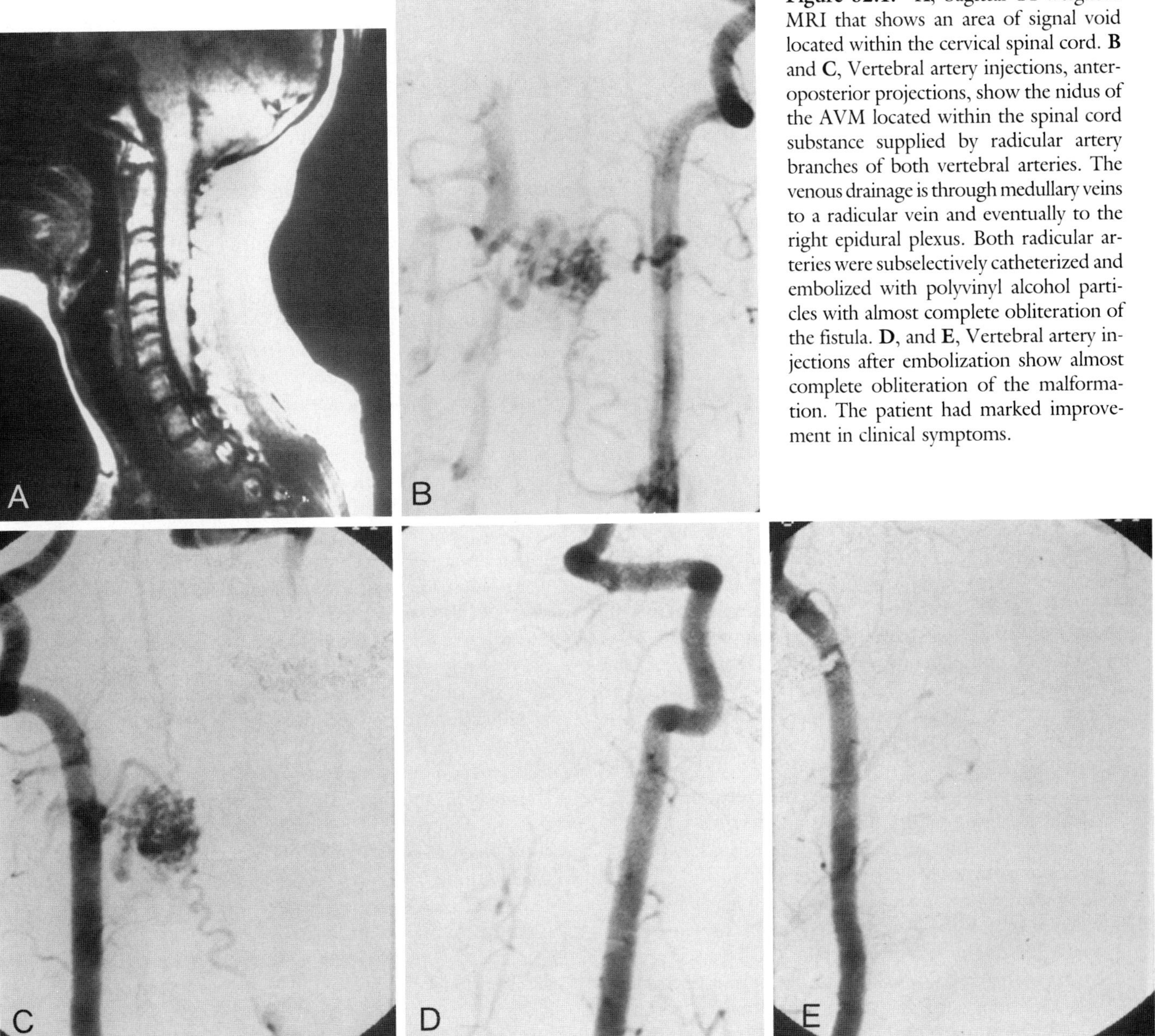

Figure 52.1. **A**, Sagittal T1-weighted MRI that shows an area of signal void located within the cervical spinal cord. **B** and **C**, Vertebral artery injections, anteroposterior projections, show the nidus of the AVM located within the spinal cord substance supplied by radicular artery branches of both vertebral arteries. The venous drainage is through medullary veins to a radicular vein and eventually to the right epidural plexus. Both radicular arteries were subselectively catheterized and embolized with polyvinyl alcohol particles with almost complete obliteration of the fistula. **D**, and **E**, Vertebral artery injections after embolization show almost complete obliteration of the malformation. The patient had marked improvement in clinical symptoms.

as opposed to their spherical counterparts inside the brain. The orientation of the fusiform axis is parallel to the axis of the spinal cord. There is evidence of hemosiderin from chronic hemorrhage at the margins as well as more recent hemorrhage within the central portion.

Periextramedullary Arteriovenous Fistulas

These recently recognized entities are direct fistulas on the surface of the spinal cord. They are generally supplied by the anterior spinal artery, lateral spinal arteries, or posterior spinal arteries, and the vast majority occur in the region of the conus. Presumably a congenital lesion, they usually present with neurologic dysfunction such as progressive paraparesis secondary to venous hypertension. Less commonly these fistulas can present with hemorrhage that usually occurs secondary to rupture of an aneurysm of a feeding artery. It may be difficult to visualize these on standard MR images. The location of the fistula on the surface of the cord can be obscured by artifacts that arise from surrounding CSF pulsations. Cardiac gating and thin sections may be essential for diagnosis. Myelography usually shows dilated feeding arteries and engorged medullary veins. Treatment can consist of surgical clipping of the fistula site or embolization with particulate or liquid adhesive agents.

SPINAL-DURAL ARTERIOVENOUS FISTULAS

These are a recently recognized entity in which the arteriovenous connection is small and localized within the dura (26). For many years these lesions were classified incorrectly as retromedullary AVMs, but with the availability of superselective angiography, the pathology has been localized to the dura itself. Generally, the feeding artery is normal in caliber and flow through these lesions is exceptionally slow. The venous drainage is to dilated radicular and medullary veins and the coronal venous plexus. Clinically, these patients present with a slowly progressive myelopathy or radiculopathy (26). Symptoms generally appear in older patients, which suggests an acquired etiology (2). If they are not treated, patients can progress to complete paraplegia or quadriparesis. The pathophysiology occurs secondary to venous stagnation from chronic venous hypertension, which results in chronic medullary ischemia. The clinical symptoms can be a slowly progressive decline in neurologic function, which, if recognized and treated, can often result in dramatic neurologic recovery. The chance of improvement after closure of the fistula is inversely related to the length of duration of the fistula. Clinical decline can be fairly abrupt in some patients, is associated with venous infarction, and has a much poorer prognosis. Occasionally, a spontaneous thrombosis can occur in the draining veins that leads to a rapid and severe neurologic decline. Although early reports suggested that MR imaging can be useful for the diagnosis of these fistulas (27), in our experience these small connections can be easily missed even with excellent quality thin-section, cardiac-gated MR images. A serpiginous area of signal void posterior to the cord that represents flow in dilated medullary veins can sometimes be seen on MR images. In addition, if gadolinium contrast medium is used, there may be subtle enhancement within the cord parenchyma (26), which presumably reflects the venous ischemia. We have seen punctate areas of increased signal intensity posterior to the cord on the MR images of several patients after the administration of gadolinium contrast medium; increased intensity may represent enhancement within the slowly flowing veins. In addition, we have seen several cases of confirmed spinal radicular artery dural fistulas that were entirely missed on good quality MR images. Therefore, MR should not be used as a screening modality for this disease, but it may be useful as a means of evaluating secondary changes such as venous infarction that may indicate a poor prognosis.

The screening method of choice for spinal radicular artery fistulas is water-soluble contrast myelography of the entire spine performed in both supine and prone positions. Because of preferential venous drainage to the retromedullary veins, these veins may be observed only in myelograms obtained in the supine position. Myelography usually shows dilatation and tortuosity of the medullary veins on the dorsum of the cord. Occasionally arterial pulsations in these veins can be observed under fluoroscopy. The spinal cord may be of normal caliber, increased caliber representing cord edema, or decreased caliber from chronic ischemic changes. The site of the fistula may be far removed from the level of clinical symptoms. If dilated medullary veins are observed on a myelogram, compete spinal angiography must be performed. In rare instances spontaneous closure of the fistula can occur. Repeat myelography shows a decrease in the caliber of the veins. Spontaneous thrombosis of the draining medullary veins can occur (Foix-Alajouanine syndrome) and is associated with a marked deterioration in neurologic function.

In many patients, the insidiousness of the presenting symptoms of pain, radiculopathy, or myelopathy commonly leads to initial misdiagnosis of ascending myelitis, transverse myelitis, or spondylosis. We have seen several patients who presented with progressive lower extremity paraparesis secondary to a dural fistula located in the cervical spine region. In addition, the fistula can be located intracranially with venous drainage inferiorly to medullary veins. Therefore, it is important to perform a complete spinal anteriographic study including selective injections of each lumbar, thoracic, internal iliac, and middle sacral artery, both vertebral arteries, thyrocervical, costocervical, and external carotid arteries until the fistula has been identified. Angiography must be of excellent quality and the films must be continued into the late venous phase because opacification of these shunts can be delayed up to several seconds after the injection. The feeding arteries are usually normal in caliber on angiograms. The location of the shunt is usually on the dura but can be on the ventral surface of the spinal cord (28). The venous drainage is by way of the coronal venous plexus to dilated medullary veins that are usually quite tortuous.

Figure 52.2**A** is a supine myelogram that shows a serpiginous filling defect located on the dorsal aspect of the spinal cord. A spinal arteriogram was obtained that showed no abnormality involving the lumbar or intercostal arteries. Selective injection of the external carotid and vertebral artery showed a dural fistula located near the anterior lip of the foramen magnum with venous drainage to dilated medullary veins (Fig. 52.2**B** through **E**). These branches were subselectively catheterized and embolized with a small injection of liquid adhesive. Control angiograms (Fig. 52.2**F** and **G**) showed that the fistula had been obliterated completely; there was marked improvement in the patient's presenting symptom, progressive lower extremity paraparesis.

A series of angiograms for an elderly female who presented with slowly progressive lower extremity paraparesis is shown in Figure 52.3. A complete spinal angiogram showed a dural fistula supplied by several radicular branches of the vertebral artery and the ascending pharyngeal artery (Fig. 52.3**A**). The ascending pharyngeal artery and radicular artery branches were occluded with particulate em-

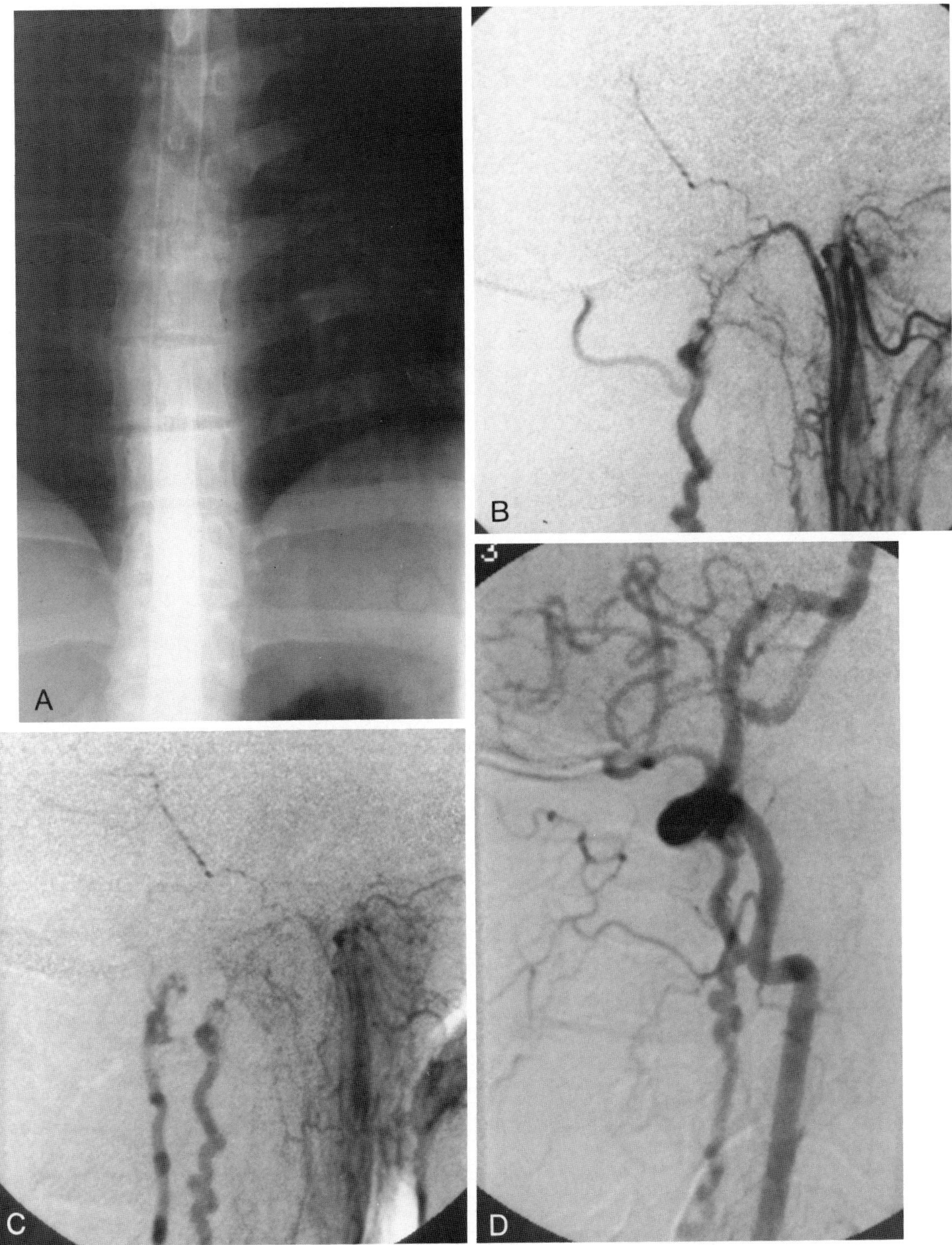

Figure 52.2. **A**, Supine myelogram that shows a serpiginous filling defect on the dorsum of the cord, representing a dilated medullary vein in a patient with slowly progressive lower extremity paraparesis. Right ascending pharyngeal artery injection, lateral projection, early arterial (**B**) and late venous (**C**) phases show a fistula located near the foramen magnum draining into dilated medullary veins on both the anterior and posterior surface of the spinal cord. Right vertebral artery injection, lateral (**D**) projection and AP (**E**) projections show the same fistula supplied by a radicular branch of the right vertebral artery. This branch was subselectively catheterized and embolized with liquid adhesives. **F**, Right vertebral injection, AP projection, after embolization shows complete closure of the fistula. **G**, Right external carotid injection, lateral projection, that shows complete obliteration of the fistula from the ascending pharyngeal artery. The patient has had marked improvement in symptoms.

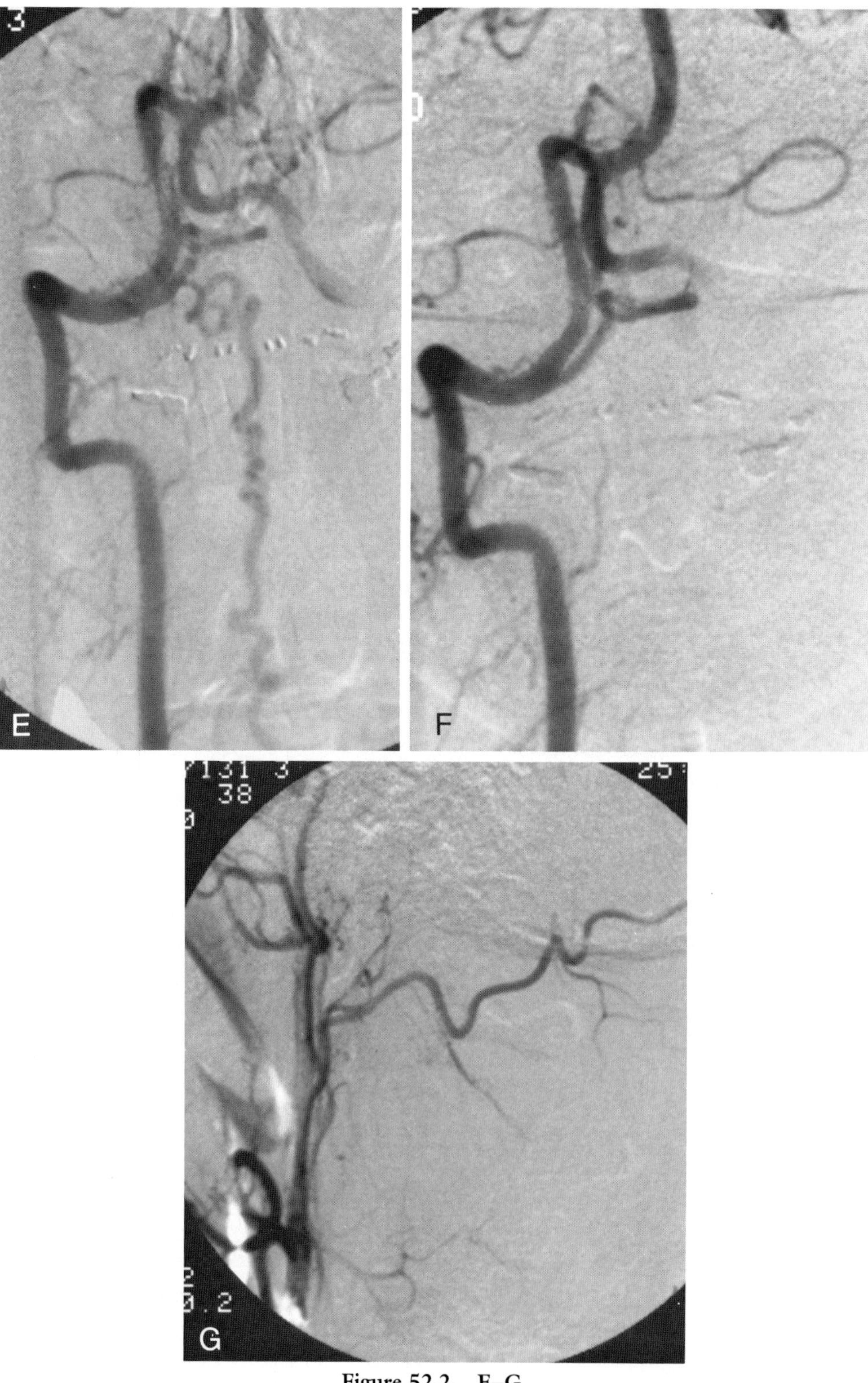

Figure 52.2. E–G

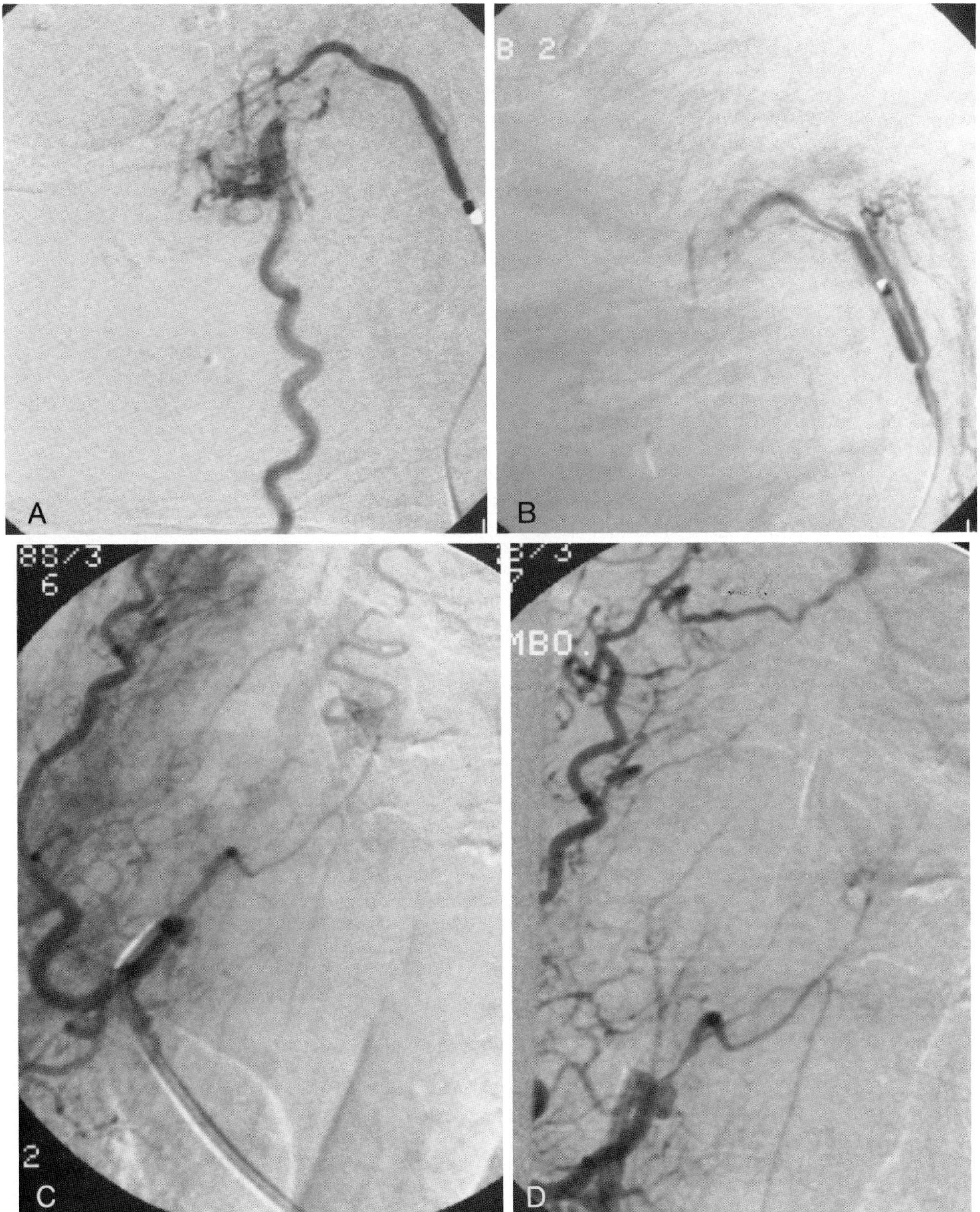

Figure 52.3. **A**, Ascending pharyngeal artery injection, lateral projection, that shows a dural fistula located on the dural surface adjacent to C2 draining into a dilated medullary vein in a patient with slowly progressive lower extremity paraparesis. The ascending pharyngeal artery was subselectively catheterized and embolized with particulate emboli with complete obliteration of the fistula **(B)**. The patient had initial improvement in her paraparesis, but 6 months later developed severe right arm pain and weakness. A follow-up angiogram showed a second dural fistula located in the C5 region supplied by the anterior spinal artery **(C)**. After subselective catheterization of this vessel and embolization with particles, there was complete closure of the fistula **(D)**.

boli (Fig. 52.3**B**), and the patient underwent surgical excision of the fistula site. The patient's neurologic condition improved initially, but 6 months later she had progression of symptoms and onset of right radicular symptoms. A follow-up angiogram showed a second, separate site arteriovenous fistula supplied by the anterior spinal artery through the right costocervical trunk (Fig. 52.3**C**). An attempt at surgical excision was unsuccessful because of the location of the ventral surface of the spinal cord. The fistula site was closed with particulate emboli in a subsequent procedure (Fig. 52.3**D**).

Both endovascular and surgical procedures can be used to treat this disease effectively. In the lumbar and thoracic region, the majority of these patients have supply to the fistula arising from intercostal or lumbar arteries not supplying the spinal cord. Endovascular treatment alone, with either particulate emboli or liquid adhesives, can produce cures. In the cervical region, however, the supply to the fistula can also involve the spinal arteries (Fig. 52.3**C**), and combined endovascular and surgical techniques may be necessary to obliterate these fistulas. One potential complication is the development of a Foix-Alajouanine syndrome in which venous thrombosis occurs after closure of the fistula (29). This may be treated with systemic anticoagulation, but the prognosis can be extremely poor.

EPIDURAL ARTERIOVENOUS MALFORMATIONS

These lesions are primarily extradural and may have drainage to either the epidural venous plexus or medullary veins (30–35). Patients harboring these lesions can present with spontaneous cervical epidural hemorrhage (34), progressive radiculopathy (35), or subarachnoid hemorrhage (32). Angiograms may show arterial supply from both vertebral arteries, costocervical arteries, or thyrocervical arteries.

An angiogram for a patient who presented with progressive radiculopathy involving the left upper extremity is shown in Figure 52.4. A series of plain films, CT scans with contrast medium, and MR images were entirely negative. After the discovery of a loud bruit over her left shoulder, selective ascending cervical angiography was performed and showed a fistula located in the epidural space with drainage to epidural veins. After complete closure of the fistula by embolization, the patient's radiculopathy resolved completely. Because of the absence of findings on MR images, CT scans, and myelograms, a high level of suspicion must be maintained if diagnosis of these lesions is to be made.

SPINAL HEMANGIOMAS

These lesions are commonly located within the vertebral body involving the thoracic or lumbar spine; in rare instances they can involve the cervical spine. The hemangioma may expand into the arch or posterior elements and encroach on the spinal cord by extension into the epidural space.

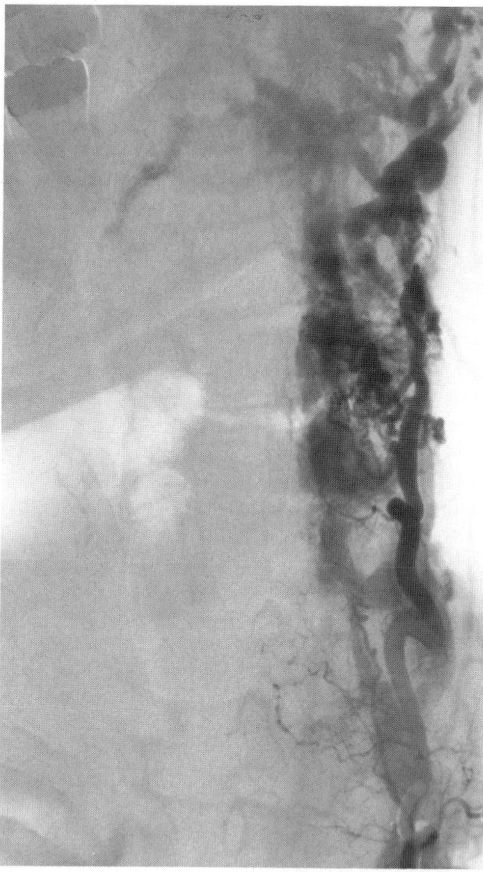

Figure 52.4. Left thyrocervical injection that shows a fistula located at the left epidural space with drainage to epidural veins in a patient who presented with severe radiculopathy but who had a negative myelogram, MR image, and CT scan.

SUMMARY

It is important to remember that no single diagnostic imaging modality is ideal for visualization of all types of AVMs involving the cervical spine region. MR imaging is an excellent screening modality for intramedullary pathology but can entirely miss spinal dural fistulas and epidural arteriovenous malformations. While myelography is the screening method of choice for detection of spinal dural arteriovenous fistulas, it can entirely overlook epidural AVMs and cavernous hemangiomas. Spinal angiography remains essential for the complete evaluation of rapidly flowing AVMs. MR imaging may be the only imaging study that can be used consistently to identify cavernous hemangiomas.

Surgical, endovascular, and combined therapies have been used to treat patients with these complicated vascular malformations and fistulas. Certain anatomic locations favor surgical excision while some lesions can be approached by transvascular techniques. Advances in microcatheter technology and the availability of new embolic agents have greatly improved the endovascular treatment of these complicated vascular abnormalities.

REFERENCES

1. Nagasawa S, Yoshida S, Ishikawa M, et al. Arteriovenous malformations of the cervical spinal cord—with special reference to CT study. No Shinkei Geka 1984;12:93–98.

2. Rosenblum B, Oldfield EH, Doppman JL, DiChiro G. Spinal arteriovenous malformations: a comparison of dural arteriovenous fistulas and intradural AVM's in 81 patients. J Neurosurg 1987;67:795–802.

3. Aminoff MJ, Logue V. Clinical features of spinal vascular malformations. Brain 1974;97:197–210.

4. Aminoff MJ, Logue V. The prognosis of patients with spinal vascular malformations. Brain 1974;97:211–218.

5. DiChiro G, Doppman JL, Dwyer AJ, et al. Tumors and arteriovenous malformations of the spinal cord; assessment using MR. Radiology 1985;156:689–697.

6. Casazza M, Bracchi M, Girotti F. Spinal myoclonus and clinical worsening after intravenous contrast medium in a patient with spinal arteriovenous malformations. AJNR 1985;6:965.

7. Djindjian R. Angiography of the spinal cord. Surg Neurol 1974;2:179–185.

8. DiChiro G, Doppman J, Ommaya AK. Selective arteriography of arteriovenous aneurysms of spinal cord. Radiology 1967;88:1065–1077.

9. Enzmann DR, Brody WR, Djang WT, et al. Intra-arterial digital subtraction spinal angiography. AJNR 1983;4:25–26.

10. Levy JM, Hessel SJ, Christensen FK, Crow JK. Digital subtraction arteriography for spinal arteriovenous malformations. AJNR 1983;4:1217–1218.

11. Yeates A, Drayer B, Heinz ER, Osborne D. Intra-arterial digital subtraction angiography of the spinal cord. Radiology 1985;155:387–390.

12. Yasargil MG, DeLong B, Guarnaschelli JJ. Complete microsurgical excision of cervical extramedullary and intramedullary vascular malformations. Surg Neurol 1975;4:211–224.

13. Tada T, Sakamoto K, Kobayashi N, Tanaka Y. Arteriovenous malformations of the spinal cord in a 17 month old child. Childs Nerv Syst 1985;1:298–301.

14. Banzhaf E, Gopel W, Banzhaf M. Cervical arteriovenous malformations of the right vertebral artery. Psychiatr Neurol Med Psychol (Leipz) 1986;38:29–32.

15. Kandel EI. Complete excision of arteriovenous malformations of the cervical cord. Surg Neurol 1980;13:135–139.

16. Gooding GA, Berger MS, Linkowski GD, Dillon WP, Weinstein PR, Boggan JE. Transducer frequency considerations in intraoperative US of the spine. Radiology 1986;160:272–273.

17. Owen MP, Brown RH, Spetzler RF, Nash CL Jr, Brodkey JS, Nulsen FE. Excision of intramedullary arteriovenous malformation using intraoperative spinal cord monitoring. Surg Neurol 1979;12:271–276.

18. Latchaw RE, Harris RD, Chou SN, Gold LH. Combined embolization and operation in the treatment of cervical arteriovenous malformations. Neurosurgery 1980;6:131–137.

19. Doppman JL, DiChiro G, Ommaya AK. Percutaneous embolization of spinal cord arteriovenous malformations. J Neurosurg 1971;34:48–55.

20. Theron J, Cosgrove R, Melanson D, Ethier R. Spinal arteriovenous malformations: advances in therapeutic embolization. Radiology 1986;158:163–169.

21. Horton JA, Latchaw RE, Gold LHA, Pang D. Emoblization of intramedullary arteriovenous malformations of the spinal cord. AJNR 1986;7:113–118.

22. Casteneda-Zuniga WR, Sanchez R, Amplatz K. Experimental observations on short and long-term effects of arterial occlusion with Ivalon. Radiology 1978;126:783–785.

23. Latchaw RE, Gold LHA. Polyvinyl foam embolization of vascular and neoplastic lesions of the head, neck, and spine. Radiology 1979;131:669–679.

24. Quisling RG, Mickle JP, Ballinger WB, Carver CC, Kaplan B. Histopathologic analysis of intraarterial polyvinyl alcohol microemboli in rat cerebral cortex. AJNR 1984;5:101–104.

25. Suh TH, Alexander L. Vascular system of the human spinal cord. Arch Neurol Psychol 1939;41:659–677.

26. Merland JJ, Riche MC, Chiras J. Intraspinal extramedullary arteriovenous fistulae draining into the medullary veins. J Neuroradiol 1980;7:271–320.

27. Masaryk TJ, Ross JS, Modic MT, Ruff RL, Selman WR, Ratcheson RA. Radiculomenigeal vascular malformations of the spine: MR imaging. Radiology 1987;164:845.

28. Djindjian M, Djindjian R, Rey A, Hurth M, Houdart R. Intradural extramedullary spinal arteriovenous malformation fed by the anterior spinal artery. Surg Neurol 1977;8:85–93.

29. Cahan LD, Higashida RT, Halbach VV, Hieshima GB. Variants of radiculomeningeal vascular malformations of the spine. J Neurosurg 1987;66:333–337.

30. Janda J, Mracek Z. Angioreticuloma of the brain stem. Simultaneous occurrence of an arteriovenous malformations in the epidural space of the cervical spinal cord. Cesk Neurol Neurochir 1978;41:397–399.

31. Kendall BE, Logue V. Spinal epidural angiomatous malformations draining into intrathecal veins. Neuroradiology 1977;13:181–189.

32. Halbach VV, Higashida RT, Hieshima GB. Treatment of vertebral arteriovenous fistulas. AJNR 1987;8:1121–1128, and AJR 1988;150:405–412.

33. Heier LA, Lee BCP. Dural spinal arteriovenous malformation with epidural venous drainage: case report. AJNR 1987;8:561.

34. Foo D, Chang VC, Rossier AB. Spontaneous cervical epidural hemorrhage, anterior cord syndrome, and familial vascular malformation: case report. Neurology 1980;30:308–311.

35. Ross D, Olsen W, Halbach VV, Rosegay H, Pitts LH. Cervical root compression by a traumatic pseudoaneurysm of the vertebral artery: case report. Neurosurgery 1988;22:414–417.

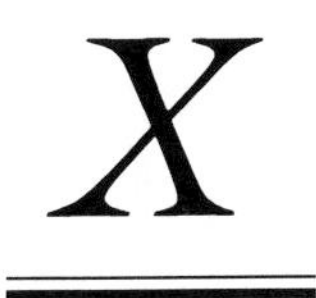

Fusion/Stabilization

53

Rheumatoid Disease of the Cervical Spine: Surgical Treatment

Stephen J. Lipson

The anatomic abnormalities of the cervical spine involved in rheumatoid arthritis (RA) are a consequence of the synovitic destruction in joints, ligaments, and bone. In joints, articular cartilage is directly destroyed, and rheumatoid pannus can reach adjacent structures. In ligaments, distention and rupture can result in instability. In bone, osteoporosis, cyst formation, and erosion can result in destruction with a loss of skeletal integrity. The inflammatory cells involved in rheumatoid inflammation at the atlantoaxial junction taken at biopsy have been shown to be the same cell types as those involved in diarthrodial peripheral joints (1). The subluxations which result from this synovitic destruction are dependent upon the specific cervical anatomy destroyed. Clinical abnormalities which result are pain and neurologic abnormality resulting from spinal cord and nerve root compression and distortion. Vertebral artery involvement can occur in the presence of cervical subluxation. Garrod (2) first described clinical involvement of the cervical spine in RA in 1890. Subluxation, particularly at the atlantoaxial joint, was identified later and is the most studied subluxation (3–5). Davis and Markley (6) in 1951 first described death caused by atlantoaxial subluxation with medullary compression.

The activity of RA in the cervical spine appears to begin early in the disease and progresses in relationship to peripheral involvement. In a prospective radiologic study of 100 patients newly presenting with RA, 83% with anterior atlantoaxial subluxation developed it within 2 years of the disease onset (7). Cervical spine subluxation has been shown to correlate with damage to the metacarpophalangeal and carpal bone (8). The degree of cervical damage strongly correlates with that of peripheral erosive disease, and subluxation is more likely in patients with progressive peripheral erosions (9). Factors correlating with the progression of atlantoaxial subluxation are a history of medical therapy with corticosteroids, seropositivity, the presence of rheumatoid subcutaneous nodules, and the presence of erosive and mutilating articular disease. The role of corticosteroids as a causative factor versus a factor correlated with the severity of the disease has never been clarified. Additionally male patients are more frequently affected by subluxations (7, 10–14).

Subluxations

Atlantoaxial subluxation (AAS) is ascribed to erosive synovitis in the atlantoaxial, atlanto-odontoid, and atlanto-occipital joints as well as the synovium-lined bursa between the odontoid and the transverse ligament (Fig. 53.1). AAS can be anterior (Fig. 53.2), posterior (Fig. 53.3), and lateral (Fig. 53.1*b*). Anterior AAS is the most common subluxation observed and in postmortem studies of RA patients has been found in 11–46% of cases (11, 15–17). The integrity of the atlantoaxial complex is dependent on the transverse, alar, and apical ligaments. Anterior subluxation of greater than 10–12 mm implies loss of the integrity in all of these ligaments (18). Most of the anterior AAS seen in RA is greater than the 3.5 mm limit of normal in adults. Overall, 43–86% of RA patients exhibit subluxations (10, 19, 20), and, in particular, anterior AAS was present in 19–71% of patients radiologically surveyed (10, 13, 21–24). Anterior AAS can be reducible, with the subluxation corrected in extension (Fig. 53.2), or unreducible, remaining fixed in position or uncorrectable to within a normal degree of subluxation.

Posterior AAS has been described, but occurs infrequently (26–29). It accounted for 6.7% of all AAS in one series and usually was not associated with cord compression (14). Erosion and/or fracture of the dens are the most common factors predisposing to posterior AAS (30). Myelopathy can be associated with posterior AAS and may be caused by a configurational abnormality of kyphotic kinking of the spinal cord (Fig. 53.3) rather than direct compression (30).

Lateral AAS can be visualized and defined as more than 2 mm subluxation of the lateral masses of the atlas on the axis (Fig. 53.1*b*). Rotational deformity probably accompanies it. Although reported (31), its incidence is probably underestimated. One series found lateral AAS to account for 21% of all AAS (14). Nonreducible head tilt was found

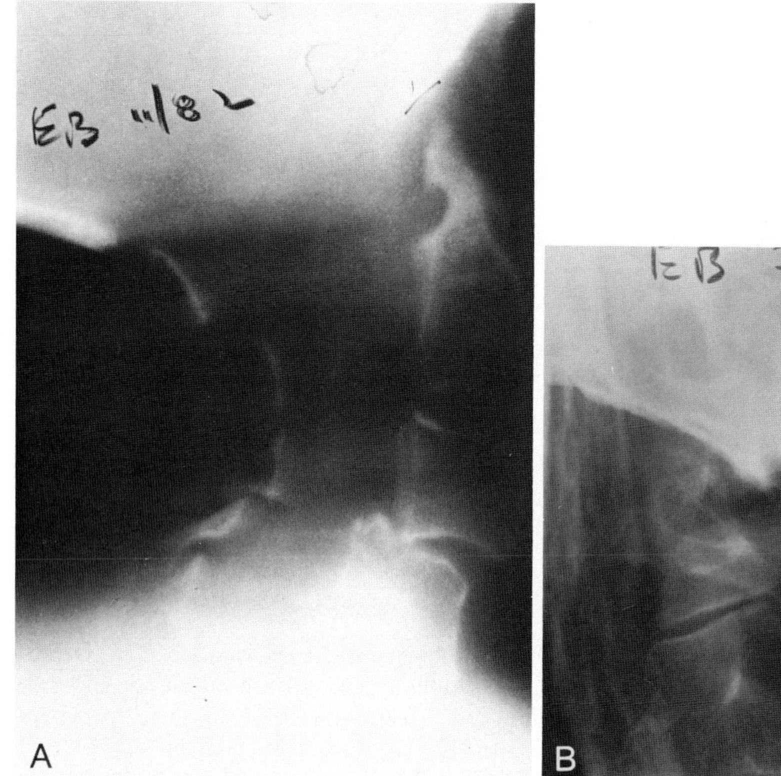

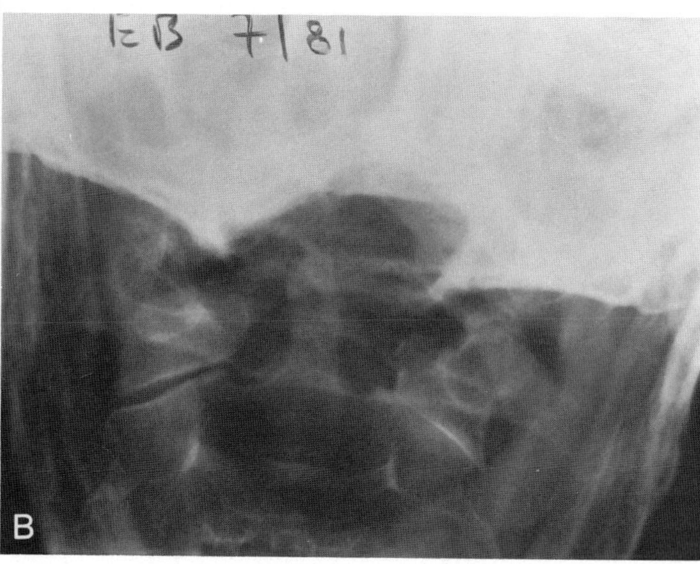

Figure 53.1. On a polytomogram (**A**), erosion of the posterior aspect of the dens is seen caused by synovitis in the transverse ligament. The apex of the dens is tapered by synovitic erosion. Concomitant subaxial subluxation is noted at C3 on C4. In **B**, the base of the dens has been eroded by synovitis laterally adjacent to the atlantoaxial lateral mass joints which have undergone lateral subluxation.

in 10% of a rheumatoid population, all with lateral AAS, but frequently combined with other deformities (32). Lateral AAS has been found more commonly in patients with spinal cord compression than in those without it (33).

Atlantoaxial impaction (AAI), also known as cranial settling, upward migration of the odontoid, pseudobasilar invagination, and vertical subluxation of the atlas, results from bone and cartilage loss in the occipitoatlantal and atlantoaxial joints. AAI has been found in 5–32% of rheumatoid patients surveyed (8, 20, 21, 34) and accounted for 22% of all upper cervical subluxations (14).

The subaxial cervical spine is affected through involvement of the facets, interspinous ligaments, and intervertebral discs (spondylodiscitis). Two pathophysiologic mechanisms leading to instability have been postulated. The first implicates the initial site of destruction is synovitis in the neurocentral joints with erosion of adjacent disc and bone leading to subluxation (35). The alternative mechanism is through primary facet arthritis and ligamentous laxity causing chronic discovertebral trauma and destructive changes (36). Additionally, the involvement of interspinous bursae with spinous process destruction and hypermobile segments is associated with disc destruction (37). Spinal cord responses to these subluxations are pachymeningitis, arachnoiditis, and medullary compression. Subaxial subluxations tend toward the C2–C3 and C3–C4 segments, typically lack osteophytes, and often are at multiple levels (39, 40), giving a stepladder appearance (Figs. 53.2 and 53.4). End-plate erosions are found in 12–15% of patients with RA (10, 38, 40). Discovertebral destruction does not always accompany subluxation. Overall, subaxial subluxations are found in 10–20% of patients (36, 38, 40). Other patterns of subaxial disease that have neurologic consequence are subluxations below higher fusions, anterior spondylodiscitis causing cord compression, intracanal rheumatoid granulations, and possibly a hyperlordotic subaxial spine (41).

CLINICAL MANIFESTATIONS AND NATURAL HISTORY

Clinical manifestations of cervical RA are pain, neurologic disturbance, and death. Pain is typically in the neck and, in particular, at the craniocervical junction, occipital headache (occipital neuralgia, Arnold's neuralgia) accompanied by stiffness and crepitance. The Sharp-Purser test, in which the flexed head is forced into extension while the spinous process of C2 is held fixed, has been positive in 20–44% of RA patients with anterior AAS (13, 21). Neurologic symptoms are multiple and can be vague. Subjective symp-

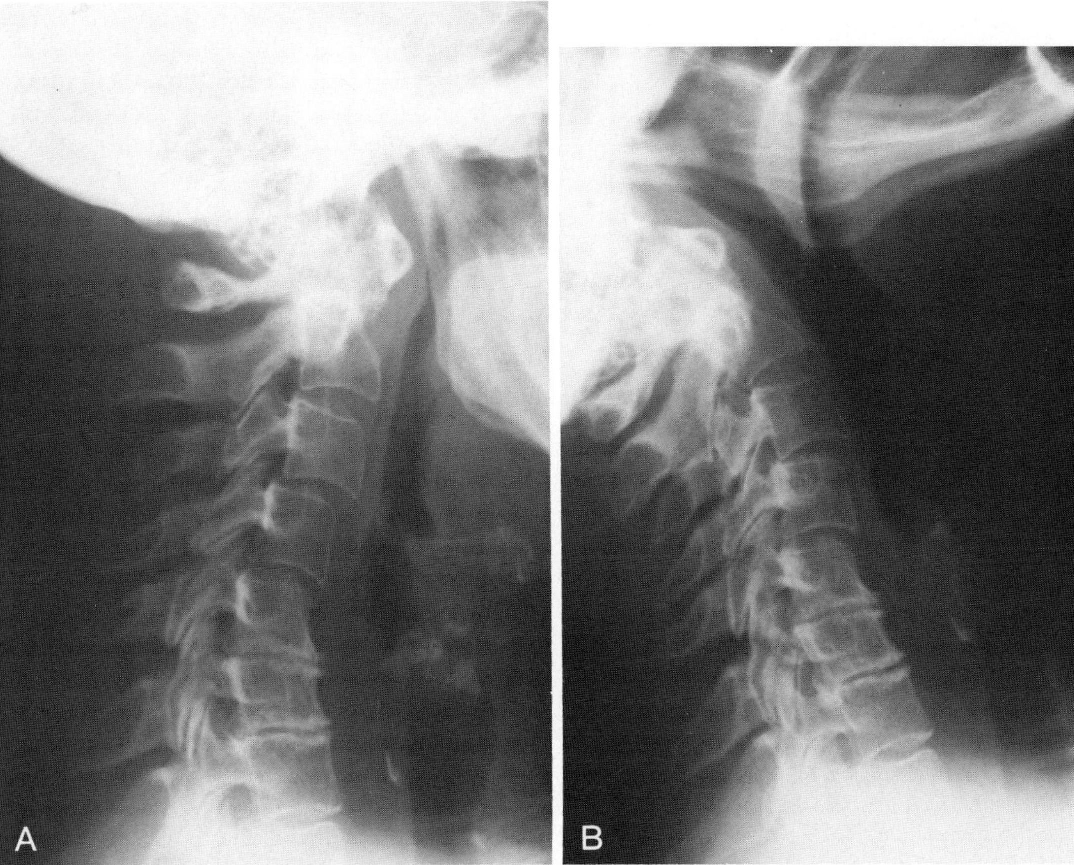

Figure 53.2. Reducible anterior atlantoaxial subluxation. In flexion, **A**, the atlantodental distance increases, then fully reduces in extension, **B**, Also noted are subaxial subluxations at C3–4 and C4–5, and, spondylodiscitis at C5–6 and C6–7.

toms of parethesias in the hands, an electric shock sensation in the body (Lhermitte's phenomenon), and a feeling of weakness or loss of endurance can occur. Objective weakness and pyramidal tract involvement with upper motor neuron signs may be found in more overt myelopathy. Vertebrobasilar insufficiency, especially in AAI, may cause loss of equilibrium, tinnitus, vertigo, dysphagia, visual disturbance, and diplopia. Bulbar disturbance may be paroxysmal and fatal. Urinary sphincter disturbance usually presents first as retention and then as urinary incontinence. Physical examination in a crippled, debilitated rheumatoid patient may be confused by peripheral rheumatoid disease causing weakness from articular involvement, tenosynovitis, tendon rupture, rheumatoid, and rheumatoid vasculitic peripheral neuropathy. Evaluation may be accomplished by a high index of suspicion for a symptomatic subluxation. Somatosensory evoked potential examination may assist in the evaluation of neurologic abnormalities when the clinical picture is not completely clear. Pain is a common finding in cervical RA, found in 40–88% of patients affected (10, 20, 24, 33). Neurologic signs are noted in 7–34% of patients (10, 13, 20).

It is necessary to examine the natural history of cervical rheumatoid disease in order to determine the likelihood of severe neurologic deterioration or death. This information underlies the decision as to whether surgical intervention is necessary and effective. Survival in patients with RA has been examined. A postmortem study (42) of 104 patients with RA revealed 11 with AAS and cord compression. Seven of the 11 experienced sudden death, and all demonstrated that the odontoid caused medullary compression. A 10% rate of fatal medullary compression was estimated. Reports indicate that survival is not influenced by subluxation, but RA patients have a significantly shorter life expectancy than the general population (12, 43). A 5-year study reported a 17% mortality rate in RA patients, 10% higher than that for the general population (20). AAS did not cause death, but subluxations did worsen in 80%, while new subluxations were noted in 27% of patient.

Existing roentgenographically confirmed subluxations can worsen. In addition to the 80% cited (20), worsening has been noted in 39–41% of patients studied (12, 14, 43). Neurologic progression is less marked and has been noted in 2–36% of patients (9, 20, 43). Once cervical myelopathy is established, mortality is common. A report on 31 patients with RA and cervical myelopathy revealed that 19 died, with 15 deaths occurring within 6 months

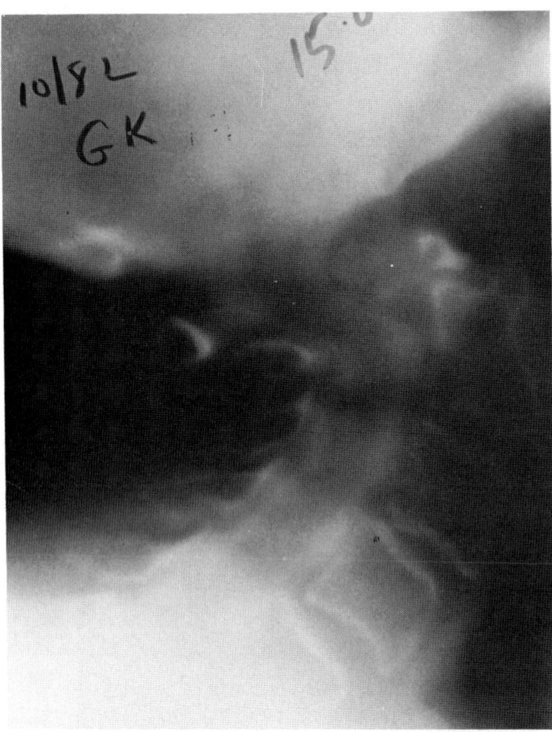

Figure 53.3. Lateral polytomography with myelographic contrast demonstrates posterior atlantoaxial subluxation via erosion and fracture of the dens. The spinal cord lies in a kinked, kyphotic configuration in this subluxation.

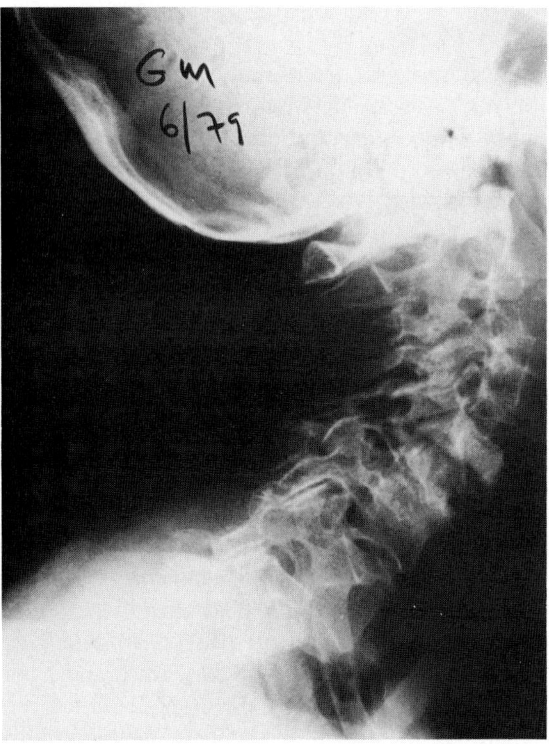

Figure 53.4. Severe subaxial subluxation at multiple levels with discovertebral destruction, anterior subluxation, and bone loss.

of presentation (44). Four deaths were of primary neurologic origin. All who were untreated died, and half of those treated with a collar died. Only fusion provided a chance for survival. Of nine RA patients with myelopathy treated nonoperatively, all died within 1 year, with four deaths arising from cord compression (45). RA patients with cervical myelopathy are at risk for a premature death, most commonly due to infection and comorbid conditions. They represent a subset of RA patients where disease severity, especially if severe extraarticular manifestations and interstitial lung disease exist, constitutes a major factor influencing survival. Interstitial lung disease identifies those patients with RA undergoing cervical spine surgery who are at greatest risk for early postoperative death (46).

RADIOLOGIC IMAGING

The importance of plain roentgenograms with flexion-extension views cannot be emphasized enough, since they permit initial assessment of involvement, localization of instabilities, and areas which require further study. On the basis of plain roentgenograms, risk factors identified that predisposed to cord compression and neurologic progression were male gender, anterior AAS greater than 9 mm, and the presence of AAI. The presence of lateral AAS is a lesser factor (14). The atlantodental distance is measured at the base of the odontoid to the base of the anterior arch of the atlas by convention and is abnormal in adults when greater than 3.5 mm. When AAI occurs, a pseudocorrection of the increased atlantodental distance occurs because the base of the atlas approaches the body of the axis. Such a decrease in the atlantodental distance should not be considered a correction of the abnormal anatomy.

On plain radiographs, AAI is measured in a variety of ways (21). McGregor's line, measuring the distance of the tip of the odontoid above a line drawn from the hard palate to the base of the occiput on a lateral view (14), has probably been the most traditional measure. The tip of the odontoid should not project more than 4.5 mm above this line. McRae's line connects the front of the foramen magnum to the back (basion to opisthion), and the odontoid should be below this line. Chamberlain's line projects from the posterior margin of the hard palate to the posterior part of the foramen magnum. The odontoid should not project more than 3 mm above this line, and 6 mm is definitely abnormal. On an open mouth odontoid view, or an anteroposterior tomogram, the Fischgold and Metzger measurement can be used. The digastric line is drawn from the base of the mastoid where it joins the base of the skull. The odontoid tip should lie 1 cm or more below this line. On plain radiographs, the skeletal outlines of the tip of the odontoid can be obscured by osteopenia, destruction, and displacement by erosive fracture. The hard palate may not be included on the film. The posterior portion of the foramen magnum may be difficult to vi-

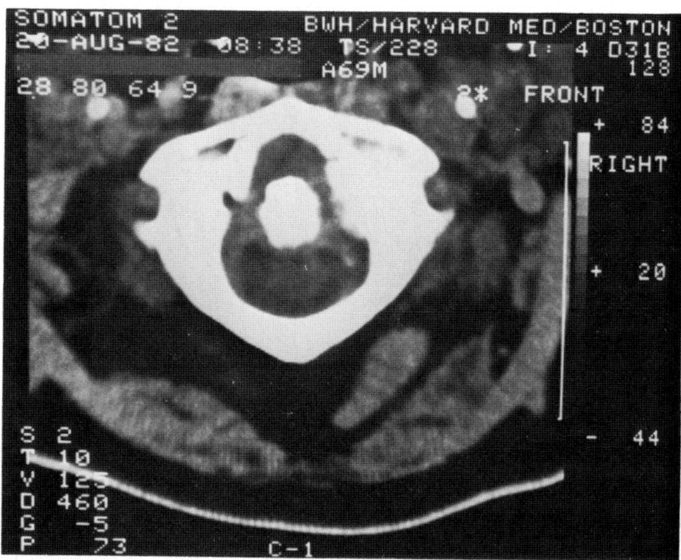

Figure 53.5. A CT scan of anterior atlantoaxial subluxation demonstrating an increased atlantodental distance and thecal sac compression.

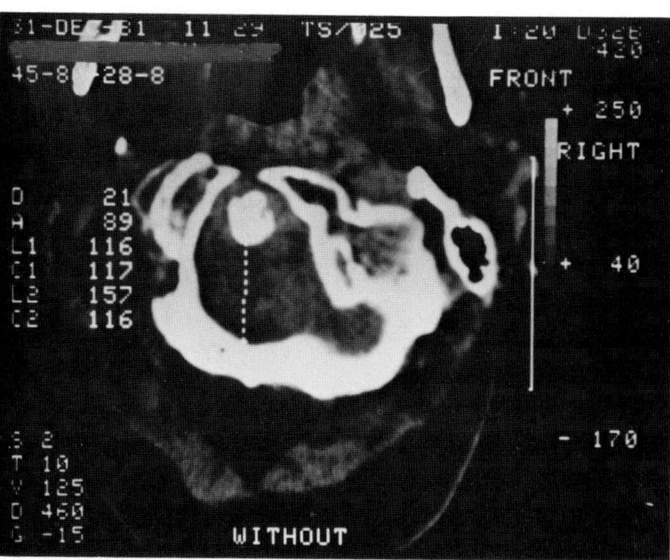

Figure 53.6. A CT scan of atlantoaxial impaction demonstrating the dens protruding inside of the foramen magnum.

sualize accurately. To avoid these problems and as a more direct measure of the loss of the height of the lateral masses of the axis, the Ranawat index can be used (47). On a lateral radiograph, a line is constructed in the midpoints of the anterior and posterior arches of the atlas. The point at the center of the pedicles of the axis is selected and a line drawn perpendicular from this point to the mid-axis line. When this line is less than 13 mm, AAI is present. The Redlund-Johnell line (48) utilizes McGregor's line and the distance from it to the caudad end-plate of the axis. This height is normally at least 34 mm in men and 29 mm in women. The method indicates AAI by loss of height in the lateral columns of the occipito-atlanto-axial complex.

Computed tomography (CT) can add valuable information by revealing the extent of erosions, spinal cord compression, and axial and sagittal relationships (Figs. 53.5 and 53.6). Bone detail, however, is superior in conventional tomography (Figs. 53.3 and 53.7) compared with sagitally reformatted CT images. Sagittal imaging with either CT or contrast-enhanced lateral tomography can demonstrate configurational changes in the spinal cord, such as in the kyphotic kinking seen in posterior AAS (Fig. 53.3) (30). The degree of medullary compression noted on the CT scan correlates with the presence of upper motor neuron signs (50). The addition of intrathecal contrast enhances the ability to demonstrate by CT the role of pannus in cord compression (51).

Magnetic resonance imaging (MRI) adds further definition to the pathologic anatomy of the cervical spine in RA. It has the advantage of requiring no contrast and can be reformatted in any plane. The craniomedullary junction and the entire length of the cervical cord can be visualized. T2-weighted images display a myelographic image demonstrating occlusion of the subarachnoid space, while T1-

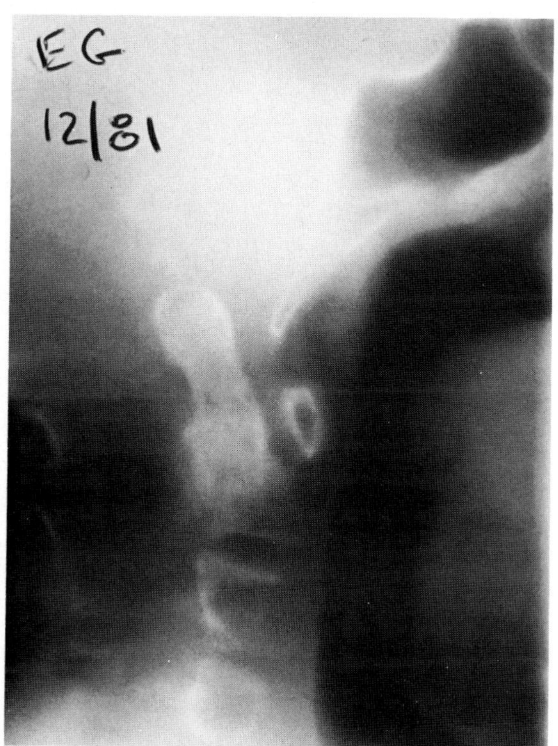

Figure 53.7. A lateral polytomogram of atlantoaxial impaction demonstrates the dens lying above the clivus inside for the foramen magnum. The base of the dens is eroded. The anterior arch of the atlas lies at the mid to lower third of the axis.

weighted images will show the cord itself. Erosion, pannus, and inflammation of soft tissues can be demonstrated (Fig. 53.8). Figure 53.9 demonstrates the use of flexion-extension MRI which can display the kinking of the spinal cord over the pannus behind the dens. The use of dynamic MRI

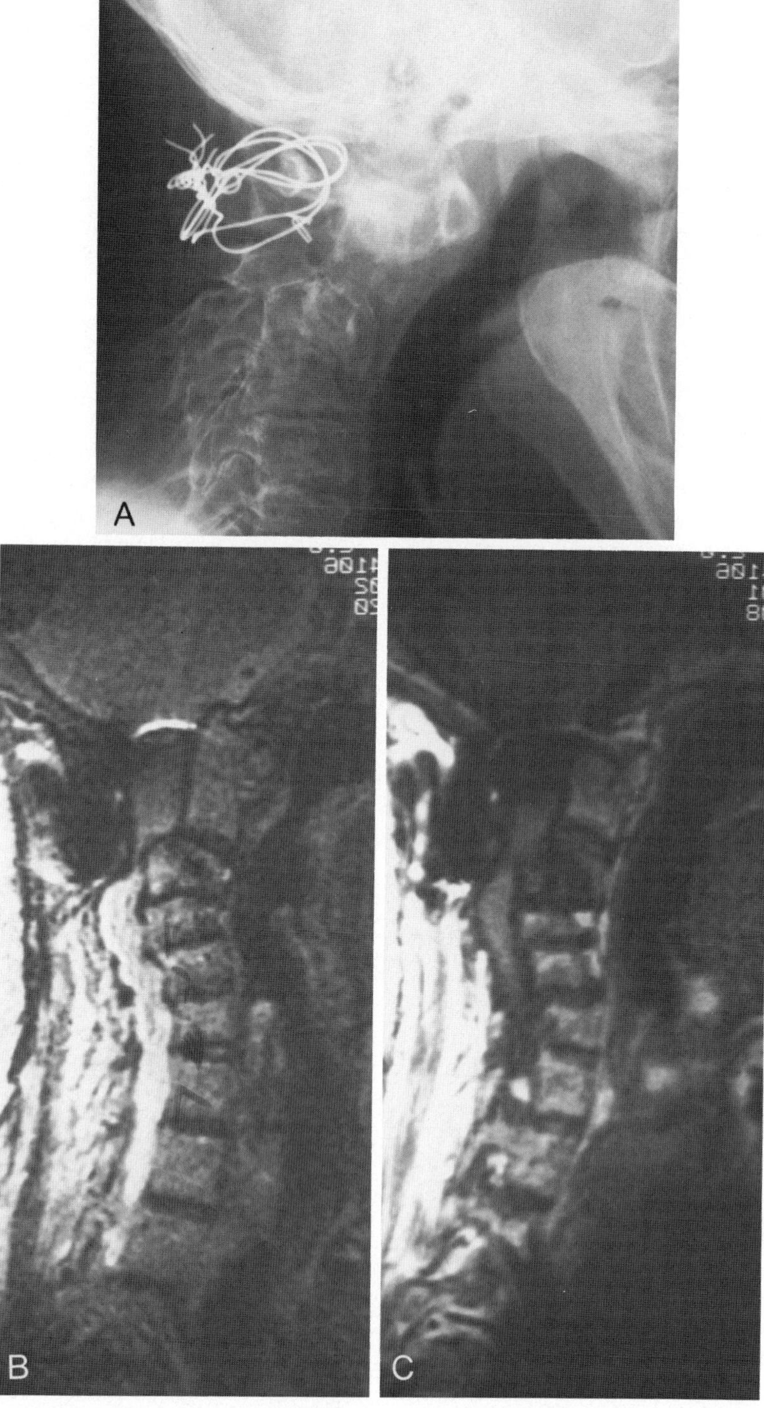

Figure 53.8. A patient with an old atlantoaxial fusion, **A**, demonstrates collapse and anterior subluxation of C3 on C4. MRI demonstrates the marked spinal cord compression on a T2-weighted image, **B**, along with the severe degree of bone destruction seen on a T1-weighted image, **C**. The metal from the wires obliterates the signal, but does not obscure the critical neuroradiologic image.

can extend the utility of this examination. Distortion of the spinal cord correlates with signs of myelopathy (52). At the cervicomedullary junction, a cervicomedullary angle of less than 135° (normal 135°–175°) correlated with clinical evidence of myelopathy (56) providing another measure for functional AAI and again indicating that cord configuration as well as compression play roles in the production of myelopathy. Figure 53.10 demonstrates the configurational change of AAI as well as the finding of an enhanced signal in the substance of the subaxial cord im-

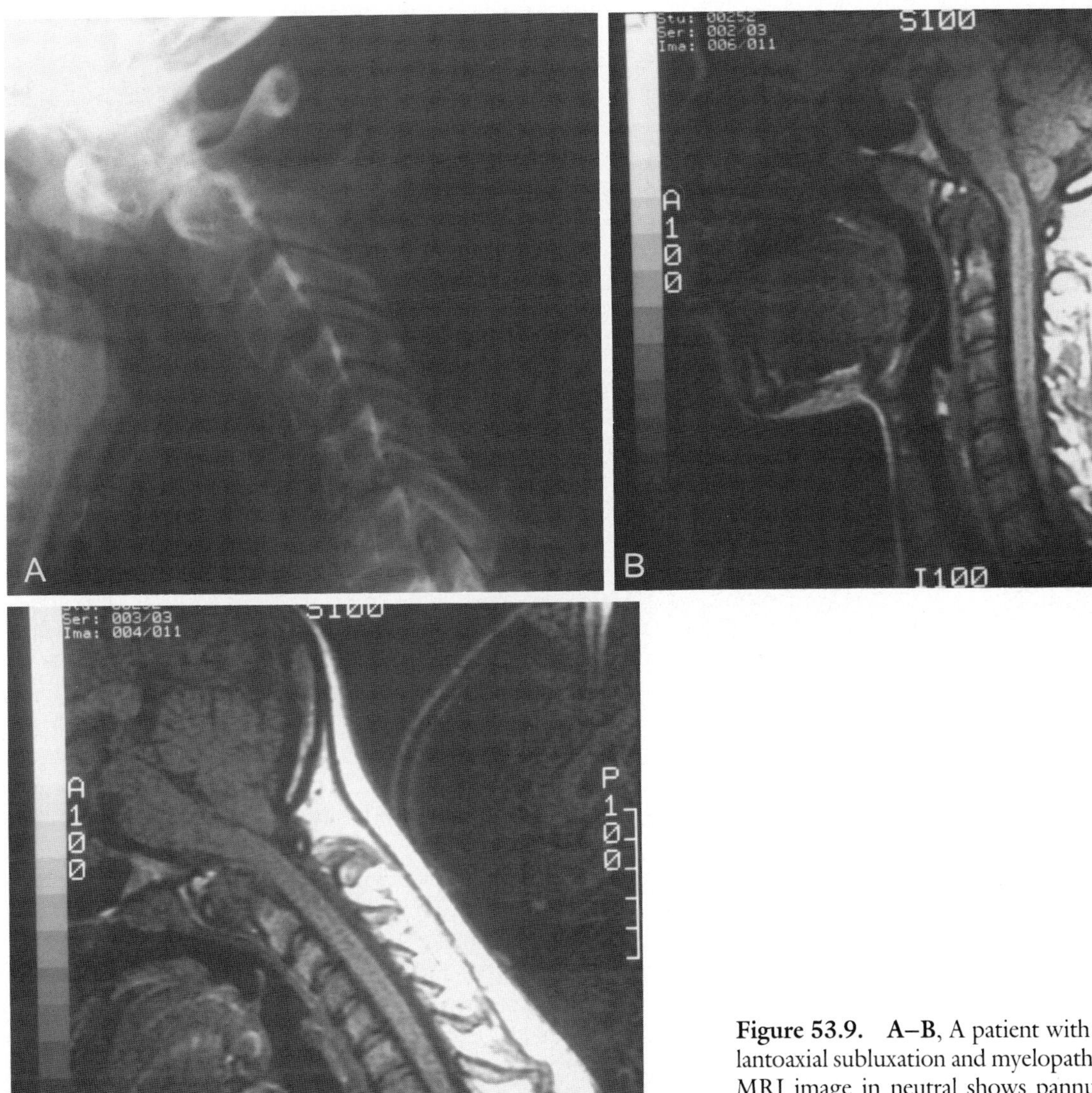

Figure 53.9. **A–B**, A patient with marked anterior atlantoaxial subluxation and myelopathy. The T2-weighted MRI image in neutral shows pannus around the dens, but no compression. By flexing the neck a dynamic MRI image shows the cord kinked over the dens and its surrounding tissue.

plicating two levels of physiologic disturbance. Demonstration of such MRI parameters may permit earlier clinical definition of the patient at risk for neurologic deterioration.

Nonsurgical Management

Since cervical spine involvement in RA appears to start early in the course of the disease and correlates with the extent and severity of the disease, early, aggressive, and continuing medical intervention is of paramount importance. The remaining nonoperative management is supportive. Cervical collars are commonly used, but no study supports their effectiveness in protecting against subluxation or neurologic progression. One study demonstrated failure to meet these goals (12). Collars are used for psychologic support, pain relief, warmth, and a feeling of stability. More rigid cervical orthoses have been shown to limit atlantoaxial motion more than soft cervical collars, but they were also shown to limit the reduction of anterior AAS by blocking extension (54). Rigid orthoses, therefore, have no special advantage. Intermittent halter cervical traction may provide comfort but will not maintain reduction of subluxations or correct myelopathy (55, 56). Pain relief can be sought anecdotally through the use of a transcutaneous nerve stimulator. Corticosteroid injection of trigger points, the greater occipital nerve, facets, and possibly, cervical epidural steroid injection, may yield some relief.

Surgical Management

The primary indication for surgical intervention is neurologic abnormality. Severe pain may also be used as an indication, and, as surgery has become safer in more recent

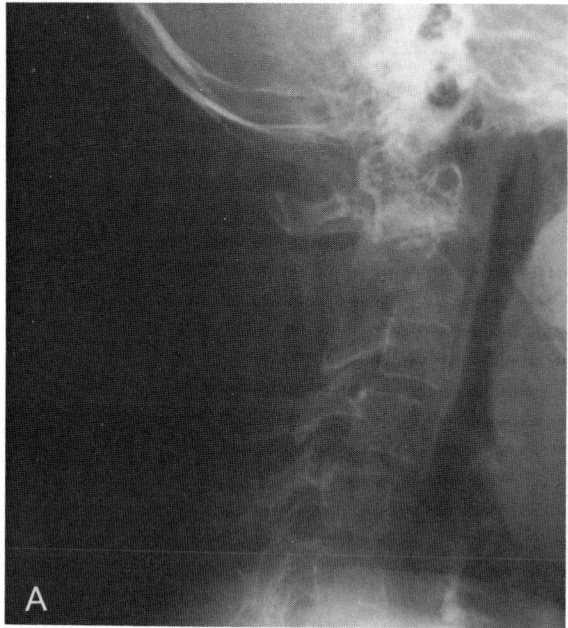

Figure 53.10. Atlantoaxial impaction and anterior subaxial subluxation at C3–4 and C4–5 are apparent on plain radiograph **A**, in a myelopathic patient. A T2-weighted MRI, **B**, shows the cord kinked over the dens with a reduced cervicomedullary angle. Although the subaxial subluxation appears reduced, the bright signal within the cord itself behind C4–5 indicates pathologic change.

times, surgeons no longer withhold surgery because of the fear of intraoperative mortality and paralysis. The presence of subluxation is not an indication for surgery since subluxations are common and do not necessarily indicate a clinical problem (20, 43). Impending neurologic deficit was introduced as an indication for surgical intervention when it was noted that once myelopathy occurred in RA patients, it could be irreversible (47). Impending neurologic deficit is defined as anterior AAS with an atlantodental distance of more than 8 mm and cord or thecal sac compression on neuroradiologic studies; or subaxial subluxation of more than 4 mm and cord or thecal sac compression on neuroradiologic studies; or AAI with compression of the brainstem or spinal cord on neuroradiologic studies (57). Impending neurologic deficit is a theoretical concept and used for asymptomatic patients with markedly abnormal radiologic studies, but it is felt that patients have a better outcome if operated upon before severe neurologic deficits occur (57). A controlled or cohort type of study is needed, especially in the area of quality of life outcome studies (58).

The major problem confronting the surgeon initially is the patient. These patients tend to be severely affected by RA; they are debilitated and crippled, have poor skin, heal wounds poorly, have osteopenic bone, making fixation of the spine difficult and bone graft mechanically inadequate with notoriously problematic rates of nonunion of fusions, and have an increased susceptibility to infection. Their airways often offer difficult management for anesthesia, and the use of fiberoptic intubation in patients with unstable and stiff necks has been a major advance. Paresis of neurologic origin, debilitation from RA, oropharyngeal swelling, poor ventilatory function from interstitial lung disease, restrictive halo-vests used postoperatively, all can combine to make the period of extubation from anesthesia perilous. Patients with cervical spine RA present a variety of preoperative, intraoperative, and postoperative challenges and incur significant surgical morbidity and mortality. Careful assessment and planning are needed when undertaking surgery.

Preoperative skeletal traction is considered necessary to reduce subluxation and myelopathic changes. Intermittent halter traction will not accomplish this goal (55, 56). Constant skeletal traction is recommended by most surgeons (45, 57, 59–61). Halo traction has been most beneficial and can be incorporated postoperatively into a halo-vest if desired. Because of debilitation, poor skin, and poor mobility, halo-vests are not found to be tolerated well by this category of RA patients. Preoperatively, a halo wheelchair is very beneficial because it allows continuous traction while the patient is sitting, as well as in bed. The halo wheelchair allows increased tolerance and comfort while avoiding the skin and infection problems of prolonged bedrest and the need for frames or special beds.

Atlantoaxial fusions are done by Gallie-type procedures (47, 60, 62) and the Brooks procedure (57). Occipitocervical fusions have evolved from the original onlay technique (63) to wired bone graft (45, 64, 65), wires and polymethylmethacrylate cement (57, 66, 67, 71), metal mesh wired in place with and without (Fig. 53.11) cement

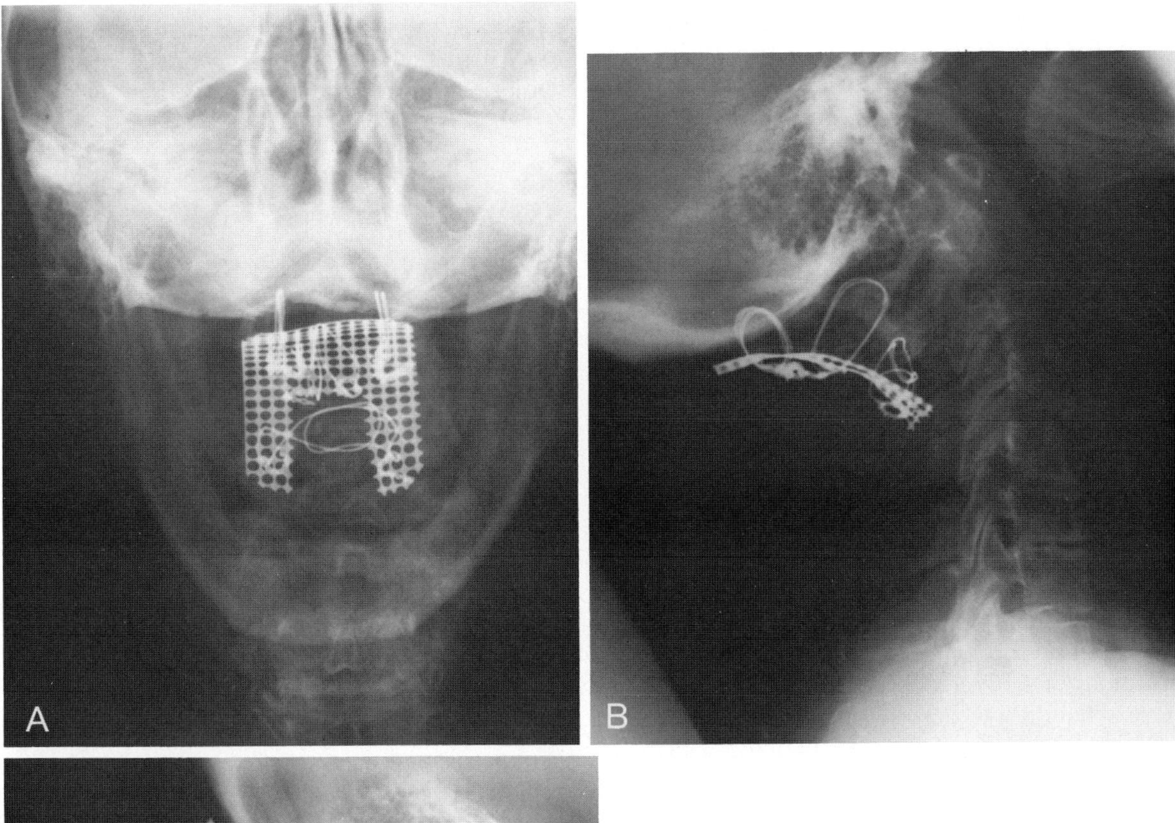

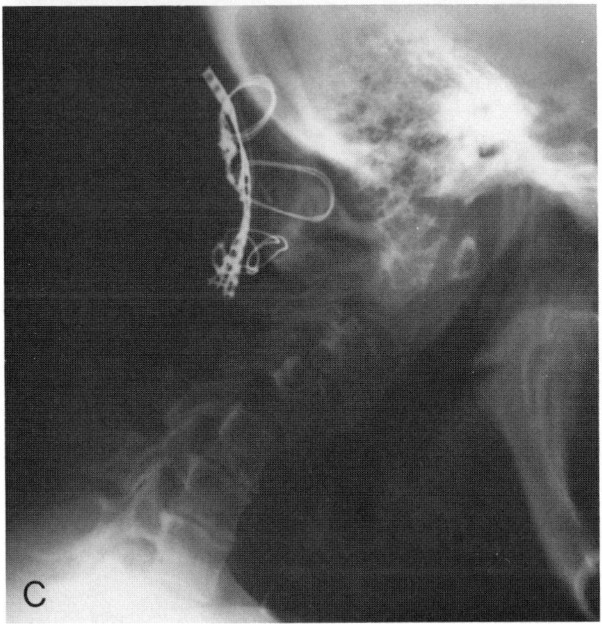

Figure 53.11. An occiptocervical fusion construct, done for atlantoaxial impaction, using metal mesh backing over bone graft. The open mouth anteroposterior view, **A**, shows the mesh with paired wires into occipital burr holes. The upper connection part lies over the occiput. The lateral views, **B**, **C**, show the occipital wires, sublaminar atlas wires, and wires into the spinous process of the axis. No motion is apparent on extension, **B**, and flexion, **C**, views. The fusion mass lies anterior to the metal mesh.

added (41, 68, 69), and contoured metal loops wired in place (70). The use of an implant may provide an immediate internal splint, allowing avoidance of a halo-vest, and provide support which cannot be achieved with the use of osteopenic bone graft. Resection of the posterior foramen magnum and posterior arch of the atlas can be accomplished at the time of fusion if necessary. For posterior fusion at the craniocervical level, nonunion rates vary from 0–50% (47, 59, 60, 62, 64, 65, 67, 68, 72, 73). Postoperative mortality is from 0–33% but the trend in the more recent reports is toward less than 10% mortality, possible due to early intervention and improved anesthetic and perioperative management (25, 47, 57, 59, 60, 62, 73–75). Neurologic improvement has been noted in 42–100% of patients (47, 57, 59, 60, 62, 65, 67, 72, 73, 76–78). Significant pain reduction is generally anticipated.

Death at a time delayed from operation is significant. Whether surgery favorably alters survival in RA is unknown. Although one study (44) suggests that survival in RA cervical myelopathy is improved by surgery, there has been no controlled study. The probability of survival in operated patients starting from the time of operation was found to be 1 year, 74%; and 5 years, 57% (46). All patients with interstitial lung disease died within 28 months of surgery. One series (75) of 32 patients and 40 operations noted an overall 57% fusion rate with 63% improvement of symptoms, and an 8% mortality rate. In their patients with severe neurologic involvement, 87% had an early death or failure, while those less neurologically involved had an 80% good result. These authors, as well as others, conclude that early diagnosis and intervention are important so as to avoid worsening myelopathy (57, 77, 78).

Transoral decompression has been advocated for irreducible anterior AAS and in situations where the pannus behind the dens causes persistent compression (54, 79, 80–82). One larger series (54, 80) comprised 14 patients where patients entering later in the series were not given tracheostomy and were nasogastrically fed in the immediate postoperative period. Immediate occipitocervical fusion followed the transoral procedure. In this study, no pharyngeal infections or immediate deaths occurred.

Complications of cervical spine surgery of any type in RA have centered on infection, wound dehiscence, nonunion, and late subaxial subluxation caudad to a fused segment (Fig. 53.8) (45, 57, 59, 68). It is believed that anatomically involved levels should be incorporated into fusions even if distal to the site of pathologic subluxation. Additionally, previously asymptomatic levels can develop subluxation below rigid segments (Fig. 53.8), so that continued long-term followup is necessary.

In the sublaxial cervical spine, subluxations are usually stabilized by wired posterior fusions. Five patterns of subaxial involvement have been observed (41). These include the usual anterior subaxial subluxation, subluxation below cephalad fusions, anterior spondylodiscitis with cord compression, compression from epidural granulations, and subaxial hyperlordosis responding to halo-traction and stabilization. Decompression and stabilization are determined by the underlying pathology elucidated by neuroradiologic studies. The role of anterior fusion for subaxial subluxation is not yet clear. Anterior fusion has been reported but lacks long-term followup (55, 83). One series reported four out of five patients without improvement, so that the procedure was not recommended (47), and in another experience of two deaths in anterior fusion (78) no enthusiasm was felt for the procedure. Anterior fusion appears to undergo resorption and collapse.

The inclusion of laminectomy in the subaxial spine has been debated, but there has been no systematic study. A report (59) of one out of five patients improving with laminectomy cast doubt on the efficacy of laminectomy along with fusion, but the authors questioned if intervention might have been too delayed. Laminectomy is always combined with fusion (41, 77). This author uses laminectomy if the subluxation is not reduced by preoperative traction. At all levels, the surgical goals are alignment of spinal configuration, decompression where necessary, and stabilization of the pathologic subluxations.

REFERENCES

1. Kontinnen Y, Sanatvirta S, Bergroth V, Sandelin J. Inflammatory involvement of cervical spine ligaments in rheumatoid arthritis. Acta Orthop Scand 1986;57:587.

2. Garrod AE. A treatise on rheumatism and rheumatoid arthritis. London: C Griffin, 1890.

3. Boger A. Ein fall von malum suboccipital rheumaticum. Arch Orthop Unfallchir 1905;3:97.

4. Ely LW. Subluxation of the atlas. A report of two cases. Arch Surg 1911;54:20.

5. Englander D. Nontraumatic occipito-atlanto-axial dislocation. Contribution to the radiology of the atlas. Br J Radiol 1942;15:341–345.

6. Davis, FW, Markley MI. Rheumatoid arthritis with death from medullary compression. Ann Intern Med 1951;35:451–454.

7. Winfield J, Cooke D, Brook AS, Corbett M. A prospective study of the radiologic changes in early rheumatoid disease. Ann Rheum Dis 1981;40:109–114.

8. Rasker JJ, Cosh JA. Radiological study of cervical spine and hand in patients with rheumatoid arthritis of 15 years duration: An assessment of the effects of corticosteroid treatment. Ann Rheum Dis 1978;37:529–535.

9. Winfield J, Young A, Williams P, Corbett M. Prospective study of the radiological changes in hands, feet, and cervical spine in adult rheumatoid disease. Ann Rheum Dis 1983;42:613–618.

10. Conlon PW, Isdale IC, Rose BS. Rheumatoid arthritis of the cervical spine. Ann Rheum Dis 1966;25:120–126.

11. Eulderink F, Meijer KAE. Pathology of the cervical spine in rheumatoid arthritis: A controlled study of 44 spines. J Pathol 1976;120:91–108.

12. Smith PH, Benn RT, Sharp J. Natural history of rheumatoid cervical luxations. Ann Rheum Dis 1972;31:431–439.

13. Stevens JC, Cartlidge NEF, Saunders M, Appleby A, Hall M, Shaw DA. Atlanto-axial subluxation and cervical myelopathy in rheumatoid arthritis, Q J Med 1971;40:391–408.

14. Weissman BN, Aliabadi P, Weinfeld MS, Thomas WH, Sosman JL. Prognostic features of atlantoaxial subluxation in rheumatoid arthritis. Radiology 1982;144:745–751.

15. Ball J. Pathology of the rheumatoid cervical spine. Ann Rheum Dis 1958;17:121.

16. Martel W, Abell MR. Fatal atlantoaxial luxation in rheumatoid arthritis. Arthritis Rheum 1963;6:224–231.

17. Mikulowski P, Wolheim FA, Rotmil P, Olsen I. Sudden death in rheumatoid arthritis with atlanto-axial dislocation. Acta Med Scand 1975;198:445–451.

18. Fielding JW, Cochran GVB, Lawsing JF, Hohl M. Tears of the transverse ligament of the atlas. A clinical and biomedical study. J Bone Joint Surg 1974;56A:1683–1691.

19. Bland JH. Rheumatoid arthritis of the cervical spine. J Rheumatol 1974;1:319–341.

20. Pellicci PM, Ranawat CS, Tsairis P, Bryan WJ. A prospective study of the progression of rheumatoid arthritis of the cervical spine. J Bone Joint Surg 1981;63A:342–346.

21. Dirheimer Y. The craniovertebral region in chronic inflammatory rheumatic diseases. Berlin: Springer-Verlag, 1977.

22. Martel W. The occipito-atlanto-axial joints in rheumatoid arthritis and ankylosing spondylitis. Am J Roentgenol 1961;86:223–240.

23. Mathews JA. Atlanto-axial subluxation in rheumatoid arthritis. Ann Rheum Dis 1969;28:260–265.

24. Sharp J, Purser DW. Spontaneous atlantoaxial dislocation in an-

kylosing spondylitis and rheumatoid arthritis. Ann Rheum Dis 1961;20:47–77.

25. Crellin RQ, MacCabe JJ, Hamilton EBD. Severe subluxation of the cervical spine in rheumatoid arthritis. J Bone Joint Surg 1970;52B:244–251.

26. Isdale JC, Corrigan AB. Backward luxation of the atlas. Ann Rheum Dis 1970;29:6–9.

27. Teigland J, Magnaes B. Rheumatoid backward dislocation of the atlas with compression of the spinal cord. Scand J Rheumatol 1980;9:253–256.

28. Verjaal A, Harder NC. Backward luxation of the atlas. Acta Radiol 1963;3:173–176.

29. Williams LE, Bland JH, Lipson RL. Cervical spine subluxations and massive osteolysis in the upper extremities in rheumatoid arthritis. Arthritis Rheum 1966;9:348–360.

30. Lipson SJ. Cervical myelopathy and posterior atlanto-axial subluxation in patients with rheumatoid arthritis. J Bone Joint Surg 1985;67A:593.

31. Burry HC. Tweed JM, Robinson RG, Howes R. Lateral subluxation of the atlanto-axial joint in rheumatoid arthritis. Ann Rheum Dis 1978;37:525–528.

32. Halla JT, Fallak S, Hardin JT. Nonreducible rotational head tilt and lateral mass collapse. A prospective study of frequency, radiographic findings, and clinical features in patients with rheumatoid arthritis. Arthritis Rheum 1982;25:1316–1324.

33. Seze S de, Dijian A, Debeyre N. Luxations altoido-axoidiennes au cours de la polyarthrite rheumatoide. Rev Rhum Mal Osteoartic 1963;30:560.

34. Morizono Y, Sakou T, Kawaida H. Upper cervical involvement in rheumatoid arthritis. Spine 1987;12:721–725.

35. Martel W. Pathogenesis of cervical discovertebral destruction in rheumatoid arthritis. Arthritis Rheum 1977;20:1217–1225.

36. Ball J, Sharp J. Rheumatoid arthritis of the cervical spine. In: Hill AGS, ed. Modern trends in rheumatology, vol 2. London: Butterworth, 1971:117–138.

37. Bywaters EGL. Rheumatoid and other diseases of the cervical interspinous bursae, and changes in the spinous processes. Ann Rheum Dis 1982;41:360–370.

38. Meikle JA, Wilkinson M. Rheumatoid involvement of the cervical spine. Ann Rheum Dis 1971;30:154–161.

39. Park WM, O'Neill MO, McCall IM. The radiology of rheumatoid involvement of the cervical spine. Skeletal Radiol 1979;4:1–7.

40. Sharp J, Purser JW, Lawrence J. Rheumatoid arthritis of the cervical spine in the adult. Ann Rheum Dis 1958; 17:303–313.

41. Lipson SJ. Patterns of rheumatoid subaxial disease causing myelopathy and strategies of management. Orthop Trans 1988;12:55.

42. Mikulowski P, Wolheim FA, Rotmil P, Olsen I. Sudden death in rheumatoid arthritis with atlanto-axial dislocation. Acta Med Scand 1975;198:445–451.

43. Isdale IC, Conlon PW. Atalnto-axial subluxation. A six year followup report. Ann Rheum Disease 1971;30:387–389.

44. Marks JS, Sharp J. Rheumatoid cervical myelopathy. Q J Med 1981;59:307–319.

45. Meijers KAE, van Beusekam GT, Luyendijk W, Duijfjes F. Dislocation of the cervical spine with cord compression in rheumatoid arthritis. J Bone Joint Surg 1974;56B:668–680.

46. Saway PA, Blackburn WD, Halla JT, Alarcon GS. Clinical characteristics affecting survival in patients with rheumatoid arthritis undergoing cervical spine surgery: a controlled study. J Rheum 1989;16:890–896.

47. Ranawat CS, O'Leary P, Pellicci P, Tsairis P, Marchisello P, Dorr L. Cervical fusion in rheumatoid arthritis. J Bone Joint Surg 1979;61A:1003–1010.

48. Redlund-Johnell I, Pettersson H. Radiographic measurements of the cranio-vertebral region. Acta Radiol 1984;25:23.

49. Braunstein EM, Weissman BNW, Seltzer SE, Sosman JL, Wang AM, Zamani A. Computed tomography and conventional radiographs of the craniocervical region in rheumatoid arthritis. Arthritis Rheum 1984;27:26–31.

50. Larrson S-E, Toolanen G, Fagerlund M. Medullary compression in rheumatoid atlanto-axial subluxation evaluated by computed tomography. Acta Orthop Scand 1986;57:262.

51. Crockard HA, Essigman WK, Stevens JM, Pozo JL, Ransford AO, Kendall BE. Surgical treatment of cervical cord compression in rheumatoid arthritis. Ann Rheum Dis 1985;44:809–816.

52. Breedveld FC, Algra PR, Vielvoye CJ, Cats A. Magnetic resonance imaging in the evaluation of patients with rheumatoid arthritis and subluxations of the cervical spine. Arthritis Rheum 1987;30:624–629.

53. Bundschuh C, Modic MT, Kearney F, Morris R, Deaf C. Rheumatoid arthritis of the cervical spine. Am J. Roentgenol 1988;151:181–187.

54. Althoff B, Goldie IF. Cervical collars in rheumatoid atlanto- axial subluxation: A radiographic comparison. Ann Rheum Dis 1980;39:485–489.

55. Hopkins JA. Cervical rheumatoid subluxation with tetraplegia. J Bone Joint Surg 1967;49B:46–51.

56. Wilson PD, Dangelmajer RC. The problem of atlantoaxial dislocation in rheumatoid arthritis. J Bone Joint Surg 1963;45A:1780.

57. Clark CR, Goetz DD, Menezes AH. Arthrodesis of the cervical spine in rheumatoid arthritis. J Bone Joint Surg 1989;71A;381–392.

58. Kaufman RL. Outcome studies, mortality versus quality of life. J Rheumatol 1989;16:857–858.

59. Conaty JP, Mongan ES. Cervical fusion in rheumatoid arthritis. J Bone Joint Surg 1981;63A:1218–1227.

60. Ferlic DC, Clayton ML, Leidholt JD, Gamble WE. Surgical treatment of the symptomatic unstable cervical spine in rheumatoid arthritis. J Bone Joint Surg 1975;57A:349–354.

61. Rana NA, Hancock DO, Taylor AR, Hill AGS. Atlanto-axial subluxation in rheumatoid arthritis. J Bone Joint Surg 1973;55B:458–470.

62. Larsson S-E, Toolanen G. Posterior fusion for atlanto-axial subluxation in rheumatoid arthritis. Spine 1986;1:525–530.

63. Newman P, Sweetnam R. Occipito-cervical fusion: an operative technique and its indications. J Bone Joint Surg 1969;51B:423–431.

64. Wertheim SB, Bohlman HH. Occipitocervical fusion. Indications, technique, and long-term results in thirteen patients. J Bone Joint Surg 1987;69A:833–836.

65. Hamblen DL. Occipito-cervical fusion. Indications, techniques, and results. J Bone Joint Surg 1967;49B:33–45.

66. Brattstrom H, Granholm L. Atlanto-axial fusion in rheumatoid arthritis. A new method of fixation with wire and bone cement. Acta Orthop Scand 1976;47:619–628.

67. Lachiewicz PF, Inglis AE, Ranawat CS. Methylmethacrylate augmentation for cervical spine arthrodesis. Orthop Trans 1987;11:7.

68. Bryan WJ, Inglis AE, Sculco TP, Ranawat CS. Methylmethacrylate stabilization for enhancement of posterior cervical arthrodesis in rheumatoid arthritis. J Bone Joint Surg 1982;64A:1045–1050.

69. Lipson SJ. Occipitocervical fusion using wired metal mesh and methacrylate backed bone graft. Orthop Trans 1985;9:141.

70. Ransford AO, Crockard HA, Pozo JL, Thomas NP, Nelson IW. Craniocervical instability treated by a contoured loop fixation. J Bone Joint Surg 1986;68B:173–177.

71. Clark CR, Keggi KJ, Panjabi MM. Methacrylate stabilization of the cervical spine. J Bone Joint Surg 1984;66A;40–46.

72. Cregan JCF. Internal fixation of the unstable rheumatoid cervical spine. Ann Rheum Dis 1966;25:242–252.

73. Thomas WH. Surgical management of the rheumatoid cervical spine. Orthop Clin North Am 1975;6:793–800.

74. Thompson RC, Meyer TJ. Posterior surgical stabilization for atlanto-axial subluxation in rheumatoid arthritis. Spine 1985;10:597–601.

75. Zoma A, Sturrock RD, Fisher WD, Freeman PA, Hamblen DL.

Surgical stabilization of the rheumatoid cervical spine. A review of indications and results. J Bone Joint Surg 1987;69B;8–12.

76. Meijers KAE, Cats A, Kremer HPH, Luyendijk W, Onvlee GJ, Thomeer RTW. Cervical myelopathy in rheumatoid arthritis. Clin Exp Rheumatol 1984;2:239–245.

77. Sanatvirta S, Slatis P, Kankaapaa U, Sandelin J, Laasonen E. Treatment of the cervical spine in rheumatoid arthritis. J Bone Joint Surg 1988;70A;658–667.

78. Heywood AWB, Learmonth ID, Thomas M. Cervical spine instability in rheumatoid arthritis. J Bone Joint Surg 1988;70B:702–707.

79. Brattstrom H, Elner A, Granholm L. Transoral surgery for myelopathy caused by rheumatoid arthritis of the cervical spine. Ann Rheum Dis 1973;32:578–581.

80. Crockard HA, Pozo JL, Ransford AO, Stevens JM, Kendall BE, Essigman WK. Transoral decompression and posterior fusion for rheumatoid atlanto-axial subluxation. J Bone Joint Surg 1986;68B:350–356.

81. Menezes AH, Van Gilder JC, Clark CR, El-Khoury G. Odontoid upward migration in rheumatoid arthritis. An analysis of 45 patients with "cranial settling." J Neurosurg 1985;63:500–509.

82. Olerud S, Sjostrom L. Dens resection in a case of vertical impression of the dens in the foramen magnum. Acta Orthop Scand 1986;57:262.

83. Lidgren L, Ljunggren B, Ratcheson RA. Reposition, anterior exposure and fusion in the treatment of myelopathy caused by rheumatoid arthritis of the cervical spine. Scan J Rheumatol 1974;3:195–198.

54

Stabilization of the Cervical Spine with Posterior Plates and Screws

Raymond Roy-Camille and Christian Mazel

Instability at the lower cervical spine level is usually due to injuries or tumors. At the upper cervical spine level, instability is usually due to tumors or degenerative diseases rather than injuries.

In our experience, the posterior approach is simple and allows for posterior fixation with plates and screws easily. This method of osteosynthesis is rigid and stable, and secondary displacement or loosening of hardware is rare.

Lower Cervical Spine Posterior Plate Fixation

Anatomy

The anatomy of the lower cervical spine is generally not well known, and when posterior fixation is performed, one can only see the posterior aspect of the posterior arches. Their shape provides information about the anterior elements (Fig. 54.1).

The posterior vertebral arch includes the spinous processes in the midline, with the lamina on both sides and the lateral articular masses (Figs. 54.2). A groove resembling a valley is located at the border between the lamina and the bulging articular mass, which can be compared to a hill. The spinal cord is anterior to the spinous process and the lamina. The vertebral artery is anterior to this valley, which is an excellent landmark. The roots at each level exit the vertebral canal horizontally via the foramina. The foramina are found at the level of the facet joint lines, a posterior marker. The plates are placed over the lateral articular masses lateral to the valley, and the screws are implanted into the masses.

These landmarks make it easy to insert the screws into the articular masses. Because of their lateral position, the screws are far from the spinal cord, and the facet joint is anterior in between the roots above and below. The screws also avoid the vertebral artery by being lateral to the valley in front of which it exists.

Instrumentation

Special plates have been designed for this type of fixation. They are premolded to fit the minimal cervical spinal lordosis. They are 2 mm thick and 1 cm wide. The holes are positioned every 13 mm, and they have 2–5 holes to enable 2–5 vertebral body fixation (Fig. 54.3). They are made out of chrome, cobalt alloy, or stainless steel. The screws are self-tapping and 3.5 mm in diameter. They are short, usually 16–18 mm long, corresponding to the thickness of the articular pillars.

Surgical Procedure

Surgery is performed through a mid-posterior approach. The patient is in the prone position and the head firmly fixed with a head-holder that enables a flexion/extension motion. A traction device, if necessary, can be attached to the operating table. Local infiltration of a Xylocaine and adrenalin solution helps to divide the muscles of the mid-

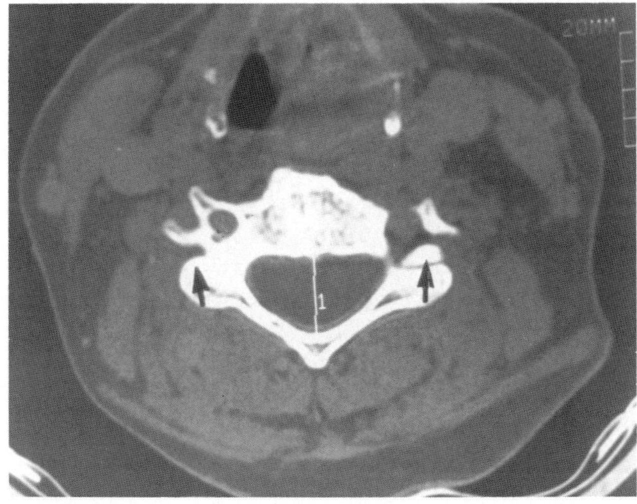

Figure 54.1. A transverse cut of the cervical spine demonstrates the position of the articular masses. The screws are lateral to the cord and the vertebral artery.

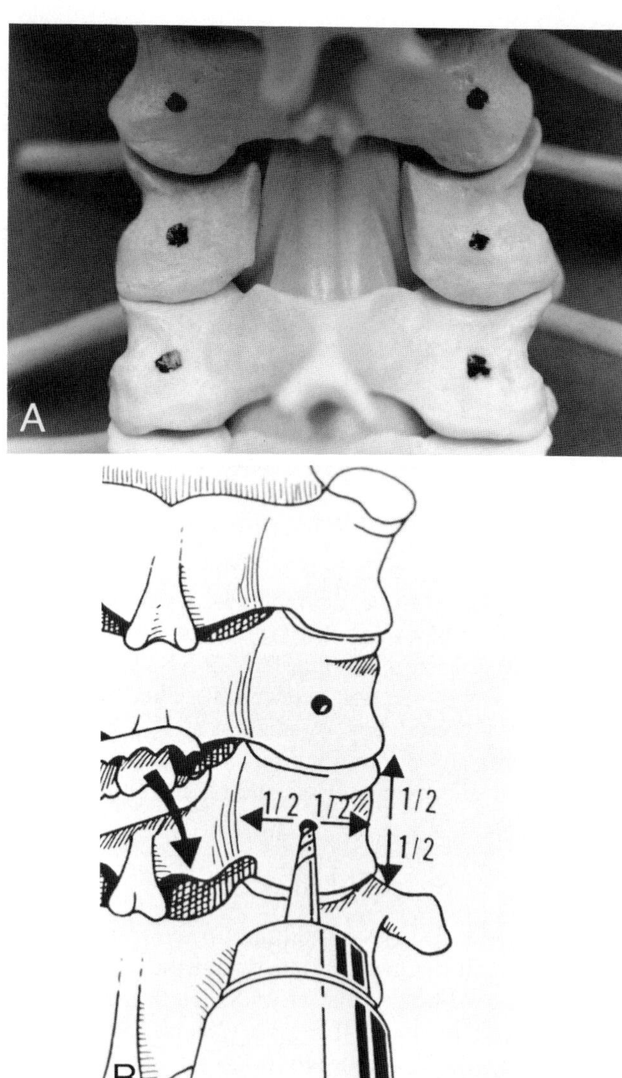

Figure 54.2. Drilling of the articular mass is performed at its center on top of the small hill lateral to the cord and the valley in front of which flows the vertebral artery.

line and diminishes bleeding. The surgical approach is achieved by reflecting the paraspinal muscles down to the lateral side of the articular masses, in order to locate the above-mentioned reference marks.

The exact position to drill and insert the screws is located at the top of the articular mass hill, exactly at its midpoint (Fig. 54.2**B**). A 2.8 mm drill bit is used for 3.5 mm screws. A special drill bit with a stop at 19 mm prevents it from penetrating too far. A slow-motor drill is utilized. The drilling direction is perpendicular to the vertebral plane, with 10° of lateral obliquity. This lateral oblique direction increases safety and ensures avoiding the vertebral artery, which is medial and anterior to the previously mentioned valley. Performed with care, no complications have occurred. The only contraindication to this plating method is severe osteopenia.

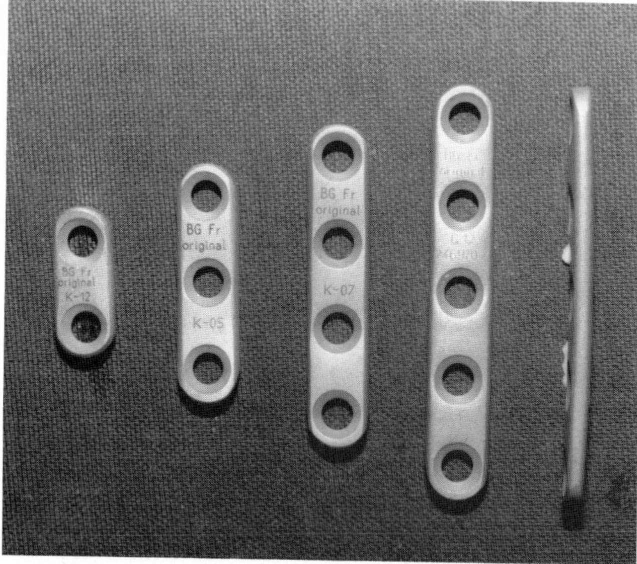

Figure 54.3. Posterior plates are designed to enable 2–5 levels of vertebral fixation.

Complementary Procedures

The posterior approach and the use of posterior plates and screws implanted into the articular masses allow for associated procedures. A laminectomy is easily performed, when necessary, because the plates are lateral to the lamina on the articular masses. A Hibbs fusion on the lamina is possible, if desired, when the lamina are maintained.

Postoperative Care

In most cases, a simple rigid collar is used for 6–12 weeks postoperatively. Ambulation is allowed on the second postoperative day.

Experimental Study

This study was performed with the assistance of R. Johnson at the V.A. Hospital in New Haven, CT. We investigated the mechanical properties of the fixation system in both flexion and extension. Two cervical vertebrae from a fresh cadaver were united posteriorly, with a symmetrical pair of two-hole plates, after removal of all ligaments and the interbody disc material. The lower vertebral body was then fixed in position. Displacement of the upper vertebral body was analyzed during motion, with displacement gauges and radiographs. The entire experiment was performed in a large glass box in order to keep a constant hydrostatic pressure in the box, and to maintain as close as possible the in vivo characteristics of the system.

The average breaking load with extension stress is 52.5 kg (515 Newtons). This represents 60% more load than necessary to dislocate two normal cervical vertebrae. These results have been compared with the other methods of cervical posterior fixation. With extension stress, a posterior wiring of the spinous process or of the articular masses is not sufficient to stabilize the spine. Fixation of the spinous processes with methylmethacrylate provides a 99% increase in stability. For a flexion stress, the posterior wiring between the spinous processes gives a 33% increase in stability. The same wiring, but around a complementary bone graft, gives a 55% increase in stability. The stability increases to 88% when the wiring passes through the articular masses. Significantly, plate fixation, gives a 92% increase in stability in flexion.

UPPER CERVICAL SPINE POSTERIOR PLATE FIXATION

Plates and screws can also be used for stabilization of the upper cervical spine. Special plates have been designed which will restore the normal angulation of the occipitocervical junction.

Anatomy of the Occipitocervical Junction

The normal occipitocervical angulation is 105° to give a normal horizontal direction to the head and eyes. Any fixation with plates must preserve this (Fig. 54.4).

The longitudinal posterior venous sinus is on the midline of the occipital bone. Lateral to the sinus, the bone is about 10–12 mm thick, with two cortices. It allows only a short screw to be inserted, but excellent fixation because of the two bone cortices at this level.

Instrumentation

To stabilize the occipitocervical junction, we use special premolded plates. Their shape is designed to restore the normal curvature of the occipitocervical junction, with a 105° angulation. They are reinforced in their middle at the apex of the curve. The occipital part of the plate is flat to prevent skin tension at this level. The fixation to the occiput is lateral to the midline and achieved usually with 13 mm-long screws (Fig. 54.5). At the cervical level, the fixation is completed with screws implanted to the articular masses as previously described. Some plates are short, going down to C4; others are longer, going down to C5.

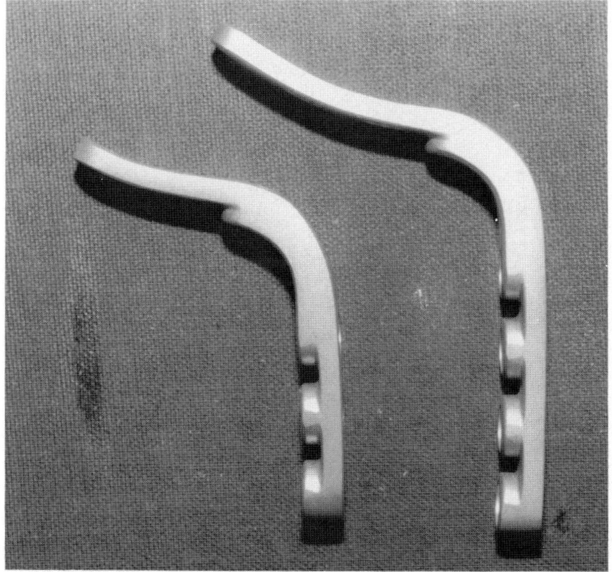

Figure 54.4. Occipitocervical plates are designed to recover normal angulation (angle is 105°). The occipital portion is thinned to avoid skin tension.

Surgical Procedure

The procedure is performed in the prone position, with the head maintained by a head holder. The position of the head over the cervical spine is evaluated with a lateral preoperative radiograph. Through a midline posterior approach, periosteum is reflected laterally on the occiput. The posterior arch of C2 is easy to find because of its bulky spinous process. The posterior arch of C1 is exposed, if necessary. The lower vertebrae with their articular masses are also exposed, and the implantation of the screws is prepared by drilling the masses down to the desired level. A 2.8 mm drill bit is used. Two plates are placed on each side of the cervical spine, first on the C3 and C4 articular masses, as usual. A screw can also be inserted into the C2 articular mass. The drilling here is done directly through the plate hole into the lower part of the C2 articular mass. At this stage, the occiput is placed against the upper part of the first plate by manipulating the head holder. The correct cervico-occipital angulation is thus ensured. The drilling of the occiput is performed through the plate holes, using a drill bit with a stop at 12 mm. A depth gauge is utilized. Two or three 12–14 mm-long screws are inserted. The second plate is secured with the same technique. The last step is fusion. Between the two plates is a large area for corticocancellous bone graft, and the graft is directly fixed to the occipital cortex with a screw. Its lower portion can be fixed by wiring to the C4 or C5 spinous process and, if desired, to the C2 spinous process. Cancellous bone is packed beneath and around the main corticocancellous graft (Fig. 54.6).

Postoperative Care

A plastic Minerva corset is worn for 3 months. Ambulation is possible in the immediate postoperative period.

C2 TRANSPEDICULAR FIXATION

First described by Robert Judet, this technique allows direct fixation of a hangman's fracture when necessary (Fig. 54.7).

Anatomy

Implanting the screw into the C2 pedicle is difficult (Fig. 54.8A). It requires a perfect working knowledge of the

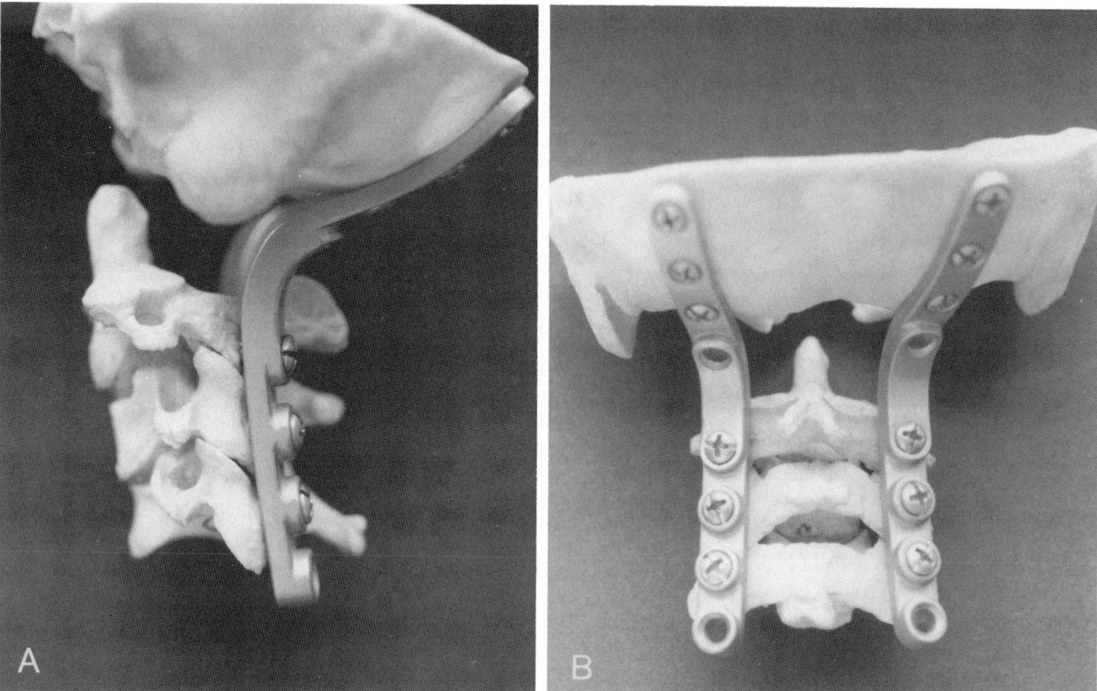

Figure 54.5. To obtain a rigid stabilization of the occipital junction, two-plate fixation is necessary. The grafts are displayed in between on the posterior arches.

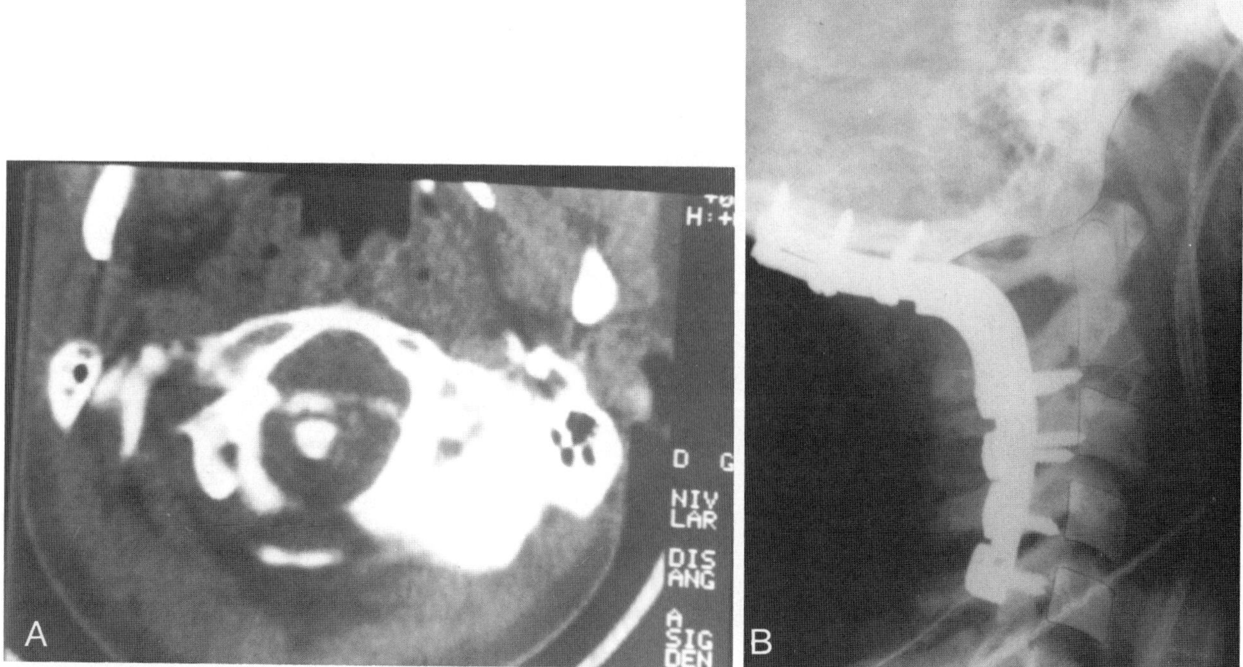

Figure 54.6. Occipitocervical fixation is rarely necessary in acute injuries. In case of the rare occipito-cervical dislocation (CT scan), it is the only way to stabilize this highly unstable injury.

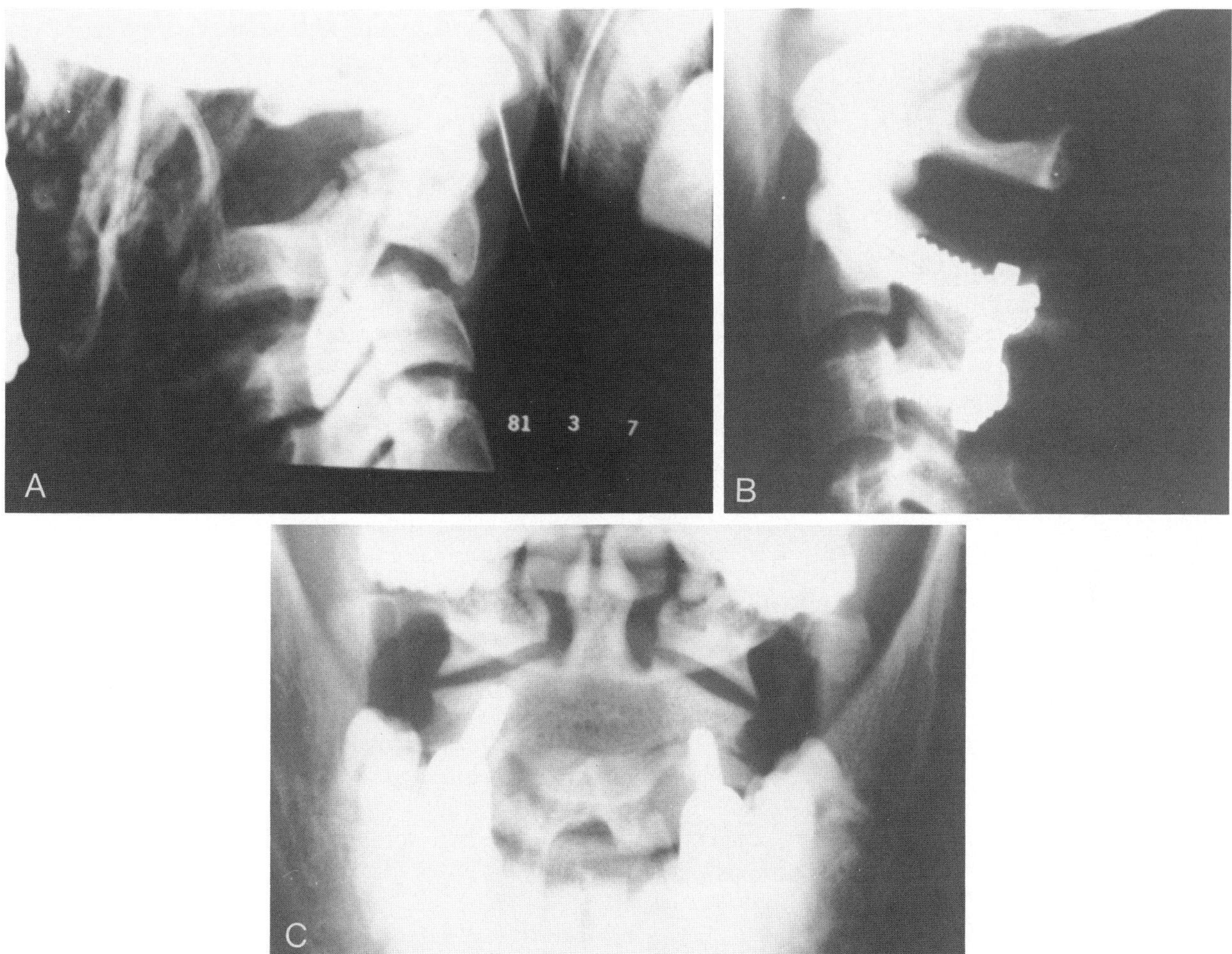

Figure 54.7. A hangman fracture with facet dislocation can only be reduced by a posterior approach. C2–3 instrumentation will provide strong, effective fixation.

anatomical landmarks to prevent vertebral artery injury. The C1 ring is normally divided into thirds; one is occupied by the odontoid process, one by the cord, and one is free. At the C2 level, the ring is still large, and no intimate contact exists between the spinal cord and the pedicles. The vertebral artery passes through the C2 articular mass, making a horizontal S-type loop. The posterior aspect of the articular mass, which is exposed via the posterior approach, can be divided into four quadrants (Fig. 54.8**B**). The vertebral artery occupies the two inferior quarters, and the upper lateral one. The upper medial quarter is where a screw can be implanted without danger. The C2 pedicle is angulated obliquely 10–15° upward and inward. A screw inserted into it must have the same direction.

Surgical Procedure

The superior border of the C2 lamina is exposed, and, as the vertebral canal is wide at this level, one can introduce a slightly curved spatula-type retractor without damage to the cord along the medial aspect of the pedicle. On the upper medial quadrant of the posterior aspect of the articular mass, the point of penetration is located, and the area is prepared with an awl. This point must be as high and medial as possible on the articular mass. From this point, the drilling is performed obliquely upward and inward 10–15°, the spatula retractor indicating the exact direction of the pedicle (Fig. 54.8**C**). The drill bit is as close as possible to the medial and upper cortex of the pedicle. Drilling is completed to a depth of 35 mm. The vertebral artery is lateral and inferior to the drill. The 35 mm-long screw can then be inserted through the fracture line of the pedicle into the vertebral body of C2.

LOWER CERVICAL SPINE INJURIES

Indications

Posterior lesions are better treated through a posterior approach, anterior lesions through an anterior one, and horizontal lesions of the mobile vertebral segment can be

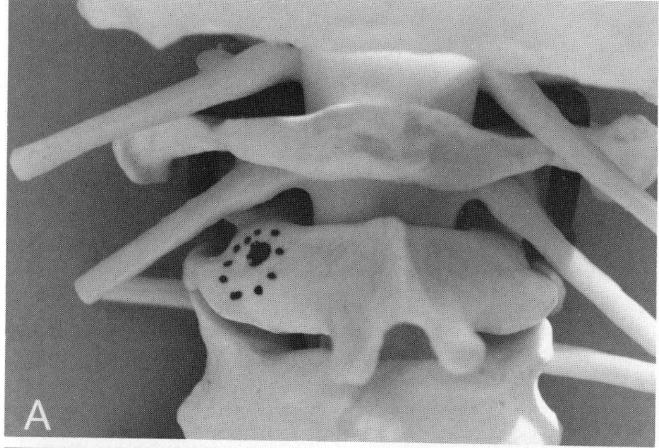

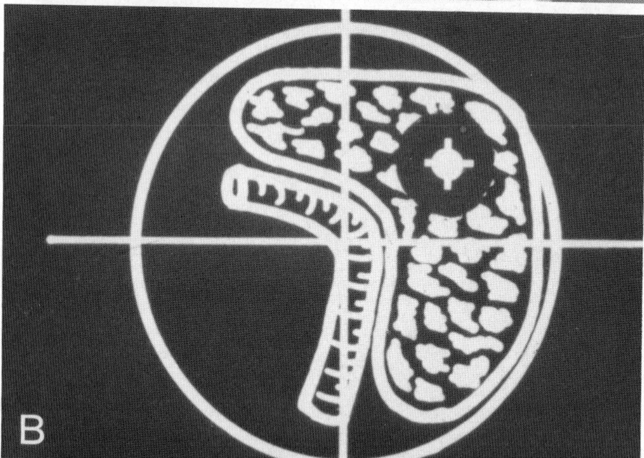

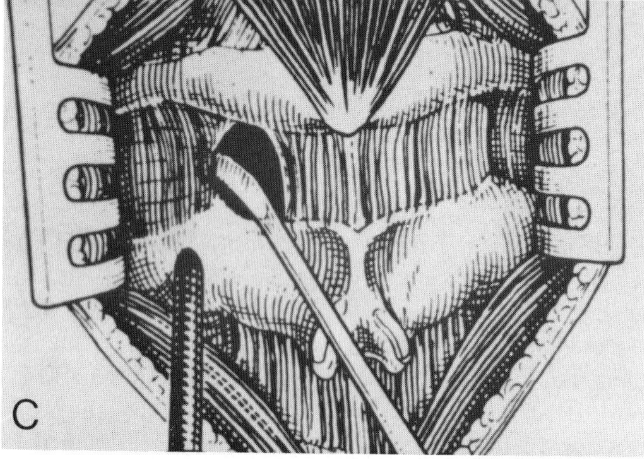

Figure 54.8. **A,** Implantation of a screw into the pedicle of C2 requires a good knowledge of its anatomy. **B,** The articular mass of C2 can be identified as a circle. The point of drilling is located on the upper medial quarter of it. **C,** Drilling must be centered down the pedicle.

treated either posteriorly or anteriorly. When there is any question concerning an approach, we utilize the posterior approach, because we are more confident in the rigid fixation of the posterior plate fixation with screws inserted in the articular masses. Most lesions in cervical spine injuries are posterior: dislocations, fractures, or fracture with dislocation of the articular facets (58% of cases). All these are best treated with our technique of posterior plating. Severe sprains are treated in the same way.

Cervical Dislocations

UNILATERAL DISLOCATIONS

In such cases, open reduction is best achieved by introducing a spatula between the laminae at the dislocated level. The first spatula is introduced near the midline close to the spinous process. While the first spatula is kept in place, a second is introduced laterally. The first is then placed farther on between the dislocated articular facets. It is then possible with a lever maneuver to achieve reduction by moving the upper articular facet backward over the lower one. Reduction is then maintained with the table head holder positioned in extension. The first posterior two-hole plate is implanted on the dislocated side, and the fixation is completed with a second plate on the opposite side. The holes are first drilled into the superior articular masses, then the lower. The upper screw is inserted through the upper hole of the plate. At that time, the lower hole usually does not line up perfectly with the second predrilled hole. It usually remains distal to the plate hole, because the reduction is not yet perfect. The second screw is inserted through the second plate hole and then into the predrilled hole through the bone, and its insertion will reduce the lower articular mass and the vertebra (Fig. 54.9).

BILATERAL DISLOCATIONS

The same reduction maneuver can be performed on both sides simultaneously, and again stabilization is achieved with two posterior two-hole plates. The fixation of a one-level dislocation with the two-hole plate is strong enough to prevent any displacement. Postoperatively, the patient will wear a simple hard collar for 6 weeks. We prefer to perform this surgical procedure on an emergency basis in the absence of any previous traction. Since open reduction gives direct visual control of the lesion, the maneuvers are precise and smooth, and posterior fixation is achieved at the same time. This all shortens the period of postoperative care. Patients without neurologic involvement ambulate on the first postoperative day, and they are usually discharged from the hospital on the 5th day after surgery.

FACET JOINT FRACTURE WITH DISLOCATION

When a facet joint fracture is combined with a dislocation, it is usually a fracture of the upper articular facet. Its displacement follows the upper cervical vertebra, and the broken fragment usually pushes into the foramen and can compress the homolateral cervical nerve root. Two problems must, therefore, be solved: the prevention or correction of a possible cervical brachialgia induced by compression of the nerve root, and fixation of the fracture/dislocation,

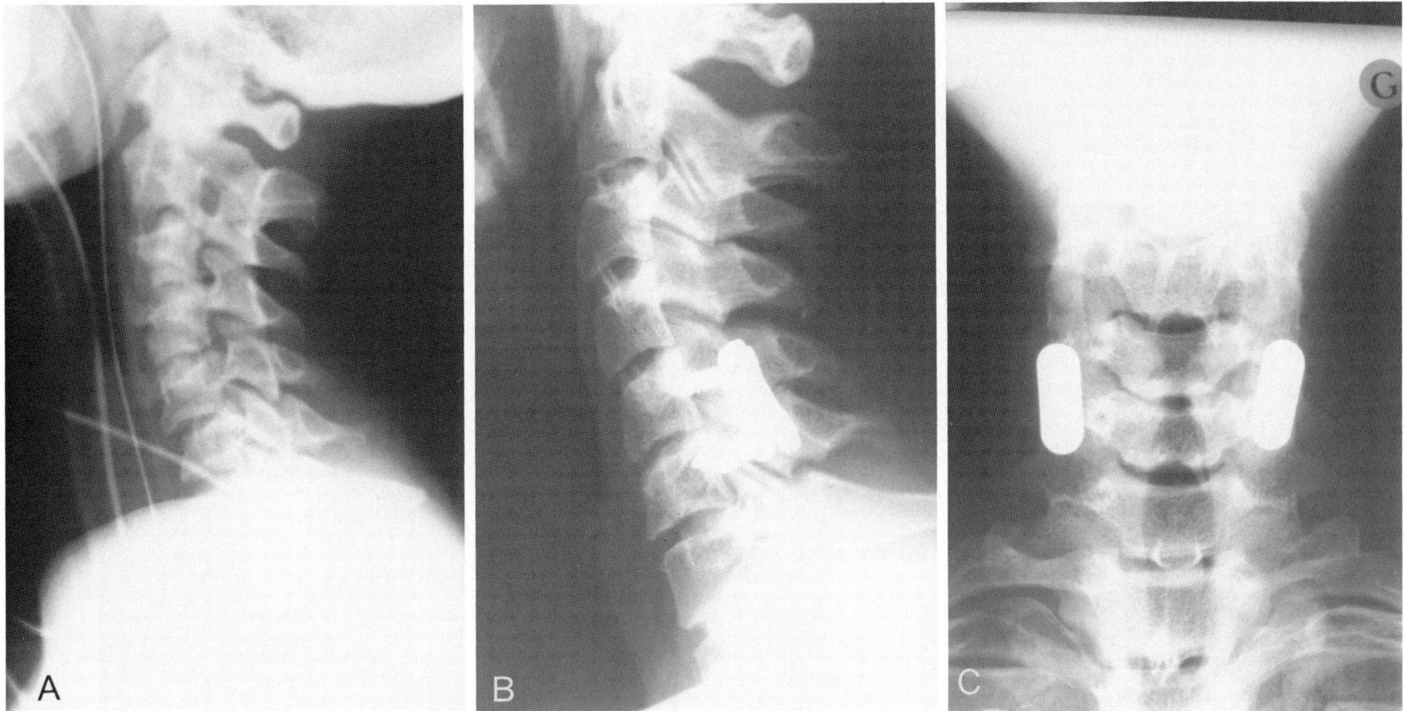

Figure 54.9. Unilateral facet dislocation. Open reduction is performed, and fixation is achieved by two-hole plates.

which is difficult, because the stability from the articular facet is missing after the reduction. The displaced compressing fragment must be removed from the foramina before performing internal fixation. This can be performed only via a posterior approach and through the broken facet joint. The fixation is then achieved with the reconstruction of the broken upper articular facet, using a special tile-shaped plate (Fig. 54.10). This very precise technique is essentially a hemiarthroplasty. The upper part of the plate is oblique and is slipped beneath the lower facet of the upper rotated vertebra. The lower part of the plate will be fixed into the inferior articular mass with a screw. At the beginning of our experience, the tile plate alone was used. We now prefer to combine a tile plate with a standard two-hole plate. The normal plate is placed over the tile plate; together, they look like a "port manteau." Fixation is achieved with a lower screw driven through the inferior holes of the two plates, and an upper screw is implanted into the articular mass of the above vertebra. A standard two-hole plate bridges the opposite side at the same level (Fig. 54.11).

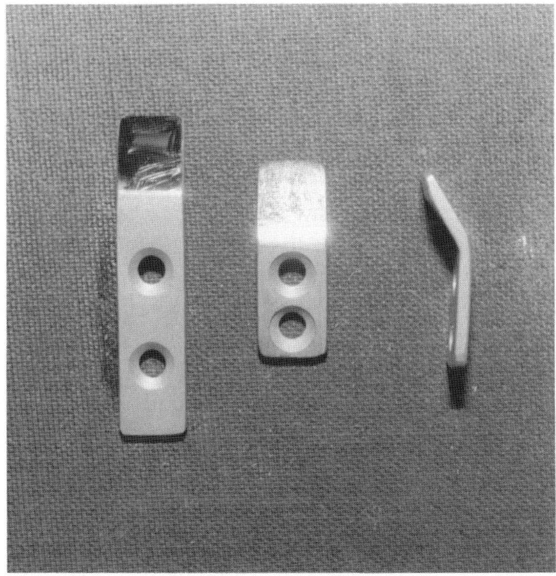

Figure 54.10. The tile plate is designed to achieve a facet arthroplasty. Long or short fixation is possible.

Separation Fracture of the Articular Mass

The diagnosis of this fracture is difficult and its stabilization often challenging. Fracture lines need to be well understood to perform the correct internal fixation (Fig. 54.12**A**, **B**, and **C**). Here, a unilateral lesion occurs, with two fracture lines separating the articular mass from the vertebra. The first line is through the pedicle, and the second through the lamina on the same side. The articular mass is thus completely free from the rest of the vertebra and can be displaced from a vertical position to a horizontal one. This induces a unilateral displacement with rotation. On the lateral x-ray, the articular mass appears horizontal and no longer parallel to the adjacent upper and lower facets, and

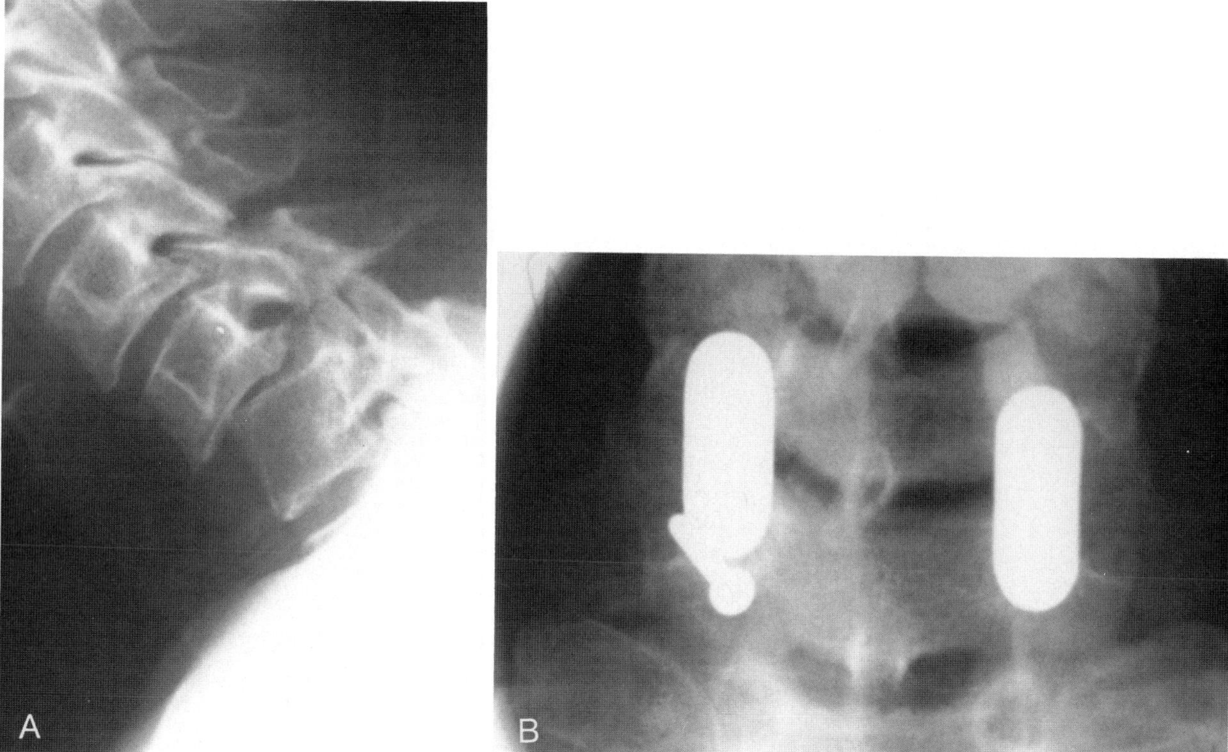

Figure 54.11. In some cases of facet fracture/dislocation, fixation of the broken facet is possible with a small screw.

oblique views are far more demonstrative. A CT scan is the test best capable of showing both fracture lines.

The ideal fixation of these fractures is difficult (Fig. 54.12**D**). From a series of 25 cases, we have demonstrated that a long, three-level "port manteau" type of internal fixation is necessary. A long tile plate is first introduced in the upper facet joint. Reduction of the horizontal articular mass is obtained by pushing the long portion of the tile plate against the spine. A three-hole cervical plate is then implanted over the top plate, improving the reduction. Another three-hole plate is implanted on the opposite side. This type of internal fixation obtains both reduction and stabilization.

TEARDROP FRACTURE

A simple teardrop fracture is most similar to a severe sprain than a fracture. The lesions involve the discs and the ligaments, and the small broken bony fragment of the vertebral body is not important. Instability comes from the severe ligamentous injury of the mobile vertebral segment. When the injury is mainly posterior, with interspinous widening and facet joint posterior opening, the surgical treatment can be performed posteriorly with posterior plates. The major problem with such fractures is to determine the exact level of instrumentation. CT scans have demonstrated the frequent existence of an anteroposterior fracture line splitting the vertebral body. In such cases, this body fracture needs fixation which will include both adjacent discs. The posterior plating reduces the displacement of the facets and, at the same time, the displacement of the posterior/inferior corner of the vertebral body from the canal. The teardrop fracture can also be approached anteriorly for a vertebrectomy and grafting. In cases without vertebral body splitting, the internal fixation will only span the injured disc level.

SEVERE SPRAINS

Severe sprains need to be suspected, because they are often undiagnosed early on. A severe sprain is the stage before the complete ligamentous disruption and dislocation of the vertebral segments. The entire mobile vertebral segment is involved by the trauma, without any bony lesion, and without any initial displacement. Induced by continuous motion of the neck, the displacement occurs progressively a few weeks or months after trauma.

Initially, a severe sprain can be diagnosed on the following: interspinous widening, facet joint subluxation, posterior disc space widening, an anterior listhesis of the upper vertebra (Fig. 54.13). Fixation with posterior plates and screws is a simple and appropriate technique for the stabilization of such injuries.

VERTEBRAL BODY FRACTURES

In a few cases, we have treated wedge body fractures with posterior plating. The reduction of the wedge is obtained

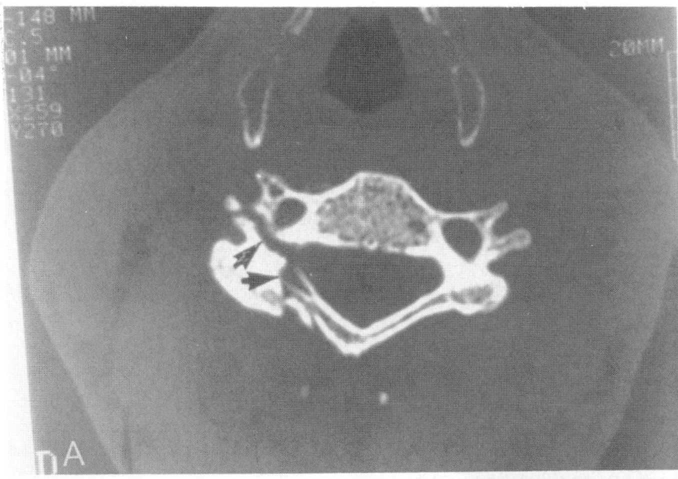

Figure 54.12. **A,** Separation fracture of the articular mass. CT scan reveals two fracture lines, one on the pedicle, and one on the lamina. **B,** AP view demonstrates a horizontal articular mass in the pedicle fracture line. **C,** On the lateral view, the articular mass is tilted forward and becomes horizontal. **D,** The port manteau fixation along with tile plate provides complete reduction and stabilization.

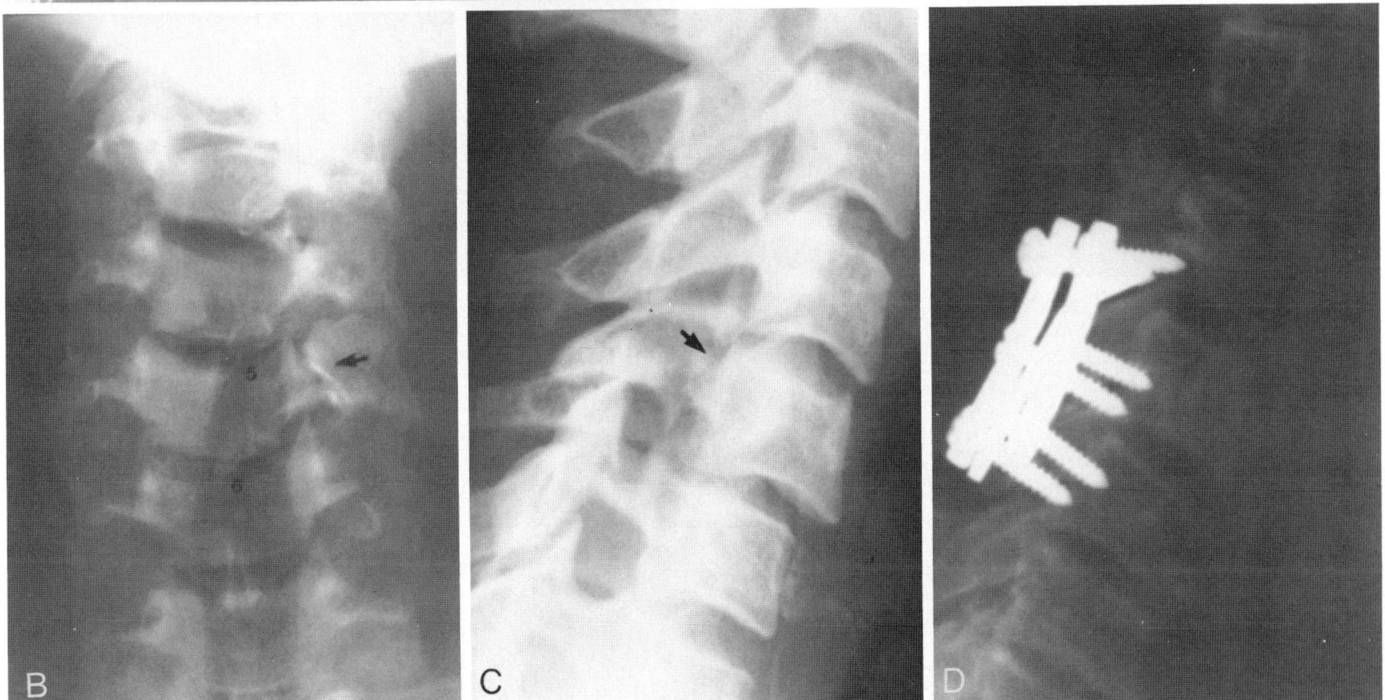

by hyperlordosis of the plate and placing the anterior longitudinal ligament under tension. Stabilization was achieved with a pair of two- or three-hole plates, bridging only the disc above the reduction or the whole vertebra.

FAILURE OF AN ANTERIOR STABILIZATION

Posterior fixation with plates and screws is a very simple and elegant method to achieve a fusion that does not succeed after failure of an anterior technique. In these cases, we usually use a posterior Hibbs fusion. The stable and rigid posterior fixation will then induce the anterior fusion.

POSTOPERATIVE CARE

Simple injuries, such as unilateral dislocations, are immobilized by a simple collar for 6 weeks. The more unstable lesions with associated fractures are immobilized for 2–3 months by a light Minerva jacket made of plastic or leather. In the case of cord injury with quadriplegia, the rigid, stable fixation induced by the plates facilitates nursing care, and, for the first days after surgery, can avoid all use of external immobilization devices.

Results

EVALUATIONS AND COMPLICATIONS OF 238 CERVICAL POSTERIOR FIXATIONS

Two hundred and nine cases (88%) out of a series of 238 cases of low cervical acute injuries healed without complications.

Mechanical Complications

A. Loss of fixation and recurrence of deformity occurred in six cases (2.2%). In four cases, revision was necessary,

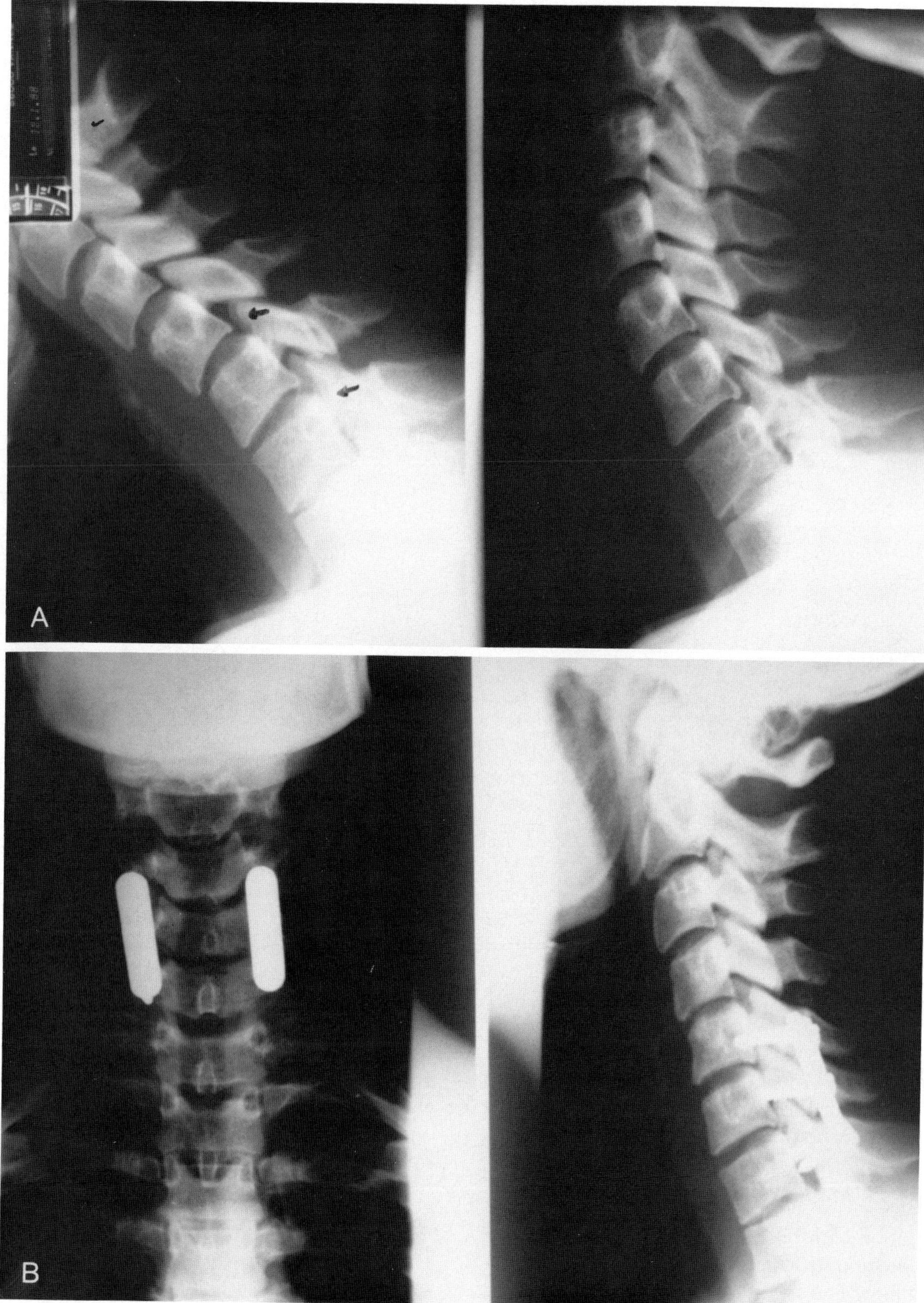

Figure 54.13. A two-level, severe ligamentous sprain. Posterior fixation enables complete restoration of anatomy.

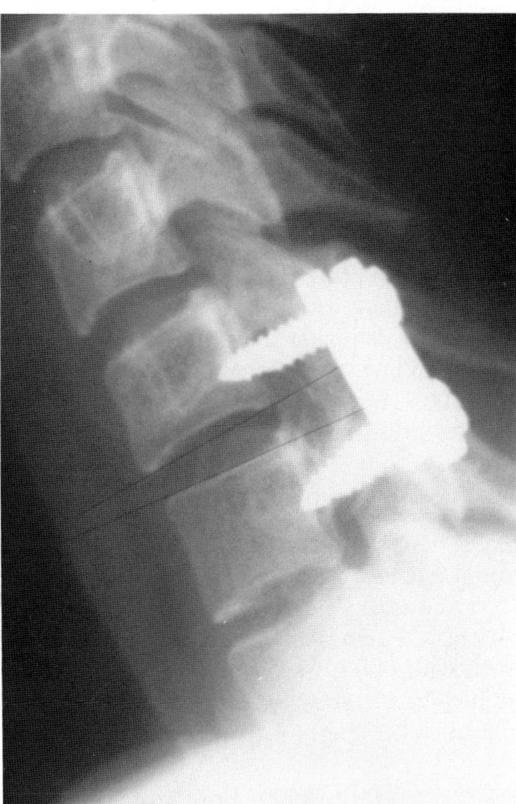

Figure 54.14. Kyphosis can be observed at the level of instrumentation. Under 10°, it must not be considered a failure of the technique.

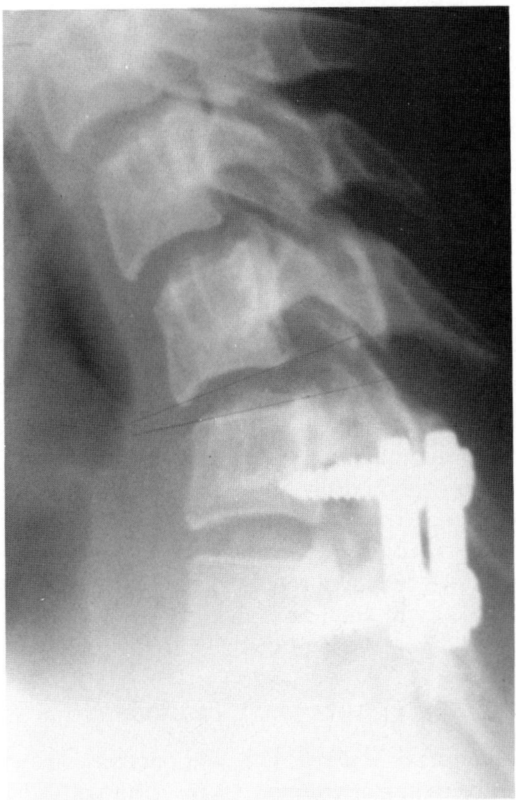

Figure 54.15. On dynamic x-rays, kyphosis of the upper adjacent disc can be disturbing. A long-term follow-up showed no cases of progression of the kyphosis.

because deformity was unacceptable. The causes were infection in two cases, a unilateral fixation in one case, and nonsymmetrical fixation in another case, and the last two cases had only partial loss of correction, and revision was not indicated.

B. Secondary kyphosis has been observed. Kyphosis at the level of the fixation has been seen. Systematic study of the disc levels involved with the fixation demonstrated the existence of a very frequent secondary kyphosis of less than 10°, which is without consequences and is very acceptable. The radiographic measurement of the disc inclination revealed such a kyphosis (Fig. 54.14).

We also observed kyphosis of more than 10°. They have been mostly seen in the cases of articular mass separation fractures (4 cases) before the use of the long "port manteau" type of fixation. In none of these cases was revision necessary.

Another type of kyphosis occurs at the adjacent disc level. The major problem is understanding its real significance. In four cases, it occurred at the adjacent level above a severe sprain. The secondary kyphosis has never been important in this series. It probably represents hypermobility occurring adjacent to a fixed disc level (Fig. 54.15).

Kyphosis of the vertebral body was observed in two cases of a misdiagnosed body fracture adjacent to the fixation.

C. Postoperative incomplete reduction — In this large series of 238 cases, 30 cases of vertebral body fractures have been treated, among them 18 have been treated only by a single posterior plate fixation. In these 18 cases, the reduction was incomplete in nine cases, and acceptable in six cases, where a retrolisthesis of less than 2 mm was present. It was not acceptable in three cases, which required an anterior approach to correct the deformity.

Associated Anterior Approaches

After the posterior plate fixation, a complementary anterior approach was necessary in nine cases in our series. This approach was indicated, either on a mechanical or a neurologic basis, and we have already discussed the three cases of incomplete reduction of a retropulsed vertebral body. There was persistent instability in four cases, and a symptomatic associated disc herniation in two cases.

Neurologic Postoperative Evaluation

The postoperative neurologic examination was directly related to the patient's initial neurologic status. Complete quadriplegia never recovered, and, in these cases, the only improvement we observed were several metameric recoveries. Of 35 cases of a complete quadriplegia, we have seen 21 metameric recoveries, one level in 13 cases, two levels in seven cases, and three levels in one case. The prognosis for incomplete quadriplegia is far better. Of 31 cases, recovery to a Frankel Grade D or E (walking possible) was observed in 85% of patients. In our series, all patients were operated on an emergency basis within the first 12 hours after trauma. These results were very similar to other series in the literature.

Neurological Complications

Implantation of screws into cervical articular masses may risk injury to the cord, the vertebral arteries and the roots. Yet we reported only four cases of neurological postoperative complications (1.6%). One case was a loss of one root level in a quadriplegic patient. It is unclear whether the fixation system really was responsible, or whether there was further necrosis of the cord secondary to trauma. Three cases had transitory root impingement. An early revision of the screws was performed, with full root recovery. We must once again emphasize that the screws must project 10° lateral during the implantation into the articular masses.

Other Complications

Two dural leaks were reported, without consequences. No cases of vertebral artery injury were reported.

Infection

In six cases, a deep wound infection occurred. Debridement was necessary in four cases, two of which were associated with loss of fixation of the plates, as mentioned. In two cases, local drainage of the infection resulted in uneventful healing.

Length of Hospital Stay

The average length of stay was 9.9 days for all patients, including postoperative complications, but not cord injuries.

Conclusion

This recent series confirms the efficacy of posterior plate cervical fixation. Eighty-eight percent of the cases healed without complications and with good anatomic results. The same basic principles must be reviewed: anatomy and landmarks in the cervical spine must be well known; fixation must be bilateral and symmetrical, even for unilateral lesions; and it must be as short as possible.

POSTERIOR PLATE FIXATION IN UPPER CERVICAL SPINE INJURIES

The stabilization of the occipitocervical junction can be achieved only posteriorly. To ensure fusion, it is necessary to have strong, rigid internal fixation, which can be obtained by the implantation of two occipito-cervical plates preserving the normal occipitocervical angulation.

Occipitocervical Dislocation

This type of dislocation is usually immediately lethal. We have seen two patients who survived, one in whom the injury had occurred 14 months prior to being seen, and another with an acute injury. A simple fusion with two plates and graft was needed for the chronic case, and a reduction with light traction, followed by fixation with two plates, for the acute case. Both cases fused uneventfully. It is important to remember the difficulty of diagnosing this dislocation, and one must use the anterior occipitocervical line on the lateral radiograph for making the diagnosis. A CT scan is the only method that clearly demonstrates this dislocation easily.

Teardrop Fracture of C2

These cases have significant instability and are associated with complex dens fractures. They have to be fixed by an occipitocervical arthrodesis. In cases not involving the dens, a simple C2–C3 stabilization is enough. This fixation is performed with two posterior plates and the screws implanted into the C2 pedicles and the C3 articular masses, as described earlier (Fig. 54.16).

Hangman's Fracture

When the fracture is stable, with minimal displacement, healing will occur with conservative treatment. In the case of an associated complete C2–3 posterior dislocation, surgical treatment is necessary to reduce and stabilize the lesion. The reduction of the posterior C2 arch is impossible with traction, but it can be achieved via a posterior approach. The fixation is then performed with two two-hole plates. The upper screw is driven into the C2 pedicles and achieves direct fixation of the fracture lines and the plate stabilizes the dislocated C2–3 dislocation.

POSTERIOR PLATE FIXATION AND CERVICAL SPINE TUMORS

In cases of malignant extradural tumors of the spine, surgery has two main goals. The less ambitious one is to decompress the cord and stabilize the spine without tumor removal. This palliative procedure improves the patient's quality of life but will not change the lethal prognosis. The more ambitious treatment goal is to perform a curative procedure, with complete tumor resection and a total spondylectomy. In cases of palliative or curative treatment, a reliable fixation system is necessary.

Cervical Spondylectomy

At the second cervical level, major problems are encountered if a total spondylectomy is indicated — namely, the vertebral arteries and the roots. Arterial carotid/vertebral bypass makes vertebral artery ligature possible. A bilateral bypass enables resection of both vertebral arteries at the

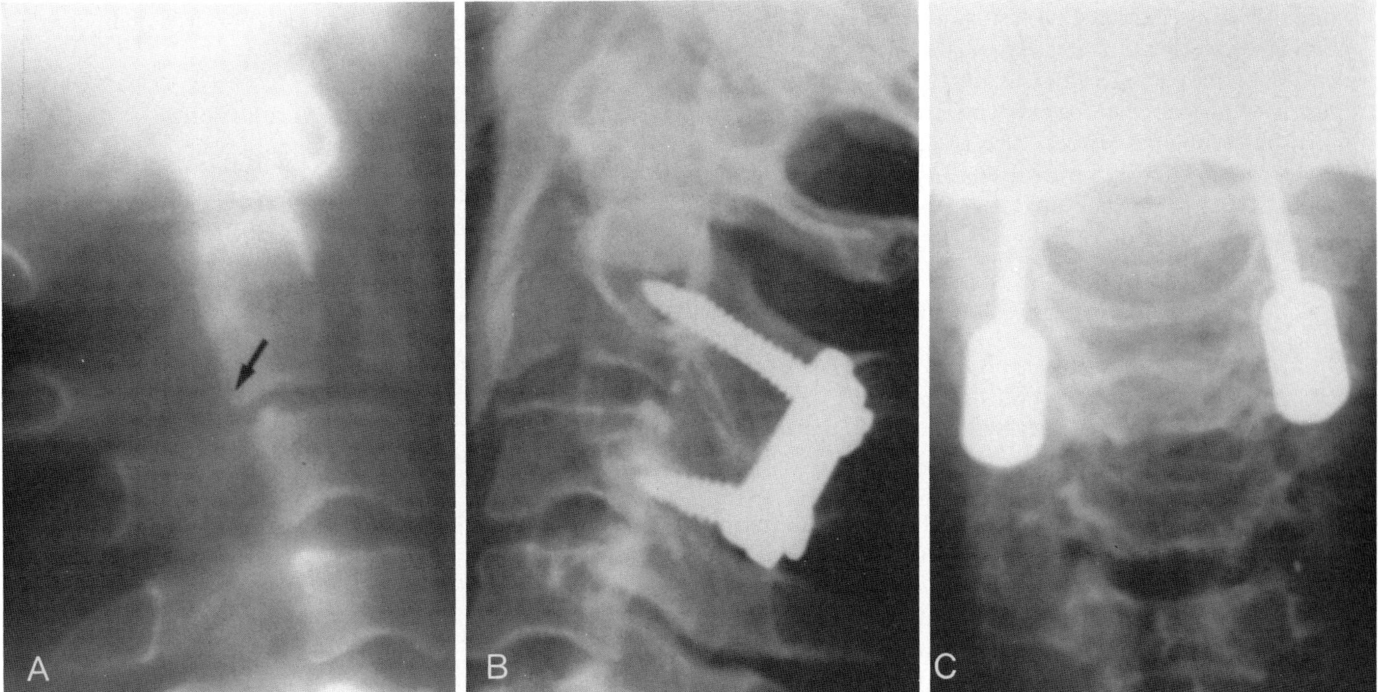

Figure 54.16. C2 teardrop fractures are rare and characterized by posterior displacement of C2. Only posterior fixation will give a good reduction and stabilization.

tumor level. Root preservation is much more difficult to perform, and, in many cases, the roots must be sacrificed with the tumor resection. Cervical spondylectomy is rarely indicated, and the procedure requires high technical skill and a double approach, anterior where the excised body is reconstructed, using a graft, and posterior, where rigid internal fixation is achieved with two long plates.

Metastatic Palliative Treatment

The goal is to give the patient palliation. Radio- and chemotherapy are utilized for the treatment of vertebral metastases, when the spine is stable. Surgery is helpful and necessary when two types of complications occur: mechanical and neurological.

Mechanical complications are due to the vertebral fragility induced by an osteolytic lesion. Trabecular microfractures are painful and lead to a collapse of the vertebral body. Stabilization of the spine is then necessary to alleviate pain and to prevent deformity. Posterior plating is very effective for this.

Neurologic complications can occur from multiple causes. An epidural tumor is most frequently responsible for cord or root compression, and evolution of the compression is usually fast. Extension of bone metastases into the canal is less frequently a cause of neurologic complication. The deformity induced by the vertebral collapse with protrusion into the vertebral canal can also be responsible for a neurologic deficit. These complications need decompression of cord and roots, and a laminectomy must be performed with exploration of the canal. Cord ischemia is rare but can be suspected when there is a sudden neurologic deficit without associated cord compression from deformity or epidural tumor. Surgery is ineffective in such cases.

Surgical Procedure

Decompression of the cord and stabilization of the spine is often necessary in emergencies involving a recent or progressive quadra- or paraplegia. In our experience, the posterior approach is effective in certain instances. Vertebral canal exploration is permitted at multiple vertebral levels and enables an easier removal of posterior and lateral epidural tumor than the anterior approach. After spinal cord decompression, the reduction of the vertebral deformity is the next step. At the cervical level, the position of lordosis of the head holder usually reduces the deformity. Fixation, the third step can be achieved by posterior plating, and, in other cases of painful metastases due to fragile vertebrae without neurologic involvement, the spine fixation may be performed alone. Then radiotherapy can be utilized on the pathologic vertebra. Special considerations have to be taken into account when considering the level of the metastases.

Upper Cervical Spine C1, C2, and C3 Metastases

The risk of a possible occipitocervical dislocation is more important than one of "compression." Treatment is, thus, limited to an occipitocervical fusion, as described. A bone graft in between the plates is not always necessary and depends on the patient's life expectancy. An iliac unicortical graft is fixed over the occiput with a direct screw, then wired to the spinous process of C4. Patients continue to wear a Minerva corset up to fusion, usually by the third month. Radiotherapy delivered over a 1 month period will not alter the evolution of the graft.

Low Cervical Spine C4–7 Metastases

The narrowness of the canal at this level explains why cord compression occurs shortly after the beginning of tumor evolution. Instability will increase this neurologic risk. In most cases, a double posterior and anterior approach is necessary (Fig. 54.17). The posterior approach is performed, first, for laminectomy and fixation of the cervical spine. The levels of the fixation are usually larger than in traumatic cases and must include one vertebra above and one below the involved vertebra. An anterior tumor resection is usually performed at the same sitting or a few days later. Reconstruction with an iliac bone graft will give a rigid, strong fixation. Fixation with a vertebral staple is often performed (Fig. 54.18). Its four self-retaining feet avoid possible loosening. Different lengths are available, ranging from 20–32 mm long. We have no experience in reconstruction utilizing methylmethacrylate or vertebral prostheses. A postoperative Minerva corset is maintained for 3 months after surgery.

Complementary Treatment

Radiotherapy and/or chemotherapy is the last step in the treatment of metastases. It depends on the histological findings. Radiotherapy is delayed until after the wound has healed, usually at 3 weeks. In cases of radiotherapy just before surgery, one may observe no wound healing and major skin problems, negating all benefit of this palliative surgery, the aim of which is the comfort of the patient. The radiation dosage is also important to prevent a post-radiation myelitis with secondary quadra- or paraplegia. The maximal dosage for the cord is 45 G-rays delivered over a 1 month period. The posterior plates are not a hindrance to radiotherapy.

Results

UPPER CERVICAL SPINE

Thirty-three cases of occipitocervical stabilization have been performed with posterior plates. In 10 cases, it was only simple fixation without bone graft. Reported deaths occurred in this group of patients only during the first 3 postoperative months. However, pain relief was achieved by this simple procedure, and no neurologic complication

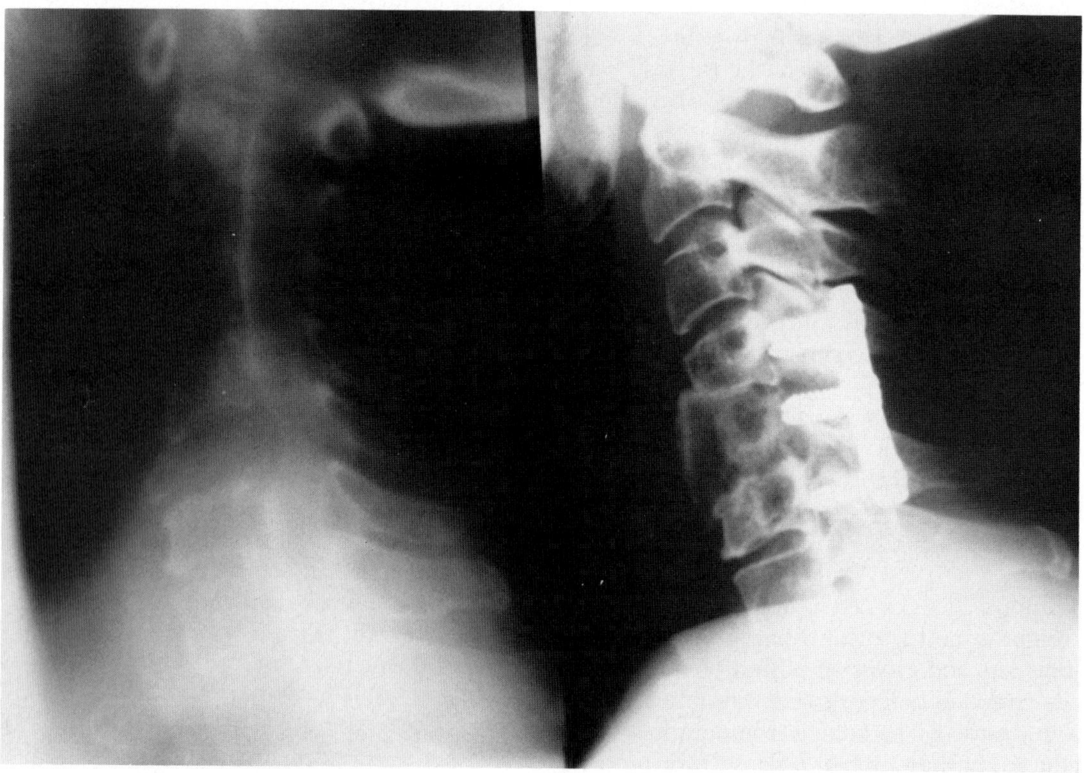

Figure 54.17. At low cervical spine levels, metastases require a posterior laminectomy and internal fixation and an anterior spondylectomy.

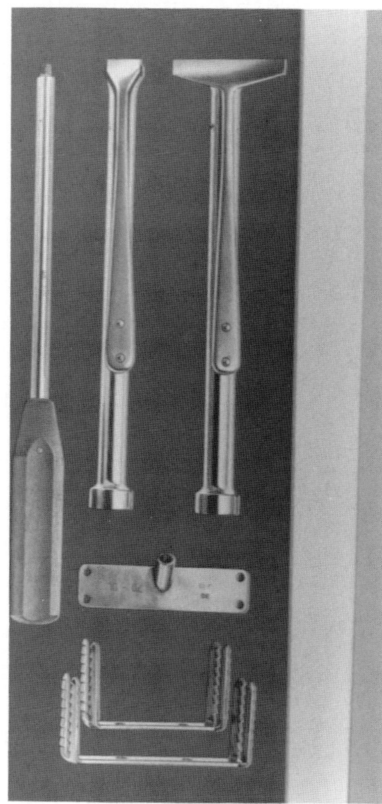

Figure 54.18. Instrumentation set for staple fixation.

occurred before death. In the other cases, the fusion rate was 94%. The major problem associated with this procedure is wound infection (two cases) and severe skin scars (four cases). The pressure of the Minerva corset was responsible for this in all cases. In fact, the Minerva must be specially designed at the occipital level and must be replaced by a collar while supine to avoid such complications. No cases of venous bleeding, dural leak during the drilling of the occiput, or root impingement by cervical screws have been reported.

LOWER CERVICAL SPINE

Thirty-eight patients with metastases were studied at the time of this retrospective study, and 22 were dead. Fifty percent died in the first 6 postoperative months. Histologic identification of the permeating tumor was the major determinant of life expectancy. Pain was completely relieved in 20 of the 21 patients living at 4 months postsurgery. Thus, good fixation of the spine is effective in relieving pain. Post-operative neurologic status is directly dependent on the initial status of the patient. In 20 patients who presented with a root impingement, eight died in the first 2 months, and the remaining 12 were improved or completely cured. In eight cases with severe cord compression, four died unchanged, three recovered and were able to walk, and only one had a complete recovery.

Reconstruction of cervical spine anatomy is dependent upon the surgical technique chosen. Our results demonstrate the necessity of a double posterior and anterior approach. Anatomy was restored in eight out of nine cases operated upon anteriorly and posteriorly, while only 11 out of 18 cases with a single posterior approach had their anatomy restored.

Other Indications for Posterior Plate Fixation in the Upper Cervical Spine

CONGENITAL MALFORMATION

These malformations are often localized in the upper cervical spine. Difficulties may arise from instability, with cord compression, usually by the odontoid process on the posterior border of the foramen magnum. In posterior plate fixation, restoring stability and normal curvature relieves cord compression, but it may be necessary, by the same posterior approach, to perform a foraminotomy.

RHEUMATOID DISEASE

In case of rheumatoid disease with progressive occipitocervical dislocation, a C1–2 fusion is usually not effective in our experience, and an occipitocervical fusion is necessary. In these steroid-dependent patients, skin healing is slow, and these patients need care to prevent local compression of the occiput at the fixation level. A large corticancellous bone graft between the two plates fuses much better than a C1–2 graft, which often resorbs spontaneously.

CORD COMPRESSION

In some patients with cord compression caused by the odontoid process (malunion, congenital deformity, rheumatoid disease), it may be necessary to remove the dens and C2 vertebral body through an anterior approach. Since this creates significant instability, stable fixation utilizing the posterior occipitocervical plating method, and bone grafting should be achieved prior to the anterior approach. Skull traction is necessary between the two surgical stages if the posterior fixation is performed after the C2 resection.

CONCLUSION

In patients with posttraumatic cervical spine instability, a posterior approach is often necessary to reduce the facets. Posterior plating and fixation are easy and effective, as demonstrated by our results. This fixation is also helpful for tumor-related instability. At the level of the upper cervical spine, the use of special occipitocervical plates increases confidence in immediate postoperative stability when an occipitocervical fusion is necessary.

55

Caspar Plating of the Cervical Spine

Ronald I. Apfelbaum

The Caspar system for anterior spinal fixation includes retractors, distractors, drill guides, trapezoidal-shaped osteosynthetic plates, and fixation screws. It is designed to ease exposure of the spine, to provide immediate stabilization after resection of bony and soft tissue elements, and to facilitate long-term stabilization. Dr. Wolfhard Caspar of West Germany developed this system which has been used in many hundreds of patients, both in the United States and Europe.

This technique is invaluable in many situations, including instability of the spine produced by trauma, when extensive pathology has destroyed the structural elements, rendering the spine unstable, or when large resections of the spinal elements are necessary, which will produce iatrogenic instability. Having this technology available allows fuller resection and treatment of anterior pathology, immediate stabilization of the spine, usually without the need for an external collar or halo-vest immobilizer, and produces the highest rate of fusion.

Operative Technique

The operative technique advocated by Dr. Caspar is a very well thought out and meticulous technique based on his extensive experience. It is well detailed and illustrated in the monograph published by Aesculap AG (1) and their American distributor, Aesculap Instrument Corporation (AIC). We will cover the basics of the technique here, but the reader is referred to that monograph for nuances and subtleties that are beyond the scope of this presentation.

The operative technique involves a unilateral anterior exposure through a horizontal incision in a natural skin crease. The initial exposure is identical to that used with the Cloward technique. We infiltrate the skin with 1:200,000 epinephrine solution to help promote hemostasis, complete hemostasis with bipolar cautery, and then elevate and incise the platysma muscle with an electrosurgical instrument. The sternocleidomastoid muscle fascia is then identified and opened sharply along the medial border of the sternocleidomastoid muscle. It is not necessary to undermine the platysma, but the sternocleidomastoid muscle fascia should be opened sharply for as long a distance as is necessary to get good exposure. This fascia limits the cranial and caudal extent of the exposure. Blunt dissection is then carried down through natural tissue planes to the prevertebral space. The path of exposure is lateral to the trachea and esophagus and medial to the carotid sheath. The recurrent laryngeal nerve is occasionally injured in this exposure. It has been suggested that a left-sided approach will lower the incidence of such injuries, but they can occur approaching it from either side. Fortunately, most recurrent laryngeal nerve palsies are temporary. If they persist, vocal cord injections can help restore normal voice volume.

Once the prevertebral space is exposed, the appropriate levels are identified fluoroscopically. It is essential that fluoroscopic guidance in the lateral plane be available to use this instrumentation safely.

The longus colli muscle is then incised in the midline and elevated from the anterior surface of the appropriate vertebral bodies with periosteal elevators. The sharp-edged retractor blades are inserted underneath these muscles and placed in the retractor blade holder. A second pair of smooth retractor blades are then placed for craniocaudal retraction and placed in a separate retractor holder orthogonal to the first one. This holds the soft tissues out of the way and provides direct visualization to the operative site (Fig. 55.1).

At this juncture, the instrumentation is similar to the earlier Cloward instrumentation. A unique feature of the Caspar set, however, is the distraction apparatus. In the Caspar system, distraction posts are placed into the vertebral bodies through a pilot drill hole. The drilling guide and drill used for this automatically limit the depth of penetration into the vertebral body to 8 mm, preventing intrusion into the spinal canal. The drill guide can be placed onto the distractor apparatus, (Fig. 55.2) allowing sequential placement of posts parallel to each other in each vertebrae. This allows parallel distraction of the vertebrae in an axial plane.

The distractor, when placed over the post, is out of the surgeon's line of vision and allows unobstructed viewing of the operative field, (Fig. 55.3) whether this is an intervertebral disc space or a corpectomy site. Multiple posts can be placed for differential distraction as desired. This is a very powerful part of the apparatus, allowing excellent distraction without impairing the surgeon's access to the field. Manipulation of the vertebral bodies to achieve normal spine alignment is also possible using the distraction posts.

The operative procedure that is undertaken, of course, depends on the pathology involved. This may involve an anterior cervical discectomy, resection of osteophytes, resection of vertebral bodies to obtain more extensive exposure and decompression of the spinal canal, and removal of pathology within the vertebral bodies on the anterior aspects of the spinal canal. Nerve roots can be decompressed bilaterally under direct visualization. At the surgeon's preference, magnified vision, either with loops or with the operating microscope, is often helpful in this stage of the procedure.

Once the pathology has been treated, a bone graft can be placed in the intervertebral spaces or in the corpectomy site. If autologous bone is to be used, we usually harvest this from the iliac crest. The Caspar system also includes a set of parallel bladed oscillating saws (Fig. 55.4) to allow removal of a very precisely sized bone graft for placement in an intervertebral disc space. These come in 1 mm increments, from 6–10 mm and allow harvesting of a tricortical graft with absolutely parallel end surfaces (Fig.

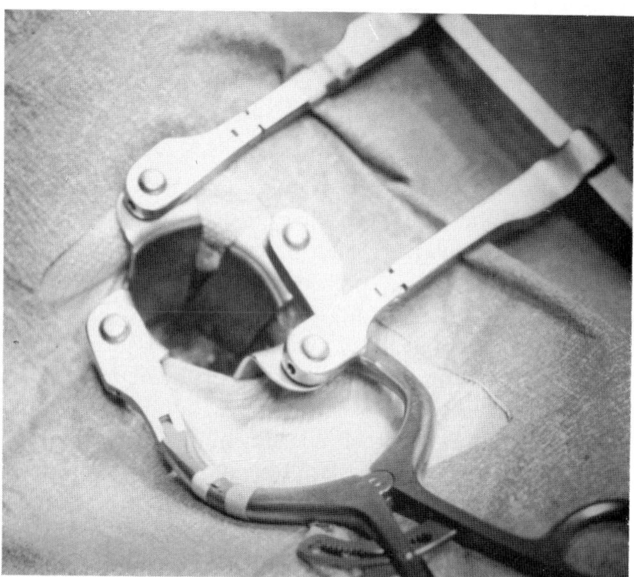

Figure 55.1. Caspar retracting system in place.

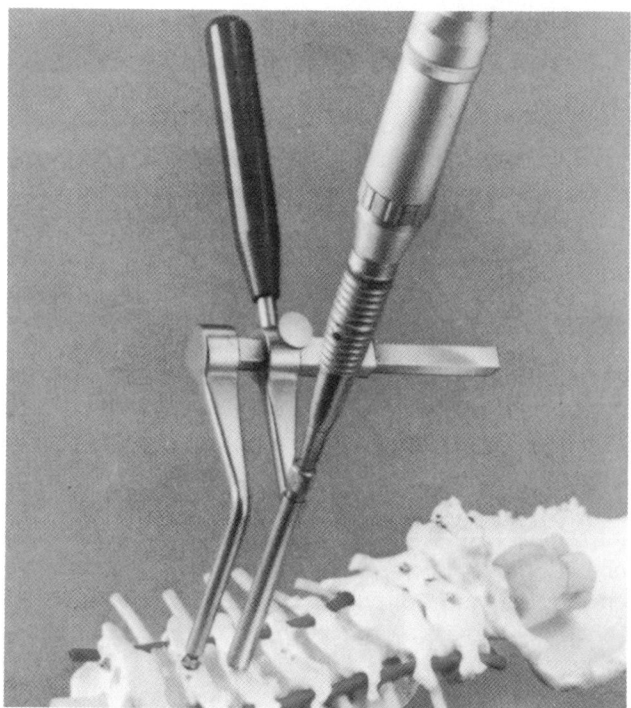

Figure 55.2. Placement of pilot hole for second distraction screw. Note that the drill guide attached to the distractor results in placement of the second screw exactly parallel to the first. With permission: Caspar W. Anterior cervical fusion and interbody stabilization with the trapecial osteosynthetic plate technique. Scientific Brochure No. 12. Tuttlingen, Germany: Aesculap, 1986.

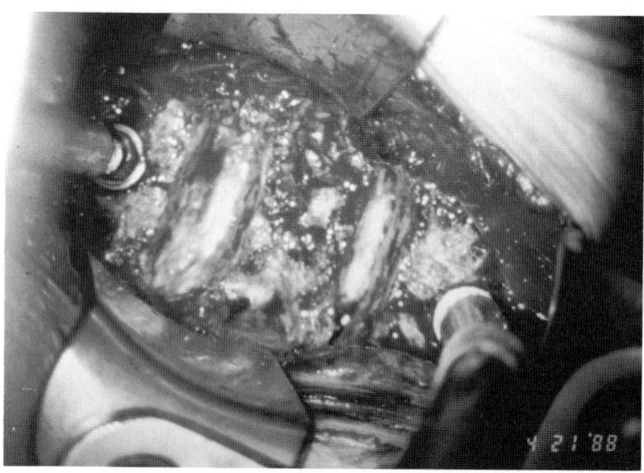

Figure 55.3. Distractor in place in a patient who is going to undergo a corpectomy and two-level discectomy. Note the clear and unobstructed view of the operative field.

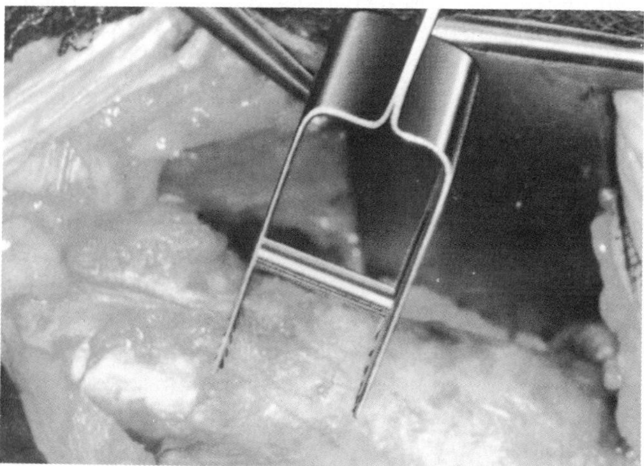

Figure 55.4. Double bladed saw used to harvest iliac crest bone graft for interbody fusion at a discectomy site. With permission: Caspar W. Anterior cervical fusion and interbody stabilization with the trapecial osteosynthetic plate technique. Scientific Brochure No. 12. Tuttlingen, Germany: Aesculap, 1986.

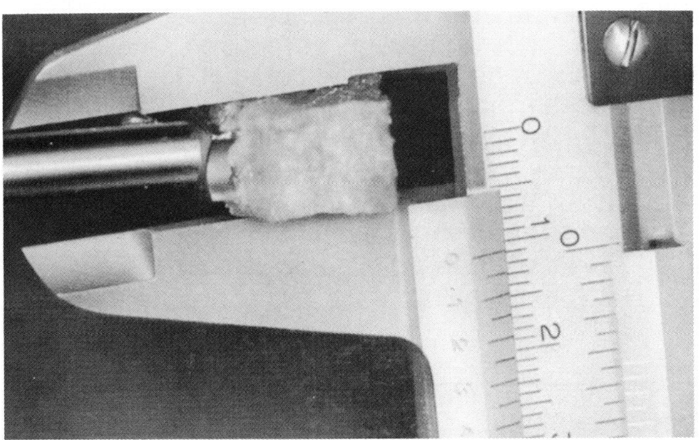

Figure 55.5. Precise graft sizing is possible using calibers. With permission: Caspar W. Anterior cervical fusion and interbody stabilization with the trapecial osteosynthetic plate technique. Scientific Brochure No. 12. Tuttlingen, Germany: Aesculap, 1986.

55.5). The recommended technique is to use a power drill to smooth the vertebral end-plate surfaces, creating parallel faces that will then accommodate the bone graft. By having parallel surfaces on the bone graft, a ramping effect, which can result in extrusion of the bone graft, is avoided. For corpectomy grafts, which are larger in dimension than the intervertebral disc grafts, single bladed oscillating saws are used to make two roughly parallel cuts. The graft is then harvested with the use of an osteotome to cut across its base and sized using the oscillating saw or power drill as is appropriate.

The Caspar plating system is then used as an internal splint, holding the spine in proper alignment and providing immediate internal stabilization while awaiting bony fusion. Plate length is determined by the patient's anatomy. It is important that the plate does not extend over nonfused segments. A proper length plate, once selected, is contoured using a plate bender to reapproximate the normal cervical lordosis. The plate is positioned over the anterior face of the vertebral bodies and secured with a series of screws that are placed through the anterior cortex of the vertebral body and engage the posterior cortex. It is extremely important that the fixation screws engage both the anterior and posterior cortex (Fig. 55.6). The screws should be placed at least 1 mm from the end plate of the vertebral bodies for maximum purchase (Fig. 55.7).

The fixation screws are placed using a special double drill guide that has depth stops that limit the penetration of the drill. The drill guide allows placement of both fixation screws through the vertebral body and directs them in a converging course from the holes in the Caspar plate toward the center of the spinal canal. This places the screw tips in the hollow concavity of the vertebral body so that penetration of a millimeter or more into the spinal canal does not result in any neural compromise. The drilling of these holes, tapping of the holes, which is done manually, and final placement of the screw *must be performed under fluoroscopic visualization* to prevent penetration beyond a

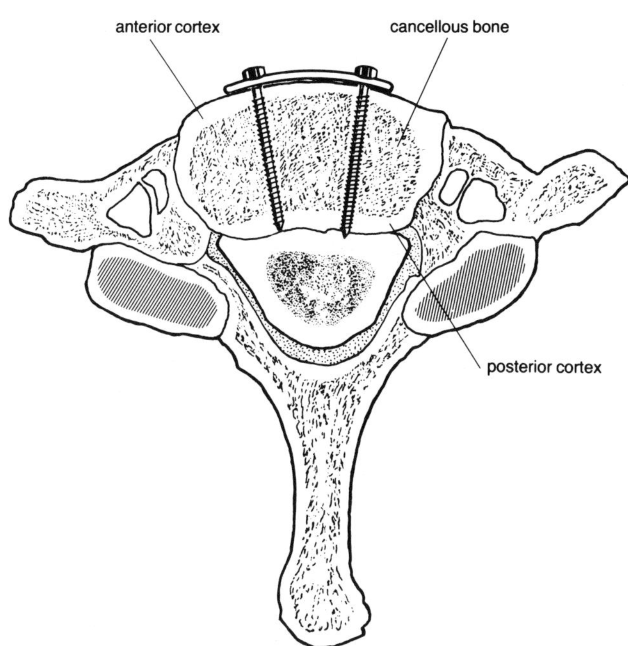

Figure 55.6. Note proper position of screws engaging both anterior and posterior vertebral cortices. A small amount of intrusion into the spinal canal is tolerable. There is a margin of safety due to the thickness of the posterior longitudinal ligament (usually 1.5 to 2 mm) and the natural concavity of the center of the vertebral body. With permission: Caspar W. Anterior cervical fusion and interbody stabilization with the trapecial osteosynthetic plate technique. Scientific Brochure No. 12. Tuttlingen, Germany: Aesculap, 1986.

safe distance into the spinal canal and injuring the neural elements. At times it may be desirable and possible to place additional screws into the same vertebral body to improve fixation. The screws must be tightened to a firm tension but not overtorqued, which will result in stripping of the screw, weaken the purchase, and may result in hardware failure. When it is necessary to incorporate multiple levels due to multisegmental disease, it may be desirable to plan the approach, if feasible, to retain two lower vertebral bodies using an intervertebral approach at that level rather than multilevel corpectomy, as this will result in stronger mechanical construct for the plating system. (Fig. 55.8).

Immediate stability can be verified by having the anesthesiologist flex and extend the patient's neck while observing the fluoroscopic image. External fixation of the spine usually has not been necessary except when the bone is felt to be osteopenic or when it has been weakened by the disease process that is being treated. If, however, contiguous multilevel corpectomies have had to be done, external fixation may be desirable to minimize the chance of hardware failure.

EXPERIENCE

Our experience with the Caspar system at the University of Utah Medical Center has continued to grow (2). We now

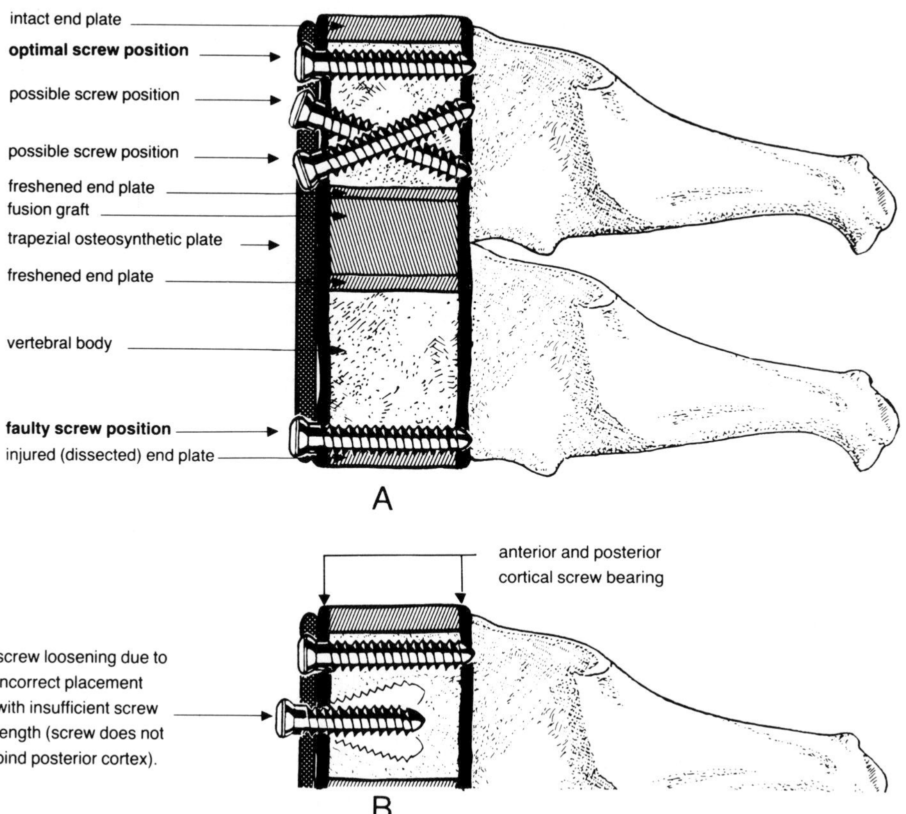

Figure 55.7. Schema of possible screw positions. As long as both anterior and posterior cortices are properly engaged and the screw is not too close the the end plate, satisfactory purchase can be obtained. With permission: Caspar W. Anterior cervical fusion and interbody stabilization with the trapecial osteosynthetic plate technique. Scientific Brochure No. 12. Tuttlingen, Germany: Aesculap, 1986.

have operated upon 100 patients in slightly less than 4 years. The primary indications included trauma in 43% of our patients, with trauma being associated with other preexisting problems in another 10%. The remaining nontraumatic conditions (as either a primary or associated diagnosis) consisted of patients who had cervical spondylosis and degenerative disc disease in 38%, failed fusions in 12%, tumor of the vertebral body in 6%, and other causes such as ossification of the posterior longitudinal ligament or swan-neck deformities in 6%. Single-level plating was accomplished in 6% and multilevel plating in 84%. Two-level fusions were most common (51%), but three-level fusions were accomplished in 28% and four-level fusions in 5%.

Motor vehicle accidents were the most common cause of trauma (55%). Of the trauma patients, 9 were neurologically intact, 16 had complete quadriplegia, 9 had partial myelopathy, 7 had radicular symptoms, and 2 presented only with neck pain. Cervical spondylosis presented with myelopathy in 62% and radiculopathy or neck pain in 38%. Failed fusion patients presented primarily with neck pain, but one third had radicular or cord symptoms as well.

The utility of this technique can be best demonstrated by several illustrative cases. First is an 18-year-old male who sustained an unstable burst fracture of the fifth cervical vertebra (Fig. 55.9) in a diving accident. He was rendered quadriplegic. He was reduced and operated upon by a posterior approach at another hospital but immediately resubluxed. He was then referred to our institution, where a corpectomy of the fifth cervical vertebra was performed, along with resection of the adjacent discs. An iliac crest corpectomy graft was placed between the fourth and sixth cervical vertebra and a Caspar plating system utilized to provide immediate stability (Fig. 55.10). The patient was immediately stable and able to be transferred promptly to the rehabilitation service. He has improved significantly but remains with a partial cord deficit.

The alternative toward management in this case would have been to place the patient in a halo. Because of his gross instability, this may not have been successful, but even if it were, it would have added encumbrances to his rehabilitation, given his weakened quadriparetic state.

Figure 55.11 illustrates the initial presentation of the oldest patient in our series, an 83-year-old gentleman with severe degenerative spondylitic changes resulting in anterolisthesis of C3 on C4, partial fusion of C4 to C5, degeneration of the C5–6 disc space, with significant posterior spurring, and severe spinal canal and spinal cord compromise due to the above-mentioned changes, particularly the dislocation at C3–4. This patient had deteriorated to the point that he was no longer ambulatory, presenting with severe quadriparesis. The patient could not be reduced in skeletal traction. The diseased segments at C5 and C6 were resected and a corpectomy graft placed from C3 to C6, augmented with Caspar plating (Fig. 55.12). This allowed us to do an excellent decompression and reconstruction of the spinal canal, restoring normal configuration and decompressing the spinal cord. Despite his advanced years and greatly weakened state, the patient tolerated the surgery well and has gone on to have a very dramatic improvement of neurologic function, regaining the ability to become ambulatory. I strongly feel that no alternative approach would have provided this degree of decompression and resulted in this type of functional recovery.

A 46-year-old female presented with severe paraparesis to the extent that she was no longer able to ambulate independently. She had been carried with the diagnosis of multiple sclerosis without confirmatory evidence. A myelogram performed at the time of her quadriparetic state (Fig. 55.13) demonstrates multilevel anterior intrusion into the spinal canal. The CT myelographic picture (Fig. 55.14) shows that there is a mass behind the vertebral body, anterior to the spinal cord, which is severely indenting the cord even beyond the extent of the spondylitic spurs which are present laterally. Because this extended over several segments and was not confined merely to the level of the interspaces, we approached this by doing a two-level corpectomy. Islands of ossification within the resected posterior longitudinal ligament were identified on histopathology. A fibular strut graft was placed between the fourth and seventh cervical vertebrae after the spinal canal had been completely decompressed (Fig. 55.15). The patient recovered completely and has no residual neurologic deficit. She participates actively in sporting activities.

Finally, Figure 55.16 shows the CT scan in a 55-year-old gentleman who presented with right arm weakness and gradually progressing myelopathy of many years duration. The patient had an osteoid osteoma, severely compromising the spinal canal, incorporating the posterior elements of the spinal canal but also extending anteriorly through the neural foramen and eroding the vertebral bodies at several levels, as can be seen on the paramedian sagittal CT reconstruction (Fig. 55.17). This patient also had a congenital fusion of the first five cervical vertebrae. We resected his tumor in two stages; first approaching this

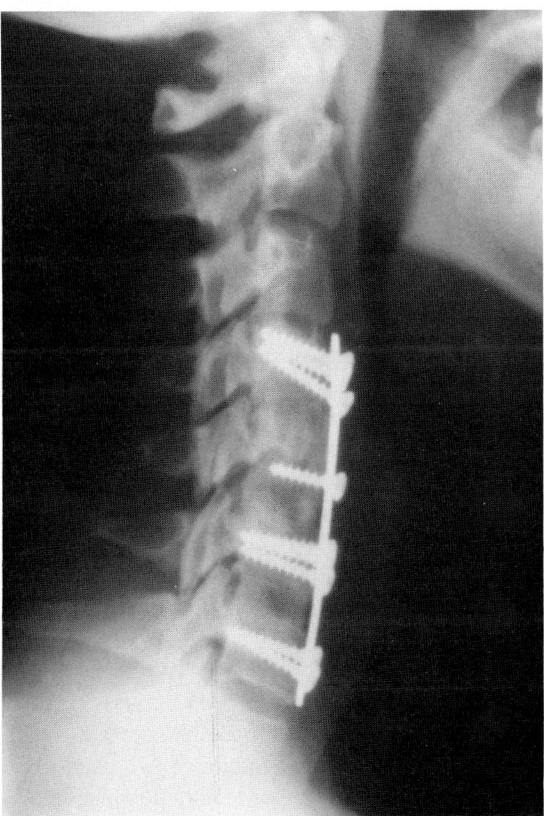

Figure 55.8. Example of a patient with multilevel cervical spondylosis. A corpectomy has been performed at C5, but at the C6–7 level the disease process has been approached through a discectomy. This allows two lower level vertebral bodies for fixation of the plate and improves the mechanical construct. This patient, therefore, had a corpectomy graft from C4 to C6 and an interbody graft from C6 to C7.

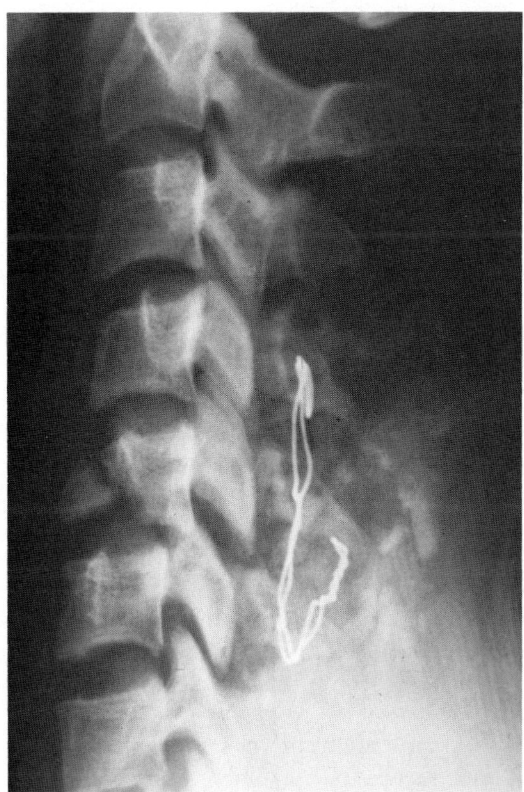

Figure 55.9. Retrolisthesis of C5 on C6, despite attempts at posterior stabilization with wire and bone, in a patient who sustained a burst fracture of C5 and severe cord compromise from a diving accident.

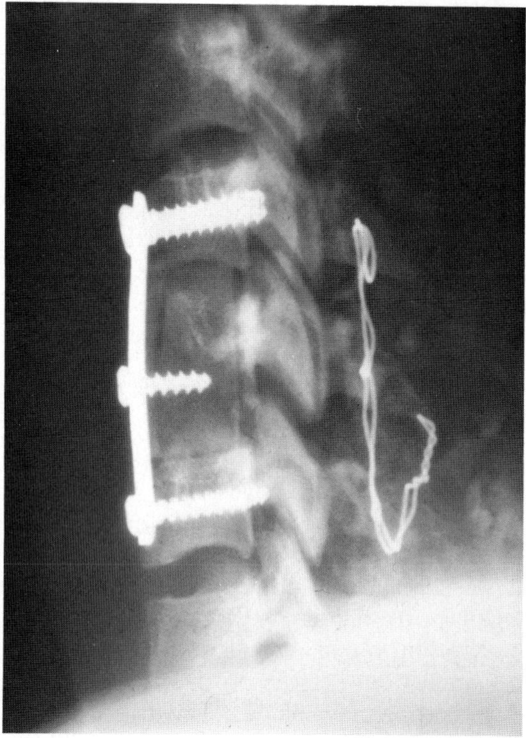

Figure 55.10. Corpectomy graft in place between C4 and C6 with stabilization by Caspar plating. Note reconstruction of normal spinal canal alignment.

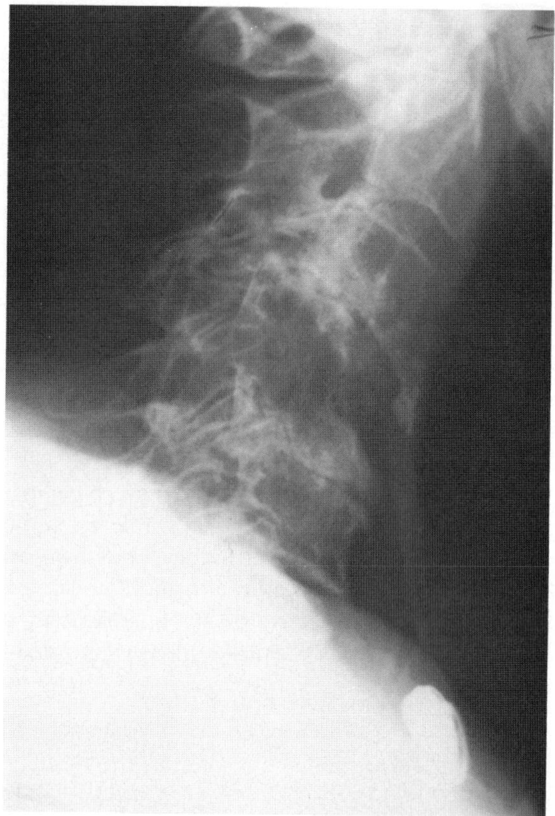

Figure 55.11. Severe degenerative spondylitic changes resulting in an anterolisthesis of C3 on C4 and spontaneous fusion of C4 and C5. The patient was severely quadriparetic.

posteriorly, doing a laminectomy and removing all the tumor within the spinal canal to decompress the spinal cord. At a second stage, the tumor within the vertebral bodies and anterior neck was resected, freeing the nerve roots in this area. This involved resection of a significant portion of the seventh cervical and first thoracic vertebra. An iliac crest bone graft was placed and the Caspar plate utilized to stabilize the spine from C6 to T2 (Fig. 55.18). The patient had immediate improvement in his myelopathic symptoms. His radicular symptoms (C8) were exacerbated by the surgery; however, over a several month period, significant improvement occurred, and the patient eventually was able to return to playing the organ, which he had not been able to do for several years. The bone graft healed without problems.

These cases demonstrate the utility of the procedure in the most common situations in which they are employed; namely, traumatic instability, extensive degenerative spondylitic disease, and structural lesions such as neoplasms of the spinal canal which produce instability of the spine or whose resection will do so.

Clinical complications in this series have been few. One of our patients who had a spine fracture and an unstable neck also suffered from AIDS. He died of respiratory failure related to the latter disease process. Another patient developed delayed esophageal erosion over a feeding tube placed for treatment of gastric cancer some 15 months after Caspar plating. Removal of the feeding tube initially resulted in satisfactory healing without any further problems, but subsequently the hardware was removed due to dysphagia. One patient had a deep wound infection postoperatively. This was treated with opening of the wound and irrigation. The hardware was not removed, and the wound healed satisfactorily after treatment with antibiotics. Seven patients experienced recurrent laryngeal nerve palsies. All were transient.

Technical complications have been more frequent. Screws backed out in 12 patients. Often this was only a turn or two and did not require any treatment other than serial observations (7/12). However, when this was associated with displacement of the plate (two patients) or displacement of the plate and graft (three patients), reoperation was usually required. Screw fractures have been observed in 4 patients but never required reoperation. Screw malpositioning has been observed in 6 patients and plate malpositioning in one. Graft settling occurred in 6 patients but only required reoperation in one. Of these 25 patients, therefore, reoperation has been required in 16. In two of these, the patients were placed in a halo brace and in two others, a collar was used following reoperation. Halo brace

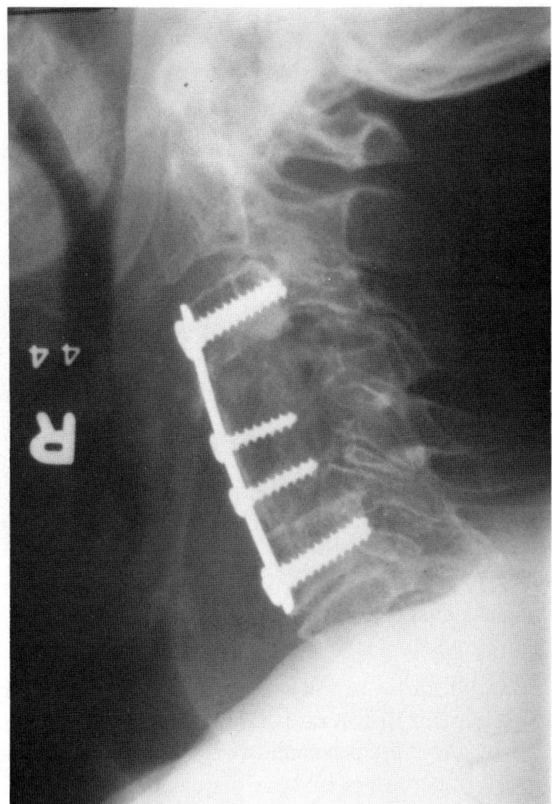

Figure 55.12. Reconstruction of the spinal canal with a corpectomy graft from C4 to C6. Caspar plating is used to stabilize the spinal column and reestablish normal spinal alignment.

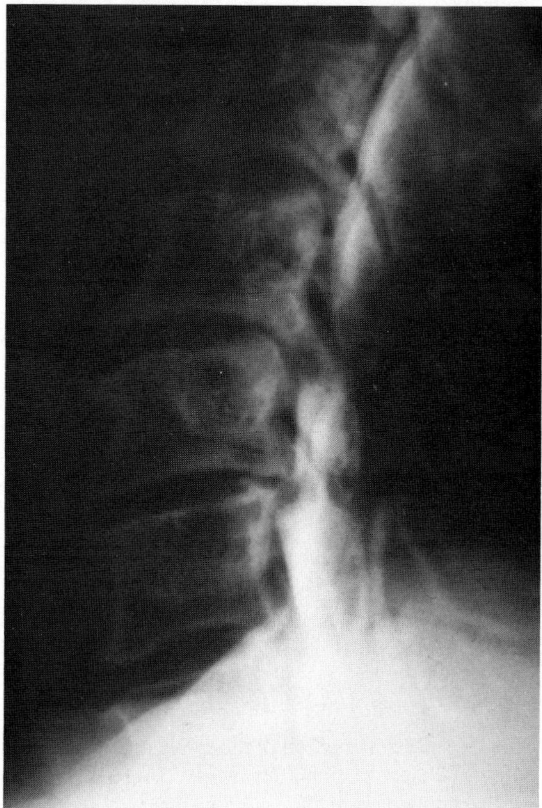

Figure 55.13. Myelogram of a 46-year-old woman with significant multilevel anterior intrusions into the spinal canal.

alone was used in 2 patients, Philadelphia collar alone in 4, and no treatment needed in 7 patients in whom the abnormality, such as a fractured screw, was noted, but the patient went on to satisfactory bone healing. Most importantly, by using this instrumentation and careful attention to detail, neither dural penetration nor cord injury by either the drill or screws has occurred.

The incidence of these technical complications seem high but is felt to be acceptable, considering the extensive nature of the surgery being performed. These patients often required extensive or multilevel resections and often were elderly with osteopenic bone. Initial analysis of these technical complications reveals a higher frequency of problems with increasing number of levels of plating, length of plate required, and more caudal position along the spinal column.

Reoperation, when required, usually has not been difficult nor produced any significant morbidity except for recurrent laryngeal nerve palsies. The latter, occurring in 2 patients, may be due to traction transmitted via the local scar tissue and suggests that unless the reoperation is performed shortly after the first procedure (i.e., one week or less) a contralateral approach might be considered.

In this group of 100 patients with follow-up averaging

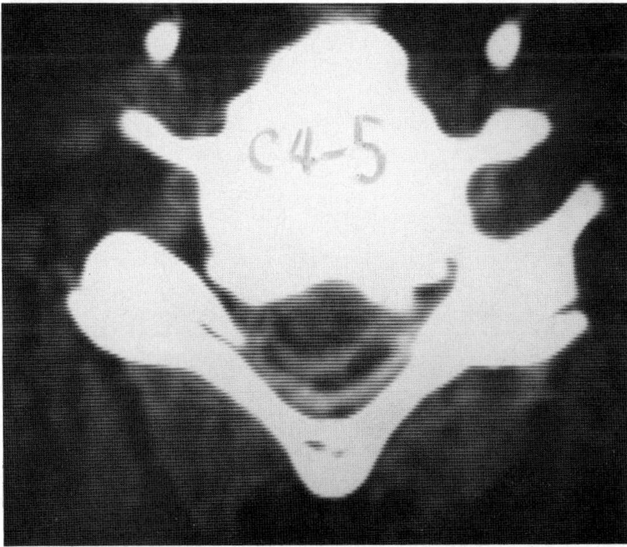

Figure 55.14. Post myelogram CT demonstrates the severe deformity of the spinal canal and dura. Note the significant midline intrusion behind the vertebral body which proved to be ossification within the posterior longitudinal ligament.

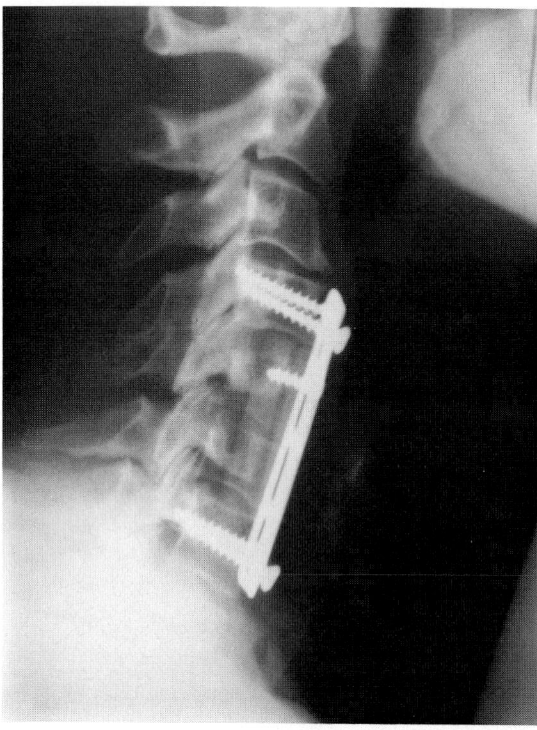

Figure 55.15. Reconstruction of the spinal canal with a fibular strut graft and Caspar plating after two level vertebrectomy and extensive decompression of the neural elements.

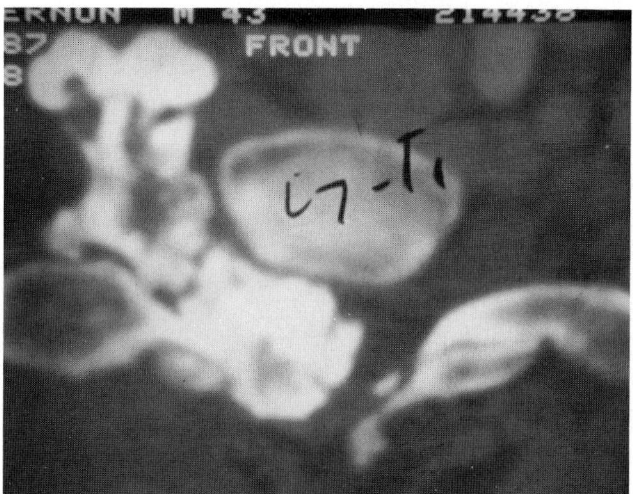

Figure 55.16. CT scan of a patient with an osteoid osteoma occupying a large portion of the spinal canal. It incorporated the posterior elements of the canal and extended through the neural foramen anteriorly.

20.3 months, there have been no failed fusions and no worsening of neurologic (cord or root) deficits.

DISCUSSION

As these results attest, the Caspar plating system has proved to be a useful adjunct to our armamentarium. It allows extensive correction of anterior cervical pathology and im-

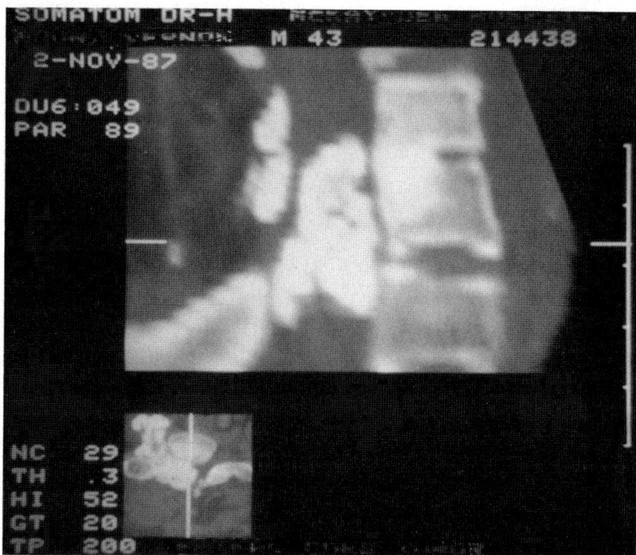

Figure 55.17. Parasagittal reconstruction of a CT scan demonstrating the multilevel extent of the disease process.

mediate stabilization of the spine. It has resulted in essentially 100 percent fusion rate. The immediate stabilization afforded by the system has allowed rapid mobilization of patients or, in patients who have major neurologic deficits, prompt transfer to appropriate rehabilitation facilities without the encumbrances in most cases of external stabilization systems such as the halo-vest.

Experimental studies have looked at the biomechanics of various types of internal stabilization systems and various procedures used to achieve stability in the cervical spine. These studies have demonstrated that the Caspar system is a very strong construct except in hyperflexion injuries with disruption of both posterior and anterior supporting structures (3). In the latter situation, posterior fusion techniques are stronger. This may not be clinically relevant, however, since use of the Caspar system in these very circumstances has resulted in as high a success rate (4) as in injuries that do not involve destruction of the anterior and posterior supporting structures. In other words, while theoretically the Caspar system is not as strong as a posterior wiring and stabilization in this particular type of injury, the clinical experience indicates that it is adequate for stabilization during the interval necessary for proper bone healing.

Research studies done on cadaver spines also cannot evaluate the loss of stability that occurs in these systems as bone absorption occurs around the fixating devices. Wires through the spinous processes or posterior elements may be more prone to loosening due to the high forces applied to a very small surface area as opposed to the Caspar system in which the load is shared by a large bone graft placed under compression and in which relatively large fixation screws (compared to the size of wiring that is used) help to dissipate these loads.

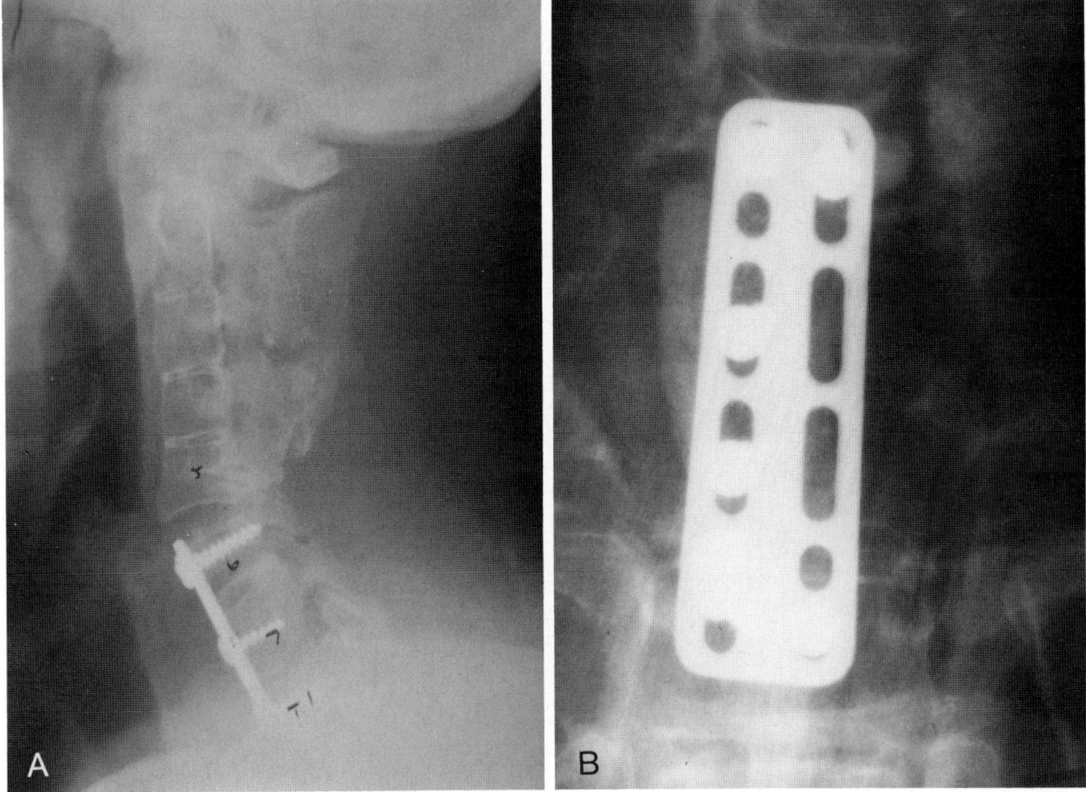

Figure 55.18. Caspar plating from C6 to T2 after resection of portions of C7 and T1. Note also the congenital blocked vertebrae from C1 to C5.

Any internal plating system, of course, is intended as a temporary adjunct to optimize bone healing. All will fail if bone healing does not occur. The fixation screws, too, must loosen as bone remodeling and resorption occur in response to the biomechanical forces on the screws. However, by temporarily reducing micromobility and holding the bone graft under compression, bone healing is facilitated. Once this occurs, the hardware, though superfluous, is stable, and no further problems, such as screw loosening, are anticipated.

The situation clinically then may be looked upon as a race between bony union and hardware failure. Failure to understand these principles, or ignoring them, such as by plating over a nonfused intervertebral disc, will almost assuredly result in failure.

CONCLUSIONS

The Caspar anterior cervical fixation system has proven to be an extremely useful part of our surgical armamentarium. It has allowed more extensive decompression of the cervical canal anteriorly than we would have been able to achieve, or would have been willing to undertake, without the ability to stabilize the spine immediately that this system provides. It has resulted in essentially 100% fusion rate of the spine with a low and acceptable rate of complications. To achieve these results, the surgeon must educate himself in the proper technique, as has been thoroughly documented by Dr. Caspar, and apply it using appropriate care.

REFERENCES

1. Caspar W. Aesculap leaflet S-039. Anterior cervical fusion and interbody stabilization with the trapezial osteosynthetic plate technique. Aesculap AG, Tuttlingen Germany, 1986.

2. Tippets RH, Apfelbaum RI. Anterior cervical fusion with the Caspar instrumentation system. Neurosurgery 1988;22:1008–1013.

3. Coe JD, Warden KE, Sutterlin CE, et al. Biomechanical evaluation of cervical spinal stabilization methods in a human cadaveric model. Spine 1989;14:1122–1131.

4. Caspar W, Barbier DD, Klara PM. Anterior cervical fusion and Caspar plate stabilization for cervical trauma. Neurosurgery 1989;25:491–501.

56

Anterior Screw Fixation for Odontoid Fractures

Ronald I. Apfelbaum

Odontoid fractures are classified as Type I, Type II, and Type III, depending on whether the fracture site is distal in the odontoid, across the neck of the odontoid, or involves the body of C2, respectively (1). Type I fractures generally are not associated with any instability, and some controversy exists whether they are true fractures rather than a separate terminal bony ossicle that has not united. They usually are incidental asymptomatic findings and require no treatment. The Type III fracture has a good record of healing and most will respond well to immobilization.

The Type II fracture is often problematic in its management. Some authors have advocated early operative intervention for these fractures (2–5), but others have recommended an initial period of conservative treatment with external immobilization (6–8). Still others recommend external immobilization if the degree of displacement is less than a certain amount (9–12). Nonunion rates with this technique, however, have varied from 7 (6) to 100 (2) percent in reported series, with other studies reporting many intermediate figures.

Dunn and Seljeskog (11) reported increased incidence of nonunion in 63 Type II odontoid fractures if the dens subluxated posteriorly, regardless of the amount of subluxation, and if the patient were over age 65. Hadley, Browner, and Sonntag (12), in their review of 40 cases of Type II odontoid fractures, found that if the displacement of the dens was 6 mm or more, the nonunion rate with external immobilization was 67% compared to a nonunion rate of 26% with lesser degrees of dislocation. In their further experience (62 patients) using these criteria, the nonunion rates were reported as 69% versus 10% (13). They could not correlate this with a direction of dislocation or patient's age. They have also identified a subtype (IIA) with a comminuted fragment at the base of the dens that is markedly unstable that they feel requires early surgical treatment. Apuzzo, et al. (10) found that greater than 4 mm dislocation resulted in a nonunion rate of 88% versus 16% for nondisplaced fractures. They also found a higher rate of nonunion in patients over age 40.

The operative technique most commonly employed for either early intervention or failure to achieve bony union with external immobilization has been posterior wiring and fusion between the arches of C1 and C2. This technique, while not perfect, has resulted in a high degree of successful union, especially when coupled with an additional period of external immobilization. The disadvantage of using this approach, however, is that it eliminates the normal rotatory motion between C1 and C2. White and Panjabi, in quantitating the normal degrees of motion of the spine, report that more than half the normal axial rotation of the spine occurs between the first and second cervical vertebrae (14) (Table 56.1).

We, therefore, are proposing an alternate technique of placing a fixation screw directly across the fracture site, reattaching the odontoid to the body of C2. This provides immediate stabilization, usually requires no external fixation, and restores normal spinal biomechanics, sparing the normal rotation between C1 and C2.

Successful attempts to achieve this have been reported by our European colleagues (15–17). Their approach, however, often involves a rather extensive neck dissection and appears to be a somewhat formidable operation. A recent report by Geisler et al. (18) using an approach similar to ours demonstrated excellent results. The technique we are proposing involves new instrumentation developed specifically for this procedure (Manufactured by Aesculap AG Instruments—Tuttlingen, Germany) which simplifies the procedure greatly, making it quick and safe.

Operative Procedure

The patient is placed supine on the operating table (Fig. 56.1). Pads are placed beneath the patient's shoulders to extend the lower neck. If the odontoid fragment is anterolisthesed and reduces with extension, an extended position is chosen for the neck. This is the ideal position and facilitates surgical exposure. If, however, the patient is retrolisthesed and can only be reduced in flexion, his head can be elevated and flexed into a neutral position. Two portable fluoroscopic units facilitate the operation (Fig. 56.2). A single unit can be used, rotating between A/P and lateral projections as necessary, but the surgeon must be sure to obtain visualization in both planes.

The approach involves a standard anterior cervical ex-

Table 56.1. Representative Values of the Range of Rotation of the Occipital-Atlanto-Axial Complex*

Unit of Complex	Type of Motion	Degrees of Motion
Occipital-atlantal joint (ocp-C1)	Flexion/Extension (± θx)	13° (Moderate)
	Lateral bending (± θz)	8° (Moderate)
	Axial rotation (± θy)	0° (*Negligible*)
Atlanto-axial joint (C1–C2)	Flexion/Extension (± θx)	10° (Moderate)
	Lateral bending (± θz)	0° (*Negligible*)
	Axial rotation (± θy)	47° (Extensive)

*Based on review of literature and authors' analysis.
With permission from: White AA, Panjabi MM. Biomechanics of the spine. Philadelphia: JB Lippincott, 1978:65.

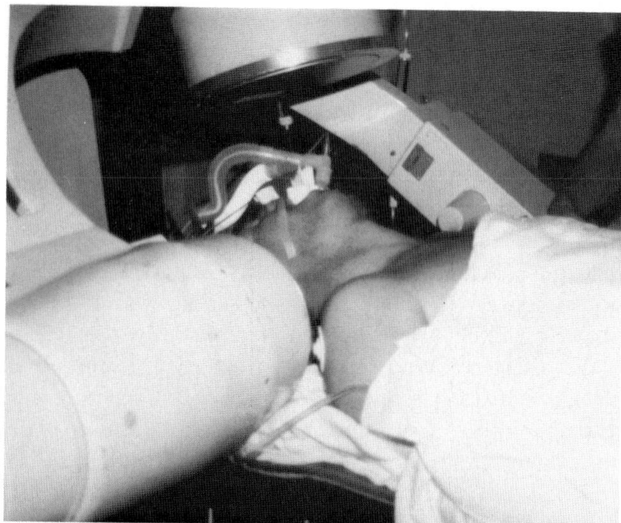

Figure 56.1. Position of the patient on operating room table with neck extended.

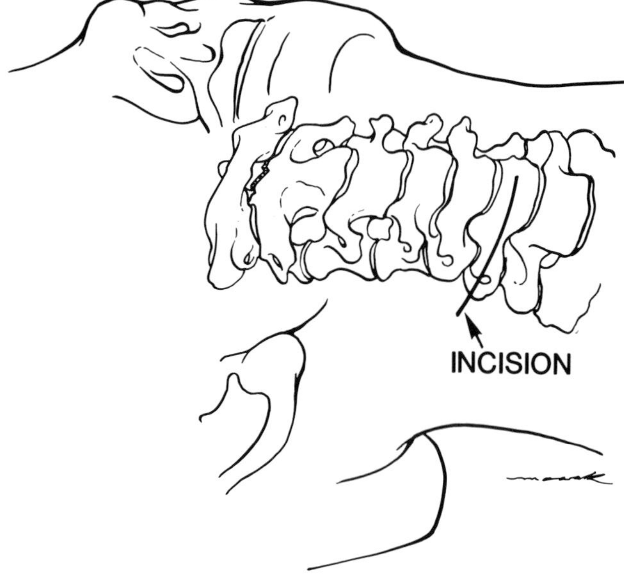

Figure 56.3. Low cervical unilateral incision.

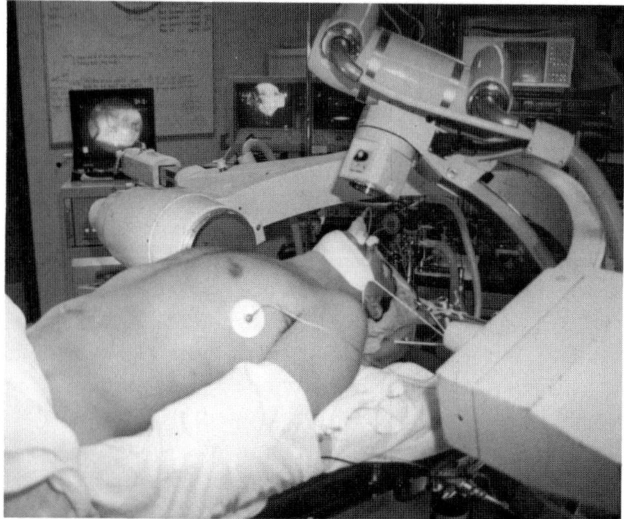

Figure 56.2. Note the use of two c-arm fluoroscopic units for AP and lateral imaging.

posure initially starting at the level of C5–6 (Fig. 56.3). The approach is similar to that used by Cloward and Caspar for gaining access to the spine at this level. A unilateral horizontal incision in a natural skin crease is chosen. The area is infiltrated with 1:200,000 epinephrine solution to facilitate hemostasis, which is completed with bipolar cautery. The platysma muscle is divided sharply and the sternocleidomastoid muscle fascia incised. Blunt dissection is then used to follow the fascial planes, medial to the carotid sheath and lateral to the trachea and esophagus, to the prevertebral space. The level is fluoroscopically identified and the longus colli muscle incised at the C5–6 level and elevated from the anterior surface of these vertebral bodies.

Caspar anterior cervical retractor blades are placed beneath the muscle belly and placed into a modified retractor blade holder. The blade holder has a series of holes in its arms that interdigitate with another retractor holder used for cephalad retraction. Once the first retractor is placed, blunt dissection in the prevertebral space allows ready access to the anterior face of the second and third cervical vertebra. An angled retractor blade (Fig. 56.4) is then inserted in this space and attached to the retractor blade holder that, as noted above, interdigitates with the lateral retractor. This system provides excellent access to the inferior edge of C2 and has the advantage that no retractor or retractor parts are present at the inferior end of the wound (Fig. 56.5). This allows the approach to C2 to be accomplished with a very low trajectory, which is necessary for proper screw placement.

A K-wire is then localized fluoroscopically at the inferior anterior edge of C2 in the midline and tapped gently into the vertebral body (Fig. 56.6). An 8-mm drill, which has a hollow inner core, is passed over the K-wire and manipulated by hand (Fig. 56.7) to create a shallow trough in the anterior face of C3 and in the annulus of the C2–3 disc. The drill is then replaced with an inner and outer drill guide system (Fig. 56.8). The two components slide over the K-wire with the inner drill guide extending to the inferior edge of C2. The outer drill guide has fixation spikes that can be gently tapped into the body of C3, holding the system in proper alignment. Once the system is thus secured, the K-wire can be removed and a drill passed through the drill guide into the starter hole made by the K-wire (Fig. 56.9). The drill is manipulated fluoroscopically and a pilot hole placed through the body of C2, across the fracture site into the odontoid fragment. As the drill is advanced, its progress is monitored on biplane fluoroscopy. When it reaches the level of the fracture site, the patient's head or the C2–C3 spine segments can be manipulated to place the odontoid fragment in normal anatomic position. The drill is advanced to the apex of the odontoid, removed, and a tap passed through the drill guide and rotated to cut threads through the bone to the tip of the odontoid (Fig. 56.10). The inner drill guide is then removed and a fixation screw passed through the outer drill guide into this tapped hole, engaging the odontoid fragment and drawing it back into close apposition with the body of C2 (Fig. 56.11).

If the patient has a chronically nonunited fracture (that is, it is not a fresh fracture), angled bisurfaced curettes may be placed, again, under fluoroscopic control, to the level

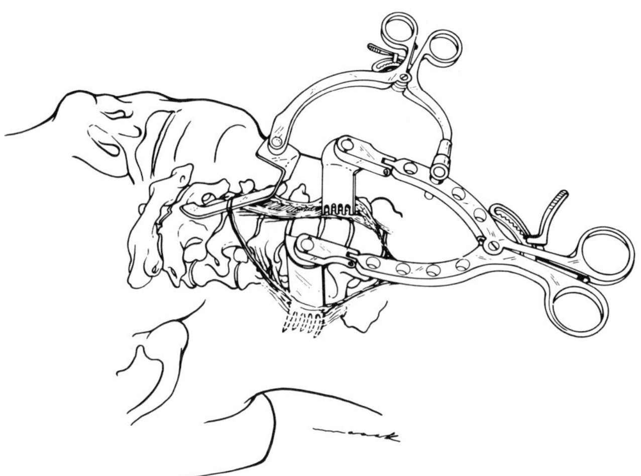

Figure 56.4. Retractor system in place.

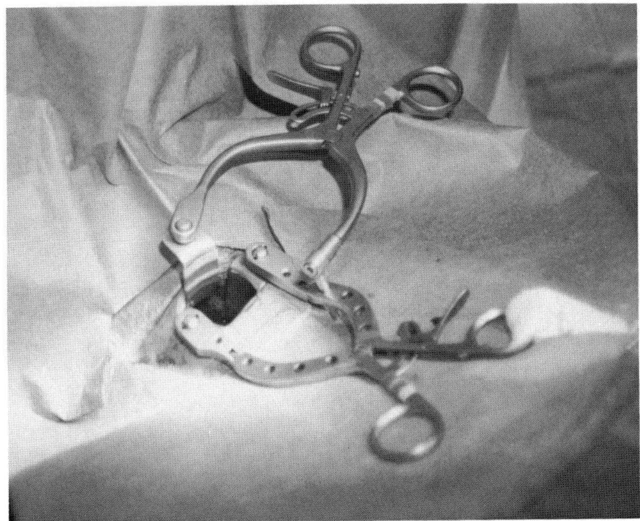

Figure 56.5. Note no obstruction inferiorly, allowing low trajectory.

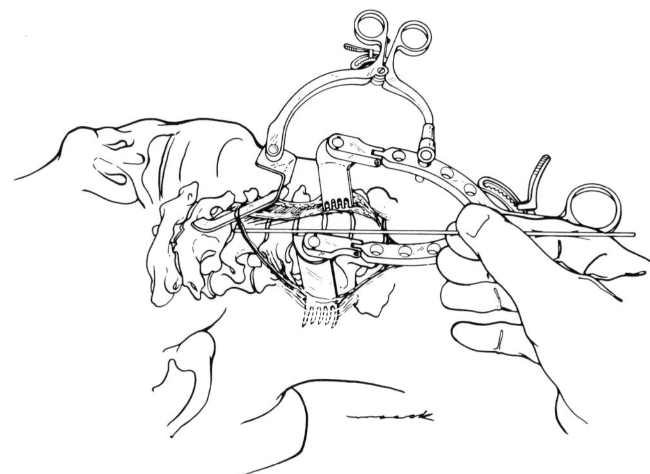

Figure 56.6. K-wire inserted into inferior edge of C2 in midline.

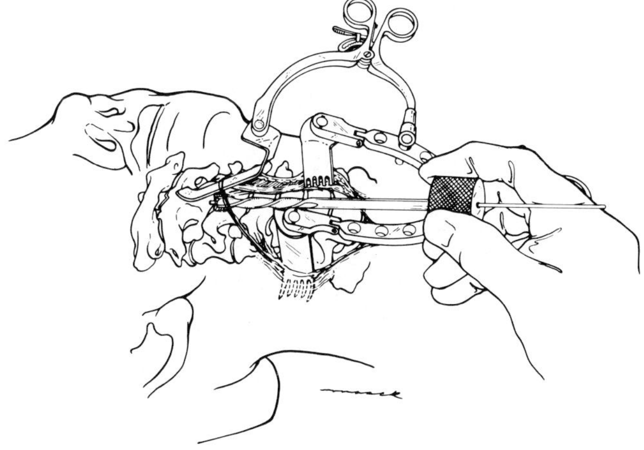

Figure 56.7. 8-mm drill placed over K-wire to incise annulus and create shallow trough in face of C3.

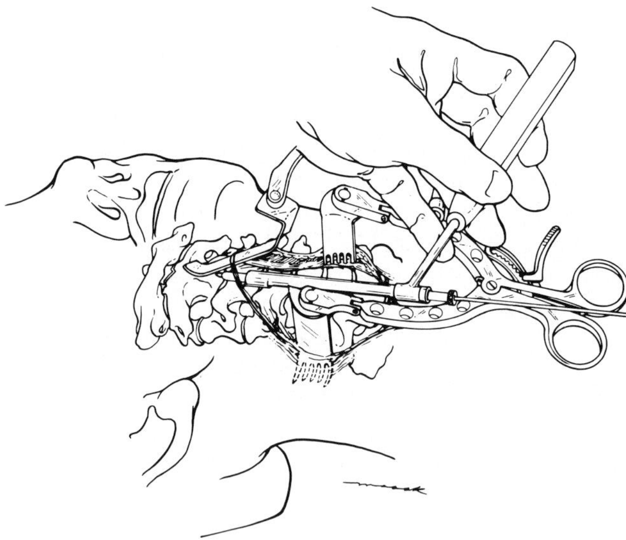

Figure 56.8. Inner and outer drill guide placed over K-wire. Note inner guide goes to inferior edge of C2; outer guide spikes secure it to C3.

of the fracture and used to curette this area before placement of the fixation screw (Fig. 56.12). This hopefully will encourage bony union.

Once the fixation screw is placed, the surgeon can immediately evaluate stability by having the patient's neck flexed and extended while monitoring the lateral fluoroscopic image. A second fixation screw may be placed if the bony anatomy is such that it will accommodate a second screw (Fig. 56.13).

The retractor system is then removed and wound closure effected in standard fashion. This technique provides immediate stability. The patient, therefore, does not require an external immobilizer, although some may prefer the use of a cervical collar for comfort for a period of time.

DISCUSSION

At this writing, we have employed this technique in 18 patients over a 41 month period. Five patients in this series had undergone previous attempts at posterior stabilization, some more than once, but did not achieve satisfactory bony

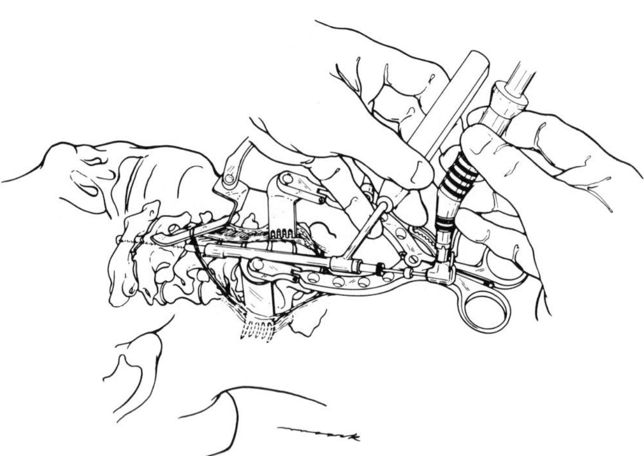

Figure 56.9. Drill being guided to apex of odontoid.

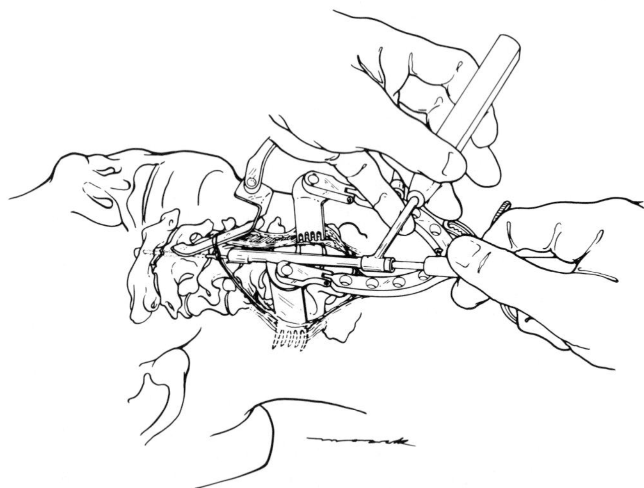

Figure 56.11. Screw placed through outer drill guide.

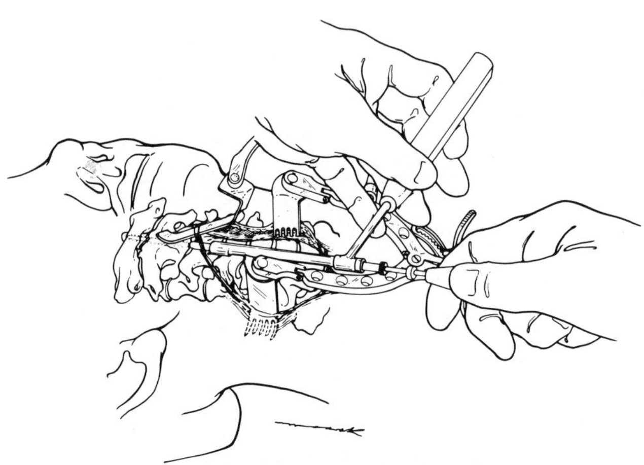

Figure 56.10. Tapping drill hole.

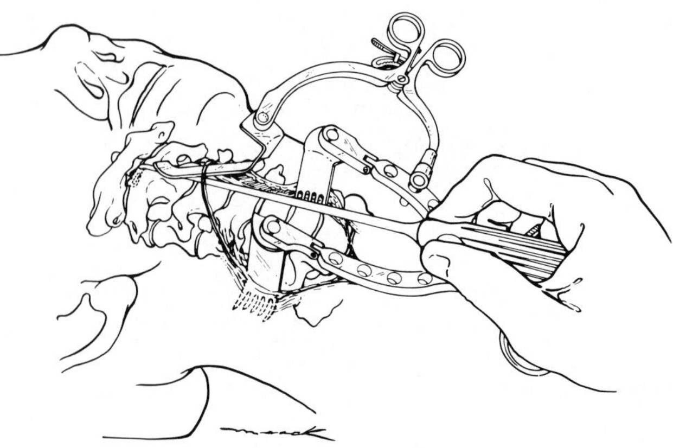

Figure 56.12. Bisurface curette freshening fracture site.

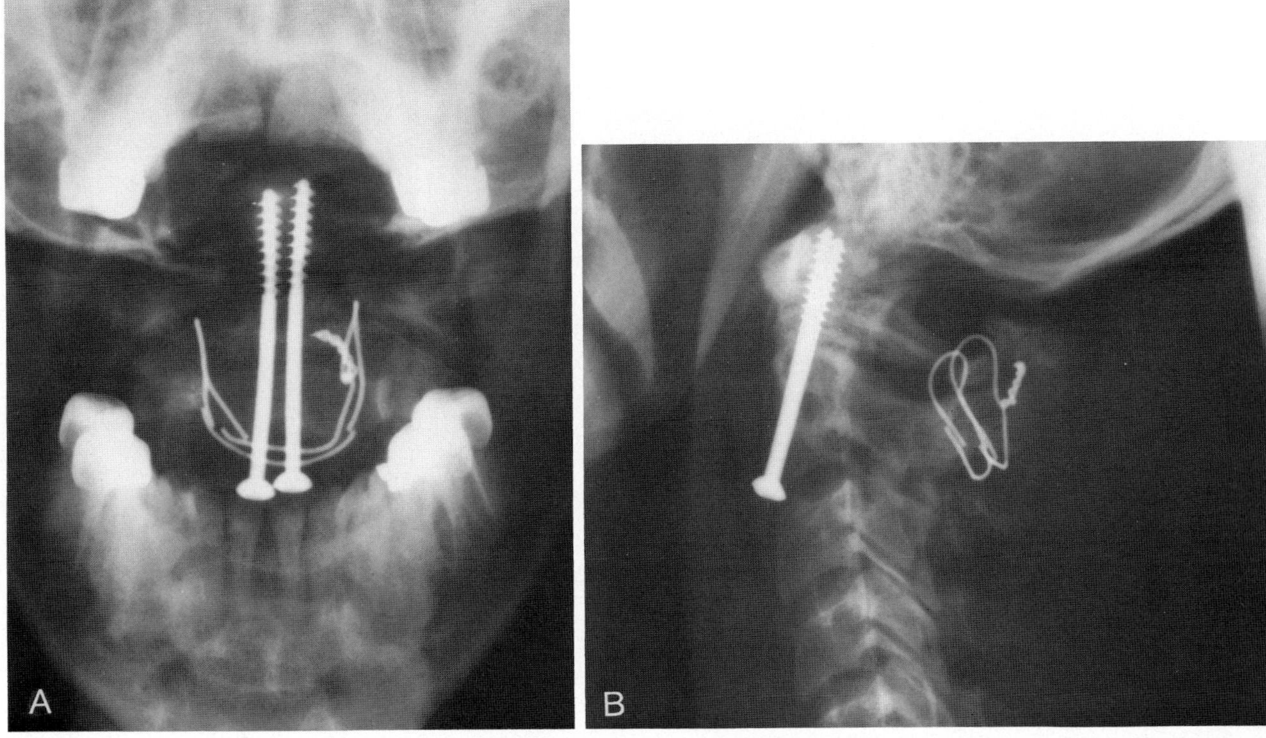

Figure 56.13. Patient with chronic nonunion of the odontoid fracture who had failed posterior wiring and bone fusion and remained unstable. Two fixation screws were placed into the odontoid.

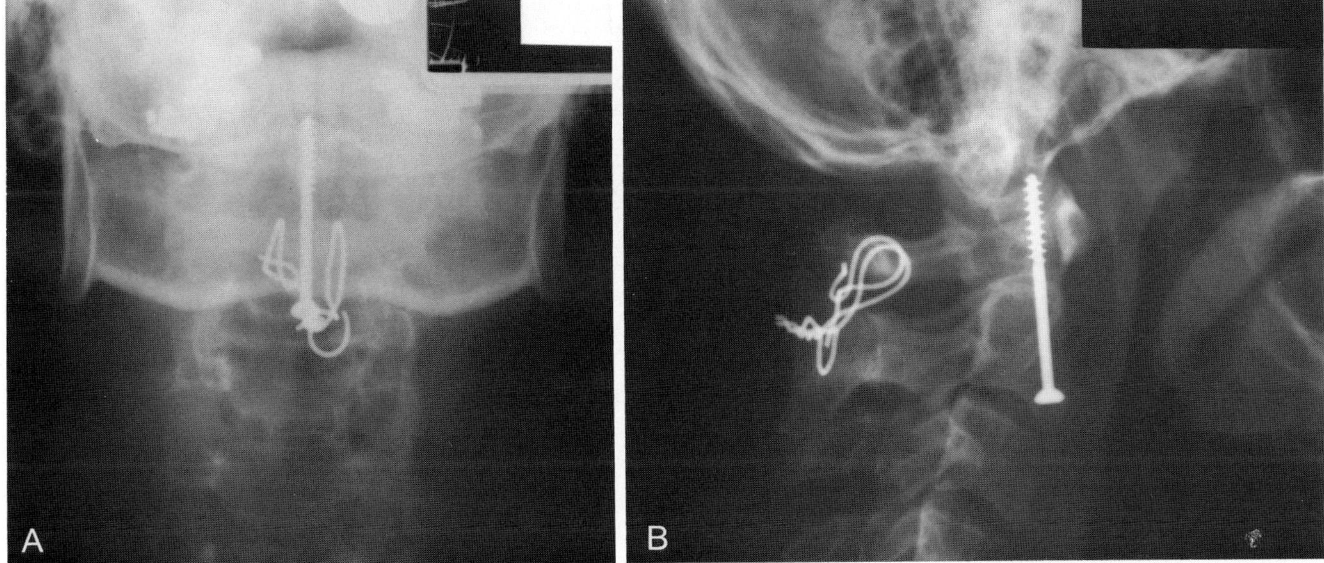

Figure 56.14. Single fixation screw used in another patient who also had failed prior attempts at posterior bone and wire fusion.

union (Fig. 56.14). In two patients, a halo-vest was used because of associated fractures in the body of C2, which raised the question of the security of the fixation screw without additional support.

Satisfactory stabilization was achieved in all these patients, and there have been no late failures. Bony union can be observed on postoperative tomograms (Fig. 56.15). When noted it was usually not well seen for 6–18 months after the procedure. There were no surgical complications.

Larson has commented (19) that the goal of our treatment should be "to return the patient to the fullest possible activity in the shortest period with the least morbidity and mortality."

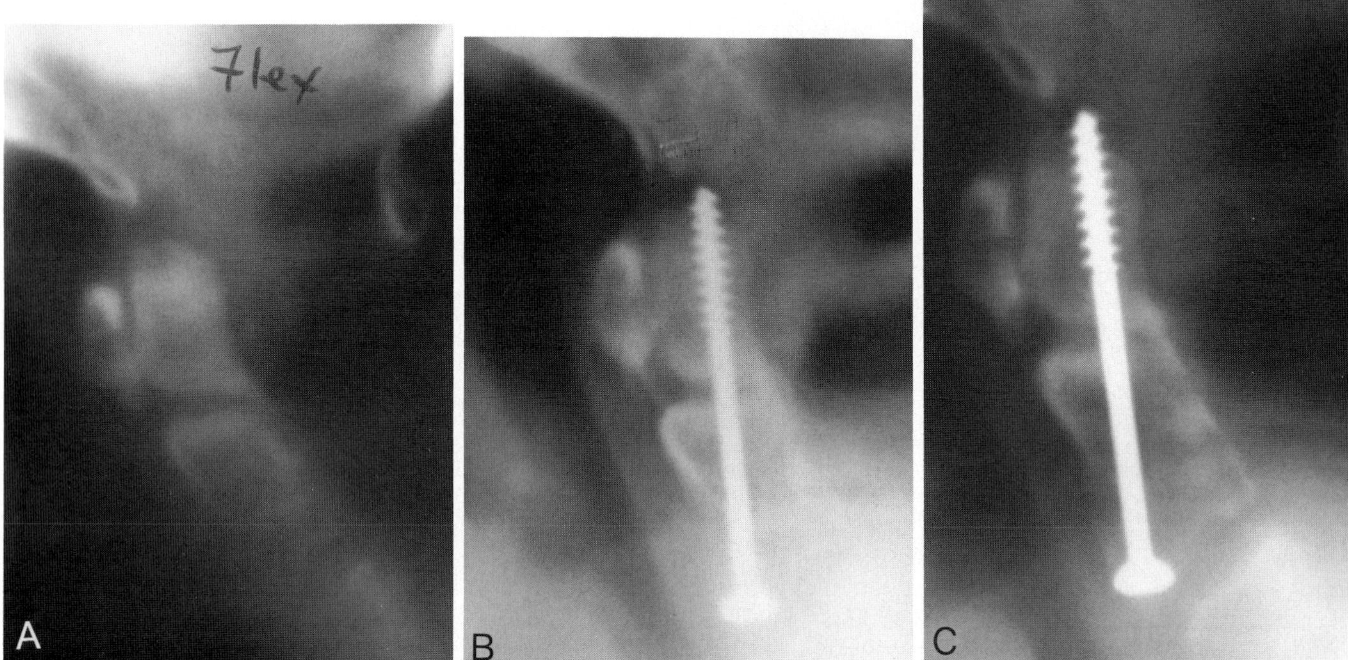

Figure 56.15. **A,** nonunited odontoid fracture which did not heal after 4 months of halo-vest immobilization (shown in position of best reduction); **B,** lateral tomogram 1 month postoperatively shows very faint bone bridging across the fracture site; **C,** at 8 months bony union has progressed nicely.

The initial satisfactory results with this technique including immediate stabilization in all patients, brief hospitalization (usually 3–5 days postoperatively), and lack of any significant morbidity associated with the procedure while preserving normal C1–2 rotatory motion appear to achieve this ideal. This leads us to suggest that this technique also might be considered in acute fractures with less than 4–5-mm displacement, if the patient is unwilling to accept external immobilization in a halo-vest or Minerva jacket. Further follow-up with a larger series of patients, however, is necessary before a firm recommendation in this regard can be made.

REFERENCES

1. Anderson LD, D'Alonzo RT. Fractures of the odontoid process of the axis. J Bone Joint Surg 1974;56-A:1663–1674.
2. Maiman DJ, Larson SJ. Management of odontoid fractures. Neurosurgery 1982;11:471–476.
3. Waddell JP, Reardon GP. Atlantoaxial arthrodesis to treat odontoid fractures. Can J Surg 1983;26:255–258.
4. Gambacorta D, Reale F. Posterior acrylic surgical fixation of odontoid fractures. Acta Neurochir 1988;43:75–78.
5. Schiess RJ, DeSaussure RL, Robertson JT. Choice of treatment of odontoid fractures. J Neurosurg 1982;57:496–499.
6. Lind B, Nordwall A, Sihlbom H. Odontoid fractures treated with halo-vest. Spine 1987;12:173–177.
7. Ekong CEU, Schwartz ML, Tator CH, et al. Odontoid fracture: management with early mobilization using the halo device. Neurosurgery 1981;9:631–637.
8. Wang GJ, Mabie KN, Whitehill R, et al. The nonsurgical management of odontoid fractures in adults. Spine 1984;9:229–230.
9. Cooper PR, Maravilla KR, Skylar FH, et al. Halo immobilization of cervical spine fractures. J Neurosurg 1979;50:603–610.
10. Apuzzo MLJ, Heiden JS, Weiss MH, et al. Acute fractures of the odontoid process. J Neurosurg 1978;48:85–91.
11. Dunn ME, Seljeskog EL. Experience in the management of odontoid process injuries: an analysis of 128 cases. Neurosurgery 1986;18:306–310.
12. Hadley MN, Browner C, Sonntag VKH. Axis fractures: a comprehensive review of management and treatment in 107 cases. Neurosurgery 1985;17:281–290.
13. Hadley MN, Browner CM, Liu SS, et al. New subtype of acute odontoid fractures (type IIA). Neurosurgery 1988;22:67–71.
14. White AA, Panjabi MM. Clinical biomechanics of the spine. Chapter 2, Kinematics of the spine. Philadelphia: JB Lippincott Co., 1978:65.
15. Bohler J. Anterior stabilization for acute fractures and non-unions of the dens. J Bone Joint Surg 1982;64-A:18–27.
16. Lesoin F, Autricque A, Franz K, et al. Transcervical approach and screw fixation for upper cervical spine pathology. Surg Neurol 1987;27:459–465.
17. Borne GM, Bedou GL, Pinaudeau M, et al. Odontoid process fracture osteosynthesis with a direct screw fixation technique in nine consecutive cases. J Neurosurg 1988;68:223–226.
18. Geisler FH, Cheng C, Poka A, et al. Anterior screw fixation of posteriorly displaced type II odontoid fractures. Neurosurgery 1989;25:30–38.
19. Larson SJ. Comments in regard to Hadley MN, Browner C, Sonntag VKH. Axis fractures: a comprehensive review of management and treatment in 107 cases. Neurosurgery 1985;17:289.

57

The Law of Medical Malpractice in Relationship to Medical and Surgical Treatment of Diseases of The Cervical Spine

Bruce G. Habian

Introduction

Legal Standards

As in all others areas of medicine, the law requires a practitioner to practice in accordance with established standards existing in the community. Common Law principles take precedence. (Reference is made herein to time-honored pattern jury instructions with regard to the topics of medical malpractice, lack of proximate cause, and informed consent).

While noncompliance with hospital regulations and community custom and practices can establish liability against the clinical practitioner, expert testimony which verbalizes (*a*) a departure(s) or deviation(s) from accepted medical and surgical standards and (*b*) proximate cause between such departure and the injury from which the patient is suffering is crucial to establishing negligence. Liability is also established for a cause of action for lack of informed consent by the same means.

Procedurally, once the "prima facie" elements of the case have been established by such testimony, the defendant physician and independent experts must persuade the jury as to their contentions concerning the standard of care and proximate cause. Theoretically and legally the plaintiff has the burden of proof on these issues. Practically, the more serious the injury that is presented to the jury, the more the burden shifts to the defense to disprove the allegations of medical negligence because of the sympathy factor.

All too often our courts are extremely lenient in the acceptance of expert testimony for the jury and lack of scrutiny with regard to the background of the witness, allowing the jury to "weigh" the testimony in light of all of the facts of the case. This author has had cases submitted to the jury wherein the departure testimony was established by general surgeons who *never* performed cervical spine surgery and merely educated themselves on these highly technical procedures by reviewing the medical literature. Unfortunately, in most jurisdictions, all that is required for the general qualifications of an adverse expert witness is a medical degree!

Sample Jury Instructions

Malpractice—Physician

A doctor's responsibilities are the same whether or not he is paid for his services. By undertaking to perform a medical service, he does not—nor does the law require him to—guarantee a good result. He is liable only for negligence.

A doctor who renders a medical service is obligated to have that reasonable degree of knowledge and ability that is expected of specialists who do that particular procedure in the community where he practices.

The law recognizes that there are differences in the abilities of doctors, just as there are in the abilities of people engaged in other activities. To practice his profession a doctor is not required to be possessed of the extraordinary knowledge and ability that belongs to a few persons of rare endowments but he is required to keep abreast of the times and to practice in accordance with the approved methods and means of treatment in general use. The standard to which he is held is measured by the degree of knowledge and ability of the average specialist in good standing in the community where he practices.

In performing a medical service the doctor is obligated to use his best judgment and to use reasonable care in the exercise of his knowledge and ability. The rule requiring him to use his best judgment does not make him liable for a mere error of judgment, provided he does what he thinks is best after careful examination. The rule of reasonable care does not require the exercise of the highest possible degree of care; it requires only that he exercise that degree of care that a reasonable prudent doctor or specialist would exercise under the same circumstances.

If a patient should sustain an injury while undergoing

medical care and that injury results from the doctor's lack of knowledge or ability, or from his failure to exercise reasonable care or to use his best judgment, then he is responsible for the injuries that are the result of his acts.

Proximate Cause

An act or omission is a proximate cause of an injury if it was a substantial factor in bringing about the injury, that is, if it had such an effect in producing the injury that reasonable men would regard it as a cause of the injury.

Malpractice—Informed Consent

A doctor who proposes to perform an operation-diagnostic procedure on a patient is under a duty to explain to the patient what it is he proposes to do, the reason for the operation-procedure and what the risks to the patient may be in performing the operation-procedure. The doctor is under a duty to advise the patient of all the facts that a reasonably prudent doctor in good standing in the community would explain before performing such an operation-procedure so that a patient who gives his consent may do so with an awareness (1) of his existing physical condition, (2) of the risks to his health or life which the operation-procedure may impose, and (3) the purpose and advantages that warrant performing the operation-procedure.

The patient should be advised whether the operation-procedure proposed is ordinarily done under the same conditions and whether other or different tests or procedures, if any, are used and the manner in which the alternative procedures are performed, and the comparative risks involved in the alternative procedure.

It is no defense that the operation-procedure which was performed was a medically sound procedure; it is still for the patient to decide whether he wished to consent to the operation-procedure.

If it is found that the doctor failed to give the plaintiff such information as a reasonably prudent physician would have given his patient to make him aware of the risks and hazards of the operation-procedure so as to enable the patient to make a decision as to whether he wishes to submit to the operation-procedure, you will find that the plaintiff's consent was not an informed consent, and the verdict must be for plaintiff. If, however, it is found that the doctor told the plaintiff all these facts which a reasonably prudent physician practicing in the community would have provided to a patient in the condition of the plaintiff at the time the consent was given, then you will find that the plaintiff gave the doctor an informed consent, you may not find that the operation-procedure was performed without the plaintiff's consent, and the verdict must be for defendant.

Much confusion exists in the minds of medical personnel between consent forms, as executed in the hospital chart and an informed consent. An unconsented to procedure, or one that is extended beyond the original scope, is considered a battery—therefore the legal necessity for an executed consent form.

"Informed" consent means just that; that prior to the procedure and independent of the signed form, the reasonable risks of the proposed treatment and the viable alternatives must be discussed with the patient. Essentially, disclosure of material facts reasonably necessary to allow the patient to make an informed choice forms the basis of the standard.

Necessity that Consent Be an Informed Consent

A medical practitioner is required reasonably to disclose to the patient, or to the person whose consent to treatment is legally required, all material facts within his knowledge relating to the proposed treatment in order that the necessary consent to treatment be based on an intelligent exercise of the judgment of the person consenting to the treatment. He must explain, in terms which a lay person can understand, the nature of any significant risks that may be encountered as a result of the treatment. Failure to so inform the patient or his proper representative is negligence. If, therefore, it is found that such disclosure was not made before the consent was obtained, one may find such failure to be negligence, which renders the practitioner liable for any injury which one finds to have resulted from the treatment administered.

Scope of Disclosure-Material Facts

A physician has a duty to disclose material facts reasonably necessary to allow the patient to form the basis of an intelligent consent. It is not incumbent on him to advise a patient as to every conceivable possibility and eventuality that may stem from his treatment. If the possibility is one that can reasonably be anticipated and falls within his expertise, then he should so inform his patient.

Consent is not properly given if the operation involves risks and results not contemplated by or explained to the patient. A nondisclosure of a possible danger is not a breach of the physician's duty in the absence of a showing that the patient's consent would have been withheld if the patient had been informed of the danger.

Evaluating Expert Testimony

Witnesses have been permitted to express opinions as to the standard of care to be expected of a medical practitioner in the defendant's position, or as to their opinion as to whether or not there has been a significant deviation from the appropriate standard of care and skill so expected (or as to the deviation, if you so find, as a legal cause of the plaintiff's injury). The fact that they have been permitted to testify should satisfy you that the laws of this state permit their testimony as competent witnesses on these matters. One should consider the nature of their qualifications, how they acquired such qualification, and the extent of their training and experience, in deliberating upon the weight or probative force which you should attach to such opinions. To put the matter another way, they have been permitted to give their expert opinion because they have, through preliminary questioning, demonstrated sufficient knowledge to express a well-formed opinion such as will probably aid you in the search for truth; but it is for you, as the triers of fact, to determine the extent to which these opinions are most worthy of credence.

Evaluating Expert Testimony—Extent of Witness' Familiarity with Controlling Standards

When one hears experts testify as to the standards of skill and care expected of the defendant practitioner in an action, it is for them to determine from this testimony whether or not the defendant, in treating the patient involved in this action, deviated from these standards. In so doing, one should consider the extent of the familiarity of each one of these expert witnesses with the standards required in such communities as that in which the defendant was practicing at the time of the alleged injury.

Case Presentations

The following history presents factual case examples demonstrating common problems facing practitioners of cervical spine surgery and clinical assessments. The case examples allow for identification of pertinent legal issues and also demonstrate how the specialties involved (emergency room physicians, general practitioners, neurologists, consultant orthopaedic surgeons and neurosurgeons, and neuroradiologists) overlap with regard to the assessment, treatment, and creation of legal problems concerning the cervical spine.

Case Study No. 1

The plaintiff, a 47-year-old male industrial structural designer, claimed to be totally disabled from pursuing his profession due to permanent cervical nerve root damage, resulting from an improperly performed spinal fusion by his orthopaedic surgeon.

The plaintiff had been involved in an automobile accident in which he sustained, among other things, a concussion and an injury to his cervical spine. The pertinent chronology immediately after the accident included no findings of cervical pathology per emergency room treatment, no findings of cervical fractures per an incomplete set of spine x-rays, and no neurologic findings prior to referral to the defendant orthopaedist for persistent cervical pain.

The orthopaedist ordered traction (unsupervised) at home and maintained extremely poor office notes concerning the historical work-up of the patient, his impressions, and the management plan. Ultimately, the orthopaedic surgeon performed a cervical fusion. The fusion was at two levels, C5–C6 and C6–C7, utilizing two bone grafts excised from the iliac crest (Cloward plug method). Immediately postoperatively the plaintiff experienced symptoms not present before the operation in the nature of radiating pain down both arms (radiculitis). The plaintiff claimed this symptomatology was consistent with irritation and compression of the nerve root exiting at the C6–C7 cervical interspace. As will be developed from this example, the plaintiff claimed that the initial operation on the cervical spine was unnecessary, given the state of the hospital record and the lack of documentation of preoperative neurologic findings. In addition, the plaintiff claimed that if the operation were necessary, it was due to the orthopaedist's improper employment of traction in further damaging the spine. The plaintiff also claimed that the operation was negligently performed with regard to the placement of the bone grafts within the contiguous levels of the cervical spine allowing for retraction of the bone plug, transection of the vertebral body bridging the two cervical levels, subluxation of the vertebrae, and the development of new neurologic signs not existing preoperatively. The plaintiff further claimed that there was an undue delay in treating the vertebral subluxation resulting from the fusion operation, causing permanent nerve root damage and hence the lack of future employability of the patient.

Less than 1 week postoperatively x-rays taken at the hospital of the cervical spine revealed a displacement (subluxation) of the plaintiff's cervical vertebrae. The radiologic report stated ". . . .vertical transection of the body of C-6 with anterior displacement and loss of joint space." The radiographs failed to demonstrate the lower graft; however, the downward angulation of the C7 spinous process established the diagnosis. Moreover, the radiology department had pinpointed the condition by drawing red lines on the original x-ray plate indicating the angulation of the C7 spinous process. Significantly, in connection with the finding of anterior displacement of the C6 vertebral body, the radiologists report noted under "impression" that there was "a disc extrusion, involving C6–C7 anteriorally."

The orthopaedist did not render any treatment for the plaintiff's cervical subluxation despite persistent symptoms and complaints of pain. The pain radiating into the shoulder became more severe: his grip became weaker and he began dropping things from his hand and experiencing weakness in his legs. The physican failed to adequately reexamine the patient with regard to those new symptoms, nor did he make a proper diagnosis. Unfortunately, the orthopaedist's office records for the postoperative office visits were entirely silent with regard to any symptomatology. Radiographs taken during postoperative visits did not visualize the lower graft. Expert testimony from the plaintiff established that it was standard care to obtain AP and lateral radiographs of the complete cervical spine to visualize the area that was not adequately seen on the orthopaedists post-operative films in view of the continued symptomatology and history. Eventually the patient consulted a neurologist who recommended another myelogram and re-directed the orthopaedist to more appropriate clinical management. The myelogram revealed significant narrowing of the spinal canal and impingement upon the lower cervical cord with extension. A neurosurgeon also reviewed the myelogram and reported that "the lower bone plug cannot be adequately visualized, but the myelogram suggested a partial block." Additional films demonstrated an incomplete block at the C6–C7 level. Due to extreme pain the patient could not assume a position to obtain an adequate lateral or swimmer's view projection. During this time period the patient's complaints of pain were documented in the hospital chart by nurses as well as by other practitioners' office records. Eventually the treating orthopaedist admitted the patient to the hospital.

The plaintiff claimed that absence of appropriate intervention by the involved practitioners in correcting his spinal malalignment would have allowed fusion in a subluxated position. Plaintiff further claimed that with the delay of more than a month and a half the symptomatology that was attempted to be relieved by subsequent operations was not relieved and hence, the permanent disability. The persistent nerve root pressure and irritation was the source of the patient's complaints. Arm pain was caused by radiculitis and inflammation of the nerve roots secondary to jamming of the articular facets which pass immediately anterior to the nerve roots. Inflammation of the articular facets as well as narrowing of the intervertebral foramen allowed for the disability.

DISCUSSION

What in reality was a serious cervical spine disorder secondary to the automobile accident, notwithstanding lack of appreciation and lack of documentation of the pathology by less than adequate emergency room x-ray studies, was made to appear as negligent orthopaedic treatment, considering the lack of adequate documentation by the physician. What in reality was an acceptable complication of the fusion of the cervical spine by means of dowels, with extrusion of the bone plugs and resultant instability, was made to appear as negligent orthopaedic treatment because of inattention to the patient postoperatively by not obtaining adequate x-ray films. The radiologist's recommendation that a complete cervical spine series should be obtained in view of the incomplete series previously taken was not heeded and created liability.

This case study presents plaintiff's theory of (1) no indication for surgery on the cervical spine; (2) creation of the pathology by improperly supervised electric traction at home necessitating treatment; (3) improperly performed surgery on the cervical spine (technique) by means of improper spacing and placing of the bone plugs; (4) inadequate postoperative examination and management so as to arrive at an appreciation of the postoperative complications; (5) significant delay and subsequent performance of surgery on the cervical spine to relieve the postoperative complications, all resulting in permanent injury to the patient.

PROOF NECESSARY FOR PLAINTIFF VERDICT

Given the multiple theories at attack by plaintiff's counsel, keep in mind that only one theory of negligence together with proximate cause must be accepted by the jury for the plaintiff to prevail. In the above-listed example, the plaintiff's claim that the operation was not warranted after the automobile accident and that the defendant orthopaedist created the pathology for the operation was not accepted by the jury. In addition the plaintiff's claim that the extrusion of the Cloward grafts and resulting instability of the spine were secondary to operative negligence was also not accepted by the jury. However, the plaintiff's claim that once the grafts had extruded, and the symptomatology became worse, with the orthopaedist delaying an assessment and treatment of the condition, this was accepted by the jury and allowed for plaintiff's recovery. In this regard, the jury was influenced by this neglect during a month's vacation by the orthopaedist (with inadequate coverage by others). Given the applicable legal standards, the plaintiff's position that the resultant delay was directly related to an irreversible radiculitis with damage to the nerve roots such as to prevent the patient from carrying on his occupation was a sustainable finding by the court.

Case Study No. 2

This plaintiff, a female in her thirties, sustained an alcohol-induced seizure while at her home in her bathroom, whereupon she passed out and fell, injuring her cervical spinal cord, With the seizure, she became incontinent of urine and had tonic/clonic movements. She arrived at the hospital by ambulance and was immediately assessed in the emergency room. Upon admission, she suffered a second seizure, again involving tonic/clonic movements. The patient was a service patient of the hospital staff. After admission, the patient's condition eventually stabilized, and she was treated with bed rest, steroids (Decadron), and an anti-convulsant (Dilantin). A neurosurgical consultation was requested. The neurosurgeon examined the patient and detected motor weakness in the upper extremities and a non-focal sensory loss in the lower extremities. After doing a complete neurological examination and reviewing the spinal radiographs, he advised conservative treatment, including a cervical soft collar. He recommended additional radiographs including flexion-extension views of the cervical spine as well as a myelogram and a post-contrast CT scan.

The neurosurgeon's impression was that the patient's clinical picture was inconsistent with any active extrinsic spinal cord compression. After reviewing the myelogram and post-contrast CT scan which demonstrated a free flow of dye, the neurosurgeon concluded that, although there was no impingement on the cord, the patient had an intramedullary contusion of the central cord for which no surgery was indicated. He was of the opinion that the patient's trauma had caused the hyperflexion injury to the cord. The patient was noted to be improving over time, and the neurosurgeon remained available for further consultation. The resident staff managing the patient never recalled the neurosurgeon for futher assessment. The notes as contained in the hospital chart were scanty and did not correlate with an improving clinical picture.

Upon completion of the myelogram the neuroradiologist reported cervical spondylosis as well as spinal stenosis extending from C3 through C6. The acute changes in the cord were secondary to congenital vertebral column narrowing combined with an acute hyperflexion injury. The neuroradiologist listed severe spinal cord compression as a final impression.

The patient remained in the hospital for several months and was discharged. Whether or not the patient improved was open to debate given the scanty notations as contained in the chart.

The patient's incontinence of urine and feces improved, she remained seizure free, and began to ambulate with the use of a four-pronged cane. Her clonus disappeared, and her grasp became stronger.

After receiving physical therapy at another institution, the patient was again seen as an outpatient in the orthopaedic clinic of the initial hospital. The patient was rehospitalized on the orthopaedic service and a second myelogram performed revealed cervical spinal stenosis and spondylosis at levels C3 through C6. On neurologic examination spasticity of the upper and lower extremities and unsustained clonus bilaterally at the ankles was noted with bilateral Babinski signs. Motor examination of the upper and lower extremities was inconsistent, but there was loss of flexion of the right foot and extension of the right wrist. The impression was that the stenosis was causing the patient's *persistent* intractable spasticity, resulting in lack of improvement. Various alternative therapies were discussed at length, and the plan was to perform a posterior laminectomy to decompress the spinal stenosis. Further discussion of a possible anterior decompression in the future was explained as well, to the patient. She was subsequently operated upon with a decompressive laminectomy carried out from C3 through C6. Post-operatively there was very little improvement noted in the patient's condition.

The plaintiff based the poor postoperative result on the failure to immediately operate upon the patient shortly after the initial trauma, claiming liability on the part of the neurosurgical consultant and the hospital staff for inadequate observation and assessment. In addition, the plaintiff claimed that the failure to perform a secondary anterior decompressive procedure after the posterior decompressive procedure allowed for persistent postoperative deficits. The plaintiff required a three-prong cane to assist her in ambulation and claimed lost earning capacity because of weakness in her upper extremities.

Discussion

In summary, the plaintiff's attorney attacked the neurosurgeon for his conservative management plan and the failure to operate for cervical stenosis causing continued spinal cord compression. The confusing and inadequate medical notes by the resident staff did not allow the defense to adequately capitalize on the fact that the patient was improving clinically. In addition, the subsequent orthopaedist's notes concerning longstanding compression of the cervical spine impacted adversely on the judgmental decision of the original neurosurgical consultant. Also, the neuroradiologist's comments of compression adversely affected the neurosurgeon's position.

The theory attacking the conservative approach was accepted by the jury. The theory to fault the orthopaedist for not performing an anterior as well as posterior decompressive procedure was rejected by the jury. The medical testimony that the earlier a severe compression of the spinal cord is relieved, the better the chance for neurologic improvement was supported by plaintiff's expert testimony as well as by deposition testimony given during the pretrial stage by the various defendants. The proximate cause argument is entirely supported by such testimony. The use of terminology such as compression, severe compression, and relief of compression by the various specialties establish cross-liabilities among them. A typical jury instruction pertaining to delay as a substantial factor in the creation and persistence of an injury is as follows:

Diagnosis—delay as a substantial factor in injury—if you find from the evidence that the defendant failed promptly to make an accurate diagnosis of the ailment of the patient involved in this action, and that this delay or failure accurately to diagnose was a substantial factor in producing the condition in respect to which this action is brought, your verdict on the question of liability should be for the plaintiff.

Conclusion

Tort law principles can have a severe impact on the physician who manages cervical spine injuries. First, many patients have an antecedent trauma, which can make impossible their complete recovery. A frank discussion with the patient addressing the limitations of the proposed care is necessary. In addition, accident victims often have less than adequate recourse to large monetary recoveries (due to inadequate insurance of an automobile driver, for example). Hence, there exists an opportunity to bring an action against a "deep pocket" hospital or physician for a compensatory award.

Second, the multiple practitioners who interact with patients who have cervical spine injuries (for example, emergency room personnel, radiologists, physical therapists, neurologists, orthopaedists, neurosurgeons, and rehabilitation specialists) can all assess the patient at different times, receive different histories, and document different impressions, consistent with their particular specialties. Conflicting medical reports can create liability scenarios for the astute patient's attorney. The physician in charge is advised to *manage* the cervical spine patient's complete care, coordinating the case with complete knowledge of the past assessments of the patient and a definitive plan for future management. Only in this fashion can the obvious pitfalls of potential litigation be adequately deflected.

Index